BRIEF CONTENTS

W9-CEJ-586

ESSENTIALS OF
MATERNITY, NEWBORN, & WOMEN'S HEALTH NURSING

ESSENTIALS OF
MATERNITY, NEWBORN, & WOMEN'S HEALTH NURSING

Second Edition

Susan Scott Ricci, ARNP, MSN, MEd

Nursing Faculty
University of Central Florida
Orlando, Florida

Former Nursing Program Director and Faculty
Lake Sumter Community College
Leesburg, Florida

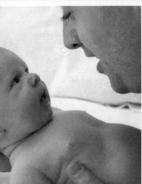
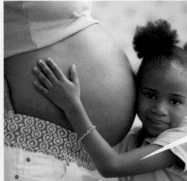
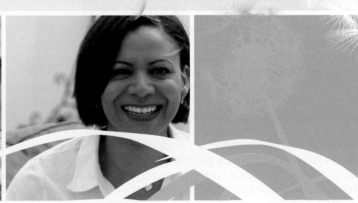

 Wolters Kluwer | Lippincott Williams & Wilkins
Health

Philadelphia · Baltimore · New York · London
Buenos Aires · Hong Kong · Sydney · Tokyo

Acquisitions Editor: Jean Rodenberger
Development Editor: Danielle DiPalma
Director of Nursing Production: Helen Ewan
Senior Production Editor: Tom Gibbons
Art Director, Design: Joan Wendt
Art Director, Illustration: Brett MacNaughton
Manufacturing Coordinator: Karin Duffield
Indexer: Katherine Pitcoff
Compositor: Circle Graphics

2nd Edition

9 8 7 6

Printed in China

Library of Congress Cataloging-in-Publication Data

Ricci, Susan Scott.
   Essentials of maternity, newborn, and women's health nursing / Susan Scott Ricci. —2nd ed.
       p. ; cn.
   Includes bibliographical references and index.
   ISBN 978-0-7817-8722-2 (cloth : alk. paper) 1. Maternity nursing. 2. Gynecologic nursing. I. Title.
   [DNLM: 1. Maternal-Child Nursing. 2. Obstetrical Nursing. 3. Pregnancy Complications—nursing. WY 157.3 R491e 2009]
   RG951.R53 2008
   618.2'0231—dc22

                                              2008029332

LWW.com

This book is dedicated to my loving husband Glenn, who has shown me the joy of learning—and living—who continues to support me in all of my professional pursuits and whose patience and understanding have meant the world to me. And also to my children, Brian and Jennifer, who have always inspired me throughout their lives.

Susan Scott Ricci

ACKNOWLEDGMENTS

I would like to thank so many people who have helped bring this textbook into being.

My appreciation goes to Jean Rodenberger for approaching me with this second project and believing that I could assist in achieving her vision. I would also like to especially thank Danielle DiPalma for her editorial expertise and for her steadfastness to this project and Erin Sweeney for gently prodding me to complete revisions. They have been ever patient through chapter drafts and revisions. In addition, I would like to thank Maryann Foley for her professional collaboration and attention to detail within the chapters. Her nursing background has been invaluable from the start. Special thanks to Sarah Kyle for her continued dedication to the vision and format of this textbook, as well as for her expert editing, and to Tom Gibbons for his skillful production of the text.

I would like to thank photographer Gus Freedman and photo producer Amy Geller for their dedicated work on the photo shoot. I would like to thank the following institutions for their help in getting the photos for this book:

UMass Memorial Health Care
The Birthplace at Wellesley
Brigham and Women's Hospital
Newton-Wellesley Hospital

Also thanks to the many nurses, midwives, doctors, and families for their participation in this book, especially Debbie Turner, Paula McGarr, Susan Martinson, Grace Jackson, and Marianne Cummings. I'm sure I have overlooked several other people who played a role in the development of this textbook, so a global appreciation is extended to the Lippincott Williams & Wilkins staff.

S.S.R.

ABOUT THE AUTHOR

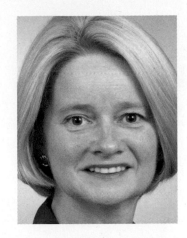

Susan Scott Ricci has a diploma from Washington Hospital Center School of Nursing, with a BSN, MSN, from Catholic University of America in Washington, D.C., an M.Ed. in Counseling from the University of Southern Mississippi, and is licensed as a Women's Health Nurse Practitioner (ARNP) from the University of Florida. She has worked in numerous women's health care settings including labor and delivery, postpartum, prenatal, and family planning ambulatory care clinics. Susan is a women's health care nurse practitioner, who has spent 30+ years in nursing education teaching in LPN, ADN, and BSN programs. She is involved in several professional nursing organizations and holds memberships in Sigma Theta Tau International Honor Society of Nursing, National Association of Ob/Gyn Nurses, Who's Who in Professional Nursing, American Nurses Association, and the Florida Council of Maternal-Child Nurses.

With Susan Scott Ricci's wealth of practical and educational experience, the time has come for her to concentrate on the "essential facts" of nursing instruction and reduce the amount of "nice to know" information that is presented to students. As an educator, she recognized the tendency for nursing educators to want to "cover the world" when teaching rather than focusing on the facts that students need to know to practice nursing. With this thought, Susan has directed her energy to the *birth* of this essentials textbook.

She recognizes that instructional time is shrinking as the world of health care is expanding exponentially. Therefore, with the valuable instructional time allotted, she has recognized the urgent need to present pertinent facts as concisely as possible to promote application of knowledge within nursing practice.

Reviewers

Marjorie L. Archer, MS, RN
Vocational Nursing Coordinator/Faculty
North Central Texas College
Gainesville, Texas

Lori Bacsalmasi, MSN, RN
Maternal/Child Faculty
Franklin Pierce University/Abrazo Health Care
Goodyear, Arizona

Virgie Barnes, RN, MSN
Professor of Nursing
Somerset Community College
Somerset, Kentucky

Linda Barren, MS, RNC
Division Head of Health Services; Assistant Professor
Oklahoma State University—Oklahoma City
Oklahoma City, Oklahoma

Kathleen Barta, EdD, RN
Associate Professor of Nursing
University of Arkansas
Fayetteville, Arkansas

Joyce Bates, RN
Faculty, Department of Nursing
Fairmont State University
Fairmont, West Virginia

Cheryl Becker, RN, MN
Chair, Health Sciences
Tenured Teaching Faculty
Bellevue Community College
Kirkland, Washington

Betty Bertrand, RNC
Instructor, LVN Program
Texarkana College
Texarkana, Texas

Nancy Bingaman, MSN
Instructor, Nursing
Monterey Peninsula College
Monterey, California

Pat Bishop, RN, MSN
Assistant Professor
Chamberlain College of Nursing
Phoenix, Arizona

Peggy Bozarth, MSN, RN, CNE
Professor
Hopkinsville Community College
Hopkinsville, Kentucky

Beverly Bradley, MSN
Coordinator, Nursing
Trident Technical College
Charleston, South Carolina

Vera C. Brancato
Associate Professor of Nursing
Kutztown University
Spring City, Pennsylvania

Marie Bright-Cobb, RNC, MSN, CNS, IBCLC
Instructor
University of Akron
Akron, Ohio

Michele Brimeyer, MSN, ARNP, WHNP-BC
Clinical Assistant Professor, College of Nursing
University of Florida
Gainesville, Florida

Patricia Burkard, MSN
Associate Professor, Nursing
Moorpark College
Moorpark, California

Deborah Campagna, RN, BSN, MSN, LCCE, FACCE
Associate Professor, Nursing
Hudson Valley Community College
Troy, New York

Diane Campbell, MSN, RN
Clinical Assistant Professor
Purdue University—West Lafayette
West Lafayette, Indiana

Darlene Cantu, RNC, MSN
Assistant Professor
San Antonio College
San Antonio, Texas
Online Faculty for the University of Phoenix
Online Faculty for Chamberlain College of Nursing

Annie M. Carson, RN, BScN
Teaching Master, Professor
Cambrian College of Applied Arts and Technology
Sudbury, Ontario, Canada

Anne Cassens, RN, MS
Nursing Faculty in Obstetrics
Normandale Community College
Bloomington, Minnesota

Anita Catlin, DNSc, FNP, FAAN
Ethics Consultant
California State University at Sonoma
Rohnert Park, California

Angelina Chambers, PhD, RN, CNM
Assistant Professor, School of Nursing
Yale University
New Haven, Connecticut

Lisa L. Courcy
Assistant Professor of Nursing
Edincott College
Beverly, Massachusetts

Catherine R. Coverston, PhD, RNC
Associate Professor, College of Nursing
Brigham Young University
Provo, Utah

Connie Daily, MSN, RN
Nursing Instructor
Shawnee Community College
Ullin, Illinois

Shelly Daily, MSNc, RN, APN
Assistant Professor
Arkansas Technical University
Russellville, Arkansas

Melissa Darnell, RN
Arkansas Technical University
Russellville, Arkansas

Karen Davis, MSN, RN, CNE, LNC
Clinical Assistant Professor, Medical Sciences
University of Arkansas
Little Rock, Arkansas

Pat Davis
Lake City Community College
School of Nursing
Lake City, Florida

Karen DeBoer, MSN, RNC, WHNP
Nursing Faculty
Macomb Community College
Clinton Township, Michigan

Carol Deresz, MSN, RNC
Assistant Professor/Clinical
University of Texas
Health Science Center at San Antonio
San Antonio, Texas

Colette Diejuste, RNC, MS
Assistant Clinical Professor
Simmons College
Boston, Massachusetts

London Draper, MSN, RN
Assistant Professor
Weber State University
Ogden, Utah

Judy Drumm, RN, MSN, EdD
Nurse Educator
Washtenaw Community College
Ann Arbor, Michigan

Theresa Dubiel, RN, MSN, Nsg Ed
Nurse Educator, School of Nursing and Health Science
Washtenaw Community College
Ann Arbor, Michigan

Patricia DuClos-Miller, MS, RN, CAN, BC
Associate Professor
Capital College
Hartford, Connecticut

Linda Dunn, DSN, RN, CCE
Professor, Capstone College of Nursing
University of Alabama
Tuscaloosa, Alabama

Pat Durham-Taylor, PhD
Professor, Nursing
Truckee Meadows Community College
Reno, Nevada

Cathy Emeis, PhD
Clinical Instructor
Beth-El College of Nursing & Health Sciences,
    University of Colorado
Colorado Springs, Colorado

Marian Farrell, PhD, APRN-BC, CRNP
Nursing Faculty
University of Scranton
Scranton, Pennsylvania

Teri Fernandez, MSN
Instructor
Yavapai College
Prescott, Arizona

Rhonda Ferrell, MSN, RN
Department Head, Health Education
James Sprunt Community College
Kenansville, North Carolina

Mary-Margaret Finney, RN, MSN, CNE
Assistant Professor, Department of Nursing
North Georgia College and State University
Dahlongea, Georgia

Alma R. Flores-Vela, MSN, RN
Nursing Faculty, College of Health Science and
    Human Service
University of Texas Pan America
Edinburg, Texas

Jamie Flower, PhD (C), MS, RN
Carolyn McKelvey-Moore School of Nursing
University of Arkansas
Fort Smith, Arkansas

Susan Frigo, RN
Naugatuck Valley Community Technical College
Waterbury, Connecticut

Mary Fuhrman, MSN, RN
East Central Regional Coordinator for the RN to BSN
    Program
College of Nursing
University of Iowa
Iowa City, Iowa

Judy Fuhrmann, RN
Cecil Community College
North East, Maryland

Sue Gabriel, EdD, MSN, MFS, RN
S.A.N.E.
Assistant Professor
Bryan LGH College of Health Sciences
Lincoln, Nebraska

Rosa E. Garces, RN, MSN
Certified Human Lactation Educator
Certified Perinatal Educator
Nursing Program Coordinator
Faculty Interamerican
University of Puerto Rico, Ponce Campus
Mercedita, Puerto Rico

Helen Gordon, MS, CNM
Assistant Clinical Professor
Duke University
School of Nursing, ABSN Program
Durham, North Carolina

Gay Goss, PhD, RN
Associate Professor of Nursing
California State University, Dominguez Hills
Carson, California

Tonia Grant, MSN, RN
CUNY at Medgar Evers College
AAS/PN Nursing Professor
School of Science, Health and Technology
Brooklyn, New York

**Julie Greenawalt, RNC, MS, MSN,
    Doctoral Candidate**
Assistant Professor, Nursing and Allied Health
    Professions
Indiana University of Pennsylvania
Indiana, Pennsylvania

Pamela Gwin, RNC
Director, Vocational Nursing Program
Brazosport College
Lake Jackson, Texas

Anna Hefner, MSN, CPNP
Director, Academic Support and Nursing Computer
    Center; Associate Professor
Azusa Pacific University
Azusa, California

Gloria Johns, PhD, MSN
Assistant Professor, Pediatric Nursing
Georgia Perimeter College
Clarkston, Georgia

Kathy Johnson, RN, BA, MA
Assistant Professor, Department of Nursing
South Dakota University
Sioux Falls, South Dakota

Linda Kapinos, RNC, MSN, IBCLC
Professor of Nursing
Capital Community College
Hartford, Connecticut

Mary F. King, RN, MS
Level III and Level IV Course Coordinator;
    Nursing Instructor
Phillips Community College of the University
    of Arkansas
Helena, Arkansas

Sandy Kluka, RN, MN, PhD
Coordinator, 4-Yr Undergraduate Nursing Program
University of Manitoba
Winnipeg, Manitoba, Canada

Karen Knowles, RN, MS
Maternal Newborn Faculty
Crouse Hospital School of Nursing
Syracuse, New York

Sue Koos, MS, RN, CNE
Professor, Health and Human Services
Heartland Community College
Normal, Illinois

Rochelle Kuhn, MS, CRNP
Pediatric Nursing Instructor
Frankford Hospital School of Nursing
Philadelphia, Pennsylvania

Diana Kunce, MS, RN
Instructor
Tarleton State University
Stephenville, Texas

Kay LaCount, BSN, MSN
Chair, Nursing
Bay De Noc Community College
Escanaba, Michigan

Robyn Leo, RN, MS
Assistant Professor of Nursing
Maternal Child Health Coordinator
Worcester State College
Worcester, Massachusetts

Kelli Lewis, BSN, MSN
Practical Nursing Instructor/Allied Health Division
Rend Lake College
Ina, Illinois

Jeanne Linhart, MS, RN
Associate Professor of Nursing
Rockland Community College
Suffern, New York

Susan Lloyd, PhD, RN, CNS
MSN Program Director
California State University—Los Angeles
Los Angeles, California

Diwana Lowe, RNC, MSN
Interim Assistant Chair, Nursing
Lawrenceville Associate Professor
Georgia Perimeter College
Lawrenceville, Georgia

Barbara Manning, MS, RN
Nursing Instructor
Northwest Mississippi Community College
Senatobia, Mississippi

Maria Marconi, RN, MS
Assistant Professor of Clinical Nursing
School of Nursing
University of Rochester
Rochester, New York

Rhonda Martin, MS, RN
Clinical Instructor in Nursing
University of Tulsa
Tulsa, Oklahoma

Ginger Meriwether, RN
Holmes Community College
Granada, Mississippi

Kathy Mix, RN,C, BSN, MS
Nursing Professor & Campus Wellness Coordinator
South Puget Sound Community College
Olympia, Washington

Cindy Morgan
University of Tennessee at Chattanooga
Chattanooga, Tennessee

Sandra G. Nadelson, PhD, MSN, MEd, RN
Associate Professor, Department of Nursing
Boise State University
Boise, Idaho

Valerie O'Dell, MSN, RN
Assistant Professor of Nursing
Youngstown State University
Youngstown, Ohio

Michelle Offutt, MSN, ARNP
Associate Professor, College of Nursing
St. Petersburg College
Pinellas Park, Florida

Cynthia Payne, RNC, WHNP-BC, CNM
Nursing Instructor
Georgia Perimeter College
Clarkston, Georgia

Gena Porter-Lankist, ARNP, MSN
Chipola Junior College
Marianna, Florida

Sherri St. Pierre, MS, APRN, PNP
Clinical Assistant Professor
Maternal/Child Health
William F. Connell School of Nursing
Boston College
Chestnut Hill, Massachusetts

Ann Schide, MSN, RN, MS, LCCE, CLNC, BSC
Assistant Professor, Nursing Program
Chattanooga State Technical Community College
Chattanooga, Tennessee

Joy Shewchuk, RN, MSN
Nursing Professor, School of Health Sciences
Humber College
Toronto, Ontario, Canada

Cordia Starling, RN, EdD
Professor/Dean, School of Nursing
Dalton State College
Dalton, Georgia

Lois Tate, RNC, EdD
Professor and Course Coordinator
Maternal Newborn Nursing
Union University Germantown Campus
Germantown, Tennessee

Rosalie Tierney-Gumaer, MSN, MPH, RN
Director, Continuing Nursing Education
Assistant Professor, Family Nursing Department
University of Texas at San Antonio
San Antonio, Texas

Maureen Tippen, RN, C, MS
Clinical Assistant Professor, Department of Nursing
University of Michigan
Flint, Michigan

Alison Trider, MS, APRN, CNM
Assistant Professor
St. Joseph College
West Hartford, Connecticut

Jennifer Visbisky, RN, MSN
Assistant Professor of Nursing
Jamestown Community College
Jamestown, New York

Daryle Wane, MS, ARNP, FNP-BC
Associate Professor of Nursing
College of Nursing
Pasco Hernando Community College
   at New Port Richey
New Port Richey, Florida

Barbara Wilson, PhD, RNC
Assistant Professor
College of Nursing and Healthcare Innovation
Arizona State University, Polytechnic Campus
Mesa, Arizona

Robin Wilson, MSN, RNC
Assistant Professor of Nursing
Lincoln Memorial University
Harrogate, Tennessee

PREFACE

This textbook is designed as a practical approach to understanding the health of women in a maternity context and the health of their newborns. Women in our society are becoming empowered to make informed and responsible choices regarding their health and that of their children, but to do so they need the encouragement and support of nurses who care for them. This textbook focuses on the reproductive issues of women throughout the lifespan and arms the student or practicing nurse with essential information to care for women and their families, to assist them to make the right choices safely, intelligently, and with confidence.

Organization

Each chapter of this textbook reviews an important dimension of a woman's general health throughout her life cycle and addresses risk factors, lifestyle choices that influence her well-being, appropriate interventions, and nursing education topics to preserve her health and that of her newborn.

The text is divided into eight units.

Unit 1: Introduction to Maternity, Newborn, and Women's Nursing

Unit 1 helps build a foundation for the student beginning the study of maternal-newborn and women's health nursing by exploring contemporary issues and trends and community-based nursing.

Unit 2: Women's Health Throughout the Lifespan

Unit 2 introduces the student to selected women's health topics, including the structure and function of the reproductive system, common reproductive concerns, sexually transmitted infections, problems of the breast, and benign disorders and cancers of the female reproductive tract. This unit encourages students to assist women in maintaining their quality of life, reducing their risk of disease, and becoming active partners with their health care professional.

Unit 3: Pregnancy

Unit 3 addresses topics related to normal pregnancy, including fetal development, genetics, and maternal adaptation to pregnancy. Nursing management during normal pregnancy is presented in a separate chapter encouraging application of basic knowledge to nursing practice. This nursing care chapter covers maternal and fetal assessment throughout pregnancy, interventions to promote self-care and minimize common discomforts, and patient education.

Unit 4: Labor and Birth

Unit 4 begins with a chapter on the normal labor and birth process, including maternal and fetal adaptations. This is followed by a chapter discussing the nurse's role during normal labor and birth, which includes maternal and fetal assessment, pharmacologic and non-pharmacologic comfort measures and pain management, and specific nursing interventions during each stage of labor and birth.

Unit 5: Postpartum Period

Unit 5 focuses on maternal adaptation during the normal postpartum period. Both physiologic and psychological aspects are explored. Paternal adaptation is also considered. This unit also focuses on related nursing management, including assessment of physical and emotional status, promoting comfort, assisting with elimination, counseling about sexuality and contraception, promoting nutrition, promoting family adaptation, and preparing for discharge.

Unit 6: The Newborn

Unit 6 covers physiologic and behavioral adaptations of the normal newborn. It also delves into nursing management of the normal newborn, including immediate assessment and specific interventions as well as ongoing assessment, physical examination, and specific interventions during the early newborn period.

Unit 7: Childbearing at Risk

Unit 7 shifts the focus to at-risk pregnancy, childbirth, and postpartum care. Pre-existing conditions of the woman, pregnancy-related complications, at-risk labor, emergencies associated with labor and birth, and medical conditions and complications affecting the postpartum woman are covered. Treatment and nursing management are presented for each medical condition. This organization allows the student to build on a solid foundation of normal material when studying the at-risk content.

Unit 8: The Newborn at Risk

Unit 8 continues to focus on at-risk content. Issues of the newborn with birth weight variations, gestational age variations, congenital conditions, and acquired disorders are explored. Treatment and nursing management are presented for each medical condition. This organization helps cement the student's understanding of the material.

Recurring Features

In order to provide the instructor and student with an exciting and user-friendly text, a number of recurring features have been developed.

Key Terms

A list of terms that are considered essential to the chapter's understanding is presented at the beginning of each chapter. Each key term appears in boldface, with the definition included in the text. Key terms may also be accessed on ThePoint.

Learning Objectives

Learning Objectives included at the beginning of each chapter guide the student in understanding what is important and why, allowing him or her to prioritize information for learning. These valuable learning tools also provide opportunities for self-testing or instructor evaluation of student knowledge and ability.

WOW

Each chapter opens with inspiring Words of Wisdom, which offer helpful, timely, or interesting thoughts. These WOW statements set the stage for each chapter and give the student valuable insight into nursing care of women and newborns.

Case Studies

Real-life scenarios present relevant maternity, newborn, and women's health information that is intended to perfect the student's caregiving skills. Questions about the scenario provide an opportunity for the student to critically evaluate the appropriate course of action.

Watch and Learn Icon

A special icon **WATCH&LEARN** throughout the book directs the student to free video clips that highlight maternity nursing care. These clips can be viewed on the Point website and also on the Student Resource CD.

Evidence-Based Practice

The consistent promotion of evidence-based practice is a key feature of the text. Throughout the chapters, pivotal questions addressed by current research have been incorporated into Evidence-Based Practice boxes, which cite studies relevant to the chapter content.

Healthy People 2010

Throughout the textbook, relevant Healthy People 2010 objectives are outlined in box format. The nursing implications or guidance provided in the box serve as a roadmap for improving the health of women, mothers, and newborns.

Teaching Guidelines

An important tool for achieving health promotion and disease prevention is health education. Throughout the textbook, Teaching Guidelines raise awareness, provide timely and accurate information, and are designed to ensure the student's preparation for educating women about various issues.

Drug Guides

Drug guide tables summarize information about commonly used medications. The actions, indications, and significant nursing implications presented assist the student in providing optimum care to women and their newborns

Common Laboratory and Diagnostic Tests

Common Laboratory and Diagnostic Tests tables in many of the chapters provide the student with a general understanding of how a broad range of disorders is diagnosed. Rather than reading the information repeatedly throughout the narrative, the student is then able to refer to the table as needed.

Common Medical Treatments

The Common Medical Treatments tables in many of the nursing management chapters provide the student with a broad awareness of how a common group of disorders is treated either medically or surgically. The tables serve as a reference point for common medical treatments.

Nursing Care Plans

Nursing Care Plans provide concrete examples of each step of the nursing process and are provided in numerous chapters. Found within the nursing process overview section of the chapter, the Nursing Care Plans summarize issue- or system-related content, thereby minimizing repetition.

Comparison Charts

These charts compare two or more disorders or other easily confused concepts. They serve to provide an explanation that clarifies the concepts for the student.

Nursing Procedures

Step-by-step Nursing Procedures are presented in a clear, concise format to facilitate competent performance of relevant procedures as well as to clarify pediatric variations when appropriate.

Consider This!

In every chapter the student is asked to *Consider This!* These first-person narratives engage the student in real-life scenarios experienced by their patients. The personal accounts evoke empathy and help the student to perfect caregiving skills. Each box ends with an opportunity for further contemplation, encouraging the student to think critically about the scenario.

Take Note!

The *Take Note!* feature draws the student's attention to points of critical emphasis throughout the chapter. This feature is often used to stress life-threatening or otherwise vitally important information.

Table, Boxes, Illustrations, and Photographs

Abundant tables and boxes summarize key content throughout the book. Additionally, beautiful illustrations and photographs help the student to visualize the content. These features allow the student to quickly and easily access information.

Key Concepts

At the end of each chapter, Key Concepts provide a quick review of essential chapter elements. These bulleted lists help the student focus on the important aspects of the chapter.

References and Websites

References and websites that were used in the development of the text are provided at the end of each chapter. These listings enable the student to further explore topics of interest. Many on-line resources are provided as a means for the student to electronically explore relevant content material. These resources can be shared with women, children, and their families to enhance patient education and support.

Chapter Worksheets

Chapter worksheets at the end of each chapter assist the student in reviewing essential concepts. Chapter worksheets include:

- **Multiple Choice Questions**—These review questions are written to test the student's ability to apply chapter material. Questions cover maternal-newborn and women's health content that the student might encounter on the national licensing exam (NCLEX).
- **Critical Thinking Exercises**—These exercises challenge the student to incorporate new knowledge with previously learned concepts and reach a satisfactory conclusion. They encourage the student to think critically, problem solve, and consider his or her own perspective on given topics.
- **Study Activities**—These interactive activities promote student participation in the learning process. This section encourages increased interaction/learning via clinical, on-line, and community activities.

Teaching–Learning Package

Instructor's Resource DVD

This valuable resource for instructors includes all the materials instructors need to teach the maternity-pediatric course, including

- PowerPoint presentations that correspond to each chapter and serve as a supplement to the instructor's course development
- A Test Generator that features hundreds of questions within a powerful tool to help the instructor create quizzes and tests
- An Image Bank that provides access to photographs and illustrations from the text in a convenient, searchable format
- Lecture Outlines for organizing classroom instruction
- Sample syllabi for setting up the maternity-pediatric nursing course
- Assignments and reading comprehension quizzes designed to test the student's understanding

Student Resource CD-ROM

The student resource CD-ROM, which is included for free in the front of the book, features video clips highlighting the developmental stages of pregnancy, vaginal labor and birth, scheduled cesarean section, breastfeeding assistance, developmental considerations, and nursing care of the child in the hospital.

The CD-ROM also includes a Spanish-English audio glossary and an NCLEX alternate item format tutorial.

ThePoint Solution

ThePoint Solution, http://thepoint.lww.com, a trademark of Wolters Kluwer Health, is a web-based course and content management system providing every resource that the instructor and student needs in one easy-to-use site. Advanced technology and superior content combine at ThePoint to allow instructors to design and deliver online and offline courses, maintain grades and class rosters, and communicate with students. Students can visit ThePoint to access supplemental multimedia resources, such as Key Concepts, Answers to Worksheets, a Glossary, and NCLEX-style student review questions to enhance their learning experience. ThePoint Solution package also includes an EBook, so students can search their text electronically, and journal articles to help students understand evidence-based practice. Students can also check the course syllabus, download content, upload assignments, and join an online study group. For instructors, a wealth of information can be found at ThePoint, all designed to make teaching easier. For example . . .

- Pre-lecture quizzes, made of five true/false and five fill-in-the-blank questions, are meant to be given at the beginning of class and help evaluate whether students are keeping up with the reading and the material it covers.
- Assignments, broken into four types—written, group, clinical, and Web—and organized by learning objective, provide opportunities for in- or after-class activities.
- Discussion topics, also organized by learning objective, allow students to critically think through scenarios and discuss their ideas with other students.
- Guided lecture notes organize the chapter objective by objective and provide references to appropriate PowerPoint slides and figures from the text.
- Sample syllabi assist instructors with setting their courses and are provided for four different course lengths: 4, 6, 8, and 10 weeks.

ThePoint . . . where teaching, learning and technology click!

Susan Scott Ricci

CONTENTS

CHAPTER *9*

Violence and Abuse 214

CHAPTER *10*

Fetal Development and Genetics 237

CHAPTER *11*

Maternal Adaptation During Pregnancy 263

CHAPTER *12*

Nursing Management During Pregnancy 288

U N I T   F O U R
LABOR AND BIRTH 333

CHAPTER *13*
Labor and Birth Process 335

CHAPTER *14*
Nursing Management During Labor
and Birth 361

CHAPTER *20*

Nursing Management of the Pregnancy at Risk: Selected Health Conditions and Vulnerable Populations 564

CHAPTER *21*

Nursing Management of Labor and Birth at Risk 610

CHAPTER *22*

Nursing Management of the Postpartum Woman at Risk 647

UNIT EIGHT
THE NEWBORN AT RISK 669

CHAPTER 23
Nursing Care of the Newborn With Special Needs 671

CHAPTER 24
Nursing Management of the Newborn at Risk: Acquired and Congenital Newborn Conditions 700

ESSENTIALS OF
MATERNITY, NEWBORN,
& WOMEN'S HEALTH NURSING

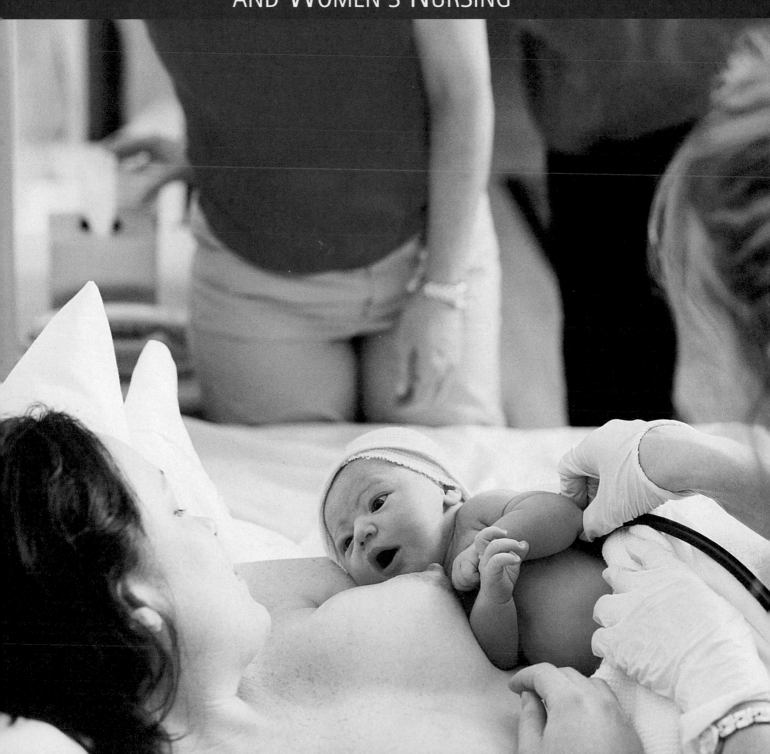

UNIT ONE

INTRODUCTION TO MATERNITY, NEWBORN,
AND WOMEN'S NURSING

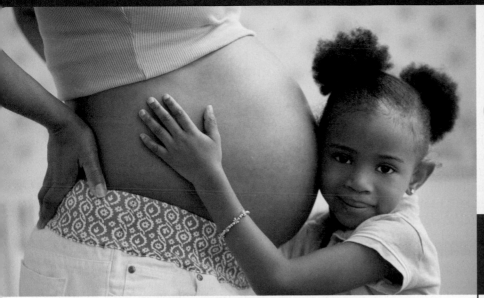

PERSPECTIVES ON MATERNAL, NEWBORN, AND WOMEN'S HEALTH CARE

KEY TERMS

case management
certified nurse midwife (CNM)
cultural competence
culture

doula
evidence-based nursing practice
family
family-centered care

fetal mortality rate
infant mortality rate
maternal mortality rate
mortality
neonatal mortality rate

LEARNING OBJECTIVES

Upon completion of the chapter, the learner will be able to:

1. Identify the key milestones in the evolution of maternal, newborn, and women's health nursing.
2. Describe the major components, concepts, and influences associated with the nursing management of women and their families.
3. Compare the past definitions of health and illness to the current definitions.
4. Identify the factors that affect maternal, newborn, and women's health.
5. Evaluate how society and culture can influence the health of women and their families.
6. Discuss the health care barriers affecting women and their families.
7. Discuss the ethical and legal issues that may arise when caring for women and their families.

Sophia Greenly, a 38-year-old woman pregnant with her third child, comes to the prenatal clinic for a routine follow-up visit. Her mother, Betty, accompanies her because Sophia's husband is out of town. Sophia lives with her husband and two children, ages 4 and 9. She works part-time as a lunch aide in the local elementary school. What factors may play a role in influencing the health of Sophia and her family?

Wow

Being pregnant and giving birth is like crossing a narrow bridge: people can accompany you to the bridge, and they can greet you on the other side, but you walk that bridge alone.

A person's ability to lead a fulfilling life and to participate fully in society depends largely on his or her health status. This is especially true for women, who commonly are responsible for not only their own health but that of others: their children and families. Thus, it is important to focus on the health of women and families. Habits and practices established during pregnancy and in early childhood can have profound effects on a person's health and illness throughout life. As a society, creating a population that cares about women and their families and promotes solid health care and lifestyle choices is crucial.

Maternal and newborn nursing encompasses a wide scope of practice typically associated with childbearing. It includes care of the woman before pregnancy, care of the woman and her fetus during pregnancy, care of the woman after pregnancy, and care of the newborn, usually during the first 6 weeks after birth. The overall goal of maternal and newborn nursing is to promote and maintain optimal health of the woman and her family.

Now more than ever, nurses contribute to nearly every health care experience. Events from birth to death, and every health care emergency in between, will likely involve the presence of a nurse. Involvement of a knowledgeable, supportive, comforting nurse often leads to a positive health care experience. Skilled nursing practice depends on a solid base of knowledge and clinical expertise delivered in a caring, holistic manner. Nurses, using their knowledge and passion, help meet the health care needs of their clients throughout the life span, whether the client is a pregnant woman, a fetus, a partner, or a woman with a health-related problems. Nurses fill a variety of roles in helping clients to live healthier lives by providing direct care, emotional support, comfort, information, advice, advocacy, support, and counseling. Nurses are often "in the trenches" advocating for issues, drawing attention to the importance of health care for the client, and dealing with the lack of resources, the lack of access to health care, and the focus on acute care rather than education and prevention.

This chapter presents a general overview of the health care of women and their families and describes the major factors affecting maternal, newborn, and women's health. Nurses need to be knowledgeable about these concepts and factors to ensure that they provide professional care.

Evolution of Maternal and Newborn Nursing

The health care of women has changed over the years due in part to changes in childbirth methods, social trends, changes in the health care system, and federal and state regulations. By reviewing historical events, nurses can gain a better understanding of the current and future status of maternal, newborn, and women's health nursing.

Early Development

Childbirth in colonial America was a difficult and dangerous experience. During the 17th and 18th centuries, women giving birth often died as a result of exhaustion, dehydration, infection, hemorrhage, or seizures (Cassidy, 2006). Approximately 50% of all children died before age 5 (Brodsky, 2006; Jolivet, 2006), compared with the 0.06% infant mortality rate of today (World Factbook, 2007).

Centuries ago, "granny midwives" handled the normal birthing process for most women. They learned their skills through an apprenticeship with a more experienced midwife. Physicians usually were called only in extremely difficult cases, and all births took place at home.

During the early 1900s, physicians attended about half the births in the United States. Midwives often cared for women who could not afford a doctor. Many women were attracted to hospitals because this showed affluence and hospitals provided pain management, which was not available in home births. In the 1950s, "natural childbirth" practices advocating birth without medication and focusing on relaxation techniques were introduced. These techniques opened the door to childbirth education classes and helped bring the father back into the picture. Both partners could participate by taking an active role in pregnancy, childbirth, and parenting (Fig. 1.1).

Current Trends

Box 1.1 shows a timeline of childbirth in America. In many ways, childbirth practices in the United States have come full circle, as we see the return of nurse midwives and doulas. The concept of women helping other women during childbirth is not new: women who labored and gave birth at home were traditionally attended to by relatives and midwives (see Evidence-Based Practice 1.1). A **certified nurse midwife** (**CNM**) has postgraduate training in the care of normal pregnancy and delivery and is certified by the American College of Nurse Midwives (ACNM). A **doula** is a birth assistant who provides emotional, physical, and educational support to the woman and family during childbirth and the postpartum period. Many nurses working in labor and birth areas today are credentialed in their specialty so that they can provide optimal care to the woman and her newborn. Childbirth choices are often based on what works best for the mother, child, and family.

Core Concepts of Maternal, Newborn, and Women's Health Nursing

Maternal, newborn, and women's health nursing focuses on providing evidence-based care to the client within the context of the family. This care involves the implementation of an interdisciplinary plan in a collaborative manner

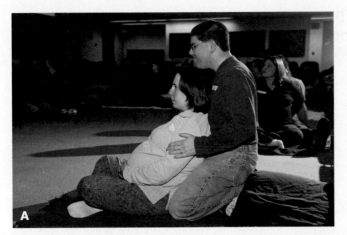
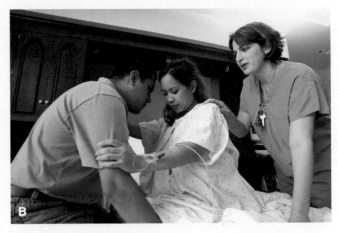

FIGURE 1.1 Today fathers and partners are welcome to take an active role in the pregnancy and childbirth experience. (**A**) A couple can participate together in childbirth education classes. (Photo by Gus Freedman) (**B**) Fathers and partners can assist the woman throughout her labor and delivery. (Photo by Joe Mitchell)

BOX 1.1 **Childbirth in America: A Time Line**

1700s   Men did not attend births, because it was considered indecent.

Women faced birth, not with joy and ecstasy, but with fear of death.

Female midwives attended the majority of all births at home.

1800s   There is a shift from using midwives to doctors among middle class women.

The word *obstetrician* was formed from the Latin, meaning "to stand before."

Puerperal (childbed) fever was occurring in epidemic proportions.

Louis Pasteur demonstrated that streptococci were the major cause of puerperal fever that was killing mothers after delivery.

The first cesarean section was performed in Boston in 1894.

The x-ray was developed in 1895 and was used to asses pelvic size for birthing purposes (Feldhusen 2003).

1900s   Twilight sleep (a heavy dose of narcotics and amnesiacs) was used on women during childbirth in the United States.

The United States was 17th out of 20 nations in infant mortality rates.

Fifty to 75% of all women gave birth in hospitals by 1940.

Nurseries were started because moms could not care for their baby for several days after receiving chloroform gas.

Dr. Grantley Dick–Reed (1933) wrote a book entitled *Childbirth Without Fear* that reduced the "fear–tension–pain" cycle women experienced during labor and birth.

Dr. Fernand Lamaze (1984) wrote a book entitled *Painless Childbirth: The Lamaze Method* that advocated distraction and relaxation techniques to minimize the perception of pain.

Amniocentesis is first performed to assess fetal growth in 1966.

In the 1970s the cesarean section rate was about 5%. By 1990 it rose to 24%, where it stands currently (Martin, 2002).

The 1970s and 1980s see a growing trend to return birthing back to the basics—nonmedicated, nonintervening childbirth.

In the late 1900s, freestanding birthing centers—LDRPs—were designed, and the number of home births began to increase.

2000s   One in four women undergo a surgical birth (cesarean).

CNMs once again assist couples at home, in hospitals, or in freestanding facilities with natural childbirths. Research shows that midwives are the safest birth attendants for most women, with lower infant mortality and maternal rates, and fewer invasive interventions such as episiotomies and cesareans (Keefe 2003).

Childbirth classes of every flavor abound in most communities.

According to the latest available data, the United States ranks 21st in the world in maternal deaths. The maternal mortality rate is approximately 7 in 1000 live births.

According to the latest available data, the United States ranks 27th in the world in infant mortality rates. The infant mortality rate is approximately 7 in 1000 live births (United Nations, 2003).

EVIDENCE-BASED PRACTICE 1.1
Women's Response to Continuous Labor Support

Throughout history, women have been helping other women in labor by providing emotional support, comfort measures, information, and advocacy. However, in recent years this practice has waned, and facilities frequently adhere to strict specific routines that may leave women feeling "dehumanized."

● Study

A study was done to assess the effects on mothers and their newborns of continuous, one-to-one intrapartum care compared to usual care. The study also evaluated routine practices and policies in the birth environment that might affect a woman's autonomy, freedom of movement, and ability to cope with labor; who the caregiver was (a staff member of the facility or not); and when the support began (early or late in labor). All published and unpublished randomized clinical trials comparing continuous support during labor with usual care were examined. One author and one research assistant used standard methods for data collection and analysis and extracted the data independently. Clinical trial authors provided additional information. The researchers used relative risk for categorical data and weighted mean difference for continuous data. Sixteen trials from 11 countries involving 13,391 women were examined.

▲ Findings

Women receiving continuous intrapartum support had a greater chance of a spontaneous vaginal delivery (including without forceps or vacuum extraction). They also had a slight decrease in the length of labor and required less analgesia during this time. These women also reported increased satisfaction with their labor and childbirth experience. Overall, the support, when provided by someone other than a facility staff member and initiated early in labor, proved to be more effective.

■ Nursing Implications

Based on this research, it is clear that women in labor benefit from one-to-one support during labor. Nurses can use the information gained from this study to educate women about the importance of having a support person during labor and delivery. Nurses can also act as client advocates in facilities where they work to foster an environment that encourages the use of support persons during the intrapartum period. The focus of nursing needs to be individualized, supportive, and collaborative with the family during their childbearing experience. In short, nurses should place the needs of the mother and her family first in providing a continuum of care.

Although the study found that support is more effective when provided by someone other than a staff member, support from an individual is the key. Assigning the same nurse to provide care to the couple throughout the birthing experience also fosters a one-to-one relationship that helps meet the couple's needs and promotes feelings of security. By meeting the couple's needs, the nurse is enhancing their birthing experience.

Hodnett, E. D., Gates, S. Hofmeyr, G. J., & Sakata, C. (2007). Continuous support for women during childbirth. *Cochrane Database of Systematic Reviews* 2007. Issue 3. Art No.: CD003766.DOI:10.1002/14651858.CD003766.pub2.

---

to ensure continuity of care that is cost-effective, quality-oriented, and outcome-focused. It involves family-centered, evidence-based, case-managed care.

Family-Centered Care

Family-centered care is the delivery of safe, satisfying, high-quality health care that focuses on and adapts to the physical and psychosocial needs of the family. It is a cooperative effort of families and other caregivers that recognizes the strength and integrity of the family. The basic principles of family-centered care are:

- Childbirth is considered a normal, healthy event in the life of a family.
- Childbirth affects the entire family, and relationships will change.
- Families are capable of making decisions about their own care if given adequate information and professional support) (Price, Noseworthy, & Thornton, 2007).

The philosophy of family-centered care recognizes the family as the constant. The health and functioning of the family affect the health of the client and other members of the family. Family members support one another well beyond the health care provider's brief time with them, such as during the childbearing process or during a child's illness. Birth is viewed as a normal life event rather than a medical procedure.

With family-centered care, support and respect for the uniqueness and diversity of families are essential, along with encouragement and enhancement of the family's strengths and competencies. It is important to create opportunities for families to demonstrate their abilities and skills. Families also can acquire new abilities and skills to maintain a sense of control. Family-centered care promotes greater family self-determination, decision-making abilities, control, and self-efficacy, thereby enhancing the client's and family's sense of empowerment. When implementing family-centered care, nurses seek caregiver input;

these suggestions and advice are incorporated into the client's plan of care as the nurse counsels and teaches the family appropriate health care interventions. Today, as nurses partner with various experts to provide high-quality and cost-effective care, one expert partnership that nurses can make is with the client's family.

The impact of family-centered care can be seen in the models of care delivery for women. From the 1980s to the present, increased access to care for all women (regardless of their ability to pay) and hospital redesigns (labor, delivery, and recovery [LDR] rooms; labor, delivery, recovery, and postpartum [LDRP] spaces) aimed at keeping families together during the childbirth experience (Fig. 1.2).

Evidence-Based, Case-Managed Care

Evidence-based nursing practice involves the use of research in establishing a plan of care and implementing that care. Evidence-based practice is a problem-solving approach to making nursing clinical decisions (Newhouse, 2006). This model of nursing practice includes the use of the best current evidence in making decisions about care. Widespread use of evidence-based practice may lead to a decrease in variation of care while at the same time increasing quality.

Modern health care focuses on an interdisciplinary plan of care designed to meet a client's physical, developmental, educational, spiritual, and psychosocial needs. This interdisciplinary collaborative type of care is termed **case management**, a collaborative process involving assessment, planning, implementation, coordination, monitoring, and evaluation. It involves the following components:

• Advocacy, communication, and resource management
• Client-focused comprehensive care across a continuum
• Coordinated care with an interdisciplinary approach
  (Foster & Heath, 2007)

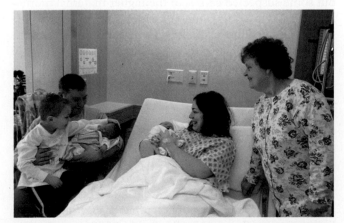

FIGURE 1.2 Providing an opportunity for the "big brother" to interact with his new siblings is an important component of family-centered nursing care.

When the nurse effectively functions in the role as a case manager, client and family satisfaction is increased, fragmentation of care is decreased, and outcome measurement for a homogenous group of clients is possible.

Think back to Sophia and her mother, Betty, who were described at the beginning of the chapter. Sophia and her husband are planning to use natural childbirth and to have their children present for the birth. While Sophia is waiting to be called for her appointment, Betty says, "Things have changed so much since I was pregnant. It's amazing what happens nowadays." Explain how things have changed in maternal and newborn health care, focusing on the concept of family-centered care.

Health Status

At one time, health was defined simply as the absence of disease; health was measured by monitoring the mortality and morbidity of a group. Over the past century, however, the focus on health has shifted to disease prevention, health promotion, and wellness. The World Health Organization defines health as "a state of complete physical, mental, and social well-being, and not merely the absence of disease or infirmity" (WHO, 2008). The definition of health is complex; it is not merely the absence of disease or an analysis of mortality and morbidity statistics.

In 1979, the Surgeon General's Report, *Healthy People*, presented a prevention agenda for the nation that identified the most significant preventable threats to the health of the United States. Through a series of reports (the current report is *Healthy People 2010: National Health Promotion and Disease Prevention Objectives*), the country now has a comprehensive, nationwide health promotion and disease prevention agenda that includes emphasis on children's health (U.S. Department of Health & Human Services [DHHS], 2000). Ten specific health indicators serve as a way to evaluate progress made in the public health arena and to coordinate the national health improvement efforts. Healthy People 2010 highlights the major health indicators of the 21st century that need to be addressed.

HEALTHY PEOPLE 2010

Major Health Concerns of the 21st Century

• Physical activity	• Mental health
• Overweight and obesity	• Injury and violence
• Tobacco use	• Environmental quality
• Substance abuse	• Immunizations
• Responsible sexual behavior	• Access to health care

Healthy People 2010 also outlines major goals intended to increase the quality and years of healthy life and to eliminate health disparities between ethnic groups by targeting the lifestyle choices and environmental conditions that cause 70% of premature deaths in the United States. Healthy People 2010 identifies specific national health goals related to maternal, infant, and child health.

Measuring health status is not a simple or convenient process. For example, some individuals with chronic illnesses do not see themselves as ill if they can control their condition through self-management. A traditional method used in this country to measure health is to examine mortality and morbidity data. Information is collected and analyzed to provide an objective description of the nation's health.

Mortality

Mortality is the incidence or number of individuals who have died over a specific period. This statistic is presented as rates per 100,000 and is calculated from a sample of death certificates. The National Center for Health Statistics, under the DHHS, collects, analyzes, and disseminates the data on America's mortality rates.

HEALTHY PEOPLE *2010*

National Health Goals—Maternal, Infant and Child Health

- Reduce fetal and infant deaths.
- Reduce maternal deaths.
- Reduce maternal illness and complications resulting from pregnancy.
- Increase the proportion of pregnant women who receive early and adequate prenatal care.
- Increase the proportion of pregnant women who attend a series of prepared childbirth classes.
- Increase the proportion of very low-birth weight (VLBW) infants born at level III hospitals or subspecialty perinatal centers.
- Reduce cesarean births among low-risk (full-term, singleton, vertex presentation) women.
- Reduce low birth weight (LBW) and VLBW.
- Reduce preterm births.
- Increase the proportion of mothers who achieve a recommended weight gain during their pregnancies.
- Increase the percentage of healthy, full-term infants who are laid down to sleep on their backs.
- Reduce the occurrence of developmental disabilities.
- Reduce the occurrence of spina bifida and other neural tube defects (NTDs).
- Increase the proportion of pregnancies begun with an optimum folic acid level.
- Increase abstinence from alcohol, cigarettes, and illicit drugs among pregnant women.
- Reduce the occurrence of fetal alcohol syndrome (FAS).
- Increase the proportion of mothers who breast-feed their babies.
- Ensure appropriate newborn bloodspot screening, follow-up testing, and referral to services.

Maternal Mortality

The **maternal mortality rate** is the number of deaths from any cause during the pregnancy cycle per 100,000 live births. In the United States, the maternal mortality rate is 7.5 (UNICEF, 2007). The federal government has pledged to improve maternal–child care outcomes and thus reduce mortality rates for women and children.

During the past several decades, mortality and morbidity have dramatically decreased as a result of an increased emphasis on hygiene, good nutrition, exercise, and prenatal care for all women. However, women are still experiencing complications at significant rates. The United States is one of the most medically and technologically advanced nations and has the highest per capita spending on health care in the world, but our current mortality rates indicate the need for improvement. For example:

- Two or three women die in the United States every day from pregnancy complications, and more than 30% of pregnant women (1.8 million women annually) experience some type of illness or injury during childbirth (Centers for Disease Control and Prevention [CDC], 2007a).
- The United States ranks 21st (in other words, below 20 other countries) in rates of maternal deaths (deaths per 100,000 live births).
- Most pregnancy-related complications are preventable. The most common are ectopic pregnancy, preterm labor, hemorrhage, emboli, hypertension, infection, stroke, diabetes, and heart disease. The leading causes of pregnancy-related mortality for the year 2003 (the last year for which data are available) are embolism (20%), hemorrhage (17%), pregnancy-related hypertension (16%), and infection (13%) (CDC, 2007a).

The maternal mortality and morbidity rates for African-American women have been three to four times higher than for whites (NCHS, 2007). Researchers do not entirely understand what accounts for this disparity, but some suspected causes of the higher maternal mortality rates for minority women include low socioeconomic status, limited or no insurance coverage, bias among health care providers (which may foster distrust), and quality of care available in the community. Language and legal barriers may also explain why some immigrant women do not receive good prenatal care.

Lack of care during pregnancy is a major factor contributing to a poor outcome. Prenatal care is well known to prevent complications of pregnancy and to support the birth of healthy infants, and not all women receive the same quality and quantity of health care during a pregnancy. More than 40% of African-American, Native American, and Latino women do not obtain prenatal care during their first trimester of pregnancy (Hollander, 2006).

The CDC has noted that the disparity in maternal mortality rates between women of color and white women represent one of the largest racial disparities among public health indicators. Eliminating racial and ethnic disparities in maternal—child health care requires enhanced efforts at preventing disease, promoting health, and delivering appropriate and timely care (CDC, 2007b). The CDC has called for more research and monitoring to understand and address racial disparities, along with increased funding for prenatal and postpartum care. Research is needed to identify causes and to design initiatives to reduce these disparities, and the CDC is calling on Congress to expand programs to provide preconception and prenatal care to underserved women.

Fetal Mortality

The **fetal mortality rate** or fetal death rate refers to the intrauterine death of a fetus who is 20 weeks of gestation or more per 1,000 live births. Fetal mortality may be attributable to maternal factors (e.g., malnutrition, disease, or preterm cervical dilation) or fetal factors (e.g., chromosomal abnormalities or poor placental attachment). Fetal mortality provides an overall picture of the quality of maternal health and prenatal care.

Neonatal and Infant Mortality

The **neonatal mortality rate** is the number of infant deaths occurring in the first 28 days of life per 1,000 live births. The **infant mortality rate** is the number of deaths occurring in the first 12 months of life. It also is documented as the number of deaths of infants younger than 1 year of age per 1,000 live births. The infant mortality rate is used as an index of the general health of a country. Generally, this statistic is one of the most significant measures of children's health. In the United States, the infant mortality rate is 6.0 (CDC, 2007b) (Fig. 1.3).

The infant mortality rate varies greatly from state to state as well as between ethnic groups. The United States has one of the highest gross national products in the world and is known for its technological capabilities, but in 2000 it ranked 27th in infant mortality rates among industrialized nations (U.S. DHHS, 2006). The main causes of early

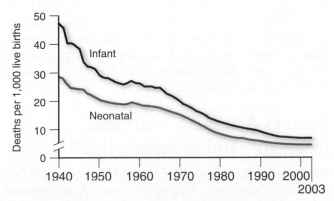

FIGURE 1.3 Infant and neonatal mortality, 1940–2003.

infant death in this country include problems occurring at birth or shortly thereafter. These include prematurity, low birthweight, congenital anomalies, sudden infant death syndrome, and respiratory distress syndrome.

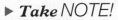

▶ *Take NOTE!*

African-American and American Indian/ Alaska Native infants have consistently had higher infant mortality rates than other ethnic groups (March of Dimes, 2006).

Congenital anomalies remain the leading cause of infant mortality in the United States. Low birthweight and prematurity are major indicators of infant health and significant predictors of infant mortality (March of Dimes, 2008). The lower the birthweight, the higher the risk of infant mortality; thus, the high incidence of low birthweight (<2,500 g) in the United States is a significant reason why its infant mortality rate is higher than that of other countries (March of Dimes, 2008).

After birth, other health promotion strategies can significantly improve an infant's health and chances of survival. Breastfeeding has been shown to reduce rates of infection in infants and to improve their long-term health. Emphasizing the importance of placing an infant on his or her back to sleep will reduce the incidence of sudden infant death syndrome. Encouraging mothers to join support groups to prevent postpartum depression and learn sound childrearing practices will improve the health of both mothers and their infants.

Morbidity

Morbidity and Women

Women today face not only diseases of genetic origin but also diseases that arise from poor personal habits. Even though women represent 51% of the population, only recently have researchers and the medical community focused on their special health needs. A recent significant study identified an urgent need to improve women's access to health insurance and health care services, place a stronger emphasis on prevention, and invest in more research on women's health (National Women's Law Center [NWLC] et al., 2007). It identified indicators of women's access to health care services, measuring the degree to which women receive preventive health care and engage in health-promoting activities (Box 1.2). The report card gave the nation an overall grade of "unsatisfactory," and not a single state received a grade of "satisfactory." Other substandard findings included the following:

• No state has focused enough attention on preventive measures, such as smoking cessation, exercise, nutrition, and screening for diseases.

- Too many women lack health insurance coverage: nationally, nearly one in seven women (14%) has no health insurance.
- No state has adequately addressed women's health needs in the areas of reproductive health, mental health, and violence against women.
- Limited research has been done on health conditions that primarily affect women and that affect women differently than men (NWLC et al., 2007).

Poor health habits can have a negative impact on all women. Smoking, drug abuse, high cholesterol levels, and obesity lead to high mortality and morbidity rates in our nation.

Major Health Issues for Women

Cardiovascular disease (CVD) is the number-one cause of death of women, regardless of racial or ethnic group. More than 500,000 women die annually in the United States of CVD—about one death per minute (Alexander et al., 2007) Women who have a heart attack are more likely than men to die. Heart attacks in women are often more difficult to diagnose than in men because of their vague and varied symptoms. Heart disease is still thought of as a "man's disease," and thus a heart attack may not be considered in the differential diagnosis when a woman presents to the emergency room. Nurses need to look beyond the obvious "crushing chest pain" textbook symptom that heralds a heart attack in men. Manifestations of heart disease differ between men and women in several other ways—for example, menopause (associated with a significant rise in coronary events); diabetes, high cholesterol levels, and left ventricular hypertrophy; and repeated episodes of weight loss and gain (increased coronary morbidity and mortality) (Framingham Heart Study [FHS], 2007).

Cancer is the second leading cause of death among women (American Cancer Society [ACS], 2008a). Women have a one-in-three lifetime risk of developing cancer, and one out of every four deaths is from cancer (Alexander et al., 2007). Although much attention is focused on cancer of the reproductive system, lung cancer is the number-one killer of women. This is largely the result of smoking and second-hand smoke. Lung cancer has no early symptoms, making early detection almost impossible. Thus, lung cancer has the lowest survival rate of any cancer: more than 90% of people who get lung cancer die of it (ACS, 2008b).

Breast cancer occurs in one in every seven women in a lifetime. It is estimated that in 2008 about 182,460 new cases of invasive breast cancer will be diagnosed among women in the United States. Women living in North America have the highest rate of breast cancer in the world. At this time there are about 2.5 million breast cancer survivors in the United States. It is the most common malignancy in women and second only to lung cancer as a cause of cancer mortality in women (ACS, 2008c). Although a positive family history of breast cancer, aging, and irregularities in the menstrual cycle at an early age are major risk factors, others risk factors include excess weight, not having children, oral contraceptive use, excessive alcohol consumption, a high-fat diet, and long-term use of hormone replacement therapy (ACS, 2008c). Breast cancer rates have dropped recently, possibly due to the decreased use of long-term hormone replacement therapy that occurred after the Women's Health Initiative (WHI) report was released in 2002 (Heiss et al., 2008). However, early detection and treatment continue to offer the best chance for a cure, and reducing the risk of cancer by decreasing avoidable risks continues to be the best preventive plan.

Women's health is a complex issue, and no single policy is going to change the overall dismal state ratings. Although progress in science and technology has helped reduce the incidence of and improve the survival rates for several diseases, women's health issues continue to have an impact on our society. By eliminating or decreasing some of the risk factors and causes for prevalent diseases and illnesses, society and science could minimize certain chronic health problems. Focusing on the causes and effects of particular illnesses could help resolve many women's health issues of today.

Factors Affecting Maternal, Newborn, and Women's Health

From conception, children are shaped by a myriad of factors such as genetics and the environment. As members of a family, they are also members of a specific population, community, culture, and society. As they learn and grow, they are affected by multiple, complex, and ever-changing influences around them. For example, dramatic demographic changes in the United States have led to shifts in majority and minority population groups. Globalization has led to an international focus on health. Access to and the types of health care available have changed due to modifications in health care delivery and financing. In addition, the United States is still grappling with issues such as immigration, poverty, homelessness, and violence.

These factors may affect the person positively, promoting healthy growth and development, or negatively, increasing the person's health risks. Nurses, especially those working with women and their families, need to understand how these influences affect the quality of nursing care and health outcomes. They must examine the impact of these variables to gain the knowledge and skills needed to plan effective care, thereby achieving the best possible outcomes.

Family

The **family** is considered the basic social unit. The way that families are defined has changed (Table 1.1). The U.S. Census Bureau (2007) defines family as a group of two or more persons related by birth, marriage, or adoption and living together. Earlier definitions of family emphasized the legal ties or genetic relationships of people living in the same household with specific roles.

The family greatly influences the development and health of its members. For example, children learn health care activities, health beliefs, and health values from their family. The family's structure, the roles assumed by family members, and social changes that affect the family's life can influence the woman's and newborn's health status. Families are unique: each one has different views and requires distinct methods for support (Fig. 1.4).

Changes in Parental Roles Over Time

Parental roles have evolved over time due to social and economic changes as well as family changes. Traditionally, the role of provider was assigned to the father. However, with increased numbers of women in the workplace and more households with two parents working, today both parents are often the providers as well as the nurturers. Technological expansion has provided parents with opportunities to work at home, allowing some parents to maintain the provider role while simultaneously fulfilling the nurturer and health manager roles. Fathers also are taking on greater responsibilities related to household management and infant and child care. Additionally, the number of single-father parent families and grandparent families is increasing.

Recall Sophia, the pregnant woman described at the beginning of the chapter. Identify the parental roles assumed by Sophia. How might these roles be different from those of her mother when she was Sophia's age?

Genetics

Genetics (the study of heredity and its variations) has implications for all stages of life and all types of diseases. The newborn's or infant's biological traits, including gender, race, some behavioral traits, and the presence of certain diseases or illnesses, are directly linked to genetic inheritance. New technologies in molecular biology and biochemistry have led to a better understanding of the mechanisms involved in hereditary transmission, including those associated with genetic disorders. These advances are leading to better diagnostic tests and better management options.

Gender

Gender is established when the sex chromosomes join. A person's gender can influence many aspects, such as physical characteristics and personal attributes, attitudes, and behaviors. Some diseases or illnesses are more common in one sex; for example, scoliosis is more common in females and color blindness in males.

Race

Race refers to the physical features that distinguish members of a particular group, such as skin color, bone structure, or blood type. Some physical features that are normal in a particular race may be considered a sign of a disorder in other races. For example, epicanthal folds (the vertical folds of skin that partially or completely cover the inner canthi of the eye) are normal in Asian children but may occur with Down syndrome or renal agenesis in other races. In addition, certain malformations and diseases are found more commonly in specific races. For example, sickle cell anemia occurs more often in African and Mediterranean population groups, and cystic fibrosis is seen more often in individuals from the Northwestern European population group.

Society

Society has a major impact on the health of women and their families. Major influences include social roles, socioeconomic status, the media, and the expanding global nature of society. Each of these may influence a person's self-concept, where he or she lives, the lifestyle he or she leads—and thus his or her health.

Social Roles

Society often prescribes specific patterns of behaviors: certain behaviors are permitted and others are prohibited.

TABLE 1.1 EXAMPLES OF FAMILY STRUCTURES IN TODAY'S SOCIETY

Nuclear family	Husband, wife, and children living in same household	May include natural or adopted children Once considered the traditional family structure; now less common due to increased divorce rates and child-rearing by unmarried persons
Binuclear family	Child who is a member of two families due to joint custody; parenting is considered a "joint venture"	Always works better when the interests of the child are put first and above the parents' needs and desires
Single-parent family	One parent is responsible for care of children.	May result from death, divorce, desertion, birth outside marriage, or adoption These families are likely to face challenges because of economic, social, and personal restraints; one person serves as homemaker, caregiver, and financial provider.
Commuter family	Adults in the family live and work apart for professional or financial reasons, often leaving the daily care of children to one parent.	Similar to single-parent family
Step- or blended family	Adults with children from previous marriages or from the new marriage	May lead to family conflict due to different expectations on the part of the child and adults; they may have different views and practices related to childcare and health
Extended family	Nuclear family and grandparents, cousins, aunts, and uncles	Need to identify decision-maker and primary caretaker of the children Popular in some cultures, such as Hispanic and Asian cultures
Same-sex family (also called homosexual or gay/lesbian family)	Adults of the same sex living together with or without children	May face negative attitudes about their "different" lifestyle
Communal family	Group of people living together to raise children and manage household; unrelated by blood or marriage	May face negative attitudes about their "different" lifestyle Need to determine the decision-maker and caretaker of the children
Foster family	A temporary family for children who are placed away from their parents to ensure their emotional and physical well-being	May include the foster family's children and other foster children in the home Foster children are more likely to have unmet health needs and chronic health problems because they may have been in a variety of health systems (AAP, 2000).
Grandparents-as-parent families	Grandparents raising their grandchildren due to the inability or absence of the parents	May increase the risk for physical, financial, and emotional stress on older adults May lead to confusion and emotional stress for child if biological parents are in and out of child's life
Adolescent families	Young parents who are still mastering the developmental tasks of their childhood	Are at greater risk for health problems in pregnancy and delivery; more likely to have premature infants, which then leads to risk of subsequent health and developmental problems Probably still need support from their family related to financial, emotional, and school issues

These social roles are often an important factor in the development of self-concept. Social roles influence a person's ideas about himself or herself. Social roles are generally carried out in groups with which the individual has intimate daily contact, such as the family, school, workplace, or peer groups.

Socioeconomic Status

Another dominant influence is a person's socioeconomic status, his or her relative position in society. This includes the family's economic, occupational, and educational levels. Low socioeconomic status typically has an adverse influence on an individual's health. Health care costs are continuing to rise, as are health insurance premiums. The family may not be able to afford food, health care, and housing; meals may be unbalanced, erratic, or insufficient. Housing may be overcrowded or have poor sanitation. These families may not understand the importance of preventive care or may simply not be able to afford it. As a result, they may be exposed to health risks such as lead poisoning or may not be immunized against communicable diseases.

Poverty

Poverty is a measurement based on the specific monetary income of a family. The poverty threshold is the dollar amount that the U.S. Census Bureau uses to determine whether a family is living in poverty. If the individual's or family's income is below the threshold, then that person or family is said to be living in poverty.

Despite the many global economic gains that have been made during the past century, poverty continues to grow and the gap between rich and poor is widening. Major gaps continue between the economic opportunities and status afforded to women and those offered to men. A disproportionate share of the burden of poverty rests on women's shoulders, and this undermines their health. However, poverty, particularly for women, is more than monetary deficiency. Women continue to lag behind men in control of cash, credit, and collateral. Other forms of impoverishment may include deficiencies in literacy, education, skills, employment opportunities, mobility, and political representation, as well as pressures on time and energy linked to their responsibilities. These poverty factors may affect a woman's health (WHO, 2007a, 2007b, 2007c).

Homelessness

Families with children are the fastest-growing segment of the homeless population. Homeless families commonly are victims of violence and may have mental health challenges. Homelessness occurs in large urban areas and midsize cities as well as suburban and rural areas.

Homelessness can have a negative impact on health and well-being in numerous ways, including:

• Mental health issues such as anxiety, depression, or aggressive behavior

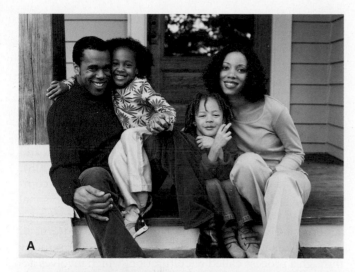
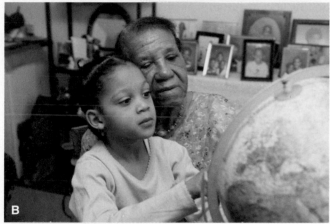
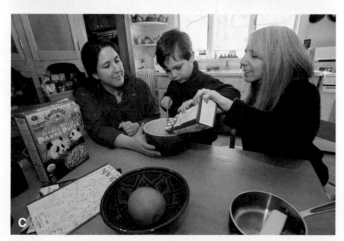

FIGURE 1.4 Nurses must take into account family dynamics when providing health care. There are many different family structures, and they influence the client's needs. (**A**) The traditional nuclear family is composed of two parents and their biological or adopted children. (**B**) The extended family includes the nuclear family plus other family members, such as grandparents, aunts, uncles, and cousins. (**C**) Gay and lesbian families comprise two people of the same sex sharing a committed relationship with or without children.

- Chronic health problems and injuries
- Nutritional deficiencies, affecting fetal growth and development
- Behaviors such as illegal substance use or unprotected sex with multiple partners
- Limited access to health care services such as preventive care, prenatal care, or dental care

Violence

Violence can occur in any setting and can involve any individual. Violence against women is a major health concern—it affects thousands of lives and costs the health care system millions of dollars. Violence affects families, women, and children of all ages, ethnic backgrounds, races, educational levels, and socioeconomic levels. Pregnancy is often a time when physical abuse starts or escalates, resulting in poorer outcomes for the mother and the baby. The nurse is responsible for assessing for and following up on any abuse.

Violence in the home environment, known as domestic violence, affects many lives in the United States. The U.S. Bureau of Justice (2006) estimates that 1 million violent crimes are committed by former spouses, boyfriends, or girlfriends each year; about 85% of the victims are women. This violence is known as intimate partner abuse, family violence, wife beating, battering, marital abuse, or partner abuse, but regardless of the term used, its effects are widespread.

Nurses serve their clients best not by trying to rescue them, but by helping them build on their strengths and providing support, thereby empowering them to help themselves. All nurses need to include "RADAR" in every client visit (Box 1.3).

Community

Community encompasses a broad range of concepts, from the nation where a person lives down to a particular neighborhood or group. The surrounding community affects many aspects of a person's health and general welfare. The quality of life within the community has a great influence on an individual's ability to develop and become a functional member of society. Community influences include the school, which is a community by itself, and peer groups. The support and assistance offered to women and their families from other areas of the community, such as school programs and community centers, can improve the individual's overall health and well-being.

Culture

Culture is a view of the world and a set of traditions that are used by a specific social group and are transmitted to the next generation. It plays a critical role with women and their families. A person's culture influences not only socialization but also his or her experiences related to health and specific health practices (Stanhope & Lancaster, 2008). Culture is a complex phenomenon involving many components, such as beliefs, values, language, time, personal space, and view of the world, all of which shape a person's actions and behavior. Individuals learn these patterns of cultural behaviors from their family and community through a process called enculturation, which involves acquiring knowledge and internalizing values. Culture influences every aspect of development and is reflected in child-bearing and child-rearing beliefs and practices designed to promote healthy adaptation.

With today's changing demographic patterns, nurses must be able to assimilate cultural knowledge into their interventions so they can care for culturally diverse women, children, and families. Nurses must be aware of the wide range of cultural traditions, values, and ethics. **Cultural competence** is the ability to apply knowledge about a client's culture so that the health care provided can be adapted to meet her needs. Nurses need to learn about general cultural groups, ethnicity, health practices and how they affect women and their health, and the changing demographics of the population. This will help them view culture as a point of congruence rather than as a potential source of conflict with clients.

Cultural Groups

A society typically includes dominant and minority groups. The dominant group, often the largest group, is the group that has the greatest authority to control values and sanctions of the society (Taylor et al., 2005). As a result, the dominant or majority culture may have the largest impact on health. The minority cultural groups may remain in their own communities and maintain some of their traditions and values while mainstreaming into American society. A culture may contain many subcultures, and geographic differences also can occur: for example, Latin Americans living in New York may be quite different from Latin Americans living in Florida. Being aware of these differences is essential in providing culturally competent care.

Nurses need to be aware of the health care values and practices that are passed along from one generation to the next. For example, the belief in folk healers relates to how the culture interprets illness and health. Some of these parts of the culture may have major influences on an individual's health. Table 1.2 highlights some major cultural groups and their common health beliefs and practices.

BOX 1.3 RADAR

R–Routinely screen every patient for abuse.
A–Ask direct, supportive, and nonjudgmental questions.
D–Document all findings.
A–Assess your client's safety.
R–Review options and provide referrals.

TABLE 1.2 BELIEFS AND PRACTICES OF SELECTED CULTURAL GROUPS

Cultural Group	Beliefs and Practices Affecting Maternal and Children's Health
African Americans	Strong extended family relationships; mother as head of household; older family members valued and respected Food as a symbol of health and wealth View of health as harmony with nature, illness as disruption in harmony Use of folk healing and home remedies common View of pregnancy as a state of wellness Emotional support during labor commonly from other women, primarily the woman's own mother Liberal use of oil on newborn's and infant's scalp and skin Belief in illnesses as natural (due to natural forces person hasn't protected self against) and unnatural (due to person or spirit) Illness commonly associated with pain Pain and suffering inevitable; relief achieved through prayers and laying on of hands Individuals vulnerable to external forces
Asian Americans	Strong loyalty to the family Family as the center, with members expected to care for one another Use of complementary modalities along with Western health care practices View of life as a cycle with everything connected to health Pain described by diverse body symptoms Health viewed as a balance between the forces of yang and yin Respect for authority emphasized View of pregnancy as a natural process and happy time for woman Little involvement of the father during labor; quiet, stoic appearance of woman during labor Protection of woman from cold forces for 30 days after birth of newborn
Arab Americans	Women subordinate to men; young individuals subordinate to older persons Family loyalty is primary Good health associated with eating properly, consuming nutritious foods, and fasting to cure disease Illness is due to inadequate diet, shifts in hot and cold, exposure of stomach while sleeping, emotional or spiritual distress, and "evil eye" Little emphasis on preventive care View of pain as unpleasant, requiring immediate control or relief Birthmarks on newborn due to unsatisfied maternal cravings Pain of labor demonstrated via facial expressions, verbalizations, and body movements; reluctant to use breathing and relaxation techniques during labor Wrapping of newborn's stomach at birth to prevent cold or wind from entering baby's body Breastfeeding often delayed for 2 to 3 days after birth Cleanliness important for prayer
Native Americans	High value on family and tribe; respect for elders Family as an extended network providing care for newborns and children Women as the verbal decision-makers View of pregnancy as a normal and natural process; entire family may be present at birth Newborn not given colostrum Celebrations to mark the stages of growth and development Use of food to celebrate life events and in healing and religious ceremonies Health as harmony with nature; illness due to disharmony, evil spirits Restoration of physical, mental, and spiritual balance through healing ceremonies View of pain as something to be tolerated
Hispanic	Family is important: father is the source of strength, wisdom, and self-confidence; mother is the caretaker and decision-maker for health; children are persons who will continue the family and culture Birthmark on baby due to unsatisfied food cravings during pregnancy Mother's legs brought together after birth of newborn to prevent air from entering uterus Possibly boisterous and loud during labor Bed rest for first 3 days postpartum; no bathing for 14 days Newborn protection from the "evil eye" Use of food for celebrations and socialization Health as God's will, maintainable with a balance of hot and cold food intake Freedom from pain indicative of good health; pain tolerated stoically due to belief that it is God's will Folk medicine practices and prayers, herbal teas and poultices for illness treatment

▶ *Take* NOTE!

Nurses can have a lifelong influence on an individual's perceptions of health and use of health services. By understanding how the woman's and family's culture influences their health practices, nurses can enhance the family's traditional practices, and different cultural practices can become sources of strength rather than areas of conflict.

▶ *Take* NOTE!

The health status of a newborn may affect his or her long-term health and development.

Nutrition

Nutrition provides the body with the calories and nutrients to sustain life and promote growth, as well as the essentials required to maintain health and prevent illness. Nutritional deficiencies or excesses are common problems in the United States, as evidenced by the persistent problem of iron-deficiency anemia and the increasing incidence of obesity. Inadequate food intake, social and cultural food practices or habits that may be nutritionally unsound, the availability of processed and nutritionally inadequate foods, lack of nutrition education in homes and schools, and the presence of illness that interferes with the ingestion, digestion, and absorption of food are factors that can affect an individual's nutrition.

During pregnancy, a woman needs additional calories to support fetal growth and development as well as to support her own needs, and an adequate intake of folic acid is important to prevent neural tube defects (Fig. 1.5). Nutrition and its effects on health status are integrated throughout this text.

Lifestyle Choices

Lifestyle choices that affect an individual's health include eating, exercise, use of tobacco, drugs, or alcohol, and methods of coping with stress. Most health problems that arise today are due to an individual's lifestyle. Poor lifestyle choices made early in life can affect the quality of life as an individual ages. The same concept of making poor choices can be applied to pregnant women and the health and well-being of the infant. Maintaining a healthy level of activity through exercise and hobbies is important for adults and children.

Environmental Exposure

Some environmental exposures can jeopardize health. In utero, the fetus can be affected by lack of maternal nutri-

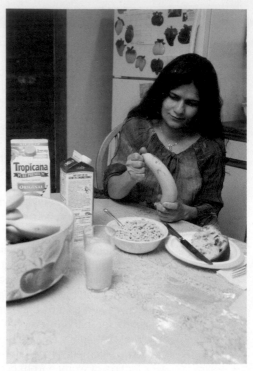

FIGURE **1.5** A pregnant client is eating a healthy meal to ensure adequate nutrition.

tion, maternal infections, or maternal use of alcohol, tobacco, and drugs. Nurses caring for pregnant women should be aware of the risks to the fetus posed by certain drugs, chemicals, and dietary agents, as well as maternal illnesses. These agents, known as teratogens, may be linked to birth defects in children. Not all drugs or agents have fetal effects, however, and research is necessary to identify the correlations between teratogens and other variables.

Stress and Coping

Disasters such as the terrorist attacks of September 11, 2001, the killings at Columbine High School, or Hurricane Katrina can have a significant impact on the well-being of women, children, and families. Stressors such as war, terrorism, violence, and natural disasters may decrease a person's coping ability. Exposure to traumatic events and violence may have long-term effects on an individual's psychosocial development and status.

Exposure to stress is not limited to disasters or traumatic events, however. Stress can also include areas such as inadequate finances, family crises, inadequate support systems, or domestic violence. Like disasters and traumatic events, the effects of these stressors can dramatically affect the health status of a woman or family.

Recall Sophia, the 38-year-old pregnant woman who has come to the prenatal clinic for a visit. While talking with the nurse, Sophia mentions that her children are very involved in activities. She says, "My husband is busy at work, so I do most of the running around. Sometimes I feel like the people at the drive-through know me by name! My husband helps out on the weekends, but during the week, it's all me." What factors may be influencing Sophia's health? How might these factors be influencing the health of her family?

Health Care Cost Containment

The health care system functions within a market setting, offering goods and services that carry a cost to health care consumers and clients. The advent of managed care has led to a trend of attempting to reduce health care costs. These efforts have led to shorter hospital stays and increased awareness on the part of nurses of the costs of supplies and services. The overall challenge is to maintain the quality of care while reducing its cost. For example, if a pregnant diabetic woman needs to go to an endocrinologist, she has very little choice except to purchase the services needed or go without care. In today's managed care environment, the woman will need to go through her "primary health care professional" or "gatekeeper" to receive a referral to a specialist. Often she must trust her primary provider to make that choice for her instead of making that decision on her own.

Although cost containment is important to restrain health care spending, such efforts should not reduce the quality or safety of care delivered. Preventive care (remember the old saying "an ounce of prevention is worth a pound of cure") has been shown to lower costs significantly. Mammograms, cervical cancer screenings, prenatal care, smoking cessation programs, and immunizations are a few examples of preventive care that yield positive outcomes and reduce overall health care costs. Using technological advances to diagnose and treat diseases early saves lives as well as money.

Nurses can be leaders in providing quality care within a limited-resource environment by emphasizing to their clients the importance of making healthy lifestyle and food choices, seeking early interventions for minor problems before they become major ones, and learning about health-related issues that affect them so they can select the best option for themselves and their families. Prevention services and health education are the cornerstones of delivering quality maternal, newborn, and women's health care.

Access to Health Care

The health care system continues to change. In the United States, changes in the health care system result from pressures coming from many directions. These changes reflect shifts in social and economic realities and the results of the biomedical and technological progress that has been made over the past several decades. The effects are felt by every individual who seeks health care in any form. The system of providing medical care in a high-tech environment has changed to providing health care in an environment with limited resources and access to services. Ways to allocate our limited health care resources continue to be the focus.

A major factor involved access to care is health insurance. People without health insurance typically cannot afford to seek health care for maintenance and prevention interventions. The "working poor" may not earn enough money to afford health insurance or medical care, and part-time workers do not always receive benefits such as health insurance.

Preventive Care Focus

The emphasis on cost reduction has also led to an emphasis on preventive care and services. Anticipatory guidance is vital during each health contact with women and their families. Education of the family includes everything from keeping the home safe to ways to prevent illness.

The Continuum of Care Emphasis

A "continuum of care" strategy is cost-effective and provides more efficient and effective services. This continuum extends from acute care settings such as hospitals to outpatient settings such as ambulatory care clinics, primary care offices, rehabilitative units, community care settings, long-term facilities, and homes. For example, the hospital stay is now integrated into a continuum that allows the client to complete therapy at home or other community settings, while re-entering the hospital for short periods for specific treatments or illnesses.

Improvements in Diagnosis and Treatments

Because of the tremendous improvements that have been made in technology and biomedicine, disorders and diseases are being diagnosed and treated earlier. The 1990s witnessed a remarkable and productive connection between genetics and various pathophysiologic processes. For example, female fetuses with congenital adrenal hyperplasia, a genetic disorder resulting in a steroid enzyme deficiency that can lead to disfiguring anatomic abnormalities, are beginning to receive treatment before birth. In addition, many genetic defects are being identified so counseling and treatment may occur early. With these improved diagnoses and treatments, nurses may now be caring for individuals who have survived situations that once would have been fatal, who are living well beyond their life expectancy for a specific illness, or who are functioning with chronic disabilities. For example, at one time women with congenital heart disease did not live long enough to become pregnant. However, with new surgical techniques to correct the defects, many of these women survive and become pregnant, progressing through their pregnancy without significant problems.

While positive and exciting, these advances and trends also pose new challenges for the health care community. For example, as health care for premature newborns improves and survival rates increase, the incidence of long-term chronic conditions such as respiratory airway dysfunction or developmental delays has also increased. As a result, nurses are faced with caring for clients at all stages along the health–illness continuum.

Empowerment of Health Care Consumers

Due to the influence of managed care, the focus on prevention, a more educated population, and technological advances, individuals and families have taken an increased responsibility for their own health. Health consumers are now better informed, and they want to play a greater role in managing health and illness. Families want information about illnesses and they want to participate in making decisions about treatment options. As client advocates valuing family-centered care, nurses are instrumental in promoting this empowerment. To do this, the nurse should respect the family's views and concerns, address all issues and concerns, consider the family members as important participants, and always include the woman and her family in the decision-making process.

Barriers to Health Care

Women are major consumers of health care services, in many cases arranging not only their own care but also that of family members. Compared with men, women have more health problems, longer life spans, and more significant reproductive health needs. Access to care can be jeopardized by lower incomes and greater responsibilities (juggling work and family). Lack of finances or transportation, language or cultural barriers, inconvenient clinic hours, and poor attitudes by health care workers often discourage clients from seeking health care.

Finances

Financial barriers are one of the most important factors that limit care. Many women have limited or no health insurance and cannot afford to pay for care. Although Medicaid covers prenatal care in most states, the paperwork and enrollment process can be so overwhelming that many women do not register. Many families do not have health insurance, do not have enough insurance to cover the services they need, or cannot pay for services.

Transportation

Getting to and from appointments can be challenging for clients who do not drive or own a car or cannot use public transportation (if there is public transportation in the area). It can be difficult for these clients to attend all recommended prenatal health care visits, especially if the woman has other small children who must be taken along on the visit. These challenges can reduce the adherence to scheduled appointments and follow-up.

Language and Culture

Language is how people communicate with each other to increase their understanding or knowledge. If a health care worker cannot speak the same language as the client or does not have a trained interpreter available, a barrier is created. The client's complaints can be misinterpreted or ignored or their significance can be misconstrued. The language barrier might prevent the client from accessing the necessary care, such as prenatal care or preventative care.

Sociocultural and ethnic factors also pose barriers to health care. These factors may involve the lack of transportation, financial situations that require both partners to work, or genetic factors. Knowledge barriers (e.g., lack of understanding of the importance of prenatal care or child health promotion) and spiritual barriers (e.g., some forms of treatment are proscribed by religions) also cross all ethnic groups.

Health Care Delivery System

The health care delivery system itself can create barriers. Eighty-five percent of employed families with insurance are covered by some type of managed health care plan or health maintenance organization (HMO). This prospective payment system based on diagnosis-related groups (DRGs) limits the amounts of health care the family may receive. This also includes Medicaid reimbursement. Due to cost-containment efforts, the trend is to discharge clients as soon as possible from the hospital and to deliver care in the home or through community-based services. Although overall insurance plans may improve access to preventive services, they may limit access to specialty care—which greatly affects clients with chronic or long-term illnesses.

Clinic hours must meet the needs of the clients, not the health care providers who work there. Evening or weekend hours might be needed to meet the schedules of working clients. Clinic personnel should evaluate the availability and accessibility of the services they offer.

Unfortunately, some health care workers exhibit negative attitudes toward poor or culturally diverse families, and this could deter these clients from seeking health care. Long delays, hurried examinations, and rude comments by staff discourage clients from returning.

▶ *Consider* THIS!

I was a 17-year-old pregnant migrant worker needing prenatal care. Although my English wasn't good, I was able to show the receptionist my "big belly" and ask for services. All the receptionist seemed interested in was a social security number and health insurance—neither of which I had. She proceeded to ask me personal questions concerning who the father was and commented on how young I looked. The receptionist then "ordered" me in a loud voice to sit down and wait for an answer by someone in the back, but never contacted anyone that I could see. It seemed to me like all eyes were on me while I found an empty seat in the waiting room. After sitting there quietly for over an hour without any attention or answer, I left.

Thoughts: Why did she leave before receiving any health care service? What must she have been feeling during her wait? Would you come back to this clinic again? Why or why not?

Legal and Ethical Issues in Maternal, Newborn, and Women's Health Care

Law and ethics are interrelated and affect all of nursing. Professional nurses must understand their scope of practice, standards of care, institutional or agency policies, and state laws. All nurses are responsible for knowing current information regarding ethics and laws related to their practice.

Several areas are of particular importance to the health care of women and their families. These include abortion, substance abuse, fetal therapy, informed consent, and confidentiality.

Abortion

Abortion was a volatile legal, social, and political issue even before *Roe v. Wade,* the 1973 Supreme Court decision that legalized abortion. Forty-nine percent of pregnancies in American women are unintended, and 40% of them are terminated by abortion (Alan Guttmacher Institute, 2007).

Abortion is one of the most common procedures performed in the United States. It has become a hotly debated political issue that separates people into two camps: pro-choice and pro-life. The pro-choice group supports the right of any woman to make decisions about her reproductive functions based on her own moral and ethical beliefs. The pro-life group feels strongly that abortion is murder and deprives the fetus of the basic right to life. Both sides will continue to debate this very emotional issue for years to come.

Medical and surgical modalities are available to terminate a pregnancy, depending on how far the pregnancy has developed. A surgical intervention can be performed up to 14 weeks' gestation; a medical intervention can be performed up to 9 weeks' gestation (Shannon & Winikoff, 2008). All women undergoing abortion need emotional support, a stable environment in which to recover, and nonjudgmental care throughout.

Abortion is a complex issue, and the controversy is not only in the public arena: many nurses struggle with the conflict between their personal convictions and their professional duty. Nurses are taught to be supportive client advocates and to interact with a nonjudgmental attitude under all circumstances. However, nurses have their own personal and political views, which may be very different from those of their clients. Nurses need to clarify their personal values and beliefs on this issue and must be able to provide nonbiased care before assuming responsibility for clients who might be in a position to consider abortion. Their decision to care for or refuse to care for such clients affects staff unity, influences staffing decisions, and challenges the ethical concept of duty (Trybulski, 2006).

The ANA's Code of Ethics for Nurses upholds the nurse's right to refuse to care for a client undergoing an abortion if the nurse ethically opposes the procedure (ANA, 2005). Nurses need to make their values and beliefs known to their managers before the situation occurs so that alternative staffing arrangements can be made. Open communication and acceptance of the personal beliefs of others can promote a comfortable working environment.

Substance Abuse

Substance abuse for any person is a problem, but when it involves a pregnant woman, substance abuse can cause fetal injury and thus has legal and ethical implications. In some instances, courts have issued jail sentences to pregnant women who caused harm to their fetuses. Many state laws require reporting evidence of prenatal drug exposure, which may lead to charges of negligence and child endangerment against the pregnant woman. This punitive approach to fetal injury raises ethical and legal questions about the degree of governmental control that is appropriate in the interests of child safety.

Fetal Therapy

Intrauterine fetal surgery is a procedure that involves opening the uterus during pregnancy, performing a surgery, and replacing the fetus in the uterus. Although the risks to the fetus and the mother are both great, fetal therapy may be used to correct anatomic lesions (Chervenak & McCullough, 2007). Some argue that medical technology should not interfere with nature, and thus this intervention should not take place. Others would argue that the surgical intervention improves the child's quality of life. For many people, these are the subjects of debates and intellectual discussions, but for nurses, these procedures may be part of their daily routine.

Nurses play an important supportive role in caring and advocating for clients and their families. As the use of technology grows, situations will surface more frequently that test a nurse's belief system. Encouraging open discussions to address emotional issues and differences of opinion among staff members is healthy and increases tolerance for differing points of view.

Informed Consent

Informed consent has four key components: disclosure, comprehension, competency, and voluntariness (Cressey, 2008). It occurs prior to initiation of the procedure or specific care and addresses the legal and ethical requirement of informing the client about the procedure. The physician or advanced practice nurse is responsible for informing the client about the procedure and obtaining consent by providing a detailed description of the procedure or treatment, its potential risks and benefits, and alternative methods available. The nurse's responsibility related to informed consent includes:

- Ensuring that the consent form is completed with signatures from the client
- Serving as a witness to the signature process
- Determining whether the client understands what she is signing by asking her pertinent questions

Although laws vary from state to state, certain key elements are associated with informed consent (Box 1.4). Nurses need to be familiar with their specific state laws as well as the policies and procedures of the health care agency where they work. Treating clients without obtaining proper consent may result in charges of assault, and the health care provider and/or facility may be held liable for any damages. Generally, only people over the age of

majority (18 years of age) can legally provide consent for health care.

Most care rendered in a health care setting is covered by the initial consent for treatment signed when the individual becomes a client at that office or clinic or by the consent to treatment signed upon admission to the hospital or other inpatient facility. Certain procedures, however, require a specific process of informed consent: major and minor surgery; invasive procedures such as amniocentesis or internal fetal monitoring; treatments placing the client at higher risk, such as chemotherapy or radiation therapy; procedures or treatments involving research; and photography involving the client.

If the client cannot provide consent, then the person closest to the client may give consent for emergency treatment. In an emergency, a verbal consent, via the telephone, may be obtained. Two witnesses must also be listening simultaneously and must sign the consent form, indicating that consent was received via telephone.

Refusal of Medical Treatment

All clients have the right to refuse medical treatment, based on the American Hospital Association's Bill of Rights. Ideally, medical care without informed consent should be used only when the client's life is in danger. Clients may refuse treatment if it conflicts with their religious or cultural beliefs. In these cases, it is important to educate the client and family about the importance of the recommended treatment without coercing or forcing the client to agree. Sometimes common ground may be reached between the family's religious or cultural beliefs and the health care team's recommendations. Communication and education are the keys in this situation.

Confidentiality

With the establishment of the Health Insurance Portability and Accountability Act (HIPAA) of 1996, the confidentiality of health care information is now mandated by law. The primary intent of the law is to protect health insurance coverage for workers and their families when they change or lose jobs. Another aspect of the law requires DHHS to establish national standards for electronic transmission of health information. The plan also addresses the security and privacy of health information. For example, no information that clearly identifies a client can be on public display, including information on a client's chart. In maternal and newborn health care, information is shared only with the client, legal partner, parents, legal guardians, or individuals as established in writing by the client or the child's parents. This law promotes the security and privacy of health care and health information for all clients. Client information should always be kept confidential in the context of the state law, as well as the institution's policies.

> **BOX 1.4** **Key Elements of Informed Consent**
>
> - The decision-maker must be of legal age in that state, with full civil rights, and must be competent (have the ability to make the decision).
> - Information is presented in a manner that is simple, concise, and appropriate to the level of education and language of the individual responsible for making the decision.
> - The decision must be voluntary, without coercion or force or under duress.
> - There must be a witness to the process of informed consent.
> - The witness must sign the consent form.

Exceptions to confidentiality exist. For example, suspicion of physical or sexual abuse and injuries caused by a weapon or criminal act must be reported to the proper authorities. Abuse cases are reported to the appropriate welfare authorities, whereas criminal acts are reported to the police. The health care provider must also follow public health laws related to reporting certain infectious diseases to the local health department (e.g., tuberculosis, hepatitis, HIV, and other sexually transmitted infections). Finally, there is a duty to warn third parties when there is a specific threat to an identifiable person. There must be a balance between confidentiality and required disclosure. If health care information must be disclosed by law, the client must be informed that this will occur (Brous, 2007).

Implications for Nurses

The health care system is intricately woven into the political and social structure of our society, and nurses should understand social, legal, and ethical health care issues so that they can play an active role in meeting the health care needs of women and their families. Nurses need to take a proactive role in advocating for and empowering their clients. For example, nurses can help women to increase control over the factors that affect health, thereby improving their health status. A woman may become empowered by developing skills not only to cope with her environment, but also to change it. Nurses also can assume this mentoring role with families, thus helping them to improve their overall health status and health outcomes.

Nurses must have a solid knowledge base about the factors affecting maternal, newborn, and women's health and barriers to health care. They can use this information to provide anticipatory guidance, health counseling, and teaching for women and their families. It also is useful in identifying high-risk groups so that interventions can be initiated early on, before problems occur.

When caring for women and their families, the nurse operates within the framework of the nursing process, which is applicable to all health care settings. Maternal, newborn, and women's health nursing is ever-changing as globalization and the exchange of information expands. Nurses must remain up to date about new technologies and treatments and integrate high-quality, evidence-based interventions into the care they provide.

■■■ Key Concepts

■ Maternal, newborn, and women's health nurses provide care using a philosophy that focuses on the family and the use of evidence-based practice in a case management environment to provide quality, cost-effective care.

■ *Healthy People 2010* presents a national set of health goals and objectives for adults and children that focus on health promotion and disease prevention.

■ One method to establish the aggregate health status of women and infants is with statistical data, such as mortality and morbidity rates.

■ The infant mortality rate is the lowest in the history of the United States, but it is still higher than that of other industrialized countries. This high rate may be due to the number of low-birthweight infants born in this country.

■ The family is considered the basic social unit. The family greatly influences the development and health of its members because members learn health care activities, health beliefs, and health values from their family.

■ Culture influences every aspect of development and is reflected in childbearing and childrearing beliefs and practices designed to promote healthy adaptation.

■ Other factors affecting the health of women and their families include health status and lifestyles, health care cost containment, improved diagnosis and treatment, and health care consumer empowerment. Finances, transportation, language, culture, and the health care delivery system can be barriers to health care.

■ Advances in science and technology have led to increased ethical dilemmas in health care.

■ All clients have the right to refuse medical treatment based on the American Hospital Association's Bill of Rights.

■ In certain states, mature minors and emancipated minors may consent to their own health care and certain health care may be provided to adolescents without parental notification, including contraception, pregnancy counseling, prenatal care, testing and treatment of sexually transmitted infections and communicable diseases (including HIV), substance abuse and mental illness counseling and treatment, and health care required as a result of a crime-related injury.

■ Nurses must be knowledgeable about the laws related to health care of women and their families in the state where they practice as well as the specific policies of their health care institution.

REFERENCES

Alexander, L. L., LaRosa, J. H., Bader, H., & Garfield, S. (2007). *New dimensions in women's health* (3rd ed.). Sudbury, MA: Jones & Bartlett Publishers.

Alan Guttmacher Institute. (2007) *Facts in brief: Induced abortion.* Available at: www.agi-usa.org/pubs/fb_induced_abortion.html.

American Cancer Society (ACS). (2008a). *Cancer facts for women.* Available at: http://www.cancer.org/docroot/ASN/content/ASN_1x_Cancer_Facts_for_Women_English_pdf.asp?sitearea=PED.

American Cancer Society (ACS). (2008b). *Overview: Lung cancer.* Available at: http://www.cancer.org/docroot/CRI/CRI_2_1x.asp?dt=15.

American Cancer Society (ACS). (2008c). *What are the key statistics for breast cancer?* Available at: http://www.cancer.org/docroot/ CRI/content/CRI_2_4_1X_What_are_the_key_statistics_for_breast_ cancer_5.asp?sitearea=.

American Nurses Association (ANA). (2005). *Code of ethics for nurses with interpretive statements.* Available at: http://nursingworld.org/ ethics/code/protected_nwcoe813.htm.

Brodsky, P. L. (2006). Childbirth. A journey through time. *International Journal of Childbirth Education, 21*(3), 10–15.

Brous, E. (2007). HIPAA vs. law enforcement: A nurse's guide to managing conflicting responsibilities. *American Journal of Nursing, 107*(8), 60–63.

Cassidy, T. (2006). *Birth: The surprising history of how we are born.* Berkeley, CA: Grove/Atlantic, Inc.

Centers for Disease Control and Prevention (CDC). (2007a). *Maternal mortality rate.* Available at: http://www.cdc.gov/NCHS/datawh/ nchsdefs/rates.htm#maternal.

Centers for Disease Control and Prevention (CDC). (2007b). *Eliminating disparities of infant mortality.* Available at: http://www.cdc.gov/ omhd/AMH/factsheets/infant.htm.

Chervenak, F., & McCullough, L. (2007). Ethics of maternal-fetal surgery. *Seminars in Fetal & Neonatal Medicine, 12*(6), 426–431.

Cressey, S. (2008). Understanding consent. *Practice Nurse, 35*(2), 38–41.

Foster, J., & Heath, A. (2007). Midwifery and the development of nursing capacity in the Dominican Republic: Caring, clinical competence, and case management. *Journal of Midwifery & Women's Health, 52*(5), 499–504.

Framingham Heart Study (FHS). (2007). *Through the looking glass: Women and heart disease.* Available at http://www.framingham.com/ heart/4stor_04.htm.

Heiss, G., Wallace, R., Anderson, G. L., et al., for the WHI Investigators. (2008). Health risks and benefits 3 years after stopping randomized treatment with estrogen and progestin. *JAMA, 299*(9), 1036–1045.

Hodnett, E. D., Gates, S., Hofmeyr, G. J., & Sakata C. (2007). Continuous support for women during childbirth. *Cochrane Database of Systematic Reviews 2007.* Issue 3. Art No.: CD003766. DOI:10.1002/14651858.CD003766.pub2.

Hollander, D. (2006). Early prenatal care does not close racial gaps in perinatal mortality. *Perspectives on Sexual & Reproductive Health, 38*(3), 174–177.

Howard, E. D. (2006). Family-centered care in the context of fetal abnormality. *Journal of Perinatal & Neonatal Nursing, 20*(3), 237–242.

Hoyert, D. L., Matthews, T. J., Menacker, F., Strobino, D. M., & Guyer, B. (2006). Annual summary of vital statistics: 2004. *Pediatrics, 117*(1), 168–183.

Jolivet, R. (2006). Nurse-midwives committed to women throughout the lifespan. *Nurse Practitioner, 9,* 10–13.

March of Dimes. (2006). *U.S. infant mortality rate fails to improve.* Available at: http://www.marchofdimes.com/15796_19840.asp.

March of Dimes. (2008). *Low birth weight and prematurity.* Available at: http://www.marchofdimes.com/professionals/14332_1153.asp

National Center for Health Statistics (NCHS). (2007). *Maternal mortality rates.* Available at: http://www.cdc.gov/NCHS/datawh/ nchsdefs/rates.htm.

National Women's Law Center, FOCUS/University of Pennsylvania, and the Lewin Group. (2007). *Making the grade on women's health: A national state-by-state report card.* Washington, DC: National Women's Law Center.

Newhouse, R. P. (2006). Examining the support for evidence-based nursing practice. *Journal of Nursing Administration, 36*(7/8), 337–340.

Price, S., Noseworthy, J., & Thornton, J. (2007). Women's experience with social presence during childbirth. *American Journal of Maternal Child Nursing, 32*(3), 184–191.

Shannon, C., & Winikoff, B. (2008). How much medical supervision is necessary for women taking mifepristone and misoprostol for early medical abortion? *Women's Health, 4*(2), 107–111.

Stanhope, M., & Lancaster, J. (2008). *Public health nursing: Population-centered health care in the community* (7th ed.). St. Louis: Mosby Elsevier.

Taylor, C., Lillis, C., & LeMone, P. (2005). *Fundamentals of nursing: The art and science of nursing care* (5th ed.). Philadelphia: Lippincott Williams & Wilkins.

Trybulski, J. (2006). Women and abortion: The past reaches into the present. *Journal of Advanced Nursing, 54*(6), 683–690.

United Nations International Children's Emergency Fund (UNICEF). (2007). *At a glance: United States of America statistics.* Available at: http://www.unicef.org/infobycountry/usa_statistics.html.

U.S. Bureau of Justice. (2006). *Crime and victims statistics.* Available at: http://www.ojp.usdoj.gov/bjs/cvict.htm.

U.S. Census Bureau. (2007). *American fact finder.* Retrieved March 22, 2007, from http://factfinder.census.gov/home/en/epss/ glossary_f.html.

U.S. Department of Health & Human Services. (2000). *Healthy people 2010.* Retrieved August 23, 2006, from http://www.healthypeople. gov/Publications/.

U.S. Department of Health and Human Services, Health Resources and Services Administration. (2006). *Women's health USA 2006.* Rockville, MD: U.S. Department of Health and Human Services.

U.S. Department of Health and Human Services, Health Resources and Services Administration, Maternal and Child Health Bureau. (2005). *Child health USA 2005.* Rockville, MD: U.S. Department of Health and Human Services.

U.S. Department of Health & Human Services, Public Health Service. (1979). *Healthy people: The Surgeon General's report on health promotion and disease prevention* (DHEW publication No. PHS 79-5507). Washington, DC: U.S. Government Printing Office.

World Factbook. (2007). *Infant mortality rate.* Washington, DC: Central Intelligence Agency.

World Health Organization. (2007a). *Statistical information system.* Available at: http://www.who.int/whosis/indicatordefinitions/en/print.html.

World Health Organization. (2007b). *Integrating poverty and gender into health programs: A sourcebook for health professionals.* Available at: http://www.wpro.who.int/publications/pub_9290612126.htm.

World Health Organization. (2007c). *Gender, health and poverty fact sheet.* Available at: www.who.int/inf-fs/en/fact251.html.

World Health Organization. (2008). *The WHO agenda.* Available at: http://www.who.int/about/agenda/en/index.html.

WEBSITES

American Heart Association: http://www.americanheart.org

Association of Reproductive Health Professionals: http://www.arhp.org

Centers for Disease Control, National Center for Injury Prevention and Control: http://www.cdc.gov/ncipc

Family Violence Prevention Fund: http://www.endabuse.org

Global Health Council: www.globalhealth.org

National Abortion Federation: http://www.prochoice.org

National Coalition Against Domestic Violence: http://www.ncadv.org

National Coalition for the Homeless: http://www.nationalhomeless.org

Planned Parenthood Federation: http://www.ppfa.org

United Nations Development Program: www.undo.org

World Health Organization (WHO): www.who.int

CHAPTER WORKSHEET

MULTIPLE CHOICE QUESTIONS

1. When preparing a presentation for a local woman's group on women's health problems, what would the nurse include as the number-one cause of mortality for women in the United States?

   a. Breast cancer

   b. Childbirth complications

   c. Injury resulting from violence

   d. Heart disease

2. Which factor would most likely be responsible for a pregnant women's failure to receive adequate prenatal care in the United States?

   a. Belief that it is not necessary in a normal pregnancy

   b. Use of denial to cope with pregnancy

   c. Lack of health insurance to cover expenses

   d. Inability to trust traditional medical practices

3. When caring for an adolescent, in which instance must the nurse share information with the parents, no matter which state care is provided in?

   a. Pregnancy counseling

   b. Depression

   c. Contraception

   d. Tuberculosis

4. Which milestone would the nurse describe as being important for providing nutritional supplementation to low-income families?

   a. Title V of the Social Security Act

   b. WIC program

   c. Medicaid Program under Title XIX

   d. Sheppard-Towner Act

5. The nurse is preparing a class about homelessness. Which factors contribute to homelessness? Select all that apply.

   ___a. Decrease in the number of people living in poverty

   ___b. Unemployment

   ___c. Exposure to abuse or neglect

   ___d. Cutbacks in public welfare programs

   ___e. Establishment of community crisis centers

CRITICAL THINKING EXERCISE

1. As a nurse working in a federally funded low-income clinic offering women's health services, you are becoming increasingly frustrated with the number of "no-shows" or appointments missed in your maternity clinic. Some clients come for their initial prenatal intake appointment and never come back. You realize that some just forget their appointments, but most don't even call to notify you. Many of the clients are high risk and thus are jeopardizing their health and the health of their future child.

   a. What changes might be helpful to address this situation?

   b. Outline what you might say at your next staff meeting to address the issue of clients making one clinic visit and then never returning.

   c. What strategies might you use to improve attendance and notification?

   d. Describe what cultural and customer service techniques might be needed.

STUDY ACTIVITIES

1. Research a current policy, bill, or issue being debated on the community, state, or national level that pertains to the health and welfare of women or their families. Summarize the major facts and supporting and opposing arguments and prepare an oral report on your findings.

2. Within your clinical group, debate the following statement: Should access to health care be a right or a privilege?

3. Visit a local community health center that offers services to women and their families from various cultures. Interview the staff about any barriers to health care that they have identified. Investigate what the staff has done to minimize these barriers.

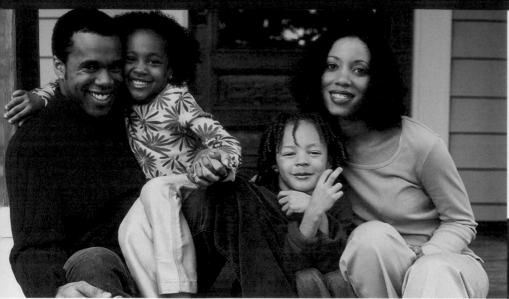

CHAPTER 2

FAMILY-CENTERED COMMUNITY-BASED CARE

KEY TERMS

community
cultural competence

epidemiology

LEARNING OBJECTIVES

Upon completion of the chapter, the learner will be able to:

1. Discuss the major components and key elements of family-centered home health care.
2. Explain the reasons for the increased emphasis on community-based care.
3. Differentiate community-based nursing from nursing in acute care settings.
4. Explain the different levels of prevention in community-based nursing, providing examples of each.
5. Give examples of cultural issues that may be faced when providing community-based nursing.
6. Provide culturally competent care to women and their families.
7. Construct strategies for integrating elements of alternative/complementary therapies and scientific health care practice.
8. Identify the variety of settings where community-based care can be provided to women and their families.
9. Outline the various roles and functions assumed by the community health nurse.
10. Demonstrate the ability to use excellent therapeutic communication skills when interacting with women and their families.
11. Explain the process of health teaching as it relates to women and their families.
12. Discuss the importance of discharge planning and case management in providing community-based care.

M aria was home a few days after giving birth to her first child. She had just changed her newborn son and placed him on his stomach for a nap when the community health nurse arrived for a postpartum visit. Because the nurse didn't speak Spanish and Maria didn't speak English, a great deal of gesturing followed. After examining Maria, the nurse then picked up her son and placed him on his back in the crib. How might the nurse have prepared for this home visit? What message did the nurse convey in changing the newborn's position?

Wow

To recognize diversity in others and respect it, we must first have some awareness of who we are.

Women and their families receive most of their health care, both well and ill care, in the community setting. During the past several years, the health care delivery system has changed dramatically. With a focus on cost containment, people are spending less time in the hospital. Clients are being discharged "sicker and quicker" from their hospital beds. The health care system has moved from reactive treatment strategies in hospitals to a proactive approach in the community. This has resulted in an increasing emphasis on health promotion and illness prevention within the community.

Nurses play an important role in the health and wellness of a community. They not only meet the health care needs of the individual but also go beyond that to implement interventions that affect the community as a whole. Nurses practice in a variety of settings within a community, such as clinics and physician offices, shelters, churches, health departments, community health centers, and homes. They promote the health of individuals, families, groups, communities, and populations and promote an environment that supports health.

This chapter describes the concepts of community and community-based nursing, addressing the varied settings where such care is provided to women and their families. The chapter also highlights the major roles and functions of community-based nurses, emphasizing their role as educators in health promotion and maintenance.

Family-Centered Care

Family-centered cares refers to the collaborative partnership among the individual, family, and caregivers to determine goals, share information, offer support, and formulate plans for health care (Chia-Chen & Thompson, 2007). Key elements in the provision of family-centered care include demonstrating interpersonal sensitivity, providing general health information and being a valuable resource, communicating specific health information, and treating people respectfully (Mullen et al., 2007). The philosophy of family-centered care recognizes the family as the constant: the health of all the family members and their functional abilities influence the health of the client and other members of the family. Family-centered care works well in all arenas of health care, from preventive care to long-term care. Family-centered care enhances the confidence of all those involved about their skills and helps to prepare individuals for assuming responsibility for their own health care needs. It is vital for the nurse to assess how much knowledge the family already has about the client's health or illness.

Using a family-centered approach is associated with positive outcomes such as decreased anxiety, improved pain management, shorter recovery times, and enhanced confidence and problem-solving skills. Communication between the health care team and the family is also improved, leading to greater satisfaction for both health care providers and health care consumers (families). Practicing true family-centered care may empower the family, strengthen family resources, and help the woman or child feel more secure throughout the process.

Community-Based Care

Community may be defined as a specific group of people, often living in a defined geographical area, who share common interests, who interact with each other, and who function collectively within a defined social structure to address common concerns (Clark, 2008). The common features of a community may be common rights and privileges as members of a certain city or common ties of identity, values, norms, culture, language, or social support. Women are caregivers to children, parents, spouses, and neighbors and provide important social support in these roles.

A person can be a part of many communities during the course of daily life. Examples might include area of residence (home, apartment, shelter), gender, place of employment (organization or home), language spoken (Spanish, Chinese, English), educational background or student status, culture (Italian, African-American, Indian), career (nurse, businesswoman, housewife), place of worship (church or synagogue), and community memberships (garden club, YMCA, support group, school PTA, youth organizations, athletic teams).

In community-based care, the community is the unit of service. The providers of care are concerned not only with the clients who present for service but also with the larger population of potential or at-risk clients.

Community Health Nursing

Community health nursing focuses on preventing illness and improving the health of populations and communities. Population is defined as a group of people who may or may not interact with each other within a defined geographical location (Clark, 2008). Community health nurses work in geographically and culturally diverse settings. They address current and potential health needs of the population or community. They promote and preserve the health of a population and are not limited to particular age groups or diagnoses. Public health nursing is a specialized area of community health nursing.

Epidemiology (the study of the causes, distribution, and control of disease in populations) can help determine the health and health needs of a population and assist in planning health services. Community health nurses perform epidemiologic investigations to help analyze and develop health policy and community health initiatives. Community health initiatives can be focused on the community as a whole or a specific target population with specific needs. *Healthy People 2010* (HP 2010) is an example of national health initiatives developed using the epidemiological process. HP 2010 ensures that health care professionals evaluate the individual as well as the community. It emphasizes the ever-present link between the individual's health and the health of the community (Clark, 2007; Zahner & Block, 2006). HP 2010 identifies two major goals: to increase the quality of life and the life expectancy of individuals of all ages and to decrease health disparities among different populations. Relevant HP 2010 objectives are highlighted throughout this text, and HP 2010 is available online at www.healthypeople.gov.

The focus of health care initiatives today is on people and their needs, strengthening their abilities to shape their own lives. The emphasis has shifted away from dependence on health professionals toward personal involvement and personal responsibility, and this gives nurses the opportunity to interact with individuals in a variety of self-help roles. Nurses in the community can be the primary force in identifying the challenges and implementing changes in women's and newborn's health for the future.

Community-Based Nursing

In the past, the only community-based roles for nurses were community health nurses or public health nurses. This is now a subset of what is considered community-based nursing. The health needs of the society and consumer demand brought about community-based and community-focused services. The movement from an illness-oriented "cure" perspective in hospitals to a focus on health promotion and primary health care in community-based settings has dramatically changed employment opportunities for today's nurses. This shift in emphasis to primary care and outpatient treatment and management will likely continue. As a result, employment growth in a variety of community-based settings can be expected for properly educated nurses.

The 2004 National Sample Survey of Registered Nurses (U.S. Department of Health and Human Services [USDHHS], Bureau of Health Professions, 2004) found the following trends in registered nurse (RN) employment settings:

- 44% of RNs work outside the hospital setting.
- The number of RNs employed in community-based settings showed a 35% increase between 2000 and 2004; this was largely the result of an increase in nurses working in home health care and managed care organizations.

Community-based nursing settings include ambulatory care, home health care, occupational health, school health, and hospice settings (Table 2.1). Clinical practice within the community may also include case management, research, quality improvement, and discharge planning. Nurses with advanced practice and experience may be employed in areas of staff development, program development, and community education.

TABLE 2.1   COMMUNITY-BASED PRACTICE SETTINGS

Setting	Description
Ambulatory care settings	Doctor's offices Health maintenance organizations (HMOs) Day surgery centers Freestanding urgent care centers Family planning clinics Mobile mammography centers
Home health care services	High-risk pregnancy/neonate care Maternal/child newborn care Skilled nursing care Hospice care
Health Department services	Maternal/child health clinics Family planning clinics Sexually transmitted infection programs Immunization clinics Substance-abuse programs Jails and prisons
Long-term care	Skilled nursing facilities Nursing homes Hospices Assisted living
Other community-based settings	Parish nursing programs Summer camps Childbirth education programs School health programs Occupational health programs

Community-Based Nursing Interventions

Nursing interventions involve any treatment that the nurse performs to enhance the client's outcome. Nursing practice in the community uses the nursing process and is similar to that in the acute care setting, because assessing, performing procedures, administering medications, coordinating services and equipment, counseling clients and their families, and teaching about care are all part of the care administered by nurses in the community. Box 2.1 highlights the most common nursing interventions used in community-based nursing practice.

Community-Based Nursing Challenges

Despite the benefits achieved by caring for families in their own homes and communities, challenges also exist. Clients are being discharged from acute care facilities very early in their recovery course and present with more health care needs than in the past. As a result, nursing care and procedures in the home and community are becoming more complex and time-consuming. Consider the example of a woman who

<table>
<tr><td>

BOX 2.1 **Community-Based Nursing Interventions**

- Health screening—detecting unrecognized or preclinical illness among individuals so they can be referred for definitive diagnosis and treatment (e.g., mammogram or Pap smear, vision and hearing checks)
- Health education programs—assisting clients in making health-related decisions about self-care, use of health resources, and social health issues such as smoking bans and motorcycle helmet laws (e.g., childbirth education or breast self-examination, drug awareness programs)
- Medication administration—preparing, giving, and evaluating the effectiveness of prescription and over-the-counter drugs (e.g., hormone replacement therapy in menopausal women)
- Telephone consultation—identifying the problem to be addressed; listening and providing support, information, or instruction; documenting advice/instructions given to concerns raised by caller (e.g., consultation for a mother with a newborn with colic, interaction with a parent whose child has a fever or is vomiting)
- Health system referral—passing along information about the location, services offered, and ways to contact agencies (e.g., referring a woman for a breast prosthesis after a mastectomy)
- Instructional—teaching an individual or a group about a medication, disease process, lifestyle changes, community resources, or research findings concerning their environment (e.g., childbirth education class, basic life support classes for parents)
- Nutritional counseling—demonstrating the direct relationship between nutrition and illness while focusing on the need for diet modification to promote wellness (e.g., Women, Infants, and Children [WIC] program; counselor interviewing a pregnant woman who has anemia)
- Risk identification—recognizing personal or group characteristics that predispose people to develop a specific health problem, and modifying or eliminating them (e.g., genetic counseling of an older pregnant woman at risk for a Down syndrome infant; genetic screening of family members for cystic fibrosis or Huntington's disease)

Dochterman, J. M., & Bulechek, G. M., & Butcher, H. K. (2007). *Nursing interventions classification* (NIC) (5th ed.). St. Louis: Elsevier Health Sciences.

</td></tr>
</table>

developed a systemic infection, a pelvic abscess, and deep vein thrombosis in her leg after a cesarean birth who is being discharged from the hospital. The nurse's primary focus of care in this situation would be to administer heparin and antibiotics intravenously rather than educating her about childcare and follow-up appointments. In the past, this woman would have remained hospitalized for treatment, but home infusion therapy is now less costly and allows the client to be discharged sooner.

This demand on the nurse's time may limit the amount of time spent on prevention measures, education, and the family's psychosocial issues. More time may be needed to help families deal with these issues and concerns. With large client caseloads, nurses may find it difficult to spend the time needed while meeting the time restrictions dictated by their health care agencies. Nurses need to plan the tasks to be accomplished (Box 2.2).

Nurses working in the community have fewer resources available to them compared with the acute care setting. Decisions often have to be made in isolation. The nurse must possess excellent assessment skills and the ability to communicate effectively with the family to be successful in carrying out the appropriate plan of care.

Nurses interested in working in community-based settings must be able to apply the nursing process in an environment that is less structured or controlled than that in acute care facilities. Nurses must be able to assimilate information well beyond the immediate physical and psychosocial needs of the client in a controlled acute care setting and deal with environmental threats, lifestyle choices, family issues, different cultural patterns, financial burdens, transportation problems, employment hazards, communication barriers, limited resources, and client acceptance and compliance.

Although opportunities for employment in community-based settings are plentiful, many positions require a baccalaureate degree. Previous medical-surgical experience in an acute care setting is typically required by home health agencies because these nurses must function fairly independently within the home environment.

The nurse must also be familiar with and respectful of many different cultures and socioeconomic levels, remaining objective in dealing with such diversity and demonstrating an understanding of and appreciation for cultural differences. Interventions must be individualized to address the cultural, social, and economic diversity among clients in their own environment (Papadopoulos, 2006).

Shift in Responsibilities From Hospital-Based to Community-Based Nursing

Community care, especially home care, is a rapidly growing service in the United States. Community-based care has been shown to be a cost-effective method for providing care. An increase in disposable income and the increased longevity of individuals with chronic and debilitating health conditions have also contributed to the continued shift of health care to the community and home setting. Technology has advanced, allowing for improved monitoring of clients in community settings and at home as well as allowing complicated procedures to be done at home, such as intravenous administration of antibiotics.

BOX 2.2   **Home Care Visitation Planning**

- Review previous interventions to eliminate unsuccessful ones.
  - Check previous home visit narrative to validate interventions.
  - Communicate with previous nurse to ask questions and clarify.
  - Formulate plan of interventions based on data received (e.g., client preference of IV placement or order of fluids).
- Prioritize client needs based on their potential to threaten the client's health status.
  - Use Maslow's hierarchy of needs to set forth a plan of care.
  - Address life-threatening physiologic issues first (e.g., an infectious process would take precedence over anorexia).
- Develop goals that reflect primary, secondary, and tertiary prevention levels.
  - *Primary prevention*—Have the patient consume adequate fluid intake to prevent dehydration.
  - *Secondary prevention*—Administer drug therapy as prescribed to contain and treat an existing infectious process.
  - *Tertiary prevention*—Instruct the client on good hand-washing technique to prevent spread and future secondary infections.
- Bear in mind the client's readiness to accept intervention and education.
  - Ascertain the client's focus and how see sees her needs.
  - Address client issues that might interfere with intervention (e.g., if the client is in pain, attempting to teach her about her care will be lost; her pain must be addressed first before she is ready to learn).
- Consider the timing of the visit to prevent interfering with other client activities.

- Schedule all visits at convenient times per client if possible (e.g., if the client has a favorite soap opera to watch, attempt to schedule around that event if at all possible).
- Reschedule a home visit if a client event comes up suddenly.
- Outline nursing activities to be completed during the scheduled visit.
  - Know the health care agency's policy and procedures for home visits.
  - Consider the time line and other visits scheduled that day.
  - Research evidence-based best practices to use in the home (e.g., if the client is fatigued, be flexible to accommodate her needs and allow for periods of rest so that she may conserve her energy).
- Obtain necessary materials/supplies before making the visit.
  - Assemble all equipment needed for any procedure in advance.
  - Secure any equipment that might be needed if a problem occurs (e.g., bring additional IV tubing and a catheter to make sure the procedure can be carried out without delay).
- Determine criteria to be used to evaluate the effectiveness of the home visit.
  - Revisit outcome goals to determine the effectiveness of the intervention.
  - Assess the client's health status to validate improvement.
  - Monitor changes in the client's behavior toward health promotion activities and disease prevention (e.g., verify/observe that the client demonstrates correct hand-washing technique after instruction and reinforcement during the home care visit).

Levels of Prevention in Community-Based Nursing

The concept of prevention is a key part of community-based nursing practice. The emphasis on health care delivery in community-based settings has moved beyond primary preventive health care (e.g., well-child checkups, routine physical examinations, prenatal care, and treatment of common acute illnesses) and now encompasses secondary and tertiary care.

Primary Prevention

The concept of primary prevention involves preventing the disease or condition before it occurs through health promotion activities, environmental protection, and specific protection against disease or injury. It encompasses a vast array of areas, including nutrition, good hygiene, sanitation, immunization, adequate shelter, smoking cessation, family planning, and the use of seat belts (Fig. 2.1; Stanhope & Lancaster, 2008).

Prevention of neural tube defects (NTDs), such as anencephaly and spina bifida, is an example of primary prevention. The use of folic acid supplementation daily for 3 months before and 3 months after conception reduces the risk of first occurrence of NTD (American College of Obstetricians and Gynecologists [ACOG], 2007). All women of childbearing age should take 0.4 mg folic acid daily as soon as they plan to become pregnant and should continue taking it throughout the pregnancy to prevent this devastating condition. Giving anticipatory guidance to parents about poison prevention and safety during play is another example of primary prevention.

Secondary Prevention

Secondary prevention is the early detection and treatment of adverse health conditions. Health screenings are the mainstay of secondary prevention. Pregnancy testing, blood pressure evaluations, cholesterol monitoring, fecal occult blood testing, breast examinations, mammography screening, hearing and vision examinations, and

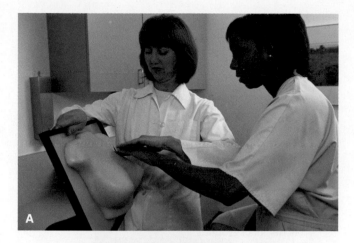

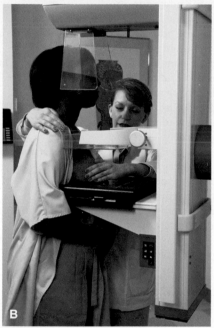

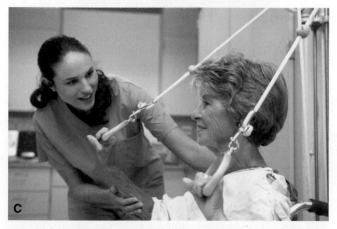

FIGURE 2.1 Levels of prevention in community-based nursing. (**A**) At the primary prevention level, the nurse provides a woman with teaching about breast self-examination. (**B**) At the secondary level of prevention, a woman undergoes a mammogram for early detection of breast problems. (**C**) At the tertiary level of prevention, a nurse assists a client with her strength exercises.

Papanicolaou (Pap) smears are examples of this level of prevention. Such interventions do not prevent the health problem but are intended for early detection and prompt treatment to prevent complications (Anderson & McFarlane, 2007).

Tertiary Prevention

Tertiary prevention is designed to reduce or limit the progression of a disease or disability. The purpose of tertiary prevention is to restore individuals to their maximum potential (Anderson & McFarlane, 2007). Tertiary prevention measures are supportive and restorative. For example, tertiary prevention efforts would focus on minimizing and managing the effects of a chronic illness such as cerebrovascular disease or the chronic effects of sexually transmitted infections (e.g., herpes, human immunodeficiency virus [HIV], and untreated syphilis). Another example would involve working with women who have suffered long-term consequences of violence. The focus of the nurse would be to maximize the woman's strengths, to help her recover from the trauma and loss, and to build support systems.

The Nurse's Role in Community-Based Preventive Care

All health professionals have a special role in health promotion, health protection, and disease prevention. Much of community nursing involves prevention, early identification, and prompt treatment of health problems and monitoring for emerging threats that might lead to health problems. Community-based nurses provide health care for women and their families at all three levels of prevention. This care often involves advocating for services to meet their needs.

Cultural Issues in Community-Based Nursing

The United States contains an ever-changing mix of cultural groups. The *Yearbook of Immigration Statistics* (United States Department of Homeland Security [USDHS], 2006) reports that the U.S. immigrant population has reached 38 million, with people arriving from every corner of the world.

▶ *Take NOTE!*

One million immigrants come to the United States each year, and more than half are of childbearing age. Latin America accounts for more than 50% of immigrants to the United States. By the year 2050, people of African, Asian, and Latino backgrounds will make up one half of our population (U.S. Census Bureau, 2007).

This growing diversity has significant implications for the health care system. For years nurses have struggled with the issues of providing optimal health care that meets the needs of women and their families from varied cultures and ethnic groups. In addition to displaying competence in technical skills, nurses must also become competent in caring for clients from varied ethnic and racial backgrounds. Adapting to different cultural beliefs and practices requires flexibility and acceptance of others' viewpoints. Nurses must listen to clients and learn about their beliefs about health and wellness. To provide culturally appropriate care to diverse populations, nurses need to know, understand, and respect culturally influenced health behaviors. Chapter 1 provides a more detailed discussion of culture and its impact on the health of women, children, and families.

Nurses must research and understand the cultural characteristics, values, and beliefs of the various people to whom they deliver care so that false assumptions and stereotyping do not lead to insensitive care. Time orientation, personal space, family orientation (patriarchal, matriarchal, or egalitarian), and language are important cultural concepts.

Culturally Competent Nursing Care

Cultural competence is defined as the knowledge, willingness, and ability to adapt health care to enhance its acceptability to and effectiveness with clients from diverse cultures (Clark, 2007). Cultural competence is a dynamic process during which nurses obtain and then apply cultural information. Nurses must look at clients through their own eyes and the eyes of clients and family members. Nurses must develop nonjudgmental acceptance of cultural differences in clients, using diversity as a strength that empowers them to achieve mutually acceptable health care goals (Kersey-Matusiak, 2006). This cultural awareness allows nurses to see the entire picture and improves the quality of care and health outcomes.

Cultural competence does not appear suddenly; it must be developed through a series of steps (Box 2.3).

Barriers to Cultural Competence

Barriers to cultural competence can be grouped into two categories: those related to providers and those related to systems (Godfrey, 2006). When a health care provider lacks knowledge of a client's cultural practices and beliefs or when the provider's beliefs differ from those of the client, the provider may be unprepared to respond when the client makes unexpected health care decisions. System-related barriers can occur if agencies that have not been designed for cultural diversity want all clients to conform to the established rules and regulations and attempt to fit everyone into the same mold.

Cultural competence does not mean replacing one's own cultural identity with another, ignoring the variability within cultural groups, or even appreciating the cultures

---

BOX 2.3 **Steps to Developing Cultural Competence**

1. Cultural Self-Awareness
   - Become aware of, appreciate, and become sensitive to the values, beliefs, customs, and behaviors that have shaped one's own culture.
   - Engage in self-exploration beyond one's own culture and "see" clients from different cultures.
   - Examine personal biases and prejudices toward other cultures.
   - Become aware of differences in personal and clients' backgrounds.
2. Cultural Knowledge
   - Learn about different cultures (e.g., books, continuing education courses, the Internet, cultural diversity conferences).
   - Become familiar with culturally/ethnically diverse groups, worldviews, beliefs, practices, lifestyles, and problem-solving strategies.
3. Cultural Skills
   - Learn how to perform a competent cultural assessment.
   - Assess each client's unique cultural values, beliefs, and practices without depending solely on written facts about specific cultural groups.
4. Cultural Encounter
   - Engage in cross-cultural interactions with people from culturally diverse backgrounds, such as attending religious services or ceremonies and participating in important family events.
   - Participate in as many cultural encounters as possible to avoid cultural stereotyping.

▶ *Consider THIS!*

Our medical mission took a team of nurse practitioners into the rural mountains of Guatemala to offer medical services to people who had never had any. One day, a distraught mother brought her 10-year-old daughter to the mission clinic, asking me if there was anything I could do about her daughter's right wrist. She had sustained a fracture a year ago and it had not healed properly. As I looked at the girl's malformed wrist, I asked if it had been splinted to help with alignment, knowing what the answer was going to be. The interpreter enlightened me by saying that this young girl would never marry and have children because of this injury. I appeared puzzled at the interpreter's prediction of this girl's future. It was later explained to me that if the girl couldn't make tortes from corn meal for her husband because of her wrist disability, she would

(continued)

▶ *Consider THIS!* (continued)

not be worthy of becoming someone's wife and thus would probably live with her parents the rest of her life.

I reminded myself during the week of the medical mission not to impose my cultural values on the women for whom I was caring and to accept their cultural mores without judgment. These silent self-reminders served me well throughout the week, for I was open to learning about their lifestyles and customs.

Thoughts: What must the young girl be feeling at the age of 10, being rejected for a disability that wasn't her fault? What might have happened if I had imposed my value system on this patient? How effective would I have been in helping her if she didn't feel accepted? This incident ripped my heart out, for this young girl will be deprived of a fulfilling family life based on a wrist disability. This is just another example of female suppression that happens all over the world—such a tragedy—and yet a part of their culture, on which nurses should not pass judgment.

being served. Instead, nurses skilled at cultural competence show a respect for difference, an eagerness to learn, and a willingness to accept multiple views of the world (Streltzer & Tseng, 2008).

Use of Complementary and Alternative Medicine

The use of complementary and alternative medicine (CAM) is not unique to a specific ethnic or cultural group: interest in CAM therapies continues to grow nationwide and will affect care of many clients. People from all walks of life and in all areas of the community use CAM. Overall, CAM use is seen more in women than men, and in people with higher educational levels. The annual out-of-pocket costs for CAM are estimated to exceed $27 billion. Prayer specifically for health reasons is the most commonly used CAM therapy (NCCAM, 2007). Research indicates that more than 43% of adults use some form of alternative practice, and one in three pregnant women use CAM therapies, some of which may be potentially harmful (Daniel, 2006).

CAM includes diverse practices, products, and health care systems that are not currently considered to be part of conventional medicine (NCCAM, 2007). *Complementary* medicine is used together with conventional medicine, such as using aromatherapy to reduce discomfort after surgery or to reduce pain during a procedure or during early labor. *Alternative* medicine is used in place of conventional medicine, such as eating a special natural diet to control nausea and vomiting or to treat cancer instead of undergoing surgery, chemotherapy, or radiation that has been recommended by a conventional doctor. *Integrative* medicine combines mainstream medical therapies and CAM therapies for which there is some scientific evidence of safety and effectiveness (NCCAM, 2007). These include acupuncture, reflexology, therapeutic touch, meditation, yoga, herbal therapies, nutritional supplements, homeopathy, naturopathic medicine, and many more used for the promotion of health and well-being (Pearson & Chesney, 2007). Table 2.2 describes selected CAM therapies and treatments.

The theoretic underpinnings of complementary and alternative health practices propose that health and illness are complex interactions of the mind, body, and spirit. It is then surmised that many aspects of clients' health experiences are not subject to traditional scientific

TABLE 2.2 **SELECTED COMPLEMENTARY AND ALTERNATIVE THERAPIES**

Therapy	Description
Aromatherapy	Use of essential oils to stimulate the sense of smell for balancing mind, body, and spirit
Homeopathy	Based on the theory of "like treats like"; helps restore the body's natural balance
Acupressure	Restoration of balance by pressing an appropriate point so self-healing capacities can take over
Feng Shui (pronounced *fung shway*)	The Chinese art of placement. Objects are positioned in the environment to induce harmony with chi.
Guided imagery	Use of consciously chosen positive and healing images along with deep relaxation to reduce stress and to help people cope
Reflexology	Use of deep massage on identified points of the foot or hand to scan and rebalance body parts that correspond with each point
Therapeutic touch	Balancing of energy by centering, invoking an intention to heal, and moving the hands from the head to the feet several inches from the skin
Herbal medicine	The therapeutic use of plants for healing and treating diseases and conditions
Spiritual healing	Praying, chanting, presence, laying on of hands, rituals, and meditation to assist in healing

methods. This field does not lend itself readily to scientific study or to investigation and therefore is not easily embraced by many hard-core scientists (Tryens et al., 2007). Much of what we consider to be alternative medicine comes from the Eastern world, folk medicine, and religious and spiritual practices. There is no unifying basic theory for the numerous treatments or modalities, except (as noted previously) that health and illness are considered to be complex interactions among the body, mind, and spirit.

Because of heightened interest in complementary treatments and their widening use, anecdotal efficacy, and growing supporting research evidence, nurses need to be sensitive to and knowledgeable enough to answer many of the questions clients ask and to guide them in a safe, objective way (Fowler & Newton, 2006). Nurses have a unique opportunity to provide services that facilitate wholeness. They need to understand all aspects of CAM, including costs, client knowledge, and drug interactions, if they are to promote holistic strategies for clients and families.

Many patients who use complementary or alternative therapies do not reveal this fact to their health care provider. Therefore, one of the nurse's most important roles during the assessment phase of the nursing process is to encourage clients to communicate their use of these therapies to eliminate the possibility of harmful interactions and contraindications with current medical therapies. When assessing clients, ask specific questions about any nonprescription medications they may be taking, including vitamins, minerals, or herbs. Clients should also be asked about any therapies they are taking that have not been ordered by their primary health care provider.

When caring for clients and their families who practice CAM, nurses need to:

- Be culturally sensitive to nontraditional treatments
- Acknowledge and respect different beliefs, attitudes, and lifestyles
- Keep an open mind, remembering that standard medical treatments do not work for all clients
- Accept CAM and integrate it if it brings comfort without harm
- Provide accurate information, not unsubstantiated opinions
- Advise clients how they can best monitor their condition using CAM
- Discourage practices only if they are harmful to the client's health
- Instruct the client to weigh the risks and benefits of CAM use
- Avoid confrontation when asking clients about CAM
- Be reflective, nonjudgmental, and open-minded about CAM

The use of complementary therapies is widespread, especially by women desiring to alleviate the nausea and vomiting of early pregnancy. Ginger tea, Sea-Bands, and vitamin B6 are typically used to treat morning sickness (Northrup, 2006). Although these may not cause any ill effects during the pregnancy, most substances ingested cross the placenta and have the potential to reach the fetus, so nurses should stress to all pregnant women that it is better to be cautious when using CAM.

Women at risk for osteoporosis are seeking alternatives to hormone replacement therapy since the Women's Health Initiative (WHI) study raised doubts about the benefit of estrogen. Some of the alternative therapies for osteoporosis include soy isoflavones, progesterone cream, magnet therapy, tai chi, and hip protectors (Kessenich, 2007). In addition, menopausal women may seek CAM therapies for hot flashes. Once again, despite many claims, most of these therapies have not undergone scientific testing and thus could place the woman at risk.

If clients are considering the use of or using CAM therapies, suggest they check with their health care provider before taking any "natural" substance. Offer clients the following instructions:

- Do not take for granted that because a substance is a natural herb or plant product, it is beneficial or harmless.
- Seek medical care when ill.
- Always inform the provider if you are taking herbs or other therapies.
- Avoid taking herbal remedies if you are pregnant or lactating.
- Be sure that any product package contains a list of all ingredients and amounts of each.
- Be aware that frequent or continual use of large doses of a CAM preparation is not advisable, and harm may result if therapies are mixed (e.g., vitamin E, garlic, and aspirin all have anticoagulant properties).
- Research CAM through resources such as books, websites, and articles (Clark & Collins, 2007).

All nurses, especially nurses working in the community, must educate themselves about the pros and cons of CAM and be prepared to discuss and help their clients make sense of it all. Expanding our consciousness by understanding and respecting diverse cultures and CAM will enable nurses to provide the best treatment for clients and their families receiving community-based care.

Community–Based Nursing Care Settings

Community-based nursing takes place in a variety of settings, including physician's offices, clinics, health departments, urgent care centers, hospital outpatient centers, churches, shelters, and clients' homes. Nurses provide well care, episodic ill care, and chronic care. They work to promote, preserve, and improve the health of the women and their families in these settings.

Due to technological advances, cost containment, and shortened hospital stays, the home is a common care setting for women and families today. Home care is geared toward the needs of the client and family. Private-duty nursing care is used when more extensive care is needed; it may be delivered hourly (several hours per day) or on a full-time, live-in basis. Periodic nursing visits may be used for intermittent interventions, such as IV antibiotic administration, follow-up client teaching, and monitoring. The goals of nursing care in the home setting include promoting, restoring, and maintaining the health of the client.

Home care focuses on minimizing the effects of the illness or disability along with providing the client with the means to care for the illness or disability at home. Nurses in the home care setting are direct care providers, educators, advocates, and case managers.

Prenatal Care

Early, adequate prenatal care has long been associated with improved pregnancy outcomes (March of Dimes, 2008). Adequate prenatal care is a comprehensive process in which any problems associated with pregnancy are identified and treated. Basic components of prenatal care are early and continuing risk assessment, health promotion, medical and psychosocial interventions, and follow-up.

Within the community setting, several services are available to provide health care for pregnant women (Box 2.4).

Not all women are aware of the community resources available to them. Most public health services are available for consultation, local hospitals have "hotlines" for questions, and public libraries have pregnancy-related resources as well as Internet access. Nurses can be a very helpful link to resources for all women regardless of their economic status.

Technologically advanced care has been shown to improve maternal and infant outcomes. Regionalized high-risk care, recommended by the American Academy of Pediatrics in the late 1970s, aimed to promote uniformity nationwide, covering the prenatal care of high-risk pregnancies and high-risk newborns. The advanced technology found in level III perinatal regional centers and community-based prenatal surveillance programs have resulted in better risk-adjusted mortality rates (Britt, Edean, & Evans, 2006; Martin & Foley, 2006). For example, fetal monitoring and ultrasound technology have traditionally been used in acute care settings to monitor the progress of many high-risk pregnancies. However, with the increased cost of hospital stays, many services were moved to outpatient facilities and into the home. The intent was to reduce health care costs and to monitor women with complications of pregnancy in the home rather than in the

---

BOX 2.4 Maternal Community Health Care Services

- State public health prenatal clinics provide access to care based on a sliding scale payment schedule or have services paid for by Medicaid.
- Federally funded community clinics typically offer a variety of services, which may include prenatal, pediatric, adult health, and dental services. A sliding scale payment schedule or Medicaid may cover costs.
- Hospital outpatient health care services offer maternal–child health services. Frequently they are associated with a teaching hospital in which medical school students, interns, and OB/GYN residents rotate through the clinic services to care for patients during their education process.
- Private OB/GYN offices are available for women with health insurance seeking care during their pregnancies. Some physicians in private practice will accept Medicaid patients as well as private patients.
- Community free clinics offer maternal–child services in some communities for women with limited economic resources (homeless, unemployed).
- Freestanding birth centers offer prenatal care for low-risk mothers as well as childbirth classes to educate couples regarding the birthing process. Most centers accept private insurance and Medicaid for reimbursement services.

- Midwifery services are available in many communities where midwives provide women's health services. They usually accept a multitude of payment plans from private pay to health insurance to Medicaid for reimbursement purposes.
- WIC provides food, nutrition counseling, and access to health services for low-income women, infants, and children. WIC is a federally funded program and is administered by each state. All persons receiving Aid to Families with Dependent Children (AFDC), food stamps, or Medicaid are automatically eligible for WIC. An estimated 45% of the infants born in the United States are served by WIC (USDA Food and Nutrition Service, 2004).
- Childbirth classes offer pregnant women and their partners a series of educational classes on childbirth preparation. Women attend them during their last trimester of pregnancy. Some classes are free and some have a fee.
- Local La Leche League groups provide mother-to-mother support for breast-feeding, nutrition, and infant care problem-solving strategies. All women who have an interest in breast-feeding are welcome to participate in the meetings, which are typically held in the home of a La Leche member.

hospital. Examples of services offered in the home setting might include:

• Infusion therapy to treat infections or combat dehydration
• Hypertension monitoring for women with gestational hypertension
• Uterine monitoring for mothers who are at high risk for preterm labor
• Fetal monitoring to evaluate fetal well-being
• Portable ultrasound to perform a biophysical profile to assess fetal well-being

As a result, home care has the potential to produce cost savings compared to inpatient care.

Labor and Birth Care

Pregnancy involves numerous choices: cloth or disposable diapers, breastfeeding or bottle feeding, doctor or midwife, and where to give birth—at a birthing center, at home, or at a hospital. Deciding where to give birth depends on the woman's pregnancy risk status. For the pregnant woman who is at high risk as a result of medical or social factors, the hospital is considered the safest place for birth. Potential complications can be addressed because medical technology, skilled professionals, and neonatal services are available. For low-risk women, a freestanding birthing center or a home birth is an option.

The choice between a birthing center, home birth, or hospital depends on the woman's preferences, her risk status, and her distance from a hospital. Some women choose an all-natural birth with no medications and no medical intervention, whereas others would feel more comfortable in a setting in which medications and trained staff are available if needed. Presenting the facts to women and allowing them to choose in collaboration with their health care provider is the nurse's role. Safety is paramount, but at the same time nurses must protect the woman's right to select birth options and should promote family-centered care in all maternity settings (see Evidence-Based Practice 2.1).

EVIDENCE-BASED PRACTICE 2.1
Home-Like Institutional Birth Settings Versus Conventional Institutional Birth Settings

Women have been giving birth to newborns in the home setting since the beginning of time; giving birth in an institution has been the norm only since the early 20th century. These institutions continue to be the primary setting for birth, but with the growing emphasis on the client as a consumer of health care and the desire for family-centered care, greater numbers of facilities are attempting to incorporate some of the home birth components into their delivery of care.

● Study
A study was done to compare the effect of care in a home-like institutional birth setting versus a conventional institutional birth setting. Two researchers using standard methods for data collection and analysis compiled information from all randomized and quasi-randomized controlled trials involving a comparison of home-like institutional and conventional institutional birth settings. In addition, the researchers evaluated eight journals and two published conference proceedings. Six trials that involved 8,677 women were included. The researchers were unable to include information related to freestanding birthing centers because they found no trials on this topic. The researchers reported the results using relative risk and 95% confidence intervals.

▲ Findings
Women giving birth in home-like institutional birth settings were less likely to receive or require intrapartum analgesia or anesthesia, less likely to have an episiotomy, and more likely to experience a spontaneous vaginal birth. They were more likely to choose the same setting for future births, they were more satisfied with intrapartum care, and they were more likely to initiate breastfeeding and continue it for the next 6 to 8 weeks. However, they also had an increased risk for vaginal or perineal tears and the risks for perinatal mortality were increased.

■ Nursing Implications
This study identified several important benefits that nurses can integrate into their practice when counseling and teaching pregnant women about birthing options. However, nurses need to stress the increased risk for perinatal mortality with this option so that women can make informed decisions about their choice of birth setting.

Nurses also can provide input about incorporating a more "home-like" atmosphere when their facilities are designing new birthing areas. In addition, nurses can advocate for the pregnant woman in labor to ensure that she has freedom to move about the birthing area, allowing her to feel more "at home."

Hodnett, D. D., Downe, S., Edwards, N., & Walsh, D. (2005). Home-like versus conventional institutional settings for birth. *Cochrane Database of Systematic Reviews* 2005. Issue 1. Art. No.: CD000012. DOI:10.1002/14651858.CD000012.pub2.

Birthing Center

A birthing center is a cross between a home birth and a hospital. Birthing centers offer a homelike setting but with close proximity to a hospital in case of complications. Midwives often are the sole care providers in freestanding birthing centers, with obstetricians as backups in case of emergencies. Birthing centers usually have fewer restrictions and guidelines for families to follow and allow for more freedom in making decisions about labor. The rates of cesarean birth and the costs are much lower than those of a hospital (Davey & Forrester-King, 2008). The normal discharge time after birth is usually measured in hours (4 to 24 hours), not days.

Birthing centers aim to provide a relaxing home environment and promote a "culture of normalcy." Birth is considered a normal physiologic process, and most centers use a non-interventional view of labor and birth. The range of services for the expectant family often includes prenatal care, childbirth education, intrapartum care, and postpartum care, including home follow-up and family planning (Fig. 2.2). One of the hallmarks of the freestanding birthing center is that it can provide truly family-centered care by approaching pregnancy and birth as a normal family event and encouraging all family members to participate. Education is often provided by such centers, encouraging families to become informed and self-reliant in the care of themselves and their families (Bainbridge, 2006).

Birthing centers provide an alternative for women who are uncomfortable with a home birth but who do not want to give birth in a hospital. Advantages of birthing centers include a non-interventional approach to obstetric care, freedom to eat and move around during labor, ability to give birth in any position, and the right to have any

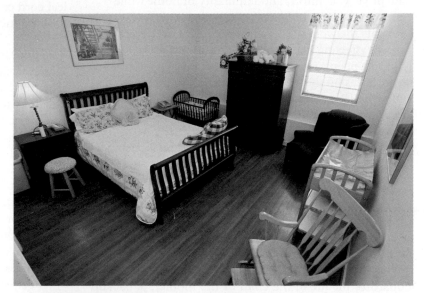

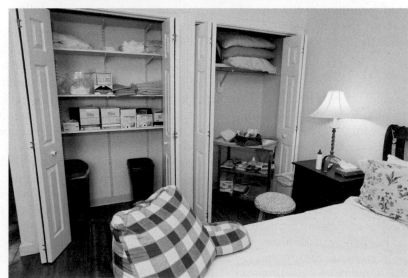

FIGURE 2.2 Birthing centers aim to provide a relaxing homelike environment and promote a culture of normality while offering a full range of health care services to the expectant family. (Photos by Gus Freedman.)

number of family and friends attend the birth. Disadvantages are that some centers have rigid screening criteria, which may eliminate healthy mothers from using birth centers; many have rigid rules concerning transporting the mother to the hospital (e.g., prolonged labor, ruptured membranes); and many have no pediatrician on staff if the newborn has special needs after birth (Lyndon, 2008).

Home Birth

For centuries women have been giving birth to babies in their home. Many feel more comfortable and relaxed when giving birth in their own environment. Women who want no medical interventions and a very family-centered birth often choose to have a home birth. Home births are recommended for pregnant women who are considered to be at low risk for complications during labor and birth. Home birth is advantageous because it:

• Is the least expensive
• Allows the woman to experience labor and birth in the privacy, comfort, and familiarity of home while surrounded by loved ones
• Permits the woman to maintain control over every aspect affecting her labor (e.g., positions, attire, support people)
• Minimizes interference and unnecessary interventions, allowing labor to progress normally
• Provides continuous one-on-one care by the midwife throughout the childbirth process
• Promotes the development of a trusting relationship with the nurse midwife (American Pregnancy Association [APA], 2007)

A home birth does have some disadvantages, including the limited availability of pain medication and danger to the mother and baby if an emergency arises (e.g., placental abruption, uterine rupture, cord prolapse, or a distressed fetus). Delay in getting to the hospital could jeopardize the life of the child or the mother. A backup plan for a health care provider and nearby hospital on standby must be established should an emergency occur (Ramsey, 2007).

Postpartum and Newborn Care

Recent reforms in health care financing have reduced hospital stays significantly for new mothers. As a result, community-based nurses play a major role in extending care beyond the hospital setting. When new mothers are discharged from the hospital, most are still experiencing perineal discomfort and uterine cramping. They may still have pain from an episiotomy. They are fatigued and may be constipated. They may feel uncertain about feeding and caring for their newborn. These new mothers need to be made aware of community resources such as telephone consultation by nurses, outpatient clinics, and home visits.

Telephone Consultation

Many hospitals offer telephone consultation services by their maternity nurses. The discharged mother is given the phone number of the nursing unit on the day of discharge and is instructed to call if she has any questions or concerns. Because the nurses on the unit are familiar with her birth history and the newborn, they are in a good position to assist her in adjusting to her new role. Although this service is usually free, not all families recognize a problem early or use this valuable informational resource.

Outpatient Clinics

Outpatient clinics offer another community-based site where the childbearing family can obtain services. Usually the mother has received prenatal care before giving birth and thus has established some rapport with the nursing staff there. The clinic staff is usually willing to answer any questions she may have about her health or that of her newborn. Appointments usually include an examination of the mother and newborn and instructions about umbilical cord care, postpartum and infant care, and nutrition for both mother and infant.

Postpartum Home Visits

Home visits offer services similar to those offered at a scheduled clinic visit, but they also give the nurse an opportunity to assess the family's adaptation and dynamics and the home environment. During the past decade, hospital stays have averaged 24 to 48 hours or less for vaginal births and 72 to 96 hours for cesarean births (Centers for Disease Control [CDC], 2007a). Federal legislation went into effect in 1998 that prohibited insurers from restricting hospital stays for mothers and newborns to less than 2 days for vaginal births or 4 days for cesarean births (CDC, 2007a). These shortened stays have reduced the time available for educating mothers about caring for themselves and their newborns.

Postpartum care in the home environment usually includes:

• Monitoring the physical and emotional well-being of the family members (Fig. 2.3)
• Identifying potential or developing complications for the mother and newborn
• Bridging the gap between discharge and ambulatory follow-up for mothers and their newborns (Goulet, D'Amour, & Pineault 2007).

High-Risk Newborn Home Care

With the reduced lengths of stay, high-risk newborns are also being cared for in community settings. High-tech care once was provided only in the hospital. Now, however, the increasing cost of complex care and the influences of managed care have brought high-tech care into the home. Families have become "health care systems" by providing physical, emotional, social, and developmental home care

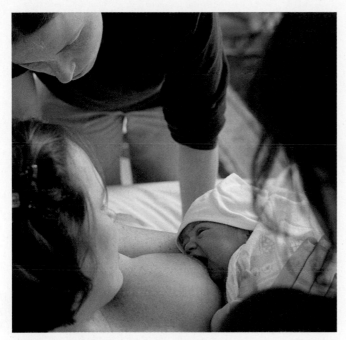

FIGURE 2.3 The nurse makes a postpartum home visit to assess the woman and her newborn. During the visit, the nurse assists the mother with breastfeeding.

for their technology-dependent infants. Suitable candidates for home care may include preterm infants who continue to need oxygen, low-birthweight infants needing nutritional or hypercaloric formulas or adjunct feeding methods (e.g., tube feedings), or infants with hydrocephalus or cerebral palsy. A wide range of equipment may be used, including mechanical ventilation, electronic apnea monitors, home oxygen equipment, intravenous infusions, respiratory nebulizers, phototherapy, and suction equipment.

All family members must work together to provide 24-hour care. The parents must negotiate with insurers for reimbursement for durable medical equipment, must be able to troubleshoot equipment problems, and must be able to manage inventories of supplies and equipment. In addition, they must be able to assess the infant for problems, determine the problem, decide when to call the nurse, pharmacist, or physical therapist, and interpret and implement prescriptions. Technology in the home requires nurses to focus on the family "home care system" to provide total care to the infant.

Nurses can play a key role in assisting families by preparing them for and increasing their confidence in caring for their infants at home. This adaptation begins before discharge from the hospital. Family members are active participants in the transition-to-home plan. Recognition of parental needs and addressing each area in the discharge plan will ease the transition to home.

Assessment of the family's preparedness is essential. The following questions can provide valuable information in this area:

- How well prepared are you to take care of your infant's physical, emotional, and equipment needs?
- How well prepared are you to obtain the home services you need for your infant?
- How well prepared are you to manage the stress of home care?

These questions convey the nurse's concern for the infant and family while obtaining a thorough assessment of the family's learning needs.

Once preparedness has been assessed, the nurse can intervene as necessary. For example, if the caretakers do not think they are prepared to maintain machinery, technology, medication, or developmental therapy, then the nurse can demonstrate the care to the family. The nurse provides instructions and hands-on experience in a supportive environment until the family's confidence increases. The nurse can also assist the family to anticipate the common problems that might occur (e.g., advising them to avoid running out of supplies, to have enough medication or special formula mixture to last throughout the weekend, and to keep backup batteries for powering machines or portable oxygen). The outcome of the preparedness assessment and intervention is that the safety of the infant is established and maintained.

Nursing for families who are using complex home care equipment requires caring for the infant and family members' physical and emotional well-being as well as providing solutions to problems they may encounter. Home health nurses need to identify, mobilize, and adapt a myriad of community resources to support the family in giving the best possible care in the home setting. Preparing families before hospital discharge, with home health nurses continuing and reinforcing that focus, will ease the burden of managing high-tech equipment in the home.

Women's Health Care

A woman's reproductive years span half her lifetime, on average. This is not a static period, but rather one that encompasses several significant stages. As her reproductive goals change, so do a woman's health care needs. Because of these changing needs, comprehensive community-centered care is critical.

Community-based women's health services have received increased emphasis during the past few decades simply because of economics. Women use more health care services than men, they make as many as 90% of health care decisions, and they represent the majority of the population (CDC, 2007b). Women spend 66 cents of every health care dollar, and 7 of the 10 most frequently performed surgeries in the United States are specific to women (Alexander et al., 2007). Examples of community-based women's health care services that can be freestanding or hospital-based include:

- Screening centers that offer mammograms, Pap smears, bone density assessments, genetic counseling, ultrasound, breast examinations, complete health risk appraisals, laboratory studies (complete blood count, cholesterol testing, thyroid testing, glucose testing for diabetes, follicle-stimulating hormone [FSH] levels), and electrocardiograms

- Educational centers that provide women's health lectures, instruction on breast self-examinations and Pap smears, and computers for research
- Counseling centers that offer various support groups: genetics, psychotherapy, substance abuse, sexual assault, and domestic violence
- Wellness centers that offer stress reduction techniques, massage therapy, guided imagery, hypnosis, smoking cessation, weight reduction, tai chi, yoga, and women's fitness/exercise classes
- Alternative/wholeness healing centers that provide acupuncture, aromatherapy, biofeedback, therapeutic touch, facials, reflexology, and herbal remedies
- Retail centers that offer specialty equipment for rental and purchase, such as breast prostheses

Women have multiple choices regarding services, settings, and health care providers. In the past most women received health care services from physicians such as obstetricians, gynecologists, and family physicians, but today nurse midwives and nurse practitioners are becoming more prevalent in providing well-women care.

Nurses who work in community-based settings need to be familiar with the many health issues commonly encountered by women within their communities. All nurses who work with women of any age in community-based settings, including the workplace, schools, practitioners' offices, and clinics, should possess a thorough understanding of the scope of women's health care and should be prepared to intervene appropriately to prevent problems and to promote health.

Roles and Functions of the Community-Based Nurse

Many nurses find the shift from acute care to community settings a challenge. With the shift in responsibilities from hospital care to community care, changes in nursing care have resulted. Nurses working in community-based settings share many of the same roles and responsibilities as their colleagues in acute care settings, but there are some differences. For example, in the community or home care setting the nurse will provide direct client care but will spend more time in the role of educator, communicator, and manager than the nurse in the acute care setting. In home care the nurse will spend a significant amount of time in the supervisory or management role.

Communicator

Effective therapeutic communication with women, children, and families is critical to the provision of quality nursing care. Client- and family-centered communication increases satisfaction with nursing care and aids in improving knowledge and health care skills (Clark, 2008).

Verbal and Nonverbal Communication

Nurses use verbal communication continuously throughout the day when interacting with their clients. Good verbal communication skills are necessary for excellent nursing assessment and teaching. Nonverbal communication, also referred to as body language, includes attending to others and active listening. When clients and families feel they are being heard, trust and rapport are established.

*R*ecall Maria, who recently was discharged from the hospital with her newborn son. How did the nurse communicate with Maria? Did the nurse's actions during the visit promote the development of trust between Maria and the nurse? What might have been done differently to foster trust?

▶ *Take* NOTE!

People of all ages desire to be listened to without interruption (Brunner, 2008).

Active listening is critical to the communication process. Listening may uncover fears or concerns that the nurse may not have discovered through questioning. By not listening, critical information may be missed. The client or family may sense that the nurse is not listening and thus may be reluctant to share further information. During the interaction, determine whether the client's verbal communication is congruent with his or her nonverbal communication.

Communication With Families

When communicating with families, be honest. Families desire to be valued and should be equal partners in the health care team. Allow family members to verbalize concerns and questions. Explain the use of equipment and the correct sequence of procedures. Help the members understand the long-term as well as short-term effects of the health treatment.

Working With an Interpreter

Attempting to communicate with a family who does not speak English can be a highly frustrating situation for health care providers. Interpreters are an invaluable aid and an essential component of client and family education. Working with an interpreter, whether in person or over the phone, requires coordination of efforts so that both the family and the interpreter understand the information to be communicated. Working as a team, the nurse questions or informs and the interpreter conveys the information completely and accurately. Box 2.5 presents tips for working with an interpreter to maximize teaching efforts.

Healthy People 2010 also addresses the topic of language differences (see Healthy People 2010). In addition, many health care facilities subscribe to Language Line (http://www.languageline.com/), which offers telephone access to interpretation of 150 languages. Numerous other interpreters, translators, and language resources are available online.

HEALTHY PEOPLE 2010

Objective	Significance
Increase the proportion of local health departments that have established culturally appropriate and linguistically competent community health promotion and disease prevention programs.	• Work with professionals and individuals from various cultures to develop materials and programs for health promotion that are culturally competent. • Ensure teaching materials are provided in the appropriate language.

Recall Maria, the woman with the newborn who is receiving home care. On the second visit to Maria's home, the nurse brought a Spanish-speaking interpreter who explained the reason for the "back to sleep" position and demonstrated to Maria several other useful positions for feeding and holding. Maria was smiling when the nurse left and asking when she would be back. What made the difference in their relationship during the second visit? What interventions demonstrate culturally competent care?

Communicating With Deaf or Hearing-Impaired Clients and Families

For hearing-impaired clients, determine the method of communication they use: lip reading, American Sign Language (ASL), another method, or some combination. If the nurse is not proficient in ASL and the client or family uses it, then an ASL interpreter must be available if another adult family member is not present for translation. According to federal law, deaf clients and deaf family members must be given the ability to communicate effectively with health care providers (Chong-Hee Lieu et al., 2007).

Direct Care Provider

The community-based nurse typically performs less direct physical care than the nurse in the acute care setting. Many times the nurse may observe the client or caregiver performing physical care tasks. Excellent assessment skills are especially important in the community care setting. The nurse often is functioning in a more autonomous role, and after data collection, the community-based nurse will often decide whether to initiate, continue, alter, or end physical nursing care. Assessment extends beyond physical assessment of the client to include the environment and the community.

The nurse provides direct care to the perinatal client, beginning with the woman's first visit to the health care provider and extending through the pregnancy and birth.

BOX 2.5   Tips for Working With Interpreters

- **Help the interpreter prepare and understand what needs to be done ahead of time.** A few minutes of preparation may save a lot of time and help communication flow more smoothly in the long run.
- **Remember, the interpreter is the "communication bridge" and not the "content expert."** The nurse's presence at teaching sessions is vital.
- **Be patient. The interpreter's timing may not match that of others involved.** It often takes longer to say in some languages what has already been said in English; therefore, plan for more time than you normally would.
- **Speak slowly and clearly.** Avoid jargon. Use short sentences and be concise. Avoid interrupting the interpreter.
- **Pause every few sentences so the interpreter can translate your information.** After 30 seconds of speaking, stop and let the interpreter express the information. Talk directly to the family, not the interpreter.
- **Give the family and the interpreter a break.** Sessions that last longer than 20 or 30 minutes are too much for anyone's attention span and concentration.
- **Express the information in two or three different ways if needed.** There may be cultural barriers as well as language and dialect differences that interfere with understanding. Interpreters may often know the correct communication protocols for the family.
- **Use an interpreter to help ensure the family can read and understand translated written materials.** The interpreter can also help answer questions and evaluate learning.
- **Avoid side conversations during sessions.** These can be uncomfortable for the family and jeopardize client–provider relationships and trust.
- **Remember, just because someone speaks another language doesn't mean that he or she will make a good interpreter.** An interpreter who has no medical background may not understand or interpret correctly, no matter how good his or her language skills are.
- **Do not use children as interpreters.** Doing so can affect family relationships, proper understanding, and compliance with health care issues.

Adapted from Weech, W. A. (1999). *Tips for using interpreters.* Foreign Service Institute of the U.S. Department of State.

In addition, the nurse provides direct care involving the following areas:

• Contraception
• Abortion
• Infertility
• Screening for sexually transmitted infections
• Preconceptual risk assessment and care

Educator

Due to shortened hospital stays and decreased admissions, providing client and family education is a key role for nurses in the community. Many times teaching begins in the community setting, especially the home. In the community-based setting, client teaching is often focused on assisting the client and family to achieve independence.

Regardless of the type of setting, nurses are in a unique position to help clients and families manage their own health care. Clients and families need to be knowledgeable about areas such as their condition, the health care management plan, and when and how to contact health care providers. With the limited time available in all health care arenas, nurses must focus on teaching goals and begin teaching at the earliest opportunity (Clark, 2008).

▶ Take NOTE!

There is no prescription more valuable than knowledge.
(C. Everett Koop, MD, Former Surgeon General of the United States)

Client education occurs when nurses share information, knowledge, and skills with clients and families, thus empowering them to take responsibility for their health care. Through client education, clients and families can overcome feelings of powerlessness and helplessness and gain the confidence and capability to be active members in their plan of care.

Overall, client and family education allows clients and families to make informed decisions, ensures the presence of basic health care skills, promotes recognition of problem situations, promotes appropriate responses to problems, and allows for questions to be answered (Clark, 2008). Client and family education is a priority and is addressed in Healthy People 2010.

▶ Take NOTE!

To cope effectively with illness, to understand and participate in decisions about treatment plans, and to maintain and improve health after treatment, clients and their families must have knowledge and skills relevant to their conditions (JCAHO, 2008).

HEALTHY PEOPLE 2010

Objective	Significance
Increase the proportion of persons appropriately counseled about health behaviors. (Developmental) Increase the proportion of health care organizations that provide client and family education; increase the proportion of clients who report that they are satisfied with the client education they receive from their health care organization.	• Assess health learning needs of women, children, and their families. • Plan health care education in collaboration with clients and their families. • Provide health education at each client encounter.

Steps of Client and Family Education

The steps of client and family education are similar to the steps of the nursing process: the nurse must assess, plan, implement, evaluate, and finally document education. Once the nurse achieves a level of comfort and experience with each of these steps, they all blend together into one harmonious whole that becomes an everyday part of nursing practice. Client education begins with the first client encounter and proceeds through discharge and beyond. Reassessment after each step or change in the process is critical to ensuring success.

Intervening to Enhance Learning

Nurses are in an excellent position to foster an environment that is conducive to learning. For example, it is entirely appropriate to say to the client, "Many people have a problem reading and remembering the information on this paper (booklet, manual). Is this ever a problem for you?" Once a problem is acknowledged, the nurse is free to adjust verbal communication techniques and written materials to assist with learning and to communicate this need to the entire interdisciplinary health care team.

Nurses implement individualized teaching techniques based on the assessment information and identified goals. In general, the following techniques can facilitate learning:

• Slow down and repeat information often.
• Speak in conversational style using plain, nonmedical language.
• "Chunk" information and teach it in small bits using logical steps.
• Prioritize information and teach "survival skills" first.
• Use visuals, such as pictures, videos, and models.
• Teach using an interactive, "hands-on" approach.

If the client or family has poor health literacy skills, learning can be fostered by the use of pictures or illustrations, videos or audio tapes, or color coding (such as medication bottles or steps of a procedure). In addition, teaching can include a "back-up" family member.

Documenting Teaching and Learning

Documenting client care and education is part of every nurse's professional practice and serves four main purposes. First and foremost, the client's medical record serves as a communication tool that the entire interdisciplinary team can use to keep track of what the client and family has learned already and what learning still needs to occur. Next, it serves to testify to the education the family has received if legal matters arise. Thirdly, it verifies standards set by the JCAHO, Centers for Medicare and Medicaid Services (CMS), and other accrediting bodies that hold health care providers accountable for client education activities. And lastly, it informs third-party payers of the goods and services that were provided for reimbursement purposes.

Documentation of client and family education is imperative. It is the only means available to ensure that the educational plan and objectives have been completed.

Discharge Planner and Case Manager

Due to the short length of stays in acute settings and the shift to community settings for clients with complex health needs, discharge planning and case management have become an important nursing role in the community. Discharge planning involves the development and implementation of a comprehensive plan for the safe discharge of a client from a health care facility and for continuing safe and effective care in the community and at home. Case management focuses on coordinating health care services while balancing quality and cost outcomes. Often clients requiring community-based care, especially home care, have complex medical needs that require an interdisciplinary team to meet their physical, psychosocial, medical, nursing, developmental, and education needs. The nurse plays an important role in initiating and maintaining the link between team members and the client to ensure that the client and family are receiving comprehensive, coordinated care.

Advocate and Resource Manager

Client advocate is another important role of the community-based nurse to ensure that the client's and family's needs are being met. Advocacy also helps ensure that the client and family have available resources and appropriate health care services. For example, the pregnant woman on bed rest at home may need help in caring for her other children, maintaining the household, or getting to her appointments. Women with complex medical needs may require financial assistance through Medicaid or Medicaid waivers (state-run programs that use federal and state money to pay for the health care of individuals with certain medical conditions). They may also need assistance in obtaining needed equipment, additional services, and transportation. Community-based nurses need a basic understanding of community, state, and federal resources to ensure that clients and their families have access to those necessary for them.

■■■ Key Concepts

- Family-centered care recognizes the concept of the family as the constant. The health and functional abilities of the family affect the health of the client and other members of the family. Family-centered care recognizes and respects family strengths and individuality, encourages referrals for family support, and facilitates collaboration. It ensures flexible, accessible, and responsive health care delivery while incorporating developmental needs and implementing policies to provide emotional and financial support to women and their families.
- Health care delivery has moved from acute care settings out into the community, with an emphasis on health promotion and illness prevention. Community health nursing focuses on preventing health problems and improving the health of populations and communities, addressing current and potential health needs of the population or community, and promoting and preserving the health of a population regardless of age or diagnosis. Community health nurses perform epidemiologic investigations to help analyze and develop health policy and community health initiatives.
- Community-based nurses focus on providing personal care to individuals and families in the community. They focus on promoting and preserving health as well as preventing disease or injury. They help women and their families cope with illness and disease. Community-based nurses are direct care providers as well as advocators and educators. They focus on minimizing barriers to allow the patient to develop to his or her full potential.
- Community-based nursing uses the nursing process in caring for clients in community settings and involves primary, secondary, and tertiary prevention levels. Nursing interventions in community-based settings include health screening, education, medication administration, telephone consultation, health system referral, instruction, nutritional counseling, and risk identification.
- Nurses working in the community need to develop cultural competence. Steps to gaining cultural competence include cultural self-awareness, cultural knowledge, cultural skills, and cultural encounters.
- Settings for community-based nursing including physicians' offices, clinics, health departments, urgent care centers, clients' homes, churches, and shelters (e.g., domestic violence shelters, homeless shelters, and disaster shelters). Nurses provide wellness care, episodic ill care, and chronic care to women and their families.
- There has been an increase in home health care due to shorter hospital stays and cost containment along with an increase in income and longevity of individuals with

chronic and debilitating health conditions. Technology also has improved, which allows clients to be monitored and to undergo complicated procedures at home.

■ Roles and functions of the community-based nurse include communicator, direct care provider, educator, discharge planner and case manager, and advocate and resource manager.

■ Open, honest communication is essential for community-based nurses. The use of an interpreter may be necessary to ensure effective communication. Maintaining confidentiality and providing privacy are key.

■ A family's knowledge related to the client's health or illness is vital. Nurses working in the community play a major role in educating women and their families.

■ Discharge planning provides a comprehensive plan for the safe discharge of a client from a health care facility and for continuing safe and effective care in the community. Case management focuses on coordinating health care services while balancing quality and cost. Both contribute to improved transition from the hospital to the community for women, their families, and the health care team.

■ Community-based nurses act as advocates and resource managers to help ensure that the client and family have the necessary resources and appropriate health care services available to them.

REFERENCES

Adams, W. G., Mann, A. M., & Bauchner, H. (2003). Use of an electronic medical record improves the quality of urban pediatric primary care. *Pediatrics, 111*(3), 626–632.

Alexander, L. L., LaRosa, J. H., Bader, H., & Garfield, S. (2007). *New dimensions in women's health* (4th ed.). Sudbury, MA: Jones and Bartlett Publishers.

American College of Obstetricians and Gynecologists (ACOG). (2007). *National Folic Acid Awareness Week.* Available at: www.acog.org.

American Pregnancy Association (APA). (2007). Birthing choices: Care providers and labor locations. Available at: http://www.americanpregnancy.org/labornbirth/birthingchoices.html.

Anderson, E. T., & McFarlane, J. (2007). *Community as partner: Theory and practice in nursing* (5th ed.). Philadelphia: Lippincott Williams & Wilkins.

Bainbridge, J. (2006). Birth centers: What price maternal choice and professional autonomy. *British Journal of Midwifery, 14*(1), 40–41.

Britt, D. W., Edean, R. D., & Evans, M. I. (2006) Matching risk and resources in high-risk pregnancies. *Journal of Maternal-Fetal Medicine, 19*(10), 645–650.

Brunner, B. (2008). Listening, communication and trust: Practitioners' perspectives of business/organizational relationships. *International Journal of Listening, 22*(1), 73–82.

Canadian Community Health Nursing Standards of Practice. (2003). *Community Health Nursing Association of Canada* [Electronic Version].

Centers for Disease Control and Prevention (CDC). (2007a). *Longer hospital stays for childbirth.* National Center for Health Statistics. Available at: www.cdc.gov/nchs/products/pubs/pubd/hestats/hospbirth.htm.

CDC. (2007b). *New study profiles women's use of health care.* Available at: www.cdc.gov/od/oc/media/pressrel/r010725.htm.

Chia-Chen, A., & Thompson, E. A. (2007). Family-centered care. *Journal for Specialists in Pediatric Nursing, 12*(2), 119–122.

Chong-Hee Lieu, C., Sadler, G., Fullerton, J., & Stohlmann, P. (2007) Communication strategies for nurses interacting with patients who are deaf. *Dermatology Nursing, 19*(6), 541–551.

Clark, C. C., & Collins, S. (2007). *A complementary and integrative practices potpourri.* Available at: http://nsweb.nursingspectrum.com/ce/ce199d.htm.

Clark, M. J. (2008). *Community health nursing: Advocacy for population health* (5th ed.). Upper Saddle River, NJ: Pearson Prentice Hall.

Clarke, P., Bowcock, M., & Gales, P. (2007). Development of an integrated care pathway for natural birth. *British Journal of Midwifery, 15*(1), 12–15.

Dale, E. (1969). *Audio-visual methods in teaching* (3rd ed.). Austin, TX: Holt, Rinehart, and Winston.

Daniel, L. (2006). Using complementary therapies in pregnancy: The debate continues. *British Journal of Midwifery, 14*(2), 95–96.

Davey, M., & Forrester-King, J. (2008). Perinatal outcomes in birth centers. *Birth: Issues in Perinatal Care, 35*(1), 85–86.

Deering, C. G., & Cody, D. J. (2002). Communicating with children and adolescents. *American Journal of Nursing, 102*(3), 34–41.

Dochterman, J. M., & Bulechek, G. M. (2004). *Nursing interventions classification* (NIC) (4th ed.). St. Louis: Mosby.

Downe, S. (2006). Normal birth focus: Engaging with the concept of unique normality in childbirth. *British Journal of Midwifery, 14*(6), 352–354.

Flores, J., & Dodier, A. (2005). HIPAA: Past, present and future implications for nurses. *Online Journal of Issues in Nursing, 10*(2), 1–12. Available at: www.nursingworld.org/ojin/topic27/tpc27_4.htm.

Fowler, S., & Newton, L. (2006). Complementary and alternative therapies: The nurse's role. *Journal of Neuroscience Nursing, 38*(4), 261–264.

Godfrey, J. R. (2006). Toward optimal health: The need for cultural competence in the healthcare of women. *Journal of Women's Health, 15*(5), 480–484.

Goulet, L., D'Amour, D., & Pineault, R. (2007). Type and timing of services following postnatal discharge: Do they make a difference? *Women & Health, 45*(4), 19–39.

Grindel, C. (2006). Fostering a nurse, client, and family partnership in care. *MedSurg Nursing, 15*(2), 58–59.

Hodnett, D. D., Downe, S., Edwards, N., & Walsh, D. (2005). Home-like versus conventional institutional settings for birth. *Cochrane Database of Systematic Reviews.* Issue 1. Art. No.: CD000012. DOI:10.1002/14651858.CD000012.pub2.

Joint Commission on Accreditation of Healthcare Organizations. (1998–2004). *Comprehensive accreditation manual for hospitals.* Oakbrook Terrace, IL: JCAHO.

Joint Commission on Accreditation of Healthcare Organizations (JCAHO). (2008). *Joint Commission standards.* Available at: http://www.jointcommission.org/Standards/

Kersey-Matusiak, G. (2006). An action plan for cultural competence. *Nursing Spectrum.* Available at: http://nsweb.nursingspectrum.com/ce/ce255.htm.

Kessenich, C. R. (2007). Alternative therapies in osteoporosis. *Nursing Spectrum.* Available at: http://nsweb.nursingspectrum.com/ce/ce282-60C.htm.

Laveist, T. (2005). *Minority populations and health: An introduction to health disparities in the U.S.* Indianapolis: Wiley & Sons.

London, F. (2004). How to prepare families for discharge in the limited time available. *Pediatric Nursing, 30*(3), 212–214, 227.

Lyndon, A. (2008). Social and environmental conditions creating fluctuating agency for safety in two urban academic birth centers. *JOGNN, 37*(1), 13–23.

Mandleco, B. (2005). *Pediatric nursing skills and procedures.* Clifton Park, NY: Thomson Delmar.

March of Dimes. (2007). *Why prenatal care?* March of Dimes Birth Defect Prevention Foundation. Available at: www.modimes.org.

March of Dimes. (2008) *Prenatal care: What you need to know.* Available at: http://www.marchofdimes.com/pnhec/159_513.asp.

Martin, S. R., & Foley, M. R. (2006), Intensive care in obstetrics: An evidence-based review. *American Journal of Obstetrics & Gynecology, 195*(3), 673–689.

Mullen, K., Conrad, L., Hoadley, G., & Iannone, D. (2007). Family-centered maternity care: One hospital's quest for excellence. *Nursing for Women's Health, 11*(3), 282–290.

National Center for Complementary and Alternative Medicine (NCCAM). (2007). *What is complementary and alternative medicine (CAM)?* Available at: http://nccam.nih.gov/health/whatiscam/.

Northrup, C. (2006). *Women's bodies, women's wisdom: Creating physical and emotional health and healing.* New York: Bantam Books.

Papadopoulos, I. (2006). *Transcultural health and social care: Development of culturally competent practitioners.* St. Louis: Elsevier Health Sciences.

Pearson, N., & Chesney, M. (2007). The CAM Education Program of the National Center for Complimentary and Alternative Medicine: An overview. *Academic Medicine: Journal of the Association of the American Medical Colleges, 82*(10), 921–926.

Ramsey, L. (2007). Birthing options: Birthing center, home, and hospitals. *PageWise.* Available at: http://ncnc.essortment.com/birthingoptions_rikm.htm.

Rice, R. (2005). *Home care nursing practice: Concepts and applications* (4th ed.). St. Louis: Elsevier Health Sciences.

Roukema, J., Los, R. K., Bleeker, S. E., van Ginneken, A. M., van der Lei, J., & Moll, H. A. (2006). Paper versus computer: Feasibility of an electronic medical record in general pediatrics. *Pediatrics, 117*(1), 15–21.

Schillinger, D. (2002). Association of health literacy with diabetes outcomes. *Journal of the American Medical Association, 288*(4), 475–482.

Sheehan, J. P. (2000). Caring for the deaf: Do you do enough? *RN, 63*(3), 69–72.

Sobo, E. J. (2004). Pediatric nurses may misjudge parent communication preferences. *Journal of Nursing Care Quality, 19*(3), 253–262.

Stanhope, M., & Lancaster, J. (2008). *Public health nursing: Population-centered health care in the community* (7th ed.). St. Louis: Mosby Elsevier.

Streltzer, J. M., & Tseng, W. S. (2008). *Cultural competence in health care: A guide for professionals.* New York: Springer-Verlag.

Tryens, E., Coulston, L., & Tlush, E. (2007). *Understanding the complexities of herbal medicine.* Available at: http://nsweb.nursingspectrum.com/ce/ce290b.htm.

U.S. Census Bureau. (2007). *The 2007 statistical abstract: The national data book.* Available at: http://www.census.gov/compendia/statab/brief.html

U.S. Department of Health and Human Services. (2000). *Healthy People 2010.* Available at: www.healthypeople.gov.

U.S. Department of Health and Human Services, Health Resources and Services Administration, Bureau of Health Professions. (2004). *National sample survey of RNs, final report.* Available at: ftp://ftp.hrsa.gov/bhpr/rnsurvey2000/rnsurvey00-1.pdf.

U.S. Department of Homeland Security (USDHS). (2006). *Yearbook of immigration statistics: 2005.* Washington, DC: U.S. Department of Homeland Security, Office of Immigration Statistics.

Weech, W. A. (1999). *Tips for using interpreters.* Foreign Service Institute of the U.S. Department of State [Online]. Available at: http://mailman1.u.washington.edu/pipermail/phsw/1999-August/000119.html.

Weiss, B. D. (2003). *Health literacy: A manual for clinicians.* Chicago: American Medical Association Foundation.

Zahner, S. J., & Block, D. E. (2006). The road to population health: Using Healthy People 2010 in nursing education. *Journal of Nursing Education, 45*(3), 105–108.

WEBSITES

Acupuncture: www.acupuncture.com
Alliance for Hispanic Health: www.hispanichealth.org
American Botanical Council: www.herbalgram.org
American Holistic Nurses Association: www.ahna.org
American Translators Association (ATA): www.atanet.org
Association for Women's Health, Obstetrics, and Neonatal Nursing: www.awhonn.org
Center for Applied Linguistics: www.cal.org
Centers for Disease Control and Prevention: www.cdc.gov
Child Health Information Center: www.childhealthinfo.com/
Holistic Health Center: www.forholistichealth.com
Institute for Family-Centered Care: www.familycenteredcare.org/
Language Line: www.languageline.com/
National Center for Homeopathy: www.homeopathic.org
NIH Complementary and Alternative Medicine: www.altmed.od.nih.gov/oam
Northwest Translators and Interpreters Society: www.notis.net
Office of Minority Health, U.S. Department of Health and Human Services: www.omhrc.gov
Transcultural Nursing Society: www.tcns.org

CHAPTER WORKSHEET

MULTIPLE CHOICE QUESTIONS

1. A community-based nurse is involved in secondary prevention activities. Which activities might be included? Select all that apply.

   a. Fecal occult blood testing

   b. Hearing screening

   c. Smoking cessation program

   d. Cholesterol testing

   e. Hygiene program

   f. Pregnancy testing

2. A woman is to undergo a colonoscopy at a freestanding outpatient surgery center. Which would the nurse identify as a major disadvantage associated with this community-based setting?

   a. Increased risk for infection

   b. Increased health care costs

   c. Need to be transferred if overnight stay is required

   d. Increased disruption of family functioning

3. When developing a teaching plan for a pregnant client with preterm labor who is to be discharged, what would the nurse do first?

   a. Decide which procedures and medications the client will be discharged on.

   b. Determine the client's learning needs and styles.

   c. Ask the client if she has ever had preterm labor before.

   d. Tell the client what the goals of the teaching session are.

4. Which action by a nurse would best demonstrate cultural competence?

   a. Being well versed in the customs and beliefs of his or her own culture

   b. Demonstrating an openness to the values and beliefs of other cultures

   c. Applying knowledge about various cultures in the practice setting

   d. Playing a role in establishing policies to address diverse cultures

5. Which factor would the nurse identify as being least likely to contribute to the rise in community-based care?

   a. Focus on illness-oriented curative care

   b. Rise in consumer disposable income

   c. Technological advances allowing complicated procedures to be performed at home

   d. Emphasis on primary care and treatment

CRITICAL THINKING EXERCISES

1. A 63-year-old woman from Saudi Arabia has become seriously ill while on a visit to the United States. It is projected that she will require a lengthy hospitalization. Describe the steps the nurse should take to communicate with and provide extensive health care teaching to this woman and her family.

2. A pregnant woman is discharged home from the hospital after admission due to preterm labor. The woman is to be on complete bed rest and will receive home health care through a local agency to assist her and her family and to monitor her health status. As the home health nurse assigned to this woman, what should your nursing assessment include?

STUDY ACTIVITIES

1. Shadow a nurse working in a community setting, such as a women's health clinic, birthing center, home care, or health department. Identify the role the nurse plays in the health of women and families in the setting and the community.

2. Arrange for a visit to a community health center that offers services to various cultural groups. Interview the staff about the strategies used to overcome communication barriers and different health care practices for the women and their families in these groups.

3. Select one of the websites listed above and explore the information provided. How could a community-based nurse use this information?

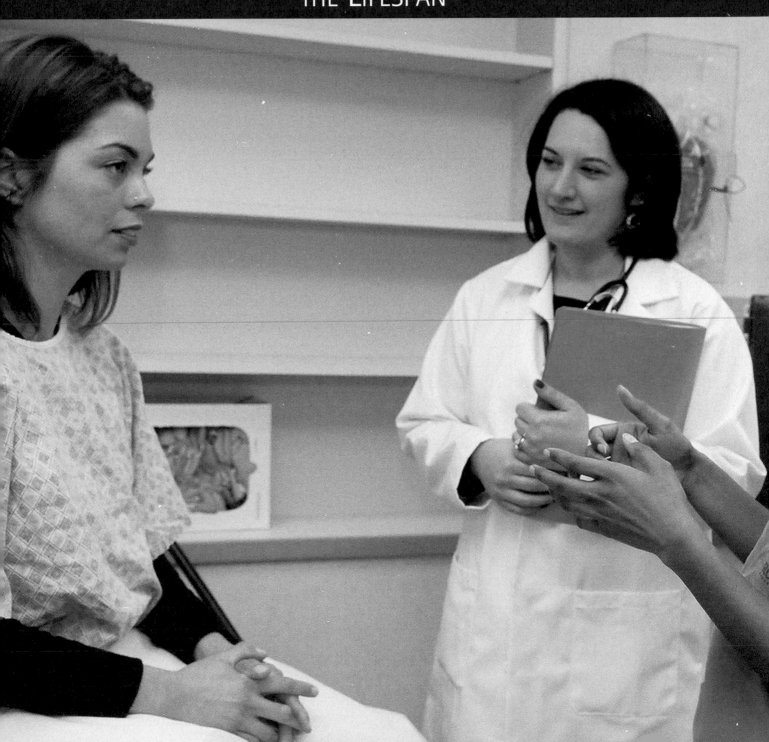

UNIT TWO

WOMEN'S HEALTH THROUGHOUT THE LIFESPAN

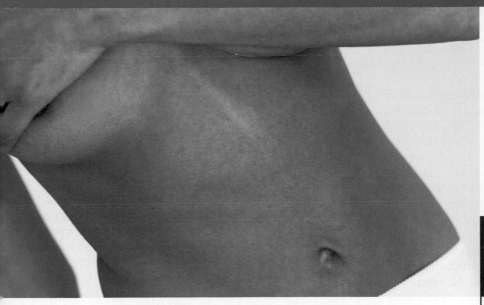

CHAPTER 3

ANATOMY AND PHYSIOLOGY OF THE REPRODUCTIVE SYSTEM

KEY TERMS

breasts	luteinizing hormone (LH)	testes
cervix	menarche	uterus
endometrium	menstruation	vagina
estrogen	ovaries	vulva
fallopian tubes	ovulation	
follicle-stimulating	penis	
hormone (FSH)	progesterone	

LEARNING OBJECTIVES

Upon completion of the chapter, the learner will be able to:

1. Define the key terms used in this chapter.
2. Explain the structure and function of the major external and internal female genital organs.
3. Outline the phases of the menstrual cycle, the dominant hormones involved, and the changes taking place in each phase.
4. Classify external and internal male reproductive structures and the function of each in hormonal regulation.

Linda, 49, started menstruating when she was 12 years old. Her menstrual periods have always been regular, but now she is experiencing irregular, heavier, and longer ones. She wonders if there is something wrong, or if this is normal.

Wow

All nurses should take care of and respect the human body, for it is a wondrous, precision machine.

The reproductive system consists of organs that function in the production of offspring. The female reproductive system produces the female reproductive cells (the eggs, or ova) and contains an organ (uterus) in which development of the fetus takes place; the male reproductive system produces the male reproductive cells (the sperm) and contains an organ (penis) that deposits the sperm within the female. Nurses need to have a thorough understanding of the anatomy and physiology of the male and female reproductive systems to be able to assess the health of these systems, to promote reproductive system health, to care for conditions that might affect the reproductive organs, and to provide client teaching concerning the reproductive system. This chapter will review the female and male reproductive systems and the menstrual cycle as it relates to reproduction.

Female Reproductive Anatomy and Physiology

The female reproductive system is composed of both external and internal reproductive organs.

External Female Reproductive Organs

The external female reproductive organs collectively are called the **vulva** (which means "covering" in Latin). The vulva serves to protect the urethral and vaginal openings and is highly sensitive to touch to increase the female's pleasure during sexual arousal (Coad & Dunstall, 2005). The structures that make up the vulva include the mons pubis, the labia majora and minora, the clitoris, the structures within the vestibule, and the perineum (Fig. 3.1).

Mons Pubis

The mons pubis is the elevated, rounded fleshy prominence over the symphysis pubis. This fatty tissue and skin is covered with pubic hair after puberty. It protects the symphysis pubis during sexual intercourse.

Labia

The labia majora (large lips), which are relatively large and fleshy, are comparable to the scrotum in males. The labia majora contain sweat and sebaceous (oil-secreting) glands; after puberty, they are covered with hair. Their function is to protect the vaginal opening. The labia minora (small lips) are the delicate hairless inner folds of skin; they can be very small or up to 2 inches wide. They lie just inside the labia majora and surround the openings to the vagina and urethra. The labia minora grow down from the anterior inner part of the labia majora on each side. They are highly vascular and abundant in nerve supply. They lubricate the vulva, swell in response to stimulation, and are highly sensitive.

Clitoris and Prepuce

The clitoris is a small, cylindrical mass of erectile tissue and nerves. It is located at the anterior junction of the labia minora. There are folds above and below the clitoris. The joining of the folds above the clitoris forms the prepuce, a hood-like covering over the clitoris; the junction below the clitoris forms the frenulum.

> ▶ *Take NOTE!*
>
> *The hood-like covering over the clitoris is the site for female circumcision, which is still practiced in some countries by some cultures.*

A rich supply of blood vessels gives the clitoris a pink color. Like the penis, the clitoris is very sensitive to touch, stimulation, and temperature and can become erect. For its small size, it has a generous blood and nerve supply.

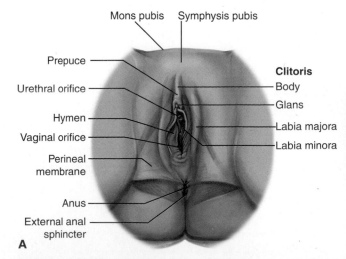

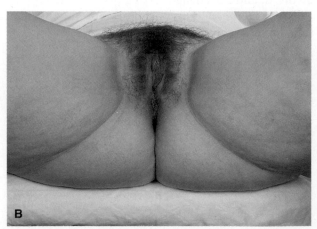

FIGURE 3.1 (**A**) The external female reproductive organs. (**B**) Normal appearance of external structures. (Photo by B. Proud.)

There are more free nerve endings of sensory reception located on the clitoris than on any other part of the body, and it is, unsurprisingly, the most erotically sensitive part of the genitalia for most females. Its function is sexual stimulation (Katz, 2007).

> ▶ **Take** NOTE!
>
> *The word "clitoris" is from the Greek word for key; in ancient times the clitoris was thought to be the key to a woman's sexuality.*

Vestibule

The vestibule is an oval area enclosed by the labia minora laterally. It is inside the labia minora and outside of the hymen and is perforated by six openings. Opening into the vestibule are the urethra from the urinary bladder, the vagina, and two sets of glands. The opening to the vagina is called the introitus, and the half-moon–shaped area behind the opening is called the fourchette. Through tiny ducts beside the introitus, Bartholin's glands, when stimulated, secrete mucus that supplies lubrication for intercourse. Skene's glands are located on either side of the opening to the urethra. They secrete a small amount of mucus to keep the opening moist and lubricated for the passage of urine (Schuiling & Likis, 2006).

The vaginal opening is surrounded by the hymen (maidenhead). The hymen is a tough, elastic, perforated, mucosa-covered tissue across the vaginal introitus. In a virgin, the hymen may completely cover the opening, but it usually encircles the opening like a tight ring. Because the degree of tightness varies among women, the hymen may tear at the first attempt at intercourse, or it may be so soft and pliable that no tearing occurs. In a woman who is not a virgin, the hymen usually appears as small tags of tissue surrounding the vaginal opening, but the presence or absence of the hymen can neither confirm nor rule out sexual experience (Mattson & Smith, 2004).

> ▶ **Take** NOTE!
>
> *Heavy physical exertion, use of tampons, or injury to the area can alter the appearance of the hymen in girls and women who have not been sexually active.*

Perineum

The perineum is the most posterior part of the external female reproductive organs. This external region is located between the vulva and the anus. It is made up of skin, muscle, and fascia. The perineum can become lacerated or incised during childbirth and may need to be repaired with sutures. Incising the perineum area to provide more space for the presenting part is called an episiotomy. Although still a common obstetric procedure, the use of episiotomy has decreased over the past 25 years. The procedure should be applied selectively rather than routinely. An episiotomy can add to postpartum discomfort and perineal trauma and can lead to fecal incontinence (Cunningham et al., 2005).

Internal Female Reproductive Organs

The internal female reproductive organs consist of the vagina, uterus, fallopian tubes, and ovaries. These structures develop and function according to the specific hormone influences that affect fertility and childbearing (Fig. 3.2).

Vagina

The **vagina** is a highly distensible musculomembranous canal situated in front of the rectum and behind the bladder. It is a tubular, fibromuscular organ lined with mucous membrane that lies in a series of transverse folds called rugae. The rugae allow for extreme dilatation of the canal during labor and birth. The vagina is a canal that connects the external genitals to the uterus. It receives the penis and the sperm ejaculated during sexual intercourse, and it serves as an exit passageway for menstrual blood and for the fetus during childbirth. The front and back walls normally touch each other so that there is no space in the vagina except when it is opened (e.g., during a pelvic examination or intercourse). In the adult, the vaginal cavity is 3 to 4 inches long. Muscles that control its diameter surround the lower third of the vagina. The upper two thirds of the vagina lies above these muscles and can be stretched easily. During a woman's reproductive years, the mucosal lining of the vagina has a corrugated appearance and is resistant to bacterial colonization. Before puberty and after menopause (if the woman is not taking estrogen), the mucosa is smooth due to lower levels of estrogen (Dorland, 2007).

The vagina has an acidic environment, which protects it against ascending infections. Antibiotic therapy, douching, perineal hygiene sprays, and deodorants upset the acid balance within the vaginal environment and can predispose women to infections.

Uterus

The **uterus** is a pear-shaped muscular organ at the top of the vagina. It lies behind the bladder and in front of the rectum and is anchored in position by eight ligaments, although it is not firmly attached or adherent to any part of the skeleton. A full bladder tilts the uterus backward; a distended rectum tilts it forward. The uterus alters its position by gravity or with change of posture, and is the size and shape of an inverted pear. It is the site of menstruation, implantation of a fertilized ovum, development of the fetus during pregnancy, and labor. Before the first pregnancy, it measures approximately 3 inches long, 2 inches wide, and 1 inch thick. After a pregnancy, the uterus remains larger than before the pregnancy. After menopause, it becomes smaller and atrophies.

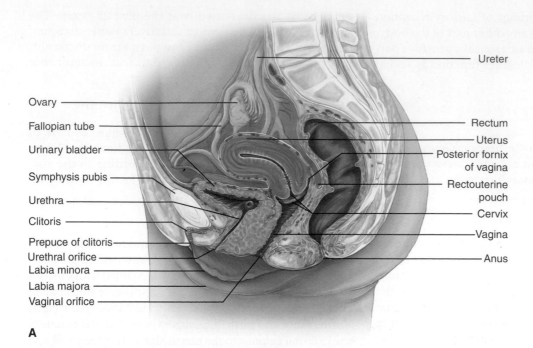

A

Ureter

Ovary

Fallopian tube

Urinary bladder

Symphysis pubis

Urethra

Clitoris

Prepuce of clitoris

Urethral orifice

Labia minora

Labia majora

Vaginal orifice

Rectum

Uterus

Posterior fornix of vagina

Rectouterine pouch

Cervix

Vagina

Anus

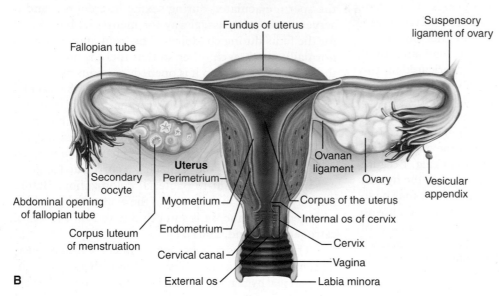

B

Fallopian tube

Fundus of uterus

Suspensory ligament of ovary

Secondary oocyte

Uterus Perimetrium

Abdominal opening of fallopian tube

Myometrium

Corpus luteum of menstruation

Endometrium

Cervical canal

External os

Ovanan ligament

Ovary

Vesicular appendix

Corpus of the uterus

Internal os of cervix

Cervix

Vagina

Labia minora

FIGURE 3.2 The internal female reproductive organs. (**A**) Lateral view. (**B**) Anterior view. (Source: Anatomical Chart Company [2001]. *Atlas of human anatomy.* Springhouse, PA: Springhouse.)

The uterine wall is relatively thick and composed of three layers: the endometrium (innermost layer), the myometrium (muscular middle layer), and the perimetrium (outer serosal layer that covers the body of the uterus). The **endometrium** is the mucosal layer that lines the uterine cavity in nonpregnant women. It varies in thickness from 0.5 mm to 5 mm and has an abundant supply of glands and blood vessels (Cunningham et al., 2005). The myometrium makes up the major portion of the uterus and is composed of smooth muscle linked by connective tissue with numerous elastic fibers. During pregnancy, the upper myometrium undergoes marked hypertrophy, but there is limited change in the cervical muscle content.

Anatomic subdivisions of the uterus include the convex portion above the uterine tubes (the fundus); the central portion (the corpus or body) between the fundus and the cervix; and the cervix, or neck, which opens into the vagina.

Cervix

The **cervix,** the lower part of the uterus, opens into the vagina and has a channel that allows sperm to enter the uterus and menstrual discharge to exit. It is composed of fibrous connective tissue. During a pelvic examination, the part of the cervix that protrudes into the upper end of the vagina can be visualized. Like the vagina, this part of the cervix is covered by mucosa, which is smooth, firm, and doughnut-shaped, with a visible central opening called the external os (Fig. 3.3). Before childbirth, the external cervical os is a small, regular, oval opening.

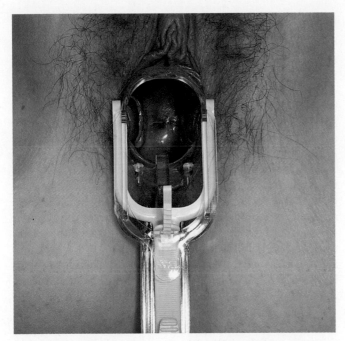

FIGURE **3.3** Appearance of normal cervix. Note: This is the cervix of a multipara female. (Photo by B. Proud.)

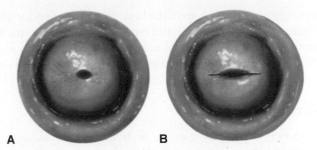

FIGURE **3.4** (**A**) Nulliparous cervical os. (**B**) Parous cervical os.

After childbirth, the opening is converted into a transverse slit that resembles lips (Fig. 3.4). Except during menstruation or ovulation, the cervix is usually a good barrier against bacteria. The cervix has an alkaline environment, which protects the sperm from the acidic environment in the vagina.

The canal or channel of the cervix is lined with mucus-secreting glands. This mucus is thick and impenetrable to sperm until just before the ovaries release an egg (**ovulation**). At ovulation, the consistency of the mucus changes so that sperm can swim through it, allowing fertilization. At the same time, the mucus-secreting glands of the cervix actually become able to store live sperm for 2 or 3 days. These sperm can later move up through the corpus and into the fallopian tubes to fertilize the egg; thus, intercourse 1 or 2 days before ovulation can lead to pregnancy. Because some women do not ovulate consistently, pregnancy can occur at varying times after the last menstrual period. The channel in the cervix is too narrow for the fetus to pass through during pregnancy, but during labor it stretches to let the newborn through.

Corpus

The corpus, or the main body of the uterus, is a highly muscular organ that enlarges to hold the fetus during pregnancy. The inner lining of the corpus (endometrium) undergoes cyclic changes as a result of the changing levels of hormones secreted by the ovaries: it is thickest during the part of the menstrual cycle in which a fertilized egg would be expected to enter the uterus and is thinnest just after menstruation. If fertilization does not take place

during this cycle, most of the endometrium is shed and bleeding occurs, resulting in the monthly period. If fertilization does take place, the embryo attaches to the wall of the uterus, where it becomes embedded in the endometrium (about 1 week after fertilization); this process is called implantation (Heffner & Schust, 2006). Menstruation then ceases during the 40 weeks (280 days) of pregnancy. During labor, the muscular walls of the corpus contract to push the baby through the cervix and into the vagina.

Fallopian Tubes

The **fallopian tubes** are hollow, cylindrical structures that extend 2 to 3 inches from the upper edges of the uterus toward the ovaries. Each tube is about 7 to 10 cm long (4 inches) and approximately 0.7 cm in diameter. The end of each tube flares into a funnel shape, providing a large opening for the egg to fall into when it is released from the ovary. Cilia (beating, hair-like extensions on cells) line the fallopian tube and the muscles in the tube's wall. The fallopian tubes convey the ovum from the ovary to the uterus and sperm from the uterus toward the ovary. This movement is accomplished via ciliary action and peristalsis. If sperm is present in the fallopian tube as a result of sexual intercourse or artificial insemination, fertilization of the ovum can occur in the distal portion of the tube. If the egg is fertilized, it will divide over a period of 4 days while it moves slowly down the fallopian tube and into the uterus.

Ovaries

The **ovaries** are a set of paired glands resembling unshelled almonds set in the pelvic cavity below and to either side of the umbilicus. They are usually pearl-colored and oblong. They are homologous to the testes. Each ovary weighs from 2 to 5 grams and is about 4 cm long, 2 cm wide, and 1 cm thick (Speroff & Fritz, 2005). The ovaries are not attached to the fallopian tubes but are suspended nearby from several ligaments, which help hold them in position. The development and the release of the ovum and the secretion of the hormones estrogen and progesterone are the two primary functions of the ovary. The ovaries link the reproductive system to the body's system of endocrine glands, as they produce the ova (eggs) and secrete, in cyclic fashion, the female sex hormones estrogen and progesterone. After an ovum matures, it passes into the fallopian tubes.

Breasts

The two mammary glands, or **breasts**, are accessory organs of the female reproductive system that are specialized to secrete milk following pregnancy. They overlie the pectoralis major muscles and extend from the second to the sixth ribs and from the sternum to the axilla. Each breast has a nipple located near the tip, which is surrounded by a circular area of pigmented skin called the areola. Each breast is composed of approximately 9 lobes (the number can range between 4 and 18), which contain glands (alveolar) and a duct (lactiferous) that leads to the nipple and opens to the outside (Fig. 3.5). The lobes are separated by dense connective and adipose tissues, which also help support the weight of the breasts (Ramsay, Kent, Hartmann & Hartmann, 2005).

During pregnancy, placental estrogen and progesterone stimulate the development of the mammary glands. Because of this hormonal activity, the breasts may double in size during pregnancy. At the same time, glandular tissue replaces the adipose tissue of the breasts.

Following childbirth and the expulsion of the placenta, levels of placental hormones (progesterone and lactogen) fall rapidly, and the action of prolactin (milk-producing hormone) is no longer inhibited. Prolactin stimulates the production of milk within a few days after childbirth, but in the interim, a dark yellow fluid called colostrum is secreted. Colostrum contains more minerals and protein, but less sugar and fat, than mature breast milk. Colostrum secretion may continue for approximately a week after childbirth, with gradual conversion to mature milk. Colostrum is rich in maternal antibodies, especially immunoglobulin A (IgA), which offers protection for the newborn against enteric pathogens.

Female Sexual Response

With sexual stimulation, tissues in the clitoris and breasts and around the vaginal orifice fill with blood and the erectile tissues swell. At the same time, the vagina begins to expand and elongate to accommodate the penis. As part of the whole vasocongestive reaction, the labia majora and minor swell and darken. As sexual stimulation intensifies, the vestibular glands secrete mucus to moisten and lubricate the tissues to facilitate insertion of the penis.

Hormones play an integral role in the female sexual response as well. Adequate estrogen and testosterone must be available for the brain to sense incoming arousal stimuli. Research indicates that estrogen preserves the vascular function of female sex organs and affects genital sensation. It also is believed to promote blood flow to these areas during stimulation. Testosterone is thought to be the hormone of sexual desire in women (McKinney, 2007).

The zenith of intense stimulation is orgasm, the spasmodic and involuntary contractions of the muscles in the region of the vulva, the uterus, and the vagina that produce a pleasurable sensation to the woman. Typically the woman feels warm and relaxed after an orgasm. Within a short time after orgasm, the two physiologic mechanisms that created the sexual response, vasocongestion and muscle contraction, rapidly dissipate.

The Female Reproductive Cycle

The female reproductive cycle is a complex process that encompasses an intricate series of chemical secretions and reactions to produce the ultimate potential for fertility and birth. The female reproductive cycle is a general term encompassing the ovarian cycle, the endometrial cycle, the hormonal changes that regulate them, and the cyclical changes in the breasts. The endometrium, ovaries, pituitary gland, and hypothalamus are all involved in the cyclic changes that help to prepare the body for fertilization. Absence of fertilization results in menstruation, the monthly shedding of the uterine lining. Menstruation

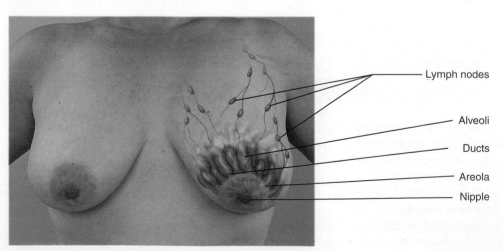

Lymph nodes

Alveoli

Ducts

Areola

Nipple

FIGURE 3.5 Anatomy of the breasts. (Photo by B. Proud.)

marks the beginning and end of each menstrual cycle. Menopause is the naturally occurring cessation of regular menstrual cycles.

Menstruation

Menstruation is the normal, predictable physiologic process whereby the inner lining of the uterus (endometrium) is expelled by the body. Typically, this occurs monthly. Menstruation has many effects on girls and women, including emotional and self-image issues. In the United States, the average age at **menarche** (the start of menstruation in females) is 12.8 years, with a range between 8 and 18. Genetics is the most important factor in determining the age at which menarche starts, but geographic location, nutrition, weight, general health, nutrition, and psychological factors are also important (Shelby & Ruocco, 2007). Pubertal events preceding the first menses have an orderly progression: thelarche, the development of breast buds; adrenarche, the appearance of pubic and then axillary hair, followed by a growth spurt; and menarche (occurring about 2 years after the start of breast development). In healthy pubertal girls, the menstrual period varies in flow heaviness and may remain irregular in occurrence for up to 2 years following menarche. After that time, the regular menstrual cycle should be established. Most women will experience 300 to 400 menstrual cycles within their lifetime (Diaz, Laufer & Breech, 2006). Normal, regular menstrual cycles vary in frequency from 21 to 36 days (with the average cycle lasting 28 days), bleeding lasts 3 to 7 days, and blood loss averages 20 to 80 mL (Schuiling & Likis, 2006). Irregular menses can be associated with irregular ovulation, stress, disease, and hormonal imbalances (Cunningham et al., 2005).

T hink back to Linda, who was introduced at the beginning of the chapter. What questions might need to be asked to assess her condition? What laboratory work might be anticipated to validate her heavier flow?

Although menstruation is a normal process, various world cultures have taken a wide variety of attitudes toward it, seeing it as everything from a sacred time to an unclean time. In a society where menstruation is viewed negatively, nurses can help women develop a more positive image of this natural physiologic process.

▶ *Take* NOTE!

Knowledge about menstruation has increased significantly and attitudes have changed since early times, when many cultures saw it as "unclean." What was once discussed only behind closed doors is discussed openly today.

Reproductive Cycle

The reproductive cycle, also referred to as the menstrual cycle, results from a functional hypothalamic–pituitary–ovarian axis and a precise sequencing of hormones that lead to ovulation. If conception doesn't occur, menses ensues. The ranges of normal menstrual cycles are as follows:

- Cycle length: 21 to 36 days
- Duration of flow: 3 to 7 days
- Amount of flow: 20 to 80 mL

The female reproductive cycle involves two cycles that occur simultaneously: the ovarian cycle, during which ovulation occurs, and the endometrial cycle, during which menstruation occurs. Ovulation divides these two cycles at midcycle. Ovulation occurs when the ovum is released from its follicle; after leaving the ovary, the ovum enters the fallopian tube and journeys toward the uterus. If sperm fertilizes the ovum during its journey, pregnancy occurs. Figure 3.6 summarizes the menstrual cycle.

Ovarian Cycle

The ovarian cycle is the series of events associated with a developing oocyte (ovum or egg) within the ovaries. While men manufacture sperm daily, often into advanced age, women are born with a single lifetime supply of ova that are released from the ovaries gradually throughout the childbearing years. In the female ovary, 2 million oocytes are present at birth, and about 400,000 follicles are still present at puberty. The excess follicles are depleted during the childbearing years, with only 400 follicles ovulated during the reproductive period (Speroff & Fritz, 2005). The ovarian cycle begins when the follicular cells (ovum and surrounding cells) swell and the maturation process starts. The maturing follicle at this stage is called a graafian follicle. The ovary raises many follicles monthly, but usually only one follicle matures to reach ovulation. The ovarian cycle consists of three phases: the follicular phase, ovulation, and the luteal phase.

Follicular Phase

This phase is so named because it is when the follicles in the ovary grow and form a mature egg. This phase starts on day 1 of the menstrual cycle and continues until ovulation, approximately 10 to 14 days later. The follicular phase is not consistent in duration because of the time variations in follicular development. These variations account for the differences in menstrual cycle lengths (Hackley, Kriebs & Rousseau, 2007). The hypothalamus is the initiator of this phase. Increasing levels of estrogen secreted from the maturing follicular cells and the continued growth of the dominant follicle cell induce proliferation of the endometrium and myometrium. This thickening of the uterine lining supports an implanted ovum if pregnancy occurs.

Prompted by the hypothalamus, the pituitary gland releases follicle-stimulating hormone (FSH), which stimulates the ovary to produce 5 to 20 immature follicles. Each follicle houses an immature oocyte or egg. The follicle that

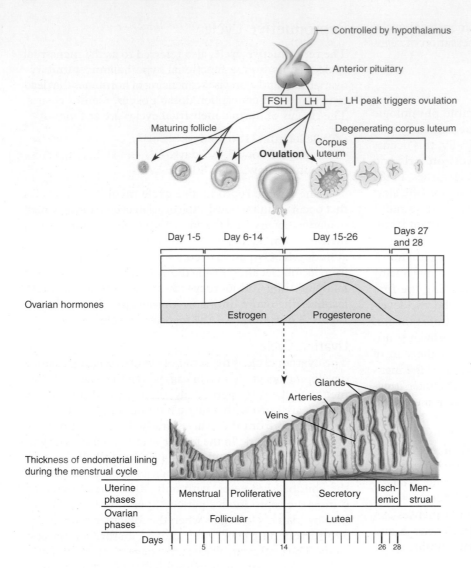

Controlled by hypothalamus

Anterior pituitary

FSH   LH — LH peak triggers ovulation

Maturing follicle

Degenerating corpus luteum

Corpus
luteum

Ovulation

Day 1-5   Day 6-14   Day 15-26   Days 27
and 28

Ovarian hormones

Estrogen   Progesterone

Glands

Arteries

Veins

Thickness of endometrial lining
during the menstrual cycle

Uterine phases	Menstrual	Proliferative	Secretory	Isch-emic	Men-strual
Ovarian phases	Follicular		Luteal		
Days	1 5	14		26 28	

FIGURE **3.6** Menstrual cycle summary based
on a 28-day (average) menstrual cycle.

is targeted to mature fully will soon rupture and expel a mature oocyte in the process of ovulation. A surge in luteinizing hormone (LH) from the anterior pituitary gland is actually responsible for affecting the final development and subsequent rupture of the mature follicle.

Ovulation

At ovulation, a mature follicle ruptures in response to a surge of LH, releasing a mature oocyte (ovum). This usually occurs on day 14 in a 28-day cycle. When ovulation occurs, there is a drop in estrogen. Typically ovulation takes place approximately 10 to 12 hours after the LH peak and 24 to 36 hours after estrogen levels peak (Speroff & Fritz, 2005). The distal ends of the fallopian tubes become active near the time of ovulation and create currents that help carry the ovum into the uterus. The lifespan of the ovum is only about 24 hours; unless it meets a sperm on its journey within that time, it will die.

During ovulation, the cervix produces thin, clear, stretchy, slippery mucus that is designed to help the sperm travel up through the cervix to meet the ovum for fertil-

ization. The one constant, whether a women's cycle is 28 days or 120 days, is that ovulation takes place 14 days before menstruation (Shelby & Ruocco, 2007).

▶ **Take** NOTE!

Some women can feel a pain on one side of the abdomen around the time the egg is released. This midcycle pain is called mittelschmerz.

Luteal Phase

The luteal phase begins at ovulation and lasts until the menstrual phase of the next cycle. It typically occurs day 15 through day 28 of a 28-day cycle. After the follicle ruptures as it releases the egg, it closes and forms a corpus luteum. The corpus luteum secretes increasing amounts of the hormone progesterone, which interacts with the endometrium to prepare it for implantation. At the beginning of the luteal phase, progesterone induces the endometrial glands to secrete glycogen, mucus, and other substances. These glands become tortuous and have large lumens due to increased secretory activity. The progesterone secreted by the corpus luteum causes the temperature of the body to rise slightly until the start of the next period. A significant increase in temperature, usually 0.5 to 1 degrees Fahrenheit, is generally seen within a day or two after ovulation has occurred; the temperature remains elevated for 12 to 16 days, until menstruation begins (Chandran, 2007). This rise in temperature can be plotted on a graph and gives an indication of when ovulation has occurred. In the absence of fertilization, the corpus luteum begins to degenerate and consequently ovarian hormone levels decrease. As estrogen and progesterone levels decrease, the endometrium undergoes involution. In a 28-day cycle, menstruation then begins approximately 14 days after ovulation in the absence of pregnancy. FSH and LH are generally at their lowest levels during the luteal phase and highest during the follicular phase.

► *Consider* THIS!

We had been married 2 years when my husband and I decided to start a family. I began thinking back to my high-school biology class and tried to remember about ovulation and what to look for. I also used the Internet to find the answers I was seeking. As I was reading, it all started to come into place. During ovulation, a woman's cervical mucus increases and she experiences a wet sensation for several days midcycle. The mucus also becomes stretchable during this time. In addition, body temperature rises slightly and then falls if no conception takes place. Armed with this knowledge, I began to check my temperature daily before arising and began to monitor the consistency of my cervical mucus. I figured that monitoring these two signs of ovulation could help me discover the best time to conceive. After 6 months of trying without results, I wondered what I was doing wrong. Did I really understand my body's reproductive activity?

What additional suggestions might the nurse offer this woman in her journey to conception? What community resources might be available to assist this couple? How does knowledge of the reproductive system help nurses take care of couples who are trying to become pregnant?

Endometrial Cycle

The endometrial cycle occurs in response to cyclic hormonal changes. The four phases of the endometrial cycle are the proliferative phase, secretory phase, ischemic phase, and menstrual phase.

Proliferative Phase

The proliferative phase starts with enlargement of the endometrial glands in response to increasing amounts of estrogen. The blood vessels become dilated and the endometrium increases in thickness dramatically from 0.5 to 5 mm in height and increases eight-fold in thickness in preparation for implantation of the fertilized ovum (Heffner & Schust, 2006). Cervical mucus becomes thin, clear, stretchy, and more alkaline, making it more favorable to sperm to enhance the opportunity for fertilization. The proliferative phase starts on about day 5 of the menstrual cycle and lasts to the time of ovulation. This phase depends on estrogen stimulation resulting from ovarian follicles, and this phase coincides with the follicular phase of the ovarian cycle.

Secretory Phase

The secretory phase begins at ovulation to about 3 days before the next menstrual period. Under the influence of progesterone released by the corpus luteum after ovulation, the endometrium becomes thickened and more vascular (growth of the spiral arteries) and glandular (secreting more glycogen and lipids). These dramatic changes are all in preparation for implantation, if it were to occur. This phase typically lasts from day 15 (after ovulation) to day 28 and coincides with the luteal phase of the ovarian cycle. The secretory phase doesn't take place if ovulation has not occurred.

Ischemic Phase

If fertilization does not occur, the ischemic phase begins. Estrogen and progesterone levels drop sharply during this phase as the corpus luteum starts to degenerate. Changes in the endometrium occur with spasm of the arterioles, resulting in ischemia of the basal layer. The ischemia leads to shedding of the endometrium down to the basal layer, and menstrual flow begins.

Menstrual Phase

The menstrual phase begins as the spiral arteries rupture secondary to ischemia, releasing blood into the uterus, and the sloughing of the endometrial lining begins. If fertilization does not take place, the corpus luteum degenerates. As a result, both estrogen and progesterone levels fall and the thickened endometrial lining sloughs away from the uterine wall and passes out via the vagina. The beginning of the menstrual flow marks the end of one menstrual cycle and the start of a new one. Most women report bleeding for an average of 3 to 7 days. The amount of menstrual flow varies, but approximately 6 to 8 ounces in volume per cycle is average (Alexander et al., 2007).

Menstrual Cycle Hormones

The menstrual cycle involves a complex interaction of hormones. The predominant hormones include gonadotropin-releasing hormone, FSH, LH, estrogen, progesterone, and prostaglandins. Box 3.1 summarizes menstrual cycle hormones.

Summary of Menstrual Cycle Hormones

- Luteinizing hormone (LH) rises and stimulates the follicle to produce estrogen.
- As estrogen is produced by the follicle, estrogen levels rise, inhibiting the output of LH.
- Ovulation occurs after an LH surge damages the estrogen-producing cells, resulting in a decline in estrogen.
- The LH surge results in establishment of the corpus luteum, which produces estrogen and progesterone.
- Estrogen and progesterone levels rise, suppressing LH output.
- Lack of LH promotes degeneration of the corpus luteum.
- Cessation of the corpus luteum means a decline in estrogen and progesterone output.
- The decline of the ovarian hormones ends their negative effect on the secretion of LH.
- LH is secreted, and the menstrual cycle begins again.

Gonadotropin-Releasing Hormone

Gonadotropin-releasing hormone (GnRH) is secreted from the hypothalamus in a pulsatile manner throughout the reproductive cycle. It pulsates slowly during the follicular phase and increases during the luteal phase. GnRH induces the release of FSH and LH to assist with ovulation.

Follicle-Stimulating Hormone

Follicle-stimulating hormone (FSH) is secreted by the anterior pituitary gland and is primarily responsible for the maturation of the ovarian follicle. FSH secretion is highest and most important during the first week of the follicular phase of the reproductive cycle.

Luteinizing Hormone

Luteinizing hormone (LH) is secreted by the anterior pituitary gland and is required for both the final maturation of preovulatory follicles and luteinization of the ruptured follicle. As a result, estrogen production declines and progesterone secretion continues. Thus, estrogen levels fall a day before ovulation, and progesterone levels begin to rise.

Estrogen

Estrogen is secreted by the ovaries and is crucial for the development and maturation of the follicle. Estrogen is predominant at the end of the proliferative phase, directly preceding ovulation. After ovulation, estrogen levels drop sharply as progesterone dominates. In the endometrial cycle, estrogen induces proliferation of the endometrial glands. Estrogen also causes the uterus to increase in size and weight because of increased glycogen, amino acids, electrolytes, and water. Blood supply is expanded as well.

Progesterone

Progesterone is secreted by the corpus luteum. Progesterone levels increase just before ovulation and peak 5 to 7 days after ovulation. During the luteal phase, progesterone induces swelling and increased secretion of the endometrium. This hormone is often called the hormone of pregnancy because of its calming effect (reduces uterine contractions) on the uterus, allowing pregnancy to be maintained.

Prostaglandins

Prostaglandins are a closely related group of oxygenated fatty acids that are produced by the endometrium, with a variety of effects throughout the body. Although they have regulatory effects and are sometimes called hormones, prostaglandins are not technically hormones because they are produced by all tissues rather than by special glands (Speroff & Fritz, 2005). Prostaglandins increase during follicular maturation and play a key role in ovulation by freeing the ovum inside the graafian follicle. Large amounts of prostaglandins are found in menstrual blood. Research is ongoing as to the various roles prostaglandins have on the menstrual cycle (Cunningham et al., 2005).

Menopause

Perimenopause and menopause are biologic markers of the transition from young adulthood to middle age. Neither of these is a symptom or disease, but rather a natural maturing of the reproductive system.

During the perimenopausal years (2 to 8 years prior to menopause) women may experience physical changes associated with decreasing estrogen levels, which may include vasomotor symptoms of hot flashes, irregular menstrual cycles, sleep disruptions, forgetfulness, irritability, mood disturbances, decreased vaginal lubrication, fatigue, vaginal atrophy, and depression (Shifren & Schiff, 2007).

Menopause refers to the cessation of regular menstrual cycles. This naturally occurring phase of every woman's life marks the end of menstruation and childbearing capacity. The average age of natural menopause—defined as 1 year without a menstrual period—is 51 (Alexander et al., 2007). As the average life expectancy for women increases, the number of women reaching and living in menopause has escalated. Most women can expect to spend more than one third of their lives beyond menopause. It is usually marked by atrophy of the breasts, uterus, fallopian tubes, and ovaries (Curran & Bachmann, 2006).

Many women pass through menopause without untoward symptoms. These women remain active and in good health with little interruption of their daily routines. Other women experience vasomotor symptoms, which give rise to sensations of heat, cold, sweating, headache, insomnia, and irritability (Kessenich, 2007). Until recently, hormone therapy was the mainstay of menopause pharmacotherapy, but with the recent results of the Women's Health Initiative trial, the use of hormone therapy has become controversial. Many women have turned to nontraditional remedies to manage their menopausal symptoms. Common herbal remedies used include Dong Quai, black cohosh, melatonin, ginseng, and St. John's wort. Research to validate their efficacy, safety, and potential harmful effects is lacking at this time, and much of the efficacy is largely anecdotal (Kessenich, 2007). Nurses can play a major role in assisting menopausal women by educating and counseling them about the multitude of options available for disease prevention, treatment for menopausal symptoms, and health promotion during this time of change in their lives. Menopause should be an opportunity for women to strive for a healthy, long life, and nurses can help to make this opportunity a reality. (See Chapter 4 for more information about menopause.)

Recall Linda, who was experiencing changes in her menstrual patterns. Which hormones might be changing, and which systems might they affect? What approach should the nurse take to enlighten Linda about what is happening to her?

Male Reproductive Anatomy and Physiology

The male reproductive system, like that of the female, consists of those organs that facilitate reproduction. The male organs are specialized to produce and maintain the male sex cells, or sperm; to transport them, along with supporting fluids, to the female reproductive system; and to secrete the male hormone testosterone. The organs of the male reproductive system include the two testes (where sperm cells and testosterone are made), the penis, the scrotum, and the accessory organs (epididymis, vas deferens, seminal vesicles, ejaculatory duct, urethra, bulbourethral glands, and prostate gland).

External Male Reproductive Organs

The penis and the scrotum form the external genitalia in the male (Fig. 3.7).

Penis

The **penis** is the organ for copulation and serves as the outlet for both sperm and urine. The skin of the penis is thin, with no hairs. The prepuce (foreskin) is a circular fold of skin that extends over the glans unless it is removed by circumcision shortly after birth. The urinary meatus, located at the tip of the penis, serves as the external opening to the urethra (Fig. 3.8). The penis is composed mostly of erectile tissue. Most of the body of the penis consists of three cylindrical spaces (sinuses) of erectile tissue. The two larger

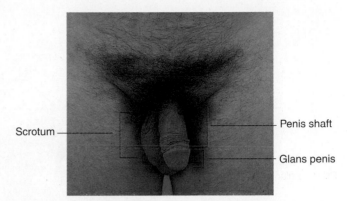

FIGURE 3.7 The external male reproductive organs. (Photo by B. Proud.)

ones, the corpora cavernosa, are side by side. The third sinus, the corpus spongiosum, surrounds the urethra. Erection results when nerve impulses from the autonomic nervous system dilate the arteries of the penis, allowing arterial blood to flow into the erectile tissues of the organ.

Scrotum

The scrotum is the thin-skinned sac that surrounds and protects the testes. The scrotum also acts as a climate-control system for the testes, because they need to be slightly cooler than body temperature to allow normal sperm development. The cremaster muscles in the scrotal wall relax or contract to allow the testes to hang farther from the body to cool or to be pulled closer to the body for warmth or protection (Ceo, 2006). A medial septum divides the scrotum into two chambers, each of which encloses a testis.

Internal Male Reproductive Organs

The internal structures include the testes, the ductal system, and accessory glands (Fig. 3.9).

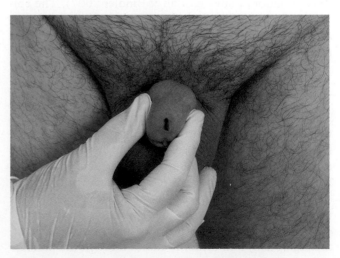

FIGURE 3.8 The urinary meatus. (Photo by B. Proud.)

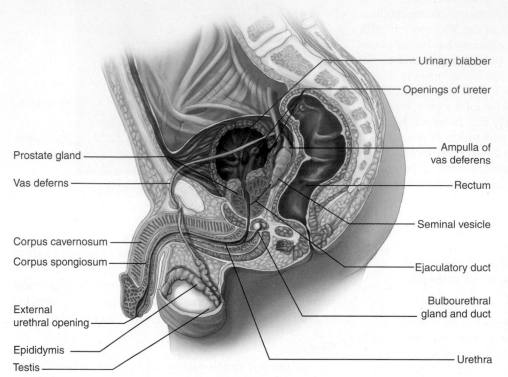

Urinary blabber

Openings of ureter

Ampulla of vas deferens

Rectum

Seminal vesicle

Ejaculatory duct

Bulbourethral gland and duct

Urethra

Prostate gland

Vas deferns

Corpus cavernosum

Corpus spongiosum

External urethral opening

Epididymis

Testis

FIGURE **3.9** Lateral view of the internal male reproductive organs. (Source: Anatomical Chart Company. [2001]. *Atlas of human anatomy*. Springhouse, PA: Springhouse.)

Testes

The **testes** are oval bodies the size of large olives that lie in the scrotum; usually the left testis hangs a little lower than the right one. The testes have two functions: producing sperm and synthesizing testosterone (the primary male sex hormone). Sperm is produced in the seminiferous tubules of the testes. Similar to the female reproductive system, the anterior pituitary releases the gonadotropins, FSH and LH. These hormones stimulate the testes to produce testosterone, which assists in maintaining spermatogenesis, increases sperm production by the seminiferous tubules, and stimulates production of seminal fluid (London, Ladewig, Ball & Bindler 2007). The epididymis, which lies against the testes, is a coiled tube almost 20 feet long. It collects sperm from the testes and provides the space and environment for sperm to mature (Fig. 3.10).

The Ductal System

The vas deferens is a cordlike duct that transports sperm from the epididymis. One such duct travels from each testis up to the back of the prostate and enters the urethra to form the ejaculatory ducts. Other structures, such as blood vessels and nerves, also travel along with each vas deferens and together form the spermatic cord. The urethra is the terminal duct of the reproductive and urinary systems, serving as a passageway for semen (fluid containing sperm) and urine. It passes through the prostate gland and the penis and opens to the outside.

Accessory Glands

The seminal vesicles, which produce nutrient seminal fluid, and the prostate gland, which produces alkaline prostatic fluid, are both connected to the ejaculatory duct leading into the urethra. The paired seminal vesicles are

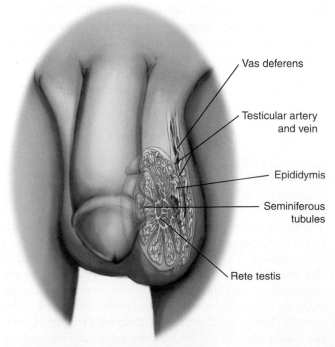

Vas deferens

Testicular artery and vein

Epididymis

Seminiferous tubules

Rete testis

FIGURE **3.10** Internal structures of a testis.

convoluted pouch-like structures lying posterior to, and at the base of, the urinary bladder in front of the rectum. They secrete an alkaline fluid that contains fructose and prostaglandins. The fructose supplies energy to the sperm on its journey to meet the ovum, and the prostaglandins assist in sperm mobility.

The prostate gland lies just under the bladder in the pelvis and surrounds the middle portion of the urethra. Usually the size of a walnut, this gland enlarges with age. The prostate and the seminal vesicles above it produce fluid that nourishes the sperm. This fluid provides most of the volume of semen, the secretion in which the sperm is expelled during ejaculation. Other fluid that makes up the semen comes from the vas deferens and from mucous glands in the head of the penis.

The bulbourethral glands (Cowper's glands) are two small structures about the size of peas, located inferior to the prostate gland. They are composed of several tubes whose epithelial linings secrete a mucus-like fluid. It is released in response to sexual stimulation and lubricates the head of the penis in preparation for sexual intercourse. Their existence is said to be constant, but they gradually diminish in size with advancing age.

Male Sexual Response

With sexual stimulation, the arteries leading to the penis dilate and increase blood flow into erectile tissues. At the same time, the erectile tissue compresses the veins of the penis, reducing blood flow away from the penis. Blood accumulates, causing the penis to swell and elongate and producing an erection. As in women, the culmination of sexual stimulation is an orgasm, a pleasurable feeling of physiologic and psychological release.

Orgasm is accompanied by emission (movement of sperm from the testes and fluids from the accessory glands) into the urethra, where it is mixed to form semen. As the urethra fills with semen, the base of the erect penis contracts, which increases pressure and forces the semen through the urethra to the outside (ejaculation). During ejaculation, the ducts of the testes, epididymis, and vas deferens contract, causing expulsion of sperm into the urethra, where the sperm mixes with the seminal and prostatic fluids. These substances, together with mucus secreted by accessory glands, form the semen, which is discharged from the urethra.

■■■ Key Concepts

■ The female reproductive system produces the female reproductive cells (the eggs, or ova) and contains an organ (uterus) where the fetus develops. The male reproductive system produces the male reproductive cells (the sperm) and contains an organ (penis) that deposits the sperm within the female.

■ The internal female reproductive organs consist of the vagina, the uterus, the fallopian tubes, and the ovaries. The external female reproductive organs make up the vulva. These include the mons pubis, the labia majora and minora, the clitoris, structures within the vestibule, and the perineum.

■ The breasts are accessory organs of the female reproductive system that are specialized to secrete milk following pregnancy.

■ The main function of the reproductive cycle is to stimulate growth of a follicle to release an egg and prepare a site for implantation if fertilization occurs.

■ Menstruation, the monthly shedding of the uterine lining, marks the beginning and end of the cycle if fertilization does not occur.

■ The ovarian cycle is the series of events associated with a developing oocyte (ovum or egg) within the ovaries.

■ At ovulation, a mature follicle ruptures in response to a surge of LH, releasing a mature oocyte (ovum).

■ The endometrial cycle is divided into four phases: the follicular or proliferative phase, the luteal or secretory phase, the ischemic phase, and the menstrual phase.

■ The menstrual cycle involves a complex interaction of hormones. The predominant hormones are gonadotropin-releasing hormone (GnRH), follicle-stimulating hormone (FSH), luteinizing hormone (LH), estrogen, progesterone, and prostaglandins.

■ The organs of the male reproductive system include the two testes (where sperm cells and testosterone are made), penis, scrotum, and accessory organs (epididymis, vas deferens, seminal vesicles, ejaculatory ducts, urethra, bulbourethral glands, and prostate gland).

REFERENCES

Alexander, L. L., LaRosa, J. H., Bader, H., & Garfield, S. (2007). *New dimensions in women's health* (4th ed.). Boston: Jones and Bartlett.

Ceo, P. D. (2006) Assessment of the male reproductive system. *Urologic Nursing, 26*(4), 290–296.

Chandran, L. (2007) Menstruation disorders. *eMedicine.* Available at: http://www.emedicine.com/ped/topic2781.htm

Coad, J., & Dunstall, M. (2005). *Anatomy and physiology for midwives* (2nd ed.). St. Louis, MO: Elsevier Health Sciences.

Cunningham, F. G., Leveno, K. J., Bloom, S. L., et al. (2005). *Williams obstetrics* (22nd ed.). New York: McGraw-Hill.

Curran, D., & Bachmann, G. (2006). Menopause. *eMedicine.* Available at: http://www.emedicine.com/med/topic3289.htm

Diaz, A., Laufer, M. R., & Breech, L. L. (2006). Menstruation in girls and adolescents: Using the menstrual cycle as a vital sign. *Pediatrics, 118*(5), 2245–2250.

Dorland, D. (2007) *Dorland's illustrated medical dictionary* (31st ed.). St. Louis, MO: Elsevier Saunders.

Hackley, B., Kriebs, J. M., & Rousseau, M. E. (2007). *Primary care of women: A guide for midwives and women's health providers.* Sudbury, MA: Jones and Bartlett Publishers.

Heffner, L. J., & Schust, D. J. (2006). *Reproductive system at a glance* (2nd ed.). Ames, IA: Blackwell Publishing Professional.

Katz, A. (2007) Sexuality and women. *Nursing for Women's Health, 11*(1), 37–43.

Kessenich, C. R. (2007). Inevitable menopause. *Nursing Spectrum.* Available at: http://nsweb.nursingspectrum.com/ce/ce232c.htm

London, M. L., Ladewig, P. W., Ball, J. W., & Bindler, R. C. (2007). *Maternal and child nursing care* (2nd ed.). Upper Saddle River, NJ: Pearson Prentice Hall.

Mattson, S., & Smith, J. E. (2004). *Core curriculum for maternal-newborn nursing* (3rd ed.). St Louis: Elsevier Saunders.

McKinney, L. N. (2007). Low libido in postmenopausal women. *Advance for Nurse Practitioners, 15*(1), 28–35.

Ramsay, D. T., Kent, J. C., Hartmann, R. A., & Hartmann, P. E. (2005). Anatomy of the lactating human breast redefined with ultrasound imaging. *Journal of Anatomy, 206*(6), 525–534.

Schuiling, K. D., & Likis, F. E. (2006). *Women's gynecologic health.* Sudbury, MA: Jones and Bartlett Publishers.

Shelby, K., & Ruocco, E. (2007). Women's hormones across the life span. *Nursing Spectrum.* Available at: http://www.nurse.com/ce/course.html?CCID=2199

Shifren, J. L., & Schiff, I. (2007). Menopause. In R. E. Rakel & E. T. Bope, eds., *Conn's current therapy 2007* (Chapter 16, pp. 1243–1244). Philadelphia: Saunders Elsevier.

Speroff, L., & Fritz, M. A. (2005). *Clinical gynecologic endocrinology and infertility* (7th ed.). Philadelphia: Lippincott Williams & Wilkins.

WEBSITES

Alan Guttmacher Institute: www.agi-usa.org
American Society for Reproductive Medicine: www.asrm.com
Kinsey Institution: www.indiana.edu/~kinsey/index.html
National Women's Health Information Center: www.4woman.gov
National Women's Health Resource Center: www.healthywomen.org
Sexuality Information of the United States: www.siecus.org
Society for Women's Health Research: www.womens-health.org

CHAPTER WORKSHEET

MULTIPLE CHOICE QUESTIONS

1. The predominant anterior pituitary hormones that orchestrate the menstrual cycle include:

   a. Thyroid-stimulating hormone (TSH)

   b. Follicle-stimulating hormone (FSH)

   c. Corticotropin-releasing hormone (CRH)

   d. Gonadotropin-releasing hormone (GnRH)

2. Which glands are located on either side of the female urethra and secrete mucus to keep the opening moist and lubricated for urination?

   a. Cowper's

   b. Bartholin's

   c. Skene's

   d. Seminal

3. What event occurs during the proliferative phase of the menstrual cycle?

   a. Menstrual flow starts

   b. Growth hormone is secreted

   c. Ovulation occurs

   d. Progesterone secretion peaks

4. Which hormone is produced in high levels to prepare the endometrium for implantation just after ovulation by the corpus luteum?

   a. Estrogen

   b. Prostaglandins

   c. Prolactin

   d. Progesterone

5. Sperm maturation and storage in the male reproductive system occurs in the:

   a. Testes

   b. Vas deferens

   c. Epididymis

   d. Seminal vesicles

CRITICAL THINKING EXERCISE

1. The school nurse was asked to speak to a 10th-grade biology class about menstruation. The teacher felt that the students don't understand this monthly event and wanted to dispel some myths about it. After the nurse explains the factors influencing the menses, one girl asks, "Could someone get pregnant if she had sex during her period?"

   a. How should the nurse respond to this question?

   b. What factor regarding the menstrual cycle was not clarified?

   c. What additional topics might this question lead to that might be discussed?

STUDY ACTIVITIES

1. Select a website from the list above and visit it to find information concerning a topic of interest regarding women's health. Be prepared to discuss it in class.

2. List the predominant hormones and their function in the menstrual cycle.

3. The ovarian cycle describes the series of events associated with the development of the _____ within the ovaries.

4. Sperm cells and the male hormone testosterone are made in which of the following structures? Select all that apply.

   a. Vas deferens

   b. Penis

   c. Scrotum

   d. Ejaculatory ducts

   e. Prostate gland

   f. Testes

   g. Seminiferous tubules

   h. Bulbourethral glands

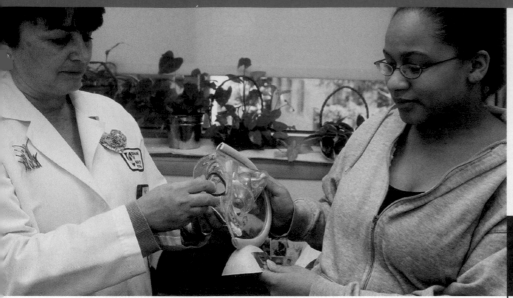

COMMON REPRODUCTIVE ISSUES

KEY TERMS

abortion
abstinence
amenorrhea
basal body temperature (BBT)
cervical cap
cervical mucus ovulation method
coitus interruptus
condoms
contraception
contraceptive sponge
Depo-Provera

diaphragm
dysfunctional uterine bleeding (DUB)
dysmenorrhea
emergency contraception (EC)
endometriosis
fertility awareness
implant
infertility
lactational amenorrhea method (LAM)
Lunelle injection

menopause
oral contraceptives
premenstrual syndrome (PMS)
Standard Days Method (SDM)
sterilization
symptothermal method
transdermal patch
tubal ligation
vaginal ring
vasectomy

LEARNING OBJECTIVES

Upon completion of the chapter, the learner will be able to:

1. Define the key terms used in this chapter.
2. Examine common reproductive concerns in terms of symptoms, diagnostic tests, and appropriate interventions.
3. Identify risk factors and outline appropriate client education needed in common reproductive disorders.
4. Compare and contrast the various contraceptive methods available and their overall effectiveness.
5. Explain the physiologic and psychological aspects of menopause.
6. Delineate the nursing management needed for women experiencing common reproductive disorders.

Izzy, a 27-year-old, presents to her health care provider complaining of progressive severe pelvic pain associated with her monthly periods. She has to take off work and "dope up" with pills to endure the pain. In addition, she has been trying to conceive for over a year without any luck.

WOW

When women bare their souls to us, we must respond without judgment.

Good health throughout the life cycle begins with the individual. Women today can expect to live well into their 80s and need to be proactive in maintaining their own quality of life. Women need to take steps to reduce their risk of disease and need to become active partners with their health care professional to identify problems early, when treatment may be most successful (Teaching Guidelines 4.1). Nurses can assist women in maintaining their quality of life by helping them to become more attuned to their body and its clues and can use the assessment period as an opportunity for teaching and counseling.

Common reproductive issues addressed in this chapter that nurses might encounter in caring for women include menstrual disorders, infertility, contraception, abortion, and menopause.

Menstrual Disorders

Many women sail through their monthly menstrual cycles with little or no concern. With few symptoms to worry about, their menses are like clockwork, starting and stopping at nearly the same time every month. For others, the menstrual cycle causes physical and emotional symptoms that initiate visits to their health care provider for consultation. The following menstruation-related conditions will be discussed in this chapter: amenorrhea, dysmenorrhea, dysfunctional uterine bleeding (DUB), premenstrual syndrome (PMS), premenstrual dysphoric disorder (PMDD), and endometriosis. To gain an understanding of menstrual disorders, it is important to know the terms used in describing them (Box 4.1).

TEACHING GUIDELINES 4.1

Tips for Being an Active Partner in Managing Your Health

- Become an informed consumer. Read, ask, and search.
- Know your family history and know factors that put you at high risk.
- Maintain a healthy lifestyle and let moderation be your guide.
- Schedule regular medical checkups and screenings for early detection.
- Ask your health care professional for a full explanation of any treatment.
- Seek a second medical opinion if you feel you need more information.
- Know when to seek medical care by being aware of disease symptoms.

BOX 4.1 Menstrual Disorder Vocabulary

- Meno = menstrual-related
- Metro = time
- Oligo = few
- A = without, none or lack of
- Rhagia = excess or abnormal
- Dys = not or pain
- Rhea = flow

▶ AMENORRHEA

Amenorrhea is the absence of menses during the reproductive years. Amenorrhea is normal in prepubertal, pregnant, and postmenopausal females. The two categories of amenorrhea are primary and secondary amenorrhea. Primary amenorrhea is defined as either:

1. Absence of menses by age 14, with absence of growth and development of secondary sexual characteristics, or
2. Absence of menses by age 16, with normal development of secondary sexual characteristics (Bielak & Harris, 2006)

Ninety-eight percent of American girls menstruate by age 16 (Krantz, 2007a, 2007b). Secondary amenorrhea is the absence of menses for three cycles or 6 months in women who have previously menstruated regularly.

Etiology

There are multiple causes of primary amenorrhea:

- Extreme weight gain or loss
- Congenital abnormalities of the reproductive system
- Stress from a major life event
- Excessive exercise
- Eating disorders (anorexia nervosa or bulimia)
- Cushing's disease
- Polycystic ovary syndrome
- Hypothyroidism
- Turner syndrome
- Imperforate hymen
- Chronic illness
- Pregnancy
- Cystic fibrosis
- Congenital heart disease (cyanotic)
- Ovarian or adrenal tumors (Master-Hunter & Heiman, 2006)

Causes of secondary amenorrhea might include:

- Pregnancy
- Breastfeeding

- Emotional stress
- Pituitary, ovarian, or adrenal tumors
- Depression
- Hyperthyroid or hypothyroid conditions
- Malnutrition
- Hyperprolactinemia
- Rapid weight gain or loss
- Chemotherapy or radiation therapy to the pelvic area
- Vigorous exercise, such as long-distance running
- Kidney failure
- Colitis
- Use of tranquilizers or antidepressants
- Postpartum pituitary necrosis (Sheehan syndrome)
- Early menopause (Bielak & Harris, 2006)

Therapeutic Management

Therapeutic intervention depends on the cause of the amenorrhea. The treatment of primary amenorrhea involves the correction of any underlying disorders and estrogen replacement therapy to stimulate the development of secondary sexual characteristics. If a pituitary tumor is the cause, it might be treated with drug therapy, surgical resection, or radiation therapy. Surgery might be needed to correct any structural abnormalities of the genital tract. Therapeutic interventions for secondary amenorrhea may include:

- Cyclic progesterone, when the cause is anovulation, or oral contraceptives
- Bromocriptine to treat hyperprolactinemia
- Nutritional counseling to address anorexia, bulimia, or obesity
- Gonadotropin-releasing hormone (GnRH), when the cause is hypothalamic failure
- Thyroid hormone replacement, when the cause is hypothyroidism (Schuiling & Likis, 2006)

Nursing Assessment

Nursing assessment for the young girl or woman experiencing amenorrhea includes a thorough health history and physical examination and several laboratory and diagnostic tests.

Health History and Physical Examination

A thorough history and physical examination is needed to determine the etiology. The history should include questions about the women's menstrual history; past illnesses; hospitalizations and surgeries; obstetric history; use of prescription and over-the-counter drugs; recent or past lifestyle changes; and history of present illness, with an assessment of any bodily changes.

The physical examination should begin with an overall assessment of the woman's nutritional status and general health. A sensitive and gentle approach to the pelvic examination is critical in young women. Height and weight should be taken, along with vital signs. Hypothermia,

bradycardia, hypotension, and reduced subcutaneous fat may be observed in women with anorexia nervosa. Facial hair and acne might be evidence of androgen excess secondary to a tumor. The presence or absence of axillary and pubic hair may indicate adrenal and ovarian hyposecretion or delayed puberty. A general physical examination may uncover unexpected findings that are indirectly related to amenorrhea. For example, hepatosplenomegaly, which may suggest a chronic systemic disease or an enlarged thyroid gland, might point to a thyroid disorder as well as a reason for amenorrhea (Nelson & Bakalov, 2006).

Laboratory and Diagnostic Tests

Common laboratory tests that might be ordered to determine the cause of amenorrhea include:

- Karyotype (might be positive for Turner syndrome)
- Ultrasound to detect ovarian cysts
- Pregnancy test to rule out pregnancy
- Thyroid function studies to determine thyroid disorder
- Prolactin level (an elevated level might indicate a pituitary tumor)
- Follicle-stimulating hormone (FSH) level (an elevated level might indicate ovarian failure)
- Luteinizing hormone (LH) level (an elevated level might indicate gonadal dysfunction)
- 17-ketosteroids (an elevated level might indicate an adrenal tumor)
- Laparoscopy to detect polycystic ovary syndrome
- CT scan of head if a pituitary tumor is suspected (Pagana & Pagana, 2007)

Nursing Management

Counseling and education are primary interventions and appropriate nursing roles. Address the diverse causes of amenorrhea, the relationship to sexual identity, possible infertility, and the possibility of a tumor or a life-threatening disease. In addition, inform the woman about the purpose of each diagnostic test, how it is performed, and when the results will be available to discuss with her. Sensitive listening, interviewing, and presenting treatment options are paramount to gain the woman's cooperation and understanding.

Nutritional counseling is also vital in managing this disorder, especially if the woman has findings suggestive of an eating disorder. Although not all causes can be addressed by making lifestyle changes, emphasize maintaining a healthy lifestyle (Teaching Guidelines 4.2).

▶ DYSMENORRHEA

Dysmenorrhea refers to painful menstruation. This condition has also been termed cyclic perimenstrual pain (CPPD) (Taylor, 2005). The term **dysmenorrhea** is derived from

TEACHING GUIDELINES 4.2

Tips for Maintaining a Healthy Lifestyle

- Balance energy expenditure with energy intake.
- Modify your diet to maintain ideal weight.
- Avoid excessive use of alcohol and mood-altering or sedative drugs.
- Avoid cigarette smoking.
- Identify areas of emotional stress and seek assistance to resolve them.
- Balance work, recreation, and rest.
- Maintain a positive outlook regarding the diagnosis and prognosis.
- Participate in ongoing care to monitor any medical conditions.
- Maintain bone density through:
  - Calcium intake (1,200 to 1,500 mg daily)
  - Weight-bearing exercise (30 minutes or more daily)
  - Hormone therapy

Source: Nelson & Bakalov, 2006.

the Greek words "dys," meaning difficult, painful, or abnormal, and "rrhea," meaning flow. It may affect more than half of menstruating women (Smith, 2006). Uterine contractions occur during all periods, but in some women these cramps can be frequent and very intense. Dysmenorrhea is categorized as primary or secondary.

Etiology

Primary dysmenorrhea is caused by increased prostaglandin production by the endometrium in an ovulatory cycle. This hormone causes contraction of the uterus, and levels tend to be higher in women with severe menstrual pain than women who experience mild or no menstrual pain. These levels are highest during the first 2 days of menses, when symptoms peak (Doty & Attaran, 2006). This results in increased rhythmic uterine contractions from vasoconstriction of the small vessels of the uterine wall. This condition usually begins within a few years of the onset of ovulatory cycles at menarche.

Secondary dysmenorrhea is painful menstruation due to pelvic or uterine pathology. It may be caused by endometriosis, adenomyosis, fibroids, pelvic infection, an intrauterine device, cervical stenosis, or congenital uterine or vaginal abnormalities. Adenomyosis involves the ingrowth of the endometrium into the uterine musculature. Endometriosis involves ectopic implantation of endometrial tissue in other parts of the pelvis. It occurs most commonly in the third or fourth decades of life and affects 10% of women of reproductive age (Hompes &

Mijatovic, 2007). Endometriosis is the most common cause of secondary dysmenorrhea and is associated with pain beyond menstruation, dyspareunia, and infertility (Speroff & Fritz, 2005). Treatment is directed toward removing the underlying pathology.

Think back to Izzy from the chapter opener. Is her pelvic pain complaint a common one with women?

Therapeutic Management

Therapeutic intervention is directed toward pain relief and building coping strategies that will promote a productive lifestyle. Treatment measures usually include treating infections if present; suppressing the endometrium if endometriosis is suspected by administering low-dose oral contraceptives; administering prostaglandin inhibitors to reduce the pain; administering Depo-Provera; and initiating lifestyle changes. Table 4.1 lists selected treatment options for dysmenorrhea.

Nursing Assessment

As with any gynecologic complaint, a thorough focused history and physical examination is needed to make the diagnosis of primary or secondary dysmenorrhea. In primary dysmenorrhea, the history usually reveals the typical cramping pain with menstruation, and the physical examination is completely normal. In secondary dysmenorrhea, the history discloses cramping pain starting after 25 years old with a pelvic abnormality, a history of infertility, heavy menstrual flow, irregular cycles, and little response to nonsteroidal anti-inflammatory drugs (NSAIDs), oral contraceptives, or both (Harel, 2006).

Health History and Clinical Manifestations

Note past medical history, including any chronic illnesses and family history of gynecologic concerns. Determine medication and substance use, such as prescription medications, contraceptives, anabolic steroids, tobacco, and marijuana, cocaine, or other illegal drugs. A detailed sexual history is essential to assess for inflammation and scarring (adhesions) secondary to pelvic inflammatory disease (PID). Women with a previous history of PID, sexually transmitted infections (STIs), multiple sexual partners, or unprotected sex are at increased risk.

During the initial interview, the nurse might ask some of the following questions to assess the woman's history of dysmenorrhea:

- "At what age did you start your menstrual cycles?"
- "Have your cycles always been painful, or did the pain start recently?"
- "When in your cycle do you experience the pain?"
- "How would you describe the pain you feel?"

TABLE 4.1 TREATMENT OPTIONS FOR DYSMENORRHEA

Therapy Options	Dosage	Comments
Nonsteroidal anti-inflammatory agents (NSAIDs)		
Ibuprofen (Ibuprin, Advil, Motrin)	400–800 mg TID	Take with meals. Don't take with aspirin. Avoid alcohol. Watch for signs of GI bleeding.
Naproxen (Anaprox, Naprelan, Naprosyn, Aleve)	250–500 mg TID	Same as above
Hormonal contraceptives		
Low-dose oral contraceptives	Taken daily (42/7 days; 63/7 or 84/7)	Take active pills for an extended time to reduce number of monthly cycles (Archer, 2006).
Depo-medroxyproges-terone (DMPA), Depo-Provera	150 mg IM every 12 wks	Within 9–12 months of DMPA therapy, 75% of women will be amenorrheic (Schuiling & Likis, 2006).
Lifestyle changes		Gives sense of control over life
Daily exercise		
Limit salty foods		
Weight loss		
Smoking cessation		
Relaxation techniques		

- "Are you sexually active?"
- "What impact does your cycle have on your physical and social activity?"
- "When was the first day of your last menstrual cycle?"
- "Was the flow of your last menstrual cycle a normal amount for you?"
- "Do your cycles tend to be heavy or last longer than 5 days?"
- "Are your cycles generally regular and predictable?"
- "What have you done to relieve your discomfort? Is it effective?"
- "Has there been a progression of symptom severity?"
- "Do you have any other symptoms?"

Assess for clinical manifestations of dysmenorrhea. Affected women experience sharp, intermittent spasms of pain, usually in the suprapubic area. Pain may radiate to the back of the legs or the lower back. Pain usually develops within hours of the start of menstruation and peaks as the flow becomes heaviest during the first day or two of the cycle (Edmundson & Erogul, 2006). Systemic symptoms of nausea, vomiting, diarrhea, fatigue, fever, headache, or dizziness are fairly common. Explore the history for physi-

cal symptoms of bloating, water retention, weight gain, headache, muscle aches, abdominal pain, food cravings, or breast tenderness.

Physical Examination

The physical examination performed by the health care provider centers on the bimanual pelvic examination. This examination is done during the nonmenstrual phase of the cycle. Explain to the woman how it is to be performed, especially if is her first pelvic examination. Prepare the woman in the examining room by offering her a cover gown to put on and covering her lap with a privacy sheet on the examination table. Remain in the examining room throughout the examination to assist the health care provider with any procedures or specimens and to offer the woman reassurance.

Laboratory and Diagnostic Tests

Common laboratory tests that may be ordered to determine the cause of dysmenorrhea might include:

- Complete blood count to rule out anemia
- Urinalysis to rule out a bladder infection

- Pregnancy test (human chorionic gonadotropin level) to rule out pregnancy
- Cervical culture to exclude STI
- Erythrocyte sedimentation rate to detect an inflammatory process
- Stool guaiac to exclude gastrointestinal bleeding or disorders
- Pelvic and/or vaginal ultrasound to detect pelvic masses or cysts
- Diagnostic laparoscopy and/or laparotomy to visualize pathology that may account for the symptoms

W̶hat diagnostic tests might be ordered to diagnose Izzy's pelvic pain?

Nursing Management

Educating the client about the normal events of the menstrual cycle and the etiology of her pain is paramount in achieving a successful outcome. Explaining the normal menstrual cycle will teach the woman the correct terms so she can communicate her symptoms more accurately and will help dispel myths. Provide the woman with monthly graphs or charts to record menses, the onset of pain, the timing of medication, relief afforded, and coping strategies used. This involves the woman in her care and provides objective information so that therapy can be modified if necessary.

The nurse should explain in detail the dosing regimen and the side effects of the medication therapy selected. Commonly prescribed drugs include NSAIDs such as ibuprofen (Motrin), naproxen (Naprosyn), and Advil. They alleviate dysmenorrhea symptoms by decreasing intrauterine pressure and inhibiting prostaglandin synthesis, thus reducing pain (Skidmore-Roth, 2007). If pain relief is not achieved in two to four cycles, a low-dose combination oral contraceptive may be initiated. Client teaching and counseling should include information about how to take pills, side effects, and danger signs to watch for.

Encourage the woman to apply a heating pad or warm compress to alleviate menstrual cramps. Additional lifestyle changes that the woman can make to restore some sense of control and active participation in her care are listed in Teaching Guidelines 4.3.

▶ DYSFUNCTIONAL UTERINE BLEEDING

Dysfunctional uterine bleeding (DUB) is a disorder that occurs most frequently in women at the beginning and end of their reproductive years. Defined as irregular, abnormal bleeding that occurs with no identifiable anatomic

TEACHING GUIDELINES 4.3

Tips to Manage Dysmenorrhea

- Exercise to increase endorphins and suppress prostaglandin release.
- Limit salty foods to prevent fluid retention.
- Increase water consumption to serve as a natural diuretic.
- Increase fiber intake with fruits and vegetables to prevent constipation.
- Use heating pads or warm baths to increase comfort.
- Take warm showers to promote relaxation.
- Sip on warm beverages, such as decaffeinated green tea.
- Keep legs elevated while lying down or lie on side with knees bent.
- Use stress management techniques to reduce emotional stress.
- Practice relaxation techniques to enhance ability to cope with pain.
- Stop smoking and decrease alcohol use.

Source: Nasir, 2007.

pathology, it affects 33% to 50% of women (Rackow & Arici, 2007). It is frequently associated with anovulatory cycles, which are common for the first year after menarche and later in life as women approach menopause.

The pathophysiology of DUB is related to a hormone disturbance. With anovulation, estrogen levels rise as usual in the early phase of the menstrual cycle. In the absence of ovulation, a corpus luteum never forms and progesterone is not produced. The endometrium moves into a hyperproliferative state, ultimately outgrowing its estrogen supply. This leads to irregular sloughing of the endometrium and excessive bleeding (Aeby & Frattarelli, 2006). If the bleeding is heavy enough and frequent enough, anemia can result.

DUB is similar to several other types of uterine bleeding disorders and sometimes overlaps these conditions. They include:

- Menorrhagia (abnormally long, heavy periods)
- Oligomenorrhea (bleeding occurs at intervals of more than 35 days)
- Metrorrhagia (bleeding between periods)
- Menometrorrhagia (bleeding occurs at irregular intervals with heavy flow lasting more than 7 days)
- Polymenorrhea (too frequent periods)

Etiology

The possible causes of DUB may include:

- Adenomyosis
- Pregnancy

- Hormonal imbalance
- Fibroid tumors (see Chapter 7)
- Endometrial polyps or cancer
- Endometriosis
- Intrauterine device (IUD)
- Polycystic ovary syndrome
- Morbid obesity
- Steroid therapy
- Hypothyroidism
- Blood dyscrasias/clotting disorder

Therapeutic Management

Treatment of DUB depends on the cause of the bleeding and the age of the client. When known, the underlying cause of the disorder is treated. Otherwise, the goal of treatment is to relieve the symptoms so that uterine bleeding does not interfere with a woman's normal activities or cause anemia (Dodds & Sinert, 2006).

Management of DUB might include medical care with pharmacotherapy or insertion of an IUD. Oral contraceptives are used for cycle regulation as well as contraception. They help prevent the risks associated with prolonged unopposed estrogen stimulation of the endometrium. NSAIDs and the levonorgestrel-releasing IUD (Mirena) decrease menstrual blood loss significantly (Lethaby, Cooke & Rees, 2006). The drug categories used in the treatment of DUB are:

- Estrogens: cause vasospasm of the uterine arteries to decrease bleeding
- Progestins: used to stabilize an estrogen-primed endometrium
- Oral contraceptives: regulate the cycle and suppress the endometrium
- NSAIDs: inhibit prostaglandins
- Levonorgestrel-20 Intrauterine System: suppresses endometrial growth
- Iron salts: replenish iron stores lost during heavy bleeding

If the client does not respond to medical therapy, surgical intervention might include dilation and curettage (D&C), endometrial ablation, or hysterectomy. Endometrial ablation is an alternative to hysterectomy. A thermal balloon or a laser is used to ablate the tissue, producing improvement in 90% of women (Speroff & Fritz, 2005).

Nursing Assessment

A thorough history should be taken to differentiate between DUB and other conditions that might cause vaginal bleeding, such as pregnancy and pregnancy-related conditions (abruptio placentae, ectopic pregnancy, abortion, or placenta previa); systemic conditions such as Cushing disease, blood dyscrasias, liver disease, renal disease, or thyroid disease; and genital tract pathology such as infections, tumors, or trauma (Hackley, Kriebs & Rousseau, 2007).

Assess for clinical manifestations of DUB, which commonly include vaginal bleeding between periods, irregular menstrual cycles (usually less than 28 days between cycles), infertility, mood swings, hot flashes, vaginal tenderness, variable menstrual flow ranging from scanty to profuse, obesity, acne, and diabetes. Signs of polycystic ovary syndrome might be present, since it is associated with unopposed estrogen stimulation, elevated androgen levels, and insulin resistance and is a common cause of anovulation (Torpy, 2007).

Measure orthostatic blood pressure and orthostatic pulse; a drop in pressure or pulse rate may occur with anemia. The health care provider, with the nurse assisting, performs a pelvic examination to identify any structural abnormalities.

Common laboratory tests that may be ordered to determine the cause of DUB include:

- Complete blood count to detect anemia
- Prothrombin time (PT) to detect blood dyscrasias
- Pregnancy test to rule out a spontaneous abortion or ectopic pregnancy
- Thyroid-stimulating hormone (TSH) level to screen for hypothyroidism
- Transvaginal ultrasound to measure endometrium
- Pelvic ultrasound to view any structural abnormalities
- Endometrial biopsy to check for intrauterine pathology
- D&C for diagnostic evaluation

Nursing Management

Educate the client about normal menstrual cycles and the possible reasons for her abnormal pattern. Inform the woman about treatment options. Do not simply encourage the woman to "live with it": complications such as infertility can result from lack of ovulation; severe anemia can occur secondary to prolonged or heavy menses; and endometrial cancer can occur associated with prolonged buildup of the endometrial lining without menstrual bleeding (Rackow & Arici, 2007). Instruct her about any prescribed medications and potential side effects. For example, if high-dose estrogens are prescribed, the woman may experience nausea. Teach her to take antiemetics as prescribed and encourage her to eat small, frequent meals to alleviate nausea. Adequate follow-up and evaluation for women who do not respond to medical management is essential. See Nursing Care Plan 4.1: Overview of a Woman With Dysfunctional Uterine Bleeding (DUB).

▶ PREMENSTRUAL SYNDROME

Premenstrual syndrome (PMS) describes a wide range of recurrent symptoms that occur during the luteal phase or last half of the menstrual cycle and resolve with the onset of menstruation (Braverman & Neinstein,

Nursing Care Plan 4.1

OVERVIEW OF A WOMAN WITH DYSFUNCTIONAL UTERINE BLEEDING (DUB)

Stacy, a 52-year-old obese woman, comes to her gynecologist with the complaint of heavy erratic bleeding. Her periods were fairly regular until about 4 months ago, and since that time they have been unpredictable, excessive, and prolonged. Stacy reports she is tired all the time, can't sleep, and feels "out of sorts" and anxious. She is fearful she has cancer.

NURSING DIAGNOSIS: Fear related to current signs and symptoms possibly indicating a life-threatening condition

Outcome Identification and Evaluation
The client will acknowledge her fears as evidenced by statements made that fear and anxiety have been lessened after explanation of diagnosis.

Interventions: Reducing Fear and Anxiety
- Distinguish between anxiety and fear to determine appropriate interventions.
- Check complete blood count and assess for possible anemia secondary to excessive bleeding to determine if fatigue is contributing to anxiety and fear. Fatigue occurs because the oxygen-carrying capacity of the blood is reduced.
- Reassure client that symptoms can be managed to help address her current concerns.
- Provide client with factual information and explain what to expect to assist client with identifying fears and help in her coping with her condition.
- Provide symptom management to reduce concerns associated with the cause of bleeding.
- Teach client about early manifestations of fear and anxiety to aid in prompt recognition and to minimize escalation of anxiety.
- Assess client's use of coping strategies in the past and reinforce use of effective ones to help control anxiety and fear.
- Instruct client in relaxation methods, such as deep breathing exercises and imagery, to provide her with additional methods for controlling anxiety and fear.

NURSING DIAGNOSIS: Deficient knowledge related to perimenopause and its management

Outcome Identification and Evaluation
The client will demonstrate understanding of her symptoms as evidenced by making health-promoting lifestyle choices, verbalizing appropriate health care practices, and adhering to measures to comply with therapy.

Interventions: Providing Patient Education
- Assess client's understanding of perimenopause and its treatment to provide a baseline for teaching and developing a plan of care.
- Review instructions about prescribed procedures and recommendations for self-care, frequently obtaining feedback from the client to validate adequate understanding of information.
- Outline link between anovulatory cycles and excessive buildup of uterine lining in perimenopausal women to assist client in understanding the etiology of her bleeding.
- Provide written material with pictures to promote learning and help client visualize what is occurring to her body during perimenopause.
- Inform client about the availability of community resources and make appropriate referrals as needed to provide additional education and support.
- Document details of teaching and learning to allow for continuity of care and further education, if needed.

2007). The American College of Obstetricians and Gynecologists (ACOG) defines premenstrual syndrome as "the cyclic occurrence of symptoms that are sufficiently severe to interfere with some aspects of life, and that appear with consistent and predictable relationship to menses" (ACOG, 2000). A woman experiencing PMS may have a wide variety of seemingly unrelated symptoms; for that reason, it is difficult to define and more challenging to diagnose. PMS affects millions of women during their reproductive years: up to 85% of menstruating women report having one or more premenstrual symptoms, and up to 10% report disabling, incapacitating symptoms

(Campagne & Campagne, 2007). The exact cause of PMS is not known. It is thought to be related to the interaction between hormonal events and neurotransmitter function, specifically serotonin. Not all women respond to serotonin reuptake inhibitors (SSRIs), however, which implies that other mechanisms may be involved (Braverman & Neinstein, 2007).

As defined by the American Psychological Association, premenstrual dysphoric disorder (PMDD) is a more severe variant of PMS. Experts compare the difference between PMS and PMDD to the difference between a mild tension headache and a migraine (Giulio & Reissing, 2006). PMDD markedly interferes with work and school, or with social activities and relationships with others.

Therapeutic Management

Treatment of PMS is often frustrating for both patients and health care providers. Clinical outcomes can be expected to improve as a result of recent consensus on the diagnostic criteria for PMS and PMDD, data from clinical trials, and the availability of evidence-based clinical guidelines.

The management of PMS or PMDD requires a multidimensional approach because these conditions are not likely to have a single cause, and they appear to affect multiple systems within a woman's body; therefore, they are not likely to be amenable to treatment with a single therapy. To reduce the negative impact of premenstrual disorders on a woman's life, education, along with reassurance and anticipatory guidance, are needed for women to feel they have some control over their condition.

▶ **Take** NOTE!

Because there are no diagnostic tests that can reliably determine the existence of PMS or PMDD, it is the woman herself who must decide that she needs help during this time of the month. The woman must embrace multiple therapies and become an active participant in her treatment plan to find the best level of symptom relief.

Therapeutic interventions for PMS and PMDD address the symptoms because the exact cause of this condition is still unknown. Treatments may include vitamin supplements, diet changes, exercise, lifestyle changes, and medications (Box 4.2). Medications used in treating PMDD may include antidepressant and antianxiety drugs, diuretics, anti-inflammatory medications, analgesics, synthetic androgen agents, oral contraceptives, or GNrH agonists to regulate menses (Pavlovich-Danis, 2007).

BOX 4.2 Treatment Options for PMS and PMDD

- Lifestyle changes:
  Reduce stress.
  Exercise three to five times each week.
  Eat a balanced diet and increase water intake.
  Decrease caffeine intake.
  Stop smoking.
  Limit intake of alcohol.
  Attend a PMS/women's support group.
- Vitamin and mineral supplements
  Multivitamin daily
  Vitamin E, 400 units daily
  Calcium, 1,200 mg daily
  Magnesium, 200 to 400 mg daily
- Medications
  NSAIDs taken a week prior to menses
  Oral contraceptives (low dose)
  Antidepressants (SSRIs)
  Anxiolytics (taken during luteal phase)
  Diuretics to remove excess fluid
  Progestins
  Gonadotropin-releasing hormone (GnRH agonists)
  Danazol (androgen hormone inhibits estrogen production)

Many women use dietary supplements and herbal remedies for their menstrual health and treating their bleeding disorders, although there has been little research to demonstrate their efficacy. Some alternative therapies used might include calcium, magnesium, vitamin B6, evening primrose oil, vitex agnus castus, ginkgo biloba, viburnum, dandelion, stinging nettle, burdock, raspberry leaf, skullcap, and St. John's wort (Canning, Waterman & Dye, 2006). Although research hasn't validated alternative therapy's efficacy, it is important for the nurse to be aware of the alternative products that many women choose to use.

Nursing Assessment

Although little consensus exists in the medical literature and among researchers about what constitutes PMS and PMDD, the physical and psychological symptoms are very real. The extent to which the symptoms debilitate or incapacitate a woman is highly variable.

There are more than 200 symptoms assigned to PMS, but irritability, tension, and dysphoria are the most prominent and consistently described (Moreno & Giesel, 2006). To establish the diagnosis of PMS, elicit a description of cyclic symptoms occurring before the woman's menstrual period. The woman should chart her symptoms daily for two cycles. These data will help demonstrate symptoms clustering around the luteal phase of ovulation, with resolution after bleeding starts. Ask the woman to bring her list of symptoms to the next appointment. Symptoms can be categorized using the following:

- A: anxiety: difficulty sleeping, tenseness, mood swings, clumsiness
- C: craving: headache, cravings for sweets, salty foods, chocolate
- D: depression: feelings of low self-esteem, anger, easily upset
- H: hydration: weight gain, abdominal bloating, breast tenderness
- O: other: hot flashes or cold sweats, nausea, change in bowel habits, aches or pains, dysmenorrhea, acne breakout (Pavlovich-Danis, 2007)

The ACOG diagnostic criteria for PMS consist of having at least one of the following affective and somatic symptoms during the 5 days before menses in each of the three previous cycles:

- Affective symptoms: depression, angry outbursts, irritability, anxiety
- Somatic symptoms: breast tenderness, abdominal bloating, edema, headache
- Symptoms relieved from days 4 to 13 of the menstrual cycle (ACOG, 2000)

In PMDD, the main symptoms are mood disorders such as depression, anxiety, tension, and persistent anger or irritability. Physical symptoms such as headache, joint and muscle pain, lack of energy, bloating, and breast tenderness are also present (Hsiao & Liu, 2007). It is estimated that 20% to 40% of reproductive-age women experience premenstrual symptoms that meet the ACOG criteria for PMS and up to 10% meet the diagnostic criteria for PMDD (Futterman & Rapkin, 2006).

According to the American Psychiatric Association, a woman must have at least five of the typical symptoms to be diagnosed with PMDD (Andoisek & Rapkin, 2007). These must occur during the week before and a few days after the onset of menstruation and must include one or more of the first four symptoms:

1. Affective lability: sadness, tearfulness, irritability
2. Anxiety and tension
3. Persistent or marked anger or irritability
4. Depressed mood, feelings of hopelessness
5. Difficulty concentrating
6. Sleep difficulties
7. Increased or decreased appetite
8. Increased or decreased sexual desire
9. Chronic fatigue
10. Headache
11. Constipation or diarrhea
12. Breast swelling and tenderness (Htay & Aung, 2006)

Nursing Management

Educate the client about the management of PMS or PMDD. Advise her that lifestyle changes often result in significant symptom improvement without pharmacotherapy. Encourage women to eat a balanced diet that includes nutrient-rich foods to avoid hypoglycemia and associated mood swings. Encourage adolescent girls to participate in aerobic exercise three times a week to promote a sense of well-being, decrease fatigue, and reduce stress. Administer calcium (1,200 to 1,600 mg/day), magnesium (400 to 800 mg/day), and vitamin B6 (50 to 100 mg/day) as prescribed. In some studies, these nutrients have been shown to decrease the intensity of PMS symptoms. NSAIDs may be useful for painful physical symptoms and spironolactone (Aldactone) may help with bloating and water retention. Herbs such as Vitex (chaste tree berry), evening primrose, and SAM-e may be recommended; although not harmful, not all herbs have enough clinical or research evidence to document their safety or efficacy (Schuiling & Likis, 2006).

A recent research study proposes calcium (1,600 mg/day) and vitamin D (400 IU/day) supplementation in adolescents and women in an effort to prevent PMS (Clayton, 2008).

Explain the relationship between cyclic estrogen fluctuation and changes in serotonin levels and how the different management strategies help maintain serotonin levels, thus improving symptoms. It is important to rule out other conditions that might cause erratic or dysphoric behavior. If the initial treatment regimen does not work, explain to the woman that she should return for further testing. Behavioral counseling and stress management might help women regain control during these stressful periods. Reassuring the woman that support and help are available through many community resources/support groups can be instrumental in her acceptance of this monthly disorder. Nurses can be a very calming force for many women experiencing PMS or PMDD.

▶ **Take** NOTE!

Adolescents and women who experience more extensive emotional symptoms with PMS should be evaluated for PMDD, as they may require antidepressant therapy.

▶ ENDOMETRIOSIS

Endometriosis is one of the most common gynecologic diseases, affecting more than 5.5 million women in the United States. In this condition, bits of functioning endometrial tissue are located outside of their normal site, the uterine cavity. This endometrial tissue is commonly found attached to the ovaries, fallopian tubes, the outer surface of the uterus, the bowels, the area between the vagina and the rectum (rectovaginal septum), and the pelvic side wall (Fig. 4.1). The places where the tissue attaches are called implants, or lesions. Endometrial tissue found outside the uterus responds to hormones released during the menstrual cycle in the same way as endometrial lining within the uterus.

At the beginning of the menstrual cycle, when the lining of the uterus is shed and menstrual bleeding begins, these abnormally located implants swell and bleed also. In short, the woman with endometriosis experiences several "mini-periods" throughout her abdomen, wherever this endometrial tissue exists.

Think back to Izzy, with her progressive pelvic pain and infertility concerns. After a pelvic examination, her health care provider suspects she has endometriosis.

Etiology and Risk Factors

It is not currently known why endometrial tissue becomes transplanted and grows in other parts of the body. Several theories exist, but to date none has been scientifically proven. However, several factors that increase a woman's risk of developing endometriosis have been identified:

- Increasing age
- Family history of endometriosis in a first-degree relative
- Short menstrual cycle (less than 28 days)
- Long menstrual flow (more than 1 week)
- Young age of menarche (younger than 12)
- Few (one or two) or no pregnancies (Speroff & Fritz, 2005)

Therapeutic Management

Therapeutic management of the client with endometriosis needs to take into consideration the following factors: severity of symptoms, desire for fertility, degree of disease, and the client's therapy goals. The aim of therapy is to suppress levels of estrogen and progesterone, which cause the endometrium to grow. Treatment can include surgery or medication (Table 4.2).

Nursing Assessment

Nurses encounter women with endometriosis in a variety of settings: community health settings, schools, clinics, day surgical centers, and hospitals. Health care professionals must not trivialize or dismiss the concerns of these women, because early recognition is essential to preserve fertility.

Health History

Obtain a health history and elicit a description of signs and symptoms to determine risk factors. Endometriosis is often asymptomatic, but it can be a severe and debilitating condition. It typically is chronic and progressive. Assess the client for clinical manifestations, which include:

- Infertility
- Pain before and during menstrual periods
- Pain during or after sexual intercourse
- Painful urination
- Depression
- Fatigue
- Painful bowel movements
- Chronic pelvic pain
- Hypermenorrhea (heavy menses)
- Pelvic adhesions

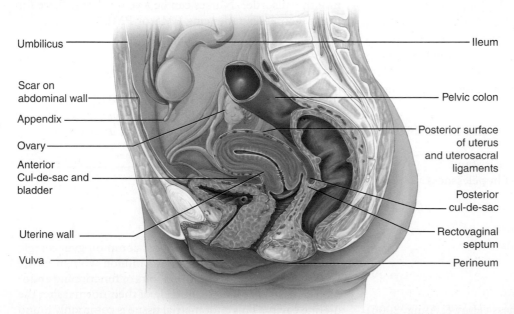

Umbilicus — Ileum
Scar on abdominal wall —
Appendix — Pelvic colon
Ovary —
Anterior Cul-de-sac and bladder — Posterior surface of uterus and uterosacral ligaments
Uterine wall — Posterior cul-de-sac
Vulva — Rectovaginal septum
Perineum

FIGURE **4.1** Common sites of endometriosis formation.

TABLE 4.2 TREATMENT OPTIONS FOR ENDOMETRIOSIS

Therapy Options	Comment
Surgical intervention	
Conservative surgery	Removal of implants/lesions using laser, cautery, or small surgical instruments. This intervention will reduce pain and allows pregnancy to occur in the future.
Definitive surgery	Abdominal hysterectomy, with or without bilateral salpingo-oophorectomy. Will eliminate pain but will leave a woman unable to become pregnant in the future.
Medication therapy	
NSAIDs	First-line treatment to reduce pain; taken early when premenstrual symptoms are first felt
Oral contraceptives	Suppresses cyclic hormonal response of the endometrial tissue
Progestogens	Used to cast off the endometrial cells and thus destroy them
Antiestrogens	Suppresses a woman's production of estrogen, thus stopping the menstrual cycle and preventing further growth of endometrium
Gonadotropin-releasing hormone analogues (GnRH-a)	Suppresses endometriosis by creating a temporary pseudomenopause
Danazol (Danacrine)	A synthetic androgen (male sex hormone) used typically as a second-line treatment of endometriosis. Disrupts the action of the pituitary gland by suppressing the output of some hormones, thus reducing estrogen, halting menstruation, and resulting in the growth of facial hair and acne.

• Irregular and more frequent menses
• Premenstrual vaginal spotting (Schuiling & Likis, 2006)

The two most common symptoms are infertility and pain. Endometriosis occurs in 38% of infertile women and in 71% to 87% of women with chronic pelvic pain (Aeby & Hraoka, 2006). About 30% to 40% of women with this condition are infertile, making it one of the top three causes of female infertility (NICHD, 2006).

What are the two most common symptoms experienced by women with endometriosis? Is Izzy's profile typical? As a nurse, what would be your role in Izzy's continued workup?

Physical Examination and Laboratory and Diagnostic Tests

The pelvic examination typically correlates with the extent of the endometriosis. The usual finding is nonspecific pelvic tenderness. The hallmark finding is the presence of tender nodular masses on the uterosacral ligaments, the posterior uterus, or the posterior cul-de-sac (Saul & Dave, 2006).

After a thorough history and a pelvic examination, the health care practitioner may suspect endometriosis, but the only certain method of diagnosing it is by seeing it. Pelvic or transvaginal ultrasound is used to assess pelvic organ structures. However, a laparoscopy is needed to diagnose endometriosis. Laparoscopy is the direct visualization of the internal organs with a lighted instrument inserted through an abdominal incision. A tissue biopsy of the suspected implant taken at the same time and examined microscopically confirms the diagnosis.

Nurses can play a role by offering a thorough explanation of the condition and explaining why tests are needed to diagnose endometriosis. The nurse can set up appointments for imaging studies and laparoscopy.

Nursing Management

In addition to the interventions outlined above, the nurse should encourage the client to adopt healthy lifestyle habits with respect to diet, exercise, sleep, and stress management. Referrals to support groups and Internet resources can help the woman to understand this condition and to cope with chronic pain. A number of organizations provide information about the diagnosis and treatment of endometriosis and offer support to women and their families (Box 4.3). See Evidence-Based Practice 4.1.

After completing several diagnostic tests, Izzy is diagnosed with endometriosis. She asks you about her chances of becoming pregnant and becoming pain-free. What treatment options would you explain to Izzy? What information can you give about her future childbearing ability?

Infertility

Infertility is defined as the inability to conceive a child after 1 year of regular sexual intercourse unprotected by contraception, or the inability to carry a pregnancy to term (Covington & Burns, 2006). Secondary infertility is the inability to conceive after a previous pregnancy. Many people take the ability to conceive and produce a

---

BOX 4.3 **Organizations and Web Resources to Assist the Client With Endometriosis**

- American College of Obstetricians and Gynecologists (ACOG): www.acog.org or e-mail at resources@acog.org
- American Society of Reproductive Medicine: www.asrm.org or e-mail at asrm@asrm.org
- Center for Endometriosis Care: http://www. centerforendo.com/
- Endometriosis Association: www.endometriosisassn.org or www.KillerCramps.org
- Endometriosis Association support groups: e-mail at support@endometriosisassn.org
- NICHD Information Resource Center: www.nichd. nih.gov or e-mail at NICHDClearinghouse@ mail.nih.gov
- National Women's Health Information Center (Dept. of Health and Human Services): http://www.4women.gov

---

EVIDENCE-BASED PRACTICE 4.1
The Effectiveness of Danazol Compared to Placebo or No Treatment in the Treatment of the Symptoms and Signs (Other than Infertility) of Endometriosis in Women of Reproductive Age

● Study

Endometriosis is defined as the presence of endometrial tissue (stromal and glandular) outside the normal uterine cavity. Conventional medical and surgical treatments for endometriosis aim to remove or decrease deposits of ectopic endometrium. The observation that hyperandrogenic states (an excess of male hormone) induce atrophy of the endometrium has led to the use of androgens in the treatment of endometriosis. Danazol is one of these treatments. The efficacy of danazol is based on its ability to produce a high-androgen/low-estrogen environment (a pseudomenopause), which results in the atrophy of endometriotic implants and thus an improvement in painful symptoms.

Only four trials met the inclusion criteria, and two authors independently extracted data from these trials. All four trials compared danazol to placebo. Two trials used danazol as sole therapy and two trials used danazol as an adjunct to surgery. Although the main outcome was pain improvement, other data relating to laparoscopic scores and hormonal parameters were also collected.

▲ Findings

Treatment with danazol was effective in relieving painful symptoms related to endometriosis when compared to placebo. Laparoscopic scores were improved with danazol treatment when compared with either placebo or no treatment. Side effects were more commonly reported in the patients receiving danazol than those receiving placebo. Thus, danazol is effective in treating the symptoms and signs of endometriosis. However, its use is limited by the occurrence of androgenic side effects.

■ Nursing Implications

According to the results of the study, danazol is an effective treatment for relieving painful symptoms of endometriosis, but it has side effects. As a nurse, it is important to educate the patient about these; they may include clitoral enlargement and masculinization. In addition, the response to the drug may take several weeks or months. Women should be cautioned to report yellowing of the skin (jaundice), fluid retention, shortness of breath, and changes in vaginal bleeding. It is important to stress that there are several effective therapies to treat endometriosis if the side effects are problematic with danazol.

Source: Selak, V., Farquhar, C., Prentice, A., & Singla, A. (2006). Danazol for pelvic pain associated with endometriosis. *Cochrane Library,* Retrieved Feb. 14, 2007, from the CINAHL Plus with Full Text database.

child for granted, but infertility affects over 6 million Americans, or 15% of the reproductive-age population, according to the American Society for Reproductive Medicine (ASRM, 2007). Infertility is a widespread problem that has an emotional, social, and economic impact on couples. Nurses must recognize infertility and understand its causes and treatment options so that they can help couples understand the possibilities as well as the limitations of current therapies. Recent studies found that women wished to be treated with respect and dignity and given appropriate information and support. They wanted their distress recognized and they wanted to feel cared for and to have confidence in health care professionals in situations where outcomes were uncertain. The caring aspect of professional nursing is an essential component of meeting the special needs of these couples (Redshaw, Hockley & Davidson, 2007). Prevention of infertility through education should also be incorporated into any client–nurse interaction.

Cultural Considerations

Cross-culturally, the expectation for couples to reproduce is an accepted norm and the inability to conceive may be considered a violation of this cultural norm. In this context, infertility represents a crisis for the couple. The manner in which different cultures, ethnic groups, and religious groups perceive and manage infertility may be very different. For example, many African-Americans believe that assisted reproductive techniques are unnatural and that they remove the spiritual or divine nature of creation from conception. For this reason, they may seek spiritual rather than medical assistance when trying to conceive. The Hispanic culture believes that children validate the marriage, so families are typically large. Like the African-American culture, Hispanics are very spiritual and may consider infertility a test of faith and seek spiritual counseling.

Religion often influences cultural factors and for this reason may also be considered when pursuing treatment for infertility. In the Jewish religion procreation is felt to be an obligation and a responsibility. Roman Catholics have a very restrictive view on the use of assisted reproductive technologies since in their view procreation cannot be separated from the relationship between parents. Thus, children must be created by the physical union between husband and wife and conceived through sexual intercourse (Schenker, 2005). Nurses must be cognizant of the client's cultural and religious background and how it may dictate which, if any, reproductive treatment options are chosen. Nurses need to include this awareness in their counseling of infertile couples.

Etiology and Risk Factors

Multiple known and unknown factors affect fertility. Female-factor infertility is detected in about 40% of cases,

male-factor infertility in about 40% of cases. The remaining 20% fall into a category of combined (both male and female factors) or unexplained infertility. In women, ovarian dysfunction (40%) and tubal/pelvic pathology (40%) are the primary contributing factors to infertility (ASRM, 2007).

Risk factors for infertility include:

- For women:
  - Overweight or underweight (can disrupt hormone function)
  - Hormonal imbalances leading to irregular ovulation
  - Fibroids
  - Tubal blockages
  - Reduced oocyte quality
  - Chromosomal abnormalities
  - Congenital anomalies of the cervix and uterus
  - Immune system disorders
  - Chronic illnesses such as diabetes, thyroid disease, asthma
  - STIs
  - Age older than 27
  - Endometriosis
  - History of PID
  - Smoking and alcohol consumption
  - Multiple miscarriages
  - Psychological stress (Kelly-Weeder & O'Conner, 2006)
- For men:
  - Exposure to toxic substances (lead, mercury, x-rays)
  - Cigarette or marijuana smoke
  - Heavy alcohol consumption
  - Use of prescription drugs for ulcers or psoriasis
  - Exposure of the genitals to high temperatures (hot tubs or saunas)
  - Hernia repair
  - Frequent long-distance cycling
  - STI
  - Undescended testicles (cryptorchidism)
  - Mumps after puberty (Ficorelli & Weeks, 2007)

Therapeutic Management

The test results are presented to the couple and different treatment options are suggested. The majority of infertility cases are treated with drugs or surgery. Various ovulation-enhancement drugs and timed intercourse might be used for the woman with ovulation problems. The woman should understand the drug's benefits and side effects before consenting to take them. Depending on the type of drug used and the dosage, some women may experience multiple births. If the woman's reproductive organs are damaged, surgery can be done to repair them. Still other couples might opt for the hi-tech approaches of artificial insemination (Fig. 4.2), in vitro fertilization (IVF; Fig. 4.3), and egg donation or contract for a gestational

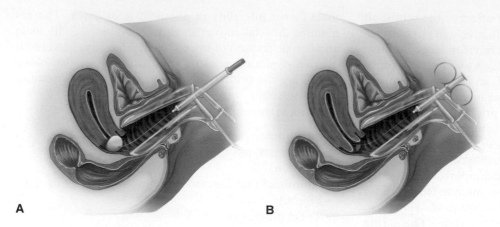

A   **B**

FIGURE 4.2 Artificial insemination. Sperm are deposited next to the cervix (**A**) or injected directly into the uterine cavity (**B**).

carrier or surrogate (Grainger, Frazier & Rowland, 2006). Table 4.3 lists selected infertility options.

Nursing Assessment

Infertile couples are under tremendous pressure and often keep the problem a secret, considering it to be very personal. The couple is often beset by feelings of inadequacy and guilt, and many are subject to pressures from both family and friends. As their problem becomes more chronic, they may begin to blame one another, with consequent marital discord. Seeking help is often a very difficult step for them, and it may take a lot of courage to discuss something about which they feel deeply embarrassed or upset. The nurse working in this specialty setting must be aware of the conflict and problems couples present with and must be very sensitive to their needs.

A full medical history should be taken from both partners, along with a physical examination. The data needed for the infertility evaluation are very sensitive and of a personal nature, so the nurse must use very professional interviewing skills.

There are numerous causes of and contributing factors to infertility, so it is important to use the process of elimination, determining what problems don't exist to better comprehend the problems that do exist. At the first visit, a plan of investigation is outlined and a complete health history is taken. This first visit forces many couples to confront the reality that their desired pregnancy may not occur naturally. Alleviate some of the anxiety associated with diagnostic testing by explaining the timing and reasons for each test.

Assessing Male Factors

The initial screening evaluation for the male partner should include a reproductive history and a semen analysis. From the male perspective, three things must happen for conception to take place: there must be an adequate number of sperm; those sperm must be healthy and mature; and the sperm must be able to penetrate and fertilize the egg. Normal males need to have more than 20 million sperm per milliliter with greater than 50% motility (WHO, 2007). Semen analysis is the most important indicator of male fertility. The man should abstain from

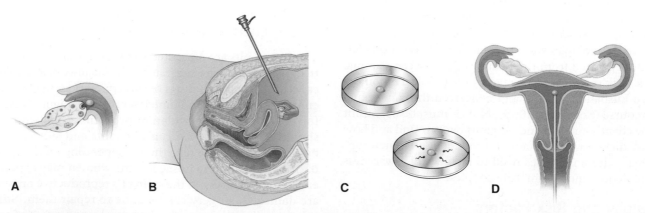

A   **B**   **C**   **D**

FIGURE 4.3 Steps involved in in vitro fertilization. (**A**) Ovulation. (**B**) Capture of the ova (done here intra-abdominally). (**C**) Fertilization of ova and growth in culture medium. (**D**) Insertion of fertilized ova into uterus.

CHAPTER 4 COMMON REPRODUCTIVE ISSUES 77

TABLE 4.3 SELECTED TREATMENT OPTIONS FOR INFERTILITY

Procedure	Comments	Nursing Considerations
Fertility drugs		
Clomiphene citrate (Clomid)	A nonsteroidal synthetic antiestrogen used to induce ovulation	Nurse can advise the couple to have intercourse every other day for 1 week starting after day 5 of medication.
Human menopausal gonadotropin (HMG); Pergonal	Induces ovulation by direct stimulation of ovarian follicle	Same as above
Artificial insemination	The insertion of a prepared semen sample into the cervical os or intrauterine cavity Enables sperm to be deposited closer to improve chances of conception Husband or donor sperm can be used	Nurse needs to advise couple that the procedure might need to be repeated if not successful the first time.
Assisted reproductive technologies*		
In vitro fertilization (IVF)	Oocytes are fertilized in the lab and transferred to the uterus. Usually indicated for tubal obstruction, endometriosis, pelvic adhesions, and low sperm counts	Nurse advises woman to take medication to stimulate ovulation so the mature ovum can be retrieved by needle aspiration.
Gamete intrafallopian transfer (GIFT)	Oocytes and sperm are combined and immediately placed in the fallopian tube so fertilization can occur naturally. Requires laparoscopy and general anesthesia, which increases risk	Nurse needs to inform couple of risks and have consent signed.
Intracytoplasmic sperm injection (ICSI)	One sperm is injected into the cytoplasm of the oocyte to fertilize it. Indicated for male factor infertility.	Nurse needs to inform the male that sperm will be aspirated by a needle through the skin into the epididymis.
Donor oocytes or sperm	Eggs or sperm are retrieved from a donor and the eggs are inseminated; resulting embryos are transferred via IVF. Recommended for women older than 40 and those with poor-quality eggs.	Nurse needs to support couple in their ethical/religious discussions prior to deciding.
Gestational carrier (surrogacy)	Laboratory fertilization takes place and embryos are transferred to the uterus of another woman, who will carry the pregnancy. Medical-legal issues have resulted over the "true ownership" of the resulting infant.	Nurse should encourage an open discussion regarding implications of this method with the couple.

*When other options have been exhausted, these are considered.

sexual activity for 24 to 48 hours before giving the sample. For a semen examination, the man is asked to produce a specimen by ejaculating into a specimen container and delivering it to the laboratory for analysis within 1 to 2 hours. When the specimen is brought to the laboratory, it is analyzed for volume, viscosity, number of sperm, sperm viability, motility, and sperm shape. If semen parameters are normal, no further male evaluation is necessary (Quallich, 2006).

The physical examination routinely includes:

• Assessment for appropriate male sexual characteristics, such as body hair distribution, development of the Adam's apple, and muscle development

- Examination of the penis, scrotum, testicles, epididymis, and vas deferens for abnormalities (e.g., nodules, irregularities, varicocele)
- Assessment for normal development of external genitalia (small testicles)
- Performance of a digital internal examination of the prostate to check for tenderness or swelling (DeMasters, 2004)

Assessing Female Factors

The initial assessment of the woman should include a thorough history of factors associated with ovulation and the pelvic organs. Diagnostic tests to determine female infertility may include:

- Assessment of ovarian function
  - Menstrual history: regularity of cycles
  - Ovulation predictor kits used midcycle
  - Urinary LH level
  - Clomiphene citrate challenge test
  - Endometrial biopsy to document luteal phase
- Assessment of pelvic organs
  - Papanicolaou (Pap) smear to rule out cervical cancer or inflammation
  - Cervical culture to rule out Chlamydia infection
  - Postcoital testing to evaluate sperm–cervical mucus interaction
  - Ultrasound to assess pelvic structures
  - Hysterosalpingography to visualize structural defects
  - Laparoscopy to visualize pelvic structures and diagnose endometriosis

Laboratory and Diagnostic Testing

The diagnostic procedures that should be done during an infertility workup should be guided by the couple's history. They generally proceed from less to more invasive tests.

Home Ovulation Predictor Kits

Home ovulation predictor kits contain monoclonal antibodies specific for LH and use the ELISA test to determine the amount of LH present in the urine. A significant color change from baseline indicates the LH surge and presumably the most fertile day of the month for the woman.

Clomiphene Citrate Challenge Test

The clomiphene citrate challenge test is used to assess a woman's ovarian reserve (ability of her eggs to become fertilized). FSH levels are drawn on cycle day 3 and on cycle day 10 after the woman has taken 100 mg clomiphene citrate on cycle days 5 through 9. If the FSH level is greater than 15, the result is considered abnormal and the likelihood of conception with her own eggs is very low (Schuiling & Likis, 2006).

Endometrial Biopsy

Another assessment of ovulation that indicates whether the secretion of progesterone is adequate is an endometrial biopsy. A strip of endometrial tissue is removed just before menstruation. Histologic documentation of secretory endometrial development implies that ovulation has taken place. An endometrium that does not conform to the normal histologic pattern indicates a defect in the luteal phase.

Postcoital Testing

Postcoital testing is done to assess the receptivity of the cervical mucus to sperm. Cervical mucus from the woman is examined 2 to 8 hours after intercourse during the expected time of ovulation, and the number of live, motile sperm present is assessed. Cervical mucus is also evaluated for stretchability (spinnbarkeit) and consistency (Alexander et al., 2007). The results are described in Comparison Chart 4.1.

Hysterosalpingogram

In a hysterosalpingogram, 3 to 10 mL of an opaque contrast medium is slowly injected through a catheter into the endocervical canal so that the uterus and tubes can be visualized during fluoroscopy and radiography. If the fallopian tubes are patent, the dye will ascend upward to distend the uterus and the tubes and will spill out into the peritoneal cavity (Fig. 4.4).

Laparoscopy

A laparoscopy is usually performed early in the menstrual cycle. During the procedure, an endoscope is inserted through a small incision in the anterior abdominal wall. Visualization of the peritoneal cavity in an infertile woman may reveal endometriosis, pelvic adhesions, tubal occlusion, fibroids, or polycystic ovaries (DeSutter, 2006).

Nursing Management

Nurses play an important role in the care of infertile couples. They are pivotal educators about preventive health care. There are a number of potentially modifiable risk

COMPARISON CHART 4.1 **NORMAL VERSUS ABNORMAL POSTCOITAL TEST RESULTS**

Normal	Abnormal
Normal amounts of sperm are seen in the sample.	No sperm or a large percentage of dead sperm are seen in the sample.
Sperm are moving forward through the cervical mucus.	Sperm are clumped.
The mucus stretches at least 2 in (5 cm).	Mucus cannot stretch 2 in (5 cm).
The mucus dries in a fernlike pattern.	Mucus does not dry in a fernlike pattern.

Source: DeSutter, 2006.

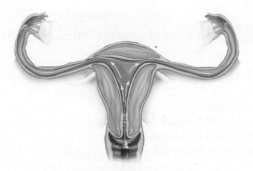

FIGURE 4.4 Insertion of a dye for a hystero-salpingogram. The contrast dye outlines the uterus and fallopian tubes on an x-ray to demonstrate patency.

factors associated with the development of impaired fertility in women, and women need to be aware of these risks to institute change. The nurse is most effective when he or she offers care and treatment in a professional manner and regards the couple as valued and respected individuals. The nurse's focus must encompass the whole person, not just the results of the various infertility studies. Throughout the entire process, the nurse's role is to provide information, anticipatory guidance, stress management, and counseling. The couple's emotional distress is usually very high, and the nurse must be able to recognize that anxiety and provide emotional support. The nurse may need to refer couples to a reproductive endocrinologist or surgeon, depending on the problem identified.

There is no absolute way to prevent infertility per se because so many factors are involved in conception. Nurses can be instrumental in educating men and women about the factors that contribute to infertility. The nurse can also outline the risks and benefits of treatments so that the couple can make an informed decision.

With advances in genetics and reproductive medicine also come a myriad of ethical, social, and cultural issues that will affect the couple's decisions. With this in mind, provide an opportunity for the couple to make informed decisions in a nondirective, nonjudgmental environment. It is important to encourage couples to remain optimistic throughout investigation and treatment. Through the use of advocacy and anticipatory guidance, assist and support couples through the diagnosis and treatment of infertility (Jenkins & Jenkins, 2006).

Finances and insurance coverage often dictate the choice of treatment. Help couples decipher their insurance coverage and help them weigh the costs of various procedures by explaining what each will provide in terms of information about their infertility problems. Assisting them to make a priority list of diagnostic tests and potential treatment options will help the couple plan their financial strategy.

Many infertile couples are not prepared for the emotional roller coaster of grief and loss during infertility treatments. Financial concerns and coping as a couple are

---

BOX 4.4 Organizations and Web Resources to Assist the Client With Infertility

- Resolve: A nationwide network of chapters dedicated to providing education, advocacy, and support for men and women facing infertility. They provide a helpline, medical referral services, and a member-to-member contact system. (http://www.resolve.org)
- American Society of Reproductive Medicine (ASRM): Provides fact sheets and other resources on infertility, treatments, insurance, and other issues (http://www.asrm.org)
- International Counsel on Infertility (INCIID): Provides information about infertility, support forums, and a directory of infertility specialists (http://www.inciid.org)
- American Fertility Association: Offers education, referrals, research, support, and advocacy for couples dealing with infertility (http://www.americaninfertility.org)
- Bertarelli Foundation: The Human Face of Infertility: Aims to promote and improve understanding of infertility by offering resources (http://www.bertarelli.edu)
- International Consumer Support for Infertility: An international network engaged in advocacy on behalf of infertile couples via fact sheets and information (http://www.icsi.ws)

---

two major areas of stress when treatment is undertaken. During the course of what may be months or even years of infertility care, it is essential to develop a holistic approach to nursing care. Stress management and anxiety reduction need to be addressed, and referral to a peer support group such as Resolve might be in order (Box 4.4).

▶ **Consider** THIS!

We had been married for 3 years and wanted to start a family, but much to our dismay nothing happened after a year of trying. I had some irregular periods and was finally diagnosed with endometriosis and put on Clomid. After 3 years of taking Clomid on and off, I went to a fertility expert. The doctor lasered the endometriosis tissue, sent air through my tubes to make sure they were patent, and put me back on Clomid, but still with no luck. Finally, 2 years later, we were put on an IVF waiting list and prayed we would have the money for the procedure when we were chosen. By then I felt a failure as a woman. We then decided that it was more important for us to be parents than it was for me to be pregnant, so we considered adoption. We tried for another year without any results.

We went to the adoption agency to fill out the paperwork for the process to begin. Our blood was

(continued)

▶ *Consider* THIS! *(continued)*

taken and we waited for an hour, wondering the whole time why it was taking so long for the results. The nurse finally appeared and handed a piece of paper to me with the word "positive" written on it. I started to cry tears of joy, for a pregnancy had started and our long journey of infertility was finally ending.

Thoughts: For many women the dream of having a child is not easily realized. Infertility can affect self-esteem, disrupt relationships, and result in depression. This couple experienced many years of frustration in trying to have a family. What help can be offered to couples during this time? What can be said to comfort the woman who feels she is a failure?

Contraception

In the United States, there are approximately 62 million women in their childbearing years, ages 15 to 44. Overall, 64% of those 60 million women use contraception, but still more than 3 million unintended pregnancies occur every year (CDC, 2006). Although numerous fertility control methods are available, the United States continues to have a higher unintended pregnancy rate than other Western countries. Every minute of every day, 10 people become infected with HIV, most through heterosexual contact; 190 women conceive an unwanted pregnancy; 1 woman dies from a pregnancy-related cause; and 40 women undergo unsafe abortions, as outlined in the UNFPA State of the World Population 2006 Report. Much of this suffering could be prevented by access to safe, efficient, appropriate, modern contraception for everyone who wants it (UNFPA, 2007).

Contraception is any method that prevents conception or childbirth. A woman's reproductive life spans almost 40 years, and throughout those years, a variety of contraceptive methods may be used. Oral contraceptives, sterilization of the female, and the male condom are the most popular methods in the United States (Alan Guttmacher Institute, 2007).

Couples must decide which method is appropriate for them to meet their changing contraceptive needs throughout their life cycles. Nurses can educate and assist couples during this selection process. This part of the chapter will outline the most common birth control methods available.

In an era when many women wish to delay pregnancy and avoid STIs, choices are difficult. There are numerous methods available today, and many more will be offered in the near future. The ideal contraceptive method for many women would have to have the following characteristics: ease of use, safety, effectiveness, minimal side effects, "naturalness," nonhormonal method, and immediate reversibility (Samra & Wood, 2006). Currently, no one contraceptive method offers everything. Box 4.5 outlines the contraceptive methods available today. Table 4.4 provides a detailed summary of each type, including information on failure rates, advantages, disadvantages, STI protection, and danger signs.

BOX 4.5 Outline of Contraceptive Methods

Reversible Methods
Behavioral
• Abstinence
• Fertility awareness
• Withdrawal (coitus interruptus)
• Lactational amenorrhea method (LAM)

Barrier
• Condom (male and female)
• Diaphragm
• Cervical cap
• Sponge

Hormonal
• Oral contraceptives
• Injectable contraceptive
• Transdermal patches
• Vaginal ring
• Implantable contraceptives
• Intrauterine systems
• Emergency contraceptives

Permanent Methods
• Tubal ligation for women
• Vasectomy for men

Types of Contraceptive Methods

Contraceptives methods can be divided into three types: behavioral methods, barrier methods, and hormonal methods.

Behavioral Methods
Behavioral methods refer to any natural contraceptive method that does not require hormones, pharmaceutical compounds, physical barriers, or surgery to prevent pregnancy. These methods require couples to take an active role in preventing pregnancy through their sexual behaviors.

Abstinence
Abstinence (not having vaginal or anal intercourse) is one of the least expensive forms of contraception and has been used for thousands of years. Basically, pregnancy cannot occur if sperm is kept out of the vagina. It also reduces the risk of contracting HIV/AIDS and other STIs, unless body fluids are exchanged through oral sex; however, some infections, like herpes and HPV, can be passed by skin-to-skin contact. There are many pleasurable

(text continues on page 86)

TABLE 4.4 **SUMMARY OF CONTRACEPTIVE METHODS**

Type	Description	Failure Rate	Pros	Cons	STI Protection	Danger Signs	Comments
Abstinence	Refrain from sexual activity	None	Costs nothing	Difficult to maintain	100%	None	Must be joint couple decision
Fertility awareness	Refrain from sex during fertile period	25%	No side effects; acceptable to most religious groups	High failure rate with incorrect use	None	None	Requires high level of couple commitment
Withdrawal (coitus interruptus)	Man withdraws before ejaculation	27%	Involves no devices and is always available	Requires considerable self-control by the man	None	None	Places woman in trusting and dependent role
Lactational amenorrhea method (LAM)	Uses lactational infertility for protection from pregnancy	1–2% chance of pregnancy in first 6 months	No cost; not coitus-linked	Temporary method; effective for only 6 months after giving birth	None	None	Mother must breastfeed infant on demand without supplementation for 6 months
Male condom	Thin sheath placed over an erect penis, blocking sperm	15%	Widely available; low cost; physiologically safe	Decreased sensation for man; interferes with sexual spontaneity; breakage risk	Provides protection against STIs	Latex allergy	Couple must be instructed on proper use of condom
Female condom	Polyurethane sheath inserted vaginally to block sperm	21%	Use controlled by woman; eliminates postcoital drainage of semen	Expensive for frequent use; cumbersome; noisy during sex act; for single use only	Provides protection against STIs	Allergy to polyurethane	Couple must be instructed on proper use of condom
Diaphragm with spermicide	Shallow latex cup with spring mechanism in its rim to hold it in place in the vagina	16%	Does not use hormone; considered medically safe; provides some protection against cervical cancer	Requires accurate fitting by health care professional; increase in UTIs	None	Allergy to latex, rubber, polyurethane, or spermicide. Report symptoms of toxic shock syndrome. Change size if excessive weight gain or loss.	Woman must be taught to insert and remove diaphragm correctly

(continued)

TABLE 4.4 **SUMMARY OF CONTRACEPTIVE METHODS** (continued)

Type	Description	Failure Rate	Pros	Cons	STI Protection	Danger Signs	Comments
Cervical cap with spermicide	Soft cup-shaped latex device that fits over base of cervix	24%	No use of hormones; provides continuous protection while in place	Requires accurate fitting by health care professional; odor may occur if left in too long	None	Irritation, allergic reaction; abnormal Pap test; risk of toxic shock syndrome	Instructions on insertion and removal must be understood by client
Sponge with spermicide	Disk-shaped polyurethane device containing a spermicide that is activated by wetting it with water	25%	Offers immediate and continuous protection for 24 hours; OTC	Can fall out of vagina with voiding; is not form-fitting in the vagina	None	Irritation, allergic reactions; toxic shock syndrome can occur if sponge left in too long	Caution woman not to leave sponge in beyond 24 hours
Oral contraceptives (combination)	A pill that suppresses ovulation by combined action of estrogen and progestin	8%	Easy to use; high rate of effectiveness; protection against ovarian and endometrial cancer	User must remember to take pill daily; possible undesirable side effects; high cost for some women; prescription needed	None	Dizziness, nausea, mood changes, high blood pressure, blood clots, heart attacks, strokes	Each woman must be assessed thoroughly to make sure she is not a smoker and does not have a history of thromboembolic disease
Oral contraceptives (progestin-only minipills)	A pill containing only progestin that thickens cervical mucus to prevent sperm from penetrating	8%	No estrogen-related side effects; may be used by lactating women; may be used by women with history of thrombophlebitis	Must be taken with meticulous accuracy; may cause irregular bleeding; less effective than combination pills	None	Irregular bleeding, weight gain, increased incidence of ectopic pregnancy	Women should be screened for history of functional ovarian cysts, previous ectopic pregnancy, hyperlipidemia prior to giving prescription

Method	Description		Advantages	Disadvantages		Side Effects	Nursing Considerations
Lunelle injectable	An injectable form of progestin and estrogen given monthly	3%	Woman will regain fertility 2–3 months after last injection; no need for daily pill taking	Must make arrangements for monthly injection; possible weight gain	None	Irregular spotting; similar to oral combination pills	Screen woman's ability to schedule monthly appointment for injection
Patch (Ortho Evra)	Transdermal patch that releases estrogen and progestin into circulation	8%	Easy system to remember; very effective	May cause skin irritation where it is placed; may fall off and not be noticed and thus provide no protection	None	Less effective in women weighing more than 200 pounds	Instruct woman to apply patch every week for 3 weeks and then not to wear one during week 4
Ring (NuvaRing)	Vaginal contraceptive ring about 2 inches in diameter that is inserted into the vagina; releases estrogen and progestin	8%	Easy system to remember; very effective	May cause a vaginal discharge; can be expelled without noticing and not offer protection	None	Similar to oral contraceptives	Instruct woman to use a backup method if ring is expelled and remains out for more than 3 hours
Depo-Provera injection	An injectable progestin that inhibits ovulation	3%	Long duration of action (3 months); highly effective; estrogen-free; may be used by smokers; can be used by lactating women	Menstrual irregularities; return visit needed every 12 weeks; weight gain, headaches, depression; return to fertility delayed up to 12 months	None	If depression is a problem, this method may increase the depression.	Inform woman that fertility is delayed after stopping the injections

(continued)

TABLE 4.4 SUMMARY OF CONTRACEPTIVE METHODS (continued)

Type	Description	Failure Rate	Pros	Cons	STI Protection	Danger Signs	Comments
Implant (Implanon)	A time-release implant (one rod) of levonorgestrel for 3 years	0.05%	Long duration of action; low dose of hormones; reversible; estrogen-free	Irregular bleeding; weight gain; breast tenderness; headaches; difficulty in removal	None	If bleeding is heavy, anemia may occur.	Before insertion, assess woman to make sure she is aware that this method will produce about 3–5 years of infertility
Intrauterine systems (IUSs)	A T-shaped device inserted into the uterus that releases copper or progesterone or levonorgestrel	1%	It is immediately and highly effective; allows for sexual spontaneity; can be used during lactation; return to fertility not impaired; requires no motivation by the user after insertion	Insertion requires a skilled professional; menstrual irregularities; prolonged amenorrhea; can be unknowingly expelled; may increase the risk of pelvic infection; user must regularly check string for placement; no protection against STIs; delay of fertility after discontinuing for possibly 6 to 12 months	None	Cramps, bleeding, pelvic inflammatory disease; infertility; perforation of the uterus	Instruct woman how to locate string to check monthly for placement

Method	Description	Effectiveness	Advantages	Disadvantages		Side effects	Patient education
Postcoital emergency contraceptives (ECs)	Combination of progestin-only pills taken within 72 hours after unprotected intercourse	80%	Provides a last chance to prevent a pregnancy	Risk of ectopic pregnancy if EC fails	None	Nausea, vomiting, abdominal pain, fatigue, headache	Inform woman that ECs do not interrupt an established pregnancy, and the sooner they are taken the more effective they are
Permanent sterilization							
Male	Sealing, tying, or cutting the vas deferens	<1%	One-time decision provides permanent sterility; short recovery time; low long-term risks	Procedures are difficult to reverse; initial cost may be high; chance of regret; some pain/discomfort after procedures	None for both	Postoperative complications: pain, bleeding, infection	Counsel both as to permanence of procedure and urge them to think it through prior to signing consent
Female	Fallopian tubes are blocked to prevent conception	<1%					

Sources: Samra, 2006; FDA, 2006; Youngkin & Davis, 2004; Hatcher, 2004.

options for sex play without intercourse ("outercourse"), such as kissing, masturbation, erotic massage, sexual fantasy, sex toys such as vibrators, and oral sex.

Many people have strong feelings about abstinence based on religious and moral beliefs. There are many good and personal reasons to choose abstinence. For some it is a way of life, while for others it is a temporary choice. Some people choose abstinence because they want to:

- Wait until they are older
- Wait for a long-term relationship
- Avoid pregnancy or STIs
- Follow religious or cultural expectations

Fertility Awareness

Fertility awareness is a natural method of contraception in which no contraceptive devices are used; instead, certain observations, techniques, and calculations are used to determine the "fertile" and the "safe" periods in a monthly menstrual cycle. There are normal physiologic changes caused by hormonal fluctuations during the menstrual cycle that can be observed and charted. This information can be used to avoid or promote pregnancy. Fertility awareness methods rely upon the following assumptions:

- A single ovum is released from the ovary 14 days before the next menstrual period. It lives approximately 24 hours.
- Sperm can live up to 5 days after intercourse. The "unsafe period" during the menstrual cycle is thus approximately 6 days: 3 days before and 3 days after ovulation. Since bodily changes start to occur before ovulation, the woman can become aware of them and not have intercourse on these days or use another method to prevent pregnancy.
- The exact time of ovulation cannot be determined, so 2 to 3 days are added to the beginning and end to avoid pregnancy.

Techniques used to determine fertility include the cervical mucus ovulation method, the basal body temperature (BBT) method, and the symptothermal method (Hatcher et al., 2004). Fertility awareness methods are moderately effective but are very unforgiving if not carried out as prescribed: not following the guidelines might cause a 27% failure or pregnancy rate per cycle (Murphy, Morgan & Likis, 2006). Fertility awareness can be used in combination with coital abstinence or barrier methods during fertile days if pregnancy is not desired.

Cervical Mucus Ovulation Method

The **cervical mucus ovulation method** is used to assess the character of the cervical mucus. Cervical mucus changes in consistency during the menstrual cycle and plays a vital role in fertilization of the egg. In the days preceding ovulation, fertile cervical mucus helps draw sperm up and into the fallopian tubes, where fertilization usually takes place. It also helps maintain the survival of sperm.

As ovulation approaches, the mucus becomes more abundant, clear, slippery, and smooth; it can be stretched between two fingers without breaking. Under the influence of estrogen, this mucus looks like egg whites. It is called spinnbarkeit mucus (Fig. 4.5). After ovulation, the cervical mucus becomes thick and dry under the influence of progesterone.

The cervical position can also be assessed to confirm changes in the cervical mucus at ovulation. Near ovulation, the cervix feels soft and is high/deep in the vagina, the os is slightly open, and the cervical mucus is copious and slippery (Hatcher et al., 2004).

This method works because the woman becomes aware of her body changes that accompany ovulation. When she notices them, she abstains from sexual intercourse or uses another method to prevent pregnancy. Each woman is an individual, so each woman's unsafe time of the month is unique and thus must be individually assessed and determined.

Basal Body Temperature

The **basal body temperature** (BBT) refers to the lowest temperature reached upon wakening. The woman takes her temperature orally before rising and records it on a chart. Preovulation temperatures are suppressed by estrogen, whereas postovulation temperatures are increased under the influence of heat-inducing progesterone. Temperatures typically rise within a day or two after ovulation and remain elevated for approximately 2 weeks (at which point bleeding usually begins). If using this method by itself, the woman should avoid unprotected intercourse until the BBT has been elevated for 3 days. Other fertility awareness methods should be used along with BBT for better results (Fig. 4.6).

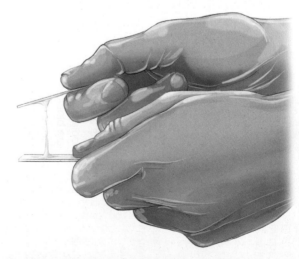

FIGURE **4.5** Spinnbarkeit is the ability of cervical mucus to stretch a distance before breaking.

Basal body temperature

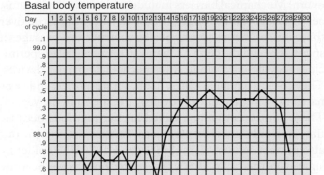

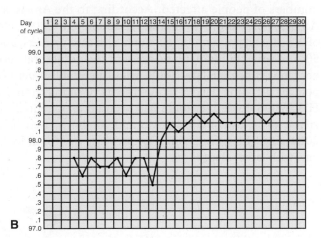

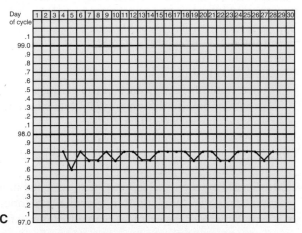

FIGURE **4.6** Basal body temperature graph. (**A**) The woman's temperature dips slightly at midpoint in the menstrual cycle, then rises sharply, an indication of ovulation. Toward the end of the cycle (the 24th day), her temperature begins to decline, indicating that progesterone levels are falling and that she did not conceive. (**B**) The woman's temperature rises at the midpoint in the cycle and remains at that elevated level past the time of her normal menstrual flow, suggesting that pregnancy has occurred. (**C**) There is no preovulatory dip and no rise of temperature anywhere during the cycle. This is the typical pattern of a woman who does not ovulate.

Symptothermal Method

The **symptothermal method** relies on a combination of techniques to recognize ovulation, including BBT, cervical mucus changes, alterations in the position and firmness of the cervix, and other symptoms of ovulation, such as increased libido, mittelschmerz, pelvic fullness or tenderness, and breast tenderness (Dirubbo, 2006). Combining all these predictors increases awareness of when ovulation occurs and increases the effectiveness of this method. A home predictor test for ovulation is also available in most pharmacies. It measures LH levels to pinpoint the day before or the day of ovulation. These tests are widely used for fertility and infertility regimens.

The Standard Days Method and the Two-Day Method

The **Standard Days Method (SDM)** and the Two-Day Method are both natural methods of contraception developed by Georgetown University Medical Center's Institute for Reproductive Health. Both methods provide women with simple, clear instructions for identifying fertile days. Women with menstrual cycles between 26 and 32 days long can use the SDM to prevent pregnancy by avoiding unprotected intercourse on days 8 through 19 of their cycles. An international clinical trial of the SDM showed that the method is more than 95% effective when used correctly (Sinai, Arevalo & Jennings, 2006). SDM identifies the 12-day "fertile window" of a woman's menstrual cycle. These 12 days takes into account the lifespan of the women's egg (about 24 hours) and the viability of the sperm (about 5 days) as well as the variation in the actual timing of ovulation from one cycle to another. For the Two-Day Method, women observe the presence or absence of cervical secretions by examining toilet paper or underwear or by monitoring their physical sensations. Every day, the woman asks two simple questions "Did I note any secretions yesterday?" and "Did I note any secretions today?" If the answer to either question is yes, she considers herself fertile and avoids unprotected intercourse. If the answers are no, she is unlikely to become pregnant from unprotected intercourse on that day (Sinai, Arevalo & Jennings, 2006).

To help women keep track of the days on which they should avoid unprotected intercourse, a string of 32 color-coded beads (CycleBeads) is used, with each bead representing a day of the menstrual cycle. Starting with the red bead, which represents the first day of her menstrual period, the woman moves a small rubber ring one bead each day. The brown beads are the days when pregnancy is unlikely, and the white beads represent her fertile days (Arevalo, 2007). This method has been used in underdeveloped countries for women with limited educational resources (Fig. 4.7).

Withdrawal (Coitus Interruptus)

In **coitus interruptus**, also known as withdrawal, a man controls his ejaculation during sexual intercourse and ejaculates outside the vagina. It is better known colloquially as

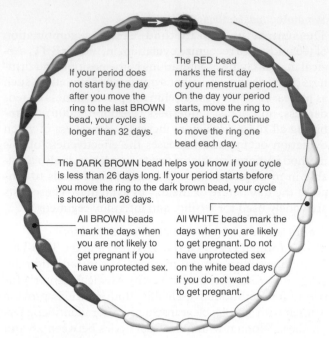

FIGURE **4.7** CycleBeads help women use the Standard Days Method.

"pulling out in time" or "being careful." It is one of the oldest and most widely used means of preventing pregnancy in the world (Murphy, Morgan & Likis, 2006). The problem with this method is that the first few drops of the true ejaculate contain the greatest concentration of sperm, and if some pre-ejaculatory fluid escapes from the urethra before orgasm, conception may result. This method requires that the woman rely solely on the cooperation and judgment of the man.

Lactational Amenorrhea Method

The **lactational amenorrhea method (LAM)** is an effective temporary method of contraception used by breastfeeding mothers. Continuous breastfeeding can postpone ovulation and thus prevent pregnancy. Breastfeeding stimulates the hormone prolactin, which is necessary for milk production, and also inhibits the release of another hormone, gonadotropin, which is necessary for ovulation.

Breastfeeding as a contraceptive method can be effective for 6 months after delivery only if a woman:

- Has not had a period since she gave birth
- Breastfeeds her baby at least six times daily on both breasts
- Breastfeeds her baby "on demand" at least every 4 hours
- Does not substitute other foods for a breast-milk meal
- Provides nighttime feedings at least every 6 hours
- Does not rely on this method after 6 months (Planned Parenthood, 2007)

Barrier Methods

Barrier contraceptives are forms of birth control that prevent pregnancy by preventing the sperm from reaching the ovum. Mechanical barriers include condoms, diaphragms, cervical caps, and sponges. These devices are placed over the penis or cervix to physically obstruct the passage of sperm through the cervix. Chemical barriers called spermicides may be used along with mechanical barrier devices. They come in creams, jellies, foam, suppositories, and vaginal films. They chemically destroy the sperm in the vagina. These contraceptives are called barrier methods because they not only provide a physical barrier for sperm, but also protect against STIs. Since the HIV/AIDS epidemic started in the early 1980s, these methods have become extremely popular.

Many of these barrier methods contain latex. Allergy to latex was first recognized in the late 1970s, and since then it has become a major health concern, with increasing numbers of people affected. According to the American Academy of Allergy, Asthma and Immunology (2007), 6% of the general population, 10% of health care workers, and 50% of spina bifida patients are sensitive to natural rubber latex. Since the late 1980s, with the establishment of policies dictating barrier requirements resulting from the HIV/AIDS epidemic, there has been an exponential increase in the use of latex gloves and condoms (Lenehan, 2004). Teaching Guidelines 4.4 provides tips for individuals with latex allergy.

TEACHING GUIDELINES 4.4

Tips for Individuals Allergic to Latex

- Symptoms of latex allergy include:
  - Skin rash, itching, hives
  - Itching or burning eyes
  - Swollen mucous membranes in the genitals
  - Shortness of breath, difficulty breathing, wheezing
  - Anaphylactic shock (OSHA, 2006)
- Use of or contact with latex condoms, cervical caps, and diaphragms is contraindicated for men and women with a latex allergy.
- If the female partner is allergic to latex, have the male partner apply a natural condom over the latex one.
- If the male partner experiences penile irritation after condom use, try different brands or place the latex condom over a natural condom.
- Use polyurethane condoms rather than latex ones.
- Use female condoms; they are made of polyurethane.
- Switch to another birth control method that isn't made with latex, such as oral contraceptives, intrauterine systems, Depo-Provera, fertility awareness, and other non-barrier methods. However, these methods do not protect against sexually transmitted infections.

Condoms

Condoms are barrier methods of contraceptives made for both males and females. The male condom is made from latex or polyurethane or natural membrane and may be coated with spermicide. Male condoms are available in many colors, textures, sizes, shapes, and thicknesses. When used correctly, the male condom is put on over an erect penis before it enters the vagina and is worn throughout sexual intercourse (Fig. 4.8). It serves as a barrier to pregnancy by trapping seminal fluid and sperm and offers protection against STIs. Condoms are not perfect barriers, though, because breakage and slippage can occur. In addition, the non-latex condoms have a higher risk of pregnancy and STIs than latex condoms (Gallo, Grimes, Lopez & Schultz, 2006).

The female condom is a polyurethane pouch inserted into the vagina. It consists of an outer and inner ring that is inserted vaginally and held in place by the pubic bone. Some women complain that the female condom is cumbersome to use and makes noise during intercourse. Female condoms are readily available, are inexpensive, and can be carried inconspicuously by the woman. The female condom was the first woman-controlled method that offered protection against pregnancy and some STIs.

Diaphragm

The **diaphragm** is a soft latex dome surrounded by a metal spring. Used in conjunction with a spermicidal jelly or cream, it is inserted into the vagina to cover the cervix (Fig. 4.9). The diaphragm may be inserted up to 4 hours before intercourse but must be left in place for at least 6 hours afterwards. Diaphragms are available in a range of sizes and styles. The diaphragm is available only by prescription and must be professionally fitted by

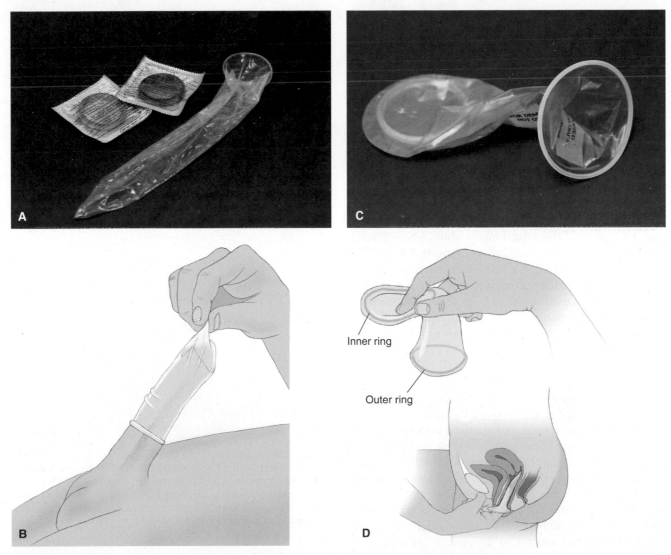

Inner ring

Outer ring

FIGURE 4.8 (**A**) Male condom. (**B**) Applying a male condom. Leaving space at the tip helps to ensure the condom will not break with ejaculation. (**C**) The female condom. (**D**) Insertion technique.

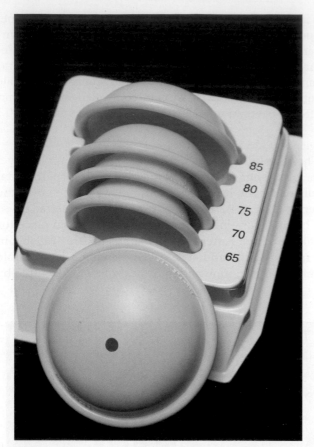

FIGURE 4.9 Sample diaphragm used for measuring.

a health care professional. Women may need to be refitted with a different-sized diaphragm after pregnancy, abdominal or pelvic surgery, or weight loss or gain of 10 pounds or more. As a general rule, diaphragms should be replaced every 1 to 2 years (Female Contraception, 2006). The woman also needs to receive thorough instruction about its use and should practice putting it in and taking it out before she leaves the medical office (Fig. 4.10). Diaphragms are user-controlled, nonhormonal methods that are needed only at the time of intercourse, but they are not effective unless used correctly.

Cervical Cap

The **cervical cap** is smaller than the diaphragm and covers only the cervix; it is held in place by suction. Caps are made from silicone or latex and are used with spermicide (Fig. 4.11). The Prentif cap and the FemCap are the only cervical cap devices approved in the United States currently (Gallo, Grimes & Schultz, 2006). The cap may be inserted up to 12 hours before intercourse and provides protection for 48 hours. The cap must be kept in the vagina for 8 hours after the final act of intercourse and should be replaced every 1 to 2 years. A refitting may also be necessary when a women experiences pregnancy, abortion, or weight changes. The dome of the cap is filled about one-third full with spermicide. Spermicide should

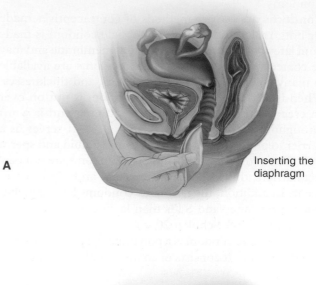

A   Inserting the diaphragm

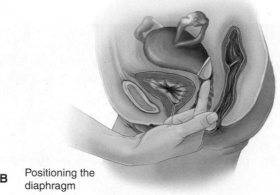

B   Positioning the diaphragm

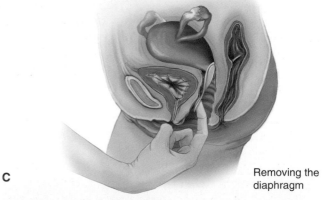

C   Removing the diaphragm

FIGURE 4.10 Application of a diaphragm. (**A**) To insert, fold the diaphragm in half, separate the labia with one hand, then insert upwards and back into the vagina. (**B**) To position, make certain the diaphragm securely covers the cervix. (**C**) To remove, hook a finger over the top of the rim and bring the diaphragm down and out.

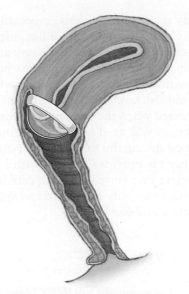

FIGURE 4.11 A cervical cap is placed over the cervix and used with a spermicidal jelly, the same as a diaphragm.

not be applied to the rim because it might interfere with the seal that must form around the cervix. The cap is available only by prescription and must be fitted by a health care professional.

Contraceptive Sponge

The **contraceptive sponge** is a nonhormonal, non-prescription device that includes both a barrier and a spermicide. When it was removed from the market in 1995, it was the most popular over-the-counter female contraceptive in America (Brucker, 2006). The manufacturer, Wyeth, stopped making the sponge rather than upgrade its manufacturing plant after the FDA found deficiencies, but the device's effectiveness and safety were never questioned. After receiving re-approval from the FDA in 2005, the contraceptive sponge is once again being marketed to women.

The contraceptive sponge is a soft polyurethane concave device that prevents pregnancy by covering the cervix and releasing spermicide. While it was less effective than several other methods and does not offer protection against STIs, the sponge achieved a wide following among women who appreciated the spontaneity with which it could be used and its easy availability. To use the sponge, the woman first wets it with water, then inserts it into the vagina with a finger, using a cord loop attachment. It can be inserted up to 24 hours before intercourse and should be left in place for at least 6 hours following intercourse. The sponge provides protection for up to 12 hours, but should not be left in for more than 30 hours after insertion to avoid the risk of toxic shock syndrome (Brucker, 2006). The sponge is a contraceptive method but does not protect against STIs.

Hormonal Methods

Several options are available to women who want long-term but not permanent protection against pregnancy. These methods of contraception work by altering the hormones within a woman's body. They rely on estrogen and progestin or progestin alone to prevent ovulation. When used consistently, these methods are a most reliable way to prevent pregnancy. Hormonal methods include oral contraceptives, injectables, implants, vaginal rings, and transdermal patches.

Oral Contraceptives

As early as 1937, scientists recognized that the injection of progesterone inhibited ovulation in rabbits and provided contraception. Breakthrough bleeding was reported in early clinical trials in women, and the role of estrogen in cycle control was launched. This established the rationale for modern combination **oral contraceptives (OCs)** that contain both estrogen and progesterone (Roederer, Blackwell & Blenning, 2006). In 1960 the FDA approved the first combination OC, Enovid-10 (150 mcg estrogen and 9 mg progesterone), for use in the United States. Today, nearly 50 combination OCs are available in the United States. The most notable change in over 40 years of OC improvement has been the lowering of the estrogen dose to as low as 20 mcg and the introduction of new progestins.

Oral contraceptives are the most popular method of nonsurgical contraception, used by approximately 18 million women in the United States (Dirubbo, 2006) (Fig. 4.12). Unlike the original OCs that women took decades ago, the new low-dose forms carry fewer health risks.

OCs, while most commonly prescribed for contraception, have long been used in the management of a wide range of conditions and have many health benefits, such as:

- Reduced incidence of ovarian and endometrial cancer
- Prevention and treatment of endometriosis
- Decreased incidence of acne and hirsutism

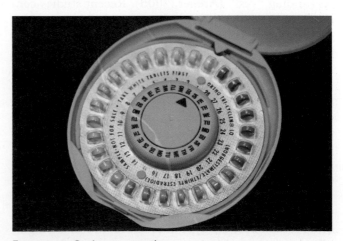

FIGURE 4.12 Oral contraceptive.

- Decreased incidence of ectopic pregnancy
- Decreased incidence of acute PID
- Reduced incidence of fibrocystic breast disease
- Decreased perimenopausal symptoms
- Increased menstrual cycle regularity
- Lower incidence of colorectal cancer
- Reduced iron-deficiency anemia by treating menorrhagia
- Reduced incidence of dysmenorrhea (Roederer, Blackwell & Blenning, 2006)

OCs work primarily by suppressing ovulation by adding estrogen and progesterone to a woman's body, thus mimicking pregnancy. This hormonal level stifles gonadotropin-releasing hormone (GnRH), which in turn suppresses FSH and LH and thus inhibits ovulation. Cervical mucus also thickens, which hinders sperm transport into the uterus. Implantation is inhibited by suppression of the maturation of the endometrium and alterations of uterine secretions (Trussell, 2004).

The combination pills are prescribed as monophasic pills, which deliver fixed dosages of estrogen and progestin, or as multiphasic ones. Multiphasic pills (e.g., biphasic and triphasic OCs) alter the amount of progestin and estrogen within each cycle. To maintain adequate hormonal levels for contraception and enhance compliance, OCs should be taken at the same time daily.

OCs that contain progestin only are called minipills. They are prescribed for women who cannot take estrogen. They work primarily by thickening the cervical mucus to prevent penetration of the sperm and make the endometrium unfavorable for implantation. Progestin-only pills must be taken at a certain time every 24 hours. Breakthrough bleeding and a higher risk of pregnancy have made these OCs less popular than combination OCs (Mishell et al., 2007).

Extended OC regimens have been used for the management of menstrual disorders and endometriosis for years but now are attracting wider attention. Surveys asking women about their willingness to reduce their menstrual cycles from 12 to 4 annually were returned with a resounding "yes!" (Archer, 2006). Recent studies confirm that the extended use of active OC pills carries the same safety profile as the conventional 28-day regimens (Anderson et al., 2006; Edelman et al., 2006; Grimes, 2006). The extended regimen consists of 84 consecutive days of active combination pills, followed by 7 days of placebo. The woman has four withdrawal-bleeding episodes a year. Seasonale, a combination OC, is on the market for women who choose to reduce the number of periods that they have. There is no physiologic requirement for cyclic hormonal withdrawal bleeds while taking OCs (Wysocki, 2007).

The balance between the benefits and the risks of OCs must be determined for each woman when she is being assessed for this type of contraceptive. It is a highly effective contraceptive when taken properly but can ag-

gravate many medical conditions, especially in women who smoke. Comparison Chart 4.2 lists advantages and disadvantages of OCs. A thorough history and pelvic examination, including a Pap smear, must be completed before the medication is prescribed and yearly thereafter. Women should also be counseled that the effectiveness of OCs is decreased when the woman is taking antibiotics; thus, the woman will need to use an alternative or secondary method during this period to prevent pregnancy.

Nurses need to provide OC users with a great deal of education before they leave the health care facility. They need to be able to identify early signs and symptoms that might indicate a problem.

▶ **Take** NOTE!

The mnemonic "ACHES" can help women remember the early warning signs that necessitate a return to the health care provider (Box 4.6).

Injectable Contraceptives

The **Lunelle injection** is a long-term reversible contraceptive for women. It contains the same hormones as the

COMPARISON CHART 4.2 **ADVANTAGES AND DISADVANTAGES OF ORAL CONTRACEPTIVES**

Advantages	Disadvantages
Regulate and shorten menstrual cycle	Offer no protection against STIs
Decrease severe cramping and bleeding	Pose slightly increased risk of breast cancer
Reduce anemia	Modest risk for vein thrombosis and pulmonary emboli
Reduce ovarian and colorectal cancer risk	
Decrease benign breast disease	Increased risk for migraine headaches
Reduce risk of endometrial cancer	Increased risk for myocardial infarction, stroke, and hypertension for women who smoke
Improve acne	
Minimize perimenopausal symptoms	
Decrease incidence of rheumatoid arthritis	May increase risk of depression
Improve PMS symptoms	User must remember to take pill daily
Protect against loss of bone density	High cost for some women

Source: Dirubbo, 2006

BOX 4.6 Early Signs of Complications for OC Users

A: Abdominal pain may indicate liver or gallbladder problems.

C: Chest pain or shortness of breath may indicate a pulmonary embolus.

H: Headaches may indicate hypertension or impending stroke.

E: Eye problems might indicate hypertension or an attack.

S: Severe leg pain may indicate a thromboembolic event

Source: Courtney, 2006.

combination OCs. It is administered once every 28 to 33 days by intramuscular injection. It provides immediate, very effective contraception if given within 5 days after the last normal menses. Its mechanism of action, contraindications, and side effects are similar to those of OCs (Murphy, Morgan & Likis, 2006).

Depo-Provera is the trade name for an injectable form of a progesterone-only contraceptive given every 12 weeks. Depo-Provera works by suppressing ovulation and the production of FSH and LH by the pituitary gland, by increasing the viscosity of cervical mucus and causing endometrial atrophy. A single injection of 150 mg into the buttocks acts like other progestin-only products to prevent pregnancy for 3 months at a time (Fig. 4.13). The primary side effect of Depo Provera is menstrual cycle disturbance.

Recent clinical studies have raised concerns about whether Depo-Provera reduces bone mineral density. This evidence has prompted the manufacturer and the FDA to issue a warning about the long-term use of Depo-Provera and bone loss (Robinson, 2005). It is not entirely clear if this loss in bone mineral density is reversible because there haven't been any long-term prospective studies in current and past users.

Transdermal Patches

A **transdermal patch**, Ortho Evra, is also available. It is a matchbox-sized patch containing hormones that are absorbed through the skin when placed on the lower abdomen, upper outer arm, buttocks, or upper torso (avoiding the breasts). The patch is applied weekly for 3 weeks, followed by a patch-free week during which withdrawal bleeding occurs. The patch delivers continuous levels of progesterone and estrogen. Transdermal absorption allows the drug to enter the bloodstream directly, avoiding rapid inactivation in the liver known as first-pass metabolism. Since estrogen and progesterone are metabolized by liver enzymes, avoiding first-pass metabolism was thought to reduce adverse effects. However, recent evidence suggests that the risk of venous thrombosis and embolism is increased with the patch (Courtney, 2006). Additional studies are underway to understand the clinical significance of these latest findings, but in the interim nurses need to focus on ongoing risk assessment and should be prepared to discuss current research findings with clients.

Compliance with combination contraceptive patch use has been shown to be significantly greater than compliance with OCs (Graziottin, 2006). The patch provides combination hormone therapy with a side effect profile similar to that of OCs. The manufacturer is currently evaluating extended regimens for the patch (Stewart et al., 2006) (Fig. 4.14).

Vaginal Rings

The contraceptive **vaginal ring**, NuvaRing, is a flexible, soft, transparent ring that is inserted by the user for a 3-week period of continuous use followed by a ring-free week to allow withdrawal bleeding (Fig. 4.15). The ring can be inserted by the woman and does not have to be

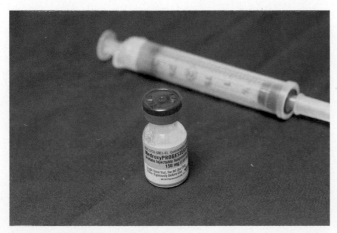

FIGURE **4.13** Injectable contraceptive.

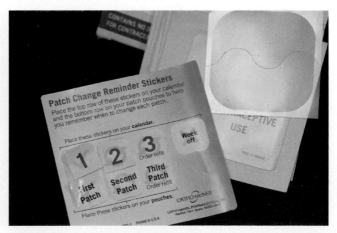

FIGURE **4.14** Transdermal patch.

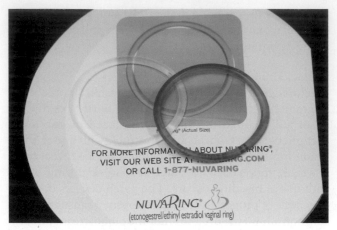

FIGURE 4.15 Vaginal ring.

fitted. The woman compresses the ring and inserts it into the vagina, behind the pubic bone, as far back as possible, but precise placement is not critical. The hormones are absorbed through the vaginal mucosa. It is left in place for 3 weeks and then removed and discarded. Effectiveness and adverse events are similar to those seen with combination OCs. Clients need to be counseled regarding timely insertion of the ring and what to do in case of accidental expulsion. This device is also being tested for extended regimens to reduce menstrual bleeding.

Implantable Contraceptives

The **implant** is a subdermal time-release method that delivers synthetic progestin. Once in place, it delivers several years of continuous, highly effective contraception. Like progestin-only pills, implants act by inhibiting ovulation and thickening cervical mucus so sperm cannot penetrate. A single-rod progestin implant (Implanon) received FDA approval in 2006 (Tolaymat & Kaunitz, 2007). The side effects are also similar to progestin-only pills: irregular bleeding, headaches, weight gain, breast tenderness, and depression. Fertility is restored quickly after it is removed. Implants require a minor surgical procedure for

both insertion and removal. The implants don't offer any protection against STIs.

Intrauterine Systems

Intrauterine systems are small plastic T-shaped objects that are placed inside the uterus to provide contraception (Fig. 4.16). They prevent pregnancy by making the endometrium of the uterus hostile to implantation of a fertilized ovum by causing a nonspecific inflammatory reaction (Hearton, 2006). Monthly periods become lighter, shorter, and less painful, making this a useful method for women with heavy, painful periods. Some implants may contain copper or progesterone to enhance their effectiveness. One or two attached strings protrude into the vagina so that the user can check for placement.

Currently there are three intrauterine systems available in the United States: the copper ParaGard-T-380A; Progestasert, a progesterone device; and the levonorgestrel intrauterine system (LNG-IUS) Mirena, a levonorgestrel-releasing device. The ParaGard-T-380A is approved for 10 years of use. The Progestasert may stay in place 1 year, then must be removed and replaced. Mirena provides intrauterine conception for up to 5 years. An advantage of these hormonally impregnated intrauterine systems is that they are relatively maintenance-free: users must consciously discontinue using them to become pregnant rather than making a daily decision to avoid conception (French et al., 2006). Box 4.7 highlights warning signs of complications.

Emergency Contraception

Unplanned pregnancy is a major health, economic, and social issue for women. Approximately half of all unplanned pregnancies end in abortion (CDC, 2006). **Emergency contraception (EC)** reduces the risk of pregnancy after unprotected intercourse or contraceptive failure such as condom breakage (Lever, 2005). It is used within 72 hours of unprotected intercourse to prevent pregnancy. The sooner ECs are taken, the more effective

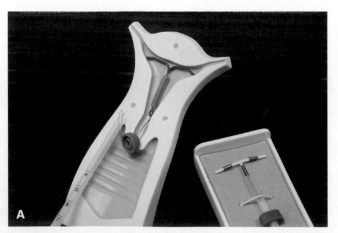

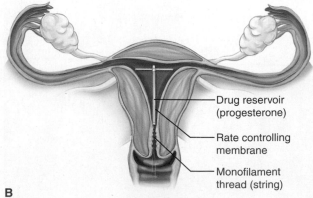

Drug reservoir (progesterone)

Rate controlling membrane

Monofilament thread (string)

A

B

FIGURE 4.16 (**A**) Intrauterine system. (**B**) An IUS in place in the uterus.

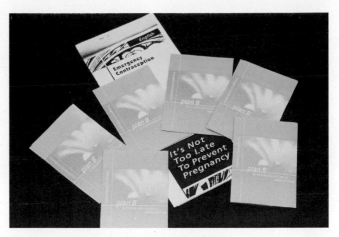

FIGURE 4.17 Emergency contraceptive kit.

they are. They reduce the risk of pregnancy for a single act of unprotected sex by almost 80% (Cheng et al., 2006). The methods available in the United States are progestin-only OCs, combination OCs, EC kit (Plan B) (Fig. 4.17), or insertion of a copper-releasing intrauterine system up to 7 days after unprotected intercourse (Lever, 2005). The FDA recently approved Plan B (levonorgestrel) to be sold over the counter to women aged 18 and older; it is still available by prescription to women younger than 18 years (U.S. Food & Drug Administration, 2006). Table 4.5 lists recommended oral medication and intrauterine regimens.

Prime points to stress concerning ECs are:

- ECs do not offer any protection against STIs or future pregnancies.
- ECs should not be used in place of regular birth control, as they are less effective.
- ECs are regular birth control pills given at higher doses and more frequently.
- ECs are contraindicated during pregnancy because they are considered to be teratogenic (Ravin, 2006).

Contrary to popular belief, ECs do not induce abortion and are not related to mifepristone or RU-486, the so-called abortion pill approved by the FDA in 2000. Mifepristone chemically induces abortion by blocking the body's progesterone receptors, which are necessary for pregnancy maintenance. ECs simply prevent embryo creation and uterine implantation from occurring in the first place. There is no evidence that ECs have any effect on an already-implanted ovum. The side effects are nausea and vomiting.

Sterilization

Sterilization is an attractive method of contraception for those who are certain they do not want any, or any more, children. **Sterilization** refers to surgical procedures intended to render the person infertile. It is one of the most popular methods of contraception in the United States and worldwide (Swica & Westhoff, 2006). More women than men undergo surgical sterilization. According to the

TABLE 4.5 EMERGENCY CONTRACEPTION (EC) OPTIONS

Product	First Dose (Within 72 Hours)	Second Dose (Taken 12 Hours Later)
Combined OCs Preven	2 tablets	2 tablets
Ovral		
Lo/Ovral, Nordette Levlen, TriLevlen	4 tablets	4 tablets
Triphasil		
Progestin-Only OCs Ovrette	20 tablets	20 tablets
Plan B	1 tablet	1 tablet
Intrauterine Devices Copper-containing IUD such as Paragard- T-380A	Inserted within 7 days after unprotected sexual episode	Can be left in for long-term contraception

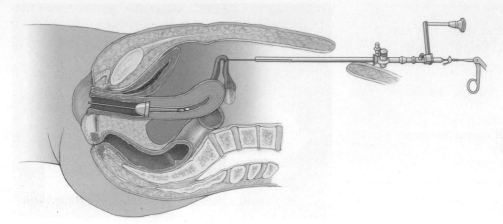

FIGURE **4.18** Laparoscopy for tubal sterilization.

CDC, approximately 18% of women undergo female sterilization in comparison to 7% of men in the United States (CDC, 2006). Sterilization should be considered a permanent end to fertility because reversal surgery is difficult, expensive, and not highly successful.

Tubal Ligation

Tubal ligation, the sterilization procedure for women, can be performed postpartum, after an abortion, or as an interval procedure unrelated to pregnancy. A laparoscope is inserted through a small subumbilical incision to provide a view of the fallopian tubes. They are grasped and sealed with a cauterizing instrument or with rings, bands, or clips or cut and tied (Fig. 4.18).

A new approach used to visualize the fallopian tubes is through the cervix instead of the abdominal incision. This procedure, called transcervical sterilization, offers several advantages over conventional tubal ligation: general anesthesia and incisions are not needed, thereby increasing safety, lowering costs, and improving access to sterilization. A tiny coil (Essure) is introduced and released into the fallopian tubes through the cervix. The coil promotes tissue growth in the fallopian tubes, and over a period of 3 months, this growth blocks the tubes (Valle, 2006). This less-invasive technique has become increasingly popular.

Vasectomy

Male sterilization is accomplished with a surgical procedure known as a **vasectomy**. It is usually performed under local anesthesia in an urologist's office, and most men can return to work and normal activities in a day or two. The procedure involves making a small incision into the scrotum and cutting the vas deferens, which carries sperm from the testes to the penis (Fig. 4.19). After vasectomy, semen no longer contains sperm. This is not immediate, though, and the man must submit semen specimens for analysis until two specimens show that no sperm is present. When the specimen shows azoospermia, the man's sterility is then confirmed (Dassow & Bennett, 2006).

Nursing Management of the Woman Choosing a Contraceptive Method

The choice of a contraceptive method is a very personal one involving many factors. What makes a woman choose one contraceptive method over another? In making contraceptive choices, couples must balance their sexual

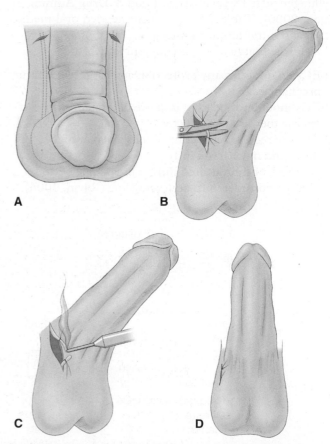

FIGURE **4.19** Vasectomy. (**A**) Site of vasectomy incisions. (**B**) The vas deferens is cut with surgical scissors. (**C**) Cut ends of the vas deferens are cauterized to ensure blockage of the passage of sperm. (**D**) Final skin suture.

lives, their reproductive goals, and each partner's health and safety. The search for a choice that satisfies all three objectives is challenging. A method that works for a sexually active teenage girl may not meet her needs later in life. Several considerations influence a person's choice of contraceptives:

• Motivation
• Cost
• Cultural and religious beliefs (Box 4.8)
• Convenience
• Effectiveness
• Side effects
• Desire for children in the future
• Safety of the method
• Comfort level with sexuality
• Protection from STIs
• Interference with spontaneity

If a contraceptive is to be effective, the woman must understand how it works, must be able to use it correctly and consistently, and must be comfortable and confident with it. If a patient cannot comply with taking a pill daily, consider a method used once a week (transdermal patches), once every 3 weeks (transvaginal ring), or once every 3 months (Depo-Provera injection). Another option may be a progesterone intrauterine device that lasts 3 to 5 years and reduces menstrual flow significantly.

Regardless of which method is chosen, the client's needs should be paramount in the discussion. The nurse can educate clients about which methods are available and their advantages and disadvantages, efficacy, cost, and safety. Counseling can help the woman choose a contraceptive method that is efficacious and fits her preferences and lifestyle.

Nursing Assessment

When assessing which contraceptive method might meet the client's needs, the nurse might ask:

• Do your religious beliefs interfere with any methods?
• Will this method interfere with your sexual pleasure?
• Are you aware of the various methods currently available?
• Is cost a major consideration, or does your insurance cover it?
• Does your partner influence which method you choose?
• Have you heard anything troubling about any of the methods?
• How comfortable are you touching your own body?
• What are your future plans for having children?

Although deciding on a contraceptive is a very personal decision between a woman and her partner, nurses can assist in this process by performing a complete health history and physical examination, and by educating the woman and her partner about necessary laboratory and diagnostic testing. Areas of focus during the nursing assessment are as follows:

• Medical history: smoking status, cancer of reproductive tract, diabetes mellitus, migraines, hypertension, thromboembolic disorder, allergies, risk factors for cardiovascular disease
• Family history: cancer, cardiovascular disease, hypertension, stroke, diabetes
• OB/GYN history: menstrual disorders, current contraceptive, previous STIs, PID, vaginitis, sexual activity
• Personal history: use of tampons and female hygiene products, plans for childbearing, comfort with touching herself, number of sexual partners and their involvement in the decision
• Physical examination: height, weight, blood pressure, breast examination, thyroid palpation, pelvic examination
• Diagnostic testing: urinalysis, complete blood count, Pap smear, wet mount to check for STIs, HIV/AIDS tests, lipid profile, glucose level

Figure 4.20 shows an example of a family planning flow record that can be used during the assessment. After collecting the assessment data above, consider the medical factors to help decide if she is a candidate for all methods or whether some should be eliminated. For example, if she reports she has multiple sex partners and has a lengthy history of various pelvic infections, she would not be a good candidate for an intrauterine system, based on her infection history. Barrier methods (male or female

---

BOX 4.8 Selected Religious Choices for Family Planning and Abortion

• Roman Catholic—Abstinence and natural family planning; no abortion
• Judaism—Family planning and abortion accepted in first trimester
• Islam—Family planning accepted; abortion only for serious reasons
• Protestant Christianity—Firmly in favor of family planning; mixed on abortion
• Buddhism—Long experience with family planning and abortion
• Hinduism—Accept both family planning and abortion
• Native American religions—Accept both family planning and abortion
• Chinese religions—Taoism and Confucianism accept both

Source: Maguire, 2004.

FAMILY PLANNING FLOW (VISIT) RECORD

Name: _____
ID #: _____
Date of Birth: _____

	Date:			Date:		
Current Method						
Reason for Visit						
LMP						
SUBJECTIVE DATA	Pt.	Comments		Pt.	Comments	
Severe headaches						
Depression						
Visual abnormalities						
Dyspnea/chest pain						
Breast changes						
SBE						
Abdominal pain						
Nausea and vomiting						
Dysuria/frequency						
Menstrual irregularities						
Vaginal discharge/infections						
Leg pain						
Surgery, injury, infections, or serious illness since last visit						
Allergic reaction						
Pregnancy plans						
Other						
OBJECTIVE DATA	Weight		B.P.	Weight		B.P.
Other						
Lab						
ASSESSMENT						
Check here if assessment continues on progress notes	O			O		
PLAN						
Type of contraceptive given						
COUNSELING/EDUCATION						
Next appointment						
SIGNATURE/TITLE						
SIGNATURE/TITLE						

O = normal   ✓ = abnormal

FIGURE 4.20 Family planning flow (visit) record.

condoms) of contraception might be recommended to this client to offer protection against STIs.

Nursing Diagnoses

A few nursing diagnoses that might be appropriate based on the nurse's assessment during the decision-making process include:

• Deficient knowledge related to:
  • Methods available
  • Side effects/safety
  • Correct use of method chosen
  • Previous myths believed
• Risk for infection related to:
  • Unprotected sexual intercourse
  • Past history of STIs
  • Methods offering protection

Nursing diagnoses applicable to the contraceptive would be:

• Health-seeking behaviors related to:
  • Perceived need for limiting number of children
  • Overall health relative to contraceptives
• Risk for ineffective health maintenance related to:
  • Not being familiar with the various contraceptive methods
  • Being unaware of high-risk sexual behavior leading to STIs
• Fear related to:
  • Not understanding the correct procedure to use
  • Unintended pregnancy occurring if not used correctly
  • General health concerning the long-term side effects

Nursing Interventions

Contraception is an important issue for all couples, and the method used should be decided by the woman and her partner jointly. Facilitate this process by establishing a trusting relationship with the client and by providing unbiased, accurate information about all methods available. As a nurse, reflect honestly on your feelings towards contraceptives while allowing the client's feelings to be central. Be aware of the practical issues involved in contraceptive use, and avoid making assumptions, making decisions on the woman's behalf, and making judgments about her and her situation. To do so, it is important to keep up to date on the latest methods available and convey this information to clients. Encourage female clients to take control of their lives by sharing information that allows them to plan their futures.

The following guidelines are helpful in counseling and educating the client or couple about contraceptives:

• Encourage the client/couple to participate in choosing a method.
• Provide client education. The client/couple must be informed users before the method is agreed upon. Education should be targeted to the client's level so it is understood. Provide step-by-step teaching and an opportunity for practice for certain methods (cervical caps, diaphragms, vaginal rings, and condoms). See Teaching Guidelines 4.5 and Figure 4.21.
• Obtain written informed consents, which are needed for intrauterine systems, implants, abortion, or sterilization. Informed consent implies that the client is making a knowledgeable, voluntary choice; has received complete information about the method, including the risks; and is free to change her mind before using the method or having the procedure (Youngkin & Davis, 2004).
• Discuss contraindications for all selected contraceptives.
• Consider the client's cultural and religious beliefs when providing care.
• Address myths and misperceptions about the methods under consideration in your initial discussion of contraceptives.

It is also important to clear up common misconceptions about contraception and pregnancy. Clearing up misconceptions will permit new learning to take hold and a better client response to whichever methods are explored and ultimately selected. Some common misconceptions include:

• Breastfeeding protects against pregnancy.
• Pregnancy can be avoided if the male partner "pulls out" before he ejaculates.
• Pregnancy can't occur during menses.
• Douching after sex will prevent pregnancy.
• Pregnancy won't happen during the first sexual experience.
• Taking birth control pills protects against STIs.
• The woman is too old to get pregnant.
• Irregular menstruation prevents pregnancy.

When discussing in detail each method of birth control, focus on specific information for each method outlined. Include information such as how this particular method works to prevent pregnancy under normal circumstances of use; the noncontraceptive benefits to overall health; advantages and disadvantages of all methods; the cost involved for each particular method; danger signs that need to be reported to the health care provider; and the required frequency of office visits needed for the particular method.

In addition, outline factors that place the client at risk for method failure. There are several reasons why there are contraceptive failures. Use Table 4.6 to provide patient education concerning a few of the reasons for contraceptive failure. Help clients who have chosen abstinence or fertility awareness methods to define the sexual activities in which they want and don't want to participate. This helps them set sexual limits or boundaries. Help them to develop communication and negotiation skills that will allow them to be successful. Supporting, encouraging, and respecting a couple's choice of abstinence is vital for nurses.

TEACHING GUIDELINES 4.5

Tips for Cervical Caps, Diaphragms, Vaginal Rings, and Condoms

Cervical Cap Insertion/Removal Technique

- It is important to be involved in the fitting process.
- To insert the cap, pinch the sides together, compress the cap dome, insert into the vagina, and place over the cervix.
- Use one finger to feel around the entire circumference to make sure there are no gaps between the cap rim and the cervix.
- After a minute or two, pinch the dome and tug gently to check for evidence of suction. The cap should resist the tug and not slide off easily.
- To remove the cap, press the index finger against the rim and tip the cap slightly to break the suction, and gently pull out the cap.
- The woman should practice inserting and removing the cervical cap three times to validate her proficiency with this device.

Client teaching and counseling regarding the cervical cap

- Fill the dome of the cap up about one-third full with spermicide cream or jelly. Do not apply spermicide to the rim, since it may interfere with the seal.
- Wait approximately 30 minutes after insertion before engaging in sexual intercourse to be sure that a seal has formed between the rim and the cervix.
- Leave the cervical cap in place for a minimum of 6 hours after sexual intercourse. It can be left in place for up to 48 hours without additional spermicide being added.
- Do not use during menses due to the potential for toxic shock syndrome. Use an alternative method such as condoms during this time.
- Inspect the cervical cap prior to insertion for cracks, holes, or tears.
- After using the cervical cap, wash it with soap and water, dry thoroughly, and store in its container.

Diaphragm Insertion/Removal Technique

- Always empty the bladder prior to inserting the diaphragm.
- Inspect diaphragm for holes or tears by holding it up to a light source, or fill it with water and check for a leak.
- Place approximately a tablespoon of spermicidal jelly or cream in the dome and around the rim of the diaphragm.
- The diaphragm can be inserted up to 6 hours prior to intercourse.

- Select the position that is most comfortable for insertion:
  - Squatting
  - Leg up, raising the nondominant leg up on a low stool
  - Reclining position, lying on her back in bed
  - Sitting forward on the edge of a chair
- Hold the diaphragm between the thumb and fingers and compress it to form a "figure-eight" shape.
- Insert the diaphragm into the vagina, directing it downward as far as it will go.
- Tuck the front rim of the diaphragm behind the pubic bone so that the rubber hugs the front wall of the vagina.
- Feel for the cervix through the diaphragm to make sure it is properly placed.
- To remove the diaphragm, insert the finger up and over the top side and move slightly to the side, breaking the suction.
- Pull the diaphragm down and out of the vagina.

Client Teaching and Counseling Regarding the Diaphragm

- Avoid the use of oil-based products such as baby oil, since this may weaken the rubber.
- Wash the diaphragm with soap and water after use and dry thoroughly.
- Place the diaphragm back into the storage case.
- The diaphragm may need to be refitted after weight loss or gain or childbirth.
- Diaphragms should not be used by women with latex allergies.

Vaginal Ring Insertion/Removal Technique and Counseling

- Each ring is used for one menstrual cycle, which consists of 3 weeks of continuous use followed by a ring-free week to allow for menses.
- No fitting is necessary—one size fits all.
- The ring is compressed and inserted into the vagina, behind the pubic bone, as far back as possible.
- Precision placement is not essential.
- Backup contraception is needed for 7 days if the ring is expelled for more than 3 hours during the 3-week period of continuous use.
- The vaginal ring is left in place for 3 weeks, then removed and discarded.
- The vaginal ring is not recommended for women with uterine prolapse or lack of vaginal muscle tone (Youngkin & Davis, 2004).

(continued)

TEACHING GUIDELINES 4.5

Tips for Cervical Caps, Diaphragms, Vaginal Rings, and Condoms (continued)

Male Condom Insertion/Removal Technique and Counseling

- Always keep the condom in its original package until ready to use.
- Store in a cool, dry place.
- Spermicidal condoms should be used if available.
- Check expiration date before using.
- Use a new condom for each sexual act.
- Condom is placed over the erect penis prior to insertion.
- Place condom on the head of the penis and unroll it down the shaft.
- Leave a half-inch of empty space at the end to collect ejaculate.
- Avoid use of oil-based products, because they may cause breakage.
- After intercourse, remove the condom while the penis is still erect.
- Discard condom after use.

Female Condom Insertion/Removal Technique and Counseling

- Practice wearing and inserting prior to first use with sexual intercourse.
- Condom can be inserted up to 8 hours before intercourse.
- Condom is intended for one-time use.
- It can be purchased over the counter—one size fits all.
- Avoid wearing rings to prevent tears; long fingernails can also cause tears.
- Spermicidal lubricant can be used if desired.
- Insert the inner ring high in the vagina, against the cervix.
- Place the outer ring on the outside of the vagina.
- Make sure the erect penis is placed inside the female condom.
- Remove the condom after intercourse. Avoid spilling the ejaculate.

After clients have chosen a method of contraception, it is important to address the following:

- Emphasize that a second method to use as a backup is always needed.
- Provide both oral and written instructions on the method chosen.
- Discuss the need for STI protection if not using a barrier method.
- Inform the client about the availability of ECs.

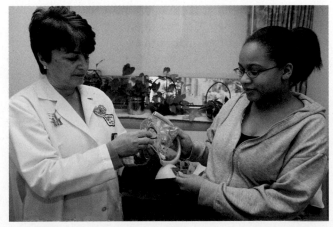

FIGURE 4.21 The nurse demonstrates insertion of a vaginal ring during client teaching.

Abortion

Abortion is defined as the expulsion of an embryo or fetus before it is viable (Alexander et al., 2007). Abortion can be a medical or surgical procedure. The purpose of abortion is to terminate a pregnancy. Surgical abortion is the most common procedure performed in the United States (approximately 1.6 million annually) and might be the most common surgical procedure in the world (Speroff & Fritz, 2005). Both medical and surgical abortions are safe and legal in the United States; an abortion is considered a woman's constitutional right based on the fundamental right to privacy (Curlin et al., 2007).

Since the landmark U.S. Supreme Court decision *Roe v. Wade* legalized abortion in 1973, debate has continued over how and when abortions are provided. Every state has laws regulating some aspects of the provision of abortion, and many have passed restrictions such as parental consent or notification requirements, mandated counseling and waiting periods, and limits on funding for abortion. Each state addresses these matters independently, and the laws that are passed or enforced are a legislative decision and a function of the political system. Although opponents of abortion continue to be very much a part of the current debates, recently they have refocused their attention on "regulation legislation" to reduce the number of abortions not medically necessary.

TABLE 4.6 **CONTRACEPTIVE PROBLEMS AND EDUCATIONAL NEEDS**

Contraceptive Failure Problem	Client Education Needed
Not following instructions for use of contraceptive correctly	Take pill the same time every day. Use condoms properly and check condition before using. Make sure diaphragm or cervical cap covers cervix completely. Check IUD for placement monthly.
Inconsistent use of contraceptive	Contraceptives must be used regularly to achieve maximum effectiveness. All it takes is one unprotected act of sexual intercourse to become pregnant. 2% to 5% of condoms will break or tear during use.
Condom broke during sex	Check expiration date. Store condoms properly. Use only a water-based lubricant. Watch for tears caused by long fingernails. Use spermicides to decrease possibility of pregnancy if failure occurs.
Use of antibiotics or other herbs taken with OCs	Use alternative methods during the antibiotic therapy, plus 7 additional days. Implement on day 1 of taking antibiotics.
Belief that you can't get pregnant during menses or that it is safe "just this one time"	It may be possible to become pregnant on almost any day of the menstrual cycle.

Surgical Abortion

Surgical abortion is usually carried out by vacuum aspiration or suction curettage. It is an ambulatory procedure done under local anesthesia. The cervix is dilated prior to surgery and then the products of conception are removed by suction evacuation. The uterus may gently be scraped by curettage to make sure that it is empty. The entire procedure lasts about 10 minutes.

HEALTHY PEOPLE 2010

Objective	Significance
Reduce pregnancies among adolescent females. Increase the proportion of sexually active, unmarried adolescents age 15–17 years who use contraception that both effectively prevents pregnancy and provides barrier protection against disease.	Would reduce number of unplanned pregnancies and girls not finishing their education. This would in turn reduce the number of single parents on state financial assistance.
Increase the proportion of young adults who have received formal instruction before turning age 18 years on reproductive health issues, including all of the following topics: birth control methods, safer sex to prevent HIB, prevention of sexually transmitted disease, and abstinence.	Awareness of contraceptive methods brings about better compliance and prevention of unintended pregnancies in this age group.
Reduce AIDS and the number of HIV infections among adolescents and adults.	Reduce the number of HIV/AIDS victims by using barrier methods to prevent the transmission of this fatal STI.
Reduce the proportion of adolescents and young adults with *Chlamydia trachomatis* infections.	Reduce the number of women with infertility issues secondary to *Chlamydia* infections.

Medical Abortion

In a medical abortion, the woman takes certain medications to induce a miscarriage to remove the products of conception. There are two methods currently used to terminate a pregnancy during the first trimester. The first method uses methotrexate (an antineoplastic agent) followed by misoprostol (a prostaglandin agent) given as a vaginal suppository or in oral form 3 to 7 days later. Methotrexate induces abortion because of its toxicity to trophoblastic tissue, the growing embryo. Misoprostol works by causing uterine contractions, which helps to expel the products of conception. This method is 90% to 98% successful in completing an abortion (Hatcher et al., 2004).

The second method used to induce first-trimester abortions involves using mifepristone (a progesterone antagonist) followed 48 hours later by misoprostol (a prostaglandin agent), which causes contractions of the uterus and expulsion of the uterine contents. Mifepristone, the generic name for RU-486, is sold under the brand names Mifeprex and Early Option. Mifepristone is a potent oral anti-progestogen; it blocks the action of progesterone that prepares the endometrium for implantation and then maintains the pregnancy. This method is 95% effective when used within 49 days after the last menstrual cycle (Hatcher et al., 2004).

Abortion is a very emotional, deeply personal issue. Give support and accurate information. If for personal, religious, or ethical reasons you feel unable to actively participate in the care of a woman undergoing an abortion, you still have the professional responsibility to ensure that the woman receives the nursing care and help she requires. This may necessitate a transfer to another area or a staffing reassignment.

Menopause

The change of life. The end of fertility. The beginning of freedom. Whatever people call it, menopause is a unique and personal experience for every woman. **Menopause** refers to the cessation of regular menstrual cycles. It is the end of menstruation and childbearing capacity. The average age of natural menopause—defined as 1 year without a menstrual period—is 51 years old (Alexander et al., 2007). With current female life expectancy at 80, this event comes in the middle of a woman's adult life.

▶ *Take* NOTE!

Humans are virtually the only species to outlive their reproductive capacities.

Menopause signals the end of an era for many women. It concludes their ability to reproduce, and some women find advancing age, altered roles, and these physiologic changes to be overwhelming events that may precipitate depression and anxiety (Kessenich, 2007). Menopause does not happen in isolation. Midlife is often experienced as a time of change and reflection. Change happens in many arenas: children are leaving or returning home, employment pressures intensify as career moves or decisions are required, elderly parents require more care or the death of a parent may have a major impact, and partners are retrenching or undergoing their own midlife crises. Women must negotiate all these changes in addition to menopause. Managing these stressful changes can be very challenging for many women as they make the transition into midlife.

A woman is born with approximately 500,000 ova, but only 300 to 400 ever mature fully to be released during the menstrual cycle. The absolute number of ova in the ovary is a major determinant of fertility. Over the course of her premenopausal life there is a steady decline in the number of immature ova. No one understands this depletion, but it does not occur in isolation. Maturing ova are surrounded by follicles that produce two major hormones: estrogen, in the form of estradiol, and progesterone. The cyclic maturation of the ovum is directed by the hypothalamus. The hypothalamus triggers a cascade of neurohormones, which act through the pituitary and the ovaries as a pulse generator for reproduction.

This hypothalamic-pituitary-ovarian axis begins to break down long before there is any sign that menopause is imminent. Some scientists believe that the pulse generator in the hypothalamus simply degenerates; others speculate that the ovary becomes more resistant to the pituitary hormone FSH and simply shuts down (Krantz, 2007b). The final act in this well-orchestrated process is amenorrhea.

As menopause approaches, more and more of the menstrual cycles become anovulatory. This period of time, usually 2 to 8 years before cessation of menstruation, is termed perimenopause (Manson, 2006). In perimenopause, the ovary begins to sputter, producing irregular and missed periods and an occasional hot flash. When menopause finally appears, viable ova are gone. Estrogen levels plummet by 90%, and estrone, produced in fat cells, replaces estradiol as the body's main form of estrogen. The major hormone produced by the ovaries during the reproductive years is estradiol; the estrogen found in postmenopausal women is estrone. Estradiol is much more biologically active than estrone (Krantz, 2007). In addition, testosterone levels decrease with menopause.

Menopause, with its dramatic decline in estrogen, affects not only the reproductive organs, but also other body systems:

- Brain: hot flashes, disturbed sleep, mood and memory problems
- Cardiovascular: lower levels of high-density lipoprotein (HDL) and increased risk of cardiovascular disease
- Skeletal: rapid loss of bone density increases the risk of osteoporosis
- Breasts: duct and glandular tissues are replaced by fat
- Genitourinary: vaginal dryness, stress incontinence, cystitis
- Gastrointestinal: less calcium is absorbed from food, increasing the risk for fractures
- Integumentary: skin becomes dry and thin, and collagen levels decrease
- Body shape: more abdominal fat; waist size swells relative to hips

Therapeutic Management

Menopause should be managed individually. In the past, despite the wide diversity of symptoms and risks, the traditional reaction was to reach for the one-size-fits-all therapy: hormone therapy. Today the medical community is changing its thinking in light of the Women's Health Initiative (WHI) study and the Heart and Estrogen/Progestin Replacement Study Follow-Up (HERS II), which reported that long-term hormone therapy (HT) increased the risks of heart attacks, strokes, and breast cancer; in short, the overall health risks of HT exceeded the benefits (Writing Group, 2002, p. 321). In addition, HT didn't protect against the development of coronary artery disease, nor did it prevent the progression of coronary artery disease, as it was previously touted to do (Shelby & O'Hair, 2007). As expected, the fallout from this study and others forced practitioners to re-evaluate their usual therapies and tailor treatment to each client's history, needs, and risk factors.

There is a universe of treatment options out there, but factors in the client's history should be the driving force when determining therapy. Women need to educate themselves about the latest research findings and collaborate with their health care provider on the right menopause therapy. The following factors should be considered in management:

- HT is not indicated to treat or prevent cardiovascular disease, according to WHI. Instead, consider lipid-lowering agents and lifestyle changes if risk or disease is present.
- HT should not be taken for more than 5 years for vasomotor symptoms. Use the lowest dose possible for any hormone therapy.
- HT is acceptable as long as there is a clear indication for use, the woman is under medical supervision, and she is aware of the risks and benefits (North American Menopause Society, 2004).
- Consider nonhormonal therapies such as bisphosphonates and selective estrogen receptor modulators (SERMs).
- Consider weight-bearing exercises, calcium, vitamin D, smoking cessation, and avoidance of alcohol to treat or prevent osteoporosis.
- Annual breast examinations and mammograms are essential.
- Local estrogen creams can be used for vaginal atrophy.
- Consider herbal therapies for symptoms (Krantz, 2007).

Although numerous symptoms have been attributed to menopause (Box 4.9), some of them are more closely related to the aging process than to estrogen deficiency. A few of the more common menopausal conditions and their management will be discussed.

Managing Hot Flashes and Night Sweats

Hot flashes and night sweats are classic signs of estrogen deficiency and the predominant complaint of perimenopausal women. A hot flash is a transient and sudden sensation of warmth that spreads over the body, particularly the neck, face, and chest. Hot flashes are caused by vasomotor instability. Nearly 85% of menopausal women experience them (Alexander et al., 2007). Hot flashes are an early and acute sign of estrogen deficiency. These flashes

---

BOX 4.9 **Common Symptoms of Menopause**

- Hot flashes or flushes of the head and neck
- Dryness in the eyes and vagina
- Personality changes
- Anxiety and/or depression
- Loss of libido
- Weight gain and water retention
- Night sweats
- Fatigue
- Irritability
- Insomnia
- Stress incontinence
- Heart palpitations

Source: Chedraui et al., 2007.

---

can be mild or extreme and can last from 2 to 30 minutes (Grady, 2006).

There are many options for treating hot flashes. Treatment must be based on symptom severity, the client's medical history, and the client's values and concerns. Although the gold standard in the treatment of hot flashes is estrogen, this is not recommended for all women. The following are suggestions for the management of hot flashes:

- Pharmacologic options
  - HT unless contraindicated
  - Androgen therapy (potentiates estrogen)
  - Estrogen and androgen combinations
  - Progestin therapy (Depo-Provera injection every 3 months)
  - Clonidine (central alpha-adrenergic agonist) weekly patch
    - Neurontin (anti-seizure) decreased hot flashes
    - Acupuncture reduced frequency of hot flashes
  - Propranolol (beta-adrenergic blocker)
  - Gabapentin (Neurontin): antiseizure drug
  - SSRIs: venlafaxine (Effexor) and sertraline (Zoloft) have shown promise
  - Vitamin E: 100 mg daily (Rubin, 2007)
- Lifestyle changes
  - Lower room temperature; use fans.
  - Wear clothing in layers for easy removal.
  - Limit caffeine and alcohol intake.
  - Drink 8 to 10 glasses of water daily.
  - Stop smoking or cut back.
  - Avoid hot drinks and spicy food.
  - Take calcium (1,200 to 1,500 mg) and vitamin D (400 to 600 IU).
  - Try relaxation techniques, deep breathing, and meditation.
  - Exercise daily, but not just before bedtime.

- Maintain a healthy weight.
- Identify stressors and learn to manage them.
- Keep a diary to identify triggers of hot flashes.
- Alternative therapies
  - Phytoestrogens: isoflavones, ligands, coumenstrols
  - Black cohosh
  - Chamomile: mild sedative to alleviate insomnia
  - Unopposed transdermal progesterone
  - Compounded bioidentical hormones
    - Estrogen
    - Progesterone
    - Testosterone
    - Dehydroepiandrosterone (DHEA)
    - Pregnenolone (Campbell, 2006)
  - Chasteberry (vitex): balances progesterone and estrogen
  - Dong quai: acts as a form of phytoestrogen
  - Ginseng: purported to improve memory
  - St. John's wort: reduces depression and fatigue
  - Valerian root: induces sleep and relaxation (AAFP, 2006)

Many women are choosing alternative treatments for managing menopausal symptoms. Because of their natural origin, women perceive that alternative treatments are safer. The interest in phytoestrogens came about because of the low prevalence of hot flashes in Asian women, which was attributed to their diet being rich in phytoestrogens (Manson, 2006). Recent studies have found that black cohosh, multibotanical herbs, and increased soy intake do not reduce the frequency or severity of menopausal hot flashes or night sweats (ACOG, 2005; Huntzinger, 2006; Newton et al., 2006; Seppa, 2007). Other remedies for easing menopausal symptoms might include red clover, motherwort, ginseng, sarsaparilla root, valerian root, L-tryptophan, calcium-magnesium, and kelp tablets (Haas, 2007). Again, research thus far has been skeptical about their efficacy, but many women report they ease their symptoms and their use has skyrocketed. While there might be some benefits to their use, evidence of the efficacy of alternative products in menopause is largely anecdotal. Small, preliminary clinical trials might demonstrate the safety of some of the nonpharmacologic products. Nurses should be aware of the purported action of these agents as well as any adverse effects or drug interactions.

Managing Urogenital Changes

Menopause can be a physically and emotionally challenging time for women. In additional to the psychological burden of leaving behind the reproductive phase of life and the stigma of an "aging" body, sexual difficulties due to urogenital changes plague most women but are frequently not addressed.

Vaginal atrophy occurs during menopause because of declining estrogen levels. These changes include thinning of the vaginal walls, an increase in pH, irritation, increased susceptibility to infection, dyspareunia, loss of lubrication with intercourse, vaginal dryness, and a decrease in sexual desire related to these changes. Decreased estrogen levels can also influence a woman's sexual function as well. Delayed clitoral reaction, decreased vaginal lubrication, diminished circulatory response during sexual stimulation, and reduced contractions during orgasm have all been linked to low estrogen levels (McKinney, 2007).

Management of these changes might include the use of estrogen vaginal tablets (Vagifem) or Premarin cream; Estring, an estrogen-releasing vaginal ring that lasts for 3 months; testosterone patches; and over-the-counter moisturizers and lubricants (Astroglide). A positive outlook on sexuality and a supportive partner are also needed to make the sexual experience enjoyable and fulfilling.

▶ **Take** NOTE!

Sexual health is an important aspect of the human experience. By keeping an open mind, listening to women, and providing evidence-based treatment options, the nurse can help improve quality of life for menopausal women.

Preventing and Managing Osteoporosis

Women are greatly affected by osteoporosis after menopause. Osteoporosis is a condition in which bone mass declines to such an extent that fractures occur with minimal trauma. Bone loss begins in the third or fourth decade of a woman's life and accelerates rapidly after menopause. It affects 8 million women, with millions more at high risk for developing it. This translates to 1 in 2 women over the age of 50 having an osteoporosis-related fracture in their lifetime (Alexander et al., 2007). This condition puts many women into long-term care, with a resulting loss of independence. Figure 4.22 shows the skeletal changes associated with osteoporosis.

Most women with osteoporosis don't know they have the disease until they sustain a fracture, usually of the wrist or hip. Risk factors include:

- Increasing age
- Postmenopausal status without hormone replacement
- Small frame, thin-boned
- Caucasian or Asian
- Impaired eyesight
- Rheumatoid arthritis
- Family history of osteoporosis
- Sedentary lifestyle
- History of treatment with:
  - Antacids with aluminum
  - Heparin
  - Steroids
  - Thyroid replacement drugs

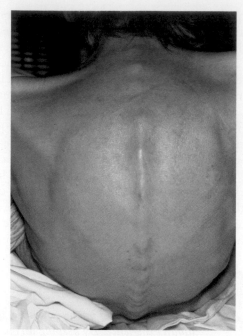

FIGURE 4.22 Skeletal changes associated with osteoporosis. (John Radcliffe Hospital/ Photo Researcher Inc.)

- Smoking and consuming alcohol
- Low calcium and vitamin D intake
- Excessive amounts of caffeine
- Anorexia nervosa or bulimia (Hansberger, 2007)

Screening tests to measure bone density are not good predictors for young women who might be at risk for developing this condition. Dual-energy x-ray absorptiometry (DXA or DEXA) is a screening test that calculates the mineral content of the bone at the spine and hip. It is highly accurate, fast, and relatively inexpensive (McNally, Kenny & Smith, 2007).

The best management for this painful, crippling, and potentially fatal disease is prevention. Women can modify many risk factors by doing the following:

- Engage in daily weight-bearing exercise, such as walking.
- Increasing calcium and vitamin D intake.
- Avoid smoking and excessive alcohol.
- Discuss your bone health with your health care provider.
- When appropriate, have a bone density test and take medication if needed (National Osteoporosis Foundation, 2007).

Medications that can help in preventing and managing osteoporosis include:

- HT (Premarin)
- SERMs (Evista)
- Calcium and vitamin D supplements (Tums)
- Bisphosphonates (Actonel or Fosamax)
- Calcitonin (Miacalcin) (Hansberger, 2007)

Preventing and Managing Cardiovascular Disease

Although cardiovascular disease is still thought of as a "man's disease," it is the major killer of postmenopausal women 50 to 75 years of age (Rosano et al., 2007). Half a million women die annually in the United States of cardiovascular disease, with strokes accounting for about 20% of the deaths (Alexander et al., 2007). This translates into approximately one death every minute. Coronary heart disease accounts for the majority of cardiovascular deaths in women, with nearly two thirds of these women dying suddenly without any previously recognized symptoms (Hackley, Kriebs & Rousseau, 2007).

For the first half of a woman's life, estrogen seems to be a protective substance for the cardiovascular system by smoothing, relaxing, and dilating blood vessels. It even helps boost HDL and lower LDL levels, helping to keep the arteries clean from plaque accumulation. But when estrogen levels plummet as women age and experience menopause, the incidence of cardiovascular disease increases dramatically.

Menopause is not the only factor that increases a woman's risk for cardiovascular disease. Lifestyle and medical history factors such as the following play a major role:

- Smoking
- Obesity
- High-fat diet
- Sedentary lifestyle
- High cholesterol levels
- Family history of cardiovascular disease
- Hypertension
- Apple-shaped body
- Diabetes

Two of the major risk factors for coronary heart disease are hypertension and dyslipidemia. Both are modifiable and can be prevented by lifestyle changes and, if needed, controlled by medication. This is why prevention is essential. In addition, women who experience early menopause lose the protection afforded by endogenous estrogen to the cardiac system and are at greater risk for more extensive atherosclerosis. Major preventive strategies include a healthy diet, increased activity, exercise, smoking cessation, decreased alcohol intake, and weight reduction.

Raising awareness of heart disease in women is an essential role for nurses. Lifestyle interventions are effective in preventing cardiovascular disease in all individuals regardless of their underlying risk (Hackley, Kriebs & Rousseau, 2007). Stressing the importance of lifestyle modifications must begin early in life and should be reinforced from the beginning of a young woman's reproductive years through menopause. Nurses are in an ideal position to teach the importance of good nutrition, healthy weight, and daily exercise before cardiovascular disease becomes clinically evident.

Nursing Assessment

Menopause is a universal and irreversible part of the overall aging process involving a woman's reproductive system. While not a disease state, menopause does place women at greater risk for the development of many conditions of aging. Nurses can help the woman become aware of her risk for postmenopausal diseases, as well as strategies to prevent them. The nurse can be instrumental in assessing risk factors and planning interventions in collaboration with the client. These might include:

- Screening for osteoporosis, cardiovascular disease, and cancer risk
  - Assessment of blood pressure to identify hypertension
  - Blood cholesterol to identify hyperlipidemia risk
  - Mammogram to find a cancerous lesion
  - Pap smear to identify cervical cancer
  - Pelvic examination to identify endometrial cancer or masses
  - Digital rectal examination to assess for colon cancer
  - Bone density testing as a baseline at menopause to identify osteopenia (low bone mass), which might lead to osteoporosis
- Assessing lifestyle to plan strategies to prevent chronic conditions:
  - Dietary intake of fat, cholesterol, and sodium
  - Weight management
  - Calcium intake
  - Use of tobacco, alcohol, and caffeine
  - Performance of breast self-examinations

Nursing Management

There is no "magic bullet" in managing menopause. Nurses can counsel women about their risks and help them to prevent disease and debilitating conditions with specific health-maintenance education. Women should make their own decisions, but the nurse should make sure they are armed with the facts to do so intelligently. Nurses can offer a thorough explanation of the menopausal process, including the latest research findings, to help women understand and make decisions about this inevitable event.

If the woman decides to use HT to control her menopausal symptoms, after being thoroughly educated, she will need frequent reassessment. There are no hard-and-fast rules that apply to meeting a woman's individual needs. The nurse can provide realistic expectations of the therapy to reduce the woman's anxiety and concern.

It is also useful to emphasize the value of friends to gain support and share information and resources. Often just talking about emotional difficulties like a death of a parent or problematic relationships helps solve problems. It also shows the woman that her emotional responses are valid.

Healthy lifestyles and stress management techniques are vital to health and longevity, and it is important to keep these on the client's agenda when discussing menopause (Staff of Boston Women's Health Book Collective, 2007).

Evidence-based interventions include lifestyle modifications, risk management therapies, and preventive drug interventions, such as the following:

- Participate actively in maintaining health.
- Exercise regularly.
- Take supplemental calcium and eat appropriately to prevent osteoporosis.
- Stop smoking to prevent lung and heart disease.
- Reduce caffeine and alcohol intake to prevent osteoporosis.
- Monitor blood pressure, lipids, and diabetes (drug therapy management).
- Use low-dose aspirin.
- Reduce dietary intake of fat, cholesterol, and sodium to prevent cardiovascular disease.
- Maintain a healthy weight for body frame.
- Perform breast self-examinations to detect breast lesions.
- Control stress (Dormire & Becker, 2007).

These life approaches may seem low-tech, but they can stave off menopause-related complications such as cardiovascular disease, osteoporosis, and depression. These tips for healthy living work well, but the client needs to be motivated to stick with them.

■■■ Key Concepts

- Establishing good health habits and avoiding risky behaviors early in life will prevent chronic conditions later on.
- There are more than 200 symptoms of PMS, and at least two different syndromes have been recognized: PMS and premenstrual dysphoric disorder (PMDD).
- Endometriosis is a condition in which bits of functioning endometrial tissue are located outside their normal site, the uterine cavity.
- Infertility is a widespread problem that has an emotional, social, and economic impact on couples.
- More than half (53%) of all unintended pregnancies occur in women who report using some method of birth control during the month of conception.
- Hormonal methods include oral contraceptives, injectables, implants, vaginal rings, and transdermal patches.
- Recent studies have shown that the extension of active oral contraceptive pills carries the same safety profile as the conventional 28-day regimens.
- Currently there are three IUSs available in the United States: the copper ParaGard-T-380A; Progestasert, a progesterone device; and the levonorgestrel intrauterine system (LNG-IUS) Mirena, a levonorgestrel-releasing device.
- Sterilization is the most popular method of contraception in the United States and worldwide.
- Menopause, with a dramatic decline in estrogen levels, affects not only the reproductive organs but also other bodily systems.

- Most women with osteoporosis do not know they have the disease until they sustain a fracture, usually of the wrist or hip.
- Half a million women die annually in the United States of cardiovascular diseases, with strokes accounting for about 20% of the deaths.
- Nurses should aim to have a holistic approach to the sexual health of women from menarche through menopause.

REFERENCES

AAFP (2006). Evidence-based complementary and alternative medicine (CAM): What should physicians know? *Medscape*. Available at: http://www.medscape.com/viewarticle/549067

ACOG Practice Bulletin (2000). Clinical management guidelines for obstetricians-gynecologists, number 15: Premenstrual syndrome. *Obstetrics & Gynecology, 95*, 1–9.

ACOG (2005). ACOG's Hormone Therapy report. *Obstetrics & Gynecology*, ACOG Task Force, (Supplement to October issue), 1–131.

Aeby, T. C., & Frattarelli, L. C. (2006). Dysfunctional uterine bleeding. *eMedicine Journal*. Available at: http://www.emedicine.com/ped/topic628.htm

Aeby, T. C., & Hraoka, M. R. (2006). Endometriosis. *Emedicine*. Available at: http://www.emedicine.com/ped/topic677.htm

Alan Guttmacher Institute (2007). Get "in the know": 20 questions about pregnancy, contraception and abortion. Available at: http://www.guttmacher.org/in-the-know/index.html

Alexander, L. L., LaRosa, J. H., Bader, H., & Garfield, S. (2007). *New dimensions in women's health* (4th ed.). Boston: Jones and Bartlett.

American Academy of Allergy, Asthma, and Immunology (AAAAI) (2007). Tips to remember: Latex allergy. Available at: http://www.aaaai.org/patients/publicedmat/tips/latexallergy.stm

American Society for Reproductive Medicine (ASRM) (2007). Frequently asked questions about infertility. Available at: http://www.asrm.org/Patients/faqs.html

Anderson, F. D., Gibbons, W., & Portman, D. (2006). Long-term study of an extended-cycle oral contraceptive (Seasonale): A 2-year multicenter open-label extension trial. *American Journal of Obstetrics & Gynecology, 195*(1), 92–96.

Andoisek, K. M., & Rapkin, A. J. (2007). Contraceptive use in women with premenstrual disorders. *USC Dialogues in Contraception, 10*(4), 4–7.

Archer, D. F. (2006). Menstrual-cycle-related symptoms: A review of the rationale for continuous use of oral contraceptives. *Contraception, 74*(5), 359–366.

Arevalo, M. (2007). CycleBeads: Easy, effective natural family planning. Available at: http://www.cyclebeads.com

Bielak, K. M., & Harris, G. S. (2006). Amenorrhea. *eMedicine*. Available at: http://www.emedicine.com/ped/topic2779.htm

Braverman, P. K., & Neinstein, L. S. (2007). Dysmenorrhea and premenstrual syndrome. In L. S. Neinstein (Ed.), *Adolescent health care, a practical guide* (5th ed., pp. 952–965). Philadelphia: Lippincott Williams & Wilkins.

Brucker, M. C. (2006). Return of the sponge: Will consumers return to a worthy old favorite? *AWHONN Lifelines, 10*(1), 74–76.

Campagne, D. M., & Campagne, G. (2007). The premenstrual syndrome revisited. *European Journal of Obstetrics & Reproductive Biology, 130*(1), 4–17.

Campbell, S. (2006) Bioidentical hormones: Achieving the perfect fit. *Advance for Nurse Practitioners, 14*(2), 25–30.

Canning, S., Waterman, M., & Dye, L. (2006). Dietary supplements and herbal remedies for premenstrual syndrome (PMS): A systematic review of the evidence for their efficacy. *Journal of Reproductive & Infant Psychology, 24*(4), 363–378.

Centers for Disease Control and Prevention (CDC) (2006). Contraceptive use. National Center for Health Statistics. Available at: http://www.cdc.gov/women/natstat/reprhlth.htm#contraception

Chedraul, P., Hidalgo, L., Chavez, D., Morocho, N., Alvarado, M., & Huc, A. (2007). Menopausal symptoms and associated risk factors among postmenopausal women screened for the metabolic syndrome. *Archives of Gynecology & Obstetrics, 275*(3), 161–168.

Cheng, L., Gulmezogulu, A. M., Van Oel, C. J., Piaggio, G., Ezcurra, E., & Van Look, P. F. A. (2006). Interventions for emergency contraception. *Cochrane Library:* CD001324, 2009357452.

Clayton, A. H. (2008). Symptoms related to the menstrual cycle: Diagnosis, prevalence, and treatment. *Journal of Psychiatric Practice, 14*(1), 13–21.

Courtney, K. (2006). The contraceptive patch: Latest developments. *AWHONN Lifelines, 10*(3), 250–253.

Covington, S., & Burns, L. H. (2006). *Infertility counseling: A comprehensive handbook for clinicians* (2nd ed.). Cambridge, UK: Cambridge University Press.

Curlin, F. A., Lawrence, R. E., Chin, M. H., & Lantos, J. D. (2007). Religion, conscience, and controversial clinical practice. *New England Journal of Medicine, 356*(6), 593–600.

Dassow, P., & Bennett, J. M. (2006). Vasectomy: An update. *American Family Physician, 74*(12), 2069–2074.

DeMasters, J. (2004). Male infertility. *Advance for Nurses, 6*(1), 19–25.

DeSutter, P. (2006). Rational diagnosis and treatment in infertility. *Best Practice & Research: Clinical Obstetrics & Gynecology, 20*(5), 647–664.

Dirubbo, N. E. (2006). Counsel your patients about contraceptive options. *Nurse Practitioner, 31*(4), 40–44.

Dodds, N., & Sinert, R. (2006). Dysfunctional uterine bleeding. *eMedicine*. Available at: http://www.emedicine.com/emerg/topic155.htm

Dormire, S., & Becker, H. (2007). Menopause health decision support for women with physical disabilities. *JOGNN, 36*(1), 97–104.

Doty, E., & Attaran, M. (2006). Managing primary dysmenorrhea. *Journal of Pediatric & Adolescent Gynecology, 19*(5), 341–344.

Edelman, A. B., Gallo, M. F., Jensen, J. T., Nichols, M. D., Schulz, K. F., & Grimes, D. A. (2006). Continuous or extended cycle versus cyclic use of combined oral contraceptives. *Cochrane Library:* CD004695

Edmundson, L. D., & Erogul, M. (2006) Dysmenorrhea. *eMedicine*. Available at: http://www.emedicine.com/emerg/topic156.htm

Female Contraception (2006). *Contraception: Female, annual report.* ADAM. Available at: http://search.ebscohost.com/login.aspx?direct=true&db=aph&AN=20517070&site=ehost-live

Ficorelli, C. T., & Weeks, B. (2007). Untangling the complexities of male infertility. *Nursing2007, 37*(1), 24–26.

French, R., Vliet, H., Cowan, F., Mansour, D., Morris, S., Hughes, D., Robinson, A., Proctor, T., Summerbell, C., Logan, S., Helmerhorst, F., & Guillebaud, J. (2006). Hormonally impregnated intrauterine systems (IUSs) versus other forms. *Cochrane Library.* CD001776: 2009357603.

Futterman, L. A., & Rapkin, A. J. (2006). Diagnosis of premenstrual disorders. *Journal of Reproductive Medicine, 51*(4), 349–358.

Gallo, M. F., Grimes, D. A., Lopez, L. M., & Schultz, K. F. (2006). Nonlatex versus latex condoms for contraception. *Cochrane Library.* Available at: www.cinahl.com/cgi-bin/refsvc?jid=3053&accno=2009358379

Gallo, M., Grimes, D., & Schultz, K. (2006). Cervical cap versus diaphragm for contraception. *Cochrane Library.* Available at: http://search.ebscohost.com/login.aspx?direct=true&db=rzh&AN=2009358282&site=ehost-live

Giulio, G. D., & Reissing, E. D. (2006). Premenstrual dysphoric disorder: Prevalence, diagnostic considerations, and controversies. *Journal of Psychosomatic Obstetrics & Gynecology, 27*(4), 201–210.

Grady, D. (2006). Management of menopausal symptoms. *New England Journal of Medicine, 355*(22), 2338–2347.

Grainger, D. A., Frazier, L. M., & Rowland, C. A. (2006) Preconception care and treatment with assisted reproductive technologies. *Maternal & Child Health*, (Supplement 10), 161–164.

Graziottin, A. (2006). A review of transdermal hormone contraception: Focus on the ethinyl estradiol/norelgestromin contraceptive patch. *Treatments in Endocrinology, 5*(6), 359–365.

Haas, E. (2007). Easing menopause symptoms naturally. *Share Guide, 89*, 29–78.

Hackley, B., Kriebs, J. M., & Rousseau, M. E. (2007). *Primary care of women: A guide for midwives and women's health providers.* Sudbury, MA: Jones and Bartlett Publishers.

Hansberger, J. (2007). Osteoporosis: Review of disease, diagnosis, and treatments for the advanced practice nurse. *Journal of Advanced Nursing Practice, 8*(1), 5–6.

Harel, Z. (2006). Dysmenorrhea in adolescents and young adults. *Journal of Pediatric & Adolescent Gynecology, 19*(6), 363–371.

Hatcher, R. A., et al. (2004). *Contraceptive technology* (18th ed.). New York: Ardent Media, Inc.

Hearton, L. (2006). Long-acting methods of reversible contraception. *Primary Health Care, 16*(4), 21–22.

Hompes, P. G., & Mijatovic, V. (2007). Endometriosis: The way forward. *Gynecological Endocrinology, 23*(1), 5–12.

Hsiao, M., & Liu, C. (2007). Unusual manifestations of premenstrual syndrome. *Psychiatry & Clinical Neurosciences, 61*(1), 120–123.

Htay, T. T., & Aung, K. (2006). Premenstrual dysphoric disorder. *Emedicine.* Available at: http://www.emedicine.com/med/topic3357.htm

Huntzinger, A. (2006). ACOG reports on compounded bioidentical hormones. *American Family Physician, 73*(12), 2242–2245.

Jenkins, G., & Jenkins, J. (2006). Issues relating to infertility. *Practice Nurse, 32*(4), 14–22.

Kelly-Weeder, S., & O'Conner, A. (2006). Modifiable risk factors for impaired fertility in women: What nurse practitioners need to know. *Journal of the American Academy of Nurse Practitioners, 18*(6), 268–276.

Kessenich, C. R. (2007). Inevitable menopause. *Nursing Spectrum.* Available at: http://www.nurse.com/ce/course.html?CCID=3183ce232.htm

Krantz, C. (2007a). Amenorrhea. In R. E. Rakel (Ed.), *Conn's current therapy 2007*. Philadelphia: Elsevier W. B. Saunders.

Krantz, C. (2007b). Menstrual cycle. In R. E. Rakel (Ed.), *Conn's current therapy 2007*. Philadelphia: Elsevier W. B. Saunders.

Lenehan, G. P. (2004). Latex allergy: Separating fact from fiction. *Travel Nursing,* pp. 12–17.

Lethaby, A., Cooke, I., & Rees, M. (2006). Progesterone/progestogen releasing intrauterine systems versus either placebo or any other medication for heavy menstrual bleeding. *Cochrane Database Systematic Review* (4), CD002126.

Lever, K. A. (2005) Emergency contraception. *AWHONN Lifelines, 9*(3), 218–225.

Manson, J. E. (2006) Perimenopause, hormones, and midlife health. *Harvard Women's Health Watch, 14*(3), 1–3.

Master-Hunter, T., & Heiman, D. L. (2006). Amenorrhea: Evaluation and treatment. *American Family Physician, 73*(8), 1374–1382.

McKinney, L. N. (2007). Low libido in postmenopausal women. *Advance for Nurse Practitioners, 15*(1), 28–36.

McNally, D. N., Kenny, A. M., & Smith, J. A. (2007), Adherence of academic geriatric practitioners to osteoporosis screening guidelines. *Osteoporosis International, 18*(2), 177–183.

Mishell, D. R., Guillebaud, J., Westoff, C., Nelson, A. L., Kaunitz, A. M., Trussell, J., & Davis, A. J. (2007). Combined hormonal contraceptive traits: Variable data collection and bleeding assessment methodologies influence study outcomes and physician perception. *Contraception, 75*(1), 4–10.

Moreno, M. A., & Giesel, A. E. (2006). Premenstrual syndrome. *Emedicine.* Available at: http://www.emedicine.com/ped/topic1890.htm

Murphy, P. A., Morgan, K., & Likis, F. E. (2006). Contraception. In K. D. Schuiling & F. E. Likis (Eds.), *Women's gynecologic health* (pp. 169–228). Sudbury, MA: Jones and Bartlett Publishers.

Nasir, L. S. (2007). Dysmenorrhea. In R. E. Rakel & E. T. Bope (Eds.), *Conn's current therapy 2007* (pp. 1238–1240). Philadelphia: Saunders.

National Institute of Child Health and Human Development (NICHD) (2006). Endometriosis. NICHD Information Resource Center, NIH Pub. No. 02-2413. Available at: http://www.nichd.nih.gov/health/topics/Endometriosis.cfm

National Osteoporosis Foundation (NOF) (2007). Steps to prevent osteoporosis. Available at: http://www.nof.org/prevention/index.htm

Nelson, L. M., & Bakalov, V. (2006). Amenorrhea. *eMedicine.* Available at: http://www.emedicine.com/med/topic117.htm

Newton, K. M., Reed, S. D., LaCroix, A. Z., Grothaus, L. C., Ehrlich, K., & Guiltinan, J. (2006). Treatment of vasomotor symptoms of menopause with black cohosh, multibotanicals, soy, hormone therapy, or placebo. A randomized trial. *Annals of Internal Medicine, 145,* 869–879.

North American Menopause Society (NAMS) (2004). Recommendations for estrogen and progesterone use in peri-menopausal and post-menopausal women. *Menopause, 11*(6), 589–600.

OSHA (2006). Latex allergy. U.S. Department of Labor, Occupational Safety & Health Administration. Available at: http://www.osha.gov/SLTC/latexallergy

Pagana, K. D., & Pagana, T. J. (2007). *Mosby's diagnostic and laboratory test reference* (8th ed.). Philadelphia: Elsevier Mosby.

Pavlovich-Danis, S. J. (2007). Cyclic upheaval: Premenstrual syndrome and premenstrual dysphoric disorder. *Nursing Spectrum.* Available at: http://www.nurse.com/ce/course.html?CCID=3297

Planned Parenthood (2007). Facts about birth control. Available at: http://www.plannedparenthood.org/bc/bcfacts4.html

Quallich, S. (2006). Examining male infertility. *Urologic Nursing, 26*(4), 277 288.

Rackow, B. W., & Arici, A. (2007). Dysfunctional uterine bleeding. In R. E. Rakel & E. T. Bope (Eds.), *Conn's current therapy 2007* (pp. 1230–1232). Philadelphia: Saunders.

Ravin, C. R. (2006). Considering contraception: What practitioners are saying. *AWHONN Lifelines, 10*(2), 122–128.

Redshaw, M., Hockley, C., & Davidson, L. L. (2007). A qualitative study of the experience of treatment for infertility among women who successfully become pregnant. *Human Reproduction, 22*(1), 295–304.

Robinson, K. (2005). Depo-Provera: New concerns—same issues? *AWHONN Lifelines, 9*(3), 214–217.

Roederer, M. W., Blackwell, J., & Blenning, C. (2006). Risks and benefits of combination contraceptives. *American Family Physician, 74*(11), 1915–1916.

Rosano, G. M., Vitale, C., Marazzi, G., Voltazzi, G., & Volterrani, M. (2007). Menopause and cardiovascular disease: The evidence. *Climacteric* (Supplement 1, 10), 19–24.

Rubin, R. (2007). A herbal menopause therapy: Get a closer look. *USA Today,* Jan. 11, 2007, p. 7.

Samra, O. M., & Wood, E. (2006). Contraception. *Emedicine.* Available at: http://www.emedicine.com/med/topic3211.htm

Saul, T., & Dave, A. K. (2006) Endometriosis. *Emedicine.* Available at: http://www.emedicine.com/EMERG/topic165.htm

Schenker, J. G. (2005). Assisted reproductive practice: Religious perspectives. *Reproductive BioMedicine, 10*(3), 310–319.

Schuiling, K. D., & Likis, F. E. (2006). *Women's gynecologic health.* Sudbury, MA: Jones and Bartlett Publishers.

Seppa, N. (2007). Putting the kibosh on black cohosh. *Science News, 171*(2), 29–30.

Shelby, K., & O'Hair, K. (2007). Hormone replacement therapy: What we know now. *Nursing Spectrum.* Available at: http://www.nurse.com/ce/course.html?CCID=2325&PageNum=3&Begin=11545

Sinai, I., Arevalo, M., & Jennings, V. (2006). Fertility awareness-based methods of family planning: Predictors of correct use. *International Family Planning Perspectives, 32*(2), 94–100.

Skidmore-Roth, L. (2007). *Mosby's drug guide for nurses* (7th ed.). St. Louis, MO: Elsevier Mosby.

Smith, R. P. (2006) Finding the best approach to dysmenorrhea. *Contemporary OB/GYN, 51*(11), 54–62.

Speroff, L., & Fritz, M. A. (2005). *Clinical gynecologic endocrinology and fertility* (7th ed.). Philadelphia: Lippincott Williams & Wilkins.

Staff of the Boston Women's Health Book Collective (2007). *Our bodies, ourselves: Menopause.* New York: Simon & Schuster Trade.

Stewart, F. H., Kaunitz, A. M., LaGuardia, K. D., Karvois, D. L., Fisher, A. C., & Friedman, A. J. (2006). Extended use of transdermal norelgestromin/ethinyl estradiol: A randomized trial. *Obstetrics & Gynecology, 105*(6), 1389–1396.

Swica, Y., & Westhoff, C. (2006). Update on new contraceptive choices. *Journal of Clinical Outcomes Management, 13*(8), 447–455.

Taylor, D. (2005). Perimenstrual symptoms and syndromes: Guidelines for symptom management and self-care. *Advanced Studies in Medicine, 5*(5), 228–241.

Tolaymat, L. L., & Kaunitz, A. M. (2007). Contraceptive methods. In R. E. Rakel & E. T. Bope (Eds.), *Conn's current therapy 2007* (pp. 882–885). Philadelphia: Saunders.

Torpy, J. M. (2007). Polycystic ovary syndrome. *JAMA, 297*(5), 554–557.

Trussell, J. (2004). Contraceptive efficacy. In R. Hatcher, et al. (Eds.), *Contraceptive technology* (18th rev. ed.). New York: Ardent Media, Inc.

UNFPA (2007). *The state of the world population 2006 report.* Available at: http://www.unfpa.org/swp/swpmain.htm

U.S. Bureau of the Census (2006). *National population estimates-characteristics.* Available at: http://eire.census.gov/popest/data/national/tables/asro/NA-EST2002-ASRO-01.php

U.S. Food & Drug Administration (FDA) (2006). FDA approves over-the-counter access for Plan B for women 18 and older; prescription remains required for those 17 and younger. *FDA News* (August 24, 2006). Available at: www.fda.gov/bbs/topics/NEWS/2006/New01436.html

Valle, R. F. (2006). Combination of tubal sterilization and endometrial ablation is safe and effective. *Fertility and Sterility, 86*(1), 152–158.

World Health Organization (WHO) (2007). Infertility in developing countries. *Reproductive Health.* Available at: http://www.who.int/reproductive-health/infertility/index.htm

Writing Group for the Women's Health Initiative Investigators (2002). Risks and benefits of estrogen plus progestin in healthy post-menopausal women: Principal results from the Women's Health Initiative randomized controlled trial. *JAMA, 288*(3), 321–333.

Wysocki, S. (2007). Clinical rationale for continuous oral contraception. *American Journal for Nurse Practitioners, 11*(3), 57–67.

Youngkin, E. Q., & Davis, M. S. (2004). *Women's health: A primary care clinical guide* (3rd ed.). New Jersey: Prentice Hall.

WEBSITES

American College of Obstetricians and Gynecologists (ACOG): (202) 863-2518, http://www.acog.org

American Psychiatric Association: (202) 682-6000, http://psych.org

American Society for Reproductive Medicine: (205) 978-5000, http://www.asrm.org

Centers for Disease Control and Prevention: (202) 329-1819, http://www.cdc.gov

Consortium for Emergency Contraceptive: http://www.cecinfo.org

Center for Reproductive Rights: http://www.crlp.org

Emergency Contraception Hotline: (888) 668-2528, http://www.not-2-late.com

Endometriosis Association: (414) 355-2200, http://www.ovf.com/endohtml.html

FDA's Office of Women's Health: http://www.fda.gov/womens

Hormone Foundation: (800) 467-6663, http://hormone.org

International Counsel on Infertility Information Dissemination: (703) 379-9178, http://www.inciid.org

National Institute of Mental Health: (301) 443-4513, http://www.nimh.nih.gov

National Women's Health Resource Center: (877) 986-9472, http://www.healthywomen.org

National Women's Information Center (NWHIC): (800) 994-9662, http://www.4women.gov

North American Menopause Society: http://www.menopause.org

Planned Parenthood Federation of America, Inc.: (800) 669-0156, http://www.plannedparenthood.org

Premenstrual Institute: (248) 624-3366, http://www.pmsinst.com

Resolve, The National Infertility Association: (617) 623-0744, http://www.resolve.org

CHAPTER WORKSHEET

MULTIPLE CHOICE QUESTIONS

1. A couple is considered infertile after how many months of trying to conceive?

   a. 6 months

   b. 12 months

   c. 18 months

   d. 24 months

2. A couple reports that their condom broke while they were having sexual intercourse last night. What would you advise to prevent pregnancy?

   a. Inject a spermicidal agent into her vagina immediately.

   b. Obtain emergency contraceptives and take them immediately.

   c. Douche with a solution of vinegar and hot water tonight.

   d. Take a strong laxative now and again at bedtime.

3. Which of the following combination contraceptives has been approved for extended continuous use?

   a. Seasonale

   b. NuvaRing

   c. Ortho Evra

   d. Mirena

4. Which of the following measures helps prevent osteoporosis?

   a. Iron supplementation

   b. Sleeping 8 hours nightly

   c. Eating lean meats only

   d. Walking 3 miles daily

5. Which of the following activities will increase a woman's risk of cardiovascular disease if she is taking oral contraceptives?

   a. Eating a high-fiber diet

   b. Smoking cigarettes

   c. Taking daily multivitamins

   d. Drinking alcohol

6. Hormone therapy taken by menopausal women reduces:

   a. Weight gain

   b. Bone density

   c. Hot flashes

   d. Heart disease

7. Throughout life, a woman's most proactive activity to promote her health would be to engage in:

   a. Consistent exercise

   b. Socialization with friends

   c. Quality quiet time with herself

   d. Consuming water

8. What comment by a woman would indicate that a diaphragm is not the best contraceptive device for her?

   a. "My husband says it is my job to keep from getting pregnant."

   b. "I have a hard time remembering to take my vitamins daily."

   c. "Hormones cause cancer and I don't want to take them."

   d. "I am not comfortable touching myself down there."

CRITICAL THINKING EXERCISE

1. Ms. London, 25, comes to your family planning clinic requesting to have an intrauterine system (IUS) inserted because "birth control pills give you cancer." In reviewing her history, you note she has been into the STI clinic three times in the past year with vaginal infections and was hospitalized for pelvic inflammatory disease (PID) last month. When you question her about her sexual history, she reports having sex with multiple partners and not always using protection.

   a. Is an IUS the most appropriate method for her? Why or why not?

   b. What myths/misperceptions will you address in your counseling session?

   c. Outline the safer sex discussion you plan to have with her.

STUDY ACTIVITIES

1. Develop a teaching plan for an adolescent with premenstrual syndrome and dysmenorrhea.

2. Arrange to shadow a nurse working in family planning for the morning. What questions does the nurse ask to ascertain the kind of family planning method that is right for each woman? What teaching goes along with each method? What follow-up care is needed? Share your findings with your classmates during a clinical conference.

3. Surf the Internet and locate three resources for infertile couples to consult that provide support and resources.

4. Sterilization is the most prevalent method of contraception used by married couples in the United States. Contact a local urologist and gynecologist to learn about the procedure involved and the cost of a male and female sterilization. Which procedure poses less risk to the person and costs less?

5. Take a field trip to a local drugstore to check out the variety and costs of male and female condoms. How many different brands did you find? What was the range of costs?

6. Noncontraceptive benefits of combined oral contraceptives include which of the following? Select all that apply.

   a. Protection against ovarian cancer

   b. Protection against endometrial cancer

   c. Protection against breast cancer

   d. Reduction in incidence of ectopic pregnancy

   e. Prevention of functional ovarian cysts

   f. Reduction in deep venous thrombosis

   g. Reduction in the risk of colorectal cancer

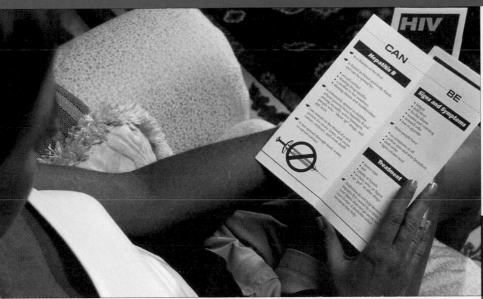

SEXUALLY TRANSMITTED INFECTIONS

KEY TERMS

bacterial vaginosis
gonorrhea
pelvic inflammatory
    disease (PID)

sexually transmitted
    infection (STI)
syphilis

trichomoniasis
vulvovaginal candidiasis

LEARNING OBJECTIVES

Upon completion of the chapter, the learner will be able to:

1. Define the key terms used in this chapter.
2. Discuss the spread and control of sexually transmitted infections.
3. Identify risk factors and outline appropriate client education needed in common sexually transmitted infections.
4. Discuss how contraceptives can play a role in the prevention of sexually transmitted infections.
5. Analyze the physiologic and psychological aspects of sexually transmitted infections.
6. Delineate the nursing management needed for women with sexually transmitted infections.

CHAPTER 5

Sandy, a 19-year-old, couldn't imagine what these "things" were that appeared "down there" in her genital area last week. She was too embarrassed to tell anyone, so she stopped by the college health service today to find out what they were.

Wow

Unconditional self-acceptance in clients is the core to reducing risky behavior and fostering peace of mind.

exually transmitted infections (STIs) are infections of the reproductive tract caused by microorganisms transmitted through vaginal, anal, or oral sexual intercourse (CDC, 2006). STIs pose a serious threat not only to women's sexual health but also to the general health and well-being of millions of people worldwide. STIs constitute an epidemic of tremendous magnitude. An estimated 65 million people live with an incurable STI, and another 15 million are infected each year (CDC, 2006). The incidence of STIs continues to rise in the United States.

STIs are biologically sexist, presenting greater risk and causing more complications among women than among men. Women are diagnosed with two thirds of the estimated 15 million new cases of STIs annually in the United States. After only a single exposure, women are twice as likely as men to acquire infections from pathogens causing gonorrhea, chlamydia infection, hepatitis B, and syphilis (Johnson-Mallard et al., 2007). STIs may contribute to cervical cancer, infertility, ectopic pregnancy, chronic pelvic pain, and death. Certain infections can be transmitted in utero to the fetus or during childbirth to the newborn (Table 5.1). STIs know no class, racial, ethnic, or social barriers—all individuals are vulnerable if exposed to the infectious organism. The problem of STIs has still not been tackled adequately on a global scale, and until this is done, numbers worldwide will continue to increase.

A special section on STIs and adolescents is presented below. This is followed by discussion of specific STIs categorized according to the CDC framework, which groups STIs according to the major symptom manifested (Box 5.1). A section on preventing STIs is included at the end of the chapter.

BOX 5.1 CDC Classification of STIs

- Infections characterized by vaginal discharge
  - Vulvovaginal candidiasis
  - Trichomoniasis
  - Bacterial vaginosis
- Infections characterized by cervicitis
  - Chlamydia
  - Gonorrhea
- Infections characterized by genital ulcers
  - Genital herpes simplex
  - Syphilis
- Pelvic inflammatory disease (PID)
- Human immunodeficiency virus (HIV)
- Human papillomavirus infection (HPV)
- Vaccine-preventable STIs
  - Hepatitis A
  - Hepatitis B
- Ectoparasitic infections
  - Pediculosis pubis
  - Scabies

Sexually Transmitted Infections and Adolescents

An estimated two thirds of all STIs occur among persons under the age of 25 (Waugh, 2007). Each year there are 4 million cases of STIs among teenagers. In the United States, teens who are sexually active experience high rates of STIs, and some groups are at higher risk, including African-American youths, abused youths, homeless youths,

TABLE 5.1   STIs AND EFFECTS ON THE FETUS OR NEWBORN

STI	Effects on Fetus or Newborn
Chlamydia	Can be infected during delivery Eye infections (neonatal conjunctivitis), pneumonia, low birthweight, preterm birth, stillbirth
Gonorrhea	Can be infected during delivery Rhinitis, vaginitis, urethritis, inflammation of sites of fetal monitoring Ophthalmia neonatorum can lead to blindness and sepsis (including arthritis and meningitis).
Herpes type II (genital herpes)	Contamination can occur during birth. Mental retardation, premature birth, low birthweight, death
Syphilis	Can be passed in utero Can result in fetal or infant death Congenital syphilis symptoms include skin ulcers, rashes, fever, weakened or hoarse cry, swollen liver and spleen, jaundice and anemia, various deformations.
Trichomoniasis	Fever, irritability, preterm birth, low birthweight
Venereal warts	May develop warts in throat (laryngeal papillomatosis); uncommon but life-threatening

young men having sex with men, and gay, lesbian, bisexual, and transgendered youths.

> ▶ **Take** NOTE!
>
> *It is estimated that before graduating from high school, 25% of adolescents will contract an STI (Pickering, 2006).*

Biological and behavioral factors place teenagers at high risk. Female adolescents are more susceptible to STIs due to their anatomy. During adolescence and young adulthood, women's columnar epithelial cells are especially sensitive to invasion by sexually transmitted organisms, such as chlamydia and gonococci, because they extend out over the vaginal surface of the cervix, where they are unprotected by cervical mucus; these cells recede to a more protected location as women age. Behaviorally, adolescent and young adults tend to think they are invincible and deny the risks of their behavior. This risky behavior exposes them to STIs and HIV/AIDS. Adolescents frequently have unprotected intercourse, they engage in partnerships of limited duration, and they face many obstacles that prevent them from using the health care system.

Nursing Assessment

Many health care providers fail to assess adolescent sexual behavior and STI risks, to screen for asymptomatic infection during clinic visits, or to counsel adolescents on STI risk reduction. Nurses need to remember that they play a key role in the detection, prevention, and treatment of STIs in adolescents. All states allow adolescents to give consent to confidential STI testing and treatment. Table 5.2 discusses clinical manifestations of common STIs in adolescents.

Nursing Management

Encourage the client to complete the antibiotic prescription (specific management for each type of STI is discussed below).

Prevention of STIs among adolescents is critical. Health care providers have a unique opportunity to provide counseling and education to their clients. Adapt the style, content, and message to the client's developmental level. Identify risk factors and risk behaviors and guide the client to develop specific individualized actions of prevention. Your interaction with the client needs to be direct and nonjudgmental.

Encourage adolescents to postpone initiation of sexual intercourse for as long as possible, but if they choose to have sexual intercourse, explain the necessity of using barrier methods, such as male and female condoms (Teaching

Guidelines 5.1). For teens who have already had sexual intercourse, the clinician can encourage abstinence at this point. If adolescents are sexually active, they should be directed to teen clinics and contraceptive options should be explained. In areas where specialized teen clinics are not available, nurses should feel comfortable discussing sexuality, safety, and contraception with teens. Encourage adolescents to minimize their lifetime number of sexual partners, to use barrier methods consistently and correctly, and to be aware of the connection between drug and alcohol use and the incorrect use of barrier methods. Table 5.3 discusses barriers to condom use and means to overcome them.

Think back to Sandy, who was introduced at the beginning of the chapter. How should the nurse handle Sandy's anxious state? What specific questions should the nurse ask Sandy to determine the source of the possible infection in her genital area?

Infections Characterized by Vaginal Discharge

Vaginitis is a generic term that means inflammation and infection of the vagina. There can be hundreds of causes for vaginitis, but more often than not the cause is infection by one of three organisms:

• Candida, a fungus
• Trichomonas, a protozoan
• Gardnerella, a bacterium

The complex balance of microbiological organisms in the vagina is a key element in the maintenance of health. Subtle shifts in the vaginal environment may allow organisms with pathologic potential to proliferate, causing infectious symptoms.

The nurse's role in managing vaginitis is one of primary prevention and education to limit recurrences of these infections. Primary prevention begins with changing the sexual behaviors that place women at risk for infection. In addition to assessing women for the common signs and symptoms and risk factors, the nurse can help women to avoid vaginitis or to prevent a recurrence by teaching them to take the precautions highlighted in Teaching Guidelines 5.2.

▶ VULVOVAGINAL CANDIDIASIS

Vulvovaginal candidiasis is one of the most common causes of vaginal discharge. It is also referred to as yeast, monilia, and a fungal infection. It is not considered an

(text continues on page 120)

TABLE 5.2 STIs COMMON IN ADOLESCENTS

Disease	Causative Organism	Transmission Mode	Diagnostic Testing	Female Symptoms	Male Symptoms	Treatment
Chlamydia Curable STI Seen frequently among sexually active adolescents and young adults Sexually active adolescents should be screened at least annually.	*Chlamydia trachomatis* (bacteria)	Vaginal, anal, oral sex, and by childbirth	Culture fluid from urethral swabs in males or endocervical swabs for females and conjunctival secretions in neonates	May be asymptomatic Dysuria Vaginal discharge (mucus or pus) Endocervicitis May lead to pelvic inflammatory disease, ectopic pregnancy, and infertility Can cause inflammation of the rectum and lining of the eye (conjunctivitis) Can infect the throat from oral sexual contact with an infected partner	May be asymptomatic Dysuria Penile discharge (mucus or pus) Urethral tingling May lead to epididymitis (inflammation of the epididymis, the tubular structure that connects the testicle with the vas deferens) and sterility Can cause inflammation of the rectum and lining of the eye (conjunctivitis) Can infect the throat from oral sexual contact with an infected partner	Azithromycin (Zithromax) Doxycycline (Vibramycin) Erythromycin (EES) Ofloxacin (Floxin) Sexual partners need evaluation, testing, and treatment also.
Gonorrhea Curable STI Client is often co-infected with *Chlamydia trachomatis*	*Neisseria gonorrhoeae* (bacteria)	Vaginal, anal, oral sex, and by childbirth	Staining samples directly for the bacterium, detection of bacterial genes or DNA in urine, and growing the bacteria in laboratory cultures More than one test may be used.	May be asymptomatic or no recognizable symptoms until serious complications such as pelvic inflammatory disease Dysuria Urinary frequency Vaginal discharge (yellow, foul) Dyspareunia Endocervicitis Arthritis May lead to pelvic inflammatory disease, ectopic pregnancy, and infertility Symptoms of rectal infection include discharge, anal itching, and occasional painful	Most produce symptoms but can be asymptomatic Dysuria Penile discharge (pus) Arthritis May lead to epididymitis and sterility Symptoms of rectal infection include discharge, anal itching, and occasional painful bowel movements with fresh blood.	Usually a single dose of one of the following: Cefiximine (Suprax) Ciprofloxacin (Cipro) Ceftriaxone (Rocephin) Ofloxacin (Floxin) Levofloxin (Levaquin) **No Floxin or Cipro if <18 years or pregnant!** Azithromycin (Zithromax) Doxycycline (Vibramycin) Usually will be treated for co-infection with chlamydia, so a combination is given (e.g., ceftriaxone and doxycycline). Sexual partners need evaluation, testing, and treatment also.

Herpes Type II (Genital Herpes)	Herpes simplex virus II (HSV II)	Having sexual contact (vaginal, oral, or anal) with someone who is shedding the herpes virus either during an outbreak or during a period with no symptoms. Can be transmitted through close skin-to-skin contact	Visual inspection and symptoms or culture. Virologic and type-specific serologic tests can tell if herpes simplex virus II is present but does not confirm genital herpes, though most providers will assume a positive HSV II means genital herpes.	bowel movements with fresh blood. Blister-like genital lesions. Dysuria. Fever, headache, muscle aches	Blister-like genital lesions. Dysuria. Fever, headache, muscle aches	Acyclovir (Zovirax). Other antivirals. DOES NOT CURE, just controls symptoms. Sexual partners benefit from evaluation and counseling. If symptomatic, they need treatment. If asymptomatic, offer testing and education.
Herpes Type II (Genital Herpes) Lifelong recurrent viral disease. Most people have not been diagnosed. There is no cure.						
Syphilis	*Treponema pallidum* (spirochete bacteria)	Sexual contact with an infected person	Blood tests. Venereal Disease Research Laboratory (VDRL), Rapid Plasma Reagin (RPR), and treponemal tests (e.g., fluorescent treponemal antibody absorbed [FTA-ABS]) can lead to a presumptive diagnosis. Darkfield examination and direct fluorescent antibody tests	Disease is divided into four stages. *Primary infection* • Chancre on place of entrance of bacteria (usually vulva or vagina but can develop in other parts of the body). *Secondary infection* • Maculopapular rash (hands & feet) • Sore throat • Lymphadenopathy • Flu-like symptoms. *Latent infection* • No symptoms • No longer contagious • Many people if not treated will suffer no further signs and symptoms.	Disease is divided into four stages. *Primary infection* • Chancre on place of entrance of bacteria (usually on penis but can develop in other parts of the body). *Secondary, latent, and tertiary infections.* All similar to female symptoms	Penicillin G inj. (if penicillin allergy, doxycycline or erythromycin). Sexual partners need evaluation and testing.

(continued)

TABLE 5.2 STIs COMMON IN ADOLESCENTS (continued)

Disease	Causative Organism	Transmission Mode	Diagnostic Testing	Female Symptoms	Male Symptoms	Treatment
			of lesion exudate or tissue provide definitive diagnosis of early syphilis.	Some people will go on to develop tertiary or late syphilis. *Tertiary infections* • Tumors of skin, bones & liver • CNS symptoms • CV symptoms • Usually not reversible at this stage		
Trichomoniasis	*Trichomonas vaginalis* (protozoan)	Vaginal intercourse with an infected partner May be picked up from direct genital contact with damp or moist objects, such as towels, wet clothing, or a toilet seat	Microscopic evaluation of vaginal secretions or culture	Many women have symptoms but some may be asymptomatic. Dysuria Urinary frequency Vaginal discharge (yellow, green, or gray & foul odor) Dyspareunia Irritation or itching of genital area	Most infected men are asymptomatic. Dysuria Penile discharge (watery, white)	Metronidazole (Flagyl) Sexual partners need evaluation, testing, and treatment also.

Venereal Warts (condylomata acuminata)	Human papillomavirus	Vaginal, anal, or oral sex with an infected partner	Visual inspection Abnormal Pap smear may indicate cervical infection of HPV.	Wart-like lesions that are soft, moist, or flesh-colored and appear on the vulva and cervix and surrounding the vagina and anus	Wart-like lesions that are soft, moist, or flesh-colored and appear on the scrotum or penis	May disappear without treatment
One of the most common STIs in the United States				Sometimes appear in clusters that resemble cauliflower-like bumps, and are either raised or flat, small or large	Sometimes appear in clusters that resemble cauliflower-like bumps, and are either raised or flat, small or large	Treatment is aimed at removing the lesions rather than HPV itself
Could lead to cancers of the cervix, vulva, vagina, anus, or penis						No optimal treatment has been identified, but there are several ways to treat them depending on size and location. Most methods rely on chemical or physical destruction of the lesion:
No cure; warts can be removed but virus remains						Imiquimod cream 20%
						Podophyllin anti-mitotic solution 0.5%
						Podofilox solution 5%
						5-fluorouracil cream
						Trichloroacetic acid (TCA)
						Small warts can be removed by:
						• Freezing (cryosurgery)
						• Burning (electro-cautery)
						• Laser treatment
						Large warts that have not responded to treatment may be removed surgically.

TEACHING GUIDELINES 5.1

Proper Condom Use

- Use latex condoms.
- Use a new condom with each act of sexual intercourse. Never reuse a condom.
- Handle condoms with care to prevent damage from sharp objects such as fingernails and teeth.
- Ensure condom has been stored in a cool, dry place away from direct sunlight. Do not store condoms in wallet or automobile or anywhere they would be exposed to extreme temperatures.
- Do not use a condom if it appears brittle, sticky, or discolored. These are signs of aging.
- Put condom on before any genital contact.
- Put condom on when penis is erect. Ensure it is placed so it will readily unroll.
- Hold the tip of the condom while unrolling. Ensure there is a space at the tip for semen to collect, but make sure no air is trapped in the tip.
- Ensure adequate lubrication during intercourse. If external lubricants are used, use only water-based lubricants such as KY jelly with latex condoms. Oil-based or petroleum-based lubricants, such as body lotion, massage oil, or cooking oil, can weaken latex condoms.
- Withdraw while penis is still erect, and hold condom firmly against base of penis.

Adapted from Pickering, L. K. (Ed.) (2006). *Red book: 2006 report of the committee on infectious diseases* (27th ed.). Elk Grove Village, IL: American Academy of Pediatrics; and Public Health Agency of Canada (2006). *Canadian guidelines on sexually transmitted infections.* Ottawa, ON: Author.

STI because Candida is a normal constituent in the vagina and becomes pathologic only when the vaginal environment becomes altered. An estimated 75% of women will have at least one episode of vulvovaginal candidiasis, and 40% to 50% will have two or more episodes in their lifetime (CDC, 2006).

Therapeutic Management

Treatment of candidiasis includes one of the following medications:

- Miconazole (Monistat) cream or suppository
- Clotrimazole (Mycelex) tablet or cream
- Terconazole (Terazol) cream or intravaginal suppository
- Fluconazole (Diflucan) oral tablet (CDC, 2006, p. 55)

Most of the above medications are used intravaginally in the form of a cream, tablet, or suppositories used for 3 to 7 days. If fluconazole (Diflucan) is prescribed, a 150-mg oral tablet is taken as a single dose.

Topical azole preparations are effective in the treatment of vulvovaginal candidiasis, relieving symptoms and producing negative cultures in 80% to 90% of women who complete therapy (CDC, 2006). If vulvovaginal candidiasis is not treated effectively during pregnancy, the newborn can develop an oral infection known as thrush during the birth process; that infection must be treated with a local azole preparation after birth.

Nursing Assessment

Assess the patient's health history for predisposing factors for vulvovaginal candidiasis, which include:

- Pregnancy
- Use of oral contraceptives with a high estrogen content
- Use of broad-spectrum antibiotics
- Diabetes mellitus
- Obesity
- Use of steroid and immunosuppressive drugs
- HIV infection
- Wearing tight, restrictive clothes and nylon underpants
- Trauma to vaginal mucosa from chemical irritants or douching

Assess the patient for clinical manifestations of vulvovaginal candidiasis. Typical symptoms, which can worsen just before menses, include:

- Pruritus
- Vaginal discharge (thick, white, curd-like)
- Vaginal soreness
- Vulvar burning
- Erythema in the vulvovaginal area
- Dyspareunia
- External dysuria

Figure 5.1 shows the typical appearance of vulvovaginal candidiasis.

Speculum examination will reveal white plaques on the vaginal walls. The vaginal pH remains within normal range. Definitive diagnosis is made by a wet smear, which reveals the filamentous hyphae and spores characteristic of a fungus when viewed under a microscope.

Nursing Management

Teach preventive measures to women with frequent vulvovaginal candidiasis infections, including:

- Reduce dietary intake of simple sugars and soda.
- Wear white, 100% cotton underpants.
- Avoid wearing tight pants or exercise clothes with spandex.
- Shower rather than taking tub baths.
- Wash with a mild, unscented soap and dry the genitals gently.
- Avoid the use of bubble baths or scented bath products.
- Wash underwear in unscented laundry detergent and hot water.

TABLE 5.3 **BARRIERS TO CONDOM USE AND MEANS TO OVERCOME THEM**

Perceived Barrier	Intervention Strategy
Decreases sexual pleasure (sensation) Note: Often perceived by those who have never used a condom.	• Encourage patient to try. • Put a drop of water-based lubricant or saliva inside the tip of the condom or on the glans of the penis before putting on the condom. • Try a thinner latex condom or a different brand or more lubrication.
Decreases spontaneity of sexual activity	• Incorporate condom use into foreplay. • Remind patient that peace of mind may enhance pleasure for self and partner.
Embarrassing, juvenile, "unmanly"	• Remind patient that it is "manly" to protect himself and others.
Poor fit (too small or too big, slips off, uncomfortable)	• Smaller and larger condoms are available.
Requires prompt withdrawal after ejaculation	• Reinforce the protective nature of prompt withdrawal and suggest substituting other postcoital sexual activities.
Fear of breakage may lead to less vigorous sexual activity.	• With prolonged intercourse, lubricant wears off and the condom begins to rub. Have a water-soluble lubricant available to reapply.
Non-penetrative sexual activity	• Condoms have been advocated for use during fellatio; unlubricated condoms may prove best for this purpose due to the taste of the lubricant. • Other barriers, such as dental dams or an unlubricated condom, can be cut down the middle to form a barrier; these have been advocated for use during certain forms of non-penetrative sexual activity (e.g., cunnilingus and anolingual sex).
Allergy to latex	• Polyurethane male and female condoms are available. • A natural skin condom can be used together with a latex condom to protect the man or woman from contact with latex.

From Public Health Agency of Canada. (2006). *Canadian guidelines on sexually transmitted infections.*

• Dry underwear in a hot dryer to kill the yeast that clings to the fabric.
• Remove wet bathing suits promptly.
• Practice good body hygiene.
• Avoid vaginal sprays/deodorants.
• Avoid wearing pantyhose (or cut out the crotch to allow air circulation).
• Use white, unscented toilet paper and wipe from front to back.
• Avoid douching (which washes away protective vaginal mucus).
• Avoid the use of super-absorbent tampons (use pads instead).

◗ TRICHOMONIASIS

Trichomoniasis is another common vaginal infection that causes a discharge. The woman may be markedly symptomatic or asymptomatic. Men are asymptomatic carriers. Although this infection is localized, there is increasing evidence of preterm birth and postpartum endometritis in women with this vaginitis (CDC, 2006). *Trichomonas vaginalis* is an ovoid, single-cell protozoan parasite that can be observed under the microscope making a jerky swaying motion.

Therapeutic Management

A single 2-gram dose of oral metronidazole (Flagyl) or tinidazole (Tindamax) for both partners is a common treatment for this infection. Sex partners of women with trichomoniasis should be treated to avoid recurrence of infection.

Nursing Assessment

Assess the patient for clinical manifestations of trichomoniasis, which include:

• A heavy yellow/green or gray frothy or bubbly discharge
• Vaginal pruritus and vulvar soreness
• Dyspareunia
• Cervix may bleed on contact
• Dysuria
• Colpitis macularis ("strawberry" look on cervix)

Figure 5.2 shows the typical appearance of trichomoniasis.

The diagnosis is confirmed when a motile flagellated trichomonad is visualized under the microscope. In addition, a vaginal pH of greater than 4.5 is a typical finding.

Nursing Management

Instruct clients to avoid sex until they and their sex partners are cured (i.e., when therapy has been completed and both partners are symptom-free) and also to avoid consuming alcohol during treatment because mixing the med-

TEACHING GUIDELINES 5.2

Preventing Vaginitis

- Avoid douching to prevent altering the vaginal environment.
- Use condoms to avoid spreading the organism.
- Avoid tights, nylon underpants, and tight clothes.
- Wipe from front to back after using the toilet.
- Avoid powders, bubble baths, and perfumed vaginal sprays.
- Wear clean cotton underpants.
- Change out of wet bathing suits as soon as possible.
- Become familiar with the signs and symptoms of vaginitis.
- Choose to lead a healthy lifestyle.

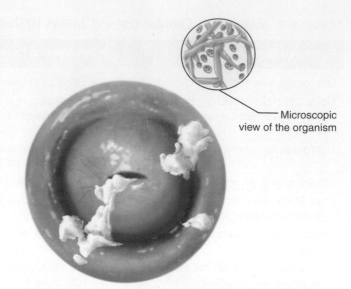

Microscopic view of the organism

FIGURE 5.1 Vulvovaginal candidiasis. (Source: The Anatomical Chart Company. [2002]. *Atlas of pathophysiology*. Springhouse, PA: Springhouse.)

ications and alcohol causes severe nausea and vomiting (CDC, 2006).

▶ BACTERIAL VAGINOSIS

A third common infection of the vagina is **bacterial vaginosis**, caused by the gram-negative bacillus *Gardnerella vaginalis*. It is the most prevalent cause of vaginal discharge or malodor, but up to 50% of women are asymptomatic. Bacterial vaginosis is a sexually associated infection characterized by alterations in vaginal flora in which lactobacilli

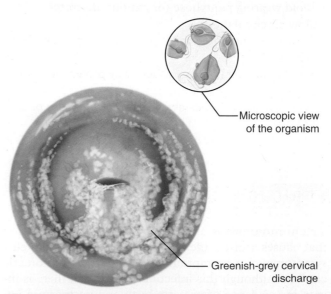

Microscopic view of the organism

Greenish-grey cervical discharge

FIGURE 5.2 Trichomoniasis. (Source: The Anatomical Chart Company. [2002]. *Atlas of pathophysiology*. Springhouse, PA: Springhouse.)

EVIDENCE-BASED PRACTICE 5.1
Interventions for Trichomoniasis in Pregnancy

● **Study**

Trichomoniasis is a very common sexually transmitted infection. Symptoms include vaginal itching and discharge. It is not clear whether pregnant women with trichomoniasis are more likely to give birth preterm or to have other pregnancy complications. The review of trials found that the drug metronidazole is effective against trichomoniasis when taken by women and their partners during pregnancy, but it may harm the baby. Of the two clinical trials reviewed, one was stopped early because women taking metronidazole were more likely to give birth preterm and have low-birthweight babies. Further research into trichomoniasis treatments for pregnant women is needed.

▲ **Findings**

Metronidazole is effective against a trichomoniasis infection during pregnancy but may increase the risk of preterm and low-birthweight babies.

■ **Nursing Implications**

The nurse's role concerning this study's results is to counsel women diagnosed with trichomoniasis during pregnancy about the potential risks of treatment. The woman should be cautioned about taking this medication if she has a previous history of preterm births, is carrying twins, or is experiencing preterm contractions. In addition, an ultrasound should validate the fetal weight linked to the gestational age to make sure it is within normal range before this medication is prescribed.

Source: Gülmezoglu A. M. (2007). Interventions for trichomoniasis in pregnancy. *Cochrane Database of Systematic Reviews* 2006, Issue 3. Art. No.: CD000220. DOI: 10.1002/14651858.CD000220.

in the vagina are replaced with high concentrations of anaerobic bacteria. The cause of the microbial alteration is not fully understood but is associated with having multiple sex partners, douching, and lack of vaginal lactobacilli (CDC, 2006). Research suggests that bacterial vaginosis is associated with preterm labor, premature rupture of membranes, chorioamnionitis, postpartum endometritis, and pelvic inflammatory disease (CDC, 2006).

Therapeutic Management

Treatment for bacterial vaginosis includes oral metronidazole (Flagyl) or clindamycin (Cleocin) cream. Treatment of the male partner has not been beneficial in preventing recurrence because sexual transmission of bacterial vaginosis has not been proven (CDC, 2006).

Nursing Assessment

Assess the patient for clinical manifestations of bacterial vaginosis. Primary symptoms are a thin, white homogeneous vaginal discharge and a characteristic "stale fish" odor. Figure 5.3 shows the typical appearance of bacterial vaginosis.

To diagnose bacterial vaginosis, three of the four criteria must be met:

• Thin, white homogeneous vaginal discharge
• Vaginal pH > 4.5
• Positive "whiff test" (secretion is mixed with a drop of 10% potassium hydroxide on a slide, producing a characteristic stale fishy odor)

• The presence of clue cells on wet-mount examination (CDC, 2006)

Nursing Management

The nurse's role is one of primary prevention and education to limit recurrences of these infections. Primary prevention begins with changing the sexual behaviors that place women at risk for infection. In addition to assessing women for common signs, symptoms, and risk factors,

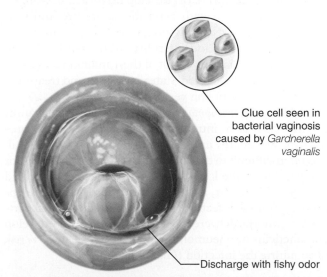

Clue cell seen in bacterial vaginosis caused by *Gardnerella vaginalis*

Discharge with fishy odor

FIGURE 5.3 Bacterial vaginosis. (Source: The Anatomical Chart Company. [2002]. *Atlas of pathophysiology*. Springhouse, PA: Springhouse.)

the nurse can help women to avoid vaginitis or to prevent a recurrence by teaching them to take the precautions highlighted in Teaching Guidelines 5.2.

Infections Characterized by Cervicitis

Cervicitis is a catchall term that implies the presence of inflammation or infection of the cervix. It is used to describe everything from symptomless erosions to an inflamed cervix that bleeds on contact and produces quantities of purulent discharge containing organisms not ordinarily found in the vagina. Cervicitis is usually caused by gonorrhea or chlamydia, as well as almost any pathogenic bacterial agent and a number of viruses. The treatment of cervicitis involves the appropriate therapy for the specific organism that has caused it.

▶ CHLAMYDIA

Chlamydia is the most common bacterial STI in the United States. The CDC estimates that there are 4 million new cases each year; the highest predictor for the infection is age. The highest rates of infection are among those ages 15 to 19, mainly because their sexual relations are often unplanned and are sometimes the result of pressure or force, and typically happen before they have the experience and skills to protect themselves. The rates are highest among this group regardless of demographics or location (CDC, 2006). The young have the most to lose from acquiring STIs, since they will suffer the consequences the longest and might not reach their full reproductive potential.

Asymptomatic infection is common among both men and women. Men primarily develop urethritis. In women, chlamydia is linked with cervicitis, acute urethral syndrome, salpingitis, ectopic pregnancy, pelvic inflammatory disease (PID), and infertility (Marrazzo & Martin, 2007). Chlamydia causes half of the 1 million recognized cases of PID in the United States each year, and treatment costs run over $1 billion yearly.

Chlamydia trachomatis is the bacterium that causes chlamydia. It is an intracellular parasite that cannot produce its own energy and depends on the host for survival. It is often difficult to detect, and this can pose problems for women due to the long-term consequences of untreated infection. Moreover, lack of treatment provides more opportunity for the infection to be transmitted to sexual partners. Newborns delivered to infected mothers may develop conjunctivitis or pneumonitis and have a 50% to 70% risk of acquiring the infection (Glasier et al., 2006).

Therapeutic Management

Antibiotics are usually used in treating this STI. The CDC treatment options for chlamydia include doxycycline (Vibromycin) 100 mg orally twice a day for 7 days or azithromycin (Zithromax) 1 gram orally in a single dose. Because of the common co-infection of chlamydia and gonorrhea, a combination regimen of ceftriaxone (Rocephin) with doxycycline or azithromycin is prescribed frequently (CDC, 2006). Additional CDC guidelines for patient management include annual screening of all sexually active women aged 20 to 25 years old; screening of all high-risk people; and treatment with antibiotics effective against both gonorrhea and chlamydia for anyone diagnosed with a gonococcal infection (CDC, 2006).

Nursing Assessment

Assess the health history for significant risk factors for chlamydia, which may include:

- Being an adolescent
- Having multiple sex partners
- Having a new sex partner
- Engaging in sex without using a barrier contraceptive (condom)
- Using oral contraceptives
- Being pregnant
- Having a history of another STI (Geisler, 2007)

Assess the client for clinical manifestations of chlamydia. The majority of women (70% to 80%) are asymptomatic (CDC, 2006). If the client is symptomatic, clinical manifestations include:

- Mucopurulent vaginal discharge
- Urethritis
- Bartholinitis
- Endometritis
- Salpingitis
- Dysfunctional uterine bleeding

The diagnosis can be made by urine testing or swab specimens collected from the endocervix or vagina. Culture, direct immunofluorescence, EIA, or nucleic acid amplification methods by polymerase chain reaction or ligase chain reaction (DNA probe, such as GenProbe or Pace2) are highly sensitive and specific when used on urethral and cervicovaginal swabs. They can also be used with good sensitivity and specificity on first-void urine specimens (Mehta, 2007). The chain reaction tests are the most sensitive and cost-effective. The CDC strongly recommends screening of asymptomatic women at high risk in whom infection would otherwise go undetected (CDC, 2006).

▶ GONORRHEA

Gonorrhea is a serious and potentially very severe bacterial infection. It is the second most commonly reported infection in the United States. Gonorrhea is highly contagious and is a reportable infection to the health department authorities. Gonorrhea increases the risk for PID, infertility, ectopic pregnancy, and HIV acquisition and transmission (CDC, 2007a, 2007b, 2007d). It is rapidly becoming more and more resistant to cure. In the United States, an estimated 600,000 new gonorrhea infections occur annually (CDC, 2006). In common with all other STIs, it is an equal-opportunity infection—no one is immune to it, regardless of race, creed, gender, age, or sexual preference.

The cause of gonorrhea is an aerobic gram-negative intracellular diplococcus, *Neisseria gonorrhoeae*. The site of infection is the columnar epithelium of the endocervix. Gonorrhea is almost exclusively transmitted by sexual activity. In pregnant women, gonorrhea is associated with chorioamnionitis, premature labor, premature rupture of membranes, and postpartum endometritis (Peterson et al., 2007). It can also be transmitted to the newborn in the form of ophthalmia neonatorum during birth by direct contact with gonococcal organisms in the cervix. Ophthalmia neonatorum is highly contagious and if untreated leads to blindness in the newborn.

Therapeutic Management

The treatment of choice for uncomplicated gonococcal infections is cefixime (Suprex) 400 mg orally in a single dose or ceftriaxone (Rocephine) 125 mg intramuscularly in a single dose. Azithromycin (Zithromax) orally or doxycycline (Vibromycin) should accompany all gonococcal treatment regimens if chlamydial infection is not ruled out (CDC, 2006). Pregnant women should not be treated with quinolones or tetracyclines. Cephalosporins or a single 2-gram intramuscular dose of spectinomycin should be used during pregnancy (CDC, 2006). To prevent gonococcal ophthalmia neonatorum, a prophylactic agent should be instilled into the eyes of all newborns; this procedure is required by law in most states. Erythromycin or tetracycline ophthalmic ointment in a single application is recommended (CDC, 2006).

Nursing Assessment

Assess the client's health history for risk factors, which may include low socioeconomic status, living in an urban area, single status, inconsistent use of barrier contraceptives, age under 20 years old, and multiple sex partners. Assess the client for clinical manifestations of gonorrhea, keeping in mind that between 50% and 90% of women infected with gonorrhea are totally symptom-free (Glasier et al., 2006). Because women are so frequently asymptomatic, they are regarded as a major factor in the spread of gonorrhea. If symptoms are present, they might include:

• Abnormal vaginal discharge
• Dysuria
• Cervicitis
• Abnormal vaginal bleeding

• Bartholin's abscess
• PID
• Neonatal conjunctivitis in newborns
• Mild sore throat (for pharyngeal gonorrhea)
• Rectal infection (asymptomatic)
• Perihepatitis (Bennett & Domachowske, 2007)

Sometimes a local gonorrhea infection is self-limiting (there is no further spread), but usually the organism ascends upward through the endocervical canal to the endometrium of the uterus, further on to the fallopian tubes, and out into the peritoneal cavity. When the peritoneum and the ovaries become involved, the condition is known as PID. The scarring to the fallopian tubes is permanent. This damage is a major cause of infertility and is a possible contributing factor in ectopic pregnancy (Mehta, 2007).

If gonorrhea remains untreated, it can enter the bloodstream and produce a disseminated gonococcal infection. This severe form of infection can invade the joints (arthritis), the heart (endocarditis), the brain (meningitis), and the liver (toxic hepatitis). Figure 5.4 shows the typical appearance of gonorrhea.

The CDC recommends screening for all women at risk for gonorrhea. Pregnant women should be screened at the first prenatal visit and again at 36 weeks of gestation. Nucleic acid hybridization tests (GenProbe) are used for diagnosis. Any woman suspected of having gonorrhea should be tested for chlamydia also because co-infection (45%) is extremely common (CDC, 2006).

Nursing Management of Chlamydia and Gonorrhea

The prevalence of chlamydia and gonorrhea is increasing dramatically, and these infections can have long-term effects on people's lives. Sexual health is an important part of a person's physical and mental health, and nurses have a professional obligation to address it. Be particularly sensitive when addressing STIs because women are often embarrassed or feel guilty. There is still a social stigma attached to STIs, so women need to be reassured about confidentiality.

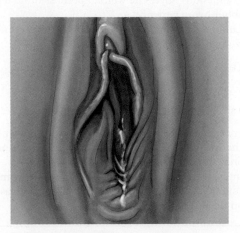

FIGURE 5.4 Gonorrhea.

The nurse's knowledge about chlamydia and gonor-rhea should include treatment strategies, referral sources, and preventive measures. It is important to be skilled at patient education and counseling and to be comfortable talking with, and advising, women diagnosed with these infections.

Provide education about risk factors for these infections. High-risk groups include single women, women younger than 25 years, African-American women, women with a history of STIs, those with new or multiple sex partners, those with inconsistent use of barrier contraception, and women living in communities with high infection rates (Bennett & Domachowske, 2007). Assessment involves taking a health history that includes a comprehensive sexual history. Ask about the number of sex partners and the use of safer sex techniques. Review previous and current symptoms. Emphasize the importance of seeking treatment and informing sex partners. The four-level P-LI-SS-IT model (Box 5.2) can be used to determine interventions for various women because it can be adapted to the nurse's level of knowledge, skill, and experience. Of utmost importance is the willingness to listen and show interest and respect in a nonjudgmental manner.

In addition to meeting the health needs of women with chlamydia and gonorrhea, the nurse is responsible for educating the public about the increasing incidence of these infections. This information should include high-risk behaviors associated with these infections, signs and symptoms, and the treatment modalities available. Stress that both of these STIs can lead to infertility and long-term sequelae. Teach safer sex practices to people in non-monogamous relationships. Know the physical and psychosocial responses to these STIs to prevent transmission and the disabling consequences.

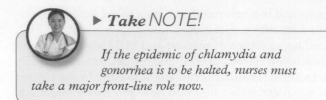

> ▶ *Take* NOTE!
>
> *If the epidemic of chlamydia and gonorrhea is to be halted, nurses must take a major front-line role now.*

Infections Characterized by Genital Ulcers

In the United States, the majority of young, sexually active patients who have genital ulcers have genital herpes, syphilis, or chancroid. The frequency of each condition differs by geographic area and patient population; however, genital herpes is the most prevalent of these diseases. More than one of these diseases can be present in a patient who has genital ulcers. All three of these diseases have been associated with an increased risk for HIV infection. Not all genital ulcers are caused by STIs.

▶ GENITAL HERPES SIMPLEX

Genital herpes is a recurrent, lifelong viral infection. The CDC estimates that 50 million Americans have genital herpes simplex (HSV) infection, with a half million new cases annually (CDC, 2006). Two serotypes of HSV have been identified: HSV-1 (not sexually transmitted) and HSV-2 (sexually transmitted). Today, approximately 10% of genital herpes infections are thought to be caused by HSV-1 and 90% by HSV-2 (Paz-Baily et al., 2007). HSV-1 causes the familiar fever blisters or cold sores on the lips, eyes, and face. HSV-2 invades the mucous membranes of the genital tract and is known as herpes genitalis. Most persons infected with HSV-2 have not been diagnosed.

The herpes simplex virus is transmitted by contact of mucous membranes or breaks in the skin with visible or nonvisible lesions. Most genital herpes infections are transmitted by individuals unaware that they have an infection. Many have mild or unrecognized infections but still shed the herpes virus intermittently. HSV is transmitted primarily by direct contact with an infected individual who is shedding the virus. Kissing, sexual contact, and vaginal delivery are means of transmission.

Having sex with an infected partner places the individual at risk for contracting HSV. After the primary outbreak, the virus remains dormant in the nerve cells for life, resulting in periodic recurrent outbreaks. Recurrent genital herpes outbreaks are triggered by precipitating factors such as emotional stress, menses, and sexual intercourse, but more than half of recurrences occur without a precipitating cause. Immunocompromised women have more

---

BOX 5.2 The P-LI-SS-IT Model

P   Permission—gives the woman permission to talk about her experience

LI   Limited Information—information given to the woman about STIs

• Factual information to dispel myths about STIs
• Specific measures to prevent transmission
• Ways to reveal information to her partners
• Physical consequences if the infections are untreated

SS   Specific Suggestions—an attempt to help women change their behavior to prevent recurrence and prevent further transmission of the STI

IT   Intensive Therapy—involves referring the woman or couple for appropriate treatment elsewhere based on their life circumstances

frequent and more severe recurrent outbreaks than normal hosts (Paz-Bailey et al., 2007).

Living with genital herpes can be difficult due to the erratic, recurrent nature of the infection, the location of the lesions, the unknown causes of the recurrences, and the lack of a cure. Further, the stigma associated with this infection may affect the individual's feelings about herself and her interaction with partners. Potential psychosocial consequences may include emotional distress, isolation, fear of rejection by a partner, fear of transmission of the disease, loss of confidence, and altered interpersonal relationships (Alexander et al., 2007).

Along with the increase in the incidence of genital herpes has been an increase in neonatal herpes simplex viral infections, which are associated with a high incidence of mortality and morbidity. The risk of neonatal infection with a primary maternal outbreak is between 30% and 50%; it is less than 1% with a recurrent maternal infection (CDC, 2006).

Therapeutic Management

No cure exists, but antiviral drug therapy helps to reduce or suppress symptoms, shedding, and recurrent episodes. Advances in treatment with acyclovir (Zovirax) 400 mg orally three times daily for 7 to 10 days, famciclovir (Famivir) 250 mg orally three times daily for 7 to 10 days, and valacyclovir (Valtrex) 1 gram orally twice daily for 7 to 10 days have resulted in an improved quality of life for those infected with HSV. However, these drugs neither eradicate latent virus nor affect the risk, frequency, or severity of recurrences after the drug is discontinued (CDC, 2006). Suppressive therapy is recommended for individuals with six or more recurrences per year. The natural course of the disease is for recurrences to be less frequent over time.

The management of genital herpes includes antiviral therapy. The safety of antiviral therapy has not been established during pregnancy. Therapeutic management also includes counseling regarding the natural history of the disease, the risk of sexual and perinatal transmission, and the use of methods to prevent further spread.

Nursing Assessment

Assess the client for clinical manifestations of HSV. Clinical manifestations can be divided into the primary episode and recurrent infections. The first or primary episode is usually the most severe, with a prolonged period of viral shedding. Primary HSV is a systemic disease characterized by multiple painful vesicular lesions, mucopurulent discharge, superinfection with candida, fever, chills, malaise, dysuria, headache, genital irritation, inguinal tenderness, and lymphadenopathy. The lesions in the primary herpes episode are frequently located on the vulva, vagina, and perineal areas. The vesicles will open and weep and finally crust over, dry, and disappear without scar formation

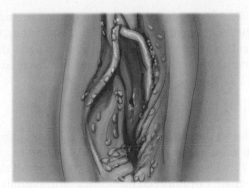

FIGURE 5.5 Genital herpes simplex.

(Fig. 5.5). This viral shedding process usually takes up to 2 weeks to complete.

Recurrent infection episodes are usually much milder and shorter in duration than the primary one. Tingling, itching, pain, unilateral genital lesions, and a more rapid resolution of lesions are characteristics of recurrent infections. Recurrent herpes is a localized disease characterized by typical HSV lesions at the site of initial viral entry. Recurrent herpes lesions are fewer in number and less painful and resolve more rapidly (Sharma & Brilliant, 2007).

Diagnosis of HSV is often based on clinical signs and symptoms and is confirmed by viral culture of fluid from the vesicle. Papanicolaou (Pap) smears are an insensitive and nonspecific diagnostic test for HSV and should not be relied on for diagnosis.

▶ SYPHILIS

Syphilis is a complex, curable bacterial infection caused by the spirochete *Treponema pallidum*. It is a serious systemic disease that can lead to disability and death if untreated. Rates of syphilis in the United States were declining, but they remain high among young adults and African-Americans in urban areas and in the south (CDC, 2006). It continues to be one of the most important STIs both because of its biological effect on HIV acquisition and transmission and because of its impact on infant health (Stoner, 2007).

The spirochete rapidly penetrates intact mucous membranes or microscopic lesions in the skin and within hours enters the lymphatic system and bloodstream to produce a systemic infection long before the appearance of a primary lesion. The site of entry may be vaginal, rectal, or oral (Ferguson & Varnado, 2006). The syphilis spirochete can cross the placenta at any time during pregnancy. One out of every 10,000 infants born in the United States has congenital syphilis (CDC, 2006). Maternal infection consequences include spontaneous abortion, prematurity, stillbirth, and multisystem failure of the heart, lungs, spleen, liver, and pancreas, as well as structural bone damage and nervous system involvement and mental retardation (Gilbert, 2007).

Therapeutic Management

Fortunately, there is effective treatment for syphilis. Penicillin G, administered by either the intramuscular or intravenous route, is the preferred drug for all stages of syphilis. For pregnant or nonpregnant women with syphilis of less than 1 year's duration, the CDC recommends 2.4 million units of benzathine penicillin G intramuscularly in a single dose. If the syphilis is of longer duration (more than 1 year) or of unknown duration, 2.4 million units of benzathine penicillin G is given intramuscularly once a week for 3 weeks. The preparations used, the dosage, and the length of treatment depend on the stage and clinical manifestations of disease (CDC, 2006). Other medications, such as doxycycline, are available if the client is allergic to penicillin.

Women should be re-evaluated at 6 and 12 months after treatment for primary or secondary syphilis with additional serologic testing. Women with latent syphilis should be followed clinically and serologically at 6, 12, and 24 months (McGregor & Richard, 2007).

Nursing Assessment

Assess the client for clinical manifestations of syphilis. Syphilis is divided into four stages: primary, secondary, latency, and tertiary. Primary syphilis is characterized by a chancre (painless ulcer) at the site of bacterial entry that will disappear within 1 to 6 weeks without intervention (Fig. 5.6). Motile spirochetes are present on darkfield examination of ulcer exudate. In addition, painless bilateral adenopathy is present during this highly infectious period. If left untreated, the infection progresses to the secondary stage. Secondary syphilis appears 2 to 6 months after the initial exposure and is manifested by flu-like symptoms and

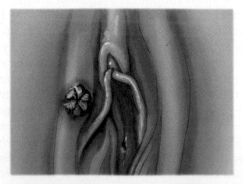

FIGURE 5.6 Chancre of primary syphilis.

a maculopapular rash of the trunk, palms, and soles. Alopecia and adenopathy are both common during this stage. In addition to rashes, secondary syphilis may present with symptoms of fever, pharyngitis, weight loss, and fatigue (Waugh, 2007). The secondary stage of syphilis lasts about 2 years. Once the secondary stage subsides, the latency period begins. This stage is characterized by the absence of any clinical manifestations of disease, although the serology is positive. This stage can last as long as 20 years. If not treated, tertiary or late syphilis occurs, with life-threatening heart disease and neurologic disease that slowly destroys the heart, eyes, brain, central nervous system, and skin.

Clients with a diagnosis of HIV or another STI should be screened for syphilis, and all pregnant women should be screened at their first prenatal visit. Darkfield microscopic examinations and direct fluorescent antibody tests of lesion exudate or tissue are the definitive methods for diagnosing early syphilis. A presumptive diagnosis can be made by using two serologic tests:

- Nontreponemal tests (Venereal Disease Research Laboratory [VDRL] and rapid plasma reagin [RPR])
- Treponemal tests (fluorescent treponemal antibody absorbed [FTA-ABS] and *T. pallidum* particle agglutination [TP-PA]) (CDC, 2006)

Nursing Management of Herpes and Syphilis

Genital ulcers from either herpes or syphilis can be devastating to women, and the nurse can be instrumental in helping her through this difficult time. Referral to a support group may be helpful. Address the psychosocial aspects of these STIs with women by discussing appropriate coping skills, acceptance of the lifelong nature of the condition (herpes), and options for treatment and rehabilitation. Teaching Guidelines 5.3 highlights appropriate teaching points for the patient with genital ulcers.

Pelvic Inflammatory Disease

Pelvic inflammatory disease refers to an inflammatory state of the upper female genital tract and nearby structures. The fallopian tubes, ovaries, or peritoneum may be involved and endometriosis may also be present. PID results from an ascending polymicrobial infection of the upper female reproductive tract, frequently caused by untreated chlamydia or gonorrhea (Fig. 5.7). An estimated 1.5 million cases are diagnosed annually, resulting in over 250,000 hospitalizations (CDC, 2006). It is a serious health problem in the United States, costing an estimated $10 billion annually in terms of hospitalizations and surgical procedures (Crossman, 2006). Complications include ectopic pregnancy, pelvic abscess, infertility, recurrent or chronic episodes of the disease, chronic abdominal pain, pelvic adhesions, and depression (Glasier et al., 2006).

Caring for Genital Ulcers

- Abstain from intercourse during the prodromal period and when lesions are present.
- Wash hands with soap and water after touching lesions to avoid autoinoculation.
- Use comfort measures such as wearing nonconstricting clothes, wearing cotton underwear, urinating in water if urination is painful, taking lukewarm sitz baths, and air-drying lesions with a hair dryer on low heat.
- Avoid extremes of temperature such as ice packs or hot pads to the genital area as well as application of steroid creams, sprays, or gels.
- Use condoms with all new or noninfected partners.
- Inform health care professionals of your condition.

Because of the seriousness of the complications of PID, an accurate diagnosis is critical.

Therapeutic Management

Treatment of PID must include empiric, broad-spectrum antibiotic coverage of likely pathogens. The client is treated on an ambulatory basis with oral antibiotics or is hospitalized and given antibiotics intravenously. The decision to hospitalize a woman is based on clinical judgment and the severity of her symptoms (e.g., severely ill with high fever or with protracted vomiting). Frequently, oral antibiotics are initiated, and if no improvement is seen within 72 hours, the woman is admitted to the hospital. Treatment then includes intravenous antibiotics, increased oral

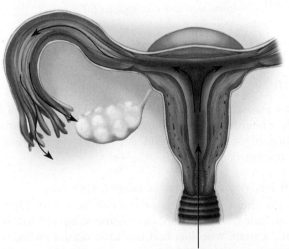

Spread of gonorrhea or chlamydia

FIGURE 5.7 Pelvic inflammatory disease. Chlamydia or gonorrhea spreads up the vagina into the uterus and then to the fallopian tubes and ovaries.

fluids to improve hydration, bed rest, and pain management. Follow-up is needed to validate that the infectious process is gone to prevent the development of chronic pelvic pain.

Nursing Assessment

Nursing assessment of the woman with PID involves a complete health history and assessment of clinical manifestations, physical examination, and laboratory and diagnostic testing.

Health History and Clinical Manifestations

Explore the client's current and past medical health history for risk factors for PID, which may include:

- Adolescence or young adulthood
- Nonwhite female
- Having multiple sex partners
- Early onset of sexual activity
- History of PID or STI
- Sexual intercourse at an early age
- Alcohol or drug use
- Having intercourse with a partner who has untreated urethritis
- Recent insertion of an intrauterine device (IUD)
- Nulliparity
- Cigarette smoking
- Engaging in sex during menses (Reyes & Abbuhl, 2007)
- Lack of consistent condom use
- Lack of contraceptive use
- Douching
- Prostitution

Assess the client for clinical manifestations of PID, keeping in mind that, because of the wide variety of clinical manifestations of PID, clinical diagnosis can be challenging. To reduce the risk of missed diagnosis, the CDC has established criteria to establish the diagnosis of PID. Minimal criteria (all must be present) are lower abdominal tenderness, adnexal tenderness, and cervical motion tenderness. Additional supportive criteria that support a diagnosis of PID are:

- Abnormal cervical or vaginal mucopurulent discharge
- Oral temperature above 101°F
- Elevated erythrocyte sedimentation rate (inflammatory process)
- Elevated C-reactive protein level (inflammatory process)
- *N. gonorrhoeae* or *C. trachomatis* infection documented (causative bacterial organism)
- White blood cells on saline vaginal smear (CDC, 2006)
- Prolonged or increased menstrual bleeding
- Dysmenorrhea
- Dysuria
- Painful sexual intercourse
- Nausea
- Vomiting

Physical Examination and Laboratory and Diagnostic Tests

Inspect the client for presence of fever (usually over 101°F) or vaginal discharge. Palpate the abdomen, noting tenderness over the uterus or ovaries. However, the only way to diagnose PID definitively is through an endometrial biopsy, transvaginal ultrasound, or laparoscopic examination.

Nursing Management

If the woman with PID is hospitalized, maintain hydration via intravenous fluids if necessary and administer analgesics as needed for pain. Semi-Fowler's positioning facilitates pelvic drainage. A key element to treatment of PID is education to prevent recurrence. Depending on the clinical setting (hospital or community clinic) where the nurse encounters the woman diagnosed with PID, a risk assessment should be done to ascertain what interventions are appropriate to prevent a recurrence. To gain the woman's cooperation, explain the various diagnostic tests needed. Discuss the implications of PID and the risk factors for the infection; her sexual partner should be included if possible. Sexual counseling should include practicing safer sex, limiting the number of sexual partners, using barrier contraceptives consistently, avoiding vaginal douching, considering another contraceptive method if she has an IUD and has multiple sexual partners, and completing the course of antibiotics prescribed (Reyes & Abbuhl, 2007). Review the serious sequelae that may occur if the condition is not treated or if the woman does not comply with the treatment plan. Ask the woman to have her partner go for evaluation and treatment to prevent a repeat infection. Provide nonjudgmental support while stressing the importance of barrier contraceptive methods and follow-up care. Teaching Guidelines 5.4 gives further information related to PID prevention.

Human Papillomavirus

Human papillomavirus (HPV) is the most common viral infection in the United States (CDC, 2007c). Genital warts

HEALTHY PEOPLE 2010

Healthy People 2010 Objectives 25–6,7	Significance
Reduce the proportion of females who have ever required treatment for pelvic inflammatory disease (PID). Reduce the proportion of childless females with fertility problems who have had a sexually transmitted disease or who have ever required treatment for pelvic inflammatory disease (PID).	Educate women that abstinence is the only way to completely avoid contracting sexually transmitted infections. Encourage women always to use condoms if participating in any sexual act. Provide an open and confidential environment so women will report symptoms and seek treatment earlier.

or condylomata (Greek for warts) are caused by HPV. Conservative estimates suggest that in the United States, approximately 20 million people have productive HPV infection, and 5.5 million Americans acquire it annually (CDC, 2007c). Clinical studies have confirmed that HPV is the cause of essentially all cases of cervical cancer, which is the fourth most common cancer in women in the United States, following lung, breast, and colorectal cancer (ACS, 2007). HPV-mediated oncogenesis is responsible for up to 95% of cervical squamous cell carcinomas and nearly all preinvasive cervical neoplasms (Gearhart & Randall, 2007). More than 30 types of HPV can infect the genital tract. HPV is most prevalent in young women between the ages of 20 and 24 years old, followed closely by the 15-to-19-year-old age group (Hackley et al., 2007).

▶ *Take NOTE!*

The lifetime risk of HPV infection is estimated to be as high as 80% in sexually active individuals.

Nursing Assessment

Nursing assessment of the woman with HPV involves a complete health history and assessment of clinical manifestations, physical examination, and laboratory and diagnostic testing.

Health History and Clinical Manifestations

Assess the client's health history for risk factors for HPV, which include having multiple sex partners, age (15 to 25), sex with a male who has had multiple sexual partners, and first intercourse at 16 or younger (Moore & Seybold, 2007). Risk factors contributing to the development of cervical cancer include smoking, few or no screenings for cervical cancer, multiple sex partners, immunosuppressed

TEACHING GUIDELINES 5.4

Preventing Pelvic Inflammatory Disease

- Advise sexually active girls and women to insist their partners use condoms.
- Discourage routine vaginal douching, as this may lead to bacterial overgrowth.
- Encourage regular sexually transmitted infection screening.
- Emphasize the importance of having each sexual partner receive antibiotic treatment.

state, long-term contraceptive use (more than 2 years), co-infection with another STI, pregnancy, nutritional deficiencies, and early onset of sexual activity (Dunne et al., 2007).

Assess the client for clinical manifestations of HPV. Most HPV infections are asymptomatic, unrecognized, or subclinical. Visible genital warts usually are caused by HPV types 6 or 11. In addition to the external genitalia, genital warts can occur on the cervix and in the vagina, urethra, anus, and mouth. Depending on the size and location, genital warts can be painful, friable, and pruritic, although most are typically asymptomatic (Fig. 5.8). The strains of HPV associated with genital warts are considered low risk for development of cervical cancer, but other HPV types (16, 18, 31, 33, and 35) have been strongly associated with cervical cancer (CDC, 2006).

Physical Examination and Laboratory and Diagnostic Tests

Clinically, visible warts are diagnosed by inspection. The warts are fleshy papules with a warty, granular surface. Lesions can grow very large during pregnancy, affecting urination, defecation, mobility, and descent of the fetus (CDC, 2006). Large lesions, which may resemble cauliflowers, exist in coalesced clusters and bleed easily.

Serial Pap smears are performed for low-risk women. These regular Pap smears will detect the cellular changes associated with HPV. The FDA has recently approved an HPV test as a follow-up for women who have an ambiguous Pap test. In addition, this HPV test may be a helpful addition to the Pap test for general screening of women age 30 and over. The HPV test is a diagnostic test that can determine the specific HPV strain, which is useful in discriminating between low-risk and high-risk HPV types. A specimen for testing can be obtained with a fluid-phase collection system such as Thin Prep. The HPV test can identify 13 of the high-risk types of HPV associated with the development of cervical cancer and can detect high-risk types of HPV even before there are any conclusive visible changes to the cervical cells. If the test is positive for the high-risk types of HPV, the woman should be referred for colposcopy.

pon physical examination, it is determined that Sandy has genital warts. The nurse finds out that Sandy engaged in high-risk behavior with a stranger she "hooked up" with recently at college. She couldn't imagine that he would give her a STI because "he looked so clean-cut." She wonders how she could possibly have genital warts. What information should be given to Sandy about STIs in general? What specific information about HPV should be stressed?

Therapeutic Management

There is currently no medical treatment or cure for HPV. Instead, therapeutic management focuses heavily on prevention through the use of the HPV vaccine and education and on the treatment of lesions and warts caused by HPV. In summer 2006, the FDA approved the HPV vaccine (Gardasil) to prevent cervical cancer. The CDC's Advisory Committee on Immunization Practices (ACIP) has recommended the vaccine for routine administration to 11- and 12-year-old girls. The ACIP also endorsed the use of Gardasil for girls as young as 9 and recommended that women between the ages of 13 and 26 receive the vaccination series, which consists of three injections over 6 months. The vaccine has been found 100% effective in preventing precancerous lesions of the cervix and genital warts (Wald, 2007). The duration of protection afforded by this vaccine, as well as its impact on long-term outcomes, is not yet known (Kennedy, 2007).

The vaccine is administered intramuscularly in three separate 0.5-mL doses. The first dose may be given to any individual 9 to 26 years old prior to infection with HPV. The second dose is administered 2 months after the first, and the third dose is given 6 months after the initial dose. The deltoid region of the upper arm or anterolateral area of the thigh may be used (Leggatt & Frazer, 2007).

If the woman doesn't receive primary prevention with the vaccine, then secondary prevention would focus on education about the importance of receiving regular Pap smears and, for women over 30, including an HPV test to determine whether the woman has a latent high-risk virus that could lead to precancerous cervical changes. Finally, treatment options for precancerous cervical lesions or genital warts caused by HPV are numerous and may include:

- Topical trichloroacetic acid (TCA) 80% to 90%
- Liquid nitrogen cryotherapy
- Topical imiquimod 5% cream (Aldara)
- Topical podophyllin 10% to 25%
- Laser carbon dioxide vaporization
- Client-applied Podofilox 0.5% solution or gel
- Simple surgical excision
- Loop electrosurgical excisional procedure (LEEP)

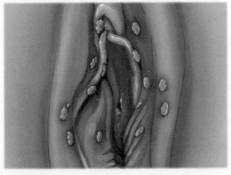

FIGURE 5.8 Genital warts.

- Intralesional interferon therapy (National Institute of Allergy and Infectious Diseases, 2007b)

The goal of treating genital warts is to remove the warts and induce wart-free periods for the client. Treatment of genital warts should be guided by the preference of the client and available resources. No single treatment has been found to be ideal for all clients, and most treatment modalities appear to have comparable efficacy. Because genital warts can proliferate and become friable during pregnancy, they should be removed using a local agent. A cesarean birth is not indicated solely to prevent transmission of HPV infection to the newborn, unless the pelvic outlet is obstructed by warts (Gearhart & Randall, 2007).

Nursing Management

An HPV infection has many implications for the woman's health, but most women are unaware of HPV and its role in cervical cancer. The average age of sexual debut is in early adolescence; therefore, it is important to target this population for use of the HPV/cervical cancer vaccine.

Key nursing roles are teaching about prevention of HPV infection and patient education and promotion of vaccines and screening tests in order to reduce the morbidity and mortality associated with cervical cancer caused by HPV infection. Teach all women that the only way to prevent HPV is to refrain from any genital contact with another individual. Although the effect of condoms in preventing HPV infection is unknown, latex condom use has been associated with a lower rate of cervical cancer. Teach women about the link between HPV and cervical cancer. Explain that, in most cases, there are no signs or symptoms of infection with HPV. Strongly encourage all young women between 9 and 26 to consider getting Gardasil, the vaccine against HPV. For all women, promote the importance of obtaining regular Pap smears and, for women over 30, suggest an HPV test to rule out the presence of a latent high-risk strain of HPV.

Education and counseling are important aspects of managing women with genital warts. Teach the woman that:

- Even after genital warts are removed, HPV still remains and viral shedding will continue.
- The likelihood of transmission to future partners and the duration of infectivity after treatment for genital warts are unknown.
- The recurrence of genital warts within the first few months after treatment is common and usually indicates recurrence rather than reinfection (CDC, 2006).

Sandy is being treated for HPV and is anxious for her "things" to disappear and never return. What education is needed to prevent further transmission from Sandy to any future sexual partners?

Vaccine-Preventable STIs: Hepatitis A and B

Hepatitis is an acute, systemic, viral infection that can be transmitted sexually. The viruses associated with hepatitis or inflammation of the liver are hepatitis A, B, C, D, E, and G. Hepatitis A (HAV) is spread via the gastrointestinal tract. It can be acquired by drinking polluted water, by eating uncooked shellfish from sewage-contaminated waters or food handled by a hepatitis carrier with poor hygiene, and from oral/anal sexual contact. Approximately 33% of the U.S. population has serologic evidence of prior hepatitis A infection; the rate increases directly with age (Wasley et al., 2007). A person with hepatitis A can easily pass the disease to others within the same household.

Hepatitis B (HBV) is transmitted through saliva, blood serum, semen, menstrual blood, and vaginal secretions (Assan & Kraszewski, 2006). In the early 2000s, transmission among heterosexual partners accounted for 40% of infections, and transmission among men who have sex with men accounted for 20% of infections. The World Health Organization (WHO) estimates the prevalence of hepatitis B worldwide is 350 million chronically infected people. Worldwide, hepatitis B has the highest death rate of any STI except HIV (WHO, 2007a). Risk factors for infection include having multiple sex partners, engaging in unprotected receptive anal intercourse, and having a history of other STIs (CDC, 2006). The most effective means to prevent the transmission of hepatitis A or B is pre-exposure immunization. Vaccines are available for the prevention of HAV and HBV, both of which can be transmitted sexually. Every person seeking treatment for an STI should be considered a candidate for hepatitis B vaccination, and some individuals (e.g., men who have sex with men, and injection-drug users) should be considered for hepatitis A vaccination (CDC, 2006).

Therapeutic Management

Unlike other STIs, HBV and HAV are preventable through immunization. HAV is usually self-limiting and does not result in chronic infection. HBV can result in serious, permanent liver damage. Treatment is generally supportive. No specific treatment for acute HBV infection exists.

Nursing Assessment

Assess the client for clinical manifestations of hepatitis A and B. Hepatitis A produces flu-like symptoms with malaise, fatigue, anorexia, nausea, pruritus, fever, and upper right quadrant pain. Symptoms of hepatitis B are similar to those of hepatitis A, but with less fever and skin involvement. The diagnosis of hepatitis A cannot be made based on clinical manifestations alone and requires serologic testing. The presence of IgM antibody to HAV is diagnostic of acute HAV infection. Hepatitis B is detected by a blood test that looks for antibodies and proteins produced by the virus and is positively diagnosed by the presence of hepatitis B surface antibody (HBsAg) (Pyrsopoulos & Reddy, 2007).

Nursing Management

Nurses should encourage all women to be screened for hepatitis when they have their annual Pap smear, or sooner if high-risk behavior is identified. Nurses should also encourage women to undergo HBV screening at their first prenatal visit and repeat screening in the last trimester for women with high-risk behaviors (Assan & Kraszewski, 2006). Nurses can also explain that hepatitis B vaccine is given to all infants after birth in most hospitals. The vaccination consists of a series of three injections given within 6 months. The vaccine has been shown to be safe and well tolerated by most recipients (CDC, 2006). Hepatitis A vaccine is strongly encouraged for children between 12 and 23 months; persons 1 year of age and older traveling to countries with a high prevalence of hepatitis A, such as Central or South America, Mexico, Asia, Africa, and eastern Europe; men who have sex with men; persons who use street drugs; and persons with chronic liver disease (CDC, 2007c). For others, hepatitis A vaccine series (two doses 6 months apart) may be started whenever a person is at risk of infection.

Ectoparasitic Infections

Ectoparasites are a common cause of skin rash and pruritus throughout the world, affecting persons of all ages, races, and socioeconomic groups. Overcrowding, delayed diagnosis and treatment, and poor public education contribute to the prevalence of ectoparasites in both industrial and nonindustrial nations. Approximately 300 million cases of ectoparasitic cases are reported worldwide each year (CDC, 2006). These infections include infestations of scabies and pubic lice. Since these parasites are easily passed from one person to another during sexual intimacy, clients should be assessed for them when receiving care for other STIs. Scabies is an intensely pruritic dermatitis caused by a mite. The female mite burrows under the skin and deposits eggs, which hatch. The lesions start as a small papule that reddens, erodes, and sometimes crusts. Diagnosis is based on history and appearance of burrows in the webs of the fingers and the genitalia (Cordoro & Wilson, 2007). Aggressive infestation can occur in immunodeficient, debilitated, or malnourished people, but healthy people do not usually suffer sequelae.

Clients with pediculosis pubis (pubic lice) usually seek treatment because of the pruritus, because of a rash brought on by skin irritation from scratching, or because they notice lice or nits in their pubic hair, axillary hair, abdominal and thigh hair, and sometimes in the eyebrows,

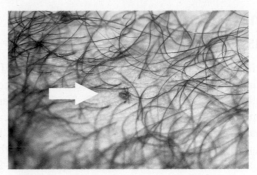

FIGURE **5.9** Pubic lice. A small brown living crab louse is seen at the base of hairs (*arrow*). (Source: Goodheart, H. [2003]. *Goodheart's photoguide of common skin disorders*. Philadelphia: Lippincott Williams & Wilkins.)

eyelashes, and beards. Infestation is usually asymptomatic until after a week or so, when bites cause pruritus and secondary infections from scratching (Fig. 5.9). Diagnosis is based on history and the presence of nits (small, shiny, yellow, oval, dewdrop-like eggs) affixed to hair shafts or lice (a yellowish, oval, wingless insect) (Wolfram, 2007).

Treatment is directed at the infested area, using permethrin cream or lindane shampoo (CDC, 2006). Bedding and clothing should be washed in hot water to decontaminate it. Sexual partners should be treated also, as well as family members who live in close contact with the infected person.

Nursing care of a woman infested with lice or scabies involves a three-tiered approach: eradicating the infestation with medication, removing nits, and preventing spread or recurrence by managing the environment. Over-the-counter products containing pyrethrins (RID, Triple X, Pronto, and Kwell) are safe for use and kill the active lice or mites. Nurses should provide education about these products (Teaching Guidelines 5.5). The nurse can follow these same guidelines to prevent the health care facility from becoming infested.

TEACHING GUIDELINES 5.5

Treating and Minimizing the Spread of Scabies and Pubic Lice

- Use the medication according to the manufacturer's instructions.
- Remove nits with a fine-toothed nit comb.
- Do not share any personal items with others or accept items from others.
- Treat objects, clothing, and bedding and wash them in hot water.
- Meticulously vacuum carpets to prevent a recurrence of infestation.

Human Immunodeficiency Virus (HIV)

An estimated 1 million people currently live with HIV and an estimated 50,000 new HIV infections have occurred annually in the United States (CDC, 2007b). In terms of epidemiology, fatality rate, and its social, legal, ethical, and political aspects, HIV/AIDS has become a public health crisis and has generated more concern than any other infectious disease in modern medical history (Mullan, 2007). To date, there is no cure for this fatal viral infection.

The HIV virus is transmitted by intimate sexual contact, by sharing needles for intravenous drug use, from mother to fetus during pregnancy, or by transfusion of blood or blood products. Men who have sex with men represent the largest proportion of new infections, followed by men and women infected through heterosexual sex (CDC, 2007b).

The number of women with HIV infection and AIDS has been increasing steadily worldwide. WHO estimates that over 25 million women are living with HIV/AIDS worldwide, accounting for approximately 50% of the 40 million adults living with HIV/AIDS (National Institute of Allergy and Infectious Diseases, 2007a). HIV disproportionately affects African-American and Hispanic women: together they represent less than 25% of all U.S. women, yet they account for more than 82% of AIDS cases in women (CDC, 2007b). Worldwide, more than 90% of all HIV infections have resulted from heterosexual intercourse. Women are particularly vulnerable to heterosexual transmission of HIV due to substantial mucosal exposure to seminal fluids. This biological fact amplifies the risk of HIV transmission when coupled with the high prevalence of nonconsensual sex, sex without condoms, and the unknown and/or high-risk behaviors of their partners (National Institute of Allergy and Infectious Diseases, 2007a). Therefore, the face of HIV/AIDS is becoming the face of young women. That shift will ultimately exacerbate the incidence of HIV because women spread it not only through sex, but also through nursing and childbirth.

AIDS is a breakdown in the immune function caused by HIV, a retrovirus. The infected person develops opportunistic infections or malignancies that become fatal. Progression from HIV infection to AIDS occurs a median of 11 years after infection (Mullan, 2007).

Twenty years have passed since HIV/AIDS began to affect our society. Since then, 50 million people have been infected by the virus, with AIDS being the fourth leading cause of death globally (CDC, 2007b). The morbidity and mortality of HIV continue to hold the attention of the medical community. While there has been a dramatic improvement in both morbidity and mortality with the use of highly active antiretroviral therapy (HAART), the incidence of HIV infection continues to rise.

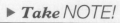

> ▶ *Take* NOTE!
>
> *More than 90% of individuals infected with HIV worldwide do not know they are infected (Dubin, 2007).*

The fetal and neonatal effects of acquiring HIV through perinatal transmission are devastating and eventually fatal. An infected mother can transmit HIV infection to her newborn before or during birth and through breastfeeding. Most cases of mother-to-child HIV transmission, the cause of more than 90% of pediatric-acquired infections worldwide, occur late in pregnancy or during delivery. Transmission rates vary from 25% in untreated non-breastfeeding populations in industrialized countries to about 40% among untreated breastfeeding populations in developing countries (National Institute of Allergy and Infectious Diseases, 2007a). Despite the dramatic reduction in perinatal transmission, hundreds of infants will be born infected with HIV.

HIV and Adolescents

The effects of HIV and AIDS on adolescents and young adults is of increasing concern, but it is difficult to get accurate data due to varying ways this population seeks health care services. Some adolescents continue to receive care through pediatricians and adult services, but many do not have access to health care. HIV infections are increasing in adolescents and young adults (13 to 24 years). Also, the proportion of adolescents diagnosed with AIDS has increased from 4% in 1999 to 6% in 2006 (NIH, 2008). At least one adolescent in the United States is infected with HIV each hour. Since it takes an average of 10 years for AIDS symptoms to appear when HIV is left untreated, it is obvious that many adults with AIDS were infected as adolescents.

Most HIV-infected adolescents are exposed to the virus though sexual intercourse. Recent data suggest that the majority of HIV-infected adolescent males are infected through sex with men. A small number of adolescent males appear to be exposed through injection of drugs or heterosexual contact. Adolescent females are mostly exposed through heterosexual contact, with a small percentage becoming infected through injected drug use (www.niaid.hih.gov/factsheets/hivadolescent.htm). African-American and Hispanic adolescents between the ages of 13 and 19 account for 66% and 21%, respectively, of reported AIDS cases in 2003. Because adolescents think they are invincible, they may delay testing, and if they test positive, they may delay treatment or refuse treatment. The inability to trace this population for medical care can lead to increased transmission of HIV.

► *Consider* THIS!

I was thinking of my carefree college days, when the most important thing was having an active sorority life and meeting guys. I had been raised by very strict parents and was never allowed to date under their watch. Since I attended an out-of-state college, I figured that my parents' outdated advice and rules no longer applied. Abruptly, my thoughts of the past were interrupted by the HIV counselor asking about my feelings concerning my positive diagnosis. What was there to say at this point? I had a lot of fun but never dreamed it would haunt me for the rest of my life, which was going to be shortened considerably now. I only wish I could turn back the hands of time and listen to my parents' advice, which somehow doesn't seem so outdated now.

Thoughts: All of us have thought back on our lives to better times and wondered how our lives would have changed if we had made better choices or gone down another path. It is a pity that we have only one chance to make good, sound decisions at times. What would you have changed in your life if given a second chance? Can you still make a change for the better now?

Clinical Manifestations

When a person is initially infected with HIV, he or she goes through an acute primary infection period for about 3 weeks. The HIV viral load drops rapidly because the host's immune system works well to fight this initial infection. The onset of the acute primary infection occurs 2 to 6 weeks after exposure. Symptoms include fever, pharyngitis, rash, and myalgia. Most people do not associate this flu-like condition with HIV infection. After initial exposure, there is a period of 3 to 12 months before seroconversion. The person is considered infectious during this time.

After the acute phase, the infected person becomes asymptomatic, but the HIV virus begins to replicate. Even though there are no symptoms, the immune system runs down. A normal person has a CD4 T-cell count of 450 to 1,200 cells per microliter. When the CD4 T-cell count reaches 200 or less, the person has reached the stage of AIDS. The immune system begins a constant battle to fight this viral invasion, but over time it falls behind. A viral reservoir occurs in T cells that can store various stages of the virus. The onset and severity of the disease correlate directly with the viral load: the more HIV virus that is present, the worse the person will feel.

As profound immunosuppression begins to occur, an opportunistic infection will occur, qualifying the person for the diagnosis of AIDS. The diagnosis is finally confirmed when the CD4 count is below 200. As of now, AIDS will eventually develop in everyone who is HIV-positive.

Because HIV over time depletes the CD4 cell population, infected people become more susceptible to opportunistic infections. Currently, the AIDS virus and response to treatment are tracked based on CD4 count rather than viral load. Untreated HIV will progress to AIDS in about 11 years, but this progression can be delayed by antiretroviral therapy (Dubin, 2007).

Diagnosis

Newly approved quick tests for HIV produce results in 20 minutes and also lower the health care worker's risk of occupational exposure by eliminating the need to draw blood. The CDC's Advancing HIV Prevention initiative, launched in 2003, has made increased testing a national priority. The initiative calls for testing to be incorporated into routine medical care and to be delivered in more nontraditional settings.

Fewer than half of adults between the ages of 18 and 64 have ever had an HIV test, according to the CDC. The agency estimates that one fourth of the million HIV-infected people in the United States do not know they are infected. This means they are not receiving treatment that can prolong their lives, and they may be unknowingly infecting others. In addition, even when people do get tested, one in three failed to return to the testing site to learn their results when there was a 2-week wait. The CDC hopes that the new "one-stop" approach to HIV testing changes that pattern. About 50,000 new HIV cases are reported each year in the United States, and that number has held steady for the past few years despite massive efforts in prevention education (CDC, 2007b).

The OraQuick Rapid HIV-1 Antibody Test detects the HIV antibody in a blood sample taken with a fingerstick or from an oral fluid sample. Both can produce results in as little as 20 minutes with more than 99% accuracy (Aaron et al., 2006). The FDA has approved two other rapid blood tests: the Reveal Rapid HIV-1 Antibody Test and the Uni-Gold Recombigen HIV Test.

Testing for HIV should be offered to anyone seeking evaluation and treatment for STIs. Counseling before and after testing is an integral part of the testing procedure. Informed consent must be obtained before an HIV test is performed. HIV infection is diagnosed by tests for antibodies against HIV-1 and HIV-2 (HIV-1/2). Antibody testing begins with a sensitive screening test (e.g., the enzyme immunoassay [ELISA]). This is a specific test for antibodies to HIV that is used to determine whether the person has been exposed to the HIV retrovirus. Reactive screening tests must be confirmed by a more specific test (e.g., the Western blot [WB]) or an immunofluorescence assay (IFA). This is a highly specific test that is used to validate a positive ELISA test finding. If the supplemental test (WB or IFA) is positive, it confirms that the person is infected with HIV and is capable of transmitting the virus to others. HIV antibody is detectable in at least 95% of people within 3 months after infection (CDC, 2006).

Therapeutic Management

The goals of HIV drug therapy are to:

- Decrease the HIV viral load below the level of detection
- Restore the body's ability to fight off pathogens
- Improve the client's quality of life
- Reduce HIV morbidity and mortality (Cressey & Lallemant, 2007)

Highly active antiretroviral therapy (HAART), which combines at least three antiretroviral drugs, has dramatically improved the prognosis of HIV/AIDS. Often treatment begins with combination HAART therapy at the time of the first infection, when the person's immune system is still intact. The current HAART therapy standard is a triple combination therapy, but some clients may be given a fourth or fifth agent.

There are obvious challenges involved in meeting these goals. The viral load can be reduced much more quickly than the T-cell count can be increased, and this disparity leaves the woman vulnerable to opportunistic infections.

Current therapy to prevent the transmission of HIV to the newborn includes a three-part regimen of having the mother take an oral antiretroviral agent at 14 to 34 weeks of gestation; it is continued throughout pregnancy. During labor, an antiretroviral agent is administered intravenously until delivery. An antiretroviral syrup is administered to the infant within 12 hours after birth.

Dramatic new treatment advances with antiretroviral medications have turned a disease that used to be a death sentence into a chronic, manageable one for individuals who live in countries where antiretroviral therapy is available. Despite these advances in treatment, however, only a minority of HIV-positive Americans who take antiretroviral medications are receiving the full benefits because they are not adhering to the prescribed regimen. Successful antiretroviral therapy requires nearly perfect adherence to a complex medication regimen; less-than-perfect adherence leads to drug resistance (Battaglioli-Denero, 2007).

Adherence is difficult because of the complexity of the regimen and the lifelong duration of treatment. A typical antiretroviral regimen may consist of three or more medications taken twice daily. Adherence is made even more difficult because of the unpleasant side effects, such as nausea and diarrhea. Women in early pregnancy already experience these, and the antiretroviral medication only exacerbates them.

Nursing Management

Nurses can play a major role in caring for the HIV-positive woman by helping her accept the possibility of a shortened life span, cope with others' reactions to a stigmatizing illness, and develop strategies to maintain her physical and emotional health. Educate the woman about changes she can make in her behavior to prevent spreading HIV to others, and refer her to appropriate community resources such as HIV medical care services, substance abuse, mental health services, and social services. See Nursing Care Plan 5.1: Overview for the Woman With HIV.

Providing Education About Drug Therapy

The goal of antiretroviral therapy is to suppress viral replication so that the viral load becomes undetectable (below 400). This is done to preserve immune function and delay disease progression but is a challenge because of the side effects of nausea and vomiting, diarrhea, altered taste, anorexia, flatulence, constipation, headaches, anemia, and fatigue. Although not everyone experiences all of the side effects, the majority do have some of them. Current research hasn't documented the long-term safety of exposure of the fetus to antiretroviral agents during pregnancy, but collection of data is ongoing.

Help to reduce the development of drug resistance and thus treatment failure by identifying the barriers to adherence; identifying these barriers can help the woman to overcome them. Some of the common barriers exist because the woman:

- Does not understand the link between drug resistance and nonadherence
- Fears revealing her HIV status by being seen taking medication
- Hasn't adjusted emotionally to the HIV diagnosis
- Doesn't understand the dosing regimen or schedule
- Experiences unpleasant side effects frequently
- Feels anxious or depressed (Dubin, 2007)

Depending on which barriers are causing nonadherence, work with the woman by educating her about the dosing regimen, helping her find ways to integrate the prescribed regimen into her lifestyle, and making referrals to social service agencies as appropriate. By addressing barriers on an individual level, the nurse can help the woman to overcome them.

Educate the woman about the prescribed drug therapy and stress that it is very important to take the regimen as prescribed. Offer suggestions about how to cope with anorexia, nausea, and vomiting by:

- Separating the intake of food and fluids
- Eating dry crackers upon arising
- Eating six small meals daily
- Using high-protein supplements (Boost, Ensure) to provide quick and easy protein and calories
- Eating "comfort foods," which may appeal when other foods don't

Promoting Compliance

Remaining compliant with drug therapy is a huge challenge for many HIV-infected people. Compliance becomes diffi-

Nursing Care Plan 5.1

OVERVIEW OF THE WOMAN WHO IS HIV-POSITIVE

Annie, a 28-year-old African-American woman, is HIV-positive. She acquired HIV through unprotected sexual contact. She has been inconsistent in taking her antiretroviral medications and presents today stating she is tired and doesn't feel well.

NURSING DIAGNOSIS: Risk for infection related to positive HIV status and inconsistent compliance with antiretroviral therapy

Outcome Identification and Evaluation

Client will remain free of opportunistic infections as evidenced by temperature within acceptable parameters and absence of signs and symptoms of opportunistic infections.

Interventions: Minimizing the Risk of Opportunistic Infections

- Assess CD4 count and viral loads *to determine disease progression* (CD4 counts <500/L and viral loads >10,000 copies/L = increased risk for opportunistic infections).
- Assess complete blood count *to identify presence of infection* (>10,000 cells/mm³ may indicate infection).
- Assess oral cavity and mucous membranes for painful white patches in mouth *to evaluate for possible fungal infection.*
- Teach client to monitor for general signs and symptoms of infections, such as fever, weakness, and fatigue, *to ensure early identification.*
- Provide information explaining the importance of avoiding people with infections when possible *to minimize risk of exposure to infections.*
- Teach importance of keeping appointments so her CD4 count and viral load can be monitored *to alert the health care provider about her immune system status.*
- Instruct her to reduce her exposure to infections via:
  - Meticulous handwashing
  - Thorough cooking of meats, eggs, and vegetables
  - Wearing shoes at all times, especially when outdoors
- Encourage a balance of rest with activity throughout the day *to prevent overexertion.*
- Stress importance of maintaining prescribed antiretroviral drug therapies *to prevent disease progression and resistance.*
- If necessary, refer Annie to a nutritionist to help her understand what constitutes a well-balanced diet with supplements *to promote health and ward off infection.*

NURSING DIAGNOSIS: Knowledge deficit related to HIV infection and possible complications

Outcome Identification and Evaluation

Client will demonstrate increased understanding of HIV infection as evidenced by verbalizing appropriate health care practices and adhering to measures to comply with therapy and reduce her risk of further exposure and reduce risk of disease progression.

Interventions: Providing Patient Education

- Assess her understanding of HIV and its treatment *to provide a baseline for teaching.*
- Establish trust and be honest with Annie; encourage her to talk about her fears and the impact of the disease *to provide an outlet for her concerns.* Encourage her to discuss reasons for her noncompliance.
- Provide a nonjudgmental, accessible, confidential, and culturally sensitive approach *to promote Annie's self-esteem and allow her to feel that she is a priority.*
- Explain measures, including safer sex practices and birth control options, to prevent disease transmission; determine her willingness to practice safer sex to protect others *to determine further teaching needs.*
- Discuss the signs and symptoms of disease progression and potential opportunistic infections *to promote early detection for prompt intervention.*
- Outline with the client the availability of community resources and make appropriate referrals as needed *to provide additional education and support.*
- Encourage Annie to keep scheduled appointments *to ensure follow-up and allow early detection of potential problems.*

cult when the same pills that are supposed to thwart the disease are making the person sick. Nausea and diarrhea are just two of the possible side effects. It is often difficult to increase the client's quality of life when so much oral medication is required. The combination medication therapy is challenging for many people, and staying compliant over a period of years is extremely difficult. Stress the importance of taking the prescribed antiretroviral drug therapies by explaining that they help prevent replication of the retroviruses and subsequent progression of the disease, as well as decreasing the risk of perinatal transmission of HIV. In addition, provide written materials describing diet, exercise, medications, and signs and symptoms of complications and opportunistic infections. Reinforce this information at each visit.

Preventing HIV Infection

The lack of information about HIV infection and AIDS causes great anxiety and fear of the unknown. It is vital to take a leadership role in educating the public about risky behaviors in the fight to control this disease. The core of HIV prevention is to abstain from sex until marriage, to be faithful, and to use condoms. This is all good advice for many women, but some simply do not have the economic and social power or choices or control over their lives to put that advice into practice. Recognize that fact, and address the factors that will give women more control over their lives by providing anticipatory guidance, giving ample opportunities to practice negotiation techniques and refusal skills in a safe environment, and encouraging the use of female condoms to protect against this deadly virus. Prevention is the key to reversing the current infection trends.

Providing Care During Pregnancy and Childbirth

Voluntary counseling and HIV testing should be offered to all pregnant women as early in the pregnancy as possible to identify HIV-infected women so that treatment can be initiated early. Once a pregnant woman is identified as being HIV-positive, she should be informed about the risk for perinatal infection. Current evidence indicates that in the absence of antiretroviral medications, 25% of infants born to HIV-infected mothers will become infected with HIV (CDC, 2007b). If women do receive a combination of antiretroviral therapies during pregnancy, however, the risk of HIV transmission to the newborn drops below 2% (National Institute of Allergy and Infectious Disease, 2007a). In addition, HIV can be spread to the infant through breastfeeding, and thus all HIV-infected pregnant women should be counseled to avoid breastfeeding and use formula instead. A recent maternal infection with HIV may raise the risk of transmission through breastfeeding to twice that of a woman with earlier established infection, owing probably to the high viral load associated with recent infection (WHO, 2007b).

In addition, the woman needs instructions on ways to enhance her immune system by following these guidelines during pregnancy:

- Getting adequate sleep each night (7 to 9 hours)
- Avoiding infections (e.g., staying out of crowds, handwashing)
- Decreasing stress in her life
- Consuming adequate protein and vitamins
- Increasing her fluid intake to 2 liters daily to stay hydrated
- Planning rest periods throughout the day to prevent fatigue

Despite the dramatic reduction in perinatal transmission, hundreds of infants will be born infected with HIV. The birth of each infected infant is a missed prevention opportunity. To minimize perinatal HIV transmission, identify HIV infection in women, preferably before pregnancy; provide information about disease prevention; and encourage HIV-infected women to follow the prescribed drug therapy.

Providing Appropriate Referrals

The HIV-infected woman may have difficulty coping with the normal activities of daily living because she has less energy and decreased physical endurance. She may be overwhelmed by the financial burdens of medical and drug therapies and the emotional responses to a life-threatening condition, as well as concern about her infant's future, if she is pregnant. A case management approach is needed to deal with the complexity of her needs during this time. Be an empathetic listener and make appropriate referrals for nutritional services, counseling, homemaker services, spiritual care, and local support groups. Many community-based organizations have developed programs to address the numerous issues regarding HIV/AIDS. The national AIDS hotline (1-800-342-AIDS) is a good resource.

Preventing Sexually Transmitted Infections

Education about safer sex practices—and the resulting increase in the use of condoms—can play a vital role in reducing STI rates all over the world. Clearly, knowledge and prevention are the best defenses against STIs. The prevention and control of STIs is based on the following concepts (CDC, 2006):

1. Education and counseling of persons at risk about safer sexual behavior
2. Identification of asymptomatic infected individuals and of symptomatic individuals unlikely to seek diagnosis and treatment
3. Effective diagnosis and treatment of infected individuals

4. Evaluation, treatment, and counseling of sex partners of people who are infected with an STI
5. Pre-exposure vaccination of people at risk for vaccine-preventable STIs

Nurses play an integral role in identifying and preventing STIs. They have a unique opportunity to educate the public about this serious public health issue by communicating the methods of transmission and symptoms associated with each condition, tracking the updated CDC treatment guidelines, and offering clients strategic preventive measures to reduce the spread of STIs.

It is not easy to discuss STI prevention when globally we are failing at it. Knowledge exists on how to prevent every single route of transmission, but the incidence continues to climb. Challenges to prevention of STIs include lack of resources and difficulty in changing the behaviors that contribute to their spread. Regardless of the challenging factors involved, nurses must continue to educate and to meet the needs of all women to promote their sexual health. Successful treatment and prevention of STIs is impossible without education. Successful teaching approaches include giving clear, accurate messages that are age-appropriate and culturally sensitive.

Primary prevention strategies include education of all women, especially adolescents, regarding the risk of early sexual activity, the number of sexual partners, and STIs. Sexual abstinence is ideal but often not practiced; therefore, the use of barrier contraception (condoms) should be encouraged (see Teaching Guidelines 5.1).

Secondary prevention involves the need for annual pelvic examinations with Pap smears for all sexually active women, regardless of age. Many women with STIs are asymptomatic, so regular screening examinations are paramount for early detection. Understanding the relationship between poor socioeconomic conditions and poor patterns of sexual and reproductive self-care is significant in disease-prevention and health-promotion strategies.

Every successful form of prevention requires a change in behavior. The nursing role in teaching and rendering quality health care is invaluable evidence that the key to reducing the spread of STIs is through behavioral change. Nurses working in these specialty areas have a responsibility to educate themselves, their clients, their families, and the community about STIs and to provide compassionate and supportive care to clients. Some strategies nurses can use to prevent the spread of STIs are detailed in Box 5.3.

Behavior Modification

Research validates that changing behaviors does result in a decrease in new STI infections, but it must encompass all levels—governments, community organizations, schools, churches, parents, and individuals (Peterson et al., 2007). Education must address ways to prevent becoming infected, ways to prevent transmitting infection, symptoms

---

BOX 5.3 **Selected Nursing Strategies to Prevent the Spread of STIs**

- Provide basic information about STI transmission.
- Outline safer sexual behaviors for people at risk for STIs.
- Refer clients to appropriate community resources to reduce risk.
- Screen asymptomatic persons with STIs.
- Identify barriers to STI testing and remove them.
- Offer pre-exposure immunizations for vaccine-preventable STIs.
- Respond honestly about testing results and options available.
- Counsel and treat sexual partners of persons with STIs.
- Educate school administrators, parents, and teens about STIs.
- Support youth development activities to reduce sexual risk-taking.
- Promote the use of barrier methods (condoms, diaphragms) to prevent the spread of STIs.
- Assist clients to gain skills in negotiating safer sex.
- Discuss reducing the number of sexual partners to reduce risk

---

of STIs, and treatment. At this point in the STI epidemic, nurses do not have time to debate the relative merits of prevention versus treatment: both are underused and underfunded, and one leads to the other. But being serious about prevention and focusing on the strategies outlined above will bring about a positive change on everyone's part.

Contraception

The spread of STIs could be prevented by access to safe, efficient, appropriate, modern contraception for everyone who wants it. Nurses can play an important role in helping women to identify their risk of STIs and to adopt preventive measures through the dual protection that contraceptives offer. Traditionally, family planning and STI services have been separate entities. Family planning services have addressed a woman's need for contraception without considering her or her partner's risk of STI; meanwhile, STI services have been heavily slanted toward men, ignoring the contraceptive needs of men and their partners.

Many women are at significant risk for unintended pregnancy and STIs, yet with this separation of services, there is limited evaluation of whether they need dual protection—that is, concurrent protection from STIs and unintended pregnancy. This lack of integration of services represents a missed opportunity to identify many at-risk women and to offer them counseling on dual protection (Hogben, 2007).

Nurses can expand their scopes in either setting by discussing dual protection by use of a male or female condom alone or by use of a condom along with a nonbarrier contraceptive. Because barrier methods are not the most effective means of fertility control, they have not been typically recommended as a method alone for dual protection. Unfortunately, the most effective pregnancy prevention methods—sterilization, hormonal methods, and intrauterine devices—do not protect against STIs. Dual-method use protects against STIs and pregnancy.

■■■ Key Concepts

- Avoiding risky sexual behaviors may preserve fertility and prevent chronic conditions later in life.

- An estimated 65 million people live with an incurable STI, and another 15 million are infected each year.

- The most reliable way to avoid transmission of STIs is to abstain from sexual intercourse (i.e., oral, vaginal, or anal sex) or to be in a long-term, mutually monogamous relationship with an uninfected partner.

- Barrier methods of contraception are recommended because they increase protection from contact with urethral discharge, mucosal secretions, and lesions of the cervix or penis.

- The high rate of asymptomatic transmission of STIs calls for teaching high-risk women the nature of transmission and how to recognize infections.

- The CDC and ACOG recommend that all women be offered group B streptococcal screening by rectovaginal culture at 35 to 37 weeks of gestation, and that colonized women be treated with intravenous antibiotics at the time of labor or ruptured membranes.

- Nurses should practice good handwashing techniques and follow standard precautions to protect themselves and their patients from STIs.

- Nurses are in an important position to promote the sexual health of all women. Nurses should make their clients and the community aware of the perinatal implications and life-long sequelae of STIs.

REFERENCES

Aaron, E., Levine, A. B., Monahan, K., & Biondo, C. P. (2006). A rapid HIV testing program for labor and delivery in an inner city teaching hospital. *AIDS Reader, 16*(1), 22–37.

Alexander, L. L., LaRosa, J. H., Bader, H., & Garfield, S. (2007). *New dimensions in women's health* (4th ed.). Sudbury, MA: Jones and Bartlett Publishers.

American Cancer Society (ACS). (2007). American Cancer Society Guideline for HPV vaccine use to prevent cervical cancer and its precursors. *CA: A Cancer Journal for Clinicians, 57*(1), 7–28.

Assan, S., & Kraszewski, S. (2006). Sexually transmitted infections: Hepatitis B. *Practice Nurse, 32*(7), 58–62.

Battaglioli-Denero, A. M. (2007). Strategies for improving adherence to therapy and long-term patient outcomes. *Journal of the Association of Nurses in AIDS Care, 18*(1), S17–22.

Bennett, N. J., & Domachowske, J. (2007). Gonorrhea. *eMedicine.* Available at: http://www.emedicine.com/PED/topic886.htm

Centers for Disease Control and Prevention (CDC). (2006). Sexually transmitted diseases treatment guidelines 2006. *MMWR, 55*(RR-11), 1–89.

Centers for Disease Control and Prevention (CDC). (2007a). Increases in gonorrhea 2000–2006. *MMWR, 56*(10), 222–225.

Centers for Disease Control and Prevention (CDC). (2007b). A glance at the HIV/AIDS epidemic. Available at: http://www.cdc.gov/hiv/resources/factsheets/print/At-A-Glance.htm

Centers for Disease Control and Prevention (CDC). (2007c). Genital HPV infection—CDC fact sheet. Available at: http://www.cdc.gov/std/HPV/STDFact-HPV.htm

Centers for Disease Control and Prevention (CDC). (2007d). Pelvic inflammatory disease—CDC fact sheet. Available at: http://www.cdc.gov/std/PID/STDFact-PID.htm

Cordoro, K. M., & Wilson, B. B. (2007). Scabies. *eMedicine.* Available at: http://www.emedicine.com/DERM/topic382.htm

Cressey, T. R., & Lallemant, M. (2007). Pharmacogenetics of antiretroviral drugs for the treatment of HIV-infected patients: An update. *Infection, Genetics & Evolution, 7*(2), 333–342.

Crossman, S. H. (2006). The challenge of pelvic inflammatory disease. *American Family Physician, 73*(5), 859–864.

Dubin, J. (2007). HIV infection and AIDS. *eMedicine.* Available at: http://www.emedicine.com/EMERG/topic253.htm

Dunne, E. F., Unger, E. R., Sternberg, M., McQuillan, G., Swan, D. C., Patel, S. S., & Markowitz, L. E. (2007). Prevalence of HPV infection among females in the United States. *JAMA, 297*(8), 813–819.

Ferguson, L. A., & Varnado, J. W. (2006) Syphilis: An old enemy still lurks. *Journal of the American Academy of Nurse Practitioners, 18,* 49–55.

Gearhart, P. A., & Randall, T. C. (2007). Human papillomavirus. *eMedicine.* Available at: http://www.emedicine.com/med/topic1037.htm

Geisler, W. M. (2007). Management of uncomplicated *Chlamydia trachomatis* infections in adolescents and adults. *Clinical Infectious Diseases, 44*(3), S77–83.

Gilbert, E. S. (2007). *Manual of high-risk pregnancy and delivery* (4th ed.). St. Louis, MO: Mosby Elsevier

Glasier, A., Gulmezoglu, A. M., Schmid, G. P., Moreno, C. G., & Van Look, P. F. A. (2006). Sexual reproductive health: A matter of life and death. *Lancet, 368*(9547), 1595–1607.

Hackley, B., Kriebs, J. M., & Rousseau, M. E. (2007). *Primary care of women: A guide for midwives and women's health providers.* Sudbury, MA: Jones and Bartlett Publishers.

Hogben, M. (2007). Partner notification for sexually transmitted disease. *Clinical Infectious Disease, 44*(3), S160–174.

Johnson-Mallard, V., Lengacher, C. A., Kromroy, J. D., Campbell, D. W., Jevitt, C. M., Daley, E., & Schmitt, K. (2007). Increasing knowledge of sexually transmitted infection risk. *Nurse Practitioner, 32*(2), 26–33.

Kennedy, M. S. (2007). In the clinical arena. *AJN, 107*(1), 22.

Leggatt, G. R., & Frazer, I. H. (2007). HPV vaccines: The beginning of the end for cervical cancer. *Current Opinion in Immunology, 19*(2), 232–238.

Marrazzo, J. M., & Martin, D. H. (2007). Management of women with cervicitis. *Clinical Infectious Diseases, 44*(3), S102–110.

McGregor, T. A., & Richard, A. J. (2007). Syphilis. *eMedicine.* Available at: http://www.emedicine.com/EMERG/topic563.htm

Mehta, S. D. (2007). Gonorrhea and chlamydia in emergency departments: Screening, diagnosis and treatment. *Current Infectious Diseases, 9*(2), 134–142.

Moore, S. L., & Seybold, V. K. (2007). HPV vaccine. *Clinical Reviews, 17*(1), 36–42.

Mullan, F. (2007). Responding to the global HIV/AIDS crisis. *Journal of the American Medical Association, 297*(7), 744–746.

National Institute of Allergy and Infectious Disease. (2006a). Chlamydia. Retrieved Sept. 15, 2007, from http://www.niaid.nih.gov/factsheets/stdclam.htm

National Institute of Allergy and Infectious Disease. (2006b). Gonorrhea. Retrieved Sept. 15, 2007, from http://www.niaid.nih.gov/factsheets/stdgon.htm

National Institute of Allergy and Infectious Diseases. (2007a). HIV infection in women. National Institutes of Health. Available at: http://www.niaid.nih.gov/factsheets/womenhiv.htm

National Institute of Allergy and Infectious Diseases. (2007b). Human papillomavirus and genital warts. National Institutes of Health. Available at: http://www.niaid.nih.gov/factsheets/stdhpv.htm

National Institute of Allergy and Infectious Disease. (2007c). Syphilis. Retrieved Sept. 15, 2007, from http://www3.niaid.nih.gov/healthscience/healthtopics/syphilis/default.htm.

National Institutes of Health (NIH). (2008). *HIV/AIDS among youth* [Online]. Available at http://www.cdc.gov/hiv/resources/factsheets/youth.htm

Paz-Bailey, G., Ramaswamy, M., Hawkes, S., & Geretti, A. (2007). Herpes simplex virus type 2: Epidemiology and management options in developing countries. *Sexually Transmitted Infections, 83*(1), 16–22.

Peterson, R., Albright, J., Garrett, J., & Curtis, K. (2007). Pregnancy and STD prevention counseling using an adaptation of motivational interviewing: A randomized controlled study. *Perspectives on Sexual & Reproductive Health, 39*(1), 21–28.

Pickering, L. K. (Ed.) (2006). *Red book: 2006 report of the committee on infectious diseases* (27th ed.). Elk Grove Village, IL: American Academy of Pediatrics.

Public Health Agency of Canada. (2006). *Canadian guidelines on sexually transmitted infections.* Ottawa, ON: Author.

Pyrsopoulos, N. T., & Reddy, K. R. (2007). Hepatitis B. *eMedicine.* Available at: http://www.emedicine.com/MED/topic992.htm

Reyes, I., & Abbuhl, S. (2007). Pelvic inflammatory disease. *eMedicine.* Available at: http://emedicine.com/emerg/topic410.htm

Sharma, R., & Brilliant, L. C. (2007). Herpes simplex. *eMedicine.* Available at: http://www.emedicine.com/EMERG/topic246.htm

Stoner, B. P. (2007). Current controversies in the management of adult syphilis. *Clinical Infectious Diseases, 44*(3), S130–146.

Wald, A. (2007). The CDC releases its HPV vaccine recommendations. *Journal Watch Women's Health.* Available at: http://womens-health.jwatch.org/cgi/content/full/2007/824/1

Wasley, A., Miller, J. T., & Finelli, L. (2007). Surveillance for active viral hepatitis—United States, 2005. *MMWR, 56*(3), 1–24.

Waugh, M. (2007). Sexual health medicine 2007. *Skinmed, 6*(2), 88–90.

Wolfram, W. (2007). Pediculosis (lice). *eMedicine.* Available at: http://www.emedicine.com/ped/topic1304.htm

World Health Organization (WHO). (2007a). Hepatitis B fact sheet. Available at: http://www.who.int/mediacentre/factsheets/fs204/en/

World Health Organization (WHO). (2007b). HIV transmission through breastfeeding. Available at: http://www.who.int/reproductive-health/docs/hiv_infantfeeding/breastfeeding.html

Workowski, K. A., & Berman, S. M. (2006). Sexually transmitted diseases treatment guidelines, 2006. *MMWR Recommendations Report, 55*(RR11), 1–94.

WEBSITES

American College of Obstetricians and Gynecologists (ACOG): (202) 863-2518, http://www.acog.org

American Psychiatric Association: (202) 682-6000, http://psych.org

American Society for Reproductive Medicine: (205) 978-5000, http://www.asrm.org

Centers for Disease Control and Prevention: (202) 329-1819, http://www.cdc.gov

CDC National AIDS hotline: 1-800-342-2437

Herpes Resource Center: www.ashastd.org/herpes/hrc

National Institute of Allergy and Infectious Disease: Human papillomavirus and genital warts, http://www.niaid.hih.gov/factsheets/stdhpv.htm

National Institute of Allergy and Infectious Disease: Chlamydia, http://www.niaid.nih.gov/factsheets/stdclam.htm

National Institute of Allergy and Infectious Disease: Gonorrhea, http://www.niaid.nih.gov/factsheets/stdgon.htm

National Institute of Allergy and Infectious Disease: Syphilis, http://www.niaid.nih.gov/factsheets/stdsyph.htm.

National Institute of Mental Health: (301) 443-4513, http://www.nimh.nih.gov

National Women's Health Resource Center: http://www.healthy-women.org

National Women's Information Center (NWHIC): 1-800-994-9662, http://www.4women.gov

Resolve, Inc. (impaired fertility): (617) 623-0744, http://www.resolve.org

Teen Source (STI information for teens): www.teensource.org

CHAPTER WORKSHEET

MULTIPLE CHOICE QUESTIONS

1. Which of the following contraceptive methods offers protection against sexually transmitted infections (STIs)?

   a. Oral contraceptives

   b. Withdrawal

   c. Latex condom

   d. Intrauterine device

2. In teaching about HIV transmission, the nurse explains that the virus cannot be transmitted by:

   a. Shaking hands

   b. Sharing drug needles

   c. Sexual intercourse

   d. Breastfeeding

3. A woman with HPV is likely to present with which nursing assessment finding?

   a. Profuse, pus-filled vaginal discharge

   b. Clusters of genital warts

   c. Single painless ulcer

   d. Multiple vesicles on genitalia

4. The nurse's discharge teaching plan for the woman with PID should reinforce which of the following potentially life-threatening complications?

   a. Involuntary infertility

   b. Chronic pelvic pain

   c. Depression

   d. Ectopic pregnancy

5. To confirm a finding of primary syphilis, the nurse would observe which of the following on the external genitalia?

   a. A highly variable skin rash

   b. A yellow-green vaginal discharge

   c. A nontender, indurated ulcer

   d. A localized gumma formation

CRITICAL THINKING EXERCISE

1. Sally, age 17, comes to the teen clinic saying that she is in pain and has some "crud" between her legs. The nurse takes her into the examining room and questions her about her symptoms. Sally states she had numerous genital bumps that had been filled with fluid, then ruptured and turned into ulcers with crusts. In addition, she has pain on urination and overall body pain. Sally says she had unprotected sex with several men when she was drunk at a party a few weeks back, but she thought they were "clean."

   a. What STI would the nurse suspect?

   b. The nurse should give immediate consideration to which of Sally's complaints?

   c. What should be the goal of the nurse in teaching Sally about STIs?

STUDY ACTIVITIES

1. Select a website at the end of the chapter to explore. Educate yourself about one specific STI thoroughly and share your expertise with your clinical group.

2. Contact your local health department and request current statistics regarding three STIs. Ask them to compare the current number of cases reported to last year's. Are they less or more? What may be some of the reasons for the change in the number of cases reported?

3. Request permission to attend a local STI clinic to shadow a nurse for a few hours. Describe the nurse's counseling role with patients and what specific information is emphasized to patients.

4. Two common STIs that appear together and commonly are treated together regardless of identification of the secondary one are _____ and _____.

5. Genital warts can be treated with which of the following? Select all that apply.

   a. Penicillin

   b. Podophyllin

   c. Imiquimod

   d. Cryotherapy

   e. Antiretroviral therapy

   f. Acyclovir

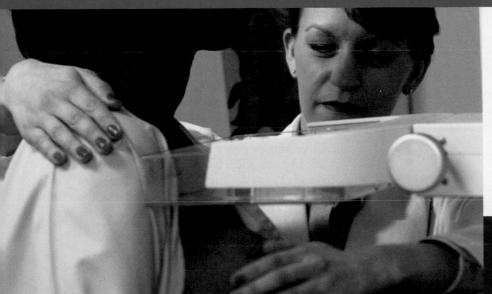

CHAPTER 6

DISORDERS OF THE BREASTS

KEY TERMS

benign breast disorder
breast cancer
breast-conserving surgery
breast self-examination
carcinoma
chemotherapy

duct ectasia
endocrine therapy
fibroadenomas
fibrocystic breast changes
intraductal papilloma
mammography

mastitis
modified radical
    mastectomy
simple mastectomy

LEARNING OBJECTIVES

Upon completion of the chapter, the learner will be able to:

1. Define the key terms used in this chapter.
2. Identify the incidence, risk factors, screening methods, and treatment modalities for benign breast conditions.
3. Outline preventive strategies for breast cancer through lifestyle changes and health screening.
4. Explain the incidence, risk factors, treatment modalities, and nursing considerations related to breast cancer.
5. Develop an educational plan to teach breast self-examination to a group of young women.

Nancy hasn't been able to sleep well since she felt the lump in her left breast over a month ago, just after her 60th birthday. She knows she is at high risk because her mother died of breast cancer, but she can't bring herself to have it checked out.

Wow

Focus on reducing fear, anxiety, pain, and aloneness in all women diagnosed with a breast disorder.

The female breast is closely linked to womanhood in American culture. Women's breasts act as physical markers for transitions from one stage of life to another, and although the primary function of the breasts is lactation, they are perceived as a symbol of beauty and sexuality.

This chapter will discuss assessments, screening procedures, and management of specific benign and malignant breast disorders. Nurses play a key role in helping women maintain breast health by education and screening. A good working knowledge of early detection techniques, diagnosis, and treatment options is essential.

Benign Breast Disorders

A **benign breast disorder** is any noncancerous breast abnormality. Though not life-threatening, benign disorders can cause pain and discomfort, and they account for a large number of visits to primary care providers.

Depending on the type of benign breast disorder, treatment might or might not be necessary. Although these disorders are benign, the emotional trauma women experience is phenomenal. Fear, anxiety, disbelief, helplessness, and depression are just a few of the reactions that a woman may have when she discovers a lump in her breast. Many women believe that all lumps are cancerous, but actually more than 90% of the lumps discovered are benign and need no treatment (Alexander et al., 2007). Patience, support, and education are essential components of nursing care.

▶ *Consider* THIS!

It was pouring down rain and I was driving alone along dark wet streets to my 8 a.m. appointment for a breast ultrasound. I recently had my annual mammogram and the radiologist thought he saw something suspicious on my right breast. I was on my way to confirm or refute his suspicions, and I couldn't keep focused on the road ahead. For the past few days I had been a basket case, fearing the worst. I was playing in my mind, what I would do if . . . ? What changes would I make in my life and how would I react when told? I have been through such personal turmoil since that doctor announced he wanted "more tests."

Thoughts: This woman is worrying and is emotionally devastated before she even has a conclusive diagnosis. Is this a typical reaction to a breast disorder? Why do women fear the worst? Many women use denial to mask their feelings and hope against hope the doctor made a mistake or misread their mammogram. How would you react if you or your sister, girlfriend, or mother were confronted with a breast disorder?

The most commonly encountered benign breast disorders in women include fibrocystic breasts, fibroadenomas, intraductal papilloma, mammary duct ectasia, and mastitis. Although these breast disorders are considered benign, fibrocystic breasts and intraductal papillomas carry a cancer risk, with prolific masses and hyperplastic changes within the breasts. Generally speaking, fibroadenomas, mastitis, and mammary duct ectasia carry little cancer risk (Sukumvanich & Borgen, 2007). Table 6-1 summarizes benign breast conditions.

▶ FIBROCYSTIC BREAST CHANGES

Fibrocystic breast changes do not refer to a disease; rather, they represent a variety of changes in the glandular and structural tissues of the breast. Because this condition affects many women at some point, it is more accurately defined as a "change" rather than a "disease." The cause of fibrocystic changes is related to the way breast tissue responds to monthly levels of estrogen and progesterone. During the menstrual cycle, hormonal stimulation of the breast tissue causes the glands and ducts to enlarge and swell. One or both breasts can be involved, and any part of the breast can become tender (Hackley, Kriebs, & Rousseau, 2007). Fibrocystic changes do not increase the risk of breast cancer for most women except when the breast biopsy shows "atypia" or abnormal breast cells. The cause for concern for many women with fibrocystic changes is that breast examinations and mammography become more difficult to interpret with multiple cysts present, and early cancerous lesions that occur may occasionally be overlooked (American Cancer Society [ACS], 2007a).

Fibrocystic breast changes are most common in women between the ages of 30 and 50. The condition is rare in postmenopausal women not taking hormone replacement therapy. According to the ACS, fibrocystic breast changes affect at least half of all women at some point in their lives and are the most common breast disorder today (ACS, 2007a).

Therapeutic Management

Management of the symptoms of fibrocystic breast changes begins with self-care. In severe cases drugs, including bromocriptine, tamoxifen, or danazol, can be used to reduce the influence of estrogen on breast tissue. However, several undesirable side effects, including masculinization, have been documented. Aspiration or surgical removal of breast lumps will reduce pain and swelling by removing the space-occupying mass.

Nursing Assessment

Nursing assessment consists of a health history, physical examination, and laboratory and diagnostic tests.

TABLE 6.1   **SUMMARY OF BENIGN BREAST DISORDERS**

Breast Condition	Nipple Discharge	Site	Characteristics/ Age of Client	Tenderness	Diagnosis & Treatment
Fibrocystic breast changes	+ or −	Bilateral; upper outer quadrant	Round, smooth Several lesions Cyclic, palpable 30 to 50 years old	+	Aspiration and biopsy Limit caffeine; ibuprofen; supportive bra
Fibroadenomas	−	Unilateral; nipple area or upper outer quadrant	Round, firm, movable Palpable, rubbery Well delineated Single lesion 15 to 30 years old	−	Mammogram "Watchful waiting" Aspiration and biopsy Surgical excision
Intraductal papilloma	+	Unilateral; near nipple	Small, wart-like Poorly delineated Nonpalpable Can become large 40 to 60 years old	+	Culture discharge Mammogram Ultrasound Surgical excision
Duct ectasia	+	Unilateral; behind nipple	Inflammation Pasty, greenish discharge Nonmobile Burning, itching Perimenopausal women	+	Mammogram Ultrasound Culture Antibiotics Surgical excision
Mastitis	−	Unilateral; outer quadrant	Wedge-shaped Warmth, redness Swelling Nipple cracked Breast engorged	+	Antibiotics Warm shower Supportive bra Breastfeeding Increase fluids

Sources: ACS, 2007a; Alexander et al., 2007; Blackburn, 2007; Sukumvanich & Borgen, 2007

Health History

Ask the woman about common clinical manifestations, which include lumpy, tender breasts, particularly during the week before menses. Changes in breast tissue produce pain by nerve irritation from edema in connective tissue and by fibrosis from nerve pinching. The pain is cyclic and frequently dissipates after the onset of menses. The pain is described as a dull, aching feeling of fullness. Masses or nodularities usually appear in both breasts and are often found in the upper outer quadrants. Some women also experience spontaneous clear to yellow nipple discharge when the breast is squeezed or manipulated.

Physical Examination

It is best to examine a woman's breast a week after menses, when swelling has subsided. Observe the breasts for fibrosis, or thickening of the normal breast tissues, which occurs in the early stages. Cysts form in the later stages and feel like multiple, smooth, well-delineated tiny pebbles or bumpy oatmeal under the skin (Fig. 6.1). On physical examination of the breasts, a few characteristics might be helpful in differentiating a cyst from a cancerous lesion. Cancerous lesions typically are fixed and painless and may cause skin retraction (pulling). Cysts tend to be mobile and tender and do not cause skin retraction in the surrounding tissue.

Laboratory and Diagnostic Tests

Mammography can be helpful in distinguishing fibrocystic changes from breast cancer. Ultrasound is a useful adjunct to mammography for breast evaluation because it helps to differentiate a cystic mass from a solid one (Aliotta & Schaeffer, 2006). Ultrasound produces images of the breasts by sending sound waves through a gel applied to the breasts. Fine-needle aspiration biopsy can also be done to differentiate a solid tumor, cyst, or malignancy. A fine-needle aspiration biopsy uses a thin needle guided by ultrasound to the mass. In a method called stereotactic needle biopsy, a computer maps the exact location of the mass using mammograms taken from two angles, and the map is used to guide the needle.

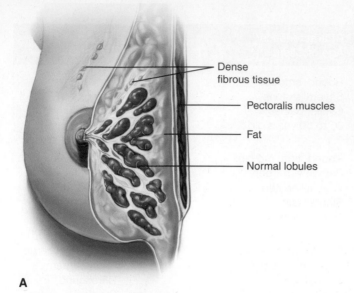

A

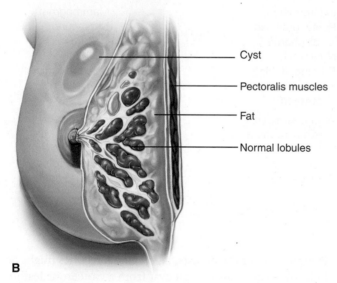

B

FIGURE 6.1 (**A**) Fibrocystic breast changes. (**B**) Cysts. (Source: The Anatomical Chart Company. [2002]. *Atlas of pathophysiology.* Springhouse, PA: Springhouse Corporation.)

Nursing Management

A nurse caring for a woman with fibrocystic breast changes can teach her about the condition, provide tips for self-care (Teaching Guidelines 6.1), suggest lifestyle changes, and demonstrate how to perform monthly breast self-examination after her menses to monitor the changes. Nursing Care Plan 6.1 presents a plan of care for a woman with fibrocystic breast changes.

▶ FIBROADENOMAS

Fibroadenomas are common benign solid breast tumors that occur in about 10% of all women and account for up

TEACHING GUIDELINES 6.1

Relieving Symptoms of Fibrocystic Breast Changes

- Wear an extra-supportive bra to prevent undue strain on the ligaments of the breasts to reduce discomfort.
- Avoid caffeine, which is a stimulant. This reduces discomfort for some women.
- Take oral contraceptives, as recommended by a health care practitioner, to stabilize the monthly hormonal levels.
- Eat a low-fat diet rich in fruits, vegetables, and grains to maintain a healthy nutritional lifestyle and ideal weight.
- Apply heat to the breasts to help reduce pain via vasodilation of vessels.
- Take diuretics, as recommended by a health care practitioner, to counteract fluid retention and swelling of the breasts.
- Reduce salt intake to reduce fluid retention and swelling in the breasts.
- Take OTC medications, such as aspirin or ibuprofen (Motrin, Advil, Nuprin), to reduce inflammation and discomfort.
- Use thiamine and vitamin E therapy. This has been found helpful for some women, but research has failed to demonstrate a direct benefit from either therapy.
- Take medications as prescribed (e.g., bromocriptine, tamoxifen, or danazol).
- Discuss the possibility of aspiration or surgical removal of breast lumps with a health care practitioner.

to half of all breast biopsies. They are the most common mass in women (Harris, 2007). They are considered hyperplastic lesions associated with an aberration of normal development and involution rather than a neoplasm. Fibroadenomas can be stimulated by external estrogen, progesterone, lactation, and pregnancy (Sukumvanich & Borgen, 2007). They are composed of both fibrous and glandular tissue and usually occur in women between 20 and 40 years of age (Alexander et al., 2007). Giant fibroadenomas account for approximately 10% of cases. These masses are frequently larger than 5 cm and occur most often in pregnant or lactating women. These large lesions may regress in size once hormonal stimulation subsides (Hackley, Kriebs, & Rousseau, 2007). Fibroadenomas are rarely associated with cancer.

Therapeutic Management

Treatment may include a period of "watchful waiting" because many fibroadenomas stop growing or shrink on their own without any treatment. Other growths may need to be

Nursing Care Plan 6.1

OVERVIEW OF THE WOMAN WITH FIBROCYSTIC BREAST CHANGES

Sheree Rollins is a 37-year-old woman who comes to the clinic for her routine check-up. During the examination, she says, "Sometimes my breasts feel so heavy and they ache a lot. I noticed a couple of lumpy areas in my breast last week just before I got my period. Is this normal? Now they feel like they're almost gone. Should I be worried?" Clinical breast examination reveals two small (pea-sized), mobile, slightly tender nodules in each breast bilaterally. No skin retraction noted. Previous mammogram revealed fibrocystic breast changes.

NURSING DIAGNOSIS: Pain related to changes in breast tissue

Outcome Identification and Evaluation
Client will demonstrate a decrease in breast pain as evidenced by a pain rating of 1 or 2 on a pain rating scale of 0 to 10 and statements that pain is lessened.

Interventions: Relieving Pain
- Ask client to rate her pain using a numeric pain rating scale *to establish a baseline.*
- Discuss with client any measures used to relieve pain *to determine effectiveness of the measures.*
- Encourage use of a supportive bra *to aid in reducing discomfort.*
- Instruct client in use of over-the-counter analgesics *to promote pain relief.*
- Advise the client to apply warm compresses or allow warm water from the shower to flow over her breasts *to promote vasodilation and subsequent pain relief.*
- Tell client to reduce her intake of salt to reduce risk of fluid retention and swelling leading *to increased pain.*

NURSING DIAGNOSIS: Deficient knowledge related to fibrocystic breast changes and appropriate care measures

Outcome Identification and Evaluation
Client will verbalize understanding of condition as evidenced by statements about the cause of breast changes and appropriate choices for lifestyle changes, and demonstration of self-care measures.

Interventions: Providing Patient Education
- Assess client's knowledge of fibrocystic breast changes *to establish a baseline for teaching.*
- Explain the role of monthly hormonal level changes and describe the signs and symptoms *to promote understanding of this condition.*
- Teach the client how to perform breast self-examination after her menstrual period *to monitor for changes.*
- Encourage client to report any changes promptly *to ensure early detection of problems.*
- Suggest client speak with her primary care provider about the use of oral contraceptives *to help stabilize monthly hormonal levels.*
- Review lifestyle choices, such as avoiding caffeine, eating a low-fat diet rich in fruits, vegetables, and grains, and adhering to screening recommendations *to promote health.*
- Discuss measures for pain relief *to minimize discomfort associated with breast changes.*

---

surgically removed if they do not regress or if they remain unchanged. Cryoablation, an alternative to surgery, can also be used to remove a tumor. In this procedure, extremely cold gas is piped into the tumor using ultrasound guidance. The tumor freezes and dies. The current trend is toward a more conservative approach to treatment after careful evaluation and continued monitoring.

Nursing Assessment

Ask the woman about clinical manifestations of fibroadenomas. These lumps are felt as firm, rubbery, well-circumscribed, freely mobile nodules that might or might not be tender when palpated.

Breast fibroadenomas are usually detected incidentally during clinical or self-examinations and are usually located in the upper outer quadrant of the breast; more than one may be present (Fig. 6.2). Several other breast lesions have similar characteristics, so every woman with a breast mass should be evaluated to exclude cancer. A clinical breast examination by a health care professional is critical. In addition, diagnostic studies include imaging studies (mammography, ultrasound, or both) and some form of biopsy, most often a fine-needle aspiration, core needle biopsy, or stereotactic needle biopsy. The core needle biopsy removes a small cylinder of tissue from the breast mass, more than the fine-needle aspiration biopsy.

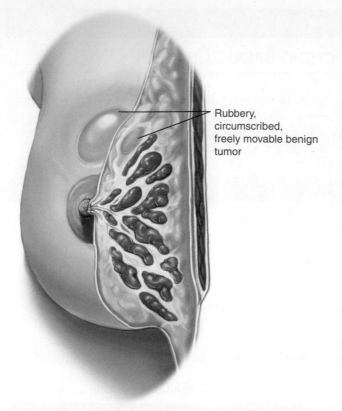

Rubbery, circumscribed, freely movable benign tumor

FIGURE 6.2 Fibroadenoma. (Source: The Anatomical Chart Company. [2002]. *Atlas of pathophysiology*. Springhouse, PA: Springhouse Corporation.)

If additional tissue needs to be evaluated, the advanced breast biopsy instrument (ABBI) is used. This instrument removes a larger cylinder of tissue for examination by using a rotating circular knife. The ABBI procedure removes more tissue than any of the other methods except a surgical biopsy (ACS, 2007b).

Nursing Management

The nurse should urge the client to return for re-evaluation in 6 months, perform monthly breast self-examinations, and return annually for a clinical breast examination.

▶ INTRADUCTAL PAPILLOMA

An **intraductal papilloma** is a benign, wart-like growth found in the mammary ducts, usually near the nipple. This benign growth is thought to be caused by a proliferation and overgrowth of ductal epithelial tissue. An intraductal papilloma is generally less than 1 cm in diameter and might not be palpable. It produces a spontaneous serous, serosanguineous, or watery nipple discharge (Graham, 2006). It mostly affects women between the ages of 40

and 60. A single duct or several ducts may be involved. Women with solitary papilloma without atypia carry a minimal increase of developing breast cancer over the general population. These women are not classified as high risk. However, the risk of subsequent breast cancer is increased by four- to fivefold in the presence of atypia (Sukumvanich & Borgen, 2007).

Therapeutic Management

Treatment consists of surgical removal of the papilloma and a part of the duct it is found in, usually through an incision at the edge of the areola. The excised papilloma and duct are sent to the pathology laboratory to rule out cancer (ACS, 2007a).

Nursing Assessment

The woman might report a feeling of fullness in the breast and may state that she can manually express a serous, serosanguineous, or watery discharge from the nipple. If the papilloma is large enough, it can be palpated in the nipple area as a soft, nontender, mobile, poorly delineated mass.

Laboratory and diagnostic testing is important to rule out cancer. The nipple discharge is evaluated for the presence of occult blood using a Hemoccult card; a blue coloration on the card indicates the presence of blood. In addition, a sample of the discharge may be sent for cytologic evaluation to screen for cancer cells. Mammography, ultrasound, or ductography (radiographic dye is instilled into a duct; it outlines the breast ductal system on radiographs) is used to diagnose or differentiate this lesion from a cancerous one. An intraductal papilloma appears as a smooth, lobulated filling defect or a solitary obstructed duct on ductography (Aliotta & Schaeffer, 2006).

Nursing Management

The nurse should advise the woman to continue monthly breast self-examinations and yearly clinical breast examinations.

▶ DUCT ECTASIA

Duct ectasia is a dilation and inflammation of the ducts behind the nipple. It is most common in perimenopausal women. This benign condition frequently occurs in women who have breastfed their children. The cause is unclear; however, chronic periductal inflammation, fibrosis, and ductal dilatation are associated factors. This condition results in noncyclic breast pain, nipple retraction, and discharge (Hackley, Kriebs, & Rousseau, 2007).

Therapeutic Management

This condition frequently improves without any specific treatment, or with warm compresses and antibiotics. If symptoms persist, the abnormal duct is removed through a local incision at the border of the areola. The tissue is sent to the pathology laboratory for evaluation.

Nursing Assessment

Assess the patient for clinical manifestations of duct ectasia. If the ducts have been chronically infected, an erythematous lesion will be present at the edge of the nipple area (ACS, 2007a). The woman may complain of nipple discharge, which can be green, brown, straw-colored, reddish, gray, or cream-colored, with the consistency of toothpaste. In addition, the woman may report a dull nipple pain, subareolar swelling, or a burning sensation accompanied by pruritus around the nipple (Richards et al., 2007).

Physical examination of the breasts might reveal subareolar redness and swelling, with mild to moderate tenderness on palpation. In addition, palpation will reveal the presence of tortuous tubular swellings beneath the areola, along with nipple retraction and dimpling in some postmenopausal women (Graham, 2006). Diagnostic and laboratory testing includes mammography, ultrasound, and cytology and testing for occult blood on a nipple discharge sample, and ductography may be used to assist in the diagnosis of this lesion.

Nursing Management

The nurse should reassure the woman that this condition is benign and should reinforce the importance of monthly self-examinations as well as annual clinical breast examinations by the woman's health care provider. This benign breast condition is typically self-limiting; the only intervention needed is reassurance.

▶ MASTITIS

Mastitis is an infection of the connective tissue in the breast that occurs primarily in lactating or engorged women. Mastitis is divided into lactational or nonlactational. The usual causative organisms for lactational mastitis are *Staphylococcus aureus, Haemophilus influenzae,* and *Haemophilus* and *Streptococcus* species, the source of which is the baby's flora. One or more of the ducts drain poorly or become blocked, resulting in bacterial growth in the retained milk (Sukumvanich & Borgen, 2007).

Nonlactational mastitis can be caused by duct ectasia, which occurs when the milk ducts become congested with secretions and debris, resulting in periductal inflammation. These women present with greenish nipple discharge, nipple retraction, and noncyclic pain.

Therapeutic Management

Management of both types of mastitis involves the use of oral antibiotics (usually a penicillinase-resistant penicillin or cephalosporin) and acetaminophen (Tylenol) for pain and fever.

Nursing Assessment

Assess the patient's health history for risk factors for mastitis, which include poor handwashing, ductal abnormalities, nipple cracks and fissures, lowered maternal defenses due to fatigue, tight clothing, poor support of pendulous breasts, failure to empty the breasts properly while breastfeeding, or missing breastfeedings.

Assess the patient for clinical manifestations of mastitis, which include flu-like symptoms of malaise, leukocytosis, fever, and chills. Physical examination of the breasts reveals increased warmth, redness, tenderness, and swelling. The nipple is usually cracked or abraded and the breast is distended with milk (Fig. 6.3). The diagnosis is made based on history and examination.

Nursing Management

Teach the woman about the etiology of mastitis and encourage her to continue to breastfeed, emphasizing that the prescribed medication is safe to take during lactation. Continued emptying of the breast or pumping improves the outcome, decreases the duration of symptoms, and decreases the incidence of breast abscess. Thus, continued breastfeeding is recommended in the presence of mastitis (Reddy et al., 2007). Instructions for the woman with mastitis are detailed in Teaching Guidelines 6.2.

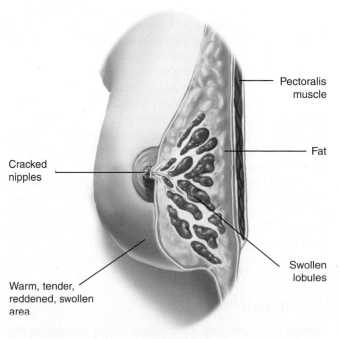

FIGURE 6.3 Mastitis.

TEACHING GUIDELINES 6.2

Caring for Mastitis

• Take medications as prescribed.
• Continue breastfeeding, as tolerated.
• Wear a supportive bra 24 hours a day to support the breasts.
• Increase fluid intake.
• Make sure infant is positioned correctly on the nipple.
• Practice good handwashing techniques.
• Apply warm compresses to the affected breast or take a warm shower before breastfeeding.
• Frequently change positions while nursing.
• Get adequate rest and nutrition to support or improve the immune system.

Sources: ACS, 2007a; Blackburn, 2007; Eglash, Plane, & Mundt, 2006.

Malignant Breast Disorders

Breast cancer is a neoplastic disease in which normal body cells are transformed into malignant ones (Opatt & Chung, 2007). It is the most common cancer in women and the second leading cause of cancer deaths (lung cancer is first) among American women. Breast cancer accounts for one of every three cancers diagnosed in the United States (ACS, 2007c). A new case is discovered every 2 minutes. It is estimated that one out of every seven women will develop the disease at some time during her life, and the mortality rate of those with breast cancer is 1 in 30 (National Cancer Institute [NCI], 2007b).

Over 200,000 cases of invasive breast cancer are diagnosed in the United States each year (ACS, 2007c). Breast cancer can also affect men, but only 1% of all individuals diagnosed with breast cancer annually are men (ACS, 2007). Because men are not routinely screened for breast cancer, the diagnosis is often delayed. The most common clinical manifestation of male breast cancer is a painless, firm, subareolar breast mass. Any suspicious breast mass in a male should undergo diagnostic biopsy. If a malignancy is diagnosed, typical treatment is mastectomy with assessment of the axillary nodes.

The cause of breast cancer, while not well understood, is thought to be a complex interaction between environment, genetic, and hormonal factors. Breast cancer is a progressive rather than a systemic disease, meaning that most cancers grow from small size with low metastatic potential to larger size and greater metastatic potential (Opatt & Chung, 2007).

Pathophysiology

Cancer is not just one disease, but rather a group of diseases that result from unregulated cell growth. Without regulation, cells divide and grow uncontrollably until they eventually form a tumor. Extensive research has determined that all cancer is the result of changes in DNA or chromosome structure that cause the mutation of specific genes. Most genetic mutations that cause cancer are acquired sporadically, which means they occur by chance and are not necessarily due to inherited mutations (Law & Alcamo, 2007). Cancer development is thought to be clonal in nature, which means that each cell is derived from another cell. If one cell develops a mutation, any daughter cell derived from that cell will have that same mutation, and this process continues until a malignant tumor forms.

Breast cancer starts in the epithelial cells that line the mammary ducts within the breast. The growth rate depends on hormonal influences, mainly estrogen and progesterone. The two major categories of breast cancer are noninvasive and invasive. Noninvasive, or in situ, breast cancers are those that have not extended beyond their duct, lobule, or point of origin into the surrounding breast tissue. Conversely, invasive, or infiltrating, breast cancers have extended into the surrounding breast tissue, with the potential to metastasize. Many researchers believe that most invasive cancers probably originate as noninvasive cancers (Underwood, 2006).

By far the most common breast cancer is invasive ductal carcinoma, which represents 85% of all cases (ACS, 2007f). **Carcinoma** is a malignant tumor that occurs in epithelial tissue; it tends to infiltrate and give rise to metastases. The incidence of this cancer peaks in the sixth decade of life (>60 years old). It spreads rapidly to axillary and other lymph nodes, even while small. Infiltrating ductal carcinoma may take various histologic forms—well differentiated and slow-growing, poorly differentiated and infiltrating, or highly malignant and undifferentiated with numerous metastases. This common type of breast cancer starts in the ducts, breaks through the duct wall, and invades the fatty breast tissue (Aliotta & Schaeffer, 2006).

Invasive lobular carcinomas, which originate in the terminal lobular units of breast ducts, account for 10% to 15% of all cases of breast cancer. The tumor is frequently located in the upper outer quadrant of the breast, and by the time it is discovered the prognosis is usually poor (Underwood, 2006). Other invasive types of cancer include tubular carcinoma (29%), which is fairly uncommon and typically occurs in women aged 55 and older. Colloid carcinoma (2% to 4%) occurs in women 60 to 70 years of age and is characterized by the presence of large pools of mucus interspersed with small islands of tumor cells. Medullary carcinoma accounts for 5% to 7% of malignant breast tumors; it occurs frequently in younger women (<50 years of age) and grows into large tumor masses. Inflammatory breast cancer (<4%) often presents with skin edema, redness, and warmth and is associated with a poor prognosis. Paget's disease (2% to 4%) originates in the nipple and typically occurs with invasive ductal carcinoma (Sukumvanich & Borgen, 2007).

Breast cancer is considered to be a highly variable disease. While the process of metastasis is a complex and poorly understood phenomenon, there is evidence to suggest that new vascularization of the tumor plays an important role in the biological aggressiveness of breast cancer (Hackley, Kriebs, & Rousseau 2007). Breast cancer metastasizes widely and to almost all organs of the body, but primarily to the bone, lungs, lymph nodes, liver, and brain. The first sites of metastases are usually local or regional, involving the chest wall or axillary supraclavicular lymph nodes or bone (ACS, 2007f).

Breast cancers are classified into three stages based on:

1. Tumor size
2. Extent of lymph node involvement
3. Evidence of metastasis

The purposes of tumor staging are to determine the probability the tumor has metastasized, to decide on an appropriate course of therapy, and to assess the client's prognosis. Table 6.2 gives details and characteristics of each stage. The overall 10-year survival rate for a woman with stage I breast cancer is 80% to 90%; for a woman with stage II, it is about 50%. The outlook is not as good for women with stage III or IV disease (Alexander et al., 2007).

There is no completely accurate way to know whether the cancer has micrometastasized to distant organs, but certain tests can help determine if the cancer has spread. A bone scan can be performed to assess the bones. Magnetic resonance imaging (MRI) can be used to detect metastases to the liver, abdominal cavity, lungs, or brain.

Risk Factors

An estimated 80% of women in whom breast cancer develops have no documented risk factors (Sukumvanich & Borgen, 2007). Breast cancer is thought to develop in response to a number of related factors: aging, delayed childbearing or never bearing children, high breast density, family history of cancer, late menopause, and hormonal factors (ACS, 2007e). Other factors might contribute to breast cancer but have not been scientifically proven.

In 1970, the lifetime risk for developing breast cancer was one in ten; since then, the risk has gradually risen (NCI, 2007b). This slight increase in incidence might be explained in a variety of ways—better detection and screening tools are available, which have identified more cases; women are living to an older age, when their risk increases; and lifestyle changes in American women (having their first pregnancy at an older age, having fewer children, and using hormonal therapy to treat the symptoms of menopause) might have produced the higher numbers. Age is a significant risk factor. Because rates of breast cancer increase with age, estimates of risk at specific ages are more meaningful than estimates of lifetime risk. The estimated chances of a woman being diagnosed with breast cancer between the ages of 30 and 70 are detailed in Table 6.3.

Risk factors for breast cancer can be divided into those that cannot be changed (nonmodifiable risk factors) and those that can be changed (modifiable risk factors). Nonmodifiable risk factors (ACS, 2007e) are:

- Gender (female)
- Aging (>50 years old)
- Genetic mutations (BRCA-1 and BRCA-2 genes)
- Personal history of ovarian or colon cancer
- Increased breast density
- Family history of breast cancer (mother, sister, daughter, grandmother, or aunt)
- Personal history of breast cancer (three- to fourfold increase in risk for recurrence)
- Race (higher in Caucasian women, but African-American women are more likely to die of it)
- Previous abnormal breast biopsy (atypical hyperplasia)
- Exposure to chest radiation (radiation damages DNA)
- Previous breast radiation (12 times normal risk)
- Early menarche (<12 years old) or late onset of menopause (>55 years old), which represents increased estrogen exposure over the lifetime

Modifiable risk factors related to lifestyle choices (ACS, 2007e) include:

- Not having children at all or not having children until after age 30—this increases the risk of breast cancer by not reducing the number of menstrual cycles
- Postmenopausal use of estrogens and progestins— the Women's Health Initiative study (2002) reported increased risks with long-term (>5 years) use of hormone replacement therapy

TABLE 6.2 STAGING OF BREAST CANCER

Stage	Characteristics
0	In situ, early type of breast cancer
I	Localized tumor <1 inch in diameter
II	Tumor 1–2 inches in diameter; spread to axillary lymph nodes
III	Tumor 2 inches or larger; spread to other lymph nodes and tissues
IV	Cancer has metastasized to other body organs

Source: ACS, 2007c.

TABLE 6.3 ESTIMATED RISK OF BREAST CANCER AT SPECIFIC AGES

Age 30 to 40	1 out of 262
Age 40 to 50	1 out of 68
Age 50 to 60	1 out of 35
Age 60 to 70	1 out of 27

Modified from National Cancer Institute (NCI). (2007). Probability of breast cancer in American women. Available at: http://cis.nci.nih.gov/fact/5_6.htm

- Failing to breastfeed for up to a year after pregnancy—increases the risk of breast cancer because it does not reduce the total number of lifetime menstrual cycles
- Alcohol consumption—boosts the level of estrogen in the bloodstream
- Smoking—exposure to carcinogenic agents found in cigarettes
- Obesity and consumption of high-fat diet—fat cells produce and store estrogen, so more fat cells create higher estrogen levels
- Sedentary lifestyle and lack of physical exercise—increases body fat, which houses estrogen

The presence of risk factors, especially several of them, calls for careful ongoing monitoring and evaluation to promote early detection. Even though risk factors are important considerations, many women with newly diagnosed breast cancer have no known risk factors. While routine mammography and self-examination are prudent for everyone, these precautions may become lifesavers for at-risk individuals.

Diagnosis

There are many studies performed to make an accurate diagnosis of a malignant breast lump. Diagnostic tests may include:

- Diagnostic mammography
- Magnetic resonance mammography (MRM)
- Fine-needle aspiration
- Stereotactic needle-guided biopsy
- Sentinel lymph node biopsy
- Hormone receptor status
- DNA ploidy status
- Cell proliferative indices
- HER-2/neu genetic marker (Opatt & Chung, 2007)

Mammography

Mammography involves taking x-ray pictures of the bare breasts while they are compressed between two plastic plates. This procedure is performed to identify and characterize a breast mass and to detect an early malignancy.

EVIDENCE-BASED PRACTICE 6.1
Can a Low-Fat Diet Reduce Breast Cancer Risk in Postmenopausal Women?

The hypothesis that a low-fat diet can reduce breast cancer risk has existed for decades but has never been tested in a controlled intervention trial.

● Study
To assess the effects of a low-fat diet on breast cancer incidence, a randomized, controlled, primary prevention trial was conducted at 40 U.S. clinical centers from 1993 to 2005. A total of 48,835 postmenopausal women, aged 50 to 79 years, without prior breast cancer, including 18.6% of minority race/ethnicity, were enrolled. Women were randomly assigned to the dietary modification intervention group (40% [n = 19,541]) or the comparison group (60% [n = 29,294]). The intervention was designed to promote dietary change with the goals of reducing intake of total fat to 20% of energy and increasing consumption of vegetables and fruit to at least five servings daily and grains to at least six servings daily. Comparison group participants were not asked to make dietary changes.

Dietary fat intake was significantly lower in the dietary modification intervention group compared with the comparison group. Vegetable and fruit consumption was higher in the intervention group by at least one serving per day and a smaller, more transient difference was found for grain consumption.

▲ Findings
The number of women who developed invasive breast cancer (annualized incidence rate) over the 8-year average follow-up period was 655 (0.42%) in the intervention group and 1,072 (0.45%) in the comparison group (hazard ratio, 0.91; 95% confidence interval, 0.83–1.01 for the comparison between the two groups). Secondary analyses suggested a lower hazard ratio among adherent women, provided greater evidence of risk reduction among women who ate a high-fat diet at baseline, and suggested a dietary effect that varies by hormone receptor characteristics of the tumor. Among postmenopausal women, a low-fat diet did not result in a statistically significant reduction in invasive breast cancer risk over an 8-year average follow-up period.

■ Nursing Implications
Although the results didn't confirm that eating a low-fat diet reduces the risk of breast cancer, nurses need to counsel their patients about the other benefits derived from a low-fat diet: weight loss, lower cholesterol levels, and decreased risk for cardiovascular disease. These additional benefits should be emphasized as part of an overall healthy lifestyle.

Source: Prentice RL, Caan B, Chlebowski RT, et al. (2006). Low-fat dietary pattern and risk of invasive breast cancer: The Women's Health Initiative Randomized Controlled Dietary Modification Trial. *JAMA, 295*(6), 629–642.

A screening mammogram typically consists of four views, two per breast (Fig. 6.4). It can detect lesions as small as 0.5 cm (the average size of a tumor detected by a woman practicing occasional breast self-examination is approximately 2.5 cm) (Kubota et al., 2007). A diagnostic mammogram is performed when the woman has suspicious clinical findings on a breast examination or an abnormality has been found on a screening mammogram. A diagnostic mammogram uses additional views of the affected breast as well as magnification views. Diagnostic mammography provides the radiologist with additional detail to render a more specific diagnosis. A digital mammography, which records images in computer code instead of on x-ray film, can also be used so that images can be transmitted and easily stored.

Most women find the 10-minute mammography procedure uncomfortable but not painful. Teaching Guidelines 6.3 offers tips for a patient to follow before she undergoes this procedure.

Magnetic Resonance Mammography

MRM is a relatively new procedure that might allow for earlier detection because it can detect smaller lesions and provide finer detail. MRM is a highly accurate (>90%

TEACHING GUIDELINES 6.3

Preparing for a Screening Mammogram

- Schedule the procedure just after menses, when breasts are less tender.
- Don't use deodorant or powder the day of the procedure, because they can appear on the x-ray film as calcium spots.
- Acetaminophen (Tylenol) or aspirin can relieve any discomfort after the procedure.
- Remove all jewelry from around your neck, because the metal can cause distortions on the film image.
- Select a facility that is accredited by the American College of Radiology (ACR) to ensure appropriate credentialed staff.

sensitivity for invasive carcinoma) but costly tool. Contrast infusion is used to evaluate the rate at which the dye initially enters the breast tissue. The basis of the high sensitivity of MRM is the tumor angiogenesis (vessel growth) that accompanies a majority of breast cancers, even early ones. Malignant lesions tend to exhibit increased enhancement within the first 2 minutes (Preda et al., 2006). Currently MRM is used only as a complement to mammography and clinical breast examination because it is expensive, but it may move into the diagnostic arena in the near future (Smith, 2007).

Fine-Needle Aspiration

Fine-needle aspiration (FNA) is done to identify a solid tumor, cyst, or malignancy. It is a simple office procedure that can be performed with or without anesthesia. A small (20- to 22-gauge) needle connected to a 10-cc or larger syringe is inserted into the breast mass and suction is applied to withdraw the contents. The aspirate is then sent to the cytology laboratory to be evaluated for abnormal cells.

Stereotactic Needle–Guided Biopsy

This diagnostic tool is used to target and identify mammographically detected nonpalpable lesions in the breast. This procedure is less expensive than an excisional biopsy. The procedure takes place in a specially equipped room and generally takes about an hour. When proper placement of the breast mass is confirmed by digital mammograms, the breast is locally anesthetized and a spring-loaded biopsy gun is used to obtain two or three core biopsy tissue samples. After the procedure is finished, the biopsy area is cleaned and a sterile dressing is applied.

Sentinel Lymph Node Biopsy

The status of the axillary lymph nodes is an important prognostic indicator in early-stage breast cancer. The pres-

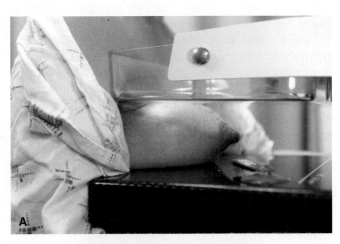

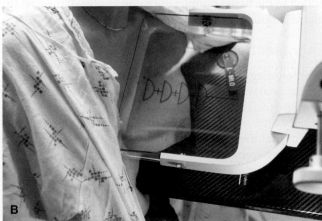

FIGURE 6.4 Mammography. (**A**) A top-to-bottom view of the breast. (**B**) A side view of the breast.

ence or absence of malignant cells in lymph nodes is highly significant: the more lymph nodes involved and the more aggressive the cancer, the more powerful chemotherapy will have to be, both in terms of the toxicity of drugs and the duration of treatment (Teal, Tabbara, & Kelly, 2007). With a sentinel lymph node biopsy, the clinician can determine whether breast cancer has spread to the axillary lymph nodes without having to do a traditional axillary lymph node dissection. Experience has shown that the lymph ducts of the breast typically drain to one lymph node first before draining through the rest of the lymph nodes under the arm. The first lymph node is called the sentinel lymph node.

This procedure can be performed under local anesthesia. A radioactive blue dye is injected 2 hours before the biopsy to identify the afferent sentinel lymph node. The surgeon usually removes one to three nodes and sends them to the pathologist to determine whether cancer cells are present. The sentinel lymph node biopsy is usually performed before a lumpectomy to make sure the cancer has not spread. Removing only the sentinel lymph node can allow women with breast cancer to avoid many of the side effects (lymphedema) associated with a traditional axillary lymph node dissection (Underwood, 2006).

Hormone Receptor Status

Normal breast epithelium has hormone receptors and responds specifically to the stimulatory effects of estrogen and progesterone. Most breast cancers retain estrogen receptors, and for those tumors estrogen will retain proliferative control over the malignant cells. It is therefore useful to know the hormone receptor status of the cancer to predict which women will respond to hormone manipulation. Hormone receptor status reveals whether the tumor is stimulated to grow by estrogen and progesterone. Tumors that have estrogen receptors are said to be "ER positive" (ER+) and tumors that do not have estrogen receptors are "ER negative" (ER–). The same terminology applies to progesterone (PR+ or PR–). ER+ and PR+ tumors have a better than 75% response to endocrine therapy in comparison to tumors that are ER+ and PR–, whose response rate is under 35%. Postmenopausal women tend to be ER+; premenopausal women tend to be ER– (Opatt & Chung, 2007). To determine hormone receptor status, a sample of breast cancer tissue obtained during a biopsy or a tumor removed surgically during a lumpectomy or mastectomy is examined by a cytologist.

DNA Ploidy Status

DNA ploidy status, which correlates with tumor aggressiveness, indicates the amount of DNA in cancer cells. Cancer cells that have the correct amount of DNA (diploid) in contrast with too much or too little DNA (aneuploid) tend not to spread. An aneuploid DNA pattern denotes a greater tendency to metastasize than a diploid one (Sukumvanich & Borgen, 2007). A sample of breast cancer tissue obtained during a biopsy or a tumor removed

surgically during a lumpectomy or mastectomy is examined for abnormal amounts of DNA. Using flow cytometry (process of counting and measuring cells), it is possible to measure the DNA content and proliferative activity of a tumor. The number of chromosome sets in the nucleus indicates the speed of cell replication and tumor growth; a high number predicts a poor outcome.

Cell Proliferative Indices

Research indicates that cell proliferation potential may have prognostic significance. Cell proliferative indices indirectly measure the rate of cell division, which is an indication of how fast the cancer is growing. Flow and image cytometry techniques are used to measure the tumor's cell cycle rate. The percentage of tumor cells in S phase (synthesis stage of cell division) of the cell cycle is assessed. S-phase percentages below 10% are considered low, and the tumor has less of a chance of spreading than one with a higher percentage. A tumor with high proliferative activity has a more aggressive metastatic potential (ACS, 2007f).

HER-2/neu Genetic Marker

Molecular and biologic factors are increasingly being used as indicators for prognosis and treatment. HER-2 is a human epidermal growth factor receptor whose biological function is associated with cell growth, resulting in loss of cell regulation and uncontrolled cell proliferation.

HER-2/neu oncoprotein is a protein that is significant, especially in large tumors. Overexpression of this protein results from an acquired genetic mutation and occurs in approximately 30% of women with metastatic breast cancer. Women whose tumors have high levels of HER-2/neu oncoprotein have a poor prognosis: they have rapid tumor progression, an increased rate of recurrence, a poor response to standard therapies, and a lower survival rate (Chernecky & Berger, 2007). The presence or absence of this oncoprotein helps determine which chemotherapy treatment will be most effective. A breast tissue sample is obtained by a fine-needle or open biopsy and treated with a material that binds to HER-2/neu oncoprotein. A dye is added to the tissue sample: the more uptake of the dye, the higher amount present (Chernecky & Berger, 2007).

Therapeutic Management

Women diagnosed with breast cancer have many treatments available to them. Generally, treatments fall into two categories: local and systemic. Local treatments are surgery and radiation therapy. Effective systemic treatments include chemotherapy, hormonal therapy, and immunotherapy.

Treatment plans are based on multiple factors, primarily on whether the cancer is invasive or noninvasive, the tumor's size and grade, the number of cancerous axillary lymph nodes, the hormone receptor status, and the ability to obtain clear surgical margins (ACS, 2007f). A combination of surgical options and adjunctive therapy is often recommended.

Another consideration in making decisions about a treatment plan is genetic testing for BRCA-1 and BRCA-2. This genetic testing became available in 1995 and can pinpoint women who have a significantly increased risk for breast and ovarian cancer: individuals with BRCA-1 and BRCA-2 mutations have a 75% lifetime risk of breast cancer and a 30% lifetime risk of ovarian cancer. Most cases of breast and ovarian cancer are sporadic in nature, but approximately 7% of breast cancers and 10% of ovarian cancers are thought to result from genetic inheritance (Kell & Burke, 2007).

Testing positive for a BRCA-1 or BRCA-2 mutation can significantly alter health care decisions. In some cases, before genetic testing was available, lumpectomy with radiation or mastectomy was the treatment most often recommended. However, if the woman is found to have a BRCA-1 mutation, she is most likely to be offered the option of contralateral prophylactic mastectomy and possible bilateral oophorectomy (Kell & Burke, 2007).

Severe psychological distress can occur as a result of genetic testing. Also, many women perceive their breasts as intrinsic to their femininity, self-esteem, and sexuality, and the risk of losing a breast can provoke extreme anxiety (Alexander et al., 2007). Nurses need to address the physical, emotional, and spiritual needs of the women they care for, as well as their families, since this mutation is inherited in an autosomal dominant fashion. Based on Mendelian genetics, first-degree relatives of affected women have a 50% risk of having inherited the mutation (Kell & Burke, 2007).

Surgical Options

Generally, the first treatment option for the woman diagnosed with breast cancer is surgery. A few women with tumors larger than 5 cm or inflammatory breast cancer may undergo neoadjuvant chemotherapy or radiotherapy to shrink the tumor before surgical removal is attempted (Opatt & Chung, 2007). The surgical options depend on the type and extent of cancer. The choices are typically either breast-conserving surgery (lumpectomy with radiation) or mastectomy with or without reconstruction. The overall survival rate with lumpectomy and radiation is about the same as that with modified radical mastectomy (ACS, 2007f). Research has shown that the survival rates in women who have had mastectomies versus those who have undergone breast-conserving surgery followed by radiation are the same. However, lumpectomy may not be an option for some women, including those:

- Who have two or more cancer sites that cannot be removed through one incision
- Whose surgery will not result in a clean margin of tissue
- Who have active connective tissue conditions (lupus or scleroderma) that make body tissues especially sensitive to the side effects of radiation
- Who have had previous radiation to the affected breast
- Whose tumors are larger than 5 cm (2 inches)
(National Comprehensive Cancer Network, 2007)

These decisions are made jointly between the woman and her surgeon. If mastectomy is chosen, either by tumor characteristics or patient preference, then discussion needs to include breast reconstruction and regional lymph node biopsy versus sentinel lymph node biopsy. The mastectomy techniques are a simple mastectomy with sentinel node biopsy or a radical mastectomy with regional node biopsy. Removal of numerous lymph nodes places the patient at high risk for lymphedema.

Breast-Conserving Surgery

Breast-conserving surgery, the least invasive procedure, is the wide local excision (or lumpectomy) of the tumor along with a 1-cm margin of normal tissue. A lumpectomy is often used for early-stage localized tumors. The goal of breast-conserving surgery is to remove the suspicious mass along with tissue free of malignant cells to prevent recurrence. The results are less drastic and emotionally less scarring to the woman. Women undergoing breast-conserving therapy receive radiation after lumpectomy with the goal of eradicating residual microscopic cancer cells to limit locoregional recurrence. In women who do not require adjuvant chemotherapy, radiation therapy typically begins 2 to 4 weeks after surgery to allow healing of the lumpectomy incision site. Radiation is administered to the entire breast at daily doses over a period of several weeks (Rao et al., 2007).

A sentinel lymph node biopsy may also be performed since the lymph nodes draining the breast are located primarily in the axilla. Theoretically, if breast cancer is to metastasize to other parts of the body, it will probably do so via the lymphatic system. If malignant cells are found in the nodes, more aggressive systemic treatment may be needed.

Mastectomy

A **simple mastectomy** is the removal of all breast tissue, the nipple, and the areola. The axillary nodes and pectoral muscles are spared. This procedure would be used for a large tumor or multiple tumors that have not metastasized to adjacent structures or the lymph system.

A **modified radical mastectomy** is another surgical option; survival rates are comparable to those of radical mastectomy, but it is more conducive to breast reconstruction and results in greater mobility and less lymphedema (Alexander et al., 2007). This procedure involves removal of breast tissue, the axillary nodes, and some chest muscles, but not the pectoralis major, thus avoiding a concave anterior chest (DiSaia & Creasman, 2007).

In conjunction with the mastectomy, lymph node surgery (removal of underarm nodes) may need to be done to reduce the risk of distant metastasis and improve a woman's chance of long-term survival. For women with a positive sentinel node biopsy, 10 to 20 underarm lymph nodes may need to be removed. Complications associated with axillary lymph node surgery include nerve damage during surgery, causing temporary numbness down the upper aspect of the arm; seroma formation followed by wound infection; restrictions in arm mobility (some women need physiotherapy); and lymphedema. In many women lymphedema can be avoided by:

- Avoiding using the affected arm for drawing blood, inserting intravenous lines, or measuring blood pressure (can cause trauma and possible infection)
- Seeking medical care immediately if the affected arm swells
- Wearing gloves when engaging in activities such as gardening that might cause injury
- Wearing a well-fitted compression sleeve to promote drainage return

Women having mastectomies must decide whether to have further surgery to reconstruct the breast. If the woman decides to have reconstructive surgery, it ideally is performed immediately after the mastectomy. The woman must also determine whether she wants the surgeon to use saline implants or natural tissue from her abdomen (TRAM flap method) or back (LAT flap method).

In the transverse rectus abdominis myocutaneous (TRAM) flap method, the rectus abdominis muscle is transferred from the abdomen via a tunnel under the skin and brought out through a new excision in the breast area. The blood supply is maintained. This tissue is used to reconstruct the breast that has been removed. In the latissimus dorsi (LAT) flap method, tissue from the latissimus dorsi muscle in the upper back is tunneled subcutaneously up to the chest area.

If reconstructive surgery is desired, the ultimate decision regarding the method will be determined by the woman's anatomy (e.g., is there sufficient fat and muscle to permit natural reconstruction) and her overall health status. Both procedures require a prolonged recovery period.

Some women opt for no reconstruction, and many of them choose to wear breast prostheses. Some prostheses are worn in the bra cup and others fit against the skin or into special pockets made into clothing.

Whether to have reconstructive surgery is an individual and very complex decision. Each woman must be presented with all of the options and then allowed to decide. The nurse can play an important role here by presenting the facts to the woman so that she can make an intelligent decision to meet her unique situation.

Adjunctive Therapy

Adjunctive therapy is supportive or additional therapy that is recommended after surgery. Adjunctive therapies include local therapy such as radiation therapy and systemic therapies using chemotherapy, hormonal therapy, and immunotherapy.

Radiation Therapy

Radiation therapy uses high-energy rays to destroy cancer cells that might have been left behind in the breast, chest wall, or underarm area after the tumor has been removed surgically. Usually serial radiation doses are given 5 days a week to the tumor site for 6 to 8 weeks postoperatively. Each treatment takes only a few minutes, but the dose is cumulative. Women undergoing breast-conserving therapy receive radiation to the entire breast after lumpectomy with the goal of eradicating residual microscopic cancer cells to reduce the chance of recurrence (Holcomb, 2006).

Side effects of traditional radiation therapy include inflammation, local edema, anorexia, swelling, and heaviness in the breast; sunburn-like skin changes in the treated area; and fatigue. Changes to the breast tissue and skin usually resolve in about a year (Willett, Czito, & Tyler, 2007). This type of therapy can be given several ways: external beam radiation, which delivers a carefully focused dose of radiation from a machine outside the body, or internal radiation, in which tiny pellets that contain radioactive material are placed into the tumor.

Several advances have taken place in the field of radiation oncology for the treatment of women with early-stage breast cancer that assist in reducing the side effects. The treatment position for external radiation has changed from supine to prone, with the arm on the affected side raised above the head, so that the treated breast hangs dependently through the opening of the treatment board. Treatment in the prone position improves dose distribution within the breast and allows for a decrease in the dose delivered to the heart, lung, chest wall, and other breast (National Comprehensive Cancer Network, 2007).

High-dose brachytherapy is another advance that is an alternative to traditional radiation treatment. A balloon catheter is used to insert radioactive seeds into the breast after the tumor is removed surgically. The seeds deliver a concentrated dose directly to the operative site; this is important because most cancer recurrences in the breast (67% to 100%) occur at or near the lumpectomy site. This allows a high dose of radiation to be delivered to a small target volume with a minimal dose to the surrounding normal tissue. This procedure takes 4 to 5 days as opposed to the 4 to 6 weeks that traditional radiation therapy takes; it also eliminates the need to delay radiation therapy to allow for wound healing. Brachytherapy is now used as a primary radiation treatment after breast-conserving surgery in selected women as an alternative to whole breast irradiation (Sanders et al., 2007). Side effects of brachytherapy include redness or discharge around catheters, fever, and infection. Daily cleansing of the catheter insertion site with a mild soap and application of an antibiotic ointment will minimize the risk of infection.

Intensity-modulated radiation therapy (IMRT) offers still another new approach to the delivery of treatment to reduce the dose within the target area while sparing surrounding normal structures. A computed tomography scan is used to create a three-dimensional model of the breast. Based on this model, a series of intensity-modulated beams are produced to the desired dose distribution to reduce radiation exposure to underlying structures. Acute toxicity is thus minimized (Willett, Czito, & Tyler, 2007). Research is ongoing to evaluate the impact of all of these advances in radiation therapy.

Chemotherapy

Chemotherapy refers to the use of drugs that are toxic to all cells and interfere with a cell's ability to reproduce. They are particularly effective against malignant cells but affect all rapidly dividing cells, especially those of the skin, the hair follicles, the mouth, the gastrointestinal tract, and the bone marrow. Breast cancer is a systemic disease in which micrometastases are already present in other organs by the time the breast cancer is diagnosed. Chemotherapeutic agents perform a systemic "sweep" of the body to reduce the chances that distant tumors will start growing.

Chemotherapy may be indicated for women with tumors larger than 1 cm, positive lymph nodes, or cancer of an aggressive type. Chemotherapy is prescribed in cycles, with each period of treatment followed by a rest period. Treatment typically lasts 3 to 6 months, depending on the dose used and the woman's health status.

Different classes of drugs affect different aspects of cell division and are used in combinations or "cocktails." The most active and commonly used chemotherapeutic agents for breast cancer include alkylating agents, anthracyclines, antimetabolites, and vinca alkaloids. Fifty or more chemotherapeutic agents can be used to treat breast cancer; however, a combination drug approach versus a single drug treatment appears to be more effective (ACS, 2007f).

Side effects of chemotherapy depend on the agents used, the intensity of dosage, the dosage schedule, the type and extent of cancer, and the client's physical and emotional status (Boehmke & Dickerson, 2006). However, typical side effects include nausea and vomiting, diarrhea or constipation, hair loss, weight loss, stomatitis, fatigue, and immunosuppression. The most serious is bone marrow suppression (myelosuppression). This causes an increased risk of infection, bleeding, and a reduced red-cell count, which can lead to anemia. Treatment of the side effects can generally be addressed through appropriate support medications such as antinausea drugs like granisetron hydrochloride (Kytril) or ondansetron (Zofran). In addition, growth-stimulating factors, such as epoetin alfa (Procrit) and filgrastim (Neupogen), help keep blood counts from dropping too low. Counts that are too low would stop or delay the use of chemotherapy.

An aggressive systemic option, when other treatments have failed or when there is a strong possibility of relapse or metastatic disease, is high-dose chemotherapy with bone marrow and/or stem cell transplant. This therapy involves the withdrawal of bone marrow before the administration of toxic levels of chemotherapeutic agents. The marrow is frozen and then returned to the client after the high-dose chemotherapy is finished. Clinical trials are still researching this experimental therapy (Guarneri et al., 2007).

Endocrine Therapy

One of estrogen's normal functions is to stimulate the growth and division of healthy cells in the breasts. However, in some women with breast cancer, this normal function contributes to the growth and division of cancer cells.

The objective of **endocrine therapy** is to block or counter the effect of estrogen. Estrogen plays a central role in the pathogenesis of cancer, and treatment with estrogen deprivation has proven to be effective (Bush, 2007). Several different drug classes are used to interfere or block estrogen receptors. They include selective estrogen receptor modulators (SERMs), estrogen receptor down-regulators, aromatase inhibitors, luteinizing hormone-releasing hormone, progestin, and biologic response modifiers (Underwood, 2006). Current recommendations for most women with ER+ breast cancer are to take a hormone-like medication—known as a SERM anti-estrogenic agent—daily for up to 5 years after initial treatment. Certain areas in the female body (breasts, uterus, ovaries, skin, vagina, and brain) contain specialized cells called hormone receptors that allow estrogen to enter the cell and stimulate it to divide. SERMs enter these same receptors and act like keys, turning off the signal for growth inside the cell (Bush, 2007). The best-known SERM is tamoxifen (Nolvadex, 20 mg daily for 5 years). Although it works well in preventing further spread of cancer, it is also associated with an increased incidence of endometrial cancer, pulmonary embolus, deep vein thrombosis, hot flashes, vaginal discharge and bleeding, stroke, and cataract formation (Bush, 2007).

A relatively new SERM is the anti-osteoporosis drug raloxifene (Evista), which has shown promising results. It has anti-estrogen effects on the breast and uterus. In a recent study involving more than 20,000 postmenopausal women at high risk for breast cancer, raloxifene worked as well as tamoxifen in preventing breast cancer, but with fewer serious adverse effects. Both drugs cut the cancer risk in half (Medical Letter, 2006). It was originally marketed solely for the prevention and treatment of osteoporosis but is now used as adjunctive breast cancer therapy.

Another class of endocrine agents, aromatase inhibitors, work by inhibiting the conversion of androgens to estrogens. Aromatase inhibitors include letozole (Femara, 2.5 mg daily), exemestane (Aromasin, 25 mg daily), and anastrozole (Arimidex, 1 mg daily for 5 years), all of which are taken orally. These are usually given to women with advanced breast cancer or cancer that recurs despite the use of tamoxifen (Holcomb, 2006).

The side effects associated with these endocrine therapies include hot flashes, bone pain, fatigue, nausea, cough, dyspnea, and headache (Hackley, Kriebs, & Rousseau, 2007). Women with hormone-sensitive cancers can live for long periods without any intervention other than hormonal manipulation, but quality-of-life issues need to be addressed in the balance between treatment and side effects.

Immunotherapy

Immunotherapy, used as an adjunct to surgery, represents an attempt to stimulate the body's natural defenses to recognize and attack cancer cells. Trastuzumab (Herceptin, 2- to 4-mg/kg intravenous infusion) is the first monoclonal antibody approved for breast cancer (National Comprehensive Cancer Network, 2007). Some tumors produce excessive amounts of HER-2/neu protein, which regulates cancer cell growth. Breast cancers that overexpress the protein HER-2/neu are associated with a more aggressive form of disease and a poorer prognosis. Trastuzumab blocks the effect of this protein to inhibit the growth of cancer cells. It can be used alone or in combination with other chemotherapy to treat clients with metastatic breast disease (Opatt & Chung, 2007). Adverse effects of trastuzumab include cardiac toxicity, vascular thrombosis, hepatic failure, fever, chills, nausea, vomiting, and pain with first infusion (Skidmore-Roth, 2007).

NURSING PROCESS FOR THE PATIENT WITH BREAST CANCER

When a woman is diagnosed with breast cancer, she faces treatment that may alter her body shape, may make her feel unwell, and may not carry a certainty of cure. Nurses can support women from the time of diagnosis, through the treatments, and through follow-up after the surgical and adjunctive treatments have been completed. Allowing patients time to ask questions and to discuss any necessary preparations for treatment is critical. As our understanding of breast disorders keeps improving, treatments continue to change. Although the goal of treatment remains improved survival, increasing emphasis is focused on prevention (Stephenson, 2007). Nurses can have an impact on early detection of breast disorders, treatment, and symptom management (Underwood, 2006). A nurse who is involved in the woman's treatment plan from the beginning can effectively offer support throughout the whole experience.

Teamwork is important in breast screening and caring for women with breast disorders. Treatment is often fragmented between the hospital and community treatment centers, which can be emotionally traumatic for the woman and her family. The advances being made in the diagnosis and treatment of breast disorders mean that guidelines are constantly changing, requiring all health care professionals to keep up to date. Informed nurses can provide support and information and, most importantly, continuity of care for the woman undergoing treatment for a breast problem.

The nurse plays a particularly important role in providing psychological support and self-care teaching to patients with breast cancer. Nurses can influence both physical and emotional recovery, which are both important aspects of care that help in improving the woman's quality of life and the ability to survive. The nurse's role should extend beyond helping clients; spreading the word in the community about screening and prevention is a big part in the ongoing fight against cancer. The community should see nurses as both educators and valued sources of credible information. This role will help improve clinical outcomes while achieving high levels of client satisfaction.

Remember Nancy from the chapter opener? Is her response typical of many women upon discovering a lump in their breast? Nancy confides her discovery of the lump and her worries to you. What advice would you give her?

Assessment

Early breast cancer has no symptoms. The earliest sign of breast cancer is often an abnormality seen on a screening mammogram before the woman or the health care professional feels it. In the woman presenting with a breast disorder, take a thorough history of the problem and explore the woman's risk factors for breast cancer. Assess the woman for clinical manifestations of breast cancer, such as changes in breast appearance and contour, which become apparent with advancing breast cancer (ACS, 2007d). These changes include:

- Continued and persistent changes in the breast
- A lump or thickening in one breast
- Persistent nipple irritation
- Unusual breast swelling or asymmetry
- A lump or swelling in the axilla
- Changes in skin color or texture
- Nipple retraction, tenderness, or discharge (Fig. 6.5)

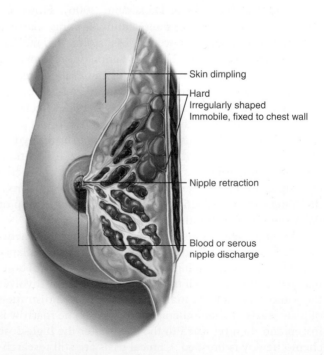

FIGURE **6.5** Malignant breast tumor.

Complete a breast examination to validate the clinical manifestations and findings of the health history and risk factor assessment. The clinical breast examination involves both inspection and palpation (Nursing Procedure 6.1). Helpful characteristics in evaluating palpable breast masses are described in Box 6.1. If a lump can be palpated, the cancer has been there for quite some time.

Be cognizant of the impact that breast cancer has on a woman's emotional state, coping ability, and quality of life. Women may experience sadness, anger, fear, and guilt as a result of breast cancer. However, despite potential negative outcomes, many women have a positive outlook for their futures and adapt to treatment modalities with a good quality of life (Holcomb, 2006). Closely monitor clients for their psychosocial adjustment to diagnosis and treatment and be able to identify those who need further psychological intervention. By giving practical advice, the nurse can help the woman adjust to her altered body image and to accept the changes to her life.

Because family members play a significant role in supporting women through breast cancer diagnosis and treatment, assess the emotional distress of both partners during the course of treatment and, if needed, make a referral for psychological counseling. By identifying interpersonal strains, negative psychosocial side effects of cancer treatment can be minimized.

Nursing Diagnosis

Appropriate nursing diagnoses for a woman with a diagnosis of breast cancer might include:

- Disturbed body image related to:
  - Loss of body part (breast)
  - Loss of femininity
  - Loss of hair due to chemotherapy
- Fear related to:
  - Diagnosis of cancer
  - Prognosis of disease
- Educational deficit related to:
  - Cancer treatment options
  - Reconstructive surgery decisions
  - Breast self-examination

Nursing Interventions

Offer information, support, and perioperative care to women diagnosed with breast cancer who are undergoing treatment. Implement health-promotion and disease-prevention strategies to minimize the risk for developing breast cancer and to promote optimal outcomes.

*R*emember Nancy, who discovered a breast lump? You offer to go with her to the doctor. After a full examination and several diagnostic tests, the results come back positive for breast cancer. What treatment options does Nancy have, and what factors need to be considered in selecting those options?

Providing Patient Education

Help the woman and her partner to prioritize the voluminous amount of information given to them so that they can make informed decisions. Explain all treatment options in detail so the patient and her family understand them. By preparing an individualized packet of information and reviewing it with the woman and her partner, the nurse can help them understand her specific type of cancer, the diagnostic studies and treatment options she may choose, and the goals of treatment. For example, nurses play an important role in educating women about the use of endocrine therapies, observing women's experiences with treatment, and communicating those observations to their primary care professionals to make dosage adjustments, in addition to contributing to the knowledge base of endocrine therapy in the treatment of breast cancer.

Providing information is a central role of the nurse in caring for the woman with a diagnosis of breast cancer. This information can be given via telephone counseling, one-to-one contact, and pamphlets. Telephone counseling with women and their partners may be an effective method to improve symptom management and quality of life (Knobf, 2007).

Providing Emotional Support

The diagnosis of cancer affects all aspects of life for a woman and her family. The threatening nature of the disease and feelings of uncertainty about the future can lead to anxiety and stress. Address the woman's needs for:

- Information about diagnosis and treatment
- Physical care while undergoing treatments
- Contact with supportive people
- Education about disease, options, and prevention measures
- Discussion and support by a caring, competent nurse

Reassure the client and her family that the diagnosis of breast cancer does not necessarily mean imminent death, a decrease in attractiveness, or diminished sexuality. Encourage the woman to express her fears and worries. Be available to listen and address the woman's concerns in an open manner to help her toward recovery. All aspects of care must include sensitivity to the patient's personal efforts to cope and heal. Some women will become involved in organizations or charities that support cancer research; they may participate in breast cancer walks to raise awareness or become a Reach for Recovery volunteer to help others. Each woman copes in her own personal manner, and all of these efforts can be positive motivators for her own healing.

To help women cope with the diagnosis of breast cancer, the American Cancer Society launched Reach to Recovery more than 30 years ago. Specially trained breast cancer survivors give women and their families opportunities to express their feelings, verbalize their fears, and get answers. Most importantly, Reach to Recovery vol-

(text continues on page 162)

Nursing Procedure 6.1

CLINICAL BREAST EXAMINATION

Purpose: To Assess Breasts for Abnormal Findings

1. Inspect the breast for size, symmetry, and skin texture and color. Inspect the nipples and areola. Ask the client to sit at the edge of the examination table, with her arms resting at her sides.

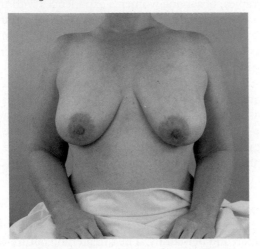

2. Inspect the breast for masses, retraction, dimpling, or ecchymosis.
   - The client places her hands on her hips.

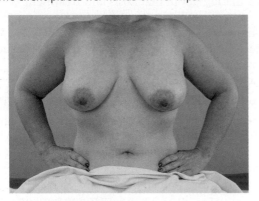

   - She then raises her arms over her head so the axillae can also be inspected.

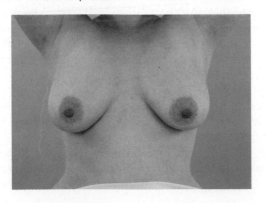

   - The client then stands, places her hands on her hips, and leans forward.

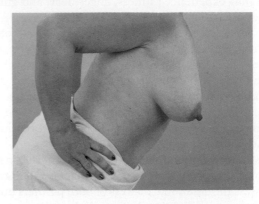

3. Palpate the breasts. Assist the client into a supine position with her arms above her head. Place a pillow or towel under the client's head to help spread the breasts. Three patterns might be used to palpate the breasts:

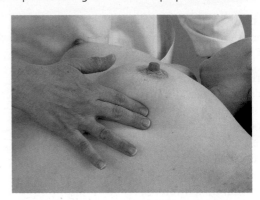

   - Spiral

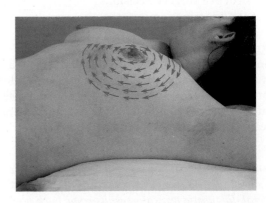

Nursing Procedure 6.1 (continued)

- Pie-shaped wedges

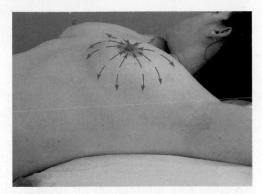

- Vertical strip

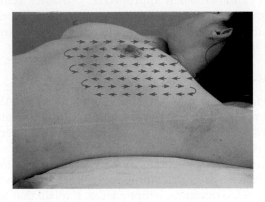

4. Compress the nipple gently between the thumb and index finger to evaluate for masses and squeeze to check for any discharge.

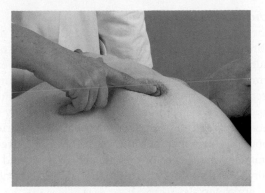

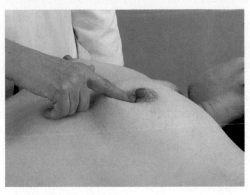

5. Palpate the axillary area for any tenderness or lymph node enlargement. Have the client sit up and move to the edge of the examination table. While supporting the client's arm, palpate downward from the armpit, palpating toward the ribs just below the breast.

Adapted from Rhoads, J. (2006). *Advanced health assessment and diagnostic reasoning.* Philadelphia: Lippincott Williams & Wilkins.

BOX 6.1 **Characteristics of Benign vs. Malignant Breast Masses**

- **Benign breast masses are described as:**
  - Frequently painful
  - Firm, rubbery mass
  - Bilateral masses
  - Induced nipple discharge
  - Regular margins (clearly delineated)
  - No skin dimpling
  - No nipple retraction
  - Mobile, not affixed to the chest wall
  - No bloody discharge

- **Malignant breast masses are described as:**
  - Hard to palpation
  - Painless
  - Irregularly shaped (poorly delineated)
  - Immobile, fixed to the chest wall
  - Skin dimpling
  - Nipple retraction
  - Unilateral mass
  - Bloody, serosanguineous, or serous nipple discharge
  - Spontaneous nipple discharge

unteers offer understanding, support, and hope through face-to-face visits or by telephone; they are proof that people can survive breast cancer and live productive lives. National contact information is 1-800-ACS-2345.

Providing Postoperative Care

For the woman who has had surgery to remove a malignant breast lump or an entire breast, excellent postoperative nursing care is crucial. Tell the woman what to expect in terms of symptoms and when they usually occur during treatment and after surgery. This allows women to anticipate these symptoms and proactively employ management strategies to improve their cancer experience. Postoperative care includes immediate postoperative care, pain management, care of the affected arm, wound care, mobility care, respiratory care, emotional care, educational needs, and referrals.

Immediate Postoperative Care

Assess the client's respiratory status by auscultating the lungs and observing the breathing pattern. Assess circulation; note vital signs, skin color, and skin temperature. Observe the client's neurologic status by evaluating the level of alertness and orientation. Monitor the wound for amount and color of drainage. Monitor the intravenous lines for patency, correct fluid, and rate. Assess the drainage tube for amount, color, and consistency of drainage.

Pain Management

Provide analgesics as needed. Reassure the woman that her pain will be controlled. Teach the woman how to communicate her pain intensity on a scale of 0 to 10, with 10 being the worst pain imaginable. Assess the client's pain level frequently and anticipate pain before assisting the woman to ambulate.

Affected Arm Care

Elevate the affected arm on a pillow to promote lymph drainage. Make sure that no treatments are performed on the affected arm, including laboratory draws, intravenous lines, blood pressures, and so on. Place a sign above the bed to warn others not to touch the affected arm.

Wound Care

Observe the wound often and empty drainage reservoirs as needed. Tell the client to report any evidence of infection early, such as fever, chills, or any area of redness or inflammation along the incision line. Also tell the client to report any increase in drainage, foul odor, or separation at the incision site.

Mobility Care

Perform active range-of-motion and arm exercises as ordered. Encourage self-care activities for successful rehabilitation. Perform dressing and drainage care; explain the care during the procedure.

Respiratory Care

Assist with turning, coughing, and deep breathing every 2 hours. Explain that this helps to expand collapsed alveoli in the lungs, promotes faster clearance of inhalation agents from the body, and prevents postoperative pneumonia and atelectasis.

Emotional Care and Referrals

Encourage the client to participate in her care. Assess her coping strategies preoperatively. Explain possible body image concerns after discharge. Promote the ACS websites, which provide the latest cancer therapy news. Encourage the client to attend local support groups for breast cancer survivors, such as Reach to Recovery, an ACS program in which trained volunteers provide support and up-to-date information for spouses, children, friends, and other loved ones. Reach to Recovery volunteers can also, when appropriate, provide a temporary breast form and give information on types of permanent prostheses, as well as lists of where those items are available in the community.

Educational Needs

Provide follow-up information about adjunctive therapy. Explain that radiation therapy may start within weeks postoperatively. Discuss chemotherapy, its side effects and cycles, home care during treatment, and future monitoring strategies. Explain hormonal therapy, including antiestrogens or aromatase inhibitors. Teach progressive arm exercises to minimize lymphedema. Explain that ongoing surveillance is needed to detect recurrence of cancer or a new primary site and that the patient will typically see the health care provider every 6 months.

Nancy underwent a mastectomy with radiation and chemotherapy. What follow-up care is needed? How can the nurse assist Nancy to cope with her uncertain future? What community resources might help her?

Implementing Health-Promotion and Disease-Prevention Strategies

In the past, most women assumed that there was little they could do to reduce their risk of developing breast cancer. However, research has found that the daily choices women make concerning breast cancer screening, diet, exercise, and other health practices have a profound impact on cancer risk. In the fight against cancer, nurses often assume a variety of roles, such as educator, counselor, advocate, and role model. Nurses can offer education about the following:

- Prevention
- Early detection
- Screening
- Dispelling myths and fears

• Self-examination techniques
• Individual risk status and strategies for risk reduction

It is important to be knowledgeable about the most current evidence-based practices and cognizant of how the media presents this information. Offer prevention strategies within the context of a woman's life. Factors such as lifestyle choices, economic status, and multiple roles need to be taken into consideration when counseling women. Advocate for healthy lifestyles and making sound choices to prevent cancer. Nurses, like all health care professionals, should offer guidance from a comprehensive perspective that acknowledges the unique needs of each individual (Banning, 2007).

Breast cancer is a frightening experience for women. Like a black cloud hanging over their heads, with little regard for any victim, breast cancer stalks women everywhere they go. Many have a close friend or relative who is battling the disease; many have watched their mothers and sisters die of this dreaded disease. Those with risk factors live with even greater anxiety and fear. No woman wants to hear those chilling words: "The biopsy is positive. You have breast cancer." Provide women with information about detection and risk factors, inform them about the new ACS screening guidelines, instruct them on breast self-examination, and outline dietary changes that might reduce their risk of breast cancer.

Awareness is the first step toward a change in habits. Raising the level of awareness about breast cancer is of paramount importance, and nurses can play an important role in health promotion, disease prevention, and education.

Breast Cancer Screening

The three components of early detection are breast self-examination, clinical breast examination, and mammography.

The ACS (2007b) has issued breast cancer screening guidelines that, for the first time, offer specific guidance for the women and greater clarification of the role of breast examinations (Table 6.4). ACS screening guidelines are revised about every 5 years to include new scientific findings and developments.

Women are exposed to multiple sources of cancer prevention information, and much of it may not be sound. Discuss the benefits, risks, and potential limitations of breast self-examination, clinical breast examination, and mammography with each woman and tailor the information to her specific risk factors (ACS, 2007b). Based on the new guidelines, make clinical judgments as to the appropriateness of recommending breast self-examination, and re-evaluate the need to teach the procedure to all women; the focus might instead be on encouraging regular mammograms (depending, of course, on the woman's individual risk factors).

TABLE 6.4 AMERICAN CANCER SOCIETY BREAST CANCER SCREENING GUIDELINES

Woman's Age	Screening Activity
20–39	Breast self-examination (BSE) is optional Clinical breast examination every 3 years
40+	BSE every month is optional Clinical breast examination every year Mammogram every year, continuing for as long as the woman is in good health

Women at increased risk (e.g., family history, genetic tendency, past history of cancer) should discuss with their health care professionals the pros and cons of starting mammography screening earlier, undergoing additional diagnostic tests (e.g., ultrasound or MRI), or increasing the frequency of examinations.

Source: ACS, 2007c.

Breast self-examination is a technique that enables a woman to detect any changes in her breasts; this could result in early cancer detection. The emphasis is now on awareness of breast changes, not just discovery of cancer. Research has shown that breast self-examination plays a small role in detecting breast cancer compared with self-awareness. However, doing breast self-examination is one way for a woman to know how her breasts normally feel so that she can notice any changes that do occur (ACS, 2007g).

There are two steps to conducting breast self-examination: visual inspection and tactile palpation. The visual part should be done in three separate positions: with the arms up behind the head, with the arms down at the sides, and bending forward. Instruct the woman to look for:

• Changes in shape, size, contour, or symmetry
• Skin discoloration or dimpling, bumps/lumps
• Sores or scaly skin
• Discharge or puckering of the nipple

In the second part, the tactile examination, the woman feels her breasts in one of three specific patterns: spiral, pie-shaped wedges, or up and down. When using any of the three patterns, the woman should use a circular rubbing motion (in dime-sized circles) without lifting the fingers. She checks not only the breasts but also between the breast and the axilla, the axilla itself, and the area above the breast up to the clavicle and across the shoulder. The pads of the three middle fingers on the right hand are used to assess the left breast; the pads of the three middle fingers on the left hand are used to assess the right breast. Instruct the woman to use three different degrees of pressure:

- Light (move the skin without moving the tissue underneath)
- Medium (midway into the tissue)
- Hard (down to the ribs)

Once the tactile examination has been completed while standing in front of a mirror, it should be repeated while lying down. Teaching Guidelines 6.4 details breast self-examination.

Nutrition

Nutrition plays a critical role in health promotion and disease prevention (Escott-Stump, 2007). Being overweight or obese is a risk factor for breast cancer in postmenopausal women (Wright, 2007). *Healthy People 2010* identified being overweight or obese as one of the 10 leading health indicators and a major health concern (USDHHS, 2000). Almost 62% of women over the age of 20 years are overweight; of these, 33.4% are obese (Smith-Warner & Stampfer, 2007). A diet high in fruits, vegetables, and high-fiber carbohydrates and low in animal fats seems to offer protection against breast cancer as well as weight control. Women who followed these dietary guidelines decreased their risk of breast cancer (Escott-Stump, 2007).

The Women's Health Initiative Dietary Modification Trial (Prentice et al., 2006) was designed to study a low-fat diet, a nutritional approach to prevention of chronic diseases. It found a marginally statistically significant reduction in breast cancer incidence among women in the low-fat dietary pattern group.

The American Institute for Cancer Research (AICR), which conducts extensive research, made the following

---

TEACHING GUIDELINES 6.4

How to Perform Breast Self-Examination

Step 1

- Stand before a mirror.
- Check both breasts for anything unusual.
- Look for discharge from the nipple and puckering, dimpling, or scaling of the skin.

The next two steps check for any changes in the contour of your breasts. As you do them, you should be able to feel your muscles tighten.

Step 2

- Watch closely in the mirror as you clasp your hands behind your head and press your hands forward.
- Note any change in the contour of your breasts.

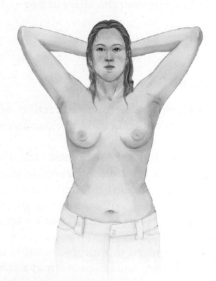

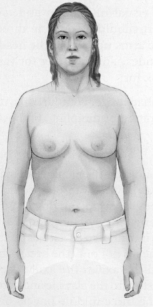

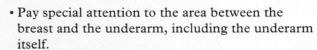

TEACHING GUIDELINES 6.4 (continued)

How to Perform Breast Self-Examination

Step 3

- Next, press your hands firmly on your hips and bow slightly toward the mirror as you pull your shoulders and elbows forward.
- Note any change in the contour of your breasts.

Some women perform the next part of the examination in the shower. Your fingers will glide easily over soapy skin, so you can concentrate on feeling for changes inside the breast.

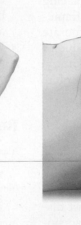

Step 4

- Raise your left arm.
- Use 3 or 4 fingers of your right hand to feel your left breast firmly, carefully, and thoroughly.
- Beginning at the outer edge, press the flat part of your fingers in small circles, moving the circles slowly around the breast.
- Gradually work toward the nipple.
- Be sure to cover the whole breast.

- Pay special attention to the area between the breast and the underarm, including the underarm itself.
- Feel for any unusual lumps or masses under the skin.
- If you have any spontaneous discharge during the month—whether or not it is during your BSE—see your doctor.
- Repeat the examination on your right breast.

Step 5

- Lie flat on your back with your left arm over your head and a pillow or folded towel under your left shoulder. (This position flattens your breast and makes it easier to check.)
- Repeat the actions of Step 4 in this position for each breast.

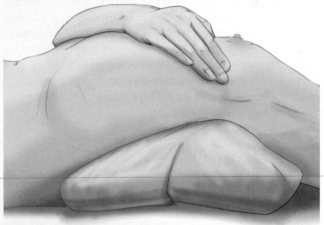

Source: American Cancer Society. (2007). *How to perform a breast self exam.* Available online at http://www.cancer.org/docroot/cri/content/cri_2_6x_how_to_perform_a_breast_self_exam_5.asp

recommendations to reduce a woman's risk for developing breast cancer:

- Engaging in daily moderate exercise and weekly vigorous physical activity
- Consuming at least five servings of fruits and vegetables daily
- Not smoking or using any tobacco products
- Keeping a maximum body mass index (BMI) of 25 and limiting weight gain to no more than 11 pounds since age 18
- Consuming seven or more daily portions of complex carbohydrates, such as whole grains and cereals

- Limiting intake of processed foods and refined sugar
- Restricting red meat intake to approximately 3 ounces daily
- Limiting intake of fatty foods, particularly those of animal origin
- Restricting intake of salted foods and use of salt in cooking (Wright, 2007)

The medical community is also starting to study the role of phytochemicals in health. The unique geographic variability of breast cancer around the world and the low rate of breast cancer in Asian compared to Western countries prompted this interest. This area of research appears hopeful for women seeking to prevent breast cancer as well as those recovering from it. Although the mechanism isn't clear, certain foods demonstrate anticancer properties and boost the immune system. Phytochemical-rich foods include:

• Green tea and herbal teas
• Garlic
• Whole grains and legumes
• Onions and leeks
• Soybeans and soy products
• Fruits (citrus, apricots, pumpkin, berries)
• Green leafy vegetables (spinach, collards, romaine)
• Colorful vegetables (carrots, squash, tomatoes)
• Cruciferous vegetables (broccoli, cabbage, cauliflower)
• Flax seeds (Escott-Stump, 2007)

Adopt a holistic approach when addressing the nutritional needs of women with breast cancer. Incorporate nutritional assessment into the general overall assessment of all women. Culturally sensitive nutritional assessment tools need to be developed and used to enhance this process. Providing examples of appropriate foods associated with the woman's current dietary habits, relating current health status to nutritional intake, and placing proposed modifications within a realistic personal framework may increase a woman's willingness to incorporate needed changes in her nutritional behavior. Be able to interpret research results and stay up to date on nutritional influences so that you can transmit this key information to the public.

■■■ Key Concepts

■ Many women believe that all lumps are cancerous, but actually more than 90% of the lumps discovered are benign and need no treatment.

■ The most commonly encountered benign breast disorders in women include fibrocystic breasts, fibroadenomas, intraductal papilloma, mammary duct ectasia, and mastitis.

■ Current research suggests that women with fibrocystic breast disease or other benign breast conditions are more likely to develop breast cancer later only if a breast biopsy shows "atypia" or abnormal breast cells.

■ Fibroadenomas are common benign solid breast tumors that can be stimulated by external estrogen, progesterone, lactation, and pregnancy.

■ An intraductal papilloma is generally less than 1 cm in diameter, not palpable, and produces a spontaneous serous, serosanguineous, or watery nipple discharge.

■ Duct ectasia is a dilation and inflammation of the ducts behind the nipple that results in noncyclic breast pain, nipple retraction, and discharge.

■ Mastitis is an infection of the connective tissue in the breast that occurs primarily in lactating or engorged women; it is divided into lactational or nonlactational types.

■ Management of both types of mastitis involves the use of oral antibiotics (usually a penicillinase-resistant penicillin or cephalosporin) and acetaminophen (Tylenol) for pain and fever.

■ Breast cancer is the most common cancer in women and the second leading cause of cancer deaths (lung cancer is first) among American women.

■ Breast cancer metastasizes widely and to almost all organs of the body, but primarily to the bone, lungs, lymph nodes, liver, and brain.

■ The etiology of breast cancer is unknown, but the disease is thought to develop in response to a number of related factors: aging, delayed childbearing or never bearing children, high breast density, family history of cancer, late menopause, and hormonal factors.

■ Breast cancer treatments fall into two categories: local and systemic. Local treatments are surgery and radiation therapy. Effective systemic treatments include chemotherapy, hormonal therapy, and immunotherapy.

■ Women perceive their breasts as intrinsic to their femininity, self-esteem, and sexuality, and the risk of losing a breast can provoke extreme anxiety.

■ Nurses can influence both physical and emotional recovery, which are both important aspects of care that help in improving the woman's quality of life and the ability to survive.

■ Providing up-to-date information and emotional support are central roles of the nurse in caring for the woman with a diagnosis of breast cancer.

REFERENCES

Alexander, L. L., LaRosa, J. H., Bader, H., & Garfield, S. (2007). *New dimensions in women's health* (4th ed.). Boston: Jones and Bartlett Publishers.

Aliotta, H. M., & Schaeffer, N. J. (2006). Breast conditions. In K. D. Schuiling & F. E. Likis (Eds.), *Women's gynecologic health* (pp. 321–342). Sudbury, MA: Jones and Bartlett Publishers.

American Cancer Society. (2007a). Benign breast conditions. Available at: http://www.cancer.org/docroot/CRI/content/CRI_2_6X_Benign_Breast_Conditions_59.a.

American Cancer Society. (2007b). Updated breast cancer screening guidelines released. Available at: http://www.cancer.org/docroot/MED/content/MED_2_1x_American_Cancer_Society_Is.

American Cancer Society. (2007c). *Cancer facts and figures 2006.* Atlanta, GA: Author.

American Cancer Society (2007d). Screening guidelines for the early detection of cancer in asymptomatic people. *Cancer prevention and early detection facts & figures 2006* (p. 31). Atlanta, GA: Author.

American Cancer Society. (2007e). What are the risk factors for breast cancer? Cancer Reference Information. Available at: http://www.cancer.org/docroot/CRI_2_4_2X_What_are_the_risk_factors_fo.

American Cancer Society. (2007f). *Breast cancer clear and simple.* Atlanta, GA: Author.

American Cancer Society (2007g). How to perform a breast self-exam. Available at: http://www.cancer.org/docroot/cri/content/cri_2_6x_how_to_perform_a_breast_self_exam_5.asp

Banning, M. (2007). Advanced breast cancer: Etiology, treatment and psychosocial features. *British Journal of Nursing, 16*(2), 86–90.

Boehmke, M. M., & Dickerson, S. S. (2006). The diagnosis of breast cancer: Transition from health to illness. *Oncology Nursing Forum, 33*(6), 1121–1127.

Bush, N. J. (2007). Advances in hormonal therapy for breast cancer. *Seminars in Oncology Nursing, 23*(1), 46–54.

Chernecky, C. C., & Berger, B. J. (2007). *Laboratory tests and diagnostic procedures* (5th ed.). Philadelphia: Elsevier Health Sciences.

DiSaia, P. J., & Creasman, W. T. (2007). *Clinical gynecologic oncology* (7th ed.). St. Louis, MO: Elsevier Health Sciences.

Eglash, A., Plane, M. B., & Mundt, M. (2006). History, physical and laboratory findings, and clinical outcomes of lactating women treated with antibiotics for chronic breast and/or nipple pain. *Journal of Human Lactation, 22*(4), 429–438.

Escott-Stump, S. (2007). *Nutrition and diagnosis-related care* (6th ed.). Philadelphia: Lippincott Williams & Wilkins.

Graham, H. (2006). Understanding benign breast conditions. *Practice Nurse, 32*(2), 29–32.

Guarneri, V., Frassoldati, A., Giovannelli, S., Borghi, F., & Conte, P. (2007). Primary systemic therapy for operable breast cancer: A review of clinical trials and perspectives. *Cancer Letters, 248*(2), 175–185.

Hackley, B., Kriebs, J. M., & Rousseau, M. E. (2007). *Primary care of women: A guide for midwives and women's health providers*. Sudbury, MA: Jones and Bartlett Publishers.

Harris, J. (2007). How to help women understand benign breast conditions. *Nursing in Practice: The Journal for Today's Primary Care Nurse,* Mar (33), 78–81.

Holcomb, S. S. (2006). Breast cancer therapy and treatment guidelines. *Nurse Practitioner, 31*(10), 59–63.

Kell, M. R., & Burke, J. P. (2007), Management of breast cancer in women with BRCA gene mutation. *British Medical Journal, 334*(7591), 437–438.

Knobf, M. T. (2007). Psychosocial responses in breast cancer survivors. *Seminars in Oncology Nursing, 23*(1), 71–83.

Kubota, K., Ogawa, Y., Nishioka, A., et al. (2007). Diagnostic accuracy of mammography, ultrasonography and magnetic resonance imaging in the detection of intraductal spread of breast cancer following neoadjuvant chemotherapy. *Oncology Reports, 17*(4), 915–918.

Law, M. P., & Alcamo, I. E. (2007). *Breast cancer*. New York: Chelsea House Publishers.

Mattson, S., & Smith, J. E. (2004). *Core curriculum for maternal-newborn nursing* (3rd ed.). St. Louis, MO: Elsevier Saunders.

Medical Letter. (2006). Raloxifene (Evista) for breast cancer prevention in postmenopausal women. *Obstetrics & Gynecology, 108*(4), 1023–1024.

National Cancer Institute. (NCI) (2007a). Breast cancer: treatment. Available at: http://cancer.gov/cancertopics/pdq/treatment/breast/healthprofessional

National Cancer Institute. (NCI) (2007b). Probability of breast cancer in American women. Available at: http://cis.nci.nih.gov/fact/5_6.htm

National Comprehensive Cancer Network (NCCN). (2007). Breast cancer treatment guidelines. NCCN patient guidelines. Available at: http://www.nccn.org/patients/patient_gls/_english/_breast/5_treatment.asp

Opatt, D. M., & Chung, C. (2007). Breast cancer. *eMedicine.* Available at: http://www.emedicine.com/plastic/topic521.htm

Ottoboni, A., & Ottoboni, F. (2007). Low-fat diet and chronic disease prevention: The Women's Health Initiative and its reception. *Journal of American Physicians & Surgeons, 12*(1), 10–13.

Preda, L., Villa, G., Rizzo, S., Bazzi, L., Origgi, D., Cassano, E., & Bellomi, M. (2006). Magnetic resonance mammography in the evaluation of recurrence at the prior lumpectomy site after conservative surgery and radiotherapy. *Breast Cancer Research, 8*(5), R53–55.

Prentice, R. L., Caan, B., Chlebowski, R. T., et al. (2006). Low-fat dietary pattern and risk of invasive breast cancer: The Women's Health Initiative Randomized Controlled Dietary Modification Trial. *JAMA, 295*(6), 629–642.

Rao, V. S., Garimella, V., Hwang, M., & Drew, P. (2007). Management of early breast cancer in the elderly. *International Journal of Cancer, 120*(6), 1155–1160.

Reddy, P., Chao, Q., Zembower, T., Noskin, G., & Bolon, M. (2007). Postpartum mastitis and community-acquired methicillin-resistant *Staphylococcus aureus. Emerging Infectious Diseases, 13*(2), 298–301.

Richards, T., Hunt, A., Courtney, S., & Umeh, H. (2007). Nipple discharge: A sign of breast cancer? *Annals of the Royal College of Surgeons of England, 89*(2), 124–126.

Sanders, M. E., Scroggins, T., Ampil, F. L., & Li, B. D. (2007). Accelerated partial breast irradiation in early-stage breast cancer. *Journal of Clinical Oncology, 25*(8), 996–1002.

Skidmore-Roth, L. (2007). *Mosby's drug guide for nurses with 2008 update* (7th ed.). St. Louis, MO: Elsevier Health Sciences

Smith, R. A. (2007). The evolving role of MRI in the detection and evaluation of breast cancer. *New England Journal of Medicine, 356,* 1362–1364.

Smith-Warner, S. A., & Stampfer, M. J. (2007). Fat intake and breast cancer. *Journal of the National Cancer Institute, 99*(6), 418–419.

Stephenson, J. (2007). Reducing breast cancer risk. *JAMA, 297*(11), 1182–1184.

Sukumvanich, P., & Borgen, P. (2007). Diseases of the breast. In R. E. Rakel & E. T. Bope (Eds.), *Conn's current therapy 2007* (pp. 1214–1225). Philadelphia: Saunders Elsevier.

Teal, C. B., Tabbara, S., & Kelly, T. A. (2007). Evaluation of intraoperative scrape cytology for sentinel lymph node biopsy in patients with breast cancer. *Breast Journal, 13*(2), 155–157.

Underwood, S. M. (2006). Breast cancer in African American women: Nursing essentials. *ABNF Journal,* Jan/Feb (1), 3–13.

U.S. Department of Health and Human Services (USDHHS). (2000). *Healthy people 2010.* Rockville, MD: Author.

Willett, C. G., Czito, B. G., & Tyler, D. S. (2007). Intraoperative radiation therapy. *Journal of Clinical Oncology, 25*(8), 971–977.

Wright, H. (2007). Getting physically active may increase your chances of surviving cancer. *Environmental Nutrition, 30*(3), 1–4.

Writing Group for Women's Health Initiative Investigators (WHI). (2002). Risks and benefits of estrogen plus progestin in healthy menopausal women: Principal results for the Women's Health Initiative randomized controlled trial. *JAMA, 288*(3), 321–333.

WEBSITES

American Cancer Society (ACS): 1-800-ACS-2345: http://www.cancer.org

Facing Our Risk of Cancer Empowered: www.facingourrisk.org

International Society of Nurses in Genetics: http://nursing.creighton.edu/isong

Living Beyond Breast Cancer, 1-888-753-5222: http://www.lbbc.org

National Alliance of Breast Cancer Organizations, 1-888-80-NABCO: http://www.nabco.org

National Cancer Institute (NCI), 1-800-422-6327: http://www.nci.nih.gov

Oncology Nursing Society (ONS), 1-866-257-4ONS: http://www.ons.org

Susan G. Komen Breast Cancer Foundation, 1-800-462-9273: http://www.komen.org

Y-me National Breast Cancer Organization, 1-800-221-2141: http://www.Y-me.org

CHAPTER WORKSHEET

MULTIPLE CHOICE QUESTIONS

1. Breast self-examinations involve both touching of breast tissue and:

   a. Palpation of cervical lymph nodes

   b. Firm squeezing of both breast nipples

   c. Visualizing both breasts for any change

   d. A mammogram to evaluate breast tissue

2. Which of the following is the strongest risk factor for breast cancer?

   a. Advancing age and being female

   b. High number of children

   c. Genetic mutations in BRCA-1 and BRCA-2

   d. Family history of colon cancer

3. A biopsy procedure that traces radioisotopes and blue dye from the tumor site through the lymphatic system into the axillary nodes is:

   a. Stereotactic biopsy

   b. Sentinel node biopsy

   c. Axillary dissection biopsy

   d. Advanced breast biopsy

4. The most serious potential adverse reaction from chemotherapy is:

   a. Thrombocytopenia

   b. Deep vein thrombosis

   c. Alopecia

   d. Myelosuppression

5. What suggestion would be helpful for the client experiencing painful fibrocystic breast changes?

   a. Increase her caffeine intake.

   b. Take a mild analgesic when needed.

   c. Reduce her intake of leafy vegetables.

   d. Wear a bra bigger than she needs.

6. A postoperative mastectomy client should be referred to which of the following organizations for assistance?

   a. National Organization for Women (NOW)

   b. Food and Drug Administration (FDA)

   c. March of Dimes Foundation (MDF)

   d. Reach to Recovery volunteers

CRITICAL THINKING EXERCISES

1. Mrs. Gordon, 48, presents to the women's community clinic where you work as a nurse. She is very upset and crying. She tells you that she found lumps in her breast: "I know that it's cancer and I will die." When you ask her about her problem, she says she does not check her breasts monthly and hasn't had a mammogram for years because "they're too expensive." She also describes the intermittent pain she experiences.

   a. What specific questions would you ask this client to get a clearer picture?

   b. What education is needed for this client regarding breast health?

   c. What community referrals are needed to meet this client's future needs?

2. Ruth Davis, 51, stops in at the urgent care facility with an anxious look on her face. She tells the nurse practitioner that she has green discharge coming from her right breast and discomfort intermittently. She can't understand how this would happen since she hasn't previously had any nipple discharge or pain.

   a. What benign breast condition might the nurse practitioner suspect based on her description?

   b. What specific information should the nurse practitioner give Mrs. Davis about duct ectasia?

   c. The typical treatment of this benign breast condition would include what?

STUDY ACTIVITIES

1. Discuss with a group of women what their breasts symbolize to them and to society. Do they symbolize something different to each one?

2. When a woman experiences a breast disorder, what feelings might she be experiencing and how can a nurse help her sort them out?

3. Interview a woman who has fibrocystic breast changes and find out how she manages this condition.

4. An infection of the breast connective tissue that frequently occurs in the lactating woman is

   _____.

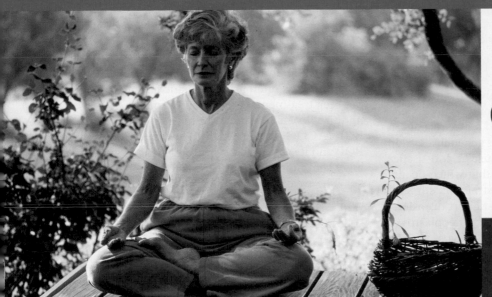

CHAPTER 7

BENIGN DISORDERS OF THE FEMALE REPRODUCTIVE TRACT

KEY TERMS

cystocele
enterocele
Kegel exercises
ovarian cyst

pelvic organ prolapse
pessary
polyps
polycystic ovary syndrome

rectocele
urinary incontinence
uterine fibroids
uterine prolapse

LEARNING OBJECTIVES

Upon completion of the chapter, the learner will be able to:

1. Define the key terms.
2. Identify the major pelvic relaxation disorders in terms of etiology, management, and nursing interventions.
3. Outline the nursing management needed for the most common benign reproductive disorders in women.
4. Discuss urinary incontinence in terms of pathology, clinical manifestations, treatment options, and effect on quality of life.
5. Compare the various benign growths in terms of their symptoms and management.
6. Discuss the emotional impact of polycystic ovarian syndrome and the nurse's role as a counselor, educator, and advocate.

Liz, a 26-year-old, overweight woman, presented to the clinic with hirsutism and facial acne and told the nurse she was concerned about her irregular menstrual periods. She also said her hair seemed to be falling out on top of her head recently. What diagnostic tests might the nurse anticipate with this patient? How can the nurse prepare Liz for them?

Wow

Women can influence their aging process by making wise lifestyle choices early on.

The incidence of several benign pelvic disorders increases as women age. For instance, women may experience pelvic support disorders related to pelvic relaxation or urinary incontinence. These disorders generally develop after years of wear and tear on the muscles and tissues that support the pelvic floor—such as that which occurs with childbearing, chronic coughing, straining, surgery, or simply aging. In addition to pelvic support disorders, woman may also experience various benign neoplasms of the reproductive tract, such as cervical polyps, uterine leiomyomas (fibroids), ovarian cysts, genital fistulas, and Bartholin's cysts. This chapter provides an overview of various pelvic support disorders and benign neoplasms, discussing the assessment, treatment, and prevention strategies for each.

Pelvic Support Disorders

Pelvic support disorders such as pelvic organ prolapse (POP) and urinary and fecal incontinence are common in aging women. The majority of the more than 13 million people in the United States who experience urinary incontinence are women with POP (Smith, 2007). Pelvic support disorders cause significant physical and psychological morbidity and can diminish women's social interactions, emotional well-being, and overall quality of life. Because pelvic support disorders increase with age, the problem will grow worse as our population ages. These disorders occur as a result of weakness of the connective tissue and muscular support of pelvic organs due to a number of factors: vaginal childbirth, obesity, lifting, chronic cough, straining at defecation secondary to constipation, and estrogen deficiency (ACOG, 2007). The bony pelvis has an exaggerated lumbar spine curve and downward tilt to it. The bladder rests on the symphysis and the posterior organs rest on the sacrum and coccyx. The pelvis holds the organs, but a woman's erect posture causes a funneling effect and constant downward pressure.

▶ PELVIC ORGAN PROLAPSE

Pelvic organ prolapse (from the Latin *prolapsus,* a slipping forth) refers to the abnormal descent or herniation of the pelvic organs from their original attachment sites or their normal position in the pelvis. POP occurs when structures of the pelvis shift and protrude into or outside of the vaginal canal. The Egyptians were the first to describe prolapse of the genital organs. Hippocrates made reference to placing a pomegranate half into the vagina to treat organ prolapse. A disorder exclusive to women, POP rarely results in severe morbidity or mortality but can affect a woman's daily activities and quality of life.

It is difficult to determine the incidence of POP, as the disorder is often asymptomatic and many women do not seek treatment. It has been estimated, however, that up to 75% of all women who have given birth experience POP (ACOG, 2007). With the aging of the population, POP and its associated symptoms are becoming increasingly common (Bartoletti, 2007).

The treatment and diagnosis of POP is challenging and problematic.

Types of Pelvic Organ Prolapse

The four most common types of genital prolapse are cystocele, rectocele, enterocele, and uterine prolapse (Fig. 7.1):

- **Cystocele** occurs when the posterior bladder wall protrudes downward through the anterior vaginal wall.
- **Rectocele** occurs when the rectum sags and pushes against or into the posterior vaginal wall.
- **Enterocele** occurs when the small intestine bulges through the posterior vaginal wall (especially common when straining).
- **Uterine prolapse** occurs when the uterus descends through the pelvic floor and into the vaginal canal. Multiparous women are at particular risk for uterine prolapse.

The extent of uterine prolapse is described in terms of degree:

- First degree: prolapse of the organ into the vaginal canal
- Second degree: cervix descends to the vaginal introitus
- Third degree: cervix is below the vaginal introitus (Berzuk, 2007)

Etiology

Anatomic support of the pelvic organs is mainly provided by the levator ani muscle complex and the connective tissue attachments of the pelvic organ fascia. Dysfunction of one or both of these components can lead to loss of support and eventually POP. Weakened pelvic floor muscles also prevent complete closure of the urethra, resulting in urine leakage during physical stress. This problem is not limited to older women: urinary incontinence has been documented in women of varying ages, including very young women (Smith, 2007).

Many risk factors for POP have been suggested, but the true cause is likely to be multifactorial. Causes might include:

- Constant downward gravity because of erect human posture
- Atrophy of supporting tissues with aging and decline of estrogen levels
- Weakening of pelvic support related to childbirth trauma
- Reproductive surgery
- Family history of POP
- Young age at first birth

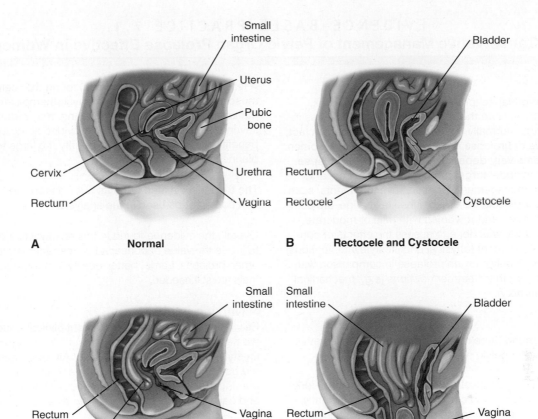

FIGURE 7.1 Types of pelvic prolapses. (**A**) Normal. (**B**) Rectocele and cystocele. (**C**) Enterocele.
(**D**) Uterine prolapse.

- Connective tissue disorders
- Infant birthweight of more than 4,500 g
- Pelvic radiation
- Increased abdominal pressure secondary to:
  - Lifting of children or heavy objects
  - Straining due to chronic constipation
  - Respiratory problems or chronic coughing
  - Obesity (Jelovsek, Maher, & Barber, 2007)

Therapeutic Management

Treatment options for POP depend on the symptoms and their effect on the woman's quality of life. Important considerations when deciding on nonsurgical or surgical options include the severity of symptoms, the woman's preferences, the woman's health status, age, and suitability for surgery, and the presence of other pelvic conditions (urinary or fecal incontinence). When surgery is being considered, the nature of the procedure and the likely outcome must be fully explained and discussed with the woman and her partner. Treatment options

for POP include Kegel exercises, estrogen replacement therapy, dietary and lifestyle modifications, use of pessaries or the Colpexin Sphere, and surgery (see Evidence-Based Practice 7.1).

Kegel Exercises

Kegel exercises strengthen the pelvic floor muscles to support the inner organs and prevent further prolapse. The purpose of pelvic floor exercises is to increase the muscle volume, which will result in a stronger muscular contraction. Kegel exercises might limit the progression of mild prolapse and alleviate mild prolapse symptoms, including low back pain and pelvic pressure. They will not, however, help severe uterine prolapse.

Hormone Replacement Therapy

Hormone replacement therapy (orally, transdermally, or vaginally) may improve the tone and vascularity of the supporting tissue in perimenopausal and menopausal women by increasing blood perfusion and the elasticity of the vaginal wall.

EVIDENCE-BASED PRACTICE 7.1
Is Conservative Management of Pelvic Organ Prolapse Effective in Women?

● Study

Pelvic organ prolapse (protrusion of the uterus, cervix, bladder, or bowel into the vagina because of weakness in the tissues that normally support them) is common; in fact, some degree of prolapse is seen in 50% of parous women. The symptoms vary depending on the type of prolapse. Treatments include surgery, mechanical devices, and conservative management. Conservative treatments, such as pelvic floor muscle training or lifestyle change, are commonly recommended for women with mild or moderate prolapse. A study was done to assess the effects of conservative management (physical and lifestyle interventions) for women with pelvic organ prolapse in comparison with no treatment or other treatment options (e.g., mechanical devices or surgery).

▲ Findings

This review found three randomized trials of conservative management for pelvic organ prolapse.

One relatively large trial of an exercise program for elderly Thai women living in the community was not sufficiently well conducted or reported to provide reliable findings.

A feasibility study (n = 47 women) found that pelvic floor muscle training, delivered by a physiotherapist to symptomatic women in an outpatient setting, may reduce the severity of prolapse. The study provided some evidence of benefit, which was sufficient to justify the large trial that is planned to follow it.

The third trial claimed benefits but was reported in a way that could not be used in the analysis.

Overall, the evidence found in this review was not sufficient to judge the value of conservative management of pelvic organ prolapse. Large, better-quality, randomized controlled trials are still needed.

■ Nursing Implications

Pelvic organ prolapse is a significant clinical issue among women of all ages, and it often results in discomfort, altered lifestyle, and urinary incontinence. Although this review did not identify a clear-cut first-line treatment, nurses can continue to stress lifestyle changes such as weight loss and daily pelvic floor strengthening exercises to improve the client's quality of life.

Hagen, S., Stark, D., Maher. C., & Adams, E. (2006). Conservative management of pelvic organ prolapse in women. *Cochrane Database of Systematic Reviews* 2006, Issue 4. Art. No.: CD003882. DOI: 10.1002/14651858.CD003882.pub3.

▶ *Take* NOTE!

Before hormone therapy is considered, a thorough medical history must be taken to assess her risk for complications (e.g., endometrial cancer, myocardial infarction, stroke, breast cancer, pulmonary emboli, and deep vein thrombosis). Because of these risks, estrogens, with or without progestins, should be given at the lowest effective dose and for the shortest duration consistent with the treatment goals and risks for the individual woman (ACOG, 2007).

Dietary and Lifestyle Modifications

Dietary and lifestyle modifications may help prevent pelvic relaxation and chronic problems later in life. Dietary habits can exacerbate the prolapse by causing constipation and consequently chronic straining. The stools of a constipated woman are hard and dry, and typically she must strain while bearing down to defecate. This straining to pass a hard stool increases intra-abdominal pressure, which over time causes the pelvic organs to prolapse. Dietary mod-

ifications can help to establish regular bowel movements without discomfort and eliminate flatus and bloating.

Pessaries

A **pessary** is a silicone or plastic device that is placed into the vagina to support the uterus, bladder, and rectum as a space-filling device, replacing normal pressure on the vaginal walls when levator ani support is unreliable (Fig. 7.2). Although there are many types and shapes, the most commonly used pessary is a firm ring that presses against the wall of the vagina and urethra to help decrease leakage and support a prolapsed vagina or uterus. Pessaries are of two main types:

• Support pessaries, which rest under the symphysis and sacrum and elevate the vagina (e.g., Ring, Gehrung, and Hodge pessaries)
• Space-occupying pessaries, which are designed to manage severe prolapse by supporting the uterus even with a lack of vaginal tone (e.g., cube, doughnut, and inflatable Gellhorn pessaries)

Indications for pessary use include uterine prolapse or cystocele, especially among elderly clients for whom surgery is contraindicated; younger women with prolapse

they do not allow for concomitant strengthening of pelvic floor musculature and they do not reduce urine leakage (Smith, 2007). The Colpexin Sphere is a polycarbonate sphere with a locator string that is fitted above the hymenal ring to support the pelvic floor muscle. The sphere is used in conjunction with pelvic floor muscle exercises, which should be performed daily.

Surgical Interventions

Surgical interventions for genital organ prolapse are designed to correct specific defects, with the goals being to restore normal anatomy and to preserve function (ACOG, 2007). Surgery is not an option for all women. Women who are at high risk of suffering recurrent prolapse after a surgical repair or who have morbid obesity, chronic obstructive pulmonary disease, or medical conditions in which general anesthesia would be risky are not good candidates for surgical repair (Bartoletti, 2007), and noninvasive treatment strategies should be discussed with them.

Surgical interventions might include anterior or posterior colporrhaphy (to repair a cystocele or rectocele) and vaginal hysterectomy (for uterine prolapse).

An anterior and posterior colporrhaphy may be effective for a first-degree prolapse. This surgical procedure tightens the anterior and posterior vaginal wall, thus repairing a cystocele or rectocele. The pubocervical fascia (supportive tissue between the vagina and bladder) is folded and sutured to bring the bladder and urethra in proper position (Lazarou & Scotti, 2007).

A vaginal hysterectomy is the treatment of choice for uterine prolapse because it removes the prolapsed organ that is bringing down the bladder and rectum with it. It can be combined with an anterior and posterior repair if a cystocele or rectocele is present.

Nursing Assessment

Nursing assessment for women with POP includes a thorough health history and physical examination and several laboratory and diagnostic tests.

Health History and Clinical Manifestations

The cause of prolapse is multifactorial, with vaginal childbirth, advancing age, and increasing body mass index as the most consistent risk factors (Jelovsek, Maher, & Barber, 2007). Assessment of risk factors (chronic straining, hysterectomy, normal aging, and abnormalities of connective tissue) in the woman's history will assist the health care provider in the diagnosis and treatment of POP. The history should include questions about:

- The woman's obstetrical history (number of pregnancies, weight of newborns, pregnancy spacing)
- Chronic respiratory condition (chronic coughing)
- Menopausal status
- Weight history (loss or gain)

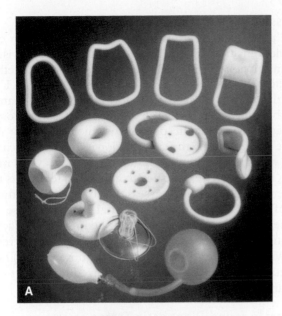

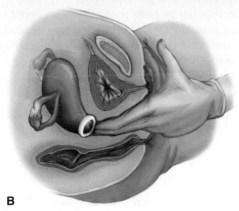

FIGURE 7.2 Examples of pessaries. (**A**) Various shapes and sizes of pessaries available. (**B**) Insertion of one type of pessary.

who plan to have additional children; and women with marked prolapse who prefer to use a pessary rather than undergo surgery (Newman, 2007). Many women use pessaries for only a short period of time and become free of symptoms. Long-term use can lead to pressure necrosis in some women; in this situation other methods of support should be explored.

Pessaries are fitted by trial and error; the woman often needs to try several sizes or styles. The largest pessary that the woman can wear comfortably is generally the most effective. The woman should be instructed to report any discomfort or difficulty with urination or defecation while wearing the pessary.

Colpexin Sphere

A new intravaginal device, the Colpexin Sphere, which became available in 2006, supports the pelvic floor muscle and facilitates rehabilitation of the pelvic floor muscles. Although pessaries may support a prolapsed pelvic organ,

- Constipation (frequency and chronicity)
- Age
- Family history (family member with POP)
- Urinary incontinence
- Previous pelvic surgeries

Assess for clinical manifestations of POP. POP is often asymptomatic, but when symptoms do occur, they are often related to the site and type of prolapse. Symptoms common to all types of prolapses are a feeling of dragging, a lump in the vagina, or something "coming down." Women with POP can present either with one symptom, such as vaginal bulging or pelvic pressure, or with several complaints, including many bladder, bowel, and pelvic symptoms. Symptoms associated with POP are summarized in Box 7.1.

Women present with varying degrees of descent. Uterine prolapse is the most troubling type of pelvic relaxation because it is often associated with concomitant defects of the vagina in the anterior, posterior, and lateral compartments (Lazarou & Scotti, 2007).

BOX 7.1 **Symptoms Associated With Pelvic Organ Prolapse**

- Urinary symptoms
  - Stress incontinence
  - Frequency (diurnal and nocturnal)
  - Urgency and urge incontinence
  - Hesitancy
  - Poor or prolonged stream
  - Feeling of incomplete emptying
- Bowel symptoms
  - Difficulty in defecation
  - Incontinence of flatus or liquid or solid stool
  - Urgency of defecation
  - Feeling of incomplete evacuation
  - Rectal protrusion or prolapse after defecation
- Sexual symptoms
  - Inability to have frequent intercourse
  - Dyspareunia
  - Lack of satisfaction or orgasm
  - Incontinence during sexual activity
- Other local symptoms
  - Pressure or heaviness in the vagina
  - Pain in the vagina or perineum
  - Low back pain after long periods of standing
  - Palpable bulge in the vaginal vault
  - Difficulty walking due to a protrusion from the vagina
  - Difficulty inserting or keeping a tampon in place
  - Vaginal-cervical mucosa hypertrophy, excoriation, ulceration, and bleeding
  - Abdominal pressure or pain (Jelovsek, Maher, & Barber, 2007; Smith, 2007)

Physical Examination

The pelvic examination performed by the health care provider includes an external genital inspection to visualize any obvious protrusion of the uterus, bladder, urethra, or vaginal wall occurring at the vaginal opening. Usually the woman is asked to perform the Valsalva maneuver (bearing down) while the examiner notes which organ prolapses first and the degree to which it occurs. Any urine leakage during the examination is important to note. The woman is asked to contract the pubococcygeal muscles (Kegel exercise); the health care provider inserts two fingers into the vagina to assess the strength and symmetry of the contraction. Since genital organ prolapse can cause urinary symptoms such as incontinence, bladder function should be assessed by determining postvoid residual with a catheter. If the woman has more than 100 mL of retained urine, she should be referred for further urodynamic evaluation and testing.

Laboratory and Diagnostic Tests

Common laboratory tests that may be ordered to determine the cause of POP might include a urinalysis to rule out a bacterial infection, urine culture to identify the specific organism if present, visualization of urine loss during the pelvic examination, and measurement of postvoid urine volume.

Nursing Management

Help the woman understand the nature of the condition, the treatment options, and the likely outcomes. Nursing considerations might include the following:

- Describe normal anatomy and causes of pelvic prolapse.
- Assess how this condition has affected the woman's life.
- Outline the options, with the advantages and disadvantages of each.
- Allow the client to make the decision that is right for her.
- Provide education.
- Schedule preoperative activities needed for surgery.
- Reassure the client that there is a solution for her symptoms.
- Provide community education about genital prolapse.

Nursing Care Plan 7.1 provides an overview of care for a woman with POP.

Encourage Pelvic Floor Muscle Training

Encourage the woman to perform Kegel exercises daily (Teaching Guidelines 7.1). Discuss current research findings and educate the woman about hormone therapy, allowing the woman to make her own decision on whether to use hormones. Controversy still exists regarding the benefits versus the risks of taking hormones, so the woman must weigh this option carefully (Luft, 2006).

Encourage Dietary and Lifestyle Modifications

Instruct clients to increase dietary fiber and fluids to prevent constipation. A high-fiber diet with an increase in

Nursing Care Plan 7.1

OVERVIEW OF A WOMAN WITH PELVIC ORGAN PROLAPSE (POP)

Katherine, a 62-year-old multiparous woman, came to her gynecologist with complaints of a chronic dragging or heavy painful feeling in her pelvis, lower backache, constipation, and urine leakage. Her symptoms increase when she stands for long periods. She hasn't had menstrual cycles for at least a decade. She tells you, "I'm not taking any of those menopausal hormones."

NURSING DIAGNOSIS: Pain related to relaxation of pelvic support and elimination difficulties

Outcome Identification and Evaluation

Client will report an acceptable level of discomfort within 1 to 2 hours of intervention as evidenced by a rating of less than 4 on a 0-to-10 pain scale.

Interventions: Providing Pain Management

- Obtain a thorough pain history, including ongoing pain experiences, methods of pain control used, what worked, what didn't, any allergies to pain medications, and the effect of pain on her activities of daily living *to provide a baseline and enable a systematic approach to pain management.*
- Assess the location, frequency, severity, duration, precipitating factors, and aggravating/alleviating factors *to identify characteristics of the client's pain to plan appropriate interventions.*
- Educate client about any medications prescribed (correct dosage, route, side effects, and precautions) *to increase the client's understanding of the therapy and promote compliance.*
- Assess problematic elimination patterns *to identify underlying factors from which to plan appropriate prevention strategies.*
- Encourage client to increase fluids and fiber in diet and increase physical activity daily *to promote peristalsis.*
- Assist client with establishing regular toileting patterns by setting aside time daily for bowel elimination *to promote regular bowel function and evacuation.*
- Urge client to avoid the routine use of laxatives *to reduce risk of compounding constipation.*

NURSING DIAGNOSIS: Knowledge deficit related to causes of structural disorders and treatment options

Outcome Identification and Evaluation

Client will demonstrate understanding of current condition and treatments as evidenced by identifying treatment options, making health-promoting lifestyle choices, verbalizing appropriate health care practices, and adhering to treatment plan.

Interventions: Provide Client Education

- Assess client's understanding of pelvic organ prolapse and its treatment options *to provide a baseline for teaching.*
- Review information provided about surgical procedures and recommendations for healthy lifestyle, obtaining feedback frequently, *to validate client's understanding of instructions.*
- Discuss association between uterine, bladder, and rectal prolapse and symptoms *to help client understand the etiology of her symptoms and pain.*
- Have client verbalize and discuss information related to diagnosis, surgical procedure, preoperative routine, and post-operative regimen *to ensure adequate understanding and provide time for correcting or clarifying any misinformation or misconceptions.*
- Provide written material with pictures *to promote learning and help client visualize what has occurred to her body secondary to aging, weight gain, childbirth, and gravity.*
- Discuss pros and cons of hormone replacement therapy, osteoporosis prevention, and cardiovascular events common in postmenopausal women *to promote informed decision making by the client about available menopausal therapies.*
- Inform client about the availability of community resources and make appropriate referrals as needed *to provide additional education and support.*
- Document details of teaching and learning *to allow for continuity of care and further education, if needed.*

TEACHING GUIDELINES 7.1

Performing Kegel Exercises

- Squeeze the muscles in your rectum as if you are trying to prevent passing flatus.
- Stop and start urinary flow to help identify the pubococcygeus muscle.
- Tighten the pubococcygeus muscle for a count of three, and then relax it.
- Contract and relax the pubococcygeus muscle rapidly 10 times.
- Try to bring up the entire pelvic floor and bear down 10 times.
- Repeat Kegel exercises at least five times daily.

fluid intake alleviates constipation by increasing stool bulk and stimulating peristalsis. It is accomplished by replacing refined, low-fiber foods with high-fiber foods. The recommended daily intake of fiber for women is 25 g (Dudek, 2006). In addition to increasing the amount of fiber in her diet, also encourage the woman to drink eight 8-oz glasses of fluid daily and to engage in regular aerobic exercise, which promotes muscle tone and stimulates peristalsis.

Educate the client about other lifestyle changes that will assist with prolapse, such as:

- Achieve ideal weight to reduce intra-abdominal pressure and strain on pelvic organs, including pressure on the bladder.
- Wear a girdle or abdominal support to support the muscles surrounding the pelvic organs.
- Avoid lifting heavy objects to reduce the risk of increasing intra-abdominal pressure, which can push the pelvic organs downward.
- Avoid high-impact aerobics, jogging, or jumping repeatedly to minimize the risk of increasing intra-abdominal pressure, which places downward pressure on the organs.
- Give up smoking to minimize the risk for a chronic "smoker's cough," which increases intra-abdominal pressure and forces the pelvic organs downward.

Provide Teaching for Pessary Use

Educate the woman about pessary use. Discuss complications as part of the instruction. Although the pessary is a safe device, it is still a foreign body in the vagina. Because of this, the most common side effects of the pessary are increased vaginal discharge, urinary tract infections, vaginitis, and odor. This can be reduced by douching with dilute vinegar or hydrogen peroxide. Postmenopausal women with thin vaginal mucosa are susceptible to vaginal ulceration with the use of a pessary. Advise the woman to use

estrogen cream to make the vaginal mucosa more resistant to erosion and to strengthen the vaginal walls.

The woman must be capable of managing use of the pessary, either alone or with the help of a caretaker. The most common recommendations for pessary care include removing the pessary twice weekly and cleaning it with soap and water; using a lubricant for insertion; and having regular follow-up examinations every 6 to 12 months after an initial period of adjustment. Educate the woman in the care of her pessary so she feels comfortable with all aspects of care before leaving the health care facility.

Provide Perioperative Care

Prepare the woman for surgery by reinforcing the risks and benefits of surgery and describing the postoperative course. Explain that a Foley catheter will be in place for up to 1 week, and that she might not be able to urinate due to the swelling after the catheter has been removed. Provide home care instructions for the Foley catheter. She should cleanse the perineal area daily with mild soap and water, especially around where the catheter enters the urinary meatus. If the woman is provided with a leg bag to be worn during waking hours, instruct her to empty it frequently and keep it below the level of the bladder to prevent backflow. The same principles are applied to the primary Foley bag when emptying.

During the recovery period, instruct the client to avoid for several weeks activities that cause an increase in abdominal pressure, such as straining, sneezing, and coughing. In addition, advise her to avoid lifting anything heavy or straining to push anything. Explain to the woman that stool softeners and gentle laxatives might be prescribed to prevent constipation and straining with bowel movements. Pelvic rest will be prescribed until the operative area is healed in 6 weeks.

Promote Prevention Strategies

Limited data are available on ways to prevent POP. Approaches include lifestyle changes that reduce modifiable risk factors, such as losing weight, avoiding heavy lifting, and relieving constipation. Explore with the woman what factors in her lifestyle might be modified to reduce her risk of developing POP (primary prevention), or improve her quality of life after receiving treatment (secondary prevention).

▶ URINARY INCONTINENCE

Urinary incontinence is the involuntary loss of urine sufficient enough to be a social or hygiene problem (Reena, Kekre, & Kekre, 2007). This disorder affects approximately 25 million people in the United States, about 12 million of them women (Berzuk, 2007). It has been estimated that one in four women experience urinary incontinence at some time in their life, varying in severity from mild to severe (Selby, 2006). It is more common than diabetes and Alzheimer's disease, both of which receive a great deal of press attention. About half the women with incontinence have never discussed the problem with their health care provider because they feel ashamed, embarrassed, guilty, or lacking control (Wallace, 2007).

▶ *Take* NOTE!

Incontinence is preventable, treatable, and often curable. However, many women believe that loss of bladder function is a normal and expected part of aging.

Incontinence can have far-reaching effects. Some women experience anxiety, depression, social isolation, and disruptions in their self-esteem and dignity. It can cause the woman to stop working, traveling, socializing, and enjoying sexual relationships. In addition, incontinence can create a tremendous burden for caretakers and is a common reason for admission to a long-term care facility (Lemack, 2007).

The three most common types of incontinence are urge incontinence (overactive bladder caused by detrusor muscle contractions), stress incontinence (inadequate urinary sphincter function), and mixed incontinence (involves both stress and urge incontinence) (Ogundele & Silverberg, 2007). Comparison Chart 7.1 details these types.

Pathophysiology and Etiology

Urinary continence requires several factors, including effective functioning of the bladder, adequate pelvic floor muscles, neural control from the brain, and integrity of the neural connections that facilitate voluntary control.

The bladder neck and proximal urethra function as a sphincter. During urination the sphincter relaxes and the bladder empties. The ability to control urination requires the integrated function of numerous components of the lower urinary tract, which must be structurally sound and function normally. Incontinence can develop if the bladder muscles become overactive due to weakened sphincter muscles, if the bladder muscles become too weak to contract properly, or if signals from the nervous system to the urinary structures are interrupted. A major factor in women that contributes to urinary continence is the estrogen level, because this hormone helps maintain bladder sphincter tone. In perimenopausal or menopausal women, incontinence can be a problem as estrogen levels begin to decline and genitourinary changes occur. In simple terms, the bladder is the reservoir, the urethra is the seal, and the levator ani muscle is the gate that holds pressure against the outflow of urine by supporting the urethra and bladder from below. When there is a dysfunction of any of the three structures, incontinence occurs.

Contributing factors in urinary incontinence include:

• Fluid intake, especially alcohol, carbonated drinks, and caffeinated beverages
• Constipation: alters the position of the pelvic organs and puts pressure on the bladder
• Habitual "preventive" emptying: may result in training the bladder to hold only small amounts of urine
• Advancing age: age-related anatomic changes provide less pelvic support
• Pregnancy and childbirth: damage to pelvic structures during childbirth
• Obesity: increases abdominal pressure (Hines & Miller, 2006)

Therapeutic Management

Treatment options depend on the type of urinary incontinence. In general, the least invasive procedure with the

---

COMPARISON CHART 7.1   Urge Incontinence vs. Stress Incontinence

	Urge Incontinence	Stress Incontinence
Description	Precipitous loss of urine, preceded by a strong urge to void, with increased bladder pressure and detrusor contraction	Accidental leakage of urine that occurs with increased pressure on the bladder from coughing, sneezing, laughing, or physical exertion
Etiology	Causes might be neurologic, idiopathic, or infectious	Develops commonly in women in their 40s and 50s, usually as the result of weakened muscles and ligaments in the pelvis following childbirth
Signs and Symptoms	Urgency, frequency, nocturia, and a large amount of urine loss	Involuntary loss of a small amount of urine in response to physical activity that raises intra-abdominal pressure

fewest risks is the first choice for treatment. Surgery is used only if other methods have failed. There is a widespread belief that urinary incontinence is an inevitable problem of getting older and that little or nothing can be done to relieve symptoms or reverse it. Nothing is further from the truth, and attitudes must change so that women feel comfortable seeking help for this embarrassing condition.

For many women with urge incontinence, simple reassurance and lifestyle interventions might help. However, if more than simple lifestyle measures are needed, effective treatments might include:

- Bladder training to establish normal voiding intervals (every 3 to 5 hours)
- Kegel exercises to strengthen the pelvic floor musculature
- Pessary ring to support pelvic structures that have weakened
- Pharmacotherapy to reduce the urge to void. Anticholinergic agents such as oxybutynin (Ditropan) or tolterodine (Detrol) might be prescribed. The most common side effects of anticholinergic agents are dry mouth, blurred vision, constipation, nausea, dizziness, and headaches (Lemack, 2007).

For women with stress incontinence, treatment is not always a cure, but it can minimize the impact of this condition on the woman's quality of life. Some treatment options for stress incontinence might include:

- Weight loss if needed
- Avoidance of constipation
- Smoking cessation
- Kegel exercises to strengthen the pelvic floor
- Pessaries
- Weighted vaginal cones to improve the tone of pelvic floor muscles
- Periurethral injection (injecting a bulking agent [collagen] to form a bulge that brings the urethral walls closer together to achieve a better closure)
- Medications such as duloxetine (Cymbalta, Yentreve) to increase urethral sphincter contractions during the storage phase of the urination cycle
- Estrogen replacement therapy to improve bladder sphincter tone
- Surgery to correct genital prolapse and improve urethral and bladder tone

Nursing Assessment

The assessment of the incontinent woman includes a history, physical examination, laboratory tests, and possibly urodynamic testing. The onset, frequency, severity, and pattern of incontinence should be determined, as well as any associated symptoms such as frequency, dysuria, urgency, and nocturia. Incontinence may be quantified by asking the woman if she wears a pad and how often the pad is changed. A review of the woman's current medica-

tions, including over-the-counter medications, should be included in the history.

A complete physical examination should be carried out by the health care provider; it should include a neurologic assessment and pelvic and rectal examinations. The presence of associated POP should be noted because it can contribute to the woman's voiding problems and may have an impact on diagnosis and treatment. A rectal examination is done to evaluate sphincter tone and perineal sensation.

A urinalysis is performed to look for hematuria, pyuria, glucosuria, or proteinuria. A urine culture is done if there is pyuria or bacteriuria. Postvoid residual should be measured either with pelvic ultrasound or directly with a catheter. If the residual exceeds the limit set, urodynamic testing is then used to diagnose the incontinence.

Nursing Management

Incontinence can be devastating and can cause psychosocial concerns and isolation. Nurses can encourage women with troublesome symptoms to seek help. Discuss the treatment options with the client, including benefits and potential outcomes, and encourage her to select the continence treatment best for her lifestyle. Provide education about good bladder habits and strategies to reduce the incidence or severity of incontinence (Teaching Guidelines 7.2). Provide support and encouragement to ensure compliance. Remember that aging can increase the risk of incontinence,

TEACHING GUIDELINES 7.2

Managing Urinary Incontinence

- Avoid drinking too much fluid (i.e., 1.5 L total daily limit), but do not decrease your intake of fluids.
- Reduce intake of fluids and foods that are bladder irritants and precipitate urgency, such as chocolate, caffeine, sodas, alcohol, artificial sweetener, hot spicy foods, orange juice, tomatoes, and watermelon (Lemack, 2007).
- Increase fiber and fluids in your diet to reduce constipation.
- Control blood glucose levels to prevent polyuria.
- Treat chronic cough.
- Remove any barriers that delay you from reaching the toilet.
- Practice good perineal hygiene by using mild soap and water. Wipe from front to back to prevent urinary tract infections.
- Become aware of adverse drug effects.
- Take your medications as prescribed.
- Continue to do pelvic floor (Kegel) exercises.

but incontinence is not an inevitable part of aging. Review the anatomy and physiology of the urinary system and offer simple explanations to help the woman cope with urinary alterations. Therapeutic listening is important. Be aware of the courage it takes for a woman to disclose an embarrassing condition.

▶ *Consider* THIS!

Life can be complicated and embarrassing at times when we least expect it. I met a man in church who seemed interested in me, and he asked me out for coffee after Sunday services. I have been alone for 10 years and this prospect seemed exciting to me. We talked for hours over coffee and seemed to have a great deal in common, especially since both of us had lost our spouses to cancer. He asked me to go square dancing with him, since that was an activity we both had enjoyed in the past with our spouses. I hadn't been out or physically active for ages and didn't realize how my body had changed with age.

It was during the first dance that I noticed a wet sensation between my legs, which I was unable to control. I managed to continue on and pretend that all was fine, but then realized what many of my friends were talking about—stress incontinence. Not being able to control one's urine is very embarrassing and it complicates your life, but I made up my mind that it wasn't going to control me!

Thoughts: Gravity and childbirth take a toll on women's reproductive organs by bringing them downward. This woman is not going to let stress incontinence curtail her outside activity, which demonstrates a good attitude. What can be done about her embarrassing accidents? Were there any preventive strategies she could have used at an earlier age?

▶ *Take* NOTE!

Simple diet and lifestyle alterations, combined with a proper pelvic floor muscle strengthening program, can often produce significant improvements for women of all ages.

Benign Growths

The most common benign growths of the reproductive tract include cervical, endocervical, and endometrial polyps; uterine fibroids (leiomyomas); ovarian cysts; genital fistulas; and Bartholin's cysts.

▶ POLYPS

Polyps are small benign growths. The cause of polyp growth is not well understood, but they are frequently the result of infection. Polyps might be associated with chronic inflammation, an abnormal local response to increased levels of estrogen, or local congestion of the cervical vasculature (Kaminski & Hoffman, 2007). Single or multiple polyps might occur. They are most common in multiparous women. Polyps can appear anywhere but are most common on the cervix and in the uterus (Fig. 7.3).

Cervical polyps often appear after menarche. They occur in 2% to 5% of women, and approximately 2% of these polyps have cancerous changes (Verga, 2006). Endocervical polyps are commonly found in multiparous women age 40 to 60. Endocervical polyps are more common than cervical polyps, with a stalk of varied width and length. Endometrial polyps are benign tumors or localized overgrowths of the endometrium. Most endometrial polyps are solitary, and they rarely occur in women younger than 20 years of age. The incidence of these polyps rises steadily with increasing age, peaks in the fifth decade of life, and gradually declines after menopause. They are present in up to 25% of women being seen for abnormal bleeding (Verga, 2006).

Therapeutic Management

Treatment of polyps usually consists of simple removal with small forceps done on an outpatient basis, removal during hysteroscopy, or dilatation and curettage (D&C). The polyp base can be removed by laser vaporization. Because many polyps are infected, an antibiotic may be

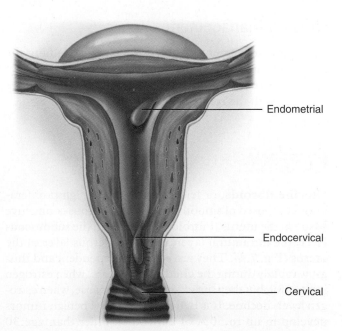

FIGURE 7.3 Cervical, endocervical, and endometrial polyps.

ordered after removal as a preventive measure or to treat early signs of infection.

Although polyps are rarely cancerous, a specimen should be sent after surgery to a pathology laboratory to exclude malignancy. A cervical biopsy typically reveals mildly atypical cells and signs of infection. Polyps rarely return after they are removed. Regularly scheduled Pap smears are suggested for women with cervical polyps to detect any future abnormal growths that may be malignant.

Nursing Assessment

Nursing assessment for a woman with polyps includes assisting with the physical examination and preparing the collected specimen to be sent to the cytologist.

Clinical Manifestations

Assess for clinical manifestations of polyps. Most endocervical polyps are cherry red, while most cervical polyps are grayish-white (Verga, 2006). Cervical and endocervical polyps are often asymptomatic, but they can produce mild symptoms such as abnormal vaginal bleeding (after intercourse or douching, between menses) or discharge. The most common clinical manifestation of endometrial polyps is metrorrhagia (irregular, acyclic uterine bleeding).

Physical Examination and Laboratory and Diagnostic Studies

Typically, cervical polyps are diagnosed when the cervix is visualized through a speculum during the woman's annual gynecologic examination (Kaminski & Hoffman, 2007). Endometrial polyps are not detected on physical examination, but rather with ultrasound or hysteroscopy (introduction of a small camera through the cervix to visualize the uterine cavity).

Nursing Management

Nursing management of polyps involves explaining the condition and the rationale for removal and giving follow-up care instructions. The nurse also assists the health care provider with the removal procedure.

▶ UTERINE FIBROIDS

Uterine fibroids, or leiomyomas, are benign proliferations composed of smooth muscle and fibrous connective tissue in the uterus. Fibroids can occur in the submucous layer, the intramural layer, or the subserous layer of the uterus (Fig. 7.4). They are estrogen-dependent and thus grow rapidly during the childbearing years, when estrogen is plentiful, but they shrink during menopause, when estrogen levels decline. It is believed that these benign tumors develop in up to 50% of all women older than age 30 (Thomason, 2007). Fibroids are the most common indi-

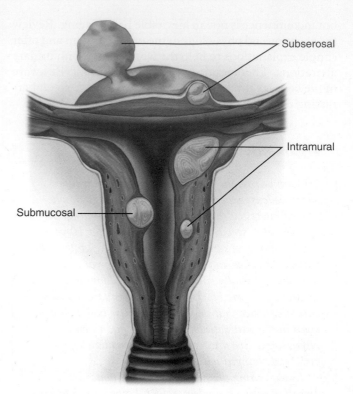

FIGURE 7.4 Submucosal, intramural, and subserosal fibroids.

cation for hysterectomy in the United States. The peak incidence occurs around the age of 45, and they are two to three times more prevalent in African-American women (Verga, 2006).

Etiology

Although the cause of fibroids is unknown, several predisposing factors have been identified, including:

• Age (late reproductive years)
• Genetic predisposition
• African-American ethnicity
• Nulliparity
• Obesity (Alexander et al., 2007)

Therapeutic Management

Treatment depends on the size of the fibroids and the woman's symptoms. There are several options, from watchful waiting to surgery.

Medical Management

The goals of medical therapy are to reduce symptoms and to reduce the tumor size. This can be accomplished with gonadotropin-releasing hormone (GnRH) agonists such as Lupron (leuprolide), Synarel (nafarelin), or Zoladex (goserelin), which induce reversible menopause, or low-dose mifepristone, a progestin antagonist. Both have produced regression and reduced the size of the tumors without surgery, but long-term therapy is expensive and not tolerated by most women. The side effects of GnRH medications include hot flashes, headaches, mood changes, vaginal dryness, musculoskeletal malaise, bone loss, and depression (Thomason, 2007). Long-term mifepristone therapy can result in endometrial hyperplasia, which increases the risk of endometrial malignancy. Once either therapy is stopped, the fibroids typically recur.

Uterine artery embolization (UAE) is an option in which polyvinyl alcohol pellets are injected into selected blood vessels via a catheter to block circulation to the fibroid, causing it to shrink and producing symptom resolution. After treatment, most fibroids are reduced by 50% within 3 months, but they might recur (Edwards et al., 2007). The failure rate is approximately 10% to 15%, and this therapy should not be performed on women desiring to retain their fertility.

Surgical Management

For women with large fibroids or severe menorrhagia, surgery is preferred over medical treatment. Surgical management might involve myomectomy, laser surgery, or hysterectomy.

Myomectomy involves removing the fibroid alone. A myomectomy is performed via laparoscopy, through an abdominal incision, or through a vaginal approach. The advantage is that only the fibroid is removed; fertility is not jeopardized because this procedure leaves the uterine muscle walls intact. Myomectomy relieves symptoms but does not affect the underlying process; thus, fibroids grow back and further treatment will be needed in the future.

Laser surgery (or electrocauterization) involves destroying small fibroids with lasers. Laser therapy can be done using a vaginal approach or laparoscopically. The laser treatment preserves the uterus, but the process may cause scarring and adhesions, thus impairing fertility (Verga, 2006). Fibroids can return after this procedure. Controversy remains as to whether laser treatment weakens the uterine wall and thus may contribute to uterine rupture in the future.

A hysterectomy is the surgical removal of the uterus. After cesarean section, it is the second most frequently performed surgical procedure for women in the United States. Approximately 600,000 hysterectomies are performed annually in the United States (CDC, 2007). The top three conditions associated with hysterectomies are fibroids, endometriosis, and uterine prolapse (CDC, 2007). A hysterectomy to remove fibroids eliminates both the symptoms and the risk of recurrence, but it also terminates the woman's ability to bear children. Three types of hysterectomy surgeries are available: vaginal hysterectomy, laparoscopically assisted vaginal hysterectomy, and abdominal hysterectomy.

In a vaginal hysterectomy, the uterus is removed through an incision in the posterior vagina. Advantages include a shorter hospital stay and recovery time and no abdominal scars. Disadvantages include a limited operating space and poor visualization of other pelvic organs.

In a laparoscopically assisted vaginal hysterectomy, the uterus is removed through a laparoscope, through which structures within the abdomen and pelvis are visualized. Small incisions are made in the abdominal wall to permit the laparoscope to enter the surgical site. Advantages include a better surgical field, less pain, lower cost, and a shorter recovery time. Disadvantages include potential injury to the bladder and the inability to remove enlarged uteruses and scar tissue.

In abdominal hysterectomy, the uterus and other pelvic organs are removed through an incision in the abdomen. This procedure allows the surgeon to visualize all pelvic organs and is typically used when a malignancy is suspected or a very large uterus is present. Disadvantages include the need for general anesthesia, a longer hospital stay and recovery period, more pain, higher cost, and a visible scar on the abdomen.

Nursing Assessment

Nursing assessment for the woman with uterine fibroids includes a thorough health history and physical examination.

Health History and Clinical Manifestations

The history should include questions about the woman's menstrual cycle, including alterations in the menstrual pattern (e.g., pain or pressure, aggravating and alleviating factors), history of infertility, and any history of spontaneous abortion, which might indicate a space-occupying uterine lesion. Ask if any female relatives have had fibroids, as there is a familial predisposition. Assess for clinical manifestations of uterine fibroids. Symptoms of fibroids depend on their size and location and may include:

• Chronic pelvic pain
• Low back pain
• Iron deficiency anemia secondary to bleeding
• Bloating
• Infertility (with large tumors)
• Dysmenorrhea
• Dyspareunia
• Urinary frequency, urgency, incontinence
• Irregular vaginal bleeding (menorrhagia)
• Feeling of heaviness in the pelvic region

Physical Examination and Laboratory and Diagnostic Studies

The bimanual examination performed by the health care provider typically shows an enlarged, irregular uterus. The uterus may be palpable abdominally if the fibroid is very large. Ultrasound may be used to confirm the diagnosis.

Nursing Management

Provide information about surgery so the woman can make an informed decision. Offer a thorough explanation of the

---

BOX 7.2 **Nursing Interventions for a Woman Undergoing a Hysterectomy**

Preoperative Care
- Instruct the patient and her family about the procedure and aftercare.
- Provide interventions to reduce anxiety (due to perceived threats to the woman's self-concept and role functioning) and fear of alteration in body image, complications, and pain. Prepare the woman so she knows what to expect throughout her perioperative experience. Explain postoperative pain management procedures that will be used. Identify the high-risk woman early to reduce her stress.
- Teach turning, deep breathing, and coughing before surgery to prevent postoperative atelectasis and respiratory complications such as pneumonia.
- Encourage the woman to discuss her feelings. Some women equate their femaleness with their reproductive capability, and loss of the uterus could evoke grieving.
- Complete all preoperative orders in a timely manner to allow for rest.

Postoperative Care
- Provide comfort measures.
- Administer analgesics promptly or use a PCA pump.
- Administer antiemetics to control nausea and vomiting per order.
- Change the client's linens and gown frequently to promote hygiene.
- Change the client's position frequently and use pillows for support to promote comfort and pain management.
- Assess the incision, the dressing, and vaginal bleeding and report if bleeding is excessive (soaking perineal pad within an hour).

- Monitor elimination and provide increased fluids and fiber to prevent constipation and straining.
- Encourage ambulation and active range-of-motion exercises when in bed to prevent thrombophlebitis and venous stasis.
- Monitor vital signs to detect early complications.
- Be comfortable discussing sexual concerns with the client.

Discharge Planning
- Advise the client to reduce her activity level to avoid fatigue, which might inhibit healing.
- Advise the client to rest when she is tired and to increase her activity level slowly.
- Educate the client on the need for pelvic rest (nothing in the vagina) for 6 weeks.
- Instruct the client to avoid heavy lifting or straining for about 6 weeks to prevent an increase in intra-abdominal pressure, which could weaken her sutures.
- Teach the client the signs and symptoms of infection.
- Advise the woman to take showers instead of tub baths to reduce the risk for infection.
- Encourage the client to eat a healthy diet with increased intake of fluids to prevent dehydration and fluid and electrolyte imbalance.
- Instruct the client to change her perineal pad frequently to prevent infection.
- Explain and schedule follow-up care appointments as needed.
- Provide information about community resources for support/help.

---

procedure and aftercare (Box 7.2). A woman undergoing a hysterectomy for the treatment of fibroids often needs special care.

▶ GENITAL FISTULAS

Genital fistulas are abnormal openings between a genital tract organ and another organ, such as the urinary tract or the gastrointestinal tract. A fistula can result from a congenital anomaly, surgical complications, Bartholin's gland abscesses, radiation, or malignancy, but the majority of fistulas that occur worldwide are related to obstetric trauma (Husain et al., 2007). During normal labor, the bladder is displaced upward into the abdomen and the anterior vaginal wall, the base of the bladder, and the urethra are compressed between the fetal head and the posterior pubis. When labor is obstructed or prolonged, this unrelieved compression causes ischemia, which causes pressure necrosis and subsequent fistula formation.

Common types of fistulas include:

- Vesicovaginal: communication between the bladder and genital tract
- Urethrovaginal: communication between the urethra and the vagina
- Rectovaginal: communication between the rectum or sigmoid colon and the vagina

The direct consequences of this damage include urinary incontinence and fecal incontinence if the rectum is involved. This tragic condition has plagued women since the beginning of history (Hamilton, Spencer, & Evans, 2007).

Therapeutic Management

Many small fistulas will heal without treatment, but large fistulas often require surgical repair; surgery may be postponed until the edema or inflammation in the surrounding tissues has dissipated. Surgical repair of fistulas is associated with a high success rate if it is done in a timely manner, but larger fistulas and those of long duration have a poorer prognosis (Kriplani et al., 2007).

Nursing Assessment

The history should include questions about any changes in the woman's urinary and bowel patterns. Assess for common signs and symptoms of fistulas, which are related to the type of fistula. If the opening involves the rectum, feces and flatus will leak through the vagina. If it involves the bladder, urine will leak from the vagina. Depending on the location and size of the fistula, the woman may or may not experience discomfort. The health care provider can detect these abnormal openings through inspection and palpation during the pelvic examination. Diagnostic or laboratory tests are generally not ordered once this condition is found.

Nursing Management

Provide guidance and support. Offer information to help the woman learn about her condition and, with appropriate intervention, to improve her quality of life. Begin by making sure the woman understands her anatomy and why she is having such symptoms. Provide a thorough explanation of the treatment options so that she can make an informed decision. Be sensitive to the woman's feeling of shame and fear about her incontinence; these feelings may be why she delayed seeking treatment. Address all of the woman's needs, both physical and emotional.

▶ BARTHOLIN'S CYSTS

A Bartholin's cyst is a swollen, fluid-filled, sac-like structure that results when one of the ducts of the Bartholin's gland becomes blocked. The cyst may become infected and an abscess may develop in the gland. The Bartholin's glands are two mucus-secreting glandular structures with duct openings bilaterally at the base of the labia minora near the opening of the vagina that provide lubrication during sexual arousal. Bartholin's cysts are the most common cystic growths in the vulva, affecting approximately 2% of women at some time in their life (Patil, Sultan, & Thakar, 2007).

Therapeutic Management

Treatment can be conservative or surgical depending on the symptoms, the size of the cyst, and whether it is infected or not. Small asymptomatic cysts do not require treatment. Sitz baths along with analgesics are used to reduce discomfort. Antibiotics are prescribed if the gland is infected. The aim of treatment for a cyst or abscess is to create a fistulous tract from the dilated duct to the outside vulva by incision and drainage (I&D). However, cysts or abscesses tend to return if this option is used.

Other treatment options beyond I&D include placement of a Word catheter to prevent closure and to allow drainage and use of a carbon dioxide laser to remove the cyst. After the Word catheter is inserted, the balloon tip is inflated and it is left in place for 4 to 6 weeks. This procedure is a safe and effective alternative to surgery (Haider et al., 2007). Treatment for a pregnant woman with a Bartholin's cyst depends on the severity of the symptoms and whether an infection is present. Surgery may be delayed until after the woman gives birth if there are no symptoms.

Nursing Assessment

Nursing assessment for the woman with a Bartholin's cyst includes a thorough health history and physical examination and laboratory and diagnostic tests.

Health History

The history should include questions about the woman's sexual practices and protective measures used. Assess for common signs and symptoms of Bartholin's cysts. The woman may be asymptomatic if the cyst is small (less than 5 cm) and not infected. If infection is present, symptoms include varying degrees of pain, especially when walking or sitting; unilateral edema; redness around the gland; and dyspareunia. Extensive inflammation may cause systemic symptoms. Abscess formation occurs when the cystic fluid becomes infected. An abscess usually develops rapidly over a 2- to 3-day period and may spontaneously rupture. A history of sudden relief of pain following profuse discharge is highly suggestive of spontaneous rupture (Schuiling & Likis, 2006).

Physical Examination and Laboratory and Diagnostic Studies

The diagnosis of Bartholin's cysts or abscesses is primarily made during a physical examination when a protruding tender labial mass is located. In women over the age of 40, there is an increased risk of malignancy, accounting for 2% to 7% of all invasive vulvar malignancies (Patil, Sultan, & Thakar, 2007). Cultures of the purulent abscess fluid and of the cervix should be obtained for *Neisseria gonorrhea* and *Chlamydia trachomatis* to rule out a sexually transmitted infection.

Nursing Management

Nurses must be aware of and knowledgeable about vulvar cysts and treatment options. The woman may be aware of a vulvar cyst secondary to the pain or may be unaware of it if it is asymptomatic. A Bartholin's cyst may be an incidental finding during a routine pelvic examination. Explain the cause of the cyst and assist with cultures if needed. Provide reassurance and support.

▶ OVARIAN CYSTS

An **ovarian cyst** is a fluid-filled sac that forms on the ovary (Fig. 7.5). These very common growths are benign 90% of the time and are asymptomatic in many women (Hackley, Kriebs, & Rousseau, 2007). Ovarian cysts occur in 30% of women with regular menses, 50% of women with irregular menses, and 6% of postmenopausal women (Verga, 2006). When the cysts grow large and exert pressure on surrounding structures, women often seek medical help.

Types of Ovarian Cysts

The most common benign ovarian cysts are follicular cysts, corpus luteum (lutein) cysts, theca-lutein cysts, and polycystic ovarian syndrome (PCOS).

Follicular Cysts

Follicular cysts are caused by the failure of the ovarian follicle to rupture at the time of ovulation. Follicular cysts seldom grow larger than 5 cm in diameter; most regress and require no treatment. They can occur at any age but are more common in reproductive-aged women and are rare after menopause. They are detected by vaginal ultrasound.

Corpus Luteum (Lutein) Cysts

A corpus luteum cyst forms when the corpus luteum becomes cystic or hemorrhagic and fails to degenerate after 14 days. These cysts might cause pain and delay the next menstrual period. A pelvic ultrasound helps to make this diagnosis. Typically these cysts appear after ovulation and resolve without intervention.

Theca-Lutein Cysts

Prolonged abnormally high levels of human chorionic gonadotropin (hCG) stimulate the development of theca-lutein cysts. Although rare, these cysts are associated with hydatidiform mole, choriocarcinoma, PCOS, and Clomid therapy.

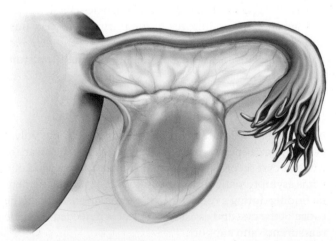

FIGURE 7.5 Ovarian cyst.

Polycystic Ovarian Syndrome

Polycystic ovary syndrome (PCOS) involves the presence of multiple inactive follicle cysts within the ovary that interfere with ovarian function. It is associated with obesity, hyperinsulinemia, elevated luteinizing hormone levels (linked to ovulation), elevated androgen levels (virilization), hirsutism (male-pattern hair growth), follicular atresia (ovarian growth failure), ovarian growth and cyst formation, anovulation (failure to ovulate), and amenorrhea (absence of menstruation or irregular periods). Recent studies also indicate that PCOS is associated with an increase in the risk of uterine fibroids (Wise et al., 2007). It is the most common endocrine disorder in reproductive-age women, affecting 1 in 15 women in the United States (Panidis & Farmakiotis, 2007).

> ▶ ***Take*** NOTE!
>
> *Careful attention should be given to this condition because affected women are at increased risk for long-term health problems such as cardiovascular disease, hypertension, dyslipidemia, type 2 diabetes (half of all women), and cancer (endometrial, breast, and ovarian) (Lorenz & Wild, 2007).*

Initially PCOS was called Stein-Leventhal syndrome after its researchers, but it is now recognized to be an anabolic syndrome (Vignesh & Mohan, 2007). Its etiology is not clearly understood, but studies suggest a genetic (autosomal-dominant) component (Speroff & Mishell, 2007).

Therapeutic Management

Treatment of ovarian cysts focuses on differentiating a benign cyst from a solid ovarian malignancy. Transvaginal ultrasound is useful in distinguishing fluid-filled cysts from solid masses. Laparoscopy may be needed to remove the cyst, if it is large and pressing on surrounding structures. For smaller cysts, monitoring with repeat ultrasounds every 3 to 6 months might be in order (Helm, 2007). Oral contraceptives are often prescribed to suppress gonadotropin levels, which may help resolve the cysts. Pain medication is also prescribed if needed.

Management of PCOS includes both drug and non-drug therapy, along with lifestyle modifications. Goals of therapy focus on reducing the production and circulating levels of androgens, protecting the endometrium against the effects of unopposed estrogens, supporting lifestyle changes to achieve ideal body weight, lowering the risk of cardiovascular disease, avoiding the effects of hyperinsulinemia on the risk of cardiovascular disease and diabetes, and inducing ovulation to achieve pregnancy if desired (see Evidence-Based Practice 7.2). Treatment modalities for PCOS are highlighted in Box 7.3.

EVIDENCE-BASED PRACTICE 7.2
Are Insulin-Sensitizing Drugs More Effective Than the Combined Oral Contraceptive Pill in Minimizing Hirsutism, Acne, Risk of Diabetes, Cardiovascular Disease, and Endometrial Cancer in PCOS?

● Study

Women with polycystic ovary syndrome (PCOS) have excessive hairiness (hirsutism), irregular periods, and acne. They are also at greater risk of developing diabetes, cardiovascular disease, and endometrial cancer. Insulin-sensitizing drugs (ISDs) have recently been advocated as a safer and more effective long-term treatment than the oral contraceptive pill (OCP) in women with PCOS. A study was conducted to assess the effectiveness and safety of ISDs versus the OCP (alone or in combination) in improving clinical, hormonal, and metabolic features of PCOS.

▲ Findings

In women with PCOS, the OCP is more effective than ISDs in improving menstrual pattern and reducing serum androgen (male hormone) levels, whereas the ISD metformin is more effective than the OCP in reducing fasting insulin levels and not increasing triglyceride levels. There is insufficient evidence in favor of either metformin or the OCP in treating hirsutism or acne, or in preventing diabetes, heart disease, or endometrial cancer. The limited data available do not support the preferential use of either ISDs or the OCP (alone or in combination) for the long-term medical management of PCOS.

■ Nursing Implications

Oral contraceptives have been the mainstay of long-term management of PCOS by decreasing LH and FSH secretion and ovarian production of androgens to reduce symptoms. This study compared the ISD metformin to the traditional therapy without conclusive results. PCOS is associated with increased insulin resistance and increased unbound androgen levels. Since this study was inconclusive, nurses can continue to counsel women to improve their lifestyle (e.g., diet, exercise, weight management) to avoid health problems later in life related to diabetes and heart disease.

Costello, M., Shrestha, B., Eden, J., Sjoblom, P., & Johnson, N. (2007). Insulin-sensitizing drugs versus the combined oral contraceptive pill for hirsutism, acne and risk of diabetes, cardiovascular disease, and endometrial cancer in polycystic ovary syndrome. *Cochrane Database of Systematic Reviews* 2007, Issue 1. Art. No.: CD005552. DOI: 10.1002/14651858.CD005552.pub2.

Nursing Assessment

Nursing assessment for the woman with PCOS includes a thorough health history and physical examination and laboratory and diagnostic tests.

Health History

The history should include questions about the woman's symptoms, including onset, location, frequency, quality, intensity, and aggravating and alleviating factors of her discomfort. Note the last menstrual period and whether or not her cycles are regular. Ask about her overall general health and any changes recently noticed, such as a change in abdominal girth without a concomitant weight gain.

Assess for common signs and symptoms of ovarian cysts. Findings might include:

- Hirsutism (face and chin, upper lip, areola, lower abdomen and perineum)
- Alopecia (frontal region and crown of head)
- Virilization (clitoral hypertrophy, deepening of voice, increased muscle mass, breast atrophy, male-pattern baldness)
- Menstrual irregularity and infertility (menorrhagia, anovulation)
- Polycystic ovaries (12 or more follicles on ovaries)
- Obesity (occurs in more than 50% of women with PCOS; occurs in abdominal region, with an increase in the waist–hip ratio)
- Insulin resistance (chronic hyperinsulinemia leads to type 2 diabetes)
- Metabolic syndrome (elevated cholesterol, triglycerides, low-density lipoprotein; risk of cardiovascular disease)
- Increased risk for endometrial cancer, ovarian cancer, breast cancer
- Psychological impact (depression, frustration, anxiety, eating disorders)
- Acne (face and shoulders) (Krantz, 2007)

BOX 7.3 Treatment Modalities for PCOS

- Oral contraceptives to treat menstrual irregularities and acne
- Mechanical hair removal (shaving, waxing, plucking, or electrolysis) to treat hirsutism
- Glucophage (metformin), which improves insulin uptake by fat and muscle cells, to treat hyperinsulinemia; thiazolinediones (Actos, Avandia) to decrease insulin resistance
- Ovulation induction agents (Clomid) to treat infertility
- Lifestyle changes (e.g., weight loss; exercise; balanced, low-fat diet)
- Referral to support groups to help improve emotional state and build self-esteem

Sources: ACOG, 2006; Dronavalli & Ehrmann, 2007; Barron & Falsetti, 2008.

Physical Examination and Laboratory and Diagnostic Studies

The physical examination includes inspection, auscultation, and palpation of the abdomen because large ovarian masses may cause visible changes in the abdomen. A complete pelvic examination is performed to assess the location, size, shape, texture, mobility, and tenderness of any palpable mass.

Diagnostic tests include a pregnancy test to rule out ectopic pregnancy. Gonorrhea and chlamydia testing is warranted if an ovarian abscess is suspected. An ultrasound may be ordered to differentiate between functional or simple ovarian cysts and a solid tumor. Additional tests may be performed depending on the findings.

Remember Liz, the client with irregular menses, facial hair, and acne? Her glucose level is elevated, multiple cysts were felt on her ovaries during the pelvic examination, and laboratory tests found elevated lipid and lipoprotein levels. What education should the nurse provide Liz regarding her PCOS diagnosis? What medications might be prescribed to address her abnormal laboratory values?

Nursing Management

Nursing care should include education about the condition, treatment options, diagnostic test arrangements, and referral for surgery if needed. Provide support and reassurance during the diagnostic period to allay anxiety in the client and her family. Reassure the woman that the majority of ovarian cysts are benign, but regardless stress the importance of follow-up care. Listen to the woman's concerns about her appearance, infertility, and facial hair growth. Offer suggestions to help the woman feel better about herself and her health.

Nurses can have a positive impact on women with PCOS through counseling and education. Provide support for women dealing with negative self-image secondary to the physical manifestations of PCOS. Through education, help the woman understand the syndrome and its associated risk factors to prevent long-term health problems. Encourage the woman to make positive lifestyle changes. Make community referrals to local support groups to help the woman build her coping skills.

Liz returns to the clinic a month later for re-evaluation of her PCOS. She has been taking metformin to reduce her insulin resistance and has followed her exercise regimen and reduced her caloric intake to lose weight, but she still complains about her facial hair and acne. What interventions might be helpful to address this problem? What medication might also be prescribed to regularize her menses and relieve the hirsutism?

■■■ Key Concepts

- Pelvic support disorders such as pelvic organ prolapse and urinary and fecal incontinence are prevalent conditions in aging women. They cause significant physical and psychological morbidity, with obvious detriment to women's social interactions, emotional well-being, and overall quality of life.
- The four most common types of genital prolapse are cystocele, rectocele, enterocele, and uterine prolapse.
- The purpose of pelvic-floor exercises is to increase the muscle volume, which will result in a stronger muscular contraction. Kegel exercises might limit the progression of mild prolapse and alleviate mild prolapse symptoms, including low back pain and pelvic pressure.
- Urinary incontinence is the involuntary loss of urine sufficient enough to be a social or hygiene problem. It affects approximately 18 million people in the United States, about 11 million of them women.
- The three most common types of incontinence are urge incontinence (overactive bladder caused by detrusor muscle contractions), stress incontinence (inadequate urinary sphincter function), and mixed incontinence (involves both stress and urge incontinence).
- The most common benign growths of the reproductive tract include cervical, endocervical, and endometrial polyps; uterine fibroids (leiomyomas); and ovarian cysts.
- PCOS involves the presence of multiple inactive follicle cysts within the ovary that interfere with ovarian function. Hyperandrogenism, insulin resistance, and chronic anovulation characterize PCOS. Careful attention should be given to this condition because women with it are at increased risk for long-term health problems such as cardiovascular disease, hypertension, dyslipidemia, type 2 diabetes, and cancer (endometrial, breast, and ovarian).

REFERENCES

Alexander, L. L., LaRosa, J. H., Bader, H., & Garfield, S. (2007). *New dimensions in women's health* (4th ed.). Sudbury, MA: Jones and Bartlett Publishers.

American College of Obstetrics and Gynecology (ACOG). (2006). ACOG Committee opinion number 351. The overweight adolescent: Prevention, treatment, and obstetric-gynecologic implications. *Obstetrics & Gynecology, 108*(5), 1337–1348.

American College of Obstetrics and Gynecology (ACOG). (2007). Pelvic organ prolapse. *Obstetrics & Gynecology, 109*(2), 461–473.

Barron, A. M., & Falsetti, D. (2008). Polycystic ovary syndrome in adolescents. *Advance for Nurse Practitioners, 16*(3), 49–54.

Bartoletti, R. (2007) Pelvic organ prolapse: A challenge for the urologist. *European Urology, 51*(4), 884–886.

Berzuk, K. (2007). A strong pelvic floor: How nurses can spread the word. *Nursing for Women's Health, 11*(1), 54–61.

Centers for Disease Control and Prevention (CDC). (2007). *Women's reproductive health: Hysterectomy.* CDC Reproductive Health. [Online] Available at: http://www.cdc.gov/reproductivehealth/WomensRH/Hysterectomy.htm.

Dronavalli, S., & Ehrmann, D. A. (2007). Pharmacologic therapy of polycystic ovary syndrome. *Clinical Obstetrics & Gynecology, 50*(1), 244–254.

Dudek, S. G. (2006). *Nutrition essentials for nursing practice* (5th ed.). Philadelphia: Lippincott Williams & Wilkins.

Edwards, R. D., Moss, J. G., Lumsden, M. A., Wu, O., & Murray, L. S. (2007). Uterine-artery embolization versus surgery for symptomatic uterine fibroids. *New England Journal of Medicine, 356*(4), 360–370.

Hackley, B., Kriebs, J. M., & Rousseau, M. E. (2007). *Primary care of women: A guide for midwives and women's health providers.* Sudbury, MA: Jones and Bartlett Publishers.

Haider, Z., Condous, G., Kirk, E., Mukri, F., & Bourne, T. (2007). The simple outpatient management of Bartholin's abscess using the Word catheter: A preliminary study. *Australian & New Zealand Journal of Obstetrics & Gynecology, 47*(2), 137–140.

Hamilton, S., Spencer, C., & Evans, A. (2007). Vagino-rectal fistula caused by Bartholin's abscess. *Journal of Obstetrics & Gynecology, 27*(3), 325–326.

Helm, C. W. (2007). Ovarian cysts. *eMedicine.* Available at: http://emedicine.com/med/topic1699.htm.

Hines, S. H., & Miller, J. M. (2006). Urinary incontinence. In K. D. Schuiling & F. E. Likis (Eds.), *Women's gynecologic health* (Chapter 24; pp. 635–658). Sudbury, MA: Jones and Bartlett Publishers.

Husain, A., Johnson, K., Glowacki, C. A., Osias, J., Wheeless, C. R., Asrat, K., Ghebrekidan, A., & Polam, M. L. (2007). Surgical management of complex obstetric fistulas in Eritrea. *Journal of Women's Health, 14*(9), 839–844.

Jelovsek, J. E., Maher, C., & Barber, M. D. (2007). Pelvic organ prolapse. *Lancet, 369*(9566), 1027–1038.

Kaminski, P., & Hoffman, M. (2007). Benign cervical lesions. *eMedicine.* Available at: http://www.emedicine.com/med/topic3297.htm.

Krantz, C. A. (2007). Amenorrhea. In R. E. Rakel & E. T. Bope (Eds.), *Conn's current therapy 2007* (Section 16, pp. 1235–1238). Philadelphia: Saunders Elsevier.

Kriplani, A., Agarwai, N., Gupta, A., & Bhatla, N. (2007). Observations on etiology and management of genital fistulas. *Archives of Gynecology & Obstetrics, 271*(1), 14–18.

Lazarou, G., & Scotti, R. J. (2007). Uterine prolapse. *eMedicine.* Available at: http://emedicine.com/med/topic3291.htm.

Lemack, G. E. (2007). Incontinence: Helping women stay in control. *Cortlandt Forum, 20*(1), 53–54.

Lorenz, L. B., & Wild, R. A. (2007). Polycystic ovarian syndrome: An evidence-based approach to evaluation and management of diabetes and cardiovascular risks for today's clinician. *Clinical Obstetrics & Gynecology, 50*(1), 226–243.

Luft, J. (2006). Pelvic organ prolapse: Current state of knowledge about this common condition. *Journal for Nurse Practitioners, 2*(3), 170–177.

Newman, D. (2007). Nonsurgical solutions for pelvic organ prolapse. *Nursing Spectrum, 16*(1), 12–13.

Ogundele, O., & Silverberg, M. A. (2007). Urinary incontinence. *eMedicine.* Available at: http://www.emedicine.com/emerg/topic791.htm.

Panidis, D., & Farmakiotis, D. (2007). Treatment of infertility in the polycystic ovary syndrome. *New England of Medicine, 356*(19), 1999–2001.

Patil, S., Sultan, A. H., & Thakar, R. (2007). Bartholin's cysts and abscesses. *Journal of Obstetrics & Gynecology, 27*(3), 241–245.

Reena, C., Kekre, A. N., & Kekre, N. (2007). Occult stress incontinence in women with pelvic organ prolapse. *International Journal of Gynecology & Obstetrics, 97*(1), 31–34.

Schuiling, K. D., & Likis, F. E. (2006). *Women's gynecologic health.* Sudbury, MA: Jones and Bartlett Publishers.

Selby, M. (2006). Dealing with incontinence. *Practice Nurse, 32*(8), 33–38.

Smith, D. A. (2007). Pelvic organ prolapse. *Advance for Nurse Practitioners, 15*(8), 39–42.

Speroff, L., & Fritz, M. A. (2005). *Clinical gynecologic endocrinology and infertility* (7th ed.). Philadelphia: Lippincott Williams & Wilkins.

Speroff, L., & Mishell, D. R. (2007). Polycystic ovary syndrome: Management and contraception. *Dialogues in Contraception, 11*(1), 5–10.

Thomason, P. (2007). Leiomyoma, uterus (fibroid). *eMedicine.* Available at: http://www.emedicine.com/radio/topic777.htm.

Verga, C. A. (2006). Benign gynecologic conditions. In K. D. Schuiling & F. E. Likis (Eds.), *Women's gynecologic health* (Chapter 22, pp. 561–594). Sudbury, MA: Jones and Bartlett Publishers.

Vignesh, J. P., & Mohan, V. (2007). Polycystic ovary syndrome: A component of metabolic syndrome? *Journal of Postgraduate Medicine, 53*(2), 128–134.

Wallace, J. D. (2007). Woman with incontinence and a history of childhood sexual abuse. *Urologic Nursing, 27*(1), 38–39.

Wise, L. A., Palmer, J. R., Stewart, E. A., & Rosenberg, L. (2007). Polycystic ovary syndrome and the risk of uterine leiomyomata. *Fertility and Sterility, 87*(5), 1108–1115.

WEBSITES

American Cancer Society: (800)-ACS-2345, www.cancer.org

American College of Obstetricians and Gynecologists: (202) 863-2518, www.acog.org

American Urological Association: (410) 727-1100, www.auanet.org

Fibroid Treatment Collective: (310) 794-6645, www.fibroid.org

Hysterectomy Educational Resource and Services (HERS): (215) 667-7757, www.ccon.com/hers

National Association for Continence: (800) 252-3337, www.nafc.org

National Women's Health Information Center: (800) 994-9662, www.4women.gov

Polycystic Ovarian Syndrome Association: www.pcossupport.org

Sexuality Information and Education Council of the United States: (212) 819-9770, www.siecus.org

CHAPTER WORKSHEET

MULTIPLE CHOICE QUESTIONS

1. When you are interviewing a patient with uterine fibroids, what subjective data would you expect to find in her history?

   a. Cyclic migraine headaches

   b. Urinary urgency

   c. Chronic pelvic pain

   d. Chronic constipation

2. Treatment options available for women with pelvic organ prolapse are:

   a. Pessaries and Kegel exercises

   b. External pelvic fixation devices

   c. Weight gain and yoga

   d. Firm panty-and-girdle garments

3. Which of the following dietary and lifestyle modifications might the nurse recommend to help prevent pelvic relaxation as women age?

   a. Eat a high-fiber diet to avoid constipation and straining.

   b. Avoid sitting for long periods; get up and walk around frequently.

   c. Limit the amount of exercise to prevent over-developing muscles.

   d. Space children a year apart to reduce wear and tear on the uterus.

4. Women with polycystic ovarian syndrome (PCOS) are at increased risk for developing which of the following long-term health problems?

   a. Osteoporosis

   b. Lupus

   c. Type 2 diabetes

   d. Migraine headaches

5. Side effects experienced by women taking gonadotropin-releasing hormone (GnRH) agonists for the treatment of fibroids closely resemble those of:

   a. Osteoporosis

   b. Osteoarthritis

   c. Depression

   d. Menopause

CRITICAL THINKING EXERCISE

1. Faith, a 42-year-old multiparous woman, presents to the women's health clinic complaining of pelvic pain, menorrhagia, and vaginal discharge. She says she has been having these problems for several months. On examination, her uterus is enlarged and irregular in shape. Her blood studies reveal anemia.

   a. What condition might Faith have, based on her symptoms?

   b. What treatment options are available to address this condition?

   c. What educational interventions should the nurse discuss with Faith?

STUDY ACTIVITIES

1. Prepare an educational session to teach women how to do Kegel exercises to prevent stress incontinence and pelvic floor relaxation.

2. In a small group, discuss the personal, social, and sexual issues that might affect a woman with pelvic organ prolapse. How might these issues affect her socialization? How might a support group help?

3. List the symptoms that a woman with uterine fibroids might have. Discuss how these symptoms might mimic a more frightening condition and why the woman might delay seeking treatment.

4. A bladder that herniates into the vagina is a

   _____.

5. A rectum that herniates into the vagina is a

   _____.

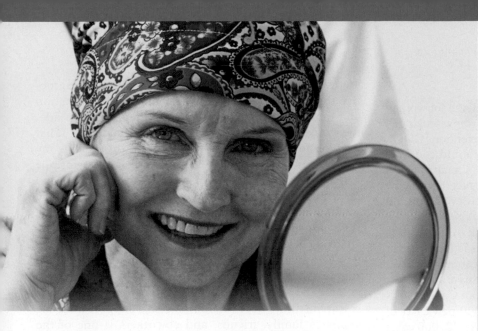

CHAPTER 8

CANCERS OF THE FEMALE REPRODUCTIVE TRACT

KEY TERMS

cervical cancer
cervical dysplasia
colposcopy
cone biopsy

cryotherapy
endometrial cancer
human papillomavirus
ovarian cancer

Papanicolaou (Pap) test
vaginal cancer
vulvar cancer

LEARNING OBJECTIVES

Upon completion of the chapter, the learner will be able to:

1. Define the key terms in the chapter.
2. Identify the major modifiable risk factors for reproductive tract cancers.
3. Discuss the risk factors, screening methods, and treatment modalities for cancers of the female reproductive tract.
4. Outline the nursing management needed for the most common malignant reproductive tract cancers in women.
5. Discuss lifestyle changes and health screenings that can reduce the risk of or prevent reproductive tract cancers.
6. List the community resources available for a woman undergoing surgery for cancer of the reproductive tract.
7. Explain the psychological distress felt by women diagnosed with cancer, and outline information that can help them to cope.

Carmella is an obese, 55-year-old woman who presents to her woman's health care provider with vaginal bleeding. She has been through menopause and wonders why she is having a period again. Her history includes infertility and hypertension. Three years ago she had a mastectomy for breast cancer, and she has been taking tamoxifen (Nolvadex) to prevent recurrent breast cancer since her surgery. What risk factors in Carmella's history might predispose her to a reproductive tract cancer? What additional information is needed to make a diagnosis?

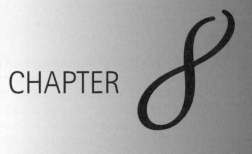

WoW

The word "cancer" can strike fear into anyone who hears it. But when it involves a reproductive organ, this fear is often magnified.

Cancer is the second leading cause of death for women in the United States, surpassed only by cardiovascular disease (Centers for Disease Control and Prevention [CDC], 2007b). Cardiovascular disease is and should continue to be a major focus of efforts in women's health. However, this should not overshadow the fact that many women between the ages of 35 and 74 are developing and dying of cancer (National Cancer Institute [NCI], 2007a). Women have a one-in-three lifetime risk of developing cancer, and one out of every four deaths is from cancer (Alexander et al., 2007). African-American women have the highest death rates from both heart disease and cancer (CDC, 2007b). According to the American Cancer Society (2008), it is estimated that over 39,000 new cases of uterine cancer (6% of all cancers) and over 22, 000 cases of ovarian cancer (3% of all cancers) will be diagnosed in 2007, with the number of estimated deaths to be over 7,000 and 15,000 respectively.

It has been estimated that in the United States half of all premature deaths, one third of acute disabilities, and one half of chronic disabilities are preventable (NCI, 2007a). Nurses need to focus their energies on screening, education, and early detection to reduce these numbers. Because cancer risk is strongly associated with lifestyle and behavior, screening programs are of particular importance for early detection. There is evidence that prevention and early detection have reduced cancer mortality rates and prevented reproductive cancers (CDC, 2007b).

This chapter begins with a nursing process overview of the care of women with reproductive cancer. It then describes selected cancers of the reproductive system—ovarian, endometrial, cervical, vaginal, and vulvar cancer. The chapter discusses the nurse's role through diagnosis, intervention, and follow-up care. Cancer management requires a multidisciplinary approach, including specialists in surgical, medical, and radiation oncology. The nurse can provide guidance and support to the client as she finds her way through the health care maze.

NURSING PROCESS OVERVIEW FOR THE WOMAN WITH CANCER OF THE REPRODUCTIVE TRACT

The word "cancer" is laden with fear and dread. These feelings may be worsened when the cancer involves a woman's reproductive tract. The diagnosis of a reproductive tract cancer can have a profound impact on a woman's sexuality because it affects the very core of her identity as a female. The loss of the reproductive body part as well as the possible loss of childbearing ability can have a significant effect on women and their partners. Nurses need to remember this impact when counseling women and their partners about cancer treatment and side effects and changes in gender roles and sexuality.

When a woman is first diagnosed with a reproductive tract cancer, two primary needs arise: information and emotional support. When the diagnosis is made, the woman typically has many questions, such as, "What is going to happen to me?", "How will this change my life?," and "Will I survive?" Nurses can play a major role in helping women find the answers to their questions and directing them to the resources they need. Two reliable sources of general cancer information are the National Cancer Institute (NCI) and the American Cancer Society (ACS). They can be reached via the Internet or by phone.

The nurse also plays a key role in offering emotional support, determining appropriate sources of support, and helping the woman use effective coping strategies. Many research studies have found that social support from the woman's family, friends, and coworkers is one of the strongest predictors of how well she will cope (Fieler & Henry, 2007). Women without a social support network may need a social work referral or may need to be guided toward support groups to receive the emotional support they need.

In addition, cancer clients have a strong need for hope. Strategies for inspiring hope may include active listening, touch, presence, and helping clients overcome communication barriers. Often it is not what nurses say or do but just their presence that counts.

Assessment

Assessment of a woman with cancer of the reproductive tract involves a thorough history and physical examination. In addition, various laboratory and diagnostic tests may be done to evaluate for a malignancy.

Health History and Physical Examination

Interview the woman carefully to determine any current or past factors that might increase her risk of cancer, such as early menarche, late menopause, sexually transmitted infections, use of hormonal agents, or infertility. Find out if the woman has a family history of cancer. Be thorough in obtaining the woman's past medical history, especially her reproductive, obstetric, and gynecologic history. Ask about her lifestyle and behaviors, including risky behaviors such as engaging in unprotected sexual intercourse or sexual intercourse with multiple partners. Find out if she has had routine or recommended screening procedures.

Ask if the woman has had any symptoms, such as abnormal vaginal bleeding or discharge or vaginal discomfort. Often the symptoms of cancer are vague and nonspecific and the woman may attribute them to another problem, such as aging, stress, or improper diet.

Perform a complete physical examination, including a review of body systems and a pelvic examination. Observe for lesions or masses in the perineal area. Note any masses when palpating the abdomen or when performing the pelvic examination.

Laboratory and Diagnostic Testing

Some of the laboratory and diagnostic tests used to help diagnose cancer of the reproductive tract are discussed in Common Laboratory and Diagnostic Tests 8.1.

Nursing Diagnoses and Related Interventions

Upon completion of a thorough assessment, the nurse might identify several nursing diagnoses, including:

- Deficient knowledge
- Disturbed body image
- Anxiety
- Fear
- Pain

Nursing goals, interventions, and evaluation for the woman with a reproductive cancer are based on the nursing diagnoses. Nursing Care Plan 8.1 may be used as a guide in planning nursing care for the woman with a reproductive cancer. It should be individualized based on the woman's symptoms and needs.

Nurses have traditionally served as advocates in the health care arena and should continue to be on the forefront of health education and diagnosis, acting as leaders in the fight against cancer. Over a half-million women in the United States will be diagnosed with cancer this year alone, and more than half will die of it. The public needs to know that not only are these deaths preventable, but many of the cancers themselves are preventable. Nurses need to work to improve the availability and quality of cancer-screening services, making them accessible to underserved and socio-economically disadvantaged clients. Through a unified effort by health care professionals, health policy experts, government agencies, health insurance companies, the

COMMON LABORATORY TESTS 8.1

Test	Explanation	Indications	Nursing Implications
Clinical breast examination	Assessment of the breast for abnormal findings; patient may discover lump herself; high-risk history for breast cancer	Identifies palpable mass, skin change, inverted nipple, or unresolved rash	• Educate client to perform breast self-examination and report any abnormalities. • Reinforce need for frequent clinical breast examinations if risk factors are present.
Mammography	Screening modality for breast cancer or any distortion in breast tissue architecture	Detects calcifications, densities, and nonpalpable cancer lesions	Stress importance of annual mammograms for all women after the age of 40 or 50, depending on their risk history.
Pap smear	Cervical cytology screening to diagnose cervical cancers	Aids in detecting abnormal cells of the cervix (from squamocolumnar junction of the cervix; most cervical cancers arise here)	Encourage all sexually active women to receive an annual pelvic examination, including a Pap smear, to promote early detection of cervical cancer.
Transvaginal ultrasound	Screening for pelvic pathology to assist in diagnosing endometrial cancers	Allows measurement of endometrial thickness to determine if endometrial biopsy is needed for postmenopausal bleeding	• Review the risk factors for the development of endometrial cancer and reason for this screening test. • Assist in preparing the patient for this examination.
CA-125	Nonspecific blood test used as a tumor marker	Elevation of marker suggests malignancy but is not specific to ovarian cancer.	• Review risk factors for ovarian cancer and explain that a series of diagnostic tests may be performed (transvaginal ultrasound, CT scan, CA-125) to assist in the diagnosis and treatment plan. • Elevated marker levels are not specific to ovarian cancer; they can be elevated in other types of cancer.

Nursing Care Plan 8.1

OVERVIEW OF A WOMAN WITH A REPRODUCTIVE TRACT CANCER

Molly, a thin 28-year-old woman, comes to the free health clinic complaining of a thin, watery vaginal discharge and spotting after sex. She says she is homeless and has lived "on the streets" for years. Molly says she has had multiple sex partners to pay for her food and cigarettes. She had an abnormal Pap smear "a while back" but didn't return to the clinic for follow-up. She hopes nothing "bad" is wrong with her because she just found a job that will allow her to get off the streets. "I'm worried that I won't be the same if there is something wrong. I don't know what I'd do if there is a problem," she tells you. Cervical cancer is suspected.

NURSING DIAGNOSIS: Anxiety related to uncertainty of diagnosis, possible diagnosis of cancer, and eventual outcome as evidenced by client's report of signs and symptoms, statements of being worried and not knowing what she would do

Outcome Identification and Evaluation

Client will demonstrate measures to cope with anxiety *as evidenced by statements acknowledging anxiety, use of positive coping strategies, and verbalization that anxiety has decreased.*

Interventions: Reducing Anxiety

- Encourage client to express her feelings and concerns *to reduce her anxiety and to determine appropriate interventions.*
- Assess the meaning of the diagnosis to the client, clarify misconceptions, and provide reliable, realistic information *to enhance her understanding of her condition, subsequently reducing her anxiety.*
- Assess client's psychological status *to determine degree of emotional distress related to diagnosis and treatment options.*
- Identify and address verbalized concerns, providing information about what to expect *to decrease uncertainty about the unknown.*
- Assess the client's use of coping mechanisms in the past and their effectiveness *to foster use of positive strategies.*
- Teach client about early signs of anxiety and help her recognize them (e.g., fast heartbeat, sweating, or feeling flushed) *to minimize escalation of anxiety.*
- Provide positive reinforcement that the client's condition can be managed *to relieve her anxiety.*

NURSING DIAGNOSIS: Deficient knowledge related to diagnosis, prevention strategies, disease course, and treatment as evidenced by client's statements about hoping nothing bad is wrong, lack of follow-up for previous abnormal Pap test, and high-risk behaviors

Outcome Identification and Evaluation

Client will demonstrate understanding of diagnosis, *as evidenced by making health-promoting lifestyle choices, verbalizing appropriate health care practices, describing condition once diagnosed, and adhering to measures to comply with therapy.*

Interventions: Providing Client Teaching

- Assess client's current knowledge about her diagnosis and proposed therapeutic regimen *to establish a baseline from which to develop a teaching plan.*
- Review contributing factors associated with development of reproductive tract cancer, including lifestyle behaviors, *to foster an understanding of the etiology of cervical cancer.*
- Review information about treatments and procedures and recommendations for healthy lifestyle, obtaining feedback frequently *to validate adequate understanding of instructions.*
- Discuss strategies, including using condoms and limiting the number of sexual partners, *to reduce the risk of transmission of STIs,* including human papillomavirus (HPV), which is associated with cervical cancer.
- Encourage client to obtain prompt treatment of any vaginal or cervical infections *to minimize the risk for cervical cancer.*
- Urge the client to have an annual Pap smear *to allow screening and early detection.*
- Describe the treatment measures used *to provide client with knowledge of what may be necessary.*
- Provide written material with pictures *to allow for client review and help her visualize what is occurring in her body.*
- Inform client about available community resources and make appropriate referrals as needed *to provide additional education and support.*
- Document details of teaching and learning *to allow for continuity of care and further education, if needed.*

Nursing Care Plan 8.1 (continued)

NURSING DIAGNOSIS: Disturbed body image related to suspected reproductive tract cancer and impact on client's sexuality and sense of self as evidenced by statement of being worried about not being the same

Outcome Identification and Evaluation

Client will verbalize or demonstrate a positive self-esteem in relation to body image as evidenced by positive statements about self, sexuality, and participation in activities with others.

Interventions: Promoting Healthy Body Image

- Assess client's use of self-criticism *to determine client's current state of coping and adjustment.*
- Determine if the client's change in body image has contributed to social isolation *to provide a direction for care.*
- Provide opportunities for client to explore her feelings related to issues of sexuality, including past behaviors that may have placed her at risk, *to minimize feelings of guilt about her condition.*
- Acknowledge the client's feelings about possible changes in her body and sexuality and her illness *to foster trust and allow client to ventilate feelings and concerns.*
- Facilitate contact with other clients with the same type of cancer *to promote sharing of feelings and decrease feelings of isolation.*
- Initiate referrals for counseling and community support groups as necessary *to assist client in gaining a positive image of herself.*

---

media, educational institutions, and women themselves, along with consistency and continuity, nurses can offer quality care to all women with cancer.

Educating to Prevent Cancer

Nurses need to provide clients with information to help prevent disease and enhance quality of life. Educate women about the importance of consistent and timely screenings to identify cancer early. Emphasize the importance of having an annual pelvic examination. Also stress the need for follow-up screenings as recommended. Provide clients with information if further diagnostic testing is required.

Nurses also play a key role in promoting cancer awareness, prevention, and control. Advocate to improve the availability of cancer-screening services and work to provide public education about risk factors for cancer.

Nurses can be instrumental in helping women to identify and change behaviors that put them at risk for various reproductive tract cancers (Teaching Guidelines 8.1). Do not limit your interventions to providing preventive education only: inform women about the consequences of doing nothing about their conditions and what the long-range outcomes might be without treatment. For example, stress the importance of visiting a health care professional if certain signs and symptoms appear:

- Blood in a bowel movement
- Unusual vaginal discharge or chronic vulvar itching
- Persistent abdominal bloating or constipation
- Irregular vaginal bleeding
- Persistent low backache not related to standing
- Elevated or discolored vulvar lesions
- Bleeding after menopause
- Pain or bleeding after sexual intercourse

Teaching the Client About Her Diagnosis

Provide information about tests that may be required to confirm or rule out the diagnosis. Review with the woman what she has been told about her diagnosis and her understanding of her condition. It is not unusual for the woman to hear the diagnosis and then become overwhelmed by the thought of cancer, blocking out whatever is said after

TEACHING GUIDELINES 8.1

Reducing Your Risk for Cancer

- Don't smoke.
- Drink alcohol only in moderation (no more than one drink daily).
- Be physically active daily.
- Eat a healthy diet.
- Stay current with immunizations.
- Reach and maintain a healthy weight.
- Take preventive medicines if needed.
- Get recommended screening tests:
  - Body mass index (BMI) to identify obesity
  - Mammogram every 1 to 2 years starting at age 40
  - Pap smear every 1 to 3 years if sexually active, between the ages of 21 and 65
  - Cholesterol checked annually starting at age 45
  - Blood pressure checked at least every 2 years
  - Diabetes test if hypertensive or hypercholesterolemic
  - Check for sexually transmitted infections (STIs) if sexually active

Sources: AHRQ, 2007; Mayo Clinic, 2008; WHO, 2008.

that. Answer any questions she may have. Go slowly and repeat the information as necessary. Use written materials to explain and reinforce the teaching. Provide information about her condition and recommended therapies. For example, if a client is undergoing surgery, discuss postoperative issues such as incision care, pain, and activity level. Instruct the client on health maintenance activities after treatment, and inform her and her family about available support resources.

Providing Emotional Support

Once the diagnosis is made, provide the woman and her family with emotional support. Validate the client's feelings and provide realistic hope, using a nonjudgmental approach and therapeutic communication skills during all interactions. Individualize the care based on the client's cultural traditions and beliefs.

Ensuring Culturally Competent Cancer Care

Cultural diversity in America is increasing, and as diverse cultures interact, conflicts inevitably ensue. These conflicts can affect health care outcomes. Providing culturally competent cancer care can improve outcomes and decrease disparities in care. Work to develop cultural competence by learning about and showing respect for all cultures. Be aware of the client's cultural background, religion, migration history, degree of acculturation, living conditions, educational level, and legal status, because each of these factors can affect the client's understanding of her diagnosis and the eventual outcome (Jenko & Moffitt, 2006).

In some cultures, sharing news of a serious illness like cancer is considered disrespectful and impolite. For example, some Europeans view such sharing as inhumane; the Asian culture views a cancer diagnosis as unnecessarily cruel. The Chinese, out of respect for aging family members, withhold discussions of serious illness to avoid causing unnecessary anxieties (Surbone, 2006). Integrate this knowledge in your care to ensure a culturally competent approach.

> ▶ *Take* NOTE!
>
> *When a diagnosis of cancer is made, assessing an individual's strengths and weaknesses from a cultural perspective will help the nurse to provide culturally competent care.*

As life becomes increasingly multilingual, multicultural, and multi-faith, learning about clients' values and cultural beliefs becomes challenging. Be willing to learn about client preferences; doing so promotes caring and nurturing.

Supporting the Pregnant Woman With Cancer

Theoretically, changes in the mother's immune system during pregnancy can increase the risk of malignancy because cell-mediated immunity, which is suppressed in pregnant women, normally protects against cancerous tumors (Blackburn, 2007). Some research has hinted at an increased rate of progression and decreased survival times in women who develop breast and cervical cancer and then become pregnant, but this generally has not been validated by research studies.

Ovarian cancer during pregnancy is rare because the disease typically occurs in older women. Because most pregnant women receive frequent medical care, including pelvic examinations, most ovarian cancers in pregnant women are found at early stages; this carries a good prognosis for both the mother and the newborn (Machado et al., 2007). Since routine screening for endometrial cancer is currently not recommended in the general population, few cases would be detected in the relatively young pregnant population (Sonoda & Barakat, 2006). Cervical cancer is more common in the pregnant population than other reproductive malignancies, and it can affect the woman's health status and the pregnancy.

Women diagnosed with any malignancy during pregnancy must confront the reality of the disease and its impact on their future fertility and live with the risk of recurrence (Roberts, Rezai, & Edmondson, 2007). The wishes of the pregnant woman and her family are of paramount importance when making decisions about continuing the pregnancy and undergoing cancer treatment. Some women will decide to terminate the pregnancy for the sake of their own health; others will undergo treatment during the pregnancy to preserve the life of the unborn child. Regardless of the woman's decision, provide support and education during treatment, birth, and beyond.

Ovarian Cancer

Ovarian cancer is malignant neoplastic growth of the ovary (Fig. 8.1). It is the eighth most common cancer among women and the fifth most common cause of cancer deaths for women in the United States. It accounts for more deaths than any other cancer of the reproductive system (ACS, 2007c). The ACS estimates that about 23,000 new cases of ovarian cancer will be diagnosed in the United States during 2007 and 15,000 deaths will occur. A woman's risk of getting ovarian cancer during her lifetime is 1.5%, or about 1 in 67. About 76% of women with ovarian cancer survive 1 year after diagnosis; only 45% survive longer than 5 years (ACS, 2007c). Older women are at highest risk. Ovarian cancer occurs most frequently in women between 55 and 75 years of age, and approximately 25% of ovarian cancer deaths occur in women between 35 and 54 years old (ACS, 2007c).

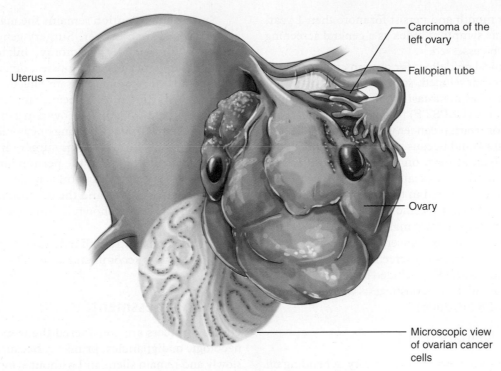

Carcinoma of the
left ovary

Fallopian tube

Uterus

Ovary

Microscopic view
of ovarian cancer
cells

FIGURE **8.1** Ovarian cancer. (The Anatomical Chart Company. [2005]. *Atlas of pathophysiology* [2nd ed.]. Philadelphia: Lippincott Williams & Wilkins.)

The most important variable influencing the prognosis is the extent of the disease. Survival depends on the stage of the tumor, grade of differentiation, gross findings at surgery, amount of residual tumor after surgery, and effectiveness of any adjunct treatment postoperatively. Many women with ovarian cancer will experience recurrence despite the best efforts of eradicating the cancer through surgery, radiation, or chemotherapy to eliminate residual tumor cells. The likelihood of long-term survival in the event of recurrence is dismal (Eaton, 2007). The 5-year survival rates (the percentage of women who live at least 5 years after their diagnosis) are shown in Table 8.1 according to stage.

TABLE 8.1   **FIVE-YEAR SURVIVAL RATES FOR OVARIAN CANCER**

Stage	Five-Year Relative Survival Rates
I	80% to 90%
II	65% to 70%
III	30% to 60%
IV	20%

American Cancer Society (ACS). (2007c). *What are the key statistics about ovarian cancer?* American Cancer Society, Inc. [Online] Available at: http://www.cancer.org/docroot/CRI/content/CRI_2_4_1X_What_are_the_key_statistics_for_ovarian_cancer_33.asp?sitearea=&level=.

Pathophysiology

Ovarian cancer, the cause of which is unknown, can originate from different cell types. Most ovarian cancers originate in the ovarian epithelium. They usually present as solid masses that have spread beyond the ovary and seeded into the peritoneum prior to diagnosis. An inherited genetic mutation is the causative factor in 5% to 10% of cases of epithelial ovarian cancer.

Screening and Diagnosis

Seventy-five percent of ovarian cancers are not diagnosed until the cancer has advanced to stage III or IV, primarily because there is still no adequate screening test. Two genes, BRCA-1 and BRCA-2, are linked with hereditary breast and ovarian cancers. Blood tests can be performed to assess DNA in white blood cells to detect mutations in the BRCA genes. These genetic markers do not predict whether the person will develop cancer; rather, they provide information regarding the risk of developing cancer: a woman who is BRCA positive may have up to an 80% chance of developing breast cancer and a 40% chance of developing ovarian cancer (Eaton, 2007).

To assist in screening, researchers have been developing an ovarian cancer symptom index that includes pelvic and abdominal pain, urinary frequency and urgency, increased abdominal size (bloating), and difficulty eating (feeling full) (Goff et al., 2007). The symptom index is considered positive if any of these symptoms occur more than 12 times a month and persist for more than 1 year. The utility of this symptom index as a general screening tool remains to be assessed.

Specific clinical guidelines for ovarian cancer screening have not been developed, so the disease is often not diagnosed until it has metastasized. The U.S. Preventive Services Task Force (USPSTF) recommends against routine screening for ovarian cancer with serum CA-125 or transvaginal ultrasound because earlier detection would have a small effect, at best, on mortality. CA-125 is a biologic tumor marker associated with ovarian cancer. Although levels are elevated in many women with ovarian cancer, CA-125 is not specific for this cancer and levels may be elevated with other malignancies (pancreatic, liver, colon, breast, and lung cancers). Currently, it is not sensitive enough to serve as a screening tool (Speroff & Fritz, 2005). The USPSTF concluded that the harm from the invasive nature of the diagnostic tests would outweigh the benefits (USPSTF, 2006).

Therapeutic Management

Treatment options for ovarian cancer vary depending on the stage and severity of the disease. Usually a laparoscopy (abdominal exploration with an endoscope) is performed for diagnosis and staging, as well as evaluation for therapy. In stage I the cancer is limited to the ovaries. In stage II the growth involves one or both ovaries, with pelvic extension. Stage III cancer has spread to the lymph nodes and other organs or structures inside the abdominal cavity. In stage IV, the cancer has metastasized to distant sites (Alexander et al., 2007). Figure 8.2 shows the likely metastatic sites for ovarian cancer.

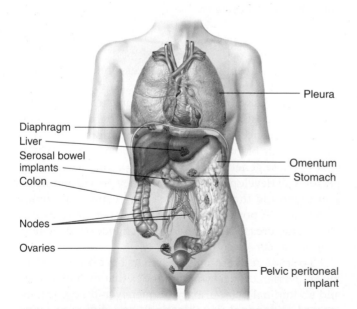

FIGURE 8.2 Common metastatic sites for ovarian cancer. (The Anatomical Chart Company. [2005]. *Atlas of pathophysiology* [2nd ed.]. Philadelphia: Lippincott Williams & Wilkins)

Surgical intervention remains the mainstay of management of ovarian cancer. Surgery generally includes a total abdominal hysterectomy, bilateral salpingo-oophorectomy, peritoneal biopsies, omentectomy, and pelvic para-aortic lymph node sampling to evaluate cancer extension (Martin, 2007). Because most women are diagnosed with advanced-stage ovarian cancer, aggressive management involving debulking or cytoreductive surgery is commonly performed. This surgery involves resecting all visible tumors from the peritoneum, taking peritoneal biopsies, sampling lymph nodes, and removing all reproductive organs and the omentum. This aggressive surgery has been shown to improve long-term survival rates.

Additional therapy with radiation may be warranted. Chemotherapy is recommended for all stages of ovarian cancer.

Nursing Assessment

Ovarian cancers are considered the worst of all the gynecologic malignancies, primarily because they develop slowly and remain silent and without symptoms until the cancer is far advanced. It has been described as "the overlooked disease" or "the silent killer" because women and health care practitioners often ignore or rationalize early symptoms. For example, women may attribute gastrointestinal problems to stress and midlife changes. However, these vague complaints may precede more obvious symptoms by months. The most common early symptoms include abdominal bloating, early satiety, fatigue, vague abdominal pain, urinary frequency, diarrhea or constipation, and unexplained weight loss or gain. The later symptoms include anorexia, dyspepsia, ascites, a palpable abdominal mass, pelvic pain, and back pain (Wallace & Sanford, 2006).

▶ *Consider* THIS!

I felt I was a lucky woman because I had been in remission from breast cancer for 12 years, and I had been given the gift of life to share with my beloved family. Recently I became ill with stomach problems: pain, indigestion, bloating, and nausea. My doctor treated me for GERD (acid reflux disease), but the symptoms persisted. I then was referred to a gastroenterologist, an urologist, and then a gynecologist, who did an ultrasound, which was negative. I received reassurance from all three that there was nothing wrong with me. As time went by, I experienced more pain, more symptoms, and increased frustration. Six months after seeing all three specialists, a repeat ultrasound revealed I had ovarian cancer, and I needed surgery as soon as possible. I underwent a complete hysterectomy

(continued)

▶ *Consider* THIS! *(continued)*

and my surgeon found I was in stage 3. Since then, I have undergone chemotherapy and participated in a clinical cancer study that wasn't successful for me, and now I am facing the fact that I am going to die soon.

Thoughts: This woman has tried everything to save her life, but, alas, time has run out for her with advanced ovarian cancer. Women diagnosed with breast cancer are at a significant risk for developing ovarian cancer later in life. Of the string of doctors she saw, one has to ponder why none ordered a CA-125 blood test with her history of breast cancer. We are haunted with the question: If they had and it was elevated, would she be in stage 3 now? I guess we will never know.

Obtain a thorough history of the woman's symptoms, including their onset, duration, and frequency. Review the woman's history for risk factors such as:

• Nulliparity
• Early menarche (before 12 years old)
• Late menopause (after 55 years old)
• Increasing age (over 50 years of age)
• High-fat diet
• Obesity
• Persistent ovulation over time
• First-degree relative with ovarian cancer
• Use of perineal talcum powder or hygiene sprays
• Older than 30 years at first pregnancy
• Positive BRCA-1 and BRCA-2 mutations
• Personal history of breast, bladder, or colon cancer
• Hormone replacement therapy for more than 10 years
• Infertility (CDC, 2007c)

Perform a complete physical examination. Inspect the abdomen, noting any distention or bloating. Palpate the abdomen. Be alert for a mass or pain on palpation. Anticipate further testing to confirm the diagnosis.

Nursing Management

The complexities of ovarian cancer make a multidisciplinary approach necessary for optimal management. With the subtle nature and high risk of recurrence and mortality of this condition, most women find it an emotionally exhausting and devastating experience. Nursing management focuses on measures to promote early detection, educate the woman about the disease and its treatments, and provide emotional support. Nurses should show a positive attitude that communicates understanding and reassurance.

Promoting Early Detection

Nurses need to ensure that women are aware of the risk factors for ovarian cancer. Urge women not to dismiss seemingly innocuous symptoms as "just a part of aging." Encourage women to describe such nonspecific complaints at health visits.

Assess the woman's family and personal history for risk factors and encourage genetic testing for women with affected family members. Outline screening guidelines for women with hereditary cancer syndrome and inform women at high risk about the appropriate screening strategies.

Urge women to have yearly bimanual pelvic examinations and a transvaginal ultrasound to allow identification of ovarian masses in their early stages. After menopause, a mass on an ovary is not a cyst: physiologic cysts can arise only from a follicle that has not ruptured or from the cystic degeneration of the corpus luteum.

▶ *Take* NOTE!

A small ovarian "cyst" found on ultrasound in an asymptomatic postmenopausal woman should arouse suspicion. Any mass or ovary palpated in a postmenopausal woman should be considered cancerous until proven otherwise (Cherry, DeGaetano, & Martin, 2007).

Educating the Client

Education is a major focus of nursing care. This teaching involves risk reduction and health promotion. Teach the woman about risk-reduction strategies; for instance, pregnancy, use of oral contraceptives, and breastfeeding reduce the risk of ovarian cancer. Instruct women to avoid using talc and hygiene sprays on their genitals. Review the lifetime risks related to BRCA-1 and BRCA-2 genes and options available should the woman test positive for these genes. Help to promote community awareness of ovarian cancer by educating the public about risk-reducing behaviors.

Instruct the woman about the importance of healthy lifestyles. Stress the importance of maintaining a healthy weight to reduce risk. Encourage women to eat a low-fat diet.

For the woman who is diagnosed with ovarian cancer, describe in simple terms the tests, treatment modalities, and follow-up needed. For example, if the woman will be having surgery, provide thorough teaching about what to expect before, during, and after surgery. Outline treatment options and the implications of choices. Assist the woman and her family to decipher the myriad of information related to staging, tests, and treatments. Teach the woman about additional treatment measures, such as radiation therapy or chemotherapy, including how to handle the common adverse effects of treatment.

Supporting the Client and Family

The diagnosis of ovarian cancer, like any cancer, can be overwhelming. In addition, the treatments and their effects can be highly stressful, both physically and emotionally. Provide one-to-one support for women facing treatment for ovarian cancer. Ovarian cancer involves the reproductive system, which has a direct impact on the woman's view of herself. Encourage open discussion of sexuality and the impact of cancer. Listen and support the woman and her family as they try to cope with this disease. Encourage the use of appropriate coping strategies to allow for the best quality of life. Try to restore hope to women with ovarian cancer, and stress treatment compliance. If appropriate, encourage participation in clinical trials to offer hope for all women. Continue to offer support to the woman and her family members as they experience sadness and grief.

Endometrial Cancer

Endometrial cancer (also known as uterine cancer) is malignant neoplastic growth of the uterine lining. It is the most common gynecologic malignancy and accounts for 6% of all cancers in women in the United States. The NCI estimates that there will be over 40,000 new cases in 2007; approximately 8,000 of these women will die (NCI, 2007b). It is uncommon before the age of 40, but as women age, their risk of endometrial cancer increases. Approximately 95% of these malignancies are carcinomas of the endometrium. Because endometrial cancer is usually diagnosed in the early stages, it has a better prognosis than cervical or ovarian cancer (ACS, 2007f).

Pathophysiology

Two mechanisms are believed to be involved in the development of endometrial cancer. A history of exposure to unopposed estrogen is the cause in 75% of women. Those that are spontaneous and are unrelated to estrogen or endometrial hyperplasia represent the other 25% of endometrial cancers.

Endometrial cancer may originate in a polyp or in a diffuse multifocal pattern. The pattern of spread partially depends on the degree of cellular differentiation. Well-differentiated tumors tend to limit their spread to the surface of the endometrium. Metastatic spread occurs in a characteristic pattern and most commonly involves the lungs, inguinal and supraclavicular nodes, liver, bones, brain, and vagina (NCI, 2007b). Early tumor growth is characterized by friable and spontaneous bleeding. Later tumor growth is characterized by myometrial invasion and growth toward the cervix (Fig. 8.3).

Adenocarcinoma of the endometrium is typically preceded by hyperplasia. Carcinoma in situ is found only on the endometrial surface. In stage I, it has spread to the muscle wall of the uterus. In stage II, it has spread to the cervix. In stage III, it has spread to the bowel or vagina, with metastases to pelvic lymph nodes. In stage IV, it has invaded the bladder mucosa, with distant metastases to the lungs, liver, and bone (Burke & Gallup, 2007).

Type I carcinomas, the most common, begin as endometrial hyperplasia and progress to carcinomas. Giving estrogen preparations without progestin for hormone replacement therapy leads to an increased risk for endometrial cancer. Type I is generally found at an earlier stage and treatment results are more favorable.

Unlike type I endometrial carcinoma, type II carcinomas appear spontaneously, are associated with a poorly differentiated cell type, and have a poor prognosis (Burke & Gallup, 2007). They account for less than 10% of all endometrial cancers but contribute to the majority of all endometrial deaths.

Screening and Diagnosis

Remember Carmella, the woman with postmenopausal bleeding? In postmenopausal women, any bleeding is abnormal and warrants further assessment. What testing would the nurse anticipate as being ordered to confirm the diagnosis? What would be the nurse's role during this testing?

Screening for endometrial cancer is not routinely done because it is not practical or cost-effective. The ACS recommends that women should be informed about the risks and symptoms of endometrial cancer at the onset of menopause and strongly encouraged to report any unexpected bleeding or spotting to their health care provider (ACS, 2007f). A pelvic examination is frequently normal in the early stages of the disease. Changes in the size, shape, or consistency of the uterus or its surrounding support structures may exist when the disease is more advanced.

An endometrial biopsy is the diagnostic procedure of choice. It can be done in the health care provider's office without anesthesia. A slender suction catheter is used to obtain a small sample of tissue for pathology. This test can detect up to 90% of cases of endometrial cancer in women with postmenopausal bleeding, depending on the technique and experience of the health care provider (Wallace & Sanford, 2006). The woman may experience mild cramping and bleeding after the procedure for about 24 hours, but typically mild pain medication will reduce this discomfort.

Transvaginal ultrasound can be used to evaluate the endometrial cavity and measure the thickness of the endometrial lining. It can be used to detect endometrial hyperplasia. If the endometrium measures less than 4 mm, then the client is at low risk for malignancy (Sonoda & Barakat, 2006).

Therapeutic Management

Typically, the stage of the disease directs treatment. It usually involves surgery with adjunct therapy based on pathologic findings. Surgery most often involves removal

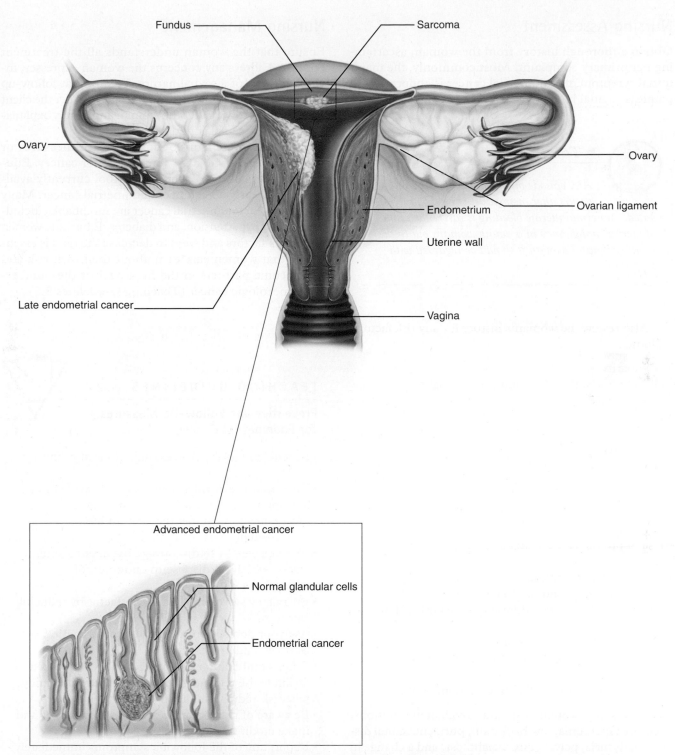

Fundus

Sarcoma

Ovary

Ovary

Ovarian ligament

Endometrium

Uterine wall

Late endometrial cancer

Vagina

Advanced endometrial cancer

Normal glandular cells

Endometrial cancer

FIGURE 8.3 Progression of endometrial cancer. (The Anatomical Chart Company. [2005]. *Atlas of pathophysiology* [2nd ed.]. Philadelphia: Lippincott Williams & Wilkins)

of the uterus (hysterectomy) and the fallopian tubes and ovaries (salpingo-oophorectomy). Removal of the tubes and ovaries is recommended because tumor cells spread early to the ovaries, and any dormant cancer cells could be stimulated to grow by ovarian estrogen. In more ad-

vanced cancers, radiation and chemotherapy are used as adjuncts to surgery. Routine surveillance intervals for follow-up care are typically every 3 to 4 months for the first 2 years, since 85% of recurrences occur in the first 3 years after diagnosis (Burke & Gallup, 2007).

Nursing Assessment

Obtain a thorough history from the woman, ascertaining her primary complaint. Most commonly, the major initial symptom of endometrial cancer is abnormal and painless vaginal bleeding.

> ▶ *Take* NOTE!
>
> *Any episode of bright-red bleeding that occurs after menopause should be investigated. Abnormal uterine bleeding is rarely the result of uterine malignancy in a young woman, but in the postmenopausal woman it should be regarded with suspicion.*

Also review the woman's history for any risk factors, including:

- Nulliparity
- Obesity (more than 50 pounds overweight)
- Liver disease
- Infertility
- Diabetes mellitus
- Hypertension
- History of pelvic radiation
- Polycystic ovary syndrome
- Infertility
- Early menarche (before 12 years old)
- High-fat diet
- Use of prolonged exogenous unopposed estrogen with an intact uterus
- Endometrial hyperplasia
- Family history of endometrial cancer
- Personal history of hereditary nonpolyposis colon cancer
- Personal history of breast or ovarian cancer
- Late onset of menopause (after age 52 years)
- Tamoxifen use
- Chronic anovulation (Tiffen & Mahon, 2006)

Assess the woman for additional manifestations, such as dyspareunia, low back pain, purulent genital discharge, dysuria, pelvic pain, weight loss, and a change in bladder and bowel habits. These may suggest advanced disease.

Perform a physical examination and assist with or perform, as appropriate, a pelvic examination. Observe for vaginal discharge. Note any changes in the size, shape, or consistency of the uterus or surrounding structures or client reports of pain during examination. Anticipate the need for transvaginal ultrasound to identify endometrial hyperplasia (usually greater than 4 mm) and endometrial biopsy to identify malignant cells.

Nursing Management

Ensure that the woman understands all the treatment options. Address any concerns the woman expresses, including those of a sexual nature. Ensure that follow-up appointments are scheduled appropriately. Refer the client to a support group. Offer the woman and family explanations and emotional support throughout.

Educate the client about preventive measures or follow-up care if she has been treated for cancer. Education may be the most important tool currently available for the early detection of endometrial cancer. Many risk factors for endometrial cancer are modifiable, including obesity, hypertension, and diabetes. Educating women about risk factors and ways to decrease the risks is essential so that women can learn about their own risk and can become partners in the fight against the number-one gynecologic cancer (Teaching Guidelines 8.2).

TEACHING GUIDELINES 8.2

Preventive and Follow-Up Measures for Endometrial Cancer

- Schedule regular pelvic examinations after the age of 21.
- Visit health care practitioner for early evaluation of any abnormal bleeding after menopause.
- Maintain a low-fat diet throughout life.
- Exercise daily.
- Manage weight to discourage hyperestrogenic states, which predispose to endometrial hyperplasia.
- Pregnancy serves as a protective factor by reducing estrogen.
- Ask your doctor about the use of combination estrogen and progestin pills.
- When combination oral contraceptives are taken to facilitate the regular shedding of the uterine lining, take risk-reduction measures.
- Be aware of risk factors for endometrial cancer and make modifications as needed.
- Report any of the following symptoms immediately:
  - Bleeding or spotting after sexual intercourse
  - Bleeding that lasts longer than a week
  - Reappearance of bleeding after 6 months or more of no menses
- After cancer therapy, schedule follow-up appointments for the next few years.
- After cancer therapy, frequently communicate with your health care provider concerning your status.
- After surgery, maintain a healthy weight.

Carmella's endometrial biopsy indicates endometrial adenocarcinoma. Her health care provider recommends surgery and adjuvant radiation therapy. How long will Carmella need to follow up after surgery? What lifestyle changes will the nurse need to stress with Carmella?

Cervical Cancer

Cervical cancer is cancer of the uterine cervix. The ACS estimates that over 12,000 cases of invasive cervical cancer will be diagnosed in the United States in 2007; approximately 3,000 of these women will die. Some researchers estimate that noninvasive cervical cancer (carcinoma in situ) is about four times more common than invasive cervical cancer. The 5-year survival rate for all stages of cervical cancer is 72% (ACS, 2007a). It is five to eight times more common in women affected with HIV or AIDS than those who do not have this virus. The probability of a woman in the United States developing cervical cancer is approximately 1 in 120, but this statistic is age-dependent; the highest incidence is in women 40 to 49 years of age (Hopkins & Sawa, 2007).

The incidence and mortality rates of cervical cancer have decreased noticeably in the past several decades, with most of the reduction attributed to the **Papanicolaou (Pap) test**, which detects cervical cancer and precancerous lesions. Cervical cancer is one of the most treatable cancers when detected at an early stage (ACS, 2007a). *Healthy People 2010* identifies two goals that address cervical cancer (Healthy People 2010 8.1; USDHHS, 2000).

HEALTHY PEOPLE 2010	
Objective	**Significance**
Reduce the death rate from cancer of the uterine cervix from 3 per 100,000 females (1998) to 2 per 100,000 females in 2010. Increase the proportion of women who received a Pap smear within the preceding 3 years from 79% to 90% by 2010.	• Will help improve mortality rates and quality of life for women, and reduce health care costs related to treatment of malignancies. • Will help to promote screening and early detection. The National Institutes of Health (NIH) reported that half of women diagnosed with invasive cervical cancer have never had a Pap smear and 10% have not had Pap smears during the past 5 years (NIH, 2007).

Pathophysiology

Cervical cancer starts with abnormal changes in the cellular lining or surface of the cervix. Typically these changes occur in the squamous–columnar junction of the cervix. Here, cylindrical secretory epithelial cells (columnar) meet the protective flat epithelial cells (squamous) from the outer cervix and vagina in what is termed the transformation zone. The continuous replacement of columnar epithelial cells by squamous epithelial cells in this area makes these cells vulnerable to take up foreign or abnormal genetic material (ACS, 2007a). Figure 8.4 shows the pathophysiology of cervical cancer.

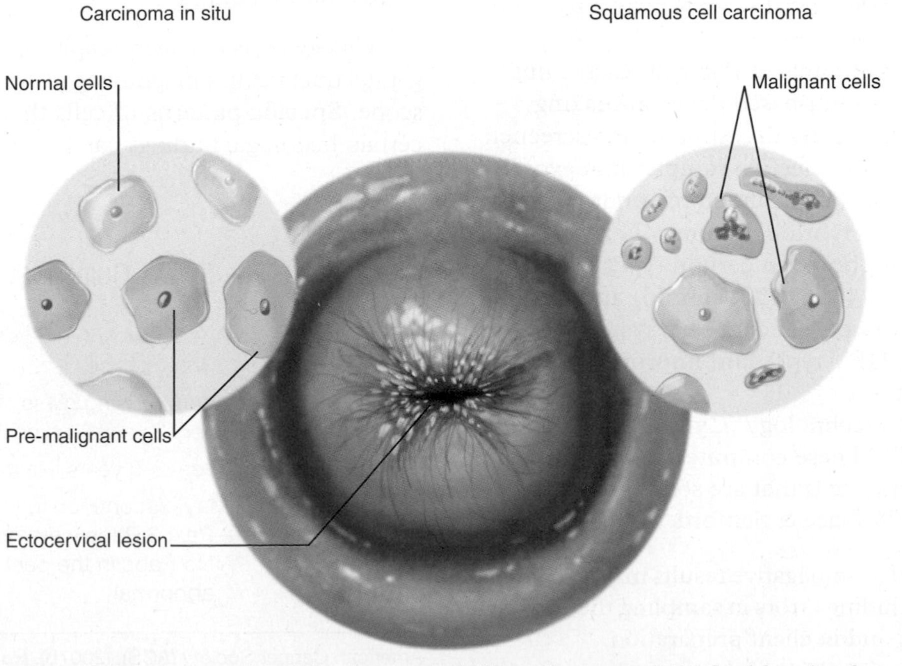

Carcinoma in situ

Squamous cell carcinoma

Normal cells

Malignant cells

Pre-malignant cells

Ectocervical lesion

FIGURE 8.4 Cervical cancer. (The Anatomical Chart Company. [2005]. *Atlas of pathophysiology* [2nd ed.]. Philadelphia: Lippincott Williams & Wilkins)

The development of cervical cancer has been linked to the **human papillomavirus (HPV)**, which is acquired through sexual activity (Torpy, 2007). More than 90% of squamous cervical cancers contain HPV DNA, and the virus is now accepted as a major causative factor in the development of cervical cancer and its precursor, **cervical dysplasia** (disordered growth of abnormal cells).

Screening and Diagnosis

Screening for cervical cancer is very effective because the presence of a precursor lesion, cervical intraepithelial neoplasia (CIN), helps determine whether further tests are needed. Lesions start as dysplasia and progress in a predictable fashion over a long period, allowing ample opportunity for intervention at a precancerous stage. Progression from low-grade to high-grade dysplasia takes an average of 9 years, and progression from high-grade dysplasia to invasive cancer takes up to 2 years (Hopkins & Sawa, 2007).

Widespread use of the Pap test (also known as a Pap smear), a procedure used to obtain cells from the cervix for cytology screening, is credited with saving tens of thousands of women's lives and decreasing deaths from cervical cancer by more than 70% (ACS, 2007a). Despite its outstanding record of success as a screening tool for cervical cancer (it detects approximately 90% of early cancer changes), the conventional Pap smear has a 20% false-negative rate. High-grade abnormalities missed by human screening are frequently detected by computerized instruments (NCI, 2007a). Thus, many technologies have been developed to improve the sensitivity and specificity of Pap testing, including:

- Thin-Prep: In this liquid-based technique, the cervical specimen is placed into a vial of preservative solution rather than on a glass slide.
- Computer-assisted automated Pap test rescreening (Autopap): An algorithm-based decision-making technology identifies slides that should be rescreened by cytopathologists by selecting samples that exceed a certain threshold for the likelihood of abnormal cells.
- HPV-DNA typing (Hybrid Capture): This system uses the association between certain types of HPV (16, 18, 31, 33, 35, 45, 51, 52, and 56) and the development of cervical cancer. This system can identify high-risk HPV types and improves detection and management.
- Computer-assisted technology (Cytyc CDS-1000, AutoCyte, AcCell): These computerized instruments can detect abnormal cells that are sometimes missed by technologists (Wallace & Sanford, 2006).

The high rate of false-negative results may also be due to other factors, including errors in sampling the cervix, in preparing the slide, and in client preparation.

Although professional medical organizations disagree as to the recommended frequency of screening for cervical cancer, the ACS 2007 guidelines suggest that women should begin annual screening for cervical cancer via a Pap test after they initiate sexual activity or at 21 years of age, whichever comes first. If three consecutive Pap smears are negative, a trained health care provider may suggest that screening can be performed less frequently. Women ages 65 to 70 with no abnormal tests in the previous 10 years may choose to stop screenings (ACS, 2007a). High-risk women should continue to have annual Pap smears throughout their life (Table 8.2).

Pap smear results are classified using the Bethesda System (Box 8.1), which provides a uniform diagnostic terminology that allows clear communication between the laboratory and the health care provider. The information provided by the laboratory is divided into three categories: specimen adequacy, general categorization of cytologic findings, and interpretation/result (ACS, 2007b).

Therapeutic Management

Treatment for abnormal Pap smears depends on the severity of the results and the health history of the woman. Therapeutic choices all involve destroying as many affected cells as possible. Box 8.2 describes treatment options.

Using the Bethesda system, the following management guidelines for abnormal Pap results were developed by the NCI to provide direction to health care providers and clients:

- ASC-US: Repeat the Pap smear in 4 to 6 months or refer for colposcopy.
- ASC-H: Refer for colposcopy without HPV testing.
- Atypical glandular cells (AGC) and adenocarcinoma in situ (AIS): Immediate colposcopy; follow-up is based on the findings.

Colposcopy is a microscopic examination of the lower genital tract using a magnifying instrument called a colposcope. Specific patterns of cells that correlate well with certain histologic findings can be visualized.

TABLE 8.2 PAP SMEAR GUIDELINES

First Pap	Age 21 or within 3 years of first sexual intercourse
Until age 30	Yearly—using glass slide method Every 2 years—using liquid-based method
Age 30–70	Every 2–3 years if last 3 Paps were normal
After age 70	May discontinue if: - Past 3 Paps were normal and - No Paps in the past 10 years were abnormal

American Cancer Society (ACS). (2007b). *How Pap test results are reported*. American Cancer Society, Inc. [Online] Available at: http://www.cancer.org/docroot/PED/content/PED_2_3X_Pap_Test.asp.

BOX 8.1 The 2001 Bethesda System for Classifying Pap Smears

Specimen Type: Conventional Pap smear vs. liquid-based

Specimen Adequacy: Satisfactory or unsatisfactory for evaluation

General Categorization: (optional)
- Negative for intraepithelial lesion or malignancy
- Epithelial cell abnormality. See interpretation/result

Automated Review: If case was examined by automated device or not

Ancillary Testing: Provides a brief description of the test methods and report results so health care provider understands

Interpretation/Result:
- Negative for intraepithelial lesion or malignancy
- Organisms: *Trichomonas vaginalis;* fungus; bacterial vaginosis; herpes simplex
- Other non-neoplastic findings: Reactive cellular changes associated with inflammation, radiation, IUDs, atrophy
- Other: Endometrial cells in a woman >40 years of age
- Epithelial cell abnormalities:
- *Squamous cell*
  - Atypical squamous cells
    - Of undetermined significance (ASC-US)
    - Cannot exclude HSIL (ASC-H)
  - Low-grade squamous intraepithelial lesion (LSIL)
    - Encompassing HPV/mild dysplasia/CIN-1
  - High-grade squamous intraepithelial lesion (HSIL)
    - Encompassing moderate and severe dysplasia CIS/CIN-2 and CIN-3
    - With features suspicious for invasion
  - Squamous cell carcinoma
- *Glandular Cell:* Atypical
  - Endocervical, endometrial, or glandular cells
    - Endocervical cells—favor neoplastic
    - Glandular cells—favor neoplastic
    - Endocervical adenocarcinoma in situ
  - Adenocarcinoma
    - Endocervical, endometrial, extrauterine
- Other malignant neoplasms (specify)

Educational Notes and Suggestions: (optional)

Sources: NIH, 2007; ACS, 2007b; Schuiling & Likis, 2006; Sherman et al., 2007.

Nursing Assessment

Obtain a thorough history and physical examination of the woman. Investigate her history for risk factors such as:

- Early age at first intercourse (within 1 year of menarche)
- Lower socioeconomic status
- Promiscuous male partners
- Unprotected sexual intercourse

BOX 8.2 Treatment Options for Cervical Cancer

- *Cryotherapy*—destroys abnormal cervical tissue by freezing with liquid nitrogen, Freon, or nitrous oxide. Studies show a 90% cure rate (Persinger & Beal, 2007). Healing takes up to 6 weeks, and the client may experience a profuse, watery vaginal discharge for 3 to 4 weeks.
- *Cone Biopsy* or *conization*—removes a cone-shaped section of cervical tissue. The base of the cone is formed by the ectocervix (outer part of the cervix) and the point or apex of the cone is from the endocervical canal. The transformation zone is contained within the cone sample. The cone biopsy is also a treatment and can be used to completely remove any precancers and very early cancers. There are two methods commonly used for cone biopsies:
  - LEEP (loop electrosurgical excision procedure) or LLETZ (large loop excision of the transformation zone)—the abnormal cervical tissue is removed with a wire that is heated by an electrical current. For this procedure, a local anesthetic is used. It is performed in the health care provider's office in approximately 10 minutes. Mild cramping and bleeding may persist for several weeks after the procedure.
  - Cold knife cone biopsy—a surgical scalpel or a laser is used instead of a heated wire to remove tissue. This procedure requires general anesthesia and is done in a hospital setting. After the procedure, cramping and bleeding may persist for a few weeks.
- *Laser therapy*—destroys diseased cervical tissue by using a focused beam of high-energy light to vaporize it (burn it off). After the procedure, the woman may experience a watery brown discharge for a few weeks. Very effective in destroying precancers and preventing them from developing into cancers.
- *Hysterectomy*—removes the uterus and cervix surgically
- *Radiation therapy*—delivered by internal radium applications to the cervix or external radiation therapy that includes lymphatics of the pelvis
- *Chemoradiation*—weekly cisplatin therapy concurrent with radiation. Investigation of this therapy is ongoing (ACS, 2007).

- Family history of cervical cancer (mother or sisters)
- Sexual intercourse with uncircumcised men
- Female offspring of mothers who took diethylstilbestrol (DES)
- Infections with genital herpes or chronic chlamydia
- Multiple sex partners
- Cigarette smoking
- Immunocompromised state
- HIV infection
- Oral contraceptive use

• Moderate dysplasia on Pap smear within past 5 years
• HPV infection (CDC, 2007b)

Question the woman about any signs and symptoms. Clinically, the first sign is abnormal vaginal bleeding, usually after sexual intercourse. Also be alert for reports of vaginal discomfort, malodorous discharge, and dysuria.

In some cases the woman is asymptomatic, with detection occurring at an annual gynecologic examination and Pap test.

Perform a physical examination. Inspect the perineal area for vaginal discharge or genital warts. Perform or assist with a pelvic examination, including the collection of a Pap smear as indicated (Nursing Procedure 8.1).

Nursing Procedure 8.1

ASSISTING WITH COLLECTION OF A PAP SMEAR

Purpose: To Obtain Cells From the Cervix for Cervical Cytology Screening

1. Explain procedure to the client (Fig. A).
2. Instruct client to empty her bladder.
3. Wash hands thoroughly.
4. Assemble equipment, maintaining sterility of equipment (Fig. B).
5. Position client on stirrups or foot pedals so that her knees fall outward.
6. Drape client with a sheet for privacy, covering the abdomen but leaving the perineal area exposed.
7. Open packages as needed.
8. Encourage client to relax.
9. Provide support to client as the practitioner obtains a sample by spreading the labia; inserting the speculum; inserting the cytobrush and swabbing the endocervix; and inserting the plastic spatula and swabbing the cervix (Fig. C–H).
10. Transfer specimen to container (Fig. I) or slide. If a slide is used, spray the fixative on the slide.
11. Place sterile lubricant on the practitioner's fingertip when indicated for the bimanual examination.
12. Wash hands thoroughly.
13. Label specimen according to facility policy.
14. Rinse reusable instruments and dispose of waste appropriately (Fig. J).
15. Wash hands thoroughly.

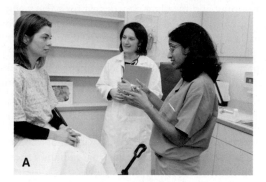

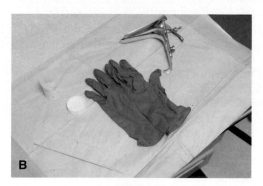

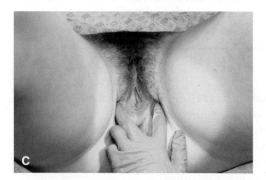

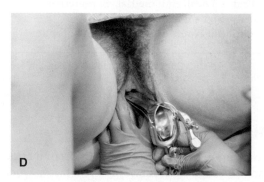

Nursing Procedure 8.1 (continued)

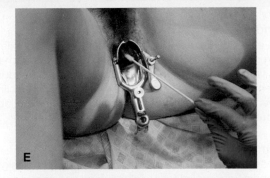

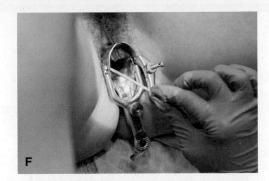

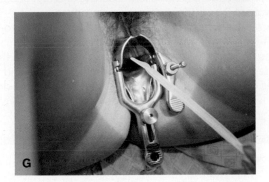

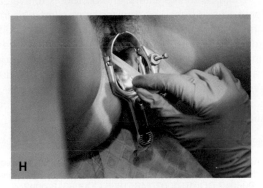

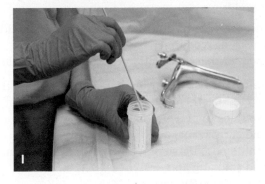

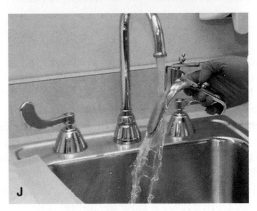

Used with permission from Klossner, N. J. (2006). *Introductory maternity nursing.* Philadelphia: Lippincott Williams & Wilkins.

> ▶ *Take* NOTE!
>
> *Suspect advanced cervical cancer in women with pelvic, back, or leg pain, weight loss, anorexia, weakness and fatigue, and fractures.*

Prepare the woman for further diagnostic testing if indicated, such as a colposcopy. In a colposcopy, the woman is placed in the lithotomy position and her cervix is cleansed with acetic acid solution. Acetic acid makes abnormal cells appear white, which is referred to as acetowhite. These white areas are then biopsied and sent to the pathologist for assessment. Although this test is not painful, has no side effects, and can be performed safely in the clinic or office setting, women may be apprehensive or anxious about it because it is done to identify and confirm potential abnormal cell growth. Provide appropriate physical and emotional preparation for this test (Evidence-Based Practice 8.1).

Nursing Management

The nurse's role involves primary prevention by educating women about risk factors and ways to prevent cervical

EVIDENCE-BASED PRACTICE 8.1
Anxiety Reduction for Women Undergoing a Colposcopy

● Study

Getting abnormal Pap smear results can be upsetting for a woman. A colposcopy is a follow-up examination that is commonly used to identify these suspicious cells and obtain a specimen for biopsy. A woman's anxiety about this examination is increased by the possibility of a cancer diagnosis. Studies have shown that anxiety can heighten discomfort, so researchers sought to discover which method of preparation for colposcopy best reduces a woman's anxiety. They conducted a detailed search of databases, clinical trial registers, and protocols to evaluate all randomized and quasi-randomized controlled trials involving interventions to reduce anxiety during colposcopy. Eleven trials involving 1,441 women were identified. The trials compared the anxiety levels of the intervention group with those of a control group. The methods used to reduce anxiety were informational leaflets, counseling, informational videos, video during colposcopy, music, and verbal information.

▲ Findings

Three methods were found to significantly reduce anxiety during colposcopy: listening to music, watching informational videos, and viewing the video during the procedure. Other methods, such as informational leaflets, counseling, and verbal information, were not found to reduce anxiety vs. control groups.

■ Nursing Implications

Nurses can use the information from this study to design appropriate strategies for client teaching and can encourage women to use these measures to reduce anxiety. For example, the nurse can suggest that the client listen to her favorite music during the procedure to help her relax. Nurses can urge women to seek agencies or settings that include these measures as part of their procedure, and nurses can work with their facilities to ensure that music, informational videos, and videotape equipment are available for use during this procedure.

Galaal, K. A., Deane, K., Sangal, S., & Lopes, A. D. (2007). Interventions for reducing anxiety in women undergoing colposcopy. *Cochrane Database of Systematic Reviews 2007,* Issue 3, Art.No.: CD006013.DOI:10.1002/14651858.CD006013.pub2.

dysplasia. Cervical cancer rates have decreased in the United States because of the widespread use of Pap testing, which can detect precancerous lesions of the cervix before they develop into cancer. Nevertheless, during 2007, an estimated 12,000 new cases will be diagnosed and approximately 3,800 women will die from cervical cancer (CDC, 2007a, 2007b; Advisory Committee on Immunization Practices [ACIP], 2007).

Gardasil, the first vaccine developed to protect girls and women from HPV, is now available. The vaccine prevents infection from four HPV types: HPV 6, 11, 16, and 18. Theses types are responsible for 70% of cervical cancers and 90% of genital warts (Snow, 2007). Clinical trials indicate that the vaccine has high efficacy in preventing persistent HPV infection, cervical cancer precursor lesions, vaginal and vulvar cancer precursor lesions, and genital warts (Bryan, 2007). The vaccine is administered by intramuscular injection, and the recommended schedule is a three-dose series with the second and third doses administered 2 and 6 months after the first dose. The recommended age for vaccination of females is 11 to 12 years old, but the vaccine can be administered to girls as young as 9 years old (Pichichero, 2007). The long-term efficacy of HPV vaccines remains to be determined. Sustained efficacy up to 4.5 years has been documented, but it could be that boosters will be needed (CDC, 2007a). However, the vaccine is not a substitute for routine cervical cancer screening, and vaccinated women should have Pap smears as recommended.

Focus primary prevention education on the following:

• Identify high-risk behaviors in clients and teach them how to reduce them:
  • Take steps to prevent STIs.
  • Avoid early sexual activity.
  • Faithfully use barrier methods of contraception.
  • Avoid smoking and drinking.
  • Receive the HPV vaccine.
• Instruct women on the importance of screening for cervical cancer by annual Pap smears. Outline the proper preparation before having a Pap smear (Teaching Guidelines 8.3). Reinforce specific guidelines for screening.

Nurses also can advocate for clients by making sure that the Pap smear is sent to an accredited laboratory for interpretation. Doing so reduces the risk of false-negative results.

Secondary prevention focuses on reducing or limiting the area of cervical dysplasia. Tertiary prevention focuses on minimizing disability or spread of cervical cancer. Explain in detail all procedures that might be needed. Encourage the client who has undergone any cervical treatment to allow the pelvic area to rest for approximately 1 month. Discuss this rest period with the client and her partner to

TEACHING GUIDELINES 8.3

Strategies to Optimize Pap Smear Results

- Schedule your Pap smear appointment about 2 weeks (10 to 18 days) after the first day of your last menses to increase the chance of getting the best sample of cervical cells without menses.
- Refrain from intercourse for 48 hours before the test because additional matter such as sperm can obscure the specimen.
- Do not douche within 48 hours before the test to prevent washing away cervical cells that might be abnormal.
- Do not use tampons, birth control foams, jellies, vaginal creams, or vaginal medications for 72 hours before the test, as they could cover up or obscure the cervical cell sample.
- Cancel your Pap appointment if vaginal bleeding occurs, because the presence of blood cells interferes with visual evaluation of the sample (Schuiling & Likis, 2006).

gain his cooperation. Outline alternatives to vaginal intercourse, such as cuddling, holding hands, and kissing. Remind the woman about any follow-up procedures that are needed and assist her with scheduling if necessary.

Throughout the process, provide emotional support to the woman and her family. During the decision-making process, the woman may be overwhelmed by the diagnosis and all the information being presented. Refer the woman and her family to appropriate community resources and support groups as indicated.

Vaginal Cancer

Vaginal cancer is malignant tissue growth arising in the vagina. It is rare, representing less than 3% of all genital cancers. The ACS estimates that in 2007, over 2,000 new cases of vaginal cancer will be diagnosed in the United States, and approximately 800 will die of this cancer (ACS, 2007d). The peak incidence of vaginal cancer occurs at 60 to 65 years of age. The prognosis of vaginal cancer depends largely on the stage of disease and the type of tumor. The overall 5-year survival rate for squamous cell carcinoma is about 42%; that for adenocarcinoma is about 78% (NCI, 2007c). Vaginal cancer can be effectively treated, and when found early it is often curable.

Pathophysiology

The etiology of vaginal cancer has not been identified. Malignant diseases of the vagina are either primary vagi-

nal cancers or metastatic forms from adjacent or distant organs. About 80% of vaginal cancers are metastatic, primarily from the cervix and endometrium. These cancers invade the vagina directly. Cancers from distant sites that metastasize to the vagina through the blood or lymphatic system are typically from the colon, kidneys, skin (melanoma), or breast. Tumors in the vagina commonly occur on the posterior wall and spread to the cervix or vulva (NCI, 2007c).

Squamous cell carcinomas that begin in the epithelial lining of the vagina account for about 85% of vaginal cancers. This type of cancer usually occurs in women over age 50. They develop slowly over a period of years, commonly in the upper third of the vagina. They tend to spread early by directly invading the bladder and rectal walls. They also metastasize through blood and lymphatics. The remaining 15% are adenocarcinomas, which differ from squamous cell carcinoma by an increase in pulmonary metastases and supraclavicular and pelvic node involvement (ACS, 2007d).

Therapeutic Management

Treatment of vaginal cancer depends on the type of cells involved and the stage of the disease. If the cancer is localized, radiation, laser surgery, or both may be used. If the cancer has spread, radical surgery might be needed, such as a hysterectomy, or removal of the upper vagina with dissection of the pelvic nodes in addition to radiation therapy.

Nursing Assessment

Begin the history and physical examination by reviewing for risk factors. Although direct risk factors for the initial development of vaginal cancer have not been identified, associated risk factors include advancing age (over 60 years old), previous pelvic radiation, exposure to diethylstilbestrol (DES) in utero, vaginal trauma, history of genital warts (HPV infection), HIV infection, cervical cancer, chronic vaginal discharge, smoking, and low socioeconomic level (ACS, 2007d).

Question the woman about any complaints. Most women with vaginal cancer are asymptomatic. Those with symptoms have painless vaginal bleeding (often after sexual intercourse), abnormal vaginal discharge, dyspareunia, dysuria, constipation, and pelvic pain (NCI, 2007c). During the physical examination, observe for any obvious vaginal discharge or genital warts, or changes in the appearance of the vaginal mucosa. Anticipate colposcopy with biopsy of suspicious lesions to confirm the diagnosis.

Nursing Management

Nursing management for this cancer is similar to that for other reproductive cancers, with emphasis on sexuality counseling and referral to local support groups. Women undergoing radical surgery need intensive counseling about the nature of the surgery, risks, potential complications, changes in physical appearance and physiologic function, and sexuality alterations.

Vulvar Cancer

Vulvar cancer is an abnormal neoplastic growth on the external female genitalia (Fig. 8.5). It is responsible for 0.6% of all malignancies in women and 4% of all female genital cancers. It is the fourth most common gynecologic cancer, after endometrial, ovarian, and cervical cancers (Naumann & Higgins, 2007). The ACS estimates that in 2007, about 4,000 cancers of the vulva will be diagnosed in the United States and over 900 women will die of this cancer (ACS, 2007e). When detected early, it is highly curable.

Vulvar cancer is found most commonly in older women in their mid-60s to 70s, but the incidence in women younger than 35 years old has increased over the past few decades. The overall 5-year survival rate when lymph nodes are not involved is 90%, but it drops to 50% to 70% when the lymph nodes have been invaded (ACS, 2007e).

Pathophysiology

Approximately 90% of vulvar tumors are squamous cell carcinomas. This type of cancer forms slowly over several years and is usually preceded by precancerous changes. These precancerous changes are termed vulvar intra-epithelial neoplasia (VIN). The two major types of VIN are classic (undifferentiated) and simplex (differentiated). Classic VIN, the more common one, is associated with HPV infection (genital warts due to types 16, 18, 31, 33, 35, and 51) and smoking (Wallace & Sanford, 2006). It typically occurs in women between 30 and 40 years old. In contrast to classic VIN, simplex VIN usually occurs in

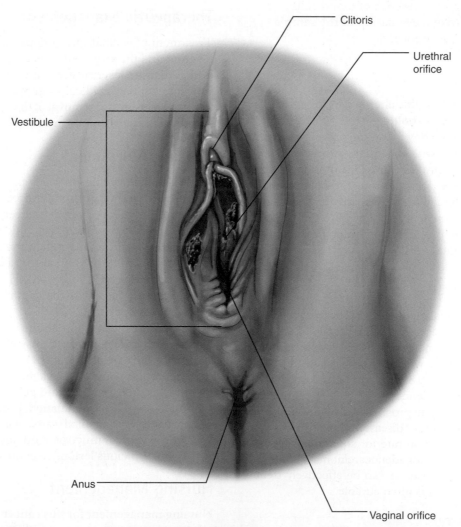

FIGURE 8.5 Vulvar cancer. (The Anatomical Chart Company. [2005]. *Atlas of pathophysiology* [2nd ed.]. Philadelphia: Lippincott Williams & Wilkins)

postmenopausal women and is not associated with HPV (Davidson, 2007).

Screening and Diagnosis

Annual vulvar examination is the most effective way to prevent vulvar cancer. Careful inspection of the vulva during routine annual gynecologic examinations remains the most productive diagnostic technique. Liberal use of biopsies of any suspicious vulvar lesion is usually necessary to make the diagnosis and to guide treatment. However, many women do not seek health care evaluation for months or years after noticing an abnormal lump or lesion.

The diagnosis of vulvar cancer is made by a biopsy of the suspicious lesion, which is usually found on the labia majora.

> ▶ *Take* NOTE!
>
> *Vulvar pruritus or a lump is present in the majority of women with vulvar cancer. Lumps should be biopsied even if the woman is asymptomatic.*

Therapeutic Management

Treatment varies depending on the extent of the disease. Laser surgery, cryosurgery, or electrosurgical incision may be used. Larger lesions may need more extensive surgery and skin grafting. The traditional treatment for vulvar cancer has been radical vulvectomy, but more conservative techniques are being used to improve psychosexual outcomes.

Nursing Assessment

Typically, no single specific clinical symptom heralds this disease, so diagnosis is often delayed significantly. Therefore, it is important to review the woman's history for risk factors such as:

- Exposure to HPV type 16
- Age over 50
- HIV infection
- VIN
- Lichen sclerosus
- Melanoma or atypical moles
- Exposure to HSV II
- Multiple sex partners
- Smoking
- History of breast cancer
- Immune suppression
- Hypertension
- Diabetes mellitus
- Obesity (ACS, 2007e)

In most cases, the woman reports persistent vulvar itching that does not improve with the use of creams or ointments. During the physical examination, observe for any masses or thickening of the vulvar area. A vulvar lump or mass most often is noted. The vulvar lesion is usually raised and may be fleshy, ulcerated, leukoplakic, or warty (Naumann & Higgins, 2007). Less commonly, the woman may present with vulvar bleeding, discharge, dysuria, and pain.

Nursing Management

Women with vulvar cancer must clearly understand their disease, treatment options, and prognosis. To accomplish this, provide information and establish effective communication with the client and her family. Act as an educator and advocate.

Teach the woman about healthy lifestyle behaviors, such as smoking cessation and measures to reduce risk factors. For example, instruct the woman how to examine her genital area, urging her to do so monthly between menstrual periods. Tell her to look for any changes in appearance (e.g., whitened or reddened patches of skin); changes in feel (e.g., areas of the vulva becoming itchy or painful); or the development of lumps, moles (e.g., changes in size, shape, or color), freckles, cuts, or sores on the vulva. Urge the woman to report these changes to the health care provider (ACS, 2007e).

Teach the woman about preventive measures such as not wearing tight undergarments and not using perfumes and dyes in the vulvar region. Also educate her about the use of barrier methods of birth control (e.g., condoms) to reduce the risk of contracting HIV, HSV, and HPV.

For the woman diagnosed with vulvar cancer, provide information and support. Discuss potential changes in sexuality if radical surgery is performed. Encourage her to communicate openly with her partner. Refer her to appropriate community resources and support groups.

▪▪▪ Key Concepts

- Women have a one-in-three lifetime risk of developing cancer, and one out of every four deaths is from cancer; thus, nurses must focus on screening and educating all women regardless of risk factors.
- The nurse plays a key role in offering emotional support, determining appropriate sources of support, and helping the woman use effective coping strategies when facing a diagnosis of cancer of the reproductive tract. Although reproductive tract cancer is rare during pregnancy, the woman's vigilance and routine screenings should continue throughout.
- A woman's sexuality and culture are inextricably interwoven, and it is essential that nurses working with

women of various cultures recognize this and remain sensitive to the vast changes that will take place when the diagnosis of cancer is made.

- Ovarian cancer is the eighth most common cancer among women and the fourth most common cause of cancer deaths for women in the United States, accounting for more deaths than any other cancer of the reproductive system.
- Ovarian cancer has been described as "the overlooked disease" or "silent killer," because women and/or health care practitioners often ignore or rationalize early symptoms. It is typically diagnosed in advanced stages.
- Unopposed endogenous and exogenous estrogens, obesity, nulliparity, menopause after the age of 52 years, and diabetes are the major etiologic risk factors associated with the development of endometrial cancer.
- The American Cancer Society (ACS) recommends that women should be informed about risks and symptoms of endometrial cancer at the onset of menopause and strongly encouraged to report any unexpected bleeding or spotting to their health care providers.
- Malignant diseases of the vagina are either primary vaginal cancers or metastatic forms from adjacent or distant organs. Vaginal cancer tumors can be effectively treated and, when found early, are often curable.
- Cervical cancer incidence and mortality rates have decreased noticeably in the past several decades, with most of the reduction attributed to the Pap test, which detects cervical cancer and precancerous lesions.
- The nurse's role involves primary prevention of cervical cancer through education of women regarding risk factors and preventive techniques to avoid cervical dysplasia.
- Diagnosis of vulvar cancer is often delayed significantly because there is no single specific clinical symptom that heralds it. The most common presentation is persistent vulvar itching that does not improve with the application of creams or ointments.

References

Advisory Committee on Immunization Practices (ACIP). (2007). Quadrivalent human papillomavirus vaccine. *MMWR*, 56(RR-2), 1–24.

Agency for Healthcare Research and Quality (AHRQ). (2007). *Women: Stay healthy at any age—Your checklist for health.* AHRQ Publications No. 07-IP005-A. Available at: http://www.ahrq.gov/ppip/healthywom.htm.

Alexander, L. L., LaRosa, J. H., Bader, H., & Garfield, S. (2007). *New dimensions in women's health* (4th ed.). Sudbury, MA: Jones and Bartlett Publishers.

American Cancer Society (ACS). (2007a). *What are the key statistics about cervical cancer?* Available at: http://www.cancer.org/docroot/CRI/content/CRI_2_4_1X_What_are_the_key_statistics_for_cervical_cancer_8.asp?sitearea=.

American Cancer Society (ACS). (2007b). *How Pap test results are reported.* Available at: http://www.cancer.org/docroot/PED/content/PED_2_3X_Pap_Test.asp.

American Cancer Society (ACS). (2007c). *What are the key statistics about ovarian cancer?* Available at: http://www.cancer.org/docroot/

CRI/content/CRI_2_4_1X_What_are_the_key_statistics_for_ovarian_cancer_33.asp?sitearea=&level=.

American Cancer Society (ACS). (2007d). *What are the key statistics about vaginal cancer?* Available at: http://www.cancer.org/docroot/CRI/content/CRI_2_4_1X_What_are_the_key_statistics_for_vaginal_cancer_55.asp?sitearea=.

American Cancer Society (ACS). (2007e). *What are the key statistics about vulvar cancer?* Available at: http://www.cancer.org/docroot/cri/content/cri_2_4_1x_what_are_the_key_statistics_for_vulvar_cancer_45.asp?sitearea=&level=.

American Cancer Society (ACS). (2007f). *Endometrial cancer.* Available at: http://www.cancer.org/docroot/CRI/CRI_2_1x.asp?rnav=criov&dt=11.

American Cancer Society (ACS). (2007g). *Cancer prevention and early detection: Cancer facts and figures 2007.* Atlanta: ACS.

American Cancer Society. (2008). *Cancer facts and figures 2007.* Atlanta: ACS.

Blackburn, S. T. (2007). *Maternal, fetal and neonatal physiology: A clinical perspective* (3rd ed.). St. Louis, MO: Saunders Elsevier.

Bryan, J. T. (2007). Developing an HPV vaccine to prevent cervical cancer and genital warts. *Vaccine*, 25(16), 3001–3006.

Burke, J. J., & Gallup, D. G. (2007). Endometrial cancer. In R. E. Rakel & E. T. Bope (Eds.), *Conn's current therapy 2007* (Section 16, pp. 1261–1264). Philadelphia: Saunders Elsevier.

Centers for Disease Control and Prevention (CDC). (2007a). Quadrivalent human papillomavirus vaccine: Recommendations of the Advisory Committee on Immunization Practices (ACIP). *MMWR*, 56(RR-2), 1–24.

Centers for Disease Control and Prevention (CDC). (2007b). *Cancer A-Z.* Available at: http://www.cdc.gov/cancer/healthdisparities/statistics/ethnic.htm.

Centers for Disease Control and Prevention (CDC). (2007c). *Ovarian cancer.* Available at: http://www.cdc.gov/cancer/ovarian/basic_info/.

Cherry, C., DeGaetano, C., & Martin, V. (2007). Ovarian cancer: Awareness is key. *Nursing Spectrum.* Available at: http://www.nurse.com/ce/print.html?CCID=3193.

Davidson, S. A. (2007). Neoplasms of the vulva. In R. E. Rakel & E. T. Bope (Eds.), *Conn's current therapy 2007* (Section 16; pp. 1268–1271). Philadelphia: Saunders Elsevier.

Eaton, L. A. (2007). Ovarian cancer. In R. E. Rakel & E. T. Bope (Eds.), *Conn's current therapy 2007* (Section 16, pp. 1259–1261). Philadelphia: Saunders Elsevier.

Fieler, V., & Henry, B. (2007). How to give psychological support to clients with cancer. *Nursing Spectrum.* Available at: http://www.nurse.com/ce/print.html?CCID=3309.

Galaal, K. A., Deane, K., Sangal, S., & Lopes, A.D. (2007). Interventions for reducing anxiety in women undergoing colposcopy. *Cochrane Database of Systematic Reviews 2007*, Issue 3, Art. No.: CD006013.DOI:10.1002/14651858.CD006013.pub2.

Goff, B. A., Mandel, L. S., Drescher, C. W., Urban, N., Gough, S., Schurman, K. M., Patras, J., Mahony, B. S., & Andersen, M. R. (2007). Development of an ovarian cancer symptom index: Possibilities for earlier detection. *Cancer*, 109(2), 221–227.

Hopkins, M. P., & Sawa, W. (2007). Cancer of the uterine cervix. In R. E. Rakel & E. T. Bope (Eds.), *Conn's current therapy 2007* (Section 16, pp. 1264–1267). Philadelphia: Saunders Elsevier.

Jenko, M., & Moffitt, S. R. (2006). Transcultural nursing principles. *Journal of Hospice and Palliative Nursing*, 8(3), 172–181.

Machado, F., Vegas, C., Leon, J., Perez, A., Sanchez, R., Parrilla, J., & Abad, L. (2007). Ovarian cancer during pregnancy: Analysis of 15 cases. *Gynecologic Oncology*, 105(2), 446–450.

Martin, V. R. (2007). Ovarian cancer: An overview of treatment options. *Clinical Journal of Oncology Nursing*, 11(2), 201–207.

Mayo Clinic. (2008). *Cancer prevention: 7 steps to reduce your risk* [Online]. Available at: http://www.mayoclinic.com/health/cancer-prevention/CA00024.

National Cancer Institute (NCI). (2007a). *Annual report on the status of cancer.* U.S. National Institutes of Health. Available at: http://www.nci.nih.gov/newscenter/pressreleases/ReportNation2007Release.

National Cancer Institute (NCI). (2007b). *Endometrial cancer: treatment.* U.S. National Institutes of Health. Available at: http://www.nci.hih.gov/cancertopics/pdq/treatment/endometrial/HealthProfessional/page1/.

National Cancer Institute (NCI). (2007c). *Vaginal cancer*. Available at: http://www.cancer.gov/cancertopics/types/vaginal/.

National Institutes of Health (NIH). (2007). *Cervical cancer: Prevention.* National Cancer Institute. Available at: http://www.nci.nih.gov/cancertopics/pdq/prevention/cervical/HealthProfessional/page2.

Naumann, R. W., & Higgins, R. V. (2007). Surgical treatment of vulvar cancer. *eMedicine.* Available at: http://www.emedicine.com/med/topic3328.htm.

Persinger, M. F., & Beal, M. W. (2007). Cervical and ovarian cancer screening. In B. Hackley, J. M. Kriebs, & M. E. Rousseau (Eds.), *Primary care of women: A guide for midwives and women's health providers.* Sudbury, MA: Jones and Bartlett Publishers.

Pichichero, M. E. (2007). Who should get the HPV vaccine? *Journal of Family Practice, 56*(3), 197–202.

Roberts, K., Rezai, N., & Edmondson, R. J. (2007). Cervical cancer in pregnancy: An assault on family and fertility. *British Journal of Midwifery, 15*(3), 1320–1326.

Schuiling, K. D., & Likis, F. E. (2006). *Women's gynecologic health.* Sudbury, MA: Jones and Bartlett Publishers.

Sherman, M. E., Dasgupta, A., Schiffman, M., Nayar, R., & Solomon, D. (2007). The Bethesda Interobserver Reproducibility Study (BIRST): A Web-based assessment of the Bethesda 2001 system for classifying cervical cytology. *Cancer, 111*(1), 15–25.

Snow, M. (2007). HPV vaccine: New treatment for an old disease. *Nursing2007, 37*(3), 67–68.

Sonoda, Y., & Barakat, R. R. (2006). Screening and the prevention of gynecologic cancer: Endometrial cancer. *Bailliere's Best Practice & Research in Clinical Obstetrics & Gynecology, 20*(2), 363–377.

Speroff, L., & Fritz, M. A. (2005). *Clinical gynecologic endocrinology and infertility* (7th ed.). Philadelphia: Lippincott Williams & Wilkins.

Surbone, A. (2006). Cultural aspects of communication in cancer care. *Recent Results in Cancer Research, 168*(1), 91–104.

Tiffen, J. M., & Mahon, S. M. (2006). Educating women regarding the early detection of endometrial cancer—What is the evidence? *Clinical Journal of Oncology Nursing, 10*(1), 102–105.

Torpy, J. M. (2007). Human papillomavirus infection. *Journal of the American Medical Association, 297*(8), 912–913.

U.S. Department of Health and Human Services (USDHHS), Public Health Service. (2000). *Healthy people 2010* (conference edition, in two volumes). Washington, DC: U.S. Government Printing Office.

U.S. Preventive Services Task Force (USPSTF). (2006). *Screening for ovarian cancer. U.S. Preventive Services Task Force Summary of Recommendations.* Available at: http://www.ahrq.gov/clinic/uspstf/uspsovar.htm.

Wallace, M., & Sanford, A. (2006). Gynecologic cancers. In K. D. Schuiling & F. E. Likis (Eds.), *Women's gynecologic health* (Chapter 23, pp. 595–633). Sudbury, MA: Jones and Bartlett Publishers.

World Health Organization (WHO). (2008). *Cancer prevention* [Online]. Available at: http://www.who.int/cancer/prevention/en/.

WEBSITES

American Cancer Society: 1-800-ACS-2345, www.cancer.org

American Urological Association: (410) 727-1100, www.auanet.org

Cancer Care, Inc.: (212) 712-8080, www.cancercare.org

Gilda Radner Familial Ovarian Cancer Registry: (800) OVARIAN, www.ovariancancer.com

Gynecologic Cancer Foundation: (800) 444-4441, www.wcn.org

Hysterectomy Educational Resource and Services (HERS): (215) 667-7757, www.ccon.com/hers

National Ovarian Cancer Coalition: (888) 682-7426. www.ovarian.org

National Women's Health Information Center: (800) 994-9662, www.4women.gov

Oncology Nursing Society (ONS): (866) 257-4ONS, www.ons.org

Ovarian Cancer Research Fund, Inc.: (800) 873-9569, www.ocrf.org

Sexuality Information and Education Counsel of the United States: (212) 819-9770, www.siecus.org

SHARE: Self-Help for Women with Breast or Ovarian Cancer: (866) 891-3431, www.sharecancersupport.org

Vulvar Health: www.vulvarhealth.org

Women's Cancer Network: (312) 644-6610, www.wcn.org

CHAPTER WORKSHEET

MULTIPLE CHOICE QUESTIONS

1. When describing ovarian cancer to a local women's group, the nurse states that ovarian cancer often is not diagnosed early because:

   a. The disease progresses very slowly.

   b. The early stages produce very vague symptoms.

   c. The disease usually is diagnosed only at autopsy.

   d. Clients don't follow up on acute pelvic pain.

2. A postmenopausal woman reports that she has started spotting again. Which of the following would the nurse do?

   a. Instruct the client to keep a menstrual diary for the next few months.

   b. Tell her not to worry, since this a common but not serious event.

   c. Have her start warm-water douches to promote healing.

   d. Anticipate that the doctor will do an endometrial biopsy.

3. Which of the following would the nurse identify as the priority psychosocial need for a women diagnosed with reproductive cancer?

   a. Clear information

   b. Hand-holding

   c. Cheerfulness

   d. Offering of hope

4. When teaching a group of women about screening and early detection of cervical cancer, the nurse would include which of the following as most effective?

   a. Fecal occult blood test

   b. CA-125 blood test

   c. Pap smear

   d. Sigmoidoscopy

5. After teaching a group of students about reproductive tract cancers, the nursing instructor determines that the teaching was successful when the students identify which of the following as the deadliest type of female reproductive cancer?

   a. Vulvar

   b. Ovarian

   c. Endometrial

   d. Cervical

CRITICAL THINKING EXERCISES

1. Tammy Scott, a 27-year-old sexually active Caucasian woman, visits the Health Department family planning clinic and requests information about the various methods available. In taking her history, the nurse learns that she started having sex at age 15 and has had multiple sex partners since then. She smokes two packs of cigarettes daily. Because she has been unemployed for a few months, her health insurance policy has lapsed. She has never previously obtained any gynecologic care.

   a. Based on her history, which risk factors for cervical cancer are present?

   b. What recommendations would you make for her, and why?

   c. What are this client's educational needs concerning health maintenance?

2. Jennifer Nappo, a 60-year-old nulliparous woman, presents to the gynecologic oncology clinic after her health care provider palpated an adnexal mass on her right ovary. In taking her history, the nurse learns that she has experienced mild abdominal bloating and weight loss for the past several months but felt fine otherwise. She was diagnosed with breast cancer 15 years ago and was treated with a lumpectomy and radiation. She has occasionally used talcum powder in her perineal area over the past 20 years.

   A transvaginal ultrasound reveals a complex mass in the right adnexa. She undergoes a total abdominal hysterectomy and bilateral salpingo-oophorectomy and lymph node biopsy. Pathology confirms a diagnosis of stage III ovarian cancer with abdominal metastasis and positive lymph nodes.

   a. Is this client's profile typical for a woman with this diagnosis?

   b. What in her history might increase her risk for ovarian cancer?

   c. What can the nurse do to increase awareness of this cancer for all women?

STUDY ACTIVITIES

1. During your surgical clinical rotation, interview a female client undergoing surgery for cancer of her reproductive organs. Ask her to recall the symptoms that brought her to the health care provider. Ask her what thoughts, feelings, and emotions went through her mind before and after her diagnosis. Finally, ask her how this experience will change her life in the future.

2. Visit an oncology and radiology treatment center to find out about the various treatment modalities available for reproductive cancers. Contrast the various treatment methods and report your findings to your class.

3. Visit one of the websites listed at the end of the chapter to explore a topic of interest concerning reproductive cancers. How correct and current is the content? What is its level? Share your assessment with your classmates.

4. Taking oral contraceptives provides protection against _____ cancer.

5. Two genes, BRCA-1 and BRCA-2, are linked with hereditary _____ and _____ cancers.

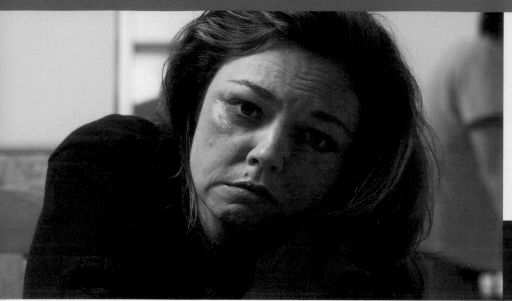

CHAPTER 9

VIOLENCE AND ABUSE

KEY TERMS

acquaintance rape
battered women
    syndrome
cycle of violence
date rape

female genital mutilation
human trafficking
incest
intimate partner
    violence

post-traumatic stress
    disorder
rape
sexual abuse
statutory rape

LEARNING OBJECTIVES

After completion of the chapter, the student should be able to:

1. Define the key terms.
2. Discuss the incidence of violence in women.
3. Outline the cycle of violence and appropriate interventions.
4. Discuss the myths and facts about violence.
5. Analyze the dynamics of rape and sexual abuse.
6. Describe the resources available to women experiencing abuse.
7. Discuss the role of the nurse who cares for abused women.

Dorothy came to the prenatal clinic with a complaint of recurring headaches. She had been in twice this week already, but insisted she be seen today and started to cry. When the nurse called her into the examination room, Dorothy's cell phone rang. She hurried to answer it and told the person on the other end that she was at the store. When the nurse asked if she was afraid at home, Dorothy answered "at times." What cues did the nurse pick up on to ask that question? How frequent is this problem in women?

Wow

After being traumatized, women can decide to stay in the shallow end of the pool or they can find support and swim in the ocean.

Violence against women is a significant health and social problem affecting virtually all societies, but often it goes unrecognized and unreported. For all the strides American women have made in the past 100 years, obliterating violence against themselves isn't one of them. Violence against women is a growing problem. In many countries it is still accepted as part of normal behavior. According to the Federal Bureau of Investigation, one third to one half of all women in the United States will experience some form of physical violence during their lifetime (FBI, 2007). Forty percent to 60 percent of murders of women in North America are committed by intimate partners (FBI, 2007). Federal funding for the problem is trickling down to local programs, but it isn't reaching victims fast enough. In the United States, there are three times more shelters for animals than for battered women (Dutton, 2007). In many cases, a victim escapes her abuser only to be turned away from a local shelter because it is full. The number of abused women is staggering: one woman is being battered every 12 seconds in the United States (CDC, 2007a).

Nurses play a major role in assessing women who have suffered some type of violence. Often, after a woman is victimized, she will complain about physical ailments that will give her the opportunity to visit a health care setting. A visit to a health care agency is an ideal time for women to be assessed for violence. Because nurses are viewed as trustworthy and sensitive about very personal subjects, women often feel comfortable in confiding or discussing these issues with them.

> ▶ **Take** *NOTE!*
>
> *Nurses will come in contact with violence and sexual abuse no matter what health care setting they work in. Nurses must be ready to ask the right questions and to act on the answers, because such action could be life-saving.*

This chapter will address two types of violence against women: intimate partner violence and sexual abuse. Both types of violence against women have devastating and costly consequences for all of society.

Intimate Partner Violence

Intimate partner violence is actual or threatened physical or sexual violence or psychological/emotional abuse. It includes threats of physical or sexual violence when the threat is used to control a person's actions (CDC, 2007a). Intimate partners include individuals who are currently in dating, cohabiting, or marital relationships, or those who have been in such relationships in the past. Some of the common terms used to describe intimate partner violence are domestic abuse, spouse abuse, domestic violence,

battering, and rape. Intimate partner violence affects a distressingly high percentage of the population and has physical, psychological, social, and economic consequences (Fig. 9.1).

A nurse may be the first health care professional to assess and identify the signs of intimate partner violence and can have a profound impact on a woman's decision to seek help. Thus, it is important for nurses to be able to identify abuse and aid the victim. Intimate partner violence can leave significant psychological scars, and a well-trained nurse can have a positive impact on the victim's mental and emotional health.

Incidence

Although estimates vary, as many as 6 million women are abused annually (CDC, 2007a). Even more shocking, 75% of the abused women initially identified in a medical setting go on to suffer repeated abuse, including homicide (CDC, 2007a). This may include physical violence, emotional abuse, sexual assault, rape, incest, or elder abuse. Each year, intimate partner violence results in an estimated 1,200 deaths and 2 million injuries among women (CDC, 2008).

Women are at risk for violence at nearly every stage of their lives. Old, young, beautiful, unattractive, married, single—no woman is completely safe from the risk of intimate partner violence. Current or former husbands or lovers kill over half of the murdered women in the United States. Intimate partner violence against women causes more serious injuries and deaths than automobile accidents, rapes, and muggings combined. The medical cost of intimate partner violence approaches $6 billion each year to pay for medical and surgical care, counseling, child care, incarceration, attorney fees, and loss of work productivity (Kelly, 2007).

Abuse occurs in both heterosexual and homosexual relationships. Violence within gay and lesbian relationships may go unreported for fear of harassment or ridicule. In addition, since gay and lesbian partnerships are not seen

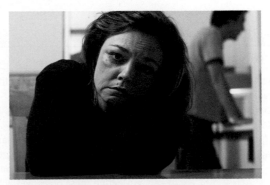

FIGURE **9.1** Intimate partner violence has significant physical, psychological, social, and economic consequences. An important role of the health care provider is to identify abusive or potentially abusive situations as soon as possible and provide support for the victim.

as legal in many states, there are few statistics gathered on incident rates.

Background

Until the mid-1970s, our society tended to legitimize a man's power and control over a woman. The U.S. legal and judicial systems considered intervention into family disputes wrong and a violation of the family's right to privacy. Intimate partner violence was often tolerated and even socially acceptable. Fortunately, attitudes and laws have changed to protect women and punish abusers. In *Healthy People 2010,* two key objectives address violence against women.

Characteristics of Intimate Partner Violence

Although more research is needed in this area, studies have found certain risk factors for intimate partner violence:

- Use and abuse of substances such as alcohol (this increases the risk of perpetration and victimization for both men and women)
- Negative affect (e.g., hostility and depression)
- History of childhood abuse
- History of antisocial behavior
- Current unemployment
- Neighborhood norms that accept violence and drug use
- Traditional gender role expectations (Herrenkohl et al., 2007)

Generation-to-Generation Continuum of Violence

Violence is a learned behavior that, without intervention, is self-perpetuating. It is a cyclical health problem. The long-term effects of violence on victims and children can be profound. Children who witness one parent abuse another are more likely to become delinquents or batterers themselves because they see abuse as an integral part of a close relationship. Thus, an abusive relationship between father and mother can perpetuate future abusive relationships. Research has found that children who witness intimate partner violence are at risk for developing psychiatric disorders, developmental problems, school failure, violence against others, and low self-esteem (Paluzzi, 2007).

Childhood maltreatment is a major health problem that is associated with a wide range of physical conditions and leads to high rates of psychiatric morbidity and social problems in adulthood. Women who were physically or sexually abused as children have an increased risk of victimization and experience adverse mental health conditions such as depression, anxiety, and low self-esteem as adults (Ferris, 2007).

In 50% to 75% of the cases when a parent is abused, the children are abused as well (Paluzzi, 2007). Exposure to violence has a negative impact on children's physical, emotional, and cognitive well-being. The cycle continues into another generation through learned responses and violent acting out. While there are always exceptions, most children deprived of their basic physical, psychological, and spiritual needs do not develop healthy personalities. They grow up with feelings of fear, inadequacy, anxiety, anger, hostility, guilt, and rage. They often lack coping skills, blame others, demonstrate poor impulse control, and generally struggle with authority. Unless this cycle is broken, more than half become abusers themselves (CDC, 2007a).

The Cycle of Violence

In an abusive relationship, the **cycle of violence** comprises three distinct phases: the tension-building phase, the acute battering phase, and the honeymoon phase (Dutton, 2007). The cyclical behavior begins with a time of tension-building arguments, progresses to violence, and settles into a making-up or calm period. This cycle of violence increases in frequency and severity as it is repeated over and over again. The cycle can cover a long or short period of time. The honeymoon phase gradually shortens and eventually disappears altogether. Abuse in relationships typically becomes accelerated and thus more dangerous over time. The abuser no longer feels the need to apologize and indulge in a honeymoon phase as the woman becomes increasingly disempowered in the relationship.

Phase 1: Tension-Building
During the first—and usually the longest—phase of the cycle, tension escalates between the couple. Excessive drinking, jealousy, or other factors might lead to name-calling, hostility, and friction. The woman might sense that her partner is reacting to her more negatively, that he is on edge and reacts heatedly to any trivial frustration. A woman often will accept her partner's building anger as legitimately directed toward her. She internalizes what she perceives as her responsibility to keep the situation from exploding. In her mind, if she does her job well, he remains calm. But if she fails, the resulting violence is her fault.

HEALTHY PEOPLE 2010

Objective	Significance
1. Reduce the rate of physical assault by current or former intimate partners. 2. Reduce the annual rate of rape or attempted rape.	• Will increase women's quality and years of healthy life • Eliminate health disparities for survivors of violence • Goal is to have 90% compliance in screening for intimate partner violence by health professionals. • Meeting these objectives will reflect the importance of early detection, intervention, and evaluation.

Available at www.healthypeople.gov/

Phase 2: Acute Battering

The second phase of the cycle is the explosion of violence. The batterer loses control both physically and emotionally. This is when the victim may be assaulted or murdered. After a battering episode, most victims consider themselves lucky that the abuse was not worse, no matter how severe their injuries. They often deny the seriousness of their injuries and refuse to seek medical treatment.

Phase 3: Honeymoon

The third phase of the cycle is a period of calm, loving, contrite behavior on the part of the batterer. He may be genuinely sorry for the pain he caused his partner. He attempts to make up for his brutal behavior and believes he can control himself and never hurt the woman he loves. The victim wants to believe that her partner really can change. She feels responsible, at least in part, for causing the incident, and she feels responsible for her partner's well-being (Box 9.1).

Types of Abuse

Abusers may use whatever it takes to control a situation from emotional abuse and humiliation to physical assault. Victims often tolerate emotional, physical, financial, and sexual abuse. Many remain in abusive relationships because they believe they deserve the abuse.

Emotional Abuse

Emotional abuse includes:

- Promising, swearing, or threatening to hit the victim
- Forcing the victim to perform degrading or humiliating acts
- Threatening to harm children, pets, or close friends
- Humiliating the woman by name-calling and insults
- Threatening to leave her and the children
- Destroying valued possessions
- Controlling the victim's every move

BOX 9.1 **Cycle of Violence**

- Phase 1: Tension-building: Verbal or minor battery occurs. Almost any subject, such as housekeeping or money, may trigger the buildup of tension. The victim attempts to calm the abuser.
- Phase 2: Acute battering: Characterized by uncontrollable discharge of tension. Violence is rarely triggered by the victim's behavior: she is battered no matter what her response.
- Phase 3: Reconciliation (honeymoon)/calm phase: The batterer becomes loving, kind, and apologetic and expresses guilt. Then the abuser works on making the victim feel responsible.

Sources: AWHONN, 2007; Aggeles, 2007; Burgess, 2007.

Physical Abuse

Physical abuse includes:

- Hitting or grabbing the victim so hard that it leaves marks
- Throwing things at the victim
- Slapping, spitting at, biting, burning, pushing, choking, or shoving the victim
- Kicking or punching the victim, or slamming her against things
- Attacking the victim with a knife, gun, rope, or electrical cord
- Controlling access to health care for injury

Financial Abuse

Financial abuse includes:

- Preventing the woman from getting a job
- Sabotaging a current job
- Controlling how all money is spent
- Failing to contribute financially

Sexual Abuse

Sexual abuse includes:

- Forcing the woman to have vaginal, oral, or anal intercourse against her will
- Biting the victim's breasts or genitals
- Shoving objects into the victim's vagina
- Forcing the victim to perform sexual acts on other people or animals

Myths and Facts About Intimate Partner Violence

There are many myths about intimate partner violence (Table 9.1). Health care providers should take steps to dispel these myths.

Abuse Profiles

Victims

Ironically, victims rarely describe themselves as abused. In **battered woman syndrome**, the woman has experienced deliberate and repeated physical or sexual assault by an intimate partner. She is terrified and feels trapped, helpless, and alone. She reacts to any expression of anger or threat by avoidance and withdrawal behavior.

Some women believe that the abuse is caused by a personality flaw or inadequacy in themselves (e.g., inability to keep the man happy). These feelings of failure are reinforced and exploited by their partners. After being told repeatedly that they are "bad," some women begin to believe it. Many victims were abused as children and may have poor self-esteem, depression, insomnia, or a history of suicide attempts, injury, or drug and alcohol abuse (Aggeles, 2007).

Abusers

Abusers come from all walks of life and often feel insecure, powerless, and helpless, feelings that are not in line with the macho image they would like to project. The abuser

TABLE 9.1 COMMON MYTHS AND FACTS ABOUT VIOLENCE

Myths	Facts
Battering of women occurs only in lower socioeconomic classes.	Violence occurs in all socioeconomic classes.
Substance abuse causes the violence.	Violence is a learned behavior and can be changed. The presence of drugs and alcohol can make a bad problem worse.
Violence occurs to only a small percentage of women.	One in four women will be victims of violence.
Women can easily choose to leave the abusive relationship.	Women stay in the abusive relationship because they feel they have no options.
Only men with mental health problems commit violence against women.	Abusers often seem normal and don't appear to suffer from personality disorders or other forms of mental illness.
Pregnant women are protected from abuse by their partners.	One in five women is physically abused during pregnancy. The effects of violence on infant outcomes can include preterm delivery, fetal distress, low birthweight, and child abuse.
Women provoke their partners to abuse them.	Women may be willing to blame themselves for someone else's bad behavior, but nobody deserves to be beaten.
Violent tendencies have gone on for generations and are accepted.	The police, justice system, and society are beginning to make domestic violence socially unacceptable.

Sources: Aggeles, 2007; AWHONN, 2007; Giardino, 2007; Kelly, 2007.

expresses his feelings of inadequacy through violence or aggression toward others (Du Plat-Jones, 2006).

Violence typically occurs at home and is usually directed toward the man's intimate partner or the children who live there. Abusers refuse to share power and choose violence to control their victims. They often exhibit child-like aggression or antisocial behaviors. They may fail to accept responsibility or blame others for their own problems. They might also have a history of substance abuse problems, mental illness, arrests, troubled relationships, obsessive jealousy, controlling behaviors, erratic employment history, and financial problems.

Violence Against Pregnant Women

Many think of pregnancy as a time of celebration and planning for the unborn child's future, but in a troubled relationship it can be a time of escalating violence. The strongest predictor of abuse during pregnancy is prior abuse (Giardino, 2007). For women who have been abused before, beatings and violence during pregnancy are "business as usual" for them.

Women are at a higher risk for violence during pregnancy. Pregnant women are vulnerable during this time, and abusers can take advantage of it. An estimated 325,000 pregnant women are abused by their partners each year (CDC, 2007a). Abuse during pregnancy poses special risks and dynamics.

Various factors may lead to battering during pregnancy, including:

- Inability of the couple to cope with the stressors of pregnancy
- Resentment toward the interference of the growing fetus and change in the woman's shape
- Doubts about paternity or the expectant mother's fidelity during pregnancy
- Perception that the baby will be a competitor
- Outside attention the pregnancy brings to the woman
- Unwanted pregnancy
- The woman's new interest in herself and her unborn baby
- Insecurity and jealousy about the pregnancy and the responsibilities it brings
- Financial burden related to expense of pregnancy and loss of income
- Stress of role transition from adult man to becoming the father of a child
- Physical and emotional changes of pregnancy that make the woman vulnerable
- Previous isolation from family and friends that limit the couple's support system

Abuse during pregnancy threatens the well-being of the mother and fetus. Physical violence may involve injuries to the head, face, neck, thorax, breasts, and abdomen (Casanueva & Martin, 2007). The mental health consequences are also significant. Several studies have confirmed the relationship between abuse and poor mental health, especially depression (Giardino, 2007). For the pregnant woman, this most often manifests itself as postpartum depression.

▶ *Take* NOTE!

Frequently the fear of harm to her unborn child will motivate a woman to escape an abusive relationship.

Women assaulted during pregnancy are at risk for:

- Injuries to themselves and the fetus
- Depression
- Chronic anxiety
- Miscarriage
- Stillbirth
- Poor nutrition
- Insomnia
- Placental abruption
- Uterine rupture
- Excessive weight gain or loss
- Smoking and substance abuse
- Delayed or no prenatal care
- Preterm labor
- Chorioamnionitis
- Vaginitis
- Sexually transmitted infections
- Urinary tract infections
- Premature and low-birthweight infants (Sharps, Laughon, & Giangrande, 2007)

Signs of abuse can emerge during pregnancy and may include poor attendance at prenatal visits, unrealistic fears, weight fluctuations, difficulty with pelvic examinations, and noncompliance with treatment.

Uncovering abuse in pregnant women requires a consistent and direct approach to every client by the nurse. Multiple assessments may enhance reporting by enabling the nurse to establish trust and rapport with the woman and identify changes in her behavior. Once abuse is discovered in a pregnant woman, interventions should include safety assessment, emotional support, counseling, referral to community services, and ongoing prenatal care (Burgess, 2007).

Violence Against Older Women

Intimate partner violence affects women of all ages, but often the literature focuses on women in the childbearing years, ignoring the problems of aging women experiencing abuse. There are laws in all 50 states requiring health care professionals to report elder or vulnerable person abuse. Estimates suggest that 500,000 to 1.5 million cases of elder abuse and neglect occur annually in the United States (Bonomi et al., 2007).

Although an injury may bring the older woman into the health care system, the physical and emotional sequelae of intimate partner violence may be more subtle: they may include depression, insomnia, chronic pain, atypical chest pain, or other kinds of somatic symptoms (Thackeray et al., 2007). Accurate detection and assess-

EVIDENCE-BASED PRACTICE 9.1
Nurse Case Management for Pregnant Women Experiencing or at Risk for Abuse

The goal of this randomized controlled trial was to determine whether individualized nursing case management can decrease stress among pregnant women at risk for abuse or in abusive relationships.

● Study
The study was conducted at two prenatal clinics in the Pacific Northwest and rural Midwest. Participants were 1,000 women who spoke English and were 13 to 23 weeks pregnant at time of recruitment. All intervention group women (n = 499) were offered an abuse video and had access to a nurse case manager 24/7. Participants at risk for abuse or in abusive relationships also received individualized nursing care management throughout the pregnancy.

▲ Findings
The most common nursing activities were providing support (38%) and assessing needs (32%). The nursing care management group received an average of 22 contacts,

most (80%) by telephone, and had a significant reduction in stress scores as measured by the Prenatal Psychosocial Profile. Compared to the control group, the differences were in the predicted direction but were not statistically different. A major finding was the choice by abused women to focus on basic needs and their pregnancies rather than the abuse, although all received safety planning.

■ Nursing Implications
Pregnant women at risk for abuse or in abusive relationships experience very stressful and complex lives. Nurses need to focus on the needs they identify, which may not be the abusive relationship.

Curry, M. A., Durham, L., Bullock, L., Bloom, T., & Davis, J. (2006). Nurse case management for pregnant women experiencing or at risk for abuse. *Journal of Obstetric, Gynecologic, and Neonatal Nursing, 35*(2), 181–192.

ment of abuse in elderly women are essential duties of all nurses.

Nursing Management

Nurses encounter thousands of abuse victims each year in their practice settings, but many victims slip through the cracks. There are many things that nurses can do to help victims. Early recognition and intervention can significantly reduce the morbidity and mortality associated with intimate partner violence. To stop the cycle of violence, nurses need to know how to assess for and identify violence and implement appropriate actions. The key is astute assessment and identification.

Assessment

Routine screening for intimate partner violence is the first way to detect abuse. The nurse should build rapport by showing an interest in the concerns of the woman, listening, and creating an atmosphere of openness. Communicating support through a nonjudgmental attitude, or telling her that no one deserves to be abused, is the first step toward establishing trust and rapport. Rather than overlooking abused women as "chronic complainers," astute nurses need to be vigilant for subtle clues of abuse.

Learning how to assess for abuse is critical. Some basic assessment guidelines follow.

Screen for Abuse During Every Health Care Visit

Screening for violence takes only a few minutes and can have an enormously positive effect on the outcome for the abused woman. Any woman could be a victim; no single sign marks a woman as an abuse victim, but the following clues may be helpful:

- Injuries: bruises, scars from blunt trauma, or weapon wounds on the face, head, and neck
- Injury sequelae: headaches, hearing loss, joint pain, sinus infections, teeth marks, clumps of hair missing, dental trauma, pelvic pain, breast or genital injuries
- Reported history of injury that is not consistent with the actual presenting problem
- Mental health problems: depression, anxiety, substance abuse, eating disorders, suicidal ideation or suicide attempts
- Frequent health care visits for chronic, stress-related disorders such as chest pain, headaches, back or pelvic pain, insomnia, and gastrointestinal disturbances
- Partner's behavior at the health care visit: appears overly solicitous or overprotective, is unwilling to leave her alone with the health care provider, answers questions for her, and attempts to control the situation (Aggeles, 2007)

Look for the following indicators of abuse:

- Previous history of assault
- Previous injuries inflicted by weapons

- Multiple medical visits for injuries or anxiety symptoms
- History of depression, substance use, or suicide attempts
- Tranquilizer or sedative use
- Sexually transmitted infections or pelvic inflammatory disease
- Bruises to the upper arm, neck and face, abdomen, or breasts
- Comments about emotional or physical abuse of "a friend"
- Hovering behavior of male partner during visit (Aggeles, 2007; Giardino, 2007)

Dorothy, who you met at the beginning of the chapter, has been frequenting the clinic with vague somatic complaints in recent weeks and admits she is sometimes afraid at home. She tells the nurse her partner doesn't want her to work, even though he was only sporadically employed at low-paying jobs. What cues in her assessment might indicate abuse? What physical signs might the nurse observe?

Isolate Patient Immediately From Family

If abuse is detected, immediately isolate the woman to provide privacy and to prevent potential retaliation from the abuser. Asking about abuse in front of the perpetrator may trigger an abusive episode during the interview or at home. Ways to ensure the woman's safety would be to take the victim to an area away from the abuser to ask questions. The assessment can take place anywhere—x-ray area, ultrasound room, elevator, ladies' room, laboratory—that is private and away from the abuser.

If abuse is detected, the nurse can do the following to enhance the nurse–client relationship:

- Educate the woman about the connection between the violence and her symptoms.
- Help the woman acknowledge what has happened to her and begin to deal with the situation.
- Offer her referrals so she can get the help that will allow her to begin to heal.

Dorothy returns to the prenatal clinic a month later with anemia, inadequate weight gain, bruises on her face and neck, and second-trimester bleeding. This time she is accompanied by her partner, who stays close to Dorothy. What questions should the nurse ask to assess the situation? Where is the appropriate location to ask these questions? What legal responsibilities does the nurse have concerning her observations?

Ask Direct or Indirect Questions About Abuse

Questions to screen for abuse should be routine and handled just like any other question. Many nurses feel uncomfortable asking questions of this nature, but broaching the subject is important even if the answer comes later. Just knowing that someone else knows about the abuse offers a victim some relief.

Ask difficult questions in an empathetic and nonthreatening manner and remain nonjudgmental in all responses and interactions. Choose the type of question that makes you most comfortable. Direct and indirect questions produce the same results. "Does your partner hit you?" or "Have you ever been or are you now in an abusive relationship?" are direct questions. If that approach feels uncomfortable, try indirect questions: "We see many women with injuries or complaints like yours and often they are being abused. Is that what is happening to you?" or "Many women in our community experience abuse from their partners. Is anything like that happening in your life?" With either approach, nurses need to maintain a nonjudgmental acceptance of whatever answer the woman offers.

The SAVE Model is a screening protocol that nurses can use when assessing women for violence (Box 9.2).

BOX 9.2 SAVE Model

SCREEN all of your patients for violence by asking:
- Do you feel safe in your home?
- Do you feel you are in control of your life?
- Have you ever been sexually or physically abused?
- Can you talk about your abuse with me now?

ASK direct questions in a nonjudgmental way:
- Begin by normalizing the topic to the woman.
- Make continuous eye contact with the woman.
- Stay calm; avoid emotional reactions to what she tells you.
- Never blame the woman, even if she blames herself.
- Don't dismiss or minimize what she tells you, even if she does.
- Wait for each answer patiently. Don't rush to the next question.
- Do not use formal, technical, or medical language.
- Use a nonthreatening, accepting approach.

VALIDATE the patient by telling her:
- You believe her story.
- You do not blame her for what happened.
- It is brave of her to tell you this.
- Help is available for her.
- Talking with you is a hopeful sign and a first big step.

EVALUATE, educate, and refer this patient by asking her:
- What type of violence was it?
- Is she now in any danger?
- How is she feeling now?
- Does she know that there are consequences to violence?
- Is she aware of community resources available to help her?

Sources: Dutton, 2007; Du Plat-Jones, 2006; Thackeray et al., 2007.

Assess Immediate Safety

The Danger Assessment Tool helps women and health care providers assess the potential for homicidal behavior in an ongoing abusive relationship. It is based on research that showed several risk factors for abuse-related murders:

- Increased frequency or severity of abuse
- Presence of firearms
- Sexual abuse
- Substance abuse
- Generally violent behavior outside of the home
- Control issues (e.g., daily chores, friends, job, money)
- Physical abuse during pregnancy
- Suicide threats or attempts (victim or abuser)
- Child abuse (Kelly, 2007)

Document and Report Your Findings

If the interview reveals a history of abuse, accurate documentation is critical because this evidence may support the woman's case in court. Documentation must include details about the frequency and severity of abuse; the location, extent, and outcome of injuries; and any treatments or interventions. When documenting, use direct quotes and be very specific: "He choked me." Describe any visible injuries, and use a body map (outline of a woman's body) to show where the injuries are. Obtain photos (with informed consent) or document her refusal if the woman declines photos. Pictures or diagrams can be worth a thousand words. Figure 9.2 shows a sample documentation form for intimate partner violence.

Laws in many states require health care providers to alert the police to any injuries that involve knives, firearms, or other deadly weapons or that present life-threatening emergencies. If assessment reveals suspicion or actual indication of abuse, you can explain to the woman that you are required by law to report it.

Nursing Diagnosis

When violence is suspected or validated, the nurse needs to formulate nursing diagnoses based on the completed assessment. Possible nursing diagnoses related to violence against women might include the following:

- Deficient knowledge related to understanding the cycle of violence and availability of resources
- Fear related to possibility of severe injury to self or children during cycle of violence
- Low self-esteem related to feelings of worthlessness
- Hopelessness related to prolonged exposure to violence
- Compromised individual and family coping related to persistence of victim–abuser relationship

Interventions

If abuse is identified, nurses can undertake interventions that can increase the woman's safety and improve her health. The goal of intervention is to enable the victim to gain control of her life. Provide sensitive, predictable care

INTIMATE PARTNER VIOLENCE DOCUMENTATION FORM

Explain to Client: The majority of what you tell me is confidential and cannot be shared with anyone without your written permission. However, I am required by law to report information pertaining to child or adult abuse and gunshot wounds or life-threatening injuries.

STEP 1–Establish total privacy to ask screening questions. Safety is the first priority. Client must be alone, or if the client has a child with her, the child must not be of verbal age. ONLY complete this form if YOU CAN assure the client's safety, privacy, and confidentiality.

STEP 2–Ask the client screening questions.

"Because abuse is so common, we are now asking all of our female clients:

Are you in a relationship in which you are being hurt or threatened, emotionally or physically?
___Yes ___ No

Do you feel unsafe at home?"
___Yes ___ No

If both screening questions are NO in STEP 2, and you are not concerned that the client may be a victim, sign and date the form in the signature block directly below. Provide information and resources as appropriate.

Signature _____ Title _____ Date _____

If both screening answers are NO and you <u>are concerned</u> that the client may be a victim, go to STEP 5. If the client answers YES to either question, proceed to STEP 3 below. Sign and date the signature block on the back of the form after completing STEP 6.

STEP 3–Assess the abuse and safety of the client and any children.

Say to client: "From the answers you have just given me, I am worried for you."

        "Has the relationship gotten worse, or is it getting scarier?"   ___Yes ___ No

        "Does your partner ever watch you closely, follow you, or stalk you?" ___Yes ___ No

Ask the following question in clinic settings only. Do not ask in home settings:

"If your partner is here with you today, are you afraid to leave with him/her?"   ___Yes ___ No

"Is there anything else you want to tell me?" _____
_____
_____
_____

                Name: _____

                ID No: _____

                Date of Birth: _____

DH 3202, 2/03
Stock Number: 5744-000-3202-2

Figure 9.2 Intimate partner violence documentation form. (Florida Department of Health) *(continued)*

"Are there children in the home?" ___Yes ___ No

If the answer to the question above is "yes," say to client: "I'm concerned for your safety and the safety of your children. You and your children deserve to be at home without feeling afraid."

"Have there been threats of abuse or direct abuse of the children?" ___Yes ___ No

STEP 4–Assess client's physical injuries and health conditions, past and present.

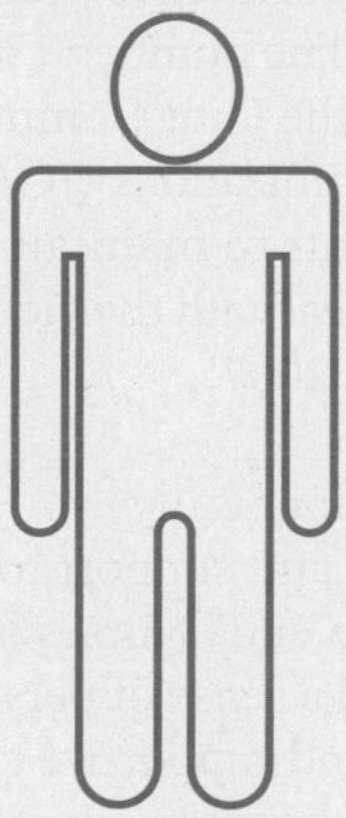

Observations/Comments/Interventions:

_____

_____

_____

_____

_____

_____

_____

_____

_____

_____

_____

_____

STEP 5–If both screening answers are NO, and you ARE CONCERNED that the client may be a victim:

a. Say to the client: "All of us know of someone at some time in our lives who is abused. So, I am providing you with information in the event you or a friend may need it in the future."

b. Document under comments in Step 6.

STEP 6–Information, referrals or reports made

Yes No

___ ___ 1. Client given domestic violence information including safety planning
___ ___ 2. Reviewed domestic violence information including safety planning
___ ___ 3. State Abuse Hotline (1-800-96-ABUSE) and State Domestic Violence
            Hotline number (1-800-500-1119) given to the client
___ ___ 4. Client called hotline during visit
___ ___ 5. Client seen by advocate during visit
___ ___ 6. Report made. If yes, to whom: _____

Comments

_____

_____

_____

_____

_____

_____

Signature _____ Title _____ Date _____

FIGURE **9.2** (continued) Intimate partner violence documentation form. (Florida Department of Health)

in an accepting setting. Offer step-by-step explanations of procedures. Provide educational materials about violence. Allow the victim to actively participate in her care and have control over all health care decisions. Pace your nursing interventions and allow the woman to take the lead. Communicate support through a nonjudgmental attitude. Carefully document assessment findings and nursing interventions.

Depending on when in the cycle of violence the nurse encounters the abused woman, goals may fall into three groups:

- Primary prevention: aimed at breaking the abuse cycle through community educational initiatives by nurses, physicians, law enforcement, teachers, and clergy
- Secondary prevention: focuses on dealing with victims and abusers in early stages, with the goal of preventing progression of abuse
- Tertiary prevention: activities are geared toward helping severely abused women and children recover and become productive members of society and rehabilitating abusers to stop the cycle of violence. These activities are typically long term and expensive.

A tool developed by Holtz and Furniss (1993)—the ABCDES—provides a framework for providing sensitive nursing interventions to abused women (Box 9.3).

Specific nursing interventions for the abused woman include educating her about community services, providing emotional support, and offering a safety plan.

BOX 9.3 The ABCDES of Caring for Abused Women

- **A** is reassuring the woman that she is not alone. The isolation by her abuser keeps her from knowing that others are in the same situation and that health care providers can help her.
- **B** is expressing the belief that violence against women is not acceptable in any situation and that it is not her fault.
- **C** is confidentiality, since the woman might believe that if the abuse is reported, the abuser will retaliate.
- **D** is documentation, which includes the following:
  1. A clear quoted statement about the abuse
  2. Accurate descriptions of injuries and the history of them
  3. Photos of the injuries (with the woman's consent)
- **E** is education about the cycle of violence and that it will escalate.
- **S** is safety, the most important aspect of the intervention, to ensure that the woman has resources and a plan of action to carry out when she decides to leave.

Educate the Woman About Community Services

A wide range of support services are available to meet the needs of victims of violence. Nurses should be prepared to help the woman take advantage of these opportunities. Services will vary by community but might include psychological counseling, legal advice, social services, crisis services, support groups, hotlines, housing, vocational training, and other community-based referrals.

Give the woman information about shelters or services even if she initially rejects it. Give the woman the National Domestic Violence hotline number: (800) 799-7233. Since 1992, guidelines from the Joint Commission on Accreditation of Healthcare Organizations (JCAHO) have required emergency departments to maintain lists of community referral agencies that deal with the victims of intimate partner violence (JCAHO, 2007).

Provide Emotional Support

Providing reassurance and support to a victim of abuse is key if the violence is to end. Nurses in all clinical settings can help victims to feel a sense of personal power and provide them with a safe and supportive environment. Appropriate action can help victims to express their thoughts and feelings in constructive ways, manage stress, and move on with their lives. Appropriate interventions are:

- Strengthen the woman's sense of control over her life by:
  - Teaching coping strategies to manage her stress
  - Assisting with activities of daily living to improve her lifestyle
  - Allowing her to make as many decisions as she can
  - Educating her about the symptoms of post-traumatic stress disorder and their basis
- Encourage the woman to establish realistic goals for herself by:
  - Teaching problem-solving skills
  - Encouraging social activities to connect with other people
- Provide support and allow the woman to grieve for her losses by:
  - Listening to and clarifying her reactions to the traumatic event
  - Discussing shock, disbelief, anger, depression, and acceptance
- Explain to the woman that:
  - Abuse is never OK. She didn't ask for it and she doesn't deserve it.
  - She is not alone and help is available.
  - Abuse is a crime and she is a victim.
  - Alcohol, drugs, money problems, depression, or jealousy does not cause violence, but these things can give the abuser an excuse for losing control and abusing her.
  - The actions of the abuser are not her fault.
  - Her history of abuse is believed.
  - Making a decision to leave an abusive relationship can be very hard and takes time.

Offer a Safety Plan

The choice to leave must rest with the victim. Nurses cannot choose a life for the victim; they can only offer choices. Leaving is a process, not an event. Victims may try to leave their abusers as many as seven or eight times before succeeding. Frequently, the final attempt to leave may result in the death of the victim. Women planning to leave an abusive relationship should have a safety plan, if possible (Teaching Guidelines 9.1).

Sexual Violence

Sexual violence is both a public health problem and a human rights violation. More than once every 3 minutes, 78 times an hour, 1,871 times a day, girls and women in America are raped (Medicine Net, 2007). Rape has been reported against females from age 6 months to 93 years, but it still remains one of the most underreported violent crimes in the United States. Estimates suggest that, somewhere in the United States, a woman is sexually assaulted every 2.5 minutes (RAINN, 2007). The National Center for Prevention and Control of Sexual Assault estimates that one out of three women will be sexually assaulted sometime in her life, and two thirds of these assaults will not be reported (CDC, 2007b). Over the course of their lives, women may experience more than one type of violence.

Sexual violence can have a variety of devastating short- and long-term effects. Women can experience psychological, physical, and cognitive symptoms that affect them daily. They can include chronic pelvic pain, headaches, backache, sexually transmitted infections, pregnancy, anxiety, denial, fear, withdrawal, sleep disturbances, guilt, nervousness, phobias, substance abuse, depression, sexual dysfunction, and post-traumatic stress disorder (CDC, 2007b). A traumatic experience not only damages a woman's sense of safety in the world, but it can also reduce her self-esteem and her ability to continue her education, to earn money and be productive, to have children and, if she has children, to nurture and protect them (Macy et al., 2007).

> ▶ **Take** NOTE!
>
> *Sexual violence has been called a "tragedy of youth." More than half of all rapes (54%) of women occur before age 18 (Medicine Net, 2007).*

Assailants, like their victims, come from all walks of life and all ethnic backgrounds; there is no typical profile. More than half are under 25, and the majority are married and leading "normal" sex lives. Why do men rape? No theory provides a satisfactory explanation. So few assailants are caught and convicted that a clear profile remains elusive. What is known is that many assailants have trouble dealing with the stresses of daily life. Such men become angry and experience feelings of powerlessness. They commit a sexual assault as an expression of power and control (Macy et al., 2007).

Sexual violence is a broad term that can be used to describe sexual abuse, incest, rape, female genital mutilation, and human trafficking.

Sexual Abuse

Sexual abuse occurs when a woman is forced to have sexual contact of any kind (vaginal, oral, or anal) without her consent. Marriage does not constitute a tacit agreement for a spouse to inflict one's demands on the other without permission. Childhood sexual abuse is any type of sexual exploitation that involves a child younger than 18 years old; it might include disrobing, nudity, masturbation, fondling, digital penetration, and intercourse (Alekseeva, 2007).

Childhood sexual abuse has a lifelong impact on its survivors. Women who were sexually abused during childhood are at a heightened risk for repeat abuse. This is because the early abuse lowers their self-esteem and their ability to protect themselves and set firm boundaries. Childhood sexual abuse is a trauma that influences the way victims form relationships, deal with adversity, cope with daily problems, relate to their children and peers, protect their health, and live. Studies have shown that the more victimization a woman experiences, the more likely it is she will be re-victimized (Kristensen & Lau, 2007).

TEACHING GUIDELINES 9.1

Safety Plan for Leaving an Abusive Relationship

- When leaving an abusive relationship, take the following items:
  - Driver's license or photo ID
  - Social security number or green card/work permit
  - Birth certificates for you and your children
  - Phone numbers for social services or women's shelter
  - The deed or lease to your home or apartment
  - Any court papers or orders
  - A change of clothing for you and your children
  - Pay stubs, checkbook, credit cards, and cash
  - Insurance cards (Du Plat-Jones, 2006; Dutton, 2007)
  - If you need to leave a domestic violence situation immediately, turn to authorities for assistance in gathering this material.
- Develop a "game plan" for leaving and rehearse it.
- Don't use phone cards—they leave a trail to follow.

EVIDENCE-BASED PRACTICE 9.2
Cognitive-Behavioral Interventions for Children Who Have Been Sexually Abused

Despite different perceptions as to what constitutes child sexual abuse, there is a consensus among clinicians and researchers that this is a substantial social problem that affects large numbers of children and young people worldwide. The effects of sexual abuse manifest themselves in a wide range of symptoms, including fear, anxiety, post-traumatic stress disorder and behavior problems such as externalizing or internalizing, or inappropriate sexual behaviors. Child sexual abuse is associated with an increased risk of psychological problems in adulthood. Knowing what is most likely to benefit children already traumatized by these events is important.

● Study
The aim of this review was to assess the efficacy of cognitive-behavioral therapy (CBT) in addressing the

immediate and longer-term sequelae of sexual abuse in children. Ten studies comprising 847 children were identified that met the inclusion criteria.

▲ Findings
The evidence suggests that CBT may have a positive impact on the sequelae of child sexual abuse, but most results were statistically nonsignificant.

● Nursing Implications
The review confirms CBT's potential for addressing the adverse consequences of child sexual abuse but highlights the tenuousness of the evidence base and the need for more carefully conducted and better reported trials.

Macdonald, G. M., Higgins, J. P. T., & Ramchandani, P. (2006). Cognitive-behavioral interventions for children who have been sexually abused. *Cochrane Database of Systematic Reviews* 2006, Issue 4. Art. No.: CD001930. DOI: 10.1002/14651858.CD001930.pub2.

Incest

Childhood sexual abuse involves any kind of sexual experience between a child and another person that violates the social taboos of family roles; children cannot yet understand these activities and cannot give informed consent (Alekseeva, 2007). **Incest** is any type of sexual exploitation between blood relatives or surrogate relatives before the victim reaches 18 years of age. Such sexual abuse is not only a crime but also a symptom of acute and irreversible family dysfunction. Survivors of incest are often tricked, coerced, or manipulated. All adults appear to be powerful to children. Perpetrators might threaten victims so that they are afraid to disclose the abuse or might tell them the abuse is their fault. Often these threats serve to silence victims.

Incestual relationships in the home endanger not only the child's intellectual and moral development, but also the health of the child. Many children don't ask for help because they don't want to expose their "secret." For this reason, just the tip of the iceberg is statistically visible—serious injuries, internal damage, sexually transmitted infections, or pregnancy. Incest can have serious long-term effects on its victims, which may include eating disorders, sexual problems in their adult life, post-traumatic stress disorder, intense guilt and shame, low self-esteem, depression, and self-destructive behavior (NCVC, 2007).

Whether an incest victim endured an isolated incident of abuse or ongoing assaults over an extended period, recovery can be painful and difficult. The recovery process begins with admission of abuse and the recognition that help and services are needed. Resources for incest victims include books, self-help groups, workshops, therapy programs, and possibly legal remedies. In addition to listening to and believing incest victims, nurses need to search for ways to prevent future generations from enduring such abuse and from continuing the cycle of abuse in their own family and relationships.

▶ *Consider THIS!*

At 53 years old, I stood and looked at myself in the mirror. The image staring back at me was one of a frightened, middle-aged, cowardly woman hiding her past. I had been sexually abused by my father for many years as a child and never told anyone. My mother knew of the abuse but felt helpless to make it stop. I married right out of high school to escape and felt I lived a "happy normal life" with my husband and three children. My children have left home and live away, and my husband recently died of a sudden heart attack. I am now experiencing dreams and thoughts about my past abuse and feeling afraid again.

Thoughts: This woman suppressed her abusive past for most of her life and now her painful experience has surfaced. What can be done to reach out to her at this point? Did her health care providers miss the "red flags" that are common to women with a history of childhood sexual abuse all those years?

> ▶ *Take* NOTE!
>
> *Childhood sexual abuse is a trauma that can affect every aspect of the victim's life.*

Rape

Rape is an expression of violence, not a sexual act. It is not an act of lust or an overzealous release of passion: it is a violent, aggressive assault on the victim's body and integrity. Rape is a legal rather than a medical term. It denotes penile penetration of the vagina, mouth, or rectum of the female or male without consent. It may or may not include the use of a weapon. **Statutory rape** is sexual activity between an adult and a person under the age of 18 and is considered to have occurred even if the underage person was willing (Kandakai & Smith, 2007). Nine out of every 10 rape victims are female (Alexander et al., 2007). Enforcement of laws, education, and community empowerment are all needed to prevent rape.

Many people believe that rape usually occurs on a dark night when a stranger assaults a provocatively dressed, promiscuous woman. They believe that rapists are sex-starved people seeking sexual gratification. Such myths and the facts are presented in Table 9.2.

Acquaintance Rape

In **acquaintance rape**, someone is forced to have sex by a person he or she knows. Rape by a coworker, a teacher, a husband's friend, or a boss is considered acquaintance rape. **Date rape**, an assault that occurs within a dating relationship or marriage without consent of one of the participants, is a form of acquaintance rape. Acquaintance and date rapes commonly occur on college campuses. One in four college women has been raped—that is, has been forced, physically or verbally, actively or implicitly, to engage in sexual activity (Elliott, 2008).

These forms of rape are physically and emotionally devastating for the victims. Research has indicated that the survivors of acquaintance rape report similar levels of depression, anxiety, complications in subsequent relationships, and difficulty attaining pre-rape levels of sexual satisfaction to what survivors of stranger rape report. Acquaintance rape remains a controversial topic because there is lack of agreement on the definition of consent (Sampson, 2007).

Although acquaintance rape and date rape do not always involve drugs, a rapist might use alcohol or other drugs to sedate his victim. In 1996 the federal government passed a law making it a felony to give an unsuspecting person a "date rape drug" with the intent of raping him or her. Even with penalties of large fines and up to 20 years in prison, the use of date rape drugs is growing (U.S. DHHS, 2007).

Date rape drugs are also known as "club drugs" because they are often used at dance clubs, fraternity parties, and all-night raves. The most common is Rohypnol (also known as roofies, forget pills, and the drop drug). It comes in the form of a liquid or pill that quickly dissolves in liquid with no odor, taste, or color. This drug is 10 times as strong as diazepam (Valium) and produces memory loss for up to 8 hours. Gamma hydroxybutyrate (GHB; called liquid ecstasy or easy lay) produces euphoria, an out-of-body high, sleepiness, increased sex drive, and memory loss. It comes in a white powder or liquid and may cause unconsciousness, depression, and coma.

TABLE 9.2 COMMON MYTHS AND FACTS ABOUT RAPE

Myths	Facts
Women who are raped get over it quickly.	It can take several years to recover emotionally and physically from rape.
Most rape victims tell someone about it.	The majority of women never tell anyone about it. In fact, almost two thirds of victims never report it to the police.
Once the rape is over, a survivor can again feel safe in her life.	The victim feels vulnerable, betrayed, and insecure afterwards.
If a woman does not want to be raped, it cannot happen.	A woman can be forced and overpowered by most men.
Women who feel guilty after having sex then say they were raped.	Few women falsely cry "rape." It is very traumatizing to be a victim.
Victims should report the violence to the police and judicial system.	Only 1% of rapists are arrested and convicted.
Women blame themselves for the rape, believing they did something to provoke the rape.	Women should never blame themselves for being the victim of someone else's violence.
Women who wear tight, short clothes are "asking for it."	No victim invites sexual assault, and what she wears is irrelevant.
Women have rape fantasies and want to be raped.	Reality and fantasy are different. Dreams have nothing to do with the brutal violation of rape.
Medication can help women forget about the rape.	Initially medication can help, but counseling is needed.

Sources: CDC, 2007b; Dutton, 2007; Medicine Net, 2007.

TEACHING GUIDELINES 9.2

Protecting Yourself Against Date Rape Drugs

- Avoid parties where alcohol is being served.
- Never leave a drink of any kind unattended.
- Don't accept a drink from someone else. Accept drinks from a bartender or in a closed container only.
- Don't drink from a punch bowl or a keg.
- If you think someone drugged you, call 911.

The third date rape drug, ketamine (known as Special K, vitamin K, or super acid), acts on the central nervous system to separate perception and sensation. Combining ketamine with other drugs can be fatal.

Date rape drugs can be very dangerous, and there are a variety of ways that women can protect themselves (Teaching Guidelines 9.2).

Rape Recovery

Rape survivors take a long time to heal from their traumatic experience. Some women never heal and never get professional counseling, but most can cope. Rape is viewed as a situational crisis that the survivor is unprepared to handle because it is an unforeseen event. Survivors typically go through four phases of recovery following rape (Table 9.3).

A significant proportion of women who are raped also experience symptoms of **post-traumatic stress disorder** (PTSD). PTSD develops when an event outside the range of normal human experience occurs that produces marked distress in the person. Symptoms of PTSD are divided into three groups:

- Intrusion (re-experiencing the trauma, including nightmares, flashbacks, recurrent thoughts)
- Avoidance (avoiding trauma-related stimuli, social withdrawal, emotional numbing)
- Hyperarousal (increased emotional arousal, exaggerated startle response, irritability)

Nursing Management

Research has found that rape survivors undergo a profound and complex trauma. The survivor should be provided with a safe and comfortable environment for a forensic examination. Nursing care of the rape survivor should focus on providing supporting care, collecting and documenting evidence, assessing for sexually transmitted infections, preventing pregnancy, and assessing for PTSD. Once initial treatment and evidence collection are completed, follow-up care should include counseling, medical treatment, and crisis intervention. There is mounting evidence that early intervention and immediate counseling speed a rape survivor's recovery. Nursing Care Plan 9.1 highlights a sample plan of care for a victim of rape.

> ▶ *Take NOTE!*
>
> *Many rape survivors seek treatment in the hospital emergency room if there are no rape crisis centers available. Unfortunately, many emergency room doctors and nurses have little training in how to treat rape survivors or in collecting evidence. To make matters worse, if they have to wait for hours in public waiting rooms, survivors may leave the hospital, never to receive treatment or supply the evidence needed to arrest and convict their assailants.*

Providing Supporting Care

Establishing a therapeutic and trusting relationship will help the survivor describe her experience. Take the woman to a secure, isolated area away from family, friends, and other patients and staff so she can be open and honest when asked about the assault. Provide a change of clothes, access to a shower and toiletries, and a private waiting area for family and friends.

Collecting and Documenting Evidence

The victim should be instructed to bring all clothing, especially undergarments, worn at the time of the assault to the medical facility. The victim should not shower or bathe before presenting for care. Typically a specially trained nurse will collect the evidence from the victim.

TABLE 9.3   FOUR PHASES OF RAPE RECOVERY

Phase	Survivor's Response
Acute phase (disorganization)	Shock, fear, disbelief, anger, shame, guilt, feelings of uncleanliness; insomnia, nightmares, and sobbing
Outward adjustment phase (denial)	Appears outwardly composed and returns to work or school; refuses to discuss the assault and denies need for counseling
Reorganization	Denial and suppression don't work, and the survivor attempts to make life adjustments by moving or changing jobs and uses emotional distancing to cope.
Integration and recovery	Survivor begins to feel safe and starts to trust others. She may become an advocate for other rape victims.

Nursing Care Plan 9.1

OVERVIEW OF THE WOMAN WHO IS A VICTIM OF RAPE

Lucia, a 20-year-old college junior, was admitted to the emergency room after police found her when a passerby called 911 to report an assault. She stated, "I think I was raped a few hours ago while I was walking home through the park." Assessment reveals the following: numerous cuts and bruises of varying sizes on her face, arms, and legs; lip swollen and cut; right eye swollen and bruised; jacket and shirt ripped and bloodied; hair matted with grass and debris; vital signs within acceptable parameters; client tearful, clutching her clothing, and trembling; perineal bruising and tearing.

NURSING DIAGNOSIS: Rape-trauma syndrome related to report of recent sexual assault

Outcome Identification and Evaluation
Client will demonstrate adequate coping skills related to effects of rape as evidenced by her ability to discuss the event, verbalize her feelings and fears, and exhibit appropriate actions to return to her pre-crisis level of functioning.

Interventions: Promoting Adequate Coping Skills
- Stay with the client *to promote feelings of safety.*
- Explain the procedures to be completed based on facility's policy *to help alleviate client's fear of the unknown.*
- Assist with physical examination for specimen collection *to obtain evidence for legal proceedings.*
- Administer prophylactic medication as ordered *to prevent pregnancy and sexually transmitted infections.*
- Provide care to wounds as ordered *to prevent infection.*
- Assist client with hygiene measures as necessary *to promote self-esteem.*
- Allow client to describe the events as much as possible *to encourage ventilation of feelings about the incident;* engage in active listening and offer nonjudgmental support *to facilitate coping and demonstrate understanding of the client's situation and feelings.*
- Help the client identify positive coping skills and personal strengths used in the past *to aid in effective decision making.*
- Assist client in developing additional coping strategies and teach client relaxation techniques *to help deal with the current crisis and anxiety.*
- Contact the rape counselor in the facility *to help the client deal with the crisis.*
- Arrange for follow-up visit with rape counselor *to provide continued care and to promote continuity of care.*
- Encourage the client to contact a close friend, partner, or family member to accompany her home *to provide support.*
- Provide the client with the telephone number of a counseling service or community support groups *to help her cope and obtain ongoing support.*
- Provide written instructions related to follow-up appointments, care, and testing *to ensure adequate understanding.*

Assessing for Sexually Transmitted Infections
As part of the assessment, a pelvic examination will be done to collect vaginal secretions to rule out any sexually transmitted infections. This examination is very emotionally stressful for most women and should be carried out very gently and sensitively.

Preventing Pregnancy
An essential element in the care of rape survivors involves offering them pregnancy prevention. After unprotected intercourse, including rape, pregnancy can be prevented by using emergency contraceptive pills, sometimes called postcoital contraception. Emergency contraceptive pills involve high doses of the same oral contraceptives that millions of women take every day. The emergency regimen consists of two doses: the first dose is taken within 72 hours of the unprotected intercourse and the second dose is taken

12 hours after the first dose or sooner. Emergency contraception works by preventing ovulation, fertilization, or implantation. It does not disrupt an established pregnancy and should not be confused with mifepristone (RU-486), a drug approved by the Food and Drug Administration for abortion in the first 49 days of gestation. Emergency contraception is most effective if the first dose is taken within 12 hours of the rape; it becomes less effective with every 12 hours of delay thereafter.

Assessing for PTSD
Nurses can begin to assess the extent to which a survivor is suffering from PTSD by asking the following questions:

- To assess the presence of intrusive thoughts:
  - Do upsetting thoughts and nightmares of the trauma bother you?

- Do you feel as though you are actually reliving the trauma?
- Does it upset you to be exposed to anything that reminds you of that event?
- To assess the presence of avoidance reactions:
  - Do you find yourself trying to avoid thinking about the trauma?
  - Do you stay away from situations that remind you of the event?
  - Do you have trouble recalling exactly what happened?
  - Do you feel numb emotionally?
- To assess the presence of physical symptoms:
  - Are you having trouble sleeping?
  - Have you felt irritable or experienced outbursts of anger?
  - Do you have heart palpitations and sweating?
  - Do you have muscle aches and pains all over?
  (Kiump, 2006)

Female Genital Mutilation

Female genital mutilation, also known as female circumcision, is a cultural practice carried out predominantly in countries of southern Africa and in some areas of the Middle East and Asia. The World Health Organization (WHO) defines female genital mutilation as all procedures involving the partial or total removal or other injury to the female genital organs, whether for cultural or other nontherapeutic purposes (WHO, 2007). More than 140 million girls are estimated to have undergone female genital mutilation and another 2 million are at risk annually, approximately 6,000 daily (WHO, 2007).

This issue has drawn increasing global attention over the past several years. Nongovernmental organizations such as Amnesty International are conducting research and campaign work on the practice. The U.S. government has taken steps to criminalize the practice in America and now considers asylum applications in light of mutilation practices in the country of origin (WHO, 2007). WHO is fighting tirelessly to eradicate this practice through advocacy, policy development, research, and training for health care providers (Zaidi et al., 2007). In fact, WHO, the United Nations Population Fund, and the United Nations Children's Fund have issued a joint plea for the eradication of the practice, saying it would be a major step forward in the promotion of human rights worldwide (WHO, 2007).

▶ *Take* NOTE!

From a Western perspective, female genital mutilation is hard to comprehend. Because it is not talked about openly in communities that practice it, women who have undergone it accept it without question and assume it is done to all girls (Wakabi 2007).

Background

Reasons for performing the ritual reflect the ideology and cultural values of each community that practices it. Some consider it a rite of passage into womanhood; others use it as a means of preserving virginity until marriage. In cultures where it is practiced, it is an important part of culturally defined gender identity. In any case, all the reasons are cultural and traditional and are not rooted in any religious texts (RAINBO, 2007). Female genital mutilation causes injury to women and does not benefit them.

Female genital mutilation is usually performed when the girl is between 4 and 10 years old, an age when she cannot give informed consent for a procedure with lifetime health consequences (WHO, 2007). In its mildest form, the clitoris is partially or totally removed. In the most extreme form, called infibulation, the clitoris, labia minora, labia majora, and the urethral and vaginal openings are cut away. The vagina is then stitched or held together, leaving a small opening for menstruation and urination. Cutting and restitching may be necessary to permit the woman to have sexual intercourse and bear children. Box 9.4 lists types of female genital mutilation procedures.

Untrained village practitioners, using no form of anesthesia, generally perform the operation. Cutting instruments may include broken glass, knives, tin lids, scissors, unspecialized razors, or other crude instruments. In addition to causing intense pain, the procedure carries with it a number of health risks, including:

- Pelvic infections
- Hemorrhage
- HIV infection
- Damage to the urethra, vagina, and anus
- Recurrent vaginitis
- Urinary tract infections
- Incontinence
- Post-traumatic stress disorder
- Panic attacks

BOX 9.4 **Four Major Types of Female Genital Mutilation Procedures**

Type I: Excision of the prepuce with or without excision of part or all of the clitoris
Type II: Excision of the clitoris and part or all of the labia minora
Type III (Infibulation): Excision of all or part of the external genitalia and stitching/narrowing of the vaginal opening
Type IV: Pricking, piercing, or incision of the clitoris or labia
   Stretching of the clitoris and/or labia
   Cauterizing by burning the clitoris and surrounding tissues
   Scraping or cutting the vaginal orifice
   Introduction of a corrosive substance into the vagina
   Placing herbs into the vagina to narrow it

Sources: WHO, 2007; Keleher & Franklin, 2008.

- Keloid formation
- Dermoid cysts
- Vulvar abscesses
- Dysmenorrhea
- Dyspareunia
- Psychosomatic illnesses
- Depression
- Feelings of betrayal
- Bitterness and anger towards family members who allowed it
- Increased morbidity and mortality during childbirth (WHO, 2007)

Nursing Management

Because of increasing migration, nurses throughout the world are increasingly exposed to women who have suffered these procedures and thus need to know about its impact on women's reproductive health. Helping women who have had one of these procedures requires good communication skills and often an interpreter, since many may not speak English. Nurses have the opportunity to educate patients by providing accurate information and positive health care experiences. Make sure that you are comfortable with your own feelings about this practice before dealing with patients. Some guidelines are as follows:

- Let the client know you are concerned and interested and want to help.
- Speak clearly and slowly, using simple, accurate terms.
- Use the term or name for this practice the recipient uses, not "female genital mutilation."
- Use pictures and diagrams to help the woman understand what you are saying.
- Be patient in allowing the client to answer questions.
- Repeat back your understanding of the client's statements.
- Always look and talk directly to the client, not the interpreter.
- Place no judgment on the cultural practice.
- Encourage the client to express herself freely.
- Maintain strict confidentiality.
- Provide culturally competent care to all women.

Human Trafficking

A girl who was just 14 years old was held captive in a tiny trailer room, where she was forced to have sex with as many as 30 men a day. On her night stand was a teddy bear that reminded her of her childhood in Mexico.

This scenario describes **human trafficking**, the enslavement of immigrants for profit in America. Human trafficking is both a global problem and a domestic problem. The United States is a major receiver of trafficked persons. Human trafficking is a modern form of slavery that affects nearly 1 million people worldwide and approximately 20,000 persons in the United States annually

(U.S. Department of State, 2007). Women and children are the primary victims of human trafficking, many in the sex trade as described above and others through forced-labor domestic servitude.

Trafficking persons is hugely profitable: one estimate places global profits at approximately $32 billion annually. Among illegal enterprises, trafficking is second only to drug dealing and is tied with the illegal arms industry in its ability to generate dollars (Jones et al., 2007).

The United States is a profitable destination country for traffickers, and these profits contribute to the development of organized criminal enterprises worldwide. According to findings of the Victims of Trafficking and Violence Protection Act of 2000:

- Victims are primarily women and children who lack education, employment, and economic opportunities in their own countries.
- Traffickers promise victims employment as nannies, maids, dancers, factory workers, sales clerks, or models in the United States.
- Traffickers transport the victims from their counties to unfamiliar destinations away from their support systems.
- Once they are here, traffickers coerce them, using rape, torture, starvation, imprisonment, threats, or physical force, into prostitution, pornography, sex trade, forced labor, or involuntary servitude.

These victims are exposed to serious and numerous health risks, such as rape, torture, HIV/AIDS, sexually transmitted infections, cervical cancer, violence, hazardous work environments, poor nutrition, and drug and alcohol addiction (Hodge & Lietz, 2007). Health care is one of the most pressing needs of these victims, and there isn't any comprehensive care available for undocumented immigrants. As a nurse it is important to be alert for trafficking victims in any setting and to recognize cues (Box 9.5).

Human trafficking is a violation of human rights. If you suspect a trafficking situation, notify local law enforcement and a regional social service organization that has experience in dealing with trafficking victims. It is imperative to reach out to these victims and stop the cycle of abuse by following through on your suspicions.

Summary

The causes of violence against women are complex. Many women will experience some type of violence in their lives, and it can have a debilitating affect on their health and future relationships. Violence frequently leaves a "legacy of pain" to future generations. Nurses can empower women and encourage them to move forward and take control of their lives. When women live in peace and security and free from violence, they have an enormous potential to contribute to their own communities and to the

BOX 9.5 **Identifying Victims of Human Trafficking**

Cues

Look beneath the surface and ask yourself: Is this person. . . .
• A female or a child in poor health?
• Foreign-born and doesn't speak English?
• Lacking immigration documents?
• Giving an inconsistent explanation of injury?
• Reluctant to give any information about self, injury, home, or work?
• Fearful of authority figure or "sponsor" if present? ("Sponsor" might not leave victim alone with health care provider.)
• Living with the employer?

Sample questions to ask the potential victim of human trafficking:
• Can you leave your job or situation if you wish?
• Can you come and go as you please?
• Have you been threatened if you try to leave?
• Has anyone threatened your family with harm if you leave?
• What are your working and living conditions?
• Do you have to ask permission to go to the bathroom, eat, or sleep?
• Is there a lock on your door so you cannot get out?
• What brought you to the United States? Are your plans the same now?
• Are you free to leave your current work or home situation?
• Who has your immigration papers? Why don't you have them?
• Are you paid for the work you do?
• Are there times you feel afraid?
• How can your situation be changed?

Sources: http://www.rainn.org/statistics.html; Jones et al., 2007.

national and global society. Violence against women is not normal, legal, or acceptable and it should never be tolerated or justified. It can and must be stopped by the entire world community.

■■■ Key Concepts

■ Violence against women is a major public health and social problem because it violates a woman's very being and causes numerous mental and physical health sequelae.

■ Every woman has the potential to become a victim of violence.

■ Several *Healthy People 2010* objectives focus on reducing the rate of physical assaults and the number of rapes and attempted rapes.

■ Abuse may be mental, physical, or sexual in nature or a combination.

■ The cycle of violence includes three phases: tension-building, acute battering, and honeymoon.

■ Many women experience post-traumatic stress disorder (PTSD) after being sexually assaulted. PTSD can inhibit a survivor from adapting or coping in a healthy manner.

■ Pregnancy can precipitate violence toward the woman to start or escalate.

■ The nurse's role in dealing with survivors of violence is to establish rapport; open up lines of communication; apply the nursing process to assess and screen all patients in all settings; and implement and intervene as appropriate.

REFERENCES

Aggeles, T. B. (2007). *Domestic violence advocacy, Florida, update.* Available at: http://nsweb.NursingSpectrum.com/ce/ce60133.html

Alekseeva, L. S. (2007). Problems of child abuse in the home. *Russian Education and Society, 49*(5), 6–18.

Alexander, L. L., LaRosa, J. H., Bader, H., & Garfield, S. (2007). *New dimensions in women's health* (4th ed.). Sudbury, MA: Jones and Bartlett Publishers.

Association of Women's Health, Obstetric and Neonatal Nurses (AWHONN). (2007). *Violence against women: Identification, screening and management of intimate partner violence.* Available at: http://www.awhonn.org.

Bonomi, A. E., Anderson, M. L., Reid, R. J., Carrell, D., Fishman, P. A., Rivara, F. P., & Thompson, R. S. (2007). Intimate partner violence in older women. *Gerontologist, 47*(1), 34–41.

Burgess, A. W. (2007) How many red flags does it take? *American Journal of Nursing, 107*(1), 28–31.

Casanueva, C. E., & Martin, S. L. (2007). Intimate partner violence during pregnancy and mother's child abuse potential. *Journal of Interpersonal Violence, 22*(5), 603–622.

Centers for Disease Control and Prevention (CDC). (2007a). *Intimate partner violence: Fact sheet.* National Center for Injury Prevention and Control. Available at: http://www.cdc.gov/ncipc/factsheets/ipvfacts.htm.

Centers for Disease Control and Prevention (CDC). (2007b). *Sexual violence: Fact sheet.* National Center for Injury Prevention and Control. Available at: http://www.cdc.gov/ncipc/factsheets/svfacts.htm.

CDC/National Center for Injury Prevention and Control. (2007). *Tips for handling domestic violence.* Available at: http://www.cdc.gov/communication/tips/domviol.htm.

Centers for Disease Control and Prevention (CDC). (2008). Adverse health conditions and health risk behaviors associated with intimate partner violence—United States. *MMWR, 57*(5), 113–117.

Du Plat-Jones, J. (2006). Domestic violence: The role of health professionals. *Nursing Standard, 21*(14), 44–48.

Dutton, D. G. (2007). *Rethinking domestic violence.* Vancouver, British Columbia, Canada: University of British Columbia Press.

Elliott, S. M. (2008). Drug-facilitated sexual assault: Educating women about the risks. *Nursing for Women's Health, 12*(1), 30–37.

Federal Bureau of Investigation (FBI). (2007). *Intimate partner violence.* Available at: http://www.ojp.usdoj.gov/bjs/pub/ascii/ipv.txt.

Ferris, L. E. (2007). Intimate partner violence. *British Medical Journal, 334*(7596), 706–707.

Giardino, E. R. (2007). Uncovering abuse in the pregnant woman. *Nursing Spectrum.* Available at: http://www.nurse.com/ce/print.html?CCID=3141.

Healthy People 2010 (2000). Available at: http://www.healthypeople.gov/document/HTML/Volume2/15Injury.htm#_Toc490549392.

Herrenkohl, T. I., Kosterman, R., Mason, W. A., & Hawkins, J. D. (2007). Youth violence trajectories and proximal characteristics of intimate partner violence. *Violence and Victims, 22*(3), 259–274.

Hodge, D. R., & Lietz, C. A. (2007). The international sexual trafficking of women and children: A review of the literature. *Journal of Women & Social Work, 22*(2), 163–174.

Holtz, H., & Furniss, K. K. (1993). The health care provider's role in domestic violence. *Trends in Health Care Law and Ethics, 15,* 519–522.

Joint Commission on Accreditation of Healthcare Organizations. (2007). *The Joint Commission accreditation manual for hospitals.* Chicago: JCAHO.

Jones, L., Engstrom, D. W., Hilliard, T., & Diaz, M. (2007). Globalization and human trafficking. *Journal of Sociology & Social Welfare, 24*(2), 107–122.

Kandakai, T. L., & Smith, L. C. (2007). Denormalizing a historical problem: Teen pregnancy, policy, and public health action. *American Journal of Health Behavior, 31*(2), 170–180.

Keleher, H., & Franklin, L. (2008). Changing gendered norms about women and girls at the level of household and community: A review of the evidence. *Global Public Health, Suppl. 1*(3), 42–57.

Kelly, P. J. (2007). Integrating intimate partner violence prevention into daily practice. *Journal of Psychosocial Nursing, 45*(4), 8–10.

Kiump, M. C. (2006). Posttraumatic stress disorder and sexual assault in women. *Journal of College Student Psychotherapy, 21*(2), 67–83.

Kristensen, E., & Lau, M. (2007). Women with a history of childhood sexual abuse. Long-term social and psychiatric aspects. *Nordic Journal of Psychiatry, 61*(2), 115–120.

Macy, R. J., Nurius, P. S., & Norris, J. (2007). Latent profiles among sexual assault survivors. *Journal of Interpersonal Violence, 22*(5), 543–565.

Medicine Net. (2007). *Sexual assault.* Available at: http://www.medicinenet.com/script/main/art.asp?articlekey=46498&pf=3.

National Center for Victims of Crime (NCVC). (2007). *Incest.* Available at: http://www.ncvc.org/ncvc/main.aspx?dbName=DocumentViewer&DocumentID=32360.

Paluzzi, P. A. (2007). Violence against women and children. In B. Hackley, J. M. Kriebs, & M. E. Rousseau (Eds.), *Primary care of women: A guide for midwives and women's health providers* (Chapter 7, pp. 193–212). Sudbury, MA: Jones and Bartlett Publishers.

Research Action and Information Network for the Bodily Integrity of Women (RAINBO). (2007). *Caring for women with circumcision: Fact sheet for physicians.* Available at: http://www.rainbo.org/factsheet.html.

Rape, Abuse, and Incest National Network (RAINN). (2007). *RAINN statistics.* Available at: http://www.rainn.org/statistics.html.

Sampson, R. (2007). *Acquaintance rape of college students.* U.S. Department of Justice COPS. Available at: http://www.cops.usdoj.gov.

Sharps, P. W., Laughon, K., & Giandrande, S. K. (2007). Intimate partner violence and the childbearing year. *Trauma, Violence & Abuse, 8*(2), 105–116.

Thackeray, J., Stelzner, S., Downs, S. M., & Miller, C. (2007). Screening for intimate partner violence. *Journal of Interpersonal Violence, 22*(6), 659–670.

U.S. Department of Health and Human Services (U.S. DHHS). (2007). *Frequently asked questions about date rape drugs.* The National Women's Health Information Center. Available at: http://www.4woman.gov/faq/rohypnol.pdf.

U.S. Department of State. (2007). *Trafficking in persons report.* U.S. Department of State Publication No. 11057, p. 7. Washington, DC: Author.

Victims of Trafficking and Violence Protection Act of 2000, Pub. Law No. 106-386 [II.R. 3244] (2000). Available at: http://ojp.gov/vawo/laws/vawo2000/stitle_a.htm.

Wakabi, W. (2007). Africa battles to make female genital mutilation history. *Lancet, 369*(9567), 1069–1070.

World Health Organization (WHO). (2007). *Female genital mutilation.* Available at: http://www.who.int/mediacentre/factsheets/fs241/en/print.html.

Zaidi, N., Khalil, A., Roberts, C., & Browne, M. (2007). Knowledge of female genital mutilation among healthcare professionals. *Journal of Obstetrics & Gynecology, 27*(2), 161–164.

WEBSITES

Boat People S.O.S., Inc.: www.bpsos.org

Center for the Prevention of Sexual and Domestic Violence: (206) 634-1903, www.cpsdv.org

Centers for Disease Control and Prevention: Intimate Partner Violence: www.cdc.gov/ncipc/factsheets/ipvfacts.htm

Coalition to Abolish Slavery and Trafficking: www.trafficked-women.org

Domestic Violence Handbook: www.domesticviolence.org

Immigrant & Refugee Community Organization: www.irco.org/irco

National Coalition Against Sexual Assault (NCADV): (303) 839-1852, www.ncadv.org

National Domestic Violence Hotline: (800) 799-SAFE (7233), www.ndvh.org

Nursing Network on Violence Against Women, International: Resources for Health Care Professionals: http://www.nnvawi.org/links.htm#professional

Protection Project: www.protectionproject.org

Rape, Abuse, and Incest National Network (RAINN): (800) 656-HOPE, www.rainn.org

SAGE Project: www.sageinc.org

Trafficking Information and Referral Hotline: (888) 373-7888, www.acf.hhs.gov/trafficking

U.S. Department of Health Human Services: aaqui@acf.hhs.gov

U.S. Department of Labor, Women's Bureau: www.dol.gov.dol/wb

Violence Against Women Office, U.S. Department of Justice: (202) 616-8894, www.raw.umn.edu

Chapter Worksheet

Multiple Choice Questions

1. The primary goal of intervention in working with abused women is to:

   a. Set up an appointment with a mental health counselor for the victim

   b. Convince them to set up a safety plan to use when they leave

   c. Help them to develop courage and financial support to leave the abuser

   d. Empower them and improve their self-esteem to regain control of their lives

2. The first phase of the abuse cycle is characterized by:

   a. The woman provokes the abuser to bring about battering

   b. Tension-building and verbal or minor battery

   c. A honeymoon period that lulls the victim into forgetting

   d. An acute episode of physical battering

3. Women recovering from abusive relationships need to learn ways to improve their:

   a. Cooking skills and provide more nutritious meals for their children

   b. Creativity so as to improve their decorating skills within the home

   c. Communication and negotiation skills to increase their assertiveness

   d. Personal appearance by losing weight and exercising more

4. Which of the following statements might empower abuse victims to take action?

   a. "You deserve better than this."

   b. "Your children deserve to grow up in a two-parent family."

   c. "Try to figure out what you do to trigger his abuse and stop it."

   d. "Give your partner more time to come to his senses about this."

Critical Thinking Exercise

1. Mrs. Boggs has three children under the age of 5 and is 6 months pregnant with her fourth child. She has made repeated unscheduled visits to your clinic with vague somatic complaints regarding the children as well as herself, but has missed several scheduled prenatal appointments. On occasion she has worn sunglasses to cover bruises around her eyes. As a nurse you sense there is something else bothering her, but she doesn't seem to want to discuss it with you. She appears sad and the children cling to her.

   a. Outline your conversation when you broach the subject of abuse with Mrs. Boggs.

   b. What is your role as a nurse in caring for a family in which you suspect abuse?

   c. What ethical/legal considerations are important in planning care for this family?

Study Activities

1. Visit the BellaOnline website for victims of violence (www.bellaonline.com). Discuss what you discovered on this site and your reactions to it.

2. Research the statistics about violence against women in your state. Are law enforcement and community interventions reducing the incidence of sexual assault and intimate partner violence?

3. Attend a dorm orientation at a local college to hear about measures in place to protect women's safety on campus. Find out the number of sexual assaults reported and what strategies the college uses to reduce this number.

4. Volunteer to spend a weekend evening at the local sheriff's department 911 hotline desk to observe the number and nature of calls received reporting domestic violence. Interview the dispatch operator about the frequency and trends of these calls.

5. Identify three community resources that could be useful to a victim of violence. Identify their sources of funding and the services they provide.

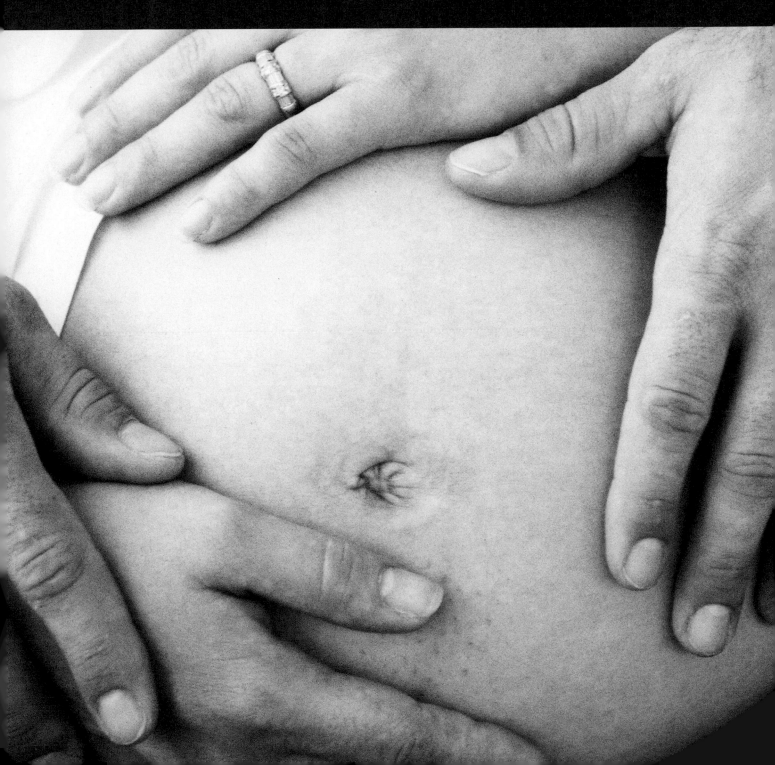

UNIT THREE

PREGNANCY

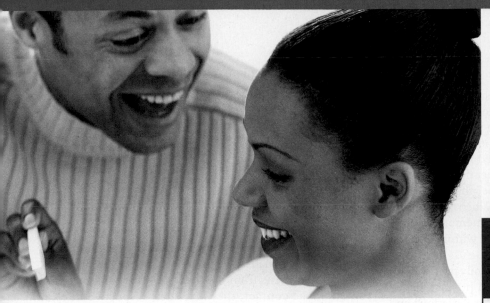

CHAPTER 10

FETAL DEVELOPMENT AND GENETICS

KEY TERMS

allele
blastocyst
embryonic stage
fertilization
fetal stage
genes
genetic counseling
genetics
genome

genotype
heterozygous
homozygous
karyotype
mosaicism
monosomies
morula
mutation
phenotype

placenta
polyploidy
preembryonic stage
trisomies
trophoblast
umbilical cord
zona pellucida
zygote

LEARNING OBJECTIVES

Upon completion of the chapter, the learner will be able to:

1. Describe the process of fertilization, implantation, and cell differentiation.
2. Explain the functions of the placenta, umbilical cord, and amniotic fluid.
3. Outline normal fetal development from conception through birth.
4. Compare the various inheritance patterns, including nontraditional patterns of inheritance.
5. Give examples of ethical and legal issues surrounding genetic testing.
6. Explain the role of the nurse in genetic counseling and genetic-related activities.

*R*obert and Kate Shafer have just received the good news that Kate's pregnancy test was positive. It had been a long and anxious 3 years of trying to start a family. Although both are elated about the prospect of becoming parents, they are also concerned about the possibility of a genetic problem because Kate is 38 years old. What might be their first step in looking into their genetic concern? As a nurse, what might raise concerns for you?

Wow

Being a nurse without awe is like food without spice. Nurses only have to witness the miracle of life to find their lost awe.

Human reproduction is one of the most intimate spheres of an individual's life. For conception to occur, a healthy ovum from the woman is released from the ovary, passes into an open fallopian tube, and starts its journey downward. Sperm from the male is deposited into the vagina and swims approximately 7 inches to meet the ovum at the outermost portion of the fallopian tube, the area where fertilization takes place (Gilbert, 2007). When one spermatozoon penetrates the ovum's thick outer membrane, pregnancy begins. All this activity takes place within a 5-hour time span.

Nurses caring for the childbearing family need to have a basic understanding of conception and prenatal development so they can identify problems or variations and can initiate appropriate interventions should any problems occur. This chapter presents an overview of fetal development, beginning with conception. It also discusses hereditary influences on fetal development and the nurse's role in genetic counseling.

Fetal Development

Fetal development during pregnancy is measured in number of weeks after fertilization. The duration of pregnancy is about 40 weeks from the time of fertilization. This equates to 9 calendar months or approximately 266 to 280 calendar days. The three stages of fetal development during pregnancy are:

1. **Preembryonic stage:** fertilization through the second week
2. **Embryonic stage:** end of the second week through the eighth week
3. **Fetal stage:** end of the eighth week until birth

Fetal circulation is a significant aspect of fetal development that spans all three stages.

Preembryonic Stage

The preembryonic stage begins with **fertilization**, also called *conception*. Fertilization is the union of ovum and sperm, which is the starting point of pregnancy. Fertilization typically occurs around 2 weeks after the last normal menstrual period in a 28-day cycle (Dillon, 2007). Fertilization requires a timely interaction between the release of the mature ovum at ovulation and the ejaculation of enough healthy, mobile sperm to survive the hostile vaginal environment through which they must travel to meet the ovum. All things considered, the act of conception is difficult at best. To say merely that it occurs when the sperm unites with the ovum is overly simple because this union requires an intricate interplay of hormonal preparation and overcoming an overwhelming number of natural barriers. A human being is truly an amazing outcome of this elaborate process.

Prior to fertilization, the ovum and the spermatozoon undergo the process of meiosis. The primary oocyte completes its first meiotic division before ovulation. The secondary oocyte begins its second meiotic division just before ovulation. Primary and secondary spermatocytes undergo meiotic division while still in the testes (Fig. 10.1).

Although each milliliter of ejaculated semen contains more than 200 million sperm, only one is able to enter the ovum to fertilize it. All others are blocked by the clear protein layer called the **zona pellucida**. The zona pellucida disappears in about 5 days. Once the sperm reaches the plasma membrane, the ovum resumes meiosis and forms a nucleus with half the number of chromosomes (23). When the nucleus from the ovum and the nucleus of the sperm make contact, they lose their respective nuclear membranes and combine their maternal and paternal chromosomes. Because each nucleus contains a haploid number of chromosomes (23), this union restores the diploid number (46). The resulting **zygote** begins the process of a new life. The genetic information from both ovum and sperm establishes the unique physical characteristics of the individual. Sex determination is also determined at fertilization and depends on whether the ovum is fertilized by a Y-bearing sperm or an X-bearing sperm. An XX zygote will become a female and an XY zygote will become a male (Fig. 10.2).

Fertilization takes place in the outer third of the ampulla of the fallopian tube. When the ovum is fertilized by the sperm (now called a zygote), a great deal of activity immediately takes place. Mitosis, or *cleavage*, occurs as the zygote is slowly transported into the uterine cavity by tubal muscular movements (Fig. 10.3). After a series of four cleavages, the 16 cells appear as a solid ball of cells or **morula**, meaning "little mulberry." The morula reaches the uterine cavity about 72 hours after fertilization (Johnson, 2007).

With additional cell division, the morula divides into specialized cells that will later form fetal structures. Within the morula, an off-center, fluid-filled space appears, transforming it into a hollow ball of cells called a **blastocyst** (Fig. 10.4). The inner surface of the blastocyst will form the embryo and amnion. The outer layer of cells surrounding the blastocyst cavity is called a **trophoblast**. Eventually, the trophoblast develops into one of the embryonic membranes, the chorion, and helps to form the placenta.

At this time, the developing blastocyst needs more food and oxygen to keep growing. The trophoblast attaches itself to the surface of the endometrium for further nourishment. Normally, implantation occurs in the upper uterus (fundus), where a rich blood supply is available. This area also contains strong muscular fibers, which clamp down on blood vessels after the placenta separates from the inner wall of the uterus. Additionally, the lining is thickest here so the placenta cannot attach so strongly that it remains

(text continues on page 240)

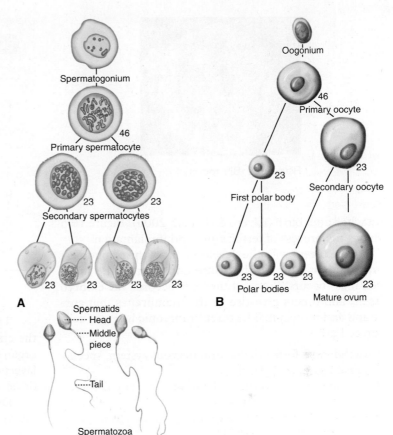

A

B

FIGURE 10.1 The formation of gametes by the process of meiosis is known as gametogenesis. (**A**) Spermatogenesis. One spermatogonium gives rise to four spermatozoa. (**B**) Oogenesis. From each oogonium, one mature ovum and three abortive cells are produced. The chromosomes are reduced to one-half the number characteristic for the general body cells of the species. In humans, the number in the body cells is 46, and that in the mature spermatozoon and secondary oocyte is 23.

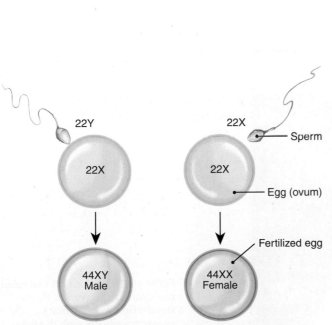

FIGURE 10.2 Inheritance of gender. Each ovum contains 22 autosomes and an X chromosome. Each spermatozoon (sperm) contains 22 autosomes and either an X chromosome or a Y chromosome. The gender of the zygote is determined at the time of fertilization by the combination of the sex chromosomes of the sperm (either X or Y) and the ovum (X).

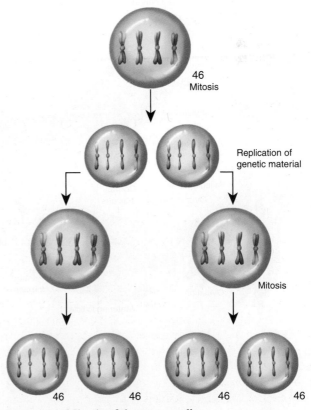

FIGURE 10.3 Mitosis of the stoma cells.

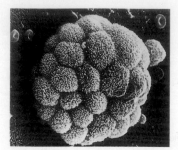

FIGURE 10.4 Blastocyst.

attached after birth (Alvero & Schlaff, 2006). Figure 10.5 shows the process of fertilization and implantation.

Concurrent with the development of the trophoblast and implantation, further differentiation of the inner cell mass occurs. Some of the cells become the embryo itself, and others give rise to the membranes that surround and protect it. The three embryonic layers of cells formed are:

1. Ectoderm—forms the central nervous system, special senses, skin, and glands
2. Mesoderm—forms the skeletal, urinary, circulatory, and reproductive organs
3. Endoderm—forms the respiratory system, liver, pancreas, and digestive system

---

BOX 10.1 **Summary of Preembryonic Development**

• Fertilization takes place in ampulla of the fallopian tube.
• Union of sperm and ovum forms a *zygote* (46 chromosomes).
• Cleavage cell division continues to form a *morula* (mass of 16 cells).
• The inner cell mass is called *blastocyst,* which forms the embryo and amnion.
• The outer cell mass is called *trophoblast,* which forms the placenta and chorion.
• Implantation occurs 7 to 10 days after conception in the endometrium.

These three layers are formed at the same time as the embryonic membranes, and all tissues, organs, and organ systems develop from these three primary germ cell layers (Dillon, 2007). Box 10.1 summarizes preembryonic development.

Despite the intense and dramatic activities going on internally to create a human life, many women are unaware that pregnancy has begun. Several weeks will pass before

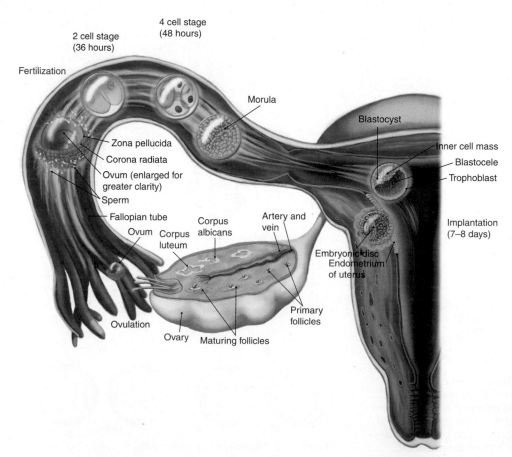

FIGURE 10.5 Fertilization and tubal transport of the zygote. From fertilization to implantation, the zygote travels through the fallopian tube, experiencing rapid mitotic division (cleavage). During the journey toward the uterus the zygote evolves through several stages, including morula and blastocyst.

even one of the presumptive signs of pregnancy—missing the first menstrual period—will take place.

Embryonic Stage

The embryonic stage of development begins at day 15 after conception and continues through week 8. Basic structures of all major body organs and the main external features are completed during this time period. Table 10.1 and Figure 10.6 summarize embryonic development.

The embryonic membranes (Fig. 10.7) begin to form around the time of implantation. The chorion consists of trophoblast cells and a mesodermal lining. It has finger-like projections called *chorionic villi* on its surface. The amnion originates from the ectoderm germ layer during the early stages of embryonic development. It is a thin

protective membrane that contains amniotic fluid. As the embryo grows, the amnion expands until it touches the chorion. These two fetal membranes form the fluid-filled amniotic sac, or bag of waters, that protects the floating embryo (Creatsas, Chrousos, & Mastorakos, 2007).

Amniotic fluid surrounds the embryo and increases in volume as the pregnancy progresses, reaching approximately a liter at term. Amniotic fluid is derived from two sources: fluid transported from the maternal blood across the amnion and fetal urine. Its volume changes constantly as the fetus swallows and voids. Sufficient amounts of amniotic fluid help maintain a constant body temperature for the fetus, permit symmetric growth and development, cushion the fetus from trauma, allow the **umbilical cord** to be relatively free from compression, and promote

TABLE 10.1 EMBRYONIC AND FETAL DEVELOPMENT

Week 3
Beginning development of brain, spinal cord, and heart
Beginning development of the gastrointestinal tract
Neural tube forms, which later becomes the spinal cord
Leg and arm buds appear and grow out from body

Week 4
Brain differentiates
Limb buds grow and develop more

4 weeks

Week 5
Heart now beats at a regular rhythm
Beginning structures of eyes and ears
Some cranial nerves are visible
Muscles innervated

Week 6
Beginning formation of lungs
Fetal circulation established
Liver produces RBCs
Further development of the brain
Primitive skeleton forms
Central nervous system forms
Brain waves detectable

Week 7
Straightening of trunk
Nipples and hair follicles form
Elbows and toes visible
Arms and legs move
Diaphragm formed
Mouth with lips and early tooth buds

Week 8
Rotation of intestines
Facial features continue to develop
Heart development complete
Resembles a human being (Ratner, 2002)

8 weeks

Weeks 9–12
Sexual differentiation continues
Buds for all 20 temporary teeth laid down
Digestive system shows activity
Head makes up nearly half the fetus size
Face and neck are well formed
Urogenital tract completes development
Red blood cells are produced in the liver
Urine begins to be produced and excreted
Fetal gender can be determined by week 12
Limbs are long and thin; digits are well formed

12 weeks

(continued)

TABLE 10.1 EMBRYONIC AND FETAL DEVELOPMENT (continued)

Weeks 13–16
A fine hair called *lanugo* develops on the head
Fetal skin is almost transparent
Bones become harder
Fetus makes active movement
Sucking motions are made with the mouth
Amniotic fluid is swallowed
Fingernails and toenails present
Weight quadruples
Fetal movement (also know as *quickening*) detected
    by mother

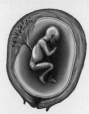

16 weeks

Weeks 17–20
Rapid brain growth occurs
Fetal heart tones can be heard with stethoscope
Kidneys continue to secrete urine into amniotic fluid
Vernix caseosa, a white greasy film, covers the fetus
Eyebrows and head hair appear
Brown fat deposited to help maintain temperature
Nails are present on both fingers and toes
Muscles are well developed

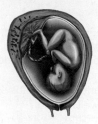

20 weeks

Weeks 21–24
Eyebrows and eyelashes are well formed
Fetus has a hand grasp and startle reflex
Alveoli forming in lungs
Skin is translucent and red
Lungs begin to produce *surfactant*

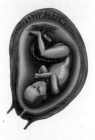

25 weeks

Weeks 25–28
Fetus reaches a length of 15 inches
Rapid brain development
Eyelids open and close
Nervous system controls some functions
Fingerprints are set
Blood formation shifts from spleen to bone marrow
Fetus usually assumes head-down position

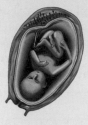

28 weeks

Weeks 29–32
Rapid increase in the amount of body fat
Increased central nervous system control over body
    functions
Rhythmic breathing movements occur
Lungs are not fully mature
Fetus stores iron, calcium, and phosphorus

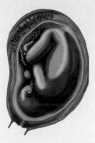

32 weeks

Weeks 33–38
Testes are in scrotum of male fetus
Lanugo begins to disappear
Increase in body fat
Fingernails reach the end of fingertips
Small breast buds are present on both sexes
Mother supplies fetus with antibodies against disease
Fetus is considered full term at 38 weeks
Fetus fills uterus (Bailey, 2003)

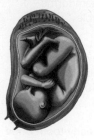

37 weeks

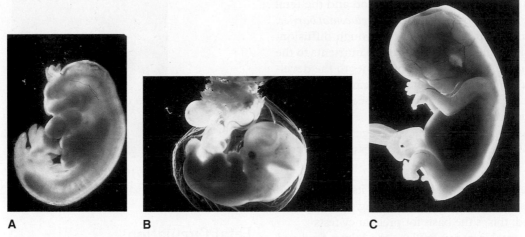

A **B** **C**

FIGURE 10.6 Embryonic development. (**A**) 4-week embryo. (**B**) 5-week embryo. (**C**) 6-week embryo.

fetal movement to enhance musculoskeletal development. Amniotic fluid is composed of 98% water and 2% organic matter. It is slightly alkaline and contains albumin, urea, uric acid, creatinine, bilirubin, lecithin, sphingomyelin, epithelial cells, vernix, and fine hair called lanugo (Johnson, 2007).

The volume of amniotic fluid is important in determining fetal well-being. It gradually fluctuates throughout the pregnancy. Alterations in amniotic fluid volume can be associated with problems in the fetus. Too little amniotic fluid (<500 mL at term), termed *oligohydramnios,* is

associated with uteroplacental insufficiency and fetal renal abnormalities. Too much amniotic fluid (>2,000 mL at term), termed *hydramnios,* is associated with maternal diabetes, neural tube defects, chromosomal deviations, and malformations of the central nervous system and/or gastrointestinal tract that prevent normal swallowing of amniotic fluid by the fetus (Gilbert, 2007).

While the placenta is developing (end of the second week), the umbilical cord is also formed from the amnion. It is the lifeline from the mother to the growing embryo. It contains one large vein and two small arteries. Wharton's jelly (a specialized connective tissue) surrounds these three blood vessels in the umbilical cord to prevent compression, which would cut off fetal blood and nutrient supply. At term, the average umbilical cord is 22 inches long and about an inch wide (Johnson, 2007).

The precursor cells of the placenta—the trophoblasts—first appear 4 days after fertilization as the outer layer of cells of the blastocyst. These early blastocyst trophoblasts differentiate into all the cells that form the **placenta**. When fully developed, the placenta serves as the interface between the mother and the developing fetus. As early as 3 days after conception, the trophoblasts make human chorionic gonadotropin (hCG), a hormone that ensures that the endometrium will be receptive to the implanting embryo. During the next few weeks the placenta begins to make hormones that control the basic physiology of the mother in such a way that the fetus is supplied with the nutrients and oxygen needed for growth. The placenta also protects the fetus from immune attack by the mother, removes waste products from the fetus, induces the mother to bring more food to the placenta, and, near the time of delivery, produces hormones that ready fetal organs for life outside the uterus (Johnson, 2007).

Theoretically, at no time during pregnancy does the mother's blood mix with fetal blood because there is no direct contact between their bloods; layers of fetal

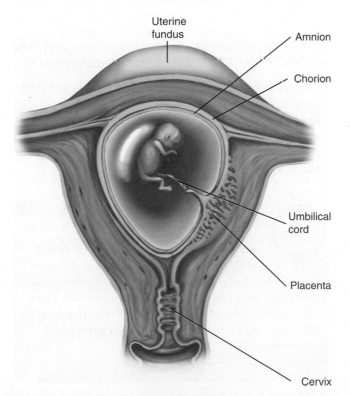

Uterine fundus

Amnion

Chorion

Umbilical cord

Placenta

Cervix

FIGURE 10.7 The embryo is floating in amniotic fluid, surrounded by the protective fetal membranes (amnion and chorion).

tissue always separate the maternal blood and the fetal blood. These fetal tissues are called the *placental barrier*. Materials can be interchanged only through diffusion. The maternal uterine arteries deliver the nutrients to the placenta, which in turn provides nutrients to the developing fetus; the mother's uterine veins carry fetal waste products away. The structure of the placenta is usually completed by week 12.

The placenta is not only a transfer organ but a factory as well. It produces several hormones necessary for normal pregnancy:

- hCG—preserves the corpus luteum and its progesterone production so that the endometrial lining of the uterus is maintained; this is the basis for pregnancy tests
- Human placental lactogen (hPL)—modulates fetal and maternal metabolism, participates in the development of maternal breasts for lactation, and decreases maternal insulin sensitivity to increase its availability for fetal nutrition
- Estrogen (estriol)—causes enlargement of a woman's breasts, uterus, and external genitalia; stimulates myometrial contractility
- Progesterone (progestin)—maintains the endometrium, decreases the contractility of the uterus, stimulates maternal metabolism and breast development, provides nourishment for the early conceptus
- Relaxin—acts synergistically with progesterone to maintain pregnancy, causes relaxation of the pelvic ligaments, softens the cervix in preparation for birth (Alvero & Schlaff, 2006)

The placenta acts as a pass-through between the mother and fetus, not a barrier. Almost everything the mother ingests (food, alcohol, drugs) passes through to the developing conceptus. This is why it is so important to advise pregnant women not to use drugs, alcohol, and tobacco, because they can be harmful to the conceptus.

During the embryonic stage, the conceptus grows rapidly as all organs and structures are forming. During this critical period of differentiation the growing embryo is most susceptible to damage from external sources, including teratogens (substances that cause birth defects, such as alcohol and drugs), infections (such as rubella or cytomegalovirus), radiation, and nutritional deficiencies.

Fetal Stage

The average pregnancy lasts 280 days from the first day of the last menstrual period. The fetal stage is the time from the end of the eighth week until birth. It is the longest period of prenatal development. During this stage, the conceptus is mature enough to be called a fetus. Although all major systems are present in their basic form, dramatic growth and refinement of all organ systems take place during the fetal period (see Table 10.1). Figure 10.8 depicts a 12- to 15-week-old fetus.

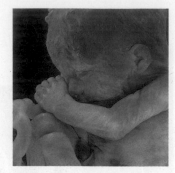

FIGURE 10.8 Fetal development: 12- to 15-week fetus.

Fetal Circulation

The circulation through the fetus during uterine life differs from that of a child or an adult. Fetal circulation involves the circulation of blood from the placenta to and through the fetus, and back to the placenta. A properly functioning fetal circulation system is essential to sustain the fetus. Before it develops, nutrients and oxygen diffuse through the extraembryonic coelom and the yolk sac from the placenta. As the embryo grows, its nutrient needs increase and the amount of tissue easily reached by diffusion increases. Thus, the circulation must develop quickly and accurately (Blackburn, 2007).

The circulatory system of the fetus functions much differently from that of a newborn. The most significant difference is that oxygen is received from the placenta during fetal life and via the lungs after birth. In addition, the fetal liver does not perform the metabolic functions that it will after birth because the mother's body performs these functions. Three shunts also are present during fetal life:

1. Ductus venosus—connects the umbilical vein to the inferior vena cava
2. Ductus arteriosus—connects the main pulmonary artery to the aorta
3. Foramen ovale—anatomic opening between the right and left atrium

▶ *Take* NOTE!

Fetal circulation functions to carry highly oxygenated blood to vital areas (e.g., heart, brain) while first shunting it away from less important ones (e.g., lungs, liver). The placenta essentially takes over the functions of the lungs and liver during fetal life. As a result, large volumes of oxygenated blood are not needed.

The oxygenated blood is carried from the placenta to the fetus via the umbilical vein. About half of this blood passes through the hepatic capillaries and the rest flows through the ductus venosus into the inferior vena cava. Blood from the vena cava is mostly deflected through the foramen ovale into the left atrium, then to the left ventricle, into the ascending aorta, and on to the head and upper body. This allows the fetal coronary circulation and the brain to receive the blood with the highest level of oxygenation.

Deoxygenated blood from the superior vena cava flows into the right atrium, the right ventricle, and then the pulmonary artery. Because of high pulmonary vascular resistance, only a small percentage (5% to 10%) of the blood in the pulmonary artery flows to the lungs; the majority is shunted through the patent ductus arteriosus and then to the descending aorta (Blackburn, 2007). The fetal lungs are essentially nonfunctional because they are filled with fluid, making them resistant to incoming blood flow. They receive only enough blood for proper nourishment. Finally, two umbilical arteries carry the unoxygenated blood from the descending aorta back to the placenta.

At birth, a dramatic change in the fetal circulatory pattern occurs. The foramen ovale, ductus arteriosus, ductus venosus, and umbilical vessels are no longer needed. With the newborn's first breath, the lungs inflate, which leads to an increase in blood flow to the lungs from the right ventricle. This increase raises the pressure in the left atrium, causing a one-way flap on the left side of the foramen ovale, called the septum primum, to press against the opening, creating a functional separation between the two atria. Blood flow to the lungs increases because blood entering the right atrium can no longer bypass the right ventricle. As a result, the right ventricle pumps blood into the pulmonary artery and on to the lungs. The ductus venosus closes with the clamping of the umbilical cord and inhibition of blood flow through the umbilical vein. The ductus arteriosus constricts partly in response to the higher arterial oxygen levels that occur after the first few breaths. This closure prevents blood from the aorta from entering the pulmonary artery (Blackburn, 2007). All of these changes leave the newborn with the typical adult pattern of circulation. Figure 10.9 shows fetal circulation.

Genetics

Genetics is the study of heredity and its variation (Brooks, 2008). According to the Centers for Disease Control and Prevention (CDC), birth defects and genetic disorders occur in about 3% of all infants born in the United States (CDC, 2007). Traditionally, genetics has been associated with making decisions about childbearing and caring for children with genetic disorders. Recently, genetic and technologic advances are expanding our understanding of how genetic changes affect human diseases such as diabetes, cancer, Alzheimer's disease, and other multifactorial diseases that are prevalent in adults (Dolan, Biermann, & Damus, 2007). Our ability to diagnose genetic conditions is more advanced than our ability to cure or treat the disorders. However, accurate diagnosis has led to improved treatment and outcomes for those affected with these disorders.

> ▶ **Take** NOTE!
>
> *Genetic science has the potential to revolutionize health care with regard to national screening programs, predisposition testing, detection of genetic disorders, and pharmacogenetics.*

Today, nurses are required to have basic skills and knowledge in genetics, genetic testing, and genetic counseling so they can assume new roles and provide information and support to women and their families.

Advances in Genetics

Recent advances in genetic knowledge and technology have affected all areas of health. These advances have increased the number of health interventions that can be undertaken with regard to genetic disorders. For example, genetic diagnosis is now possible before conception and very early in pregnancy (see Evidence-Based Practice 10.1). Genetic testing can now identify presymptomatic conditions in children and adults. Gene therapy can be used to replace or repair defective or missing genes with normal ones. Gene therapy has been used for a variety of disorders, including cystic fibrosis, melanoma, diabetes, HIV, and hepatitis (Newman & Bettinger, 2007). The potential exists for creation of increased intelligence and size through genetic intervention. Genetic agents may replace drugs, general surgery may be replaced by gene surgery, and genetic intervention may replace radiation (Erlen, 2006). It may also be used to treat many chronic illnesses.

The Human Genome Project (HGP) was an international 13-year effort to produce a comprehensive sequence of the human genome. It was started in 1990 by the Department of Energy and the National Institutes of Health and was completed in May 2003. It has brought advances to the field of genetics and genetic testing (Jenkins & Calzone, 2007). An individual's **genome** represents his or her genetic blueprint, which determines **genotype** (the gene pairs inherited from parents; the specific genetic makeup) and **phenotype** (observed outward characteristics of an individual) (Muzny et al., 2006).

A primary goal of the HGP was to translate the findings into new strategies for the prevention, diagnosis, and treatment of genetic diseases and disorders. Two key findings from the project were that all human beings are 99.9% identical at the DNA level, and approximately 30,000 genes make up the human genome (International Human Genome Sequencing Consortium, 2007). More

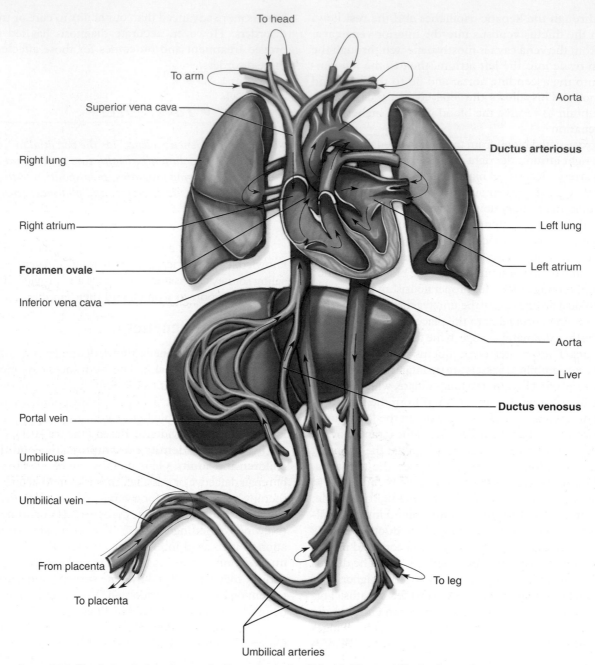

FIGURE 10.9 Fetal circulation. Arrows indicate the path of blood. The umbilical vein carries oxygen-rich blood from the placenta to the liver and through the ductus venosus. From there it is carried to the inferior vena cava to the right atrium of the heart. Some of the blood is shunted through the foramen ovale to the left side of the heart, where it is routed to the brain and upper extremities. The rest of the blood travels down to the right ventricle and through the pulmonary artery. A small portion of the blood travels to the nonfunctioning lungs, while the remaining blood is shunted through the ductus arteriosus into the aorta to supply the rest of the body.

information about the HGP may be accessed at: http://www.ornl.gov/sci/techresources/Human_Genomehome.shtml#index.

Current and potential applications for the HGP in health care include rapid and more specific diagnosis of disease, with hundreds of genetic tests available in research or clinical practice; earlier detection of genetic predisposition to disease; less emphasis on treating the symptoms of a disease and more emphasis on looking at the fundamental causes of the disease; new classes of drugs; avoidance of environmental conditions that may trigger disease; and augmentation or replacement of defective genes through gene

EVIDENCE-BASED PRACTICE 10.1
Is Preimplantation Genetic Screening Effective in Promoting Pregnancy With Assisted Reproductive Technologies?

Assisted reproductive technologies such as in vitro fertilization (IVF) and intracytoplasmic sperm injection (ICSI) involve the transfer of an embryo to the mother to achieve pregnancy. The physician selects the embryos for transfer based on specific criteria related to their structure and form. These "good-quality" embryos are then implanted in the mother in the hopes of achieving a pregnancy. Unfortunately, many women do not experience a pregnancy. The reasons for these failures are not known. One belief is that the embryos being transferred, although they meet the criteria for structure and form, may have an abnormal number of chromosomes, which affects implantation and the development of a pregnancy. Preimplantation genetic screening (PGS) is a tool being used to identify embryos of good quality with the normal number of chromosomes. Based on the screening, only these embryos are implanted; in theory, this would increase the rate of pregnancy. However, there are questions as to how effective PGS is in improving the rates of pregnancy and live birth.

● Study

Two independent authors used predetermined quality criteria to collect and analyze data from numerous databases, registers, and reference lists of articles. The researchers also gathered additional data from other authors as necessary. The researchers selected all relevant randomized controlled trials dealing with IVF or ICSI with and without PGS. The primary outcome was the live birth rate.

The researchers reviewed two randomized controlled trials, both involving IVF or ICSI with and without the use of PGS. The group without PGS was considered the control group. The trials also involved women of advanced maternal age (over age 35).

▲ Findings

Compared with the control group, the PGS group did not show significant differences in the live birth rate. There were also no significant differences in the rates of ongoing pregnancy. The researchers noted that these findings were limited by the small number of trials (two trials), the advanced maternal age, and the sample size of the one trial (39 women). Based on this study, the researchers could not find evidence to support routine use of PGS to facilitate pregnancy. They recommended more in-depth randomized trials to evaluate this technology.

■ Nursing Implications

Although the study failed to support the effectiveness of PGS, nurses need to be aware of the emerging technology and techniques associated with genetics so that they can provide women and their families with the most appropriate information about options and therapies. Nurses can incorporate information from this study in their teaching, anticipatory guidance, and counseling about options so that the couple can make the best-informed decision possible.

Twisk, M., Mastenbroek, S., van Wely, M., Heineman, M. J., Van der Veen, F,, & Repping, S. (2006). Preimplantation genetic screening for abnormal number of chromosomes (aneuploidies) in in vitro fertilization or intracytoplasmic sperm injection. *Cochrane Database of Systematic Reviews*, Issue 1. Art. No.: CD005291.DOI:10.1002/14651858.CD005291.pub2.

therapy. This new genetic knowledge and technology, along with the commercialization of this knowledge, will change both professional and parental understanding of genetic disorders.

The potential benefits of these discoveries are vast, but so is the potential for misuse. These advances challenge all health care professionals to consider the many ethical, legal, and social ramifications of genetics in human lives. In the near future, individual risk profiling based on an individual's unique genetic makeup will be used to tailor prevention, treatment, and ongoing management of health conditions. This profiling will raise issues associated with patient privacy and confidentiality related to workplace discrimination and access to health insurance. Issues of autonomy are equally problematic as society considers how to address the injustices that will inevitably surface when disease risk can be determined years before the disease occurs. Nurses will

play an important role in developing policies and providing direction and support in this arena, and to do so they will need a basic understanding of genetics, including inheritance and inheritance patterns. (For more information on the ethical, social, and legal issues surrounding human genetic research and advances, go to: http://www.ornl.gov/sci/techresources/Human_Genome/research/elsi.shtml.)

Inheritance

The nucleus within the cell is the controlling factor in all cellular activities because it contains chromosomes, long continuous strands of deoxyribonucleic acid (DNA) that carry genetic information. Each chromosome is made up of **genes**. Genes are individual units of heredity of all traits and are organized into long segments of DNA that occupy a specific location on a chromosome and determine a particular characteristic in an organism.

DNA stores genetic information and encodes the instructions for synthesizing specific proteins needed to maintain life. DNA is double-stranded and takes the form of a double helix. The side pieces of the double helix are made up of a sugar, deoxyribose, and a phosphate, occurring in alternating groups. The cross-connections or rungs of the ladder are attached to the sides and are made up of four nitrogenous bases: adenine, cytosine, thymine, and guanine. The sequence of the base pairs as they form each rung of the ladder is referred to as the genetic code (Fig. 10.10; Wright & Hastie, 2007).

Each gene has a segment of DNA with a specific set of instructions for making proteins needed by body cells for proper functioning. Genes control the types of proteins made and the rate at which they are produced (Dolan, Biermann, & Damus, 2007). Any change in gene structure or location leads to a **mutation**, which may alter the type and amount of protein produced (Fig. 10.11). Genes never act in isolation; they always interact with other genes and the environment. They are arranged in a specific linear formation along a chromosome.

The genotype, the specific genetic makeup of an individual, usually in the form of DNA, is the internally coded inheritable information. It refers to the particular **allele**, which is one of two or more alternative versions of gene at a given position or locus on a chromosome that imparts the same characteristic of that gene. For instance, each human has a gene that controls height, but there are variations of these genes, which are alleles, in accordance with the specific height for which the gene codes. A gene that controls eye color may have an allele that can produce blue eyes or an allele that produces brown eyes. The genotype, together with environmental variation that influences the individual, determines the phenotype, or the observed, outward characteristics of an individual. A human inherits two genes, one from each parent. Therefore, one allele

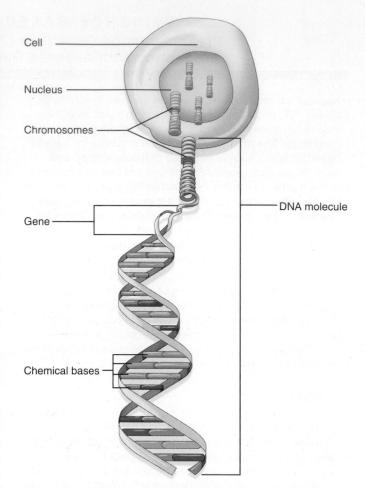

FIGURE 10.10 DNA is made up of four chemical bases. Tightly coiled strands of DNA are packaged in units called chromosomes, housed in the cell's nucleus. Working subunits of DNA are known as genes. (From the National Institute of Health and National Cancer Institute. [1995]. *Understanding gene testing* [NIH Pub. No. 96-3905]. Washington, DC: U.S. Department of Human Services.)

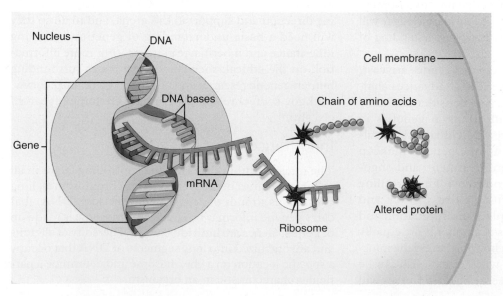

FIGURE 10.11 When a gene contains a mutation, the protein encoded by that gene will be abnormal. Some protein changes are insignificant, while others are disabling. (From the National Institutes of Health and National Cancer Institute. [1995]. *Understanding gene testing* [NIH Pub. No. 96-3905]. Washington, DC: U.S. Department of Human Services.)

comes from the mother and one from the father. These alleles may be the same for the characteristic (**homozygous**) or different (**heterozygous**). For example, WW stands for homozygous dominant; ww stands for homozygous recessive. Heterozygous would be indicated as Ww. If the two alleles differ, such as Ww, the dominant one will usually be expressed in the phenotype of the individual.

Human beings typically have 46 chromosomes. This includes 22 pairs of non-sex chromosomes or autosomes and 1 pair of sex chromosomes (two X chromosomes in females, and an X chromosome and a Y chromosome in males). Offspring receive one chromosome of each of the 23 pairs from each parent.

Regulation and expression of the thousands of human genes is very complex and is the result of many intricate interactions within each cell. Alterations in gene structure, function, transcription, translation, and protein synthesis can influence an individual's health (Wright & Hastie, 2007). Gene mutations are a permanent change in the sequence of DNA. Some mutations have no significant effect, whereas others can have a tremendous impact on the health of the individual. Several genetic disorders such as cystic fibrosis, sickle-cell disease, phenylketonuria, or hemophilia, can result from these mutations.

The pictorial analysis of the number, form, and size of an individual's chromosomes is termed the **karyotype**. This analysis commonly uses white blood cells and fetal cells in amniotic fluid. The chromosomes are numbered from the largest to the smallest, 1 to 22, and the sex chromosomes are designated by the letter X or Y. A female karyotype is designated as 46,XX and a male karyotype is designated as 46,XY. Figure 10.12 illustrates an example of a karyotyping pattern.

Patterns of Inheritance

A genetic disorder is a disease caused by an abnormality in an individual's genetic material or genome. Diagnosis of a genetic disorder is usually based on clinical signs and symptoms or on laboratory confirmation of an altered gene associated with the disorder. Accurate diagnosis can be aided by the recognition of the pattern of inheritance within a family. The pattern of inheritance is also vital to understand when teaching and counseling families about the risks in future pregnancies. Some genetic disorders occur in multiple family members, while others may occur in only a single family member. A genetic disorder is caused by completely or partially altered genetic material, while a familial disorder is more common in relatives of the affected individual but may be caused by environmental influences and not genetic alterations.

Monogenic Disorders
Patterns of inheritance demonstrate how a genetic disorder can be passed on to offspring. Principles of genetic disease

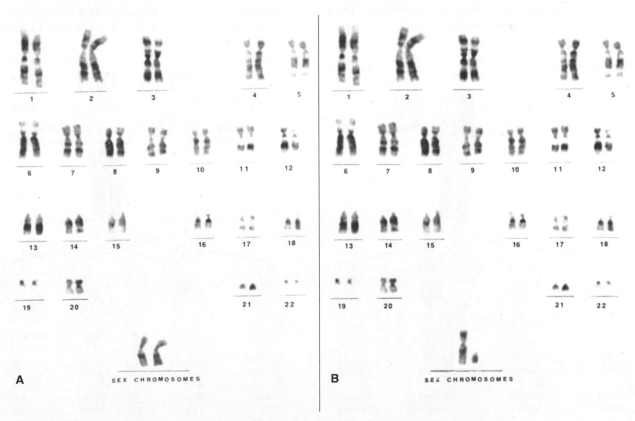

FIGURE 10.12 Karyotype pattern. (**A**) Normal female karyotype. (**B**) Normal male karyotype.

inheritance of single-gene disorders are the same principles that govern the inheritance of other traits, such as eye and hair color. These are known as Mendel's laws of inheritance, named for the genetic work of Gregor Mendel, an Austrian naturalist. These patterns occur due to a single gene being defective and are referred to as monogenic or sometimes Mendelian disorders. If the defect occurs on the autosome, the genetic disorder is termed autosomal; if the defect is on the X chromosome, the genetic disorder is termed X-linked. The defect also can be classified as dominant or recessive. Monogenic disorders include autosomal dominant, autosomal recessive, X-linked dominant, and X-linked recessive patterns.

Autosomal Dominant Inheritance Disorders

Autosomal dominant inherited disorders occur when a single gene in the heterozygous state is capable of producing the phenotype. In other words, the abnormal or mutant gene overshadows the normal gene and the individual will demonstrate signs and symptoms of the disorder. The affected person generally has an affected parent, and an affected person has a 50% chance of passing the abnormal gene to each of his or her children (Fig. 10.13). Affected individuals are present in every generation. Males and family members who are phenotypically normal (do not show signs or symptoms of the disorder) do not transmit the condition to their offspring. Females and males are equally affected and a male can pass the disorder on to his son. This male-to-male transmission is important in distinguishing autosomal dominant inheritance from X-linked inheritance. There are varying degrees of pre-

sentation among individuals in a family. Therefore, a parent with a mild form could have a child with a more severe form. Common types of genetic disorders that follow the autosomal dominant pattern of inheritance include neurofibromatosis (genetic disorders affecting the development and growth of neural cells and tissues), Huntington's disease (a genetic disorder affecting the nervous system characterized by abnormal involuntary movements and progressive dementia), achondroplasia (a genetic disorder resulting in disordered growth and abnormal body proportion), and polycystic kidney disease (a genetic disorder involving the growth of multiple, bilateral, grape-like clusters of fluid-filled cysts in the kidneys that eventually compress and replace functioning renal tissue).

Autosomal Recessive Inheritance Disorders

Autosomal recessive inherited disorders occur when two copies of the mutant or abnormal gene in the homozygous state are necessary to produce the phenotype. In other words, two abnormal genes are needed for the individual to demonstrate signs and symptoms of the disorder. These disorders are generally less common than autosomal dominant disorders (Behrman et al., 2007). Both parents of the affected person must be heterozygous carriers of the gene (clinically normal but carry the gene), and their offspring have a 25% chance of being homozygous (a 50% chance of getting the mutant gene from each parent and therefore a 25% chance of inheriting two mutant genes). If the child is clinically normal, there is a 50% chance that he or she is a carrier (Fig. 10.14). Affected individuals

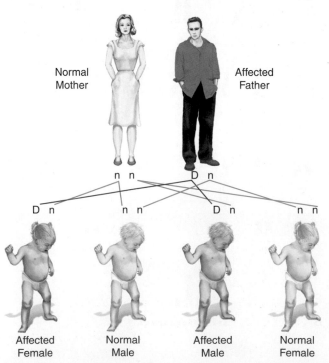

FIGURE 10.13 Autosomal dominant inheritance.

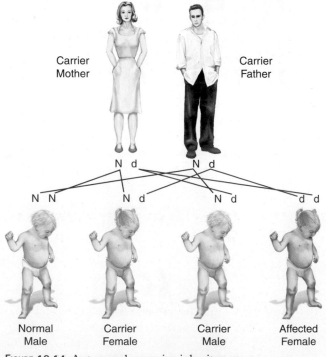

FIGURE 10.14 Autosomal recessive inheritance.

are usually present in only one generation of the family. Females and males are equally affected and a male can pass the disorder on to his son. The chance that any two parents will both be carriers of the mutant gene is increased if the couple is consanguineous (having a common ancestor). Common types of genetic disorders that follow the autosomal recessive inheritance pattern include cystic fibrosis (a genetic disorder involving generalized dysfunction of the exocrine glands), phenylketonuria (a disorder involving a deficiency in a liver enzyme that leads to the inability to process the essential amino acid phenylalanine), Tay-Sachs disease (a disorder due to insufficient activity of the enzyme hexoaminodase, which is necessary for the breakdown of certain fatty substances in the brain and nerve cells), and sickle-cell disease (a genetic disorder in which the red blood cells carry an ineffective type of hemoglobin instead of the normal adult hemoglobin).

X-linked Inheritance Disorders

X-linked inherited disorders are those associated with altered genes present on the X chromosome. They differ from autosomal disorders. If a male inherits an X-linked altered gene, he will express the condition. Since a male has only one X chromosome, all the genes on his X chromosome will be expressed (the Y chromosome carries no normal allele to compensate for the altered gene). Because females inherit two X chromosomes, they can be either heterozygous or homozygous for any allele. Therefore, X-linked disorders in females are expressed similarly to autosomal disorders.

Most X-linked disorders demonstrate a recessive pattern of inheritance. Males are more affected than females. A male has only one X chromosome and all the genes on his X chromosome will be expressed, whereas a female will usually need both X chromosomes to carry the disease. There is no male-to-male transmission (since no X chromosome from the male is transmitted to male offspring), but any man who is affected will have carrier daughters. If a woman is a carrier, there is a 50% chance that her sons will be affected and a 50% chance that her daughters will be carriers (Fig. 10.15). Common types of genetic disorders that follow X-linked recessive inheritance patterns include hemophilia (a genetic disorder involving a deficiency of one of the coagulation factors in the blood), color blindness, and Duchenne muscular dystrophy (a disorder involving progressive muscular weakness and wasting).

X-linked dominant inheritance is present if heterozygous female carriers demonstrate signs and symptoms of the disorder. All of the daughters and none of the sons of an affected male have the condition, while both male and female offspring of an affected woman have a 50% chance of inheriting and presenting with the condition (Fig. 10.16). X-linked dominant disorders are rare. The most common is hypophosphatemic (vitamin D-resistant)

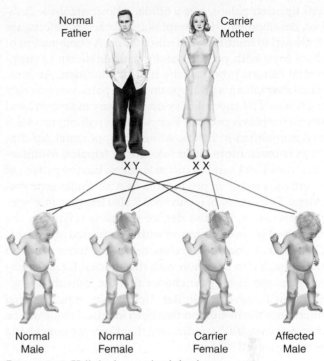

FIGURE **10.15** X-linked recessive inheritance.

rickets (a disorder involving a softening or weakening of the bones).

Multifactorial Inheritance Disorders

Multifactorial inherited disorders are thought to be caused by multiple genetic (polygenic) and environmental factors. Many of the common congenital malformations, such as

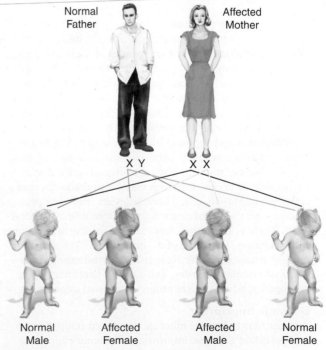

FIGURE **10.16** X-linked dominant inheritance.

cleft lip, cleft palate, spina bifida, pyloric stenosis, club-foot, developmental hip dysplasia, and cardiac defects, are attributed to multifactorial inheritance. A combination of genes from both parents, along with unknown environmental factors, produces the trait or condition. An individual may inherit a predisposition to a particular anomaly or disease. The anomalies or diseases vary in severity, and often a sex bias is present. For example, pyloric stenosis is seen more often in males, while developmental hip dysplasia is much more likely to occur in females. Multifactorial conditions tend to run in families, but the pattern of inheritance is not as predictable as with single-gene disorders. The chance of recurrence is also less than in single-gene disorders, but the degree of risk is related to the number of genes in common with the affected individual. The closer the degree of relationship, the more genes an individual has in common with the affected family member, resulting in a higher chance that the individual's off-spring will have a similar defect. In multifactorial inheritance the likelihood that both identical twins will be affected is not 100%, indicating that there are nongenetic factors involved.

Nontraditional Inheritance Patterns

Molecular studies have revealed that some genetic disorders are inherited in ways that do not follow the typical patterns of dominant, recessive, X-linked, or multifactorial inheritance. Examples of nontraditional inheritance patterns include mitochondrial inheritance and genomic imprinting (Box 10.2). As the science of molecular genetics advances and more is learned about inheritance patterns, other nontraditional patterns of inheritance may be discovered or found to be relatively common.

Chromosomal Abnormalities

In some cases of genetic disorders, the abnormality occurs due to problems with the chromosomes. Chromosomal abnormalities do not follow straightforward patterns of inheritance. Sperm and egg cells each have 23 unpaired chromosomes. When they unite during pregnancy they form a fertilized egg with 46 chromosomes. Sometimes before pregnancy begins, an error has occurred during the process of cell division, leaving an egg or sperm with too many or too few chromosomes. If this egg or sperm cell joins with a normal egg or sperm cell, the resulting embryo has a chromosomal abnormality. Chromosomal abnormalities can also occur due to an error in the structure of the chromosome. Small pieces of the chromosome may be deleted, duplicated, inverted, misplaced, or exchanged with part of another chromosome. Most chromosomal abnormalities occur due to an error in the egg or sperm. Therefore, the abnormality is present in every cell of the body. However, some abnormalities can happen after fertilization during mitotic cell division and result in **mosaicism**. Mosaicism or mosaic form refers to

---

BOX 10.2 **Nontraditional Inheritance Patterns**

Mitochondrial Inheritance
Certain diseases result from mutations in the mitochondrial DNA. Mitochondria, which are the part of the cell responsible for energy production, are inherited almost exclusively from the mother. Therefore, mitochondrial inheritance is usually passed from the mother to the offspring, regardless of the offspring's sex (differentiating mitochondrial inheritance from X-linked recessive inheritance). These mutations are often deletions and abnormalities of these disorders and are often seen in one or more specific organs, such as the brain, eye, and skeletal muscle. They are often associated with energy deficits in cells with high energy requirements, such as nerve and muscle cells. These disorders tend to be progressive, and the age of onset can vary from infancy to adulthood. There is an extreme amount of variability in symptoms within a family. Examples of disorders that follow mitochondrial inheritance include Kearns-Sayre syndrome, which is a neuromuscular disorder, and Leber's hereditary optic neuropathy, which causes progressive visual impairment.

Genomic Imprinting
Another nontraditional inheritance pattern results from a process called genomic imprinting. Genomic imprinting plays a critical role in fetal growth and development and placental functioning. In genomic imprinting, the expression of a gene is determined by its parental origin. In genomic imprinting both the maternal and paternal alleles are present, but only one is expressed; the other is inactive. Genomic imprinting does not alter the genetic sequence itself but affects the phenotype observed. In these cases the altered genes in a certain region of the genome have very different expressions depending on whether they were inherited from the mother or the father. Several human syndromes are known to be associated with defects in gene imprinting. Disorders that result from a disruption of imprinting usually involve a growth phenotype and include varying degrees of developmental problems. Common examples include Prader-Willi syndrome (a condition resulting in severe hypotonia and hyperphagia leading to obesity and mental retardation), Angelman syndrome (a neurodevelopmental disorder associated with mental retardation, jerky movements, and seizures), and Beckwith-Wiedemann syndrome (characterized by somatic overgrowth, congenital malformations, and a predisposition to embryonic neoplasia).

when the chromosomal abnormalities do not show up in every cell and only some cells or tissues carry the abnormality. In mosaic forms of the disorder, the symptoms are usually less severe than if all the cells were abnormal.

About 1 in 150 live-born infants is born with a chromosomal abnormality (March of Dimes, 2007a). These often cause major defects because they involve added or missing genes. Congenital anomalies and mental retardation are often associated with chromosomal abnormalities. These abnormalities occur on autosomal as well as sex chromosomes and can result from changes in the number of chromosomes or changes in the structure of the chromosomes.

Numerical Abnormalities

Chromosomal abnormalities of number often result due to nondisjunction, or failure of the chromosome pair to separate during cell division, meiosis, or mitosis. Few chromosomal numerical abnormalities are compatible with full-term development and most result in spontaneous abortion. One type of abnormal chromosome number is **polyploidy**. Polyploidy causes an increase in the number of haploid sets (23) of chromosomes in a cell. Triploidy refers to three whole sets of chromosomes in a single cell (in humans, a total of 69 chromosomes per cell); tetraploidy refers to four whole sets of chromosomes in a single cell (in humans, a total of 92 chromosomes per cell). Polyploidy usually results in an early spontaneous abortion and is incompatible with life.

Some numerical abnormalities do support development to term because the chromosome on which the abnormality is present carries relatively few genes (such as chromosome 13, 18, 21, or X). Two common abnormalities of chromosome number are monosomies or trisomies. In **monosomies** there is only one copy of a particular chromosome instead of the usual pair (an entire single chromosome is missing). In these cases, all fetuses spontaneously abort in early pregnancy. Survival is seen only in mosaic forms of these disorders. In **trisomies**, there are three of a particular chromosome instead of the usual two (an entire single chromosome is added). Trisomies may be present in every cell or may present in the mosaic form. The most common trisomies include trisomy 21 (Down syndrome), trisomy 18, and trisomy 13.

Trisomy 21

Down syndrome is an example of a trisomy. Individuals with Down syndrome have three copies of chromosome 21 (Fig. 10.17). Down syndrome affects 1 in 800 to 1,000 live-born babies. The risk of this and other trisomies increases with maternal age. The risk of having a baby with Down syndrome is about 1 in 1,250 for a woman at age 25, 1 in 1,000 at 30, 1 in 400 at 35, and 1 in 100 at age 40 (March of Dimes, 2007b). Individuals with Down syndrome have characteristic features that are usually identified at birth (Fig. 10.18). These common characteristics include:

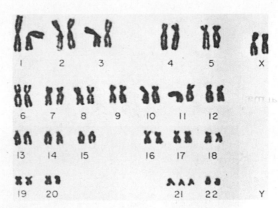

FIGURE 10.17 Karyotype of a child with Down syndrome.

- Small, low-set ears
- Hyperflexibility
- Muscle hypotonia
- Deep crease across palm (termed simian crease)
- Flat facial profile
- Small white, crescent-shaped spots on irises
- Open mouth with protruding tongue
- Broad, short fingers (Tonkin & Kirk, 2007)

The outlook for children with Down syndrome is much brighter now than it was years ago. Most children with Down syndrome have mental retardation in the mild to moderate range. With early intervention and special education, many learn to read and write, and participate in diverse childhood activities (March of Dimes, 2007b). Despite modern medical technology, the individual with Down syndrome has a shortened life span, with an average life expectancy of 55 years (March of Dimes, 2007b).

Trisomy 18 and Trisomy 13

Two other common trisomies are trisomy 18 and trisomy 13. Trisomy 18 and trisomy 13 are, respectively, the second and third most commonly diagnosed autosomal trisomies in live-born infants. These conditions are associated with a high degree of infant mortality, with most dying before their first birthday (March of Dimes, 2007a). Trisomy 18, or Edward syndrome, occurs in 1 of every 6,000 newborns (March of Dimes, 2007a), with advanced maternal age as a causative factor. Prenatally, several findings are apparent on ultrasound: intrauterine growth restriction (IUGR), hydramnios or oligohydramnios, cardiac malformations, a single umbilical artery, and decreased fetal movement. Additionally, trisomy 18 has been associated with a decrease in maternal serum levels of maternal serum alpha-fetoprotein (MSAFP) and hCG. Most affected newborns are female, with a 4:1 ratio to males. Affected newborns have 47 chromosomes (three at chromosome 18) and are characterized by severe mental retardation, growth deficiency of the cranium (microcephaly), low-set ears, small for gestational age, seizures, drooping

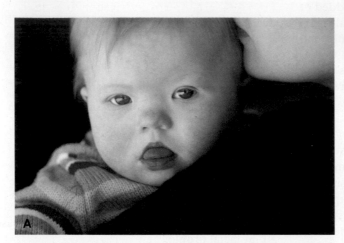

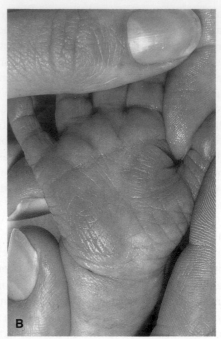

FIGURE 10.18 (A) Typical facial features of an infant with Down syndrome. (B) A simian line, a horizontal crease seen in children with Down syndrome.

eyelids, webbing of fingers, congenital heart defects, rocker-bottom feet, and severe hypotonia (National Organization for Rare Disorders, 2008). Infants with trisomy 18 have multiple anomalies that are severe, and life expectancy is greatly reduced beyond a few months.

Trisomy 13, or Patau syndrome, affects 1 of 10,000 newborns (March of Dimes, 2007a). Forty-seven chromosomes (three of chromosome 13) are present. Maternal age is also thought to be a causative factor in this genetic disorder. The common abnormalities associated with trisomy 13 are microcephaly, cardiac defects, central nervous system anomalies, cleft lip and palate, cryptorchidism, polydactyly (Fig. 10.19), severe mental retardation, severe hypotonia, and seizures. Life expectancy is only a few months for most infants with trisomy 13. Care is supportive for these infants.

Structural Abnormalities

Chromosome abnormalities of structure usually occur when there is a breakage and loss of a portion of one or

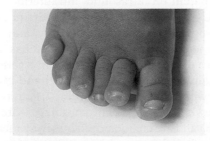

FIGURE 10.19 An infant with trisomy 13 has supernumerary digits (polydactyly).

more chromosomes, and during the repair process the broken ends are rejoined incorrectly. Structural abnormalities usually lead to having too much or too little genetic material. Altered chromosome structure can take on several forms. Deletions occur when a portion of the chromosome is missing, resulting in a loss of that chromosomal material. Duplications are seen when a portion of the chromosome is duplicated and an extra chromosomal segment is present. Clinical findings vary depending on how much chromosomal material is involved. Inversions occur when a portion of the chromosome breaks off at two points and is turned upside down and reattached; therefore, the genetic material is inverted. With inversion, there is no loss or gain of chromosomal material and carriers are phenotypically normal, but they do have an increased risk for miscarriage and chromosomally abnormal offspring. Ring chromosomes are seen when a portion of a chromosome has broken off in two places and formed a circle.

The most clinically significant structural abnormality is a translocation. This occurs when part of one chromosome is transferred to another chromosome and an abnormal rearrangement is present.

Structural abnormalities can be balanced or unbalanced. Balanced abnormalities involve the rearrangement of genetic material with neither an overall gain nor loss. Individuals who inherit a balanced structural abnormality are usually phenotypically normal but are at a higher risk for miscarriages and having chromosomally abnormal offspring. Examples of structural rearrangements that can be balanced include inversions, translocation, and ring chromosomes. Unbalanced structural abnormalities are similar to numerical abnormalities because genetic material is either gained or lost. Unbalanced structural abnormalities can encompass several genes and result in severe clinical consequences.

Cri du Chat Syndrome

Cri du chat syndrome ("cry of the cat") is caused by a missing piece of chromosome 5. It was named "cri du chat" based on the distinctive cry in newborns, which is due to a laryngeal defect. The incidence of the disorder is thought to be approximately 1 in 50,000 live births (Chen, 2007a). In addition to the cat-like, high-pitched cry in infancy, it is also associated with severe mental retardation, microcephaly, low birthweight and slow growth, hypotonia, failure to thrive, wide-set eyes, small jaw, low-set ears, and various organ malformations. No specific treatment is available for this syndrome. With contemporary interventions, the child may survive to adulthood: 75% of deaths occur during the first several months of life and almost 90% occur in the first year. Death occurs in 6% to 8% of the overall population affected with the syndrome. Pneumonia, aspiration pneumonia, congenital heart defects, and respiratory distress are the common causes of death (Chen, 2007a). Parents should be referred for genetic counseling.

Fragile X Syndrome

Fragile X syndrome, also termed Martin–Bell syndrome, is a structural abnormality involving the X chromosome, which demonstrates breaks and gaps. The syndrome is usually diagnosed by molecular DNA studies. Conservative estimates report that fragile X syndrome affects approximately 1 in 4,000 males and 1 in 8,000 females (Jewell, 2007). Typically, a female becomes the carrier and will be mildly affected. The male who receives the X chromosome that has a fragile site will exhibit the full effects of the syndrome. Fragile X syndrome is characterized by mental retardation, hyperactivity, short attention span, hand flapping, strabismus, hypotonia, speech delay, inflexible behavior, autistic-like behavior, poor eye contact, tactile defensiveness, double-jointedness, and perseverative speech (continued repetition of words or phrases). It is the most common form of male retardation (Jewell, 2007). Aside from the morbidity associated with mental retardation and cognitive/behavioral/neuropsychological problems, the life span of an individual with fragile X syndrome is unaffected. There is no cure for this disorder. Speech, occupational, and physical therapy services usually are needed, as well as special education and counseling.

Sex Chromosome Abnormalities

Chromosomal abnormalities can also involve sex chromosomes. These cases are usually less severe in their clinical effects than autosomal chromosomal abnormalities. Sex chromosome abnormalities are gender-specific and involve a missing or extra sex chromosome. They affect sexual development and may cause infertility, growth abnormalities, and possibly behavioral and learning problems. Many affected individuals lead essentially normal lives. Examples are Turner syndrome (in females) and Klinefelter's syndrome (in males).

Turner Syndrome

Turner syndrome is a common abnormality of the sex chromosome in which a portion or all of the X chromosome is missing. It affects about 1 in 2,500 newborn girls (March of Dimes, 2007a). Clinical manifestations include a low posterior hairline and webbing of the neck, short stature, broad skeletal abnormalities, a shield-like chest with widely spaced nipples, puffy feet, underdeveloped secondary sex characteristics, and infertility (Postellon, 2007). Only about a third of cases are diagnosed as newborns; the remaining two thirds are diagnosed in early adolescence when they experience primary amenorrhea. No cure exists for this syndrome. Growth hormone typically is given; hormone replacement therapy also may be used to induce puberty and stimulate continued growth. Most females with Turner syndrome are of normal intelligence and usually live essentially normal lives (Postellon, 2007).

Klinefelter Syndrome

Klinefelter syndrome is a sex chromosomal abnormality that occurs only in males. About 1 in 500 to 1,000 males born have Klinefelter syndrome (Chen, 2007b). There is an extra X chromosome (XXY) present. The extra genetic material causes abnormal development of the testicles, resulting in decreased production of sperm and male sex hormones. Clinical manifestations may include:

- Mild mental retardation
- Small testicles
- Infertility
- Long arms and legs
- Enlarged breast tissue (gynecomastia)
- Scant facial and body hair
- Decreased sex drive (libido) (Chen, 2007b)

No treatment can correct this genetic abnormality, but testosterone replacement therapy can improve symptoms resulting from the deficiency. Surgery may be done to reduce gynecomastia. Most males with Klinefelter syndrome (XXY) are diagnosed in late puberty. Infertility is common and life expectancy is normal (Chen, 2007b).

Genetic Evaluation and Counseling

Genetic counseling has been defined as an educational process that assists affected and/or at-risk individuals to understand genetic disorders, their transmission, and the options available to them in management and family planning (Behrman et al., 2007). There are a variety of reasons an individual should be referred for genetic counseling. Box 10.3 lists those who may benefit from genetic counseling. In many cases, geneticists and genetic counselors provide information to families regarding genetic diseases.

BOX 10.3 Those Who May Benefit From Genetic Counseling

- Maternal age 35 years or older when the baby is born
- Paternal age 50 years or older
- Previous child, parents, or close relatives with an inherited disease, congenital anomalies, metabolic disorders, developmental disorders, or chromosomal abnormalities
- Consanguinity or incest
- Pregnancy screening abnormality, including alpha-fetoprotein, triple screen, amniocentesis, or ultrasound
- Stillborn with congenital anomalies
- Two or more pregnancy losses
- Teratogen exposure or risk
- Concerns about genetic defects that occur frequently in their ethnic or racial group (for instance, those of African descent are most at risk for having a child with sickle-cell anemia)
- Abnormal newborn screening
- Child born with one or more major malformations in a major organ system
- Child with abnormalities of growth
- Child with developmental delay, mental retardation, blindness, or deafness

However, an experienced family physician, pediatrician, or nurse who has received special training in genetics may also provide the information.

A genetic consultation involves evaluation of an individual or a family. Its purposes are to confirm, diagnose, or rule out genetic conditions; to identify medical management issues; to calculate and communicate genetic risks to a family; to discuss ethical and legal issues; and to provide and arrange psychosocial support. Genetic counselors serve as educators and resource persons for other health care providers and the general public.

The ideal time for genetic counseling is before conception. Preconception counseling gives couples the chance to identify and reduce potential pregnancy risks, plan for known risks, and establish early prenatal care. Unfortunately, many women delay seeking prenatal care until their second or third trimester, after the crucial time of organogenesis. Therefore, it is important that preconception counseling is offered to all women as they seek health care throughout their childbearing years, especially if they are contemplating pregnancy. This requires health care providers to take a proactive role.

Preconception screening and counseling can raise serious ethical and moral issues for a couple. The results of prenatal genetic testing can lead to the decision to terminate a pregnancy, even if the results are not conclusive but indicate a strong possibility that the child will have an abnormality. The severity of the abnormality may not be known, and some may find the decision to terminate unethical. Another difficult situation that provides an example of the ethical and moral issues surrounding genetic screening and counseling involves disorders that affect only one gender of offspring. A mother may find she is a carrier of a gene for a disorder for which there is no prenatal screening test available. In these cases the couple may decide to terminate any pregnancy where the fetus is the affected sex, even though there is a 50% chance that the child will not inherit the disorder. In these situations, the choice is the couple's and information and support must be provided in a nondirective manner.

Genetic counseling is particularly important if a congenital anomaly or genetic disease has been diagnosed prenatally or if a child is born with a life-threatening congenital anomaly or genetic disease. In these cases families need information urgently so they can make immediate decisions. If a diagnosis with genetic implications is made later in life, if a couple with a family history of a genetic disorder or a previous child with a genetic disorder is planning a family, or if there is suspected teratogen exposure, urgency of information is not such an issue. In these situations, the family needs time to ponder all their options. This may involve several meetings over a longer period of time.

Genetic counseling involves gathering information regarding birth history, past medical history, and current health status as well as a family history of congenital anomalies, mental retardation, genetic diseases, reproductive history, general health, and causes of death. A detailed family history is imperative and in most cases will include the development of a pedigree, which is like a family tree (Fig. 10.20). Information is ideally gathered on three generations, but if the family history is complicated, informa-

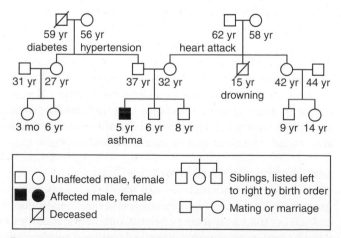

FIGURE 10.20 A pedigree is a diagram made using symbols that demonstrates the links between family members and focuses on medical and health information for each relative.

tion from more distant relatives may be needed. Families receiving genetic counseling may benefit from being told in advance that this information will be necessary; they may need to discuss these sensitive, private issues with family members to obtain the needed facts. When necessary, medical records may be requested for family members, especially those who have a genetic disorder, to help ensure accuracy of the information. Sometimes a pedigree may reveal confidential information not known by all family members, such as an adoption, a child conceived through in vitro fertilization, or a husband not being the father of a baby. Therefore, maintaining confidentiality is extremely important. After careful analysis of the data obtained, referral to a genetic counselor when indicated is appropriate.

Medical genetic knowledge has increased dramatically over the past few decades. Not only is it possible to detect specific diseases with genetic mutations, but it is also possible to test for a genetic predisposition to various diseases or conditions and certain physical characteristics. This leads to complex ethical, moral, and social issues. Maintaining client privacy and confidentiality and administering care in a nondiscriminatory manner are essential while maintaining sensitivity to cultural differences. It is essential to respect client autonomy and present information in a nondirective manner.

Nursing Roles and Responsibilities

The nurse is likely to interact with the client in a variety of ways related to genetics—taking a family history, scheduling genetic testing, explaining the purposes of all screening and diagnostic tests, answering questions, and addressing concerns raised by family members. Nurses are often the first health care providers to encounter women with preconception and prenatal issues. Nurses play an important role in beginning the preconception counseling process and referring women and their partners for further genetic testing when indicated.

An accurate and thorough family history is an essential part of preconception counseling. Nurses in any practice setting can obtain a patient's history during the initial encounter. The purpose is to gather patient and family information that may provide clues as to whether the patient has a genetic trait, inherited condition, or inherited predisposition (Erlen, 2006). At a basic level, all nurses should be able to take a family medical history to help identify those at risk for genetic conditions, and then initiate a referral when appropriate. Box 10.4 presents examples of focused assessment questions that can be used. Based on the information gathered during the history, the nurse must decide whether a referral to a genetic specialist is necessary or whether further evaluation is needed. Prenatal testing to assess for genetic risks and defects might be used to identify genetic disorders. These tests are described in Common Laboratory and Diagnostic Tests 10.1.

BOX 10.4 **Focused Health Assessment: Genetic History**

What was the cause and age of death for deceased family members?

Does any consanguinity exist between relatives?

Do any serious illnesses or chronic conditions exist? If so, what was the age of onset?

Do any female family members have a history of miscarriages, stillbirths, or diabetes?

Do any female members have a history of alcohol or drug use during pregnancy?

What were the ages of female members during childbearing, especially if older than 35?

Do any family members have mental retardation or developmental delays?

Do any family members have a known or suspected metabolic disorder such as PKU?

Do any family members have an affective disorder such as bipolar disorder?

Have any close relatives been diagnosed with any type of cancer?

What is your ethnic background (explore as related to certain disorders)?

Do any family members have a known or suspected chromosomal disorder?

Do any family members have a progressive neurologic disorder?

Source: Bradley et al., 2007.

Remember Robert and Kate Shafer? Based on the information gathered from their genetic history, they were referred to a genetic specialist. What prenatal tests might be ordered to assess their risk for genetic disorders? What would be the nurse's role related to genetic counseling?

Nurses working with families involved with genetic counseling typically have certain responsibilities. These include:

• Using interviewing and active listening skills to identify genetic concerns
• Knowing basic genetic terminology and inheritance patterns
• Explaining basic concepts of probability and disorder susceptibility
• Safeguarding the privacy and confidentiality of patients' genetic information
• Providing complete informed consent to facilitate decisions about genetic testing
• Discussing costs of genetic services and the benefits and risks of using health insurance to pay for genetic services, including potential risks of discrimination

COMMON LABORATORY AND DIAGNOSTIC TESTS 10.1 PRENATAL TESTS TO ASSESS RISK FOR GENETIC DISORDERS

Test	Description	Indication	Timing
Alpha-fetoprotein	A sample of the woman's blood is drawn to evaluate plasma protein that is produced by the fetal liver, yolk sac, and GI tract, and crosses from the amniotic fluid into the maternal blood.	Increased levels might indicate a neural tube defect, Turner syndrome, tetralogy of Fallot, multiple gestation, omphalocele, gastroschisis, or hydrocephaly. Decreased levels might indicate Down syndrome or trisomy 18.	Typically performed between 15 and 18 weeks' gestation
Amniocentesis	Amniotic fluid aspirated from the amniotic sac; safety concerns include infection, pregnancy loss, and fetal needle injuries	To perform chromosome analysis, alpha-fetoprotein, DNA markers, viral studies, karyotyping; and identify inborn errors of metabolism	Usually performed between 15 and 20 weeks' gestation to allow for adequate amniotic fluid volume to accumulate; results take 2 to 4 weeks
Chorionic villus sampling	Removal of small tissue specimen from the fetal portion of the placenta, which reflects the fetal genetic makeup; main complications include severe transverse limb defects and spontaneous pregnancy loss	To detect fetal karyotype, sickle-cell anemia, phenylketonuria, Down syndrome, Duchenne muscular dystrophy, and numerous other genetic disorders	Typically performed between 10 and 12 weeks' gestation, with results available in less than a week
Percutaneous umbilical blood sampling	Insertion of a needle directly into a fetal umbilical vessel under ultrasound guidance; two potential complications: fetal hemorrhage and risk of infection	Used for prenatal diagnosis of inherited blood disorders such as hemophilia A, karyotyping, detection of fetal infection, determination of acid–base status, and assessment and treatment of isoimmunization	Generally performed after 16 weeks' gestation
Fetal nuchal translucency (FNT)	An intravaginal ultrasound that measures fluid collection in the subcutaneous space between the skin and the cervical spine of the fetus	To identify fetal anomalies; abnormal fluid collection can be associated with genetic disorders (trisomies 13, 18, and 21), Turner syndrome, cardiac deformities, and/or physical anomalies. When the FNT is greater than 2.5 mm, the measurement is considered abnormal.	Performed between 10 and 14 weeks' gestation
Level II ultrasound/ fetal scan	Use of high-frequency sound waves to visualize the fetus	Enables early evaluation of structural changes	Typically performed after 18 weeks' gestation
Triple marker test	Serum screening test using the levels of three maternal serum markers—MSAFP, unconjugated estriol, and hCG—in combination with maternal age to calculate risk	To identify risk for Down syndrome, neural tube defects, and other chromosomal disorders. Elevated hCG combined with lower-than-normal estriol and MSAFP levels indicate increased risk for Down syndrome or other trisomy condition.	Performed between 16 and 18 weeks' gestation

Sources: Sahin & Gungor, 2008; Boyd et al., 2008; Cowan, 2008; Wynbrandt & Ludman, 2008.

- Recognizing and defining ethical, legal, and social issues
- Providing accurate information about the risks and benefits of genetic testing
- Using culturally appropriate methods to convey genetic information
- Monitoring patients' emotional reactions after receiving genetic analysis
- Providing information on appropriate local support groups
- Knowing their own limitations and making appropriate referrals (Jenkins & Calzone, 2007)

Talking with families who have recently been diagnosed with a genetic disorder or who have had a child born with congenital anomalies is very difficult. Many times the nurse may be the one who has first contact with these parents and will be the one to provide follow-up care.

Genetic disorders are significant, life-changing, and possibly life-threatening situations. The information is highly technical and the field is undergoing significant technologic advances. Nurses need an understanding of who will benefit from genetic counseling and must be able to discuss the role of the genetic counselor with families. The goal is to ensure that families at risk are aware that genetic counseling is available before they attempt to have another baby.

*B**ased on the results of their genetic tests, Robert and Kate are placed at moderate risk for having an infant with an autosomal recessive genetic disorder. The couple asks the nurse what all of this means. What information should the nurse provide about concepts of probability and disorder susceptibility for this couple? How can the nurse help this couple to make knowledgeable decisions concerning their reproductive future?*

Nurses play an essential role in providing emotional support to the family through this challenging time. This is especially important with follow-up counseling after the couple or family has been to the genetic specialist.

▶ *Take* NOTE!

Nurses need to be actively engaged with patients and their families and help them consider the facts, values, and context in which they are making decisions. Nurses need to be open and honest with families as they discuss these sensitive and emotional choices.

The nurse is in an ideal position to help families review what has been discussed during the genetic counseling sessions and to answer any additional questions they might have. Referral to appropriate agencies, support groups, and resources, such as a social worker, a chaplain, or an ethicist, is another key role when caring for families with suspected or diagnosed genetic disorders.

▶ *Consider* THIS!

As I waited for the genetic counselor to come into the room, my mind was filled with numerous fears and questions. What does an inconclusive amniocentesis really mean? What if this pregnancy produced an abnormal baby? How would I cope with a special child in my life? If only I had gone to the midwife sooner when I thought I was pregnant, but still in denial. Why did I wait so long to admit this pregnancy and get prenatal care? If only I had started to take my folic acid pills when prescribed. Why didn't I research my family's history to know of any hidden genetic conditions? What about my sister with a Down syndrome child? What must I have been thinking? I guess I could play the "what-if" game forever and never come up with answers. It was too late to do anything about this pregnancy because I was in my last trimester. I started to pray silently when the counselor opened the door. . . .

Thoughts: This woman is reviewing the last several months, looking for answers to her greatest fears. Inconclusive screenings can introduce emotional torment for many women as they wait for validating results. Are these common thoughts and fears for many women facing potential genetic disorders? What supportive interventions might the nurse offer?

■■■ Key Concepts

- Fertilization, which takes place in the outer third of the ampulla of the fallopian tube, leads to the formation of a zygote. The zygote undergoes cleavage, eventually implanting in the endometrium about 7 to 10 days after conception.
- Three embryonic layers of cells are formed: ectoderm, which forms the central nervous system, special senses, skin, and glands; mesoderm, which forms the skeletal, urinary, circulatory, and reproductive systems; and endoderm, which forms the respiratory system, liver, pancreas, and digestive system.
- Amniotic fluid surrounds the embryo and increases in volume as the pregnancy progresses, reaching approximately a liter by term.
- At no time during pregnancy is there any direct connection between the blood of the fetus and the blood of the mother, so there is no mixing of blood. A specialized connective tissue known as Wharton's jelly surrounds the three blood vessels in the umbilical cord to prevent compression, which would choke off the blood supply and nutrients to the growing life inside.

■ The placenta protects the fetus from immune attack by the mother, removes waste products from the fetus, induces the mother to bring more food to the placenta, and, near the time of delivery, produces hormones that mature fetal organs in preparation for life outside the uterus.

■ The purpose of fetal circulation is to carry highly oxygenated blood to vital areas (heart and brain) while first shunting it away from less vital ones (lungs and liver).

■ Humans have 46 paired chromosomes that are found in all cells of the body, except the ovum and sperm cells, which have just 23 chromosomes. Each person has a unique genetic constitution, or genotype.

■ Research from the Human Genome Project has provided a better understanding of the genetic contribution to disease.

■ Genetic disorders can result from abnormalities in patterns of inheritance or chromosomal abnormalities involving chromosomal number or structure.

■ Autosomal dominant inheritance occurs when a single gene in the heterozygous state is capable of producing the phenotype. Autosomal recessive inheritance occurs when two copies of the mutant or abnormal gene in the homozygous state are necessary to produce the phenotype. X-linked inheritance disorders are those associated with altered genes present on the X chromosome. They can be dominant or recessive. Multifactorial inheritance is thought to be caused by multiple gene and environmental factors.

■ In some cases of genetic disorders, a chromosomal abnormality occurs. Chromosomal abnormalities do not follow straightforward patterns of inheritance. These abnormalities occur on autosomal as well as sex chromosomes and can result from changes in the number of chromosomes or changes in the structure of the chromosomes.

■ Genetic counseling involves evaluation of an individual or a family. Its purpose is to confirm, diagnose, or rule out genetic conditions, identify medical management issues, calculate and communicate genetic risks to a family, discuss ethical and legal issues, and assist in providing and arranging psychosocial support.

■ Legal, ethical, and social issues that can arise related to genetic testing include the privacy and confidentiality of genetic information, who should have access to personal genetic information, psychological impact and stigmatization due to individual genetic differences, use of genetic information in reproductive decision making and reproductive rights, and whether testing be performed if no cure is available.

■ Preconception screening and counseling can raise serious ethical and moral issues for a couple. The results of prenatal genetic testing can lead to the decision to terminate a pregnancy.

■ Nurses play an important role in beginning the preconception counseling process and referring women and their partners for further genetic information when indicated. Many times the nurse is the one who has first contact with these women and will be the one to provide follow-up care.

■ Nurses need to have a solid understanding of who will benefit from genetic counseling and must be able to discuss the role of the genetic counselor with families, ensuring that families at risk are aware that genetic counseling is available before they attempt to have another baby.

■ Nurses play an essential role in providing emotional support and referrals to appropriate agencies, support groups, and resources when caring for families with suspected or diagnosed genetic disorders. Nurses can assist patients with their decision making by referring them to a social worker, a chaplain, or an ethicist.

REFERENCES

Alvero, R., & Schlaff, W. D. (2006). *Reproductive endocrinology and infertility: The requisites in obstetrics and gynecology.* St. Louis: Mosby.

Behrman, R. E., Kliegman, R. M., & Jenson, H. B. (2007). *Nelson's textbook of pediatrics* (18th ed.). Philadelphia: Elsevier Health Sciences.

Blackburn, S. T. (2007). *Maternal, fetal and neonatal physiology* (3rd ed.). Philadelphia: Saunders.

Boyd, P., DeVigan C., Khoshnood, B., Loane, M., Garne, E., & Dolk, H. (2008). Survey of prenatal screening policies in Europe for structural malformations and chromosome anomilies, and their impact on detection and termination rates for neural tube defects and Down's Syndrome. *BJOG: An International Journal of Obstetrics & Gynecology, 115*(6), 689–696.

Bradley, L., Kloza, E., Haddow, P., Beauregard, L., Johnson J., & Haddow, J. (2007). A genetic history questionnaire-based system in primary prenatal care to screen for selected fetal disorders. *Genetic Testing, 11*(3), 291–295.

Brooks, M. L. (2008). *Exploring medical language.* St. Louis: Mosby.

Centers for Disease Control and Prevention (CDC). (2007). *Frequently asked questions about birth defects.* Available at: http://www.cdc.gov/ncbddd/bd/faq1.htm#Whatisabirthdefect.

Chen, H. (2007a). Cri du chat syndrome. *eMedicine.* Available at: http://www.emedicine.com/ped/TOPIC504.HTM.

Chen, H. (2007b). Klinefelter syndrome. *eMedicine.* Available at: http://www.emedicine.com/ped/TOPIC1252.HTM.

Cowan, R. S. (2008). *Heredity and hope: The case for genetic screening.* Cambridge, MA: Harvard University Press.

Creatsas, G., Chrousos, G. P., & Mastorakos, G. (2007). *Women's health and disease: Gynecologic and reproductive issues.* Malden, MA: Blackwell Publishers.

Dillon, P. M. (2007). *Nursing health assessment: A critical thinking, case studies approach* (2nd ed.). Philadelphia: F. A. Davis.

Dolan, S., Biermann, J., & Damus, K. (2007). Genomics for health in preconception and prenatal periods. *Journal of Nursing Scholarship, 39*(1), 4–9.

Erlen, J. A. (2006). Genetic testing and counseling: Selected ethical issues. *Orthopedic Nursing, 25*(6), 423–427.

Gilbert, E. S. (2007). *Manual of high-risk pregnancy and delivery* (4th ed.). St. Louis: Mosby.

Human Genome Management Information System. (2006). *Human Genome Project information.* Available at: http://www.ornl.gov/sci/techresources/Human_Genome/home.shtml#index.

International Human Genome Sequencing Consortium. (2007). *NIH launches Human Microbiome Project.* Available at: http://www.genome.gov/26524200

Jenkins, J., & Calzone, K. A. (2007). Establishing the essential nursing competencies for genetics and genomics. *Journal of Nursing Scholarship, 39*(1), 10–16.

Jewell, J. (2007). Fragile X syndrome. *eMedicine.* Available at: http://www.emedicine.com/ped/TOPIC800.HTM.

Johnson, M. H. (2007). *Essential reproduction* (6th ed.). Malden, MA: Blackwell Publishers.

March of Dimes. (2007a). *Quick reference and fact sheets: Chromosomal abnormalities.* Retrieved on March 12, 2008, from http://search.marchofdimes.com/cgi-bin/MsmGo.exe?grab_id= 3&page_id=14876672&query=down+syndrome&hiword=DOW NER+DOWNERS+DOWNI+DOWNIE+DOWNING+DOWN S+SYNDROM+SYNDROMES+down+syndrome+.

March of Dimes. (2007b). *Quick reference and fact sheets: Down syndrome.* Retrieved on March 12, 2008, from http://search. marchofdimes.com/cgi-bin/MsmGo.exe?grab_id=3&page_id= 15204352&query=Down+syndrome+and+life+expectancy&hiword= DOWNER+DOWNERS+DOWNI+DOWNIE+DOWNING+ DOWNS+Down+EXPECTANT+LIFES+SYNDROM+ SYNDROMES+and+expectancy+life+syndrome+.

March of Dimes. (2007c). *Recommended newborn screening tests: 29 disorders.* Retrieved April 23, 2007, from http://www. marchofdimes.com/professionals/14332_15455.asp.

Muzny, D., Scherer, S., Kaul, R., Wang, J., Yu, J., Sudbrak, R., et al. (2006). The DNA sequence, annotation and analysis of human chromosomes. *Nature, 440*(7088), 1194–1198.

National Organization for Rare Disorders (NORD). (2008). Trisomy 18 syndrome. Retrieved on March 12, 2008, from http://www.rarediseases.org/search/rdbdetail_abstract.html? disname=Trisomy%2018%20Syndrome.

Sahin, N., & Gungor, I. (2008). Congenital anomalies: Parents' anxiety and women's concerns before prenatal testing and women's opinions toward the risk factors. *Journal of Clinical Nirsing, 17*(6), 827–836.

Newman, C. M., & Bettinger, T. (2007). Gene therapy progress and prospects. *Gene Therapy, 14*(6), 465–475.

Postellon, D. (2007). Turner syndrome. *eMedicine.* Available at http://www.emedicine.com/ped/TOPIC2330.HTM.

Tonkin, E., & Kirk, M. (2007). Genetics: Your nursing role. *Primary Health Care, 17*(8), 15–18.

Twisk, M., Mastenbroek, S., van Wely, M., Heineman, M. J., Van der Veen, F., & Repping, S. (2006). Preimplantation genetic screening for abnormal number of chromosomes (aneuploidies) in in vitro fertilization or intracytoplasmic sperm injection. *Cochrane Database of Systematic Reviews,* Issue 1. Art. No.: CD005291.DOI:10.1002/ 14651858.CD005291.pub2.

Wright, A., & Hastie, N. (2007). *Genes and common diseases.* New York: Cambridge University Press.

Wynbrandt, J., & Ludman, M. (2008). *Encyclopedia of genetic disorders and birth defects* (3rd ed.). New York: Facts on File, Inc.

WEBSITES

American Society of Human Genetics: www.faseb.org/genetics/ashg/ ashgmenu.htm

CDC, Office of Genetics: www.cdc.gov/genetics/activities/ogdp.htm

Gene Clinics: www.geneclinics.org

Gene Tests: www.genetests.org

Genetic Alliance: www.geneticalliance.org

Human Genome Project of the U.S. Department of Energy: www.ornl.gov/hgmis

International Society of Nurses in Genetics: www.nursing.creighton.edu/isong

March of Dimes: www.marchofdimes.com

National Coalition for Health Professional Education in Genetics: www.nchpeg.org

National Human Genome Research Institute: www.nhgri.gov

Virtual Library on Genetics: www.ornl.gov/TechResources/ Human_Genome/genetics.html

Visible Embryo: www.visembryo.ucsf.edu

CHAPTER WORKSHEET

MULTIPLE CHOICE QUESTIONS

1. After teaching a group of students about fertilization, the instructor determines that the teaching was successful when the group identifies which as the usual site of fertilization?

   a. Fundus of the uterus

   b. Endometrium of the uterus

   c. Upper portion of fallopian tube

   d. Follicular tissue of the ovary

2. A client comes to the clinic for pregnancy testing. The nurse explains that the test detects the presence of which hormone?

   a. hPL

   b. hCG

   c. FSH

   d. TSH

3. The nurse is counseling a couple, one of whom is affected by an autosomal dominant disorder. They express concerns about the risk of transmitting the disorder. What is the best response by the nurse regarding the risk that their baby may have the disease?

   a. "You have a one in four (25%) chance."

   b. "The risk is 12.5%, or a one in eight chance."

   c. "The chance is 100%."

   d. "Your risk is 50%, or a one in two chance."

4. What is the first step in determining a couple's risk for a genetic disorder?

   a. Observing the patient and family over time

   b. Conducting extensive psychological testing

   c. Obtaining a thorough family health history

   d. Completing an extensive exclusionary list

5. A nurse is working in a women's health clinic. Genetic counseling would be most appropriate for the woman who:

   a. Just had her first miscarriage at 10 weeks

   b. Is 30 years old and planning to conceive

   c. Has a history that reveals a close relative with Down syndrome

   d. Is 18 weeks pregnant with a normal triple screen result

CRITICAL THINKING EXERCISE

1. Mr. and Mrs. Martin wish to start a family, but they can't agree on something important: Mr. Martin wants his wife to be tested for cystic fibrosis (CF) to see if she is a carrier. Mr. Martin had a brother with CF and watched his parents struggle with the hardship and the expense of caring for him for years, and he doesn't want to experience it in his own life. Mr. Martin has found out he is a CF carrier. Mrs. Martin doesn't want to have the test because she figures that once a baby is in their arms, they will be glad, no matter what.

   a. What information/education should this couple consider before deciding whether to have the test?

   b. How can you assist this couple in their decision-making process?

   c. What is your role in this situation if you don't agree with their decision?

STUDY ACTIVITIES

1. Obtain the video "Miracle of Life," which shows conception and fetal development. What are your impressions? Is the title of this video realistic?

2. Select one of the websites listed above to explore the topic of genetics. Critique the information presented. Was it understandable to a layperson? What specifically did you learn? Share your findings with your classmates during a discussion group.

3. Draw your own family pedigree, identifying inheritance patterns. Share it with your family to validate its accuracy. What did you discover about your family's past health?

4. Select one of the various prenatal screening tests (alpha-fetoprotein, amniocentesis, chorionic villus sampling, or fetal nuchal translucency) and research it in depth. Role-play with another nursing student how you would explain its purpose, the procedure, and potential findings to an expectant couple at risk for a fetal abnormality.

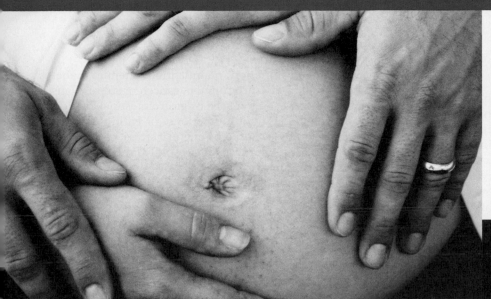

CHAPTER 11

MATERNAL ADAPTATION DURING PREGNANCY

KEY TERMS

ballottement
Braxton Hicks contractions
Chadwick's sign
dietary reference intakes (DRIs)

Goodell's sign
Hegar's sign
linea nigra
physiologic anemia of pregnancy

pica
quickening
trimester

LEARNING OBJECTIVES

Upon completion of the chapter, the learner will be able to:

1. Define the key terms used in this chapter.
2. Differentiate between subjective (presumptive), objective (probable), and diagnostic (positive) signs of pregnancy.
3. Explain maternal physiologic changes that occur during pregnancy.
4. Summarize the nutritional needs of the pregnant woman and her fetus.
5. Identify the emotional and psychological changes that occur during pregnancy.

M arva, age 17, appeared at the health department clinic complaining that she had a stomach virus and needed to be seen today. When the nurse asked her additional questions about her illness, Marva reported that she had been sick to her stomach and "beat tired" for days. She had stopped eating to avoid any more nausea and vomiting.

Wow

When a woman discovers that she is pregnant, she must remember to protect and nourish the fetus by making wise choices.

Pregnancy is a normal life event that involves considerable physical and psychological adjustments for the mother. A pregnancy is divided into three **trimesters** of 13 weeks each (Arenson & Drake, 2007). Within each trimester, numerous adaptations take place that facilitate the growth of the fetus. The most obvious are physical changes to accommodate the growing fetus. However, pregnant women also undergo psychological changes as they prepare for parenthood.

Signs and Symptoms of Pregnancy

Traditionally, signs and symptoms of pregnancy have been grouped into the following categories: presumptive, probable, and positive (Box 11.1). The only signs that can determine a pregnancy with 100% accuracy are positive signs.

What additional information is necessary to complete the assessment of Marva, the 17-year-old with nausea and vomiting? What diagnostic tests might be done to confirm the nurse's suspicion that she is pregnant?

Subjective (Presumptive) Signs

Presumptive signs are those signs experienced by the woman herself. The most obvious presumptive sign of pregnancy is the absence of menstruation. Skipping a period is not a reliable sign of pregnancy by itself, but if it is accompanied by consistent nausea, fatigue, breast tenderness, and urinary frequency, pregnancy would seem very likely.

Presumptive changes are the least reliable indicators of pregnancy because any one of them can be caused by conditions other than pregnancy (Walsh, 2007). For example, amenorrhea can be caused by early menopause,

endocrine dysfunction, malnutrition, anemia, diabetes mellitus, long-distance running, cancer, or stress. Nausea and vomiting can be caused by gastrointestinal disorders, food poisoning, acute infections, or eating disorders. Fatigue could be caused by anemia, stress, or viral infections. Breast tenderness may result from chronic cystic mastitis, premenstrual changes, or the use of oral contraceptives. Urinary frequency could have a variety of causes other than pregnancy, such as infection, cystocele, structural disorders, pelvic tumors, or emotional tension (Frieden & Chan, 2007).

▶ **Consider** THIS!

Jim and I decided to start our family, so I stopped taking the Pill 3 months ago. One morning when I got out of bed to take the dog out, I felt queasy and light-headed. I sure hoped I wasn't coming down with the flu. By the end of the week, I was feeling really tired and started taking naps in the afternoon. In addition, I seemed to be going to the bathroom frequently, despite not drinking much fluid. When my breasts started to tingle and ache, I decided to make an appointment with my doctor to see what "illness" I had contracted.

After listening to my list of physical complaints, the office nurse asked me if I might be pregnant. My eyes opened wide: I had somehow missed the link between my symptoms and pregnancy. I started to think about when my last period was, and it had been 2 months ago. The office ran a pregnancy test and much to my surprise it was positive!

Thoughts: Many women stop contraceptives in an attempt to achieve pregnancy but miss the early signs

(continued)

BOX 11.1 **Signs and Symptoms of Pregnancy**

Presumptive (Time of Occurrence)	Probable (Time of Occurrence)	Positive (Time of Occurrence)
Fatigue (12 wk)	Braxton Hicks contractions (16–28 wk)	Ultrasound verification of embryo or fetus (4–6 wk)
Breast tenderness (3–4 wk)	Positive pregnancy test (4–12 wk)	Fetal movement felt by experienced clinician (20 wk)
Nausea and vomiting (4–14 wk)	Abdominal enlargement (14 wk)	Auscultation of fetal heart tones via Doppler (10–12 wk)
Amenorrhea (4 wk)	Ballottement (16–28 wk)	
Urinary frequency (6–12 wk)	Goodell's sign (5 wk)	
Hyperpigmentation of the skin (16 wk)	Chadwick's sign (6–8 wk)	
Fetal movements (quickening; 16–20 wk)	Hegar's sign (6–12 wk)	
Uterine enlargement (7–12 wk)		
Breast enlargement (6 wk)		

Sources: Blackburn, 2007; Frieden and Chan, 2007; Torgersen and Curran 2006.

Objective (Probable) Signs

Probable signs of pregnancy are those that are apparent on physical examination by a health care professional. Common probable signs of pregnancy include softening of the lower uterine segment or isthmus (Hegar's sign), softening of the cervix (Goodell's sign), and a bluish-purple coloration of the vaginal mucosa and cervix (Chadwick's sign). Other probable signs include changes in the shape and size of the uterus, abdominal enlargement, Braxton Hicks contractions, and **ballottement** (the examiner pushes against the woman's cervix during a pelvic examination and feels a rebound from the floating fetus).

Along with these physical signs, pregnancy tests are also considered a probable sign of pregnancy. Several pregnancy tests are available (Table 11.1). The tests vary in sensitivity, specificity, and accuracy and are influenced by the length of gestation, specimen concentration, presence of blood, and the presence of some drugs (Likes & Rittenhouse, 2007).

Human chorionic gonadotropin (hCG) is the earliest biochemical marker for pregnancy, and many pregnancy tests are based on the recognition of hCG or a beta subunit of hCG. hCG levels in normal pregnancy usually double every 48 to 72 hours until they peak approx-

imately 60 to 70 days after fertilization; they then decrease to a plateau at 100 to 130 days of pregnancy (Likes & Rittenhouse, 2007).

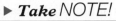

▶ **Take** NOTE!

This elevation of hCG corresponds to the morning sickness period of approximately 6 to 12 weeks during early pregnancy.

Home pregnancy tests are available over the counter and have become quite popular since their introduction in 1975. These tests are very sensitive, cost-effective, and faster than traditional laboratory pregnancy tests. Enzyme-linked immunosorbent assay (ELISA) technology is the basis for most home pregnancy tests.

Although probable signs suggest pregnancy and are more reliable than presumptive signs, they still are not 100% reliable in confirming a pregnancy. For example, uterine tumors, polyps, infection, and pelvic congestion can cause changes to uterine shape, size, and consistency. And although pregnancy tests are used to establish the diagnosis of pregnancy when the physical signs are still inconclusive, they are not completely reliable, because conditions other than pregnancy (e.g., ovarian cancer, choriocarcinoma, hydatidiform mole) can also elevate hCG levels.

Positive Signs

Usually within 2 weeks after a missed period, enough subjective symptoms are present so that a woman can be reasonably sure she is pregnant. However, an experienced health care professional can confirm her suspicions by

TABLE 11.1 **SELECTED PREGNANCY TESTS**

Type	Specimen	Example	Remarks
Agglutination inhibition tests	Urine	Pregnosticon, Gravindex	If hCG is present in urine, agglutination does not occur, which is positive for pregnancy; reliable 14–21 days after conception; 95% accurate in diagnosing pregnancy
Immunoradiometric assay	Blood serum	Neocept, Pregnosis	Measures ability of blood sample to inhibit the binding of radiolabeled hCG to receptors; reliable 6–8 days after conception; 99% accurate in diagnosing pregnancy
Enzyme-linked immunosorbent assay (ELISA)	Blood serum or urine	Over-the-counter home/ office pregnancy tests; precise	Uses an enzyme to bond with hCG in the urine if present; reliable 4 days after implantation; 99% accurate if hCG specific

Sources: Hackley, Kriebs, & Rousseau, 2007; Likes & Rittenhouse, 2007.

identifying positive signs of pregnancy. The positive signs of pregnancy confirm that a fetus is growing in the uterus. Visualizing the fetus by ultrasound, palpating for fetal movements, and hearing a fetal heartbeat are all signs that make the pregnancy a certainty.

Once pregnancy is confirmed, the health care professional will set up a schedule of prenatal visits to assess the woman and her fetus throughout the entire pregnancy. Assessment and education begins at the first visits and continues throughout the pregnancy (see Chapter 12).

Remember Marva, who thought she had a stomach virus? Her pregnancy test was positive. On questioning by the nurse, she acknowledged missing two menstrual periods and being sexually active with her boyfriend without using protection. What is the nurse's role at this point with Marva? What instructions might be given to her while she waits for her first prenatal visit?

Physiologic Adaptations During Pregnancy

Every system of a woman's body changes during pregnancy to accommodate the needs of the growing fetus, and with startling rapidity. The physical changes of pregnancy can be uncomfortable, although every woman reacts uniquely.

Reproductive System Adaptations

Significant changes occur throughout the woman's body during pregnancy to accommodate the growing human being within her. Many have a protective role for maternal homeostasis and are essential to meet the demands of both the mother and the fetus. Many adaptations are reversible after the woman gives birth, but some persist for life.

Uterus

During the first few months of pregnancy, estrogen stimulates uterine growth, and the uterus undergoing a tremendous increase in size, weight, length, width, depth, volume, and overall capacity throughout pregnancy. The weight of the uterus increases from 70 g to about 1100 g at term; its capacity increases from 10 mL to 5000 mL or more at term (Levano, Cunningham, Alexander, et al., 2007). The uterine walls thin to 1.5 cm or less; from a solid globe, the uterus becomes a hollow vessel.

Uterine growth occurs as a result of both hyperplasia and hypertrophy of the myometrial cells, which do not increase much in number but do increase in size. Blood vessels elongate, enlarge, dilate, and sprout new branches to support and nourish the growing muscle tissue, and the increase in uterine weight is accompanied by a large increase in uterine blood flow necessary to perfuse the uterine muscle and accommodate the growing fetus (Frieden & Chan, 2007).

Uterine contractility is enhanced as well. Spontaneous, irregular, and painless contractions, called **Braxton Hicks contractions**, begin during the first trimester. These contractions continue throughout pregnancy, becoming especially noticeable during the last month, when they function to thin out or efface the cervix before birth (see Chapter 12 for more information).

Changes in the uterus occurring during the first 6 to 8 weeks of gestation produce some of the typical findings, including a positive **Hegar's sign**. This softening and compressibility of the lower uterine segment results in exaggerated uterine anteflexion during the early months of pregnancy, which adds to urinary frequency (Arenson & Drake, 2007).

The uterus remains in the pelvic cavity for the first 3 months of pregnancy, after which it progressively ascends into the abdomen (Fig. 11.1). As the uterus grows, it presses on the urinary bladder and causes the increased frequency of urination experienced during early pregnancy. In addition, the heavy gravid uterus in the last trimester can fall back against the inferior vena cava in the supine position, resulting in vena cava compression, which reduces venous return and decreases cardiac output and blood pressure, with increasing orthostatic stress. This occurs when the woman changes her position from recumbent to sitting to standing. This acute hemodynamic change, termed supine hypotensive syndrome, causes the woman

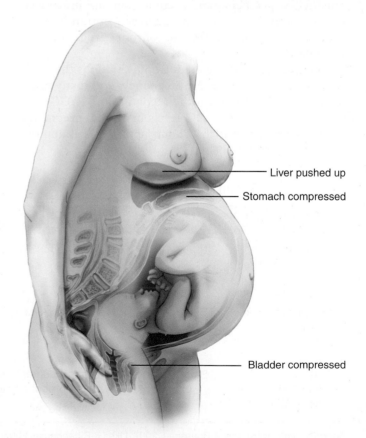

— Liver pushed up

— Stomach compressed

— Bladder compressed

FIGURE 11.1 The growing uterus in the abdomen.

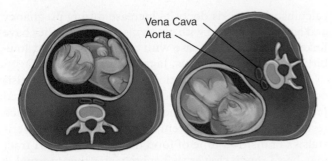

Supine position   Side-lying position

FIGURE 11.2 Supine hypotensive syndrome.

to experience symptoms of weakness, lightheadedness, nausea, dizziness, or syncope (Fig. 11.2). These changes are reversed when the woman is in the left lateral position, which displaces the uterus to the left and off the vena cava.

The uterus, which starts as a pear-shaped organ, becomes ovoid as length increases over width. By 20 weeks' gestation, the fundus, or top of the uterus, is at the level of the umbilicus and measures 20 cm. A monthly measurement of the height of the top of the uterus in centimeters, which corresponds to the number of gestational weeks, is commonly used to date the pregnancy.

> ▶ *Take* NOTE!
>
> *Fundal height can be typical of gestational weeks between 18 and 32 weeks, but after 36 weeks' gestation, this measurement is no longer reliable because of the beginning of fetal descent.*

The fundus reaches its highest level, at the xiphoid process, at approximately 36 weeks. Between 38 to 40 weeks, fundal height drops as the fetus begins to descend and engage into the pelvis. Because it pushes against the diaphragm, many women experience shortness of breath. By 40 weeks, the fetal head begins to descend and engage in the pelvis, which is termed *lightening*. For the woman who is pregnant for the first time, lightening usually occurs approximately 2 weeks before the onset of labor; for the woman who is experiencing her second or subsequent pregnancy, it usually occurs at the onset of labor. Although breathing becomes easier because of this descent, the pressure on the urinary bladder now increases and women experience urinary frequency again.

Cervix

Between weeks 6 and 8 of pregnancy, the cervix begins to soften (**Goodell's sign**) due to vasocongestion. Along with the softening, the endocervical glands increase in size and number and produce more cervical mucus. Under the influence of progesterone, a thick mucus plug is formed that blocks the cervical os and protects the opening from bacterial invasion. At about the same time, increased vascularization of the cervix causes **Chadwick's sign**. Cervical ripening (softening, effacement, and increased distensibility) begins about 4 weeks before birth. Ripening is an inflammatory process and is not dependent on uterine contractions (Blackburn, 2007).

Vagina

During pregnancy, there is increased vascularity because of the influences of estrogen, resulting in pelvic congestion and hypertrophy of the vagina in preparation for the distention needed for birth. The vaginal mucosa thickens, the connective tissue begins to loosen, the smooth muscle begins to hypertrophy, and the vaginal vault begins to lengthen (Frieden & Chan, 2007).

Vaginal secretions become more acidic, white, and thick. Most women experience an increase in a whitish vaginal discharge, called leukorrhea, during pregnancy. This is normal except when it is accompanied by itching and irritation, possibly suggesting *Candida albicans*, a monilial vaginitis, which is a very common occurrence in this glycogen-rich environment (Mashburn, 2006). Monilial vaginitis is a benign fungal condition that is uncomfortable for the woman, but it can be transmitted from an infected mother to her newborn at birth. Neonates develop an oral infection known as thrush, which presents as white patches on the mucous membranes of their mouths. It is self-limiting and is treated with local antifungal agents.

Ovaries

The increased blood supply to the ovaries causes them to enlarge until approximately the 12th to 14th week of gestation. The ovaries are not palpable after that time because the uterus fills the pelvic cavity. Ovulation ceases during pregnancy because of the elevated levels of estrogen and progesterone, which block secretion of follicle-stimulating hormone (FSH) and luteinizing hormone (LH) from the anterior pituitary. The ovaries are very active in hormone production to support the pregnancy until about weeks 6 to 7, when the corpus luteum regresses and the placenta takes over the major production of progesterone.

Breasts

The breasts increase in fullness, become tender, and grow larger throughout pregnancy under the influence of estrogen and progesterone. The breasts become highly vascular, and veins become visible under the skin. The nipples become larger and more erect. Both the nipples and the areola become deeply pigmented, and tubercles of Montgomery (sebaceous glands) become prominent. These sebaceous glands keep the nipples lubricated for breastfeeding.

Changes that occur in the connective tissue of the breasts, along with the tremendous growth, lead to striae (stretch marks) in approximately half of all pregnant women (Graham, 2007). Initially they appear as pink to purple lines on the skin, but they eventually fade to a silver color. Although they become less conspicuous in time, they never completely disappear.

Creamy, yellowish breast fluid called colostrum can be expressed by the third trimester. This fluid provides nourishment for the breastfeeding newborn during the first few days of life (see Chapters 15 and 16 for more information).

Table 11.2 summarizes reproductive system adaptations.

General Body System Adaptations

In addition to changes in the reproductive system, the pregnant woman also experiences changes in virtually every other body system in response to the growing fetus.

Gastrointestinal System

The gastrointestinal (GI) system begins in the oral cavity and ends at the rectum. During pregnancy, the gums become hyperemic, swollen, and friable and tend to bleed easily. This change is influenced by estrogen and increased proliferation of blood vessels and circulation to the mouth. In addition, the saliva produced in the mouth becomes more acidic. Some women complain about excessive salivation, termed ptyalism, which may be caused by the decrease in unconscious swallowing by the woman when nauseated (Cunningham et al., 2005). Dental plaque, calculus, and debris deposits increase during pregnancy and are all associated with gingivitis. Recent studies have linked periodontal disease with preterm birth and low-birthweight risk (Pretorius, Jagatt, & Lamont, 2007).

Smooth muscle relaxation and decreased peristalsis occur related to the influence of progesterone. Elevated progesterone levels cause smooth muscle relaxation, which results in delayed gastric emptying and decreased peristalsis. Transition time of food throughout the GI tract may be so much slower that more water than normal is reabsorbed, leading to bloating and constipation. Constipation can also result from low-fiber food choices, reduced fluid intake, use of iron supplements, decreased activity level, and intestinal displacement secondary to a growing uterus. Constipation, increased venous pressure, and the pressure of the gravid uterus contribute to the formation of hemorrhoids.

The slowed gastric emptying combined with relaxation of the cardiac sphincter allows reflux, which causes heartburn. Acid indigestion or heartburn (pyrosis) seems to be a universal problem for pregnant women. It is caused by regurgitation of the stomach contents into the upper esophagus and may be associated with the generalized relaxation of the entire digestive system. Over-the-counter antacids will usually relieve the symptoms, but they should be taken with the health care provider's knowledge and only as directed.

The emptying time of the gallbladder is prolonged secondary to the smooth muscle relaxation from progesterone. Hypercholesterolemia can follow, increasing the risk of gallstone formation. Other risk factors for

TABLE 11.2 **SUMMARY OF REPRODUCTIVE SYSTEM ADAPTATIONS**

Reproductive Organ	Adaptations
Uterus	Size increases 20 times that of nonpregnant size. Capacity increases by 2,000 times to accommodate the developing fetus. Weight increases from 2 oz to approximately 2 lb at term. Uterine growth occurs as a result of both hyperplasia and hypertrophy of the myometrial cells. Increased strength and elasticity allow uterus to contract and expel fetus during birth.
Cervix	Increases in mass, water content, and vascularization Changes from a relatively rigid to a soft, distensible structure that allows the fetus to be expelled Under the influence of progesterone, a thick mucus plug is formed, which blocks the cervical os and protects the developing fetus from bacterial invasion.
Vagina	Increased vascularity because of estrogen influences, resulting in pelvic congestion and hypertrophy Increased thickness of mucosa, along with an increase in vaginal secretions to prevent bacterial infections
Ovaries	Increased blood supply to the ovaries causes them to enlarge until approximately the 12th to 14th week of gestation, when the placenta takes over their function. Ovulation ceases during pregnancy because of the elevated levels of estrogen and progesterone.
Breasts	Breast changes begin soon after conception; they increase in size and areolar pigmentation. The tubercles of Montgomery enlarge and become more prominent, and the nipples more erect. The blood vessels become more prominent, and blood flow to the breast doubles.

gallbladder disease include obesity, Hispanic ethnicity, and increasing maternal age (Ko, 2006).

Nausea and vomiting, better known as morning sickness, plagues about 50% to 80% of pregnant women (Lane, 2007). Although it occurs most often in the morning, the nauseated feeling can last all day in some women. The highest incidence of morning sickness is between 6 and 12 weeks. The physiologic basis for morning sickness is still debatable. It has been linked to the high levels of hCG, high levels of circulating estrogens, reduced stomach acidity, and the lowered tone and motility of the digestive tract (Lane, 2007).

Cardiovascular System

Cardiovascular changes occur early during pregnancy to meet the demands of the enlarging uterus and the placenta for more blood and more oxygen. Perhaps the most striking cardiac alteration occurring during pregnancy is the increase in blood volume.

Blood Volume

Blood volume increases by approximately 1,500 mL, or 50% above nonpregnant levels (Cunningham et al., 2005). The increase is made up of 1,000 mL plasma plus 450 mL red blood cells (RBCs). It begins at weeks 10 to 12, peaks at weeks 32 to 34, and decreases slightly at week 40.

▶ *Take NOTE!*

The rise in blood volume correlates directly with fetal weight.

This increase in blood volume is needed to provide adequate hydration of fetal and maternal tissues, to supply blood flow to perfuse the enlarging uterus, and to provide a reserve to compensate for blood loss at birth and during postpartum (Martin & Foley, 2006). This increase is also necessary to meet the increased metabolic needs of the mother and to meet the need for increased perfusion of other organs, especially the woman's kidneys, because she is excreting waste products for herself and the fetus.

Cardiac Output and Heart Rate

Cardiac output is the product of stroke volume and heart rate. It increases from 30% to 50% over the nonpregnant rate by the 32nd week of pregnancy and declines to about a 20% increase at 40 weeks' gestation. The increase in cardiac output is associated with an increase in venous return and greater right ventricular output, especially in the left lateral position (Blackburn, 2007). Heart rate increases by 10 to 15 bpm between 14 and 20 weeks of gestation, and this persists to term. There is slight hypertrophy or enlargement of the heart during pregnancy. This is probably to accommodate the increase in blood volume and cardiac output. The heart works harder and pumps more blood to supply the oxygen needs of the fetus as well as those of the mother. Both heart rate and venous return are increased in pregnancy, contributing to the increase in cardiac output seen throughout gestation. A woman with preexisting heart disease may become symptomatic and begin to decompensate during the time the blood volume peaks. Close monitoring is warranted during 28 to 35 weeks' gestation.

Blood Pressure

Blood pressure, especially the diastolic pressure, declines slightly during pregnancy as a result of peripheral vasodilation caused by progesterone. It reaches a low point at midpregnancy and thereafter increases to prepregnant levels until term (Blackburn, 2007). During the first trimester, blood pressure typically remains at the prepregnancy level. During the second trimester, the blood pressure decreases 5 to 10 mmHg and thereafter returns to first-trimester levels (Blackburn, 2007). Any significant rise in blood pressure during pregnancy should be investigated to rule out gestational hypertension.

Blood Components

The number of RBCs also increases throughout pregnancy to a level 25% to 33% higher than nonpregnant values, depending on the amount of iron available. This increase is necessary to transport the additional oxygen required during pregnancy. Although there is an increase in RBCs, there is a greater increase in the plasma volume as a result of hormonal factors and sodium and water retention. Because the plasma increase exceeds the increase of RBC production, normal hemoglobin and hematocrit values decrease. This state of hemodilution is referred to as **physiologic anemia of pregnancy**. Changes in RBC volume are due to increased circulating erythropoietin and accelerated RBC production. The rise in erythropoietin in the last two trimesters is stimulated by progesterone, prolactin, and human placental lactogen (Blackburn, 2007).

Iron requirements during pregnancy increase because of the demands of the growing fetus and the increase in maternal blood volume. The fetal tissues take predominance over the mother's tissues with respect to use of iron stores. With the accelerated production of RBCs, iron is necessary for hemoglobin formation, the oxygen-carrying component of RBCs.

▶ *Take NOTE!*

Many women enter pregnancy with insufficient iron stores and thus need supplementation to meet the extra demands of pregnancy.

Both fibrin and plasma fibrinogen levels increase, along with various blood-clotting factors. These factors make pregnancy a hypercoagulable state. These changes, coupled with venous stasis secondary to venous pooling, which occurs during late pregnancy after long periods of standing in the upright position with the pressure exerted by the uterus on the large pelvic veins, contribute to slowed venous return, pooling, and dependent edema. These factors also increase the woman's risk for venous thrombosis (Martin & Foley, 2006).

Respiratory System

The growing uterus and the increased production of the hormone progesterone cause the lungs to function differently during pregnancy. During the pregnancy, the amount of space available to house the lungs decreases as the uterus puts pressure on the diaphragm and causes it to shift upward by 4 cm above its usual position. The growing uterus does change the size and shape of the thoracic cavity, but diaphragmatic excursion increases, chest circumference increases by 2 to 3 in, and the transverse diameter increases by an inch, allowing a larger tidal volume, as evidenced by deeper breathing (Blackburn, 2007). Tidal volume or the volume of air inhaled increases gradually by 30 to 40% (from 500 to 700 mL) as the pregnancy progresses. As a result of these changes, the women's breathing becomes more diaphragmatic than abdominal (Torgersen & Curran, 2006).

A pregnant woman breathes faster and more deeply because she and the fetus need more oxygen. Oxygen consumption increases during pregnancy as airway resistance and lung compliance remain unchanged. Changes in the structures of the respiratory system take place to prepare the body for the enlarging uterus and increased lung volume (Alexander et al., 2007). As muscles and cartilage in the thoracic region relax, the chest broadens, with a conversion from abdominal breathing to thoracic breathing. This leads to a 50% increase in air volume per minute. All these structural alterations are temporary and revert back to their prepregnant state at the end of the pregnancy.

Increased vascularity of the respiratory tract is influenced by increased estrogen levels, leading to congestion. This congestion gives rise to nasal and sinus stuffiness, epistaxis (nosebleed), and changes in the tone and quality of the woman's voice (Martin & Foley, 2006).

Renal/Urinary System

The renal system must handle the effects of increased maternal intravascular and extracellular volume and metabolic waste products as well as excretion of fetal wastes. The predominant structural change in the renal system during pregnancy is dilation of the renal pelvis and uterus. Changes in renal structure occur from hormonal influences of estrogen and progesterone, pressure from an enlarging uterus, and an increase in maternal blood volume.

Like the heart, the kidneys work harder throughout the pregnancy. Changes in kidney function occur to accommodate a heavier workload while maintaining a stable electrolyte balance and blood pressure. As more blood flows to the kidneys, the glomerular filtration rate (GFR) increases, leading to an increase in urine flow and volume, substances delivered to the kidneys, and filtration and excretion of water and solutes (Jeyabalan & Lain, 2007).

Anatomically, the kidneys enlarge during pregnancy. Each kidney increases in length and weight as a result of hormonal effects that cause increased tone and decreased motility of the smooth muscle. The renal pelvis becomes dilated. The ureters (especially the right ureter) elongate, widen, and become more curved above the pelvic rim as early as the 10th gestational week (Jeyabalan & Lain, 2007). Progesterone is thought to cause both these changes because of its relaxing influence on smooth muscle.

Blood flow to the kidneys increases by 50% to 80% as a result of the increase in cardiac output. This in turn leads to an increase in the GFR by as much as 40% to 60% starting during the second trimester. This elevation continues until birth (Blackburn, 2007).

The activity of the kidneys normally increases when a person lies down and decreases on standing. This difference is amplified during pregnancy, which is one reason a pregnant woman feels the need to urinate frequently while trying to sleep. Late in the pregnancy, the increase in kidney activity is even greater when the woman lies on her side rather than her back. Lying on the side relieves the pressure that the enlarged uterus puts on the vena cava carrying blood from the legs. Subsequently, venous return to the heart increases, leading to increased cardiac output. Increased cardiac output results in increased renal perfusion and glomerular filtration (Fitzgerald & Graziano, 2007).

Musculoskeletal System

Changes in the musculoskeletal system are progressive, resulting from the influence of hormones, fetal growth, and maternal weight gain. Pregnancy is characterized by changes in posture and gait. By the 10th to 12th week of pregnancy, the ligaments that hold the sacroiliac joints and the pubis symphysis in place begin to soften and stretch, and the articulations between the joints widen and become more movable (Frieden & Chan, 2007). The relaxation of the joints peaks by the beginning of the third trimester. The purpose of these changes is to increase the size of the pelvic cavity and to make delivery easier.

The postural changes of pregnancy—an increased swayback and an upper spine extension to compensate for the enlarging abdomen—coupled with the loosening of the sacroiliac joints may result in lower back pain. The woman's center of gravity shifts forward, requiring a realignment of the spinal curvatures. An increase in the normal lumbosacral curve (lordosis) occurs and a compensatory curvature in the cervicodorsal area develops

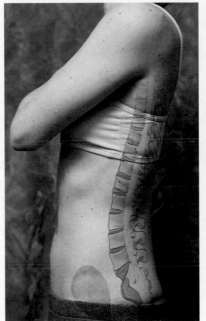
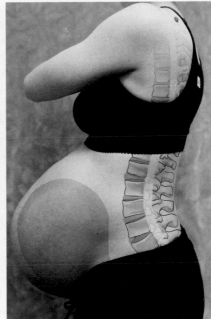

A. Early pregnancy   **B.** Late pregnancy

FIGURE 11.3 Postural changes during (**A**) the first trimester and (**B**) the third trimester.

to assist her in maintaining her balance (Fig. 11.3). In addition, relaxation and increased mobility of joints occur because of the hormones progesterone and relaxin, which lead to the characteristic "waddle gait" that pregnant women demonstrate toward term. Increased weight gain can add to this discomfort by accentuating the lumbar and dorsal curves (Torgersen & Curran, 2006).

Integumentary System

The skin of pregnant women undergoes hyperpigmentation primarily as a result of estrogen, progesterone, and melanocyte-stimulating hormone levels. These changes are mainly seen on the nipples, areola, umbilicus, perineum, and axilla. Although many integumentary changes disappear after giving birth, some only fade. Many pregnant women express concern about stretch marks, skin color changes, and hair loss. Unfortunately, little is known about how to avoid these changes.

Complexion changes are not unusual. The increased pigmentation that occurs on the breasts and genitalia also develops on the face to form the "mask of pregnancy," or facial melasma. It occurs in up to 70% of pregnant women. There is a genetic predisposition toward melasma, which is exacerbated by the sun; it tends to recur in subsequent pregnancies. This blotchy, brownish pigment covers the forehead and cheeks in dark-haired women. Most fade as the hormones subside at the end of the pregnancy, but some may linger. The skin in the middle of the abdomen may develop a pigmented line called **linea nigra**, which extends from the umbilicus to the pubic area (Fig. 11.4).

Striae gravidarum, or stretch marks, are irregular reddish streaks that appear on the abdomen, breasts, and buttocks in about half of pregnant women. Striae are most prominent by 6 to 7 months. They result from reduced connective tissue strength resulting from the elevated adrenal steroid levels and stretching of the structures secondary to growth (Tunzi & Gray, 2007). They are more common in younger women, women with larger infants, and women with higher body mass indices. Nonwhites and women with a history of breast or thigh striae or a family history of striae gravidarum also are at higher risk (Osman et al., 2007).

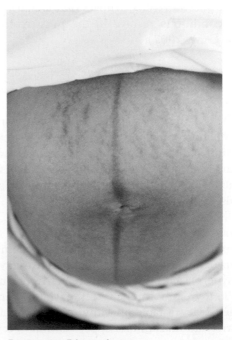

FIGURE 11.4 Linea nigra.

Vascular changes during pregnancy manifested in the integumentary system include varicosities of the legs, vulva, and perineum. Varicose veins commonly are the result of distention, instability, and poor circulation secondary to prolonged standing or sitting and the heavy gravid uterus placing pressure on the pelvic veins, preventing complete venous return. Interventions to reduce the risk of developing varicosities include:

- Elevating both legs when sitting or lying down
- Avoiding prolonged standing or sitting; changing position frequently
- Resting in the left lateral position
- Walking daily for exercise
- Avoiding tight clothing or knee-high hosiery
- Wearing support hose if varicosities are a preexisting condition to pregnancy

Another skin manifestation, believed to be secondary to vascular changes and high estrogen levels, is the appearance of small blood vessels called vascular spiders. They may appear on the neck, thorax, face, and arms. They are especially obvious in white women and typically disappear after childbirth (Tunzi & Gray, 2007). Palmar erythema is a well-delineated pinkish area on the palmar surface of the hands. This integumentary change is also related to elevated estrogen levels (Tunzi & Gray, 2007).

The hair on many women's heads may appear thicker during pregnancy. This is because higher hormone levels prevent normal hair loss. During pregnancy hair tends to stay in the resting phase longer than usual, most hairs are in the resting phase at any one time and fewer hairs fall out each day, causing hair to seem thicker and fuller. Nails typically grow faster during pregnancy. Pregnant women may experience increased brittleness and transverse grooves on the nails, but most of these conditions resolve in the postpartum period (Tunzi & Gray, 2007).

Endocrine System

The endocrine system undergoes many changes during pregnancy because hormonal changes are essential in meeting the needs of the growing fetus. Hormonal changes play a major role in controlling the supplies of maternal glucose, amino acids, and lipids to the fetus. Although estrogen and progesterone are the main hormones involved in pregnancy changes, other endocrine glands and hormones also change during pregnancy.

Thyroid Gland

The thyroid gland enlarges slightly and becomes more active during pregnancy as a result of increased vascularity and hyperplasia. Increased gland activity results in an increase in thyroid hormone secretion starting during the first trimester; levels taper off within a few weeks after birth and return to normal limits (Poppe, Velkeniers, & Glinoer, 2007). With an increase in the secretion of thyroid hormones, the basal metabolic rate (BMR; the amount of oxygen consumed by the body over a unit of time in milliliters per minute) progressively increases by 25%, along with heart rate and cardiac output (Blackburn, 2007).

Pituitary Gland

The pituitary gland, also known as the hypophysis, is a small, oval gland about the size of a pea that is connected to the hypothalamus by a stalk called the infundibulum. During pregnancy, the pituitary gland enlarges; it returns to normal size after birth.

The anterior lobe of the pituitary is glandular tissue and produces multiple hormones. The release of these hormones is regulated by releasing and inhibiting hormones produced by the hypothalamus. Some of these anterior pituitary hormones induce other glands to secrete their hormones. The increase in blood levels of the hormones produced by the final target glands (e.g., the ovary or thyroid) inhibits the release of anterior pituitary hormones. Changes in levels of pituitary hormones are discussed in the following paragraphs.

FSH and LH secretion are inhibited during pregnancy, probably as a result of hCG produced by the placenta and corpus luteum, and the increased secretion of prolactin by the anterior pituitary gland. Levels remain decreased until after delivery.

Thyroid-stimulating hormone (TSH) is reduced during the first trimester but usually returns to normal for the remainder of the pregnancy. Decreased TSH is thought to be one of the factors, along with elevated hCG levels, associated with morning sickness, nausea, and vomiting during the first trimester.

Growth hormone (GH) is an anabolic hormone that promotes protein synthesis. It stimulates most body cells to grow in size and divide, facilitating the use of fats for fuel and conserving glucose. During pregnancy, there is a decrease in the number of GH-producing cells and a corresponding decrease in GH blood levels. The action of human placental lactogen (hPL) is thought to decrease the need for and use of GH.

During pregnancy, prolactin is secreted in pulses and increases ten-fold to promote breast development and the lactation process. High levels of progesterone secreted by the placenta inhibit the direct influence of prolactin on the breast during pregnancy, thus suppressing lactation. At birth, as soon as the placenta is expelled and there is a drop in progesterone, lactogenesis can begin (Cunningham et al., 2005).

Melanocyte-stimulating hormone (MSH), another anterior pituitary hormone, increases during pregnancy. For many years, its increase was thought to be responsible for many of the skin changes of pregnancy, particularly changes in skin pigmentation (e.g., darkening of the areola, melasma, and linea nigra). However, currently it is thought that the skin changes are due to estrogen (and possibly progesterone) as well as the increase in MSH.

The two hormones oxytocin and antidiuretic hormone (ADH) released by the posterior pituitary are actually synthesized in the hypothalamus. They migrate along nerve fibers to the posterior pituitary and are stored until stimulated to be released into the general circulation.

Oxytocin is released by the posterior pituitary gland, and its production gradually increases as the fetus matures (Ochedalski et al., 2007). Oxytocin is responsible for uterine contractions, both before and after delivery. The muscle layers of the uterus (myometrium) become more sensitive to oxytocin near term. Toward the end of a term pregnancy, levels of progesterone decline and contractions that were previously suppressed by progesterone begin to occur more frequently and with stronger intensity. This change in the hormonal levels is believed to be one of the initiators of labor.

Oxytocin is responsible for stimulating the uterine contractions that bring about delivery. Contractions lead to cervical thinning and dilation. They also exert pressure, helping the fetus to descend in the pelvis for eventual delivery. After delivery, oxytocin secretion continues, causing the myometrium to contract and helping to constrict the uterine blood vessels, decreasing the amount of vaginal bleeding after delivery.

Oxytocin is also responsible for milk ejection during breastfeeding. Stimulation of the breasts through sucking or touching stimulates the secretion of oxytocin from the posterior pituitary gland. Oxytocin causes contraction of the myoepithelial cells in the lactating mammary gland. With breastfeeding, "after pains" often occur, which signals that oxytocin is being released.

Vasopressin (ADH) functions to inhibit or prevent the formation of urine via vasoconstriction, which results in increased blood pressure. Vasopressin also exhibits an antidiuretic effect and plays an important role in the regulation of water balance (Fitzgerald & Graziano, 2007).

Pancreas

The pancreas is an exocrine organ, supplying digestive enzymes and buffers, and an endocrine organ. The endocrine pancreas consists of the islets of Langerhans, which are groups of cells scattered throughout, each containing four cell types. One of the cell types is the beta cell, which produces insulin. Insulin lowers blood glucose by increasing the rate of glucose uptake and utilization by most body cells. The growing fetus needs significant amounts of glucose, amino acids, and lipids. Even during early pregnancy the fetus makes demands on the maternal glucose stores. Ideally, hormonal changes of pregnancy help meet fetal needs without putting the mother's metabolism out of balance.

A woman's insulin secretion works on a "supply-versus-demand" mode. As the demand to meet the needs of pregnancy increases, more insulin is secreted. Maternal insulin does not cross the placenta, so the fetus must produce his or her own supply to maintain glucose con-

BOX 11.2 Pregnancy, Insulin, and Glucose

- During early pregnancy, there is a decrease in maternal glucose levels because of the heavy fetal demand for glucose. The fetus is also drawing amino acids and lipids from the mother, decreasing the mother's ability to synthesize glucose. Maternal glucose is diverted across the placenta to assist the growing embryo/fetus during early pregnancy, and thus levels decline in the mother. As a result, maternal glucose concentrations decline to a level that would be considered "hypoglycemic" in a nonpregnant woman. During early pregnancy there is also a decrease in maternal insulin production and insulin levels.
- The pancreas is responsible for the production of insulin, which facilitates entry of glucose into cells. Although glucose and other nutrients easily cross the placenta to the fetus, insulin does not. Therefore, the fetus must produce its own insulin to facilitate the entry of glucose into its own cells.
- After the first trimester, hPL from the placenta and steroids (cortisol) from the adrenal cortex act against insulin. hPL acts as an antagonist against maternal insulin, and thus more insulin must be secreted to counteract the increasing levels of hPL and cortisol during the last half of pregnancy.
- Prolactin, estrogen, and progesterone are also thought to oppose insulin. As a result, glucose is less likely to enter the mother's cells and is more likely to cross over the placenta to the fetus (Cunningham et al., 2005).

trol (Box 11.2 gives information about pregnancy, glucose, and insulin).

During the first half of pregnancy, much of the maternal glucose is diverted to the growing fetus, and thus the mother's glucose levels are low. hPL and other hormonal antagonists increase during the second half of pregnancy. Therefore, the mother must produce more insulin to overcome the resistance by these hormones.

If the mother has normal beta cells of the islets of Langerhans, there is usually no problem meeting the demands for extra insulin. However, if the woman has inadequate numbers of beta cells, she may be unable to produce enough insulin and will develop glucose intolerance during pregnancy. If the woman has glucose intolerance, she is not able to meet the increasing demands and her blood glucose level increases.

Adrenal Glands

Pregnancy does not cause much change in the size of the adrenal glands themselves, but there are changes in some secretions and activity. One of the key changes is the marked increase in cortisol secretion, which regulates carbohydrate and protein metabolism and is helpful in times of stress. Although pregnancy is considered a normal condition, it is a time of stress for a woman's body. Cortisol increases in response to increased estrogen levels throughout pregnancy and returns to normal levels within 6 weeks postpartum (Blackburn, 2007).

During the stress of pregnancy, cortisol:

- Helps keep up the level of glucose in the plasma by breaking down noncarbohydrate sources, such as amino and fatty acids, to make glycogen. Glycogen, stored in the liver, is easily broken down to glucose when needed so that glucose is available in times of stress.
- Breaks down proteins to repair tissues and manufacture enzymes
- Has anti-insulin, anti-inflammatory, and antiallergic actions
- Is needed to make the precursors of adrenaline, which the adrenal medulla produces and secretes (Cunningham et al., 2005)

Aldosterone, also secreted by the adrenal glands, is increased during pregnancy. It normally regulates absorption of sodium from the distal tubules of the kidney. During pregnancy, progesterone allows salt to be "wasted" (or lost) in the urine. Aldosterone is produced in increased amounts by the adrenal glands as early as 15 weeks of pregnancy (Jeyabalan & Lain, 2007).

Prostaglandin Secretion During Pregnancy

Prostaglandins are not protein or steroid hormones; they are chemical mediators, or "local" hormones. Although hormones circulate in the blood to influence distant tissues, prostaglandins act locally on adjacent cells. The fetal membranes of the amniotic sac—the amnion and chorion—are both believed to be involved in the production of prostaglandins. Various maternal and fetal tissues, as well as the amniotic fluid itself, are considered to be sources of prostaglandins, but details about their composition and sources are limited. It is widely believed that prostaglandins play a part in softening the cervix and initiating and/or maintaining labor, but the exact mechanism is unclear.

Placental Secretion

The placenta has a feature possessed by no other endocrine organ—the ability to form protein and steroid hormones. Very early during pregnancy, the placenta begins to produce the following hormones:

- hCG
- hPL
- Relaxin
- Progesterone
- Estrogen

Table 11.3 summarizes the role of these hormones.

Immune System

The immune system is made up of organs and specialized cells whose primary purpose is to defend the body from foreign substances (antigens) that may cause tissue injury or disease. The mechanisms of innate and adaptive immunity work cooperatively to prevent, control, and eradicate foreign antigens in the body.

A general enhancement of innate immunity (inflammatory response and phagocytosis) and suppression of adaptive immunity (protective response to a specific foreign antigen) takes place during pregnancy. These immunologic alterations help prevent the mother's immune system from rejecting the fetus (foreign body), increase her risk of developing certain infections such as urinary tract infections, and influence the course of chronic disorders such as autoimmune diseases. Some chronic conditions worsen (diabetes) while others seem to stabilize (asthma) during pregnancy, but this is individualized and not predictable. In general, immune function in pregnant women is similar to immune function in nonpregnant women.

*M*arva returns for her first prenatal appointment and tells the nurse that her whole body is "out of sorts." She is overwhelmed and feels poorly. Outline the bodily changes Marva can expect each trimester to help her understand the adaptations taking place. What guidance can the nurse give Marva to help her understand the changes of pregnancy?

Table 11.4 summarizes the general body systems adaptations to pregnancy.

Changing Nutritional Needs of Pregnancy

Healthy eating during pregnancy enables optimal gestational weight gain and reduces complications, both of which are associated with positive birth outcomes. During pregnancy, maternal nutritional needs change to meet the demands of the pregnancy. Healthy eating can help ensure that adequate nutrients are available for both mother and fetus.

Nutritional intake during pregnancy has a direct effect on fetal well-being and birth outcome. Inadequate nutritional intake, for example, is associated with preterm birth, low birthweight, and congenital anomalies. Excessive nutritional intake is connected with fetal macrosomia (>4,000 g), leading to a difficult birth, neonatal hypoglycemia, and continued obesity in the mother (Blackburn, 2007).

Since the requirements for so many nutrients increase during pregnancy, pregnant women should take a vitamin and mineral supplement daily. Prenatal vitamins are prescribed routinely as a safeguard against a less-than-optimal diet. In particular, iron and folic acid need to be supplemented because their increased requirements during pregnancy are usually too great to be met through diet alone

TABLE 11.3 **PLACENTAL HORMONES**

Hormone	Description
hCG	• Responsible for maintaining the maternal corpus luteum, which secretes progesterone and estrogens, with synthesis occurring before implantation • Production by fetal trophoblast cells until the placenta is developed sufficiently to take over that function • Basis for early pregnancy tests because it appears in the maternal bloodstream soon after implantation • Production peaks at 8 weeks and then gradually declines.
hPL (also known as human chorionic somatomammotropin [hCS])	• Preparation of mammary glands for lactation and involved in the process of making glucose available for fetal growth by altering maternal carbohydrate, fat, and protein metabolism • Antagonist of insulin because it decreases tissue sensitivity or alters the ability to use insulin • Increase in the amount of circulating free fatty acids for maternal metabolic needs and decrease in maternal metabolism of glucose to facilitate fetal growth
Relaxin	• Secretion by the placenta as well as the corpus luteum during pregnancy • Thought to act synergistically with progesterone to maintain pregnancy • Increase in flexibility of the pubic symphysis, permitting the pelvis to expand during delivery • Dilation of the cervix, making it easier for the fetus to enter the vaginal canal; thought to suppress the release of oxytocin by the hypothalamus, thus delaying the onset of labor contractions (Blackburn, 2007)
Progesterone	• Often called the "hormone of pregnancy" because of the critical role it plays in supporting the endometrium of the uterus • Supports the endometrium to provide an environment conducive to fetal survival • Produced by the corpus luteum during the first few weeks of pregnancy and then by the placenta until term • Initially, causes thickening of the uterine lining in anticipation of implantation of the fertilized ovum. From then on, it maintains the endometrium, inhibits uterine contractility, and assists in the development of the breasts for lactation (Graham, 2007).
Estrogen	• Promotes enlargement of the genitals, uterus, and breasts, and increases vascularity, causing vasodilatation. • Relaxation of pelvic ligaments and joints (Blackburn, 2007) • Associated with hyperpigmentation, vascular changes in the skin, increased activity of the salivary glands, and hyperemia of the gums and nasal mucous membranes (Tunzi & Gray, 2007) • Aids in developing the ductal system of the breasts in preparation for lactation (Graham, 2007)

(Blackburn, 2007). Iron and folic acid are needed to form new blood cells for the expanded maternal blood volume and to prevent anemia. Folic acid is essential before pregnancy and in the early weeks of pregnancy to prevent neural tube defects in the fetus. For most pregnant women, supplements of 30 mg of ferrous iron and 600 mcg of folic acid per day are recommended by the **dietary reference intakes (DRIs)** (Institute of Medicine [IOM], 2006a, 2006b, 2006c, 2006d, 2006e, 2006f). Women with a previous history of a fetus with a neural tube defect are often prescribed a higher dose.

There is an abundance of conflicting advice about nutrition during pregnancy and what is good or bad to eat. Overall, the following guidelines are helpful:

• Increase your consumption of fruits and vegetables.
• Replace saturated fats with unsaturated ones.
• Avoid hydrogenated or partially hydrogenated fats.

• Use reduced-fat spreads and dairy products instead of full-fat ones.
• Eat at least two servings of fish weekly, with one of them being an oily fish.
• Consume at least 2 quarts of water daily (Arenson & Drake, 2007).

In the months before conception, food choices are key. The foods and vitamins consumed can ensure that the woman and her fetus will have the nutrients that are essential for the very start of pregnancy.

While most women recognize the importance of healthy eating during pregnancy, some find it challenging to achieve. Many women say they have little time and energy to devote to meal planning and preparation. Another barrier to healthy eating is conflicting messages from various sources, resulting in a lack of clear, reliable, and relevant information. Moreover, many women

TABLE 11.4   SUMMARY OF GENERAL BODY SYSTEM ADAPTATIONS

System	Adaptation
Gastrointestinal system	*Mouth and pharynx:* Gums become hyperemic, swollen, and friable and tend to bleed easily. Saliva production increases. *Esophagus:* Decreased lower esophageal sphincter pressure and tone, which increases the risk of developing heartburn *Stomach:* Decreased tone and mobility with delayed gastric emptying time, which increases the risk of gastroesophageal reflux and vomiting. Decreased gastric acidity and histamine output, which improves symptoms of peptic ulcer disease. *Intestines:* Decreased intestinal tone motility with increased transit time, which increases risk of constipation and flatulence *Gallbladder:* Decreased tone and motility, which may increase risk of gallstone formation
Cardiovascular system	*Blood volume:* Marked increase in plasma (50%) and RBCs (25% to 33%) compared to nonpregnant values. Causes hemodilution, which is reflected in a lower hematocrit and hemoglobin. *Cardiac output and heart rate:* CO increases from 30% to 50% over the nonpregnant rate by the 32nd week of pregnancy. The increase in CO is associated with an increase in venous return and greater right ventricular output, especially in the left lateral position. Heart rate increases by 10 to 15 bpm between 14 and 20 weeks of gestation, and this increase persists to term. *Blood pressure:* Diastolic pressure decreases typically 10 to 15 mmHg to reach its lowest point by mid-pregnancy; it then gradually returns to nonpregnant baseline values by term. *Blood components:* The number of RBCs increases throughout pregnancy to a level 25% to 33% higher than nonpregnant values. Both fibrin and plasma fibrinogen levels increase, along with various blood-clotting factors. These factors make pregnancy a hypercoagulable state.
Respiratory system	Enlargement of the uterus shifts the diaphragm up to 4 cm above its usual position. As muscles and cartilage in the thoracic region relax, the chest broadens, with conversion from abdominal breathing to thoracic breathing. This leads to a 50% increase in air volume per minute. Tidal volume, or the volume of air inhaled, increases gradually by 30% to 40% (from 500 to 700 mL) as the pregnancy progresses.
Renal/Urinary system	The renal pelvis becomes dilated. The ureters (especially the right ureter) elongate, widen, and become more curved above the pelvic rim. Bladder tone decreases and bladder capacity doubles by term. GFR increases 40% to 60% during pregnancy. Blood flow to the kidneys increases by 50% to 80% as a result of the increase in cardiac output.
Musculoskeletal system	Distention of the abdomen with growth of the fetus tilts the pelvis forward, shifting the center of gravity. The woman compensates by developing an increased curvature (lordosis) of the spine. Relaxation and increased mobility of joints occur because of the hormones progesterone and relaxin, which lead to the characteristic "waddle gait" that pregnant women demonstrate toward term.
Integumentary system	Hyperpigmentation of the skin is the most common alteration during pregnancy. The most common areas include the areola, genital skin, axilla, inner aspects of the thighs, and linea nigra. Striae gravidarum, or stretch marks, are irregular reddish streaks that may appear on the abdomen, breasts, and buttocks in about half of pregnant women. The skin in the middle of the abdomen may develop a pigmented line called linea nigra, which extends from the umbilicus to the pubic area. Melasma ("mask of pregnancy") occurs in 45% to 70% of pregnant women. It is characterized by irregular, blotchy areas of pigmentation on the face, most commonly on the cheeks, chin, and nose.
Endocrine system	Controls the integrity and duration of gestation by maintaining the corpus luteum via hCG secretion; production of estrogen, progesterone, hPL, and other hormones and growth factors via the placenta; release of oxytocin (by the posterior pituitary gland), prolactin (by the anterior pituitary), and relaxin (by the ovary, uterus, and placenta).
Immune system	A general enhancement of innate immunity (inflammatory response and phagocytosis) and suppression of adaptive immunity (protective response to a specific foreign antigen) takes place during pregnancy. These immunologic alterations help prevent the mother's immune system from rejecting the fetus (foreign body), increase her risk of developing certain infections, and influence the course of chronic disorders such as autoimmune diseases.

are eating less in an effort to control their weight, putting them at greater risk of inadequate nutrient intake.

Nutritional Requirements During Pregnancy

Pregnancy is one of the most nutritionally demanding periods of a woman's life. Gestation involves rapid cell division and organ development, and an adequate supply of nutrients is essential to support this tremendous fetal growth.

Most women are usually motivated to eat properly during pregnancy for the sake of the fetus. The Food and Nutrition Board of the National Research Council has made recommendations for nutrient intakes for people living in the United States. The DRIs are more comprehensive than previous nutrient guidelines issued by the board. They have replaced previous recommendations because they are not limited to preventing deficiency diseases; rather, the DRIs incorporate current concepts about the role of nutrients and food components in reducing the risk of chronic disease, developmental disorders, and other related problems. The DRIs can be used to plan and assess diets for healthy people (Dudek, 2006).

These dietary recommendations also include information for women who are pregnant or lactating, because growing fetal and maternal tissues require increased quantities of essential dietary components. For example, the current DRIs suggest an increase in the pregnant woman's intake of protein from 60 to 80 g per day, iron from 18 to 27 g per day, and folate from 400 to 600 mcg per day, along with an increase of 300 calories per day over the recommended intake of 1,800 to 2,200 calories for nonpregnant women (IOM, 2006a, 2006b, 2006c, 2006d, 2006e, 2006f) (Table 11.5).

For a pregnant woman to meet recommended DRIs, it is important for her to eat according to the USDA's Food Guide Pyramid (Fig. 11.5). The 2005 Dietary Guidelines for Americans are the basis for federal nutrition policy. The Food Guide Pyramid provides guidance to help implement these guidelines. A summary of the new guidelines is as follows:

• Eat a variety of food from all food groups using portion control.
• Increase intake of vitamins, minerals, and dietary fiber.
• Lower intake of saturated fats, trans fats, and cholesterol.
• Consume adequate synthetic folic acid from supplements or from fortified foods.
• Increase intake of fruits, vegetables, and whole grains.
• Balance calorie intake with exercise to maintain ideal healthy weight (USDA, 2005).

An eating plan that follows the pyramid should provide sufficient nutrients for a healthy pregnancy. Except

TABLE 11.5 **DIETARY RECOMMENDATIONS FOR THE PREGNANT AND LACTATING WOMAN**

Nutrient	Nonpregnant Women	Pregnant Woman	Lactating Woman
Calories	2,200	2,500	2,700
Protein	60 g	80 g	80 g
Water/fluids	6–8 glasses daily	8 glasses daily	8 glasses daily
Vitamin A	700 mcg	770 mcg	1,300 mcg
Vitamin C	75 mg	85 mg	120 mg
Vitamin D	5 mcg	5 mcg	5 mcg
Vitamin E	15 mcg	15 mcg	19 mcg
B1 (thiamine)	1.1 mg	1.5 mg	1.5 mg
B2 (riboflavin)	1.1 mg	1.4 mg	1.6 mg
B3 (niacin)	14 mg	18 mg	17 mg
B6 (pyridoxine)	1.3 mg	1.9 mg	2 mg
B12 (cobalamin)	2.4 mcg	2.6 mcg	2.8 mcg
Folate	400 mcg	600 mcg	500 mcg
Calcium	1,000 mg	1,000 mg	1,000 mg
Phosphorus	700 mg	700 mg	700 mg
Iodine	150 mcg	220 mcg	290 mcg
Iron	18 mg	27 mg	9 mg
Magnesium	310 mg	350 mg	310 mg
Zinc	8 mg	11 mg	12 mg

Sources: Institute of Medicine, 2006a, 2006b, 2006c, 2006d, 2006e, 2006f.

MyPyramid Plan for Moms

Food Group	1st Trimester	2nd and 3rd Trimesters	What counts as 1 cup or 1 ounce?	Remember to...
	Eat this amount from each group daily.*			
Fruits 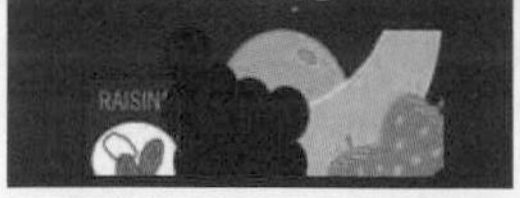	2 cups	2 cups	1 cup fruit or juice, ½ cup dried fruit	*Focus on fruits*—Eat a variety of fruit.
Vegetables 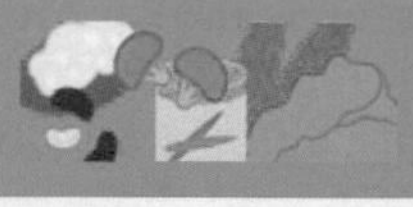	2½ cups	3 cups	1 cup raw or cooked vegetables or juice, 2 cups raw leafy vegetables	*Vary your veggies*—Eat more dark green and orange vegetables and cooked dry beans.
Grains 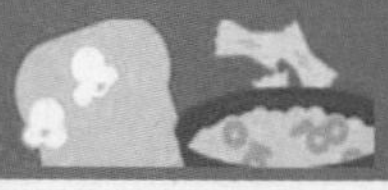	6 ounces	8 ounces	1 slice bread; ½ cup cooked pasta, rice, cereal; 1 ounce ready-to-eat cereal	*Make half your grains whole*—Choose whole instead of refined grains.
Meat and Beans 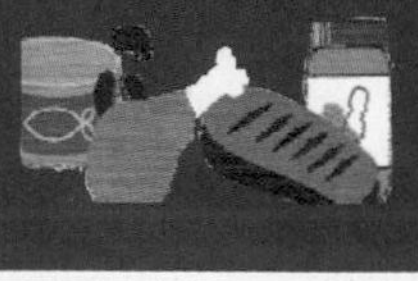	5½ ounces	6½ ounces	1 ounce lean meat, poultry, fish; 1 egg; ¼ cup cooked dry beans; ½ ounce nuts; 1 tablespoon peanut butter	*Go lean with protein*—Choose low-fat or lean meats and poultry.
Milk 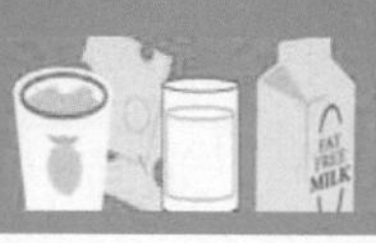	3 cups	3 cups	1 cup milk, 8 ounces yogurt, 1½ ounces cheese, 2 ounces processed cheese	*Get your calcium-rich foods*—Go low-fat or fat-free when you choose milk, yogurt, and cheese.

*These amounts are for an average pregnant woman. You may need more or less than the average. Check with your doctor to make sure you are gaining weight as you should.

FIGURE 11.5 Food Guide Pyramid for pregnancy.

for iron, folic acid, and calcium, most of the nutrients a woman needs during pregnancy can be obtained by making healthy food choices. However, a vitamin and mineral supplement is generally prescribed.

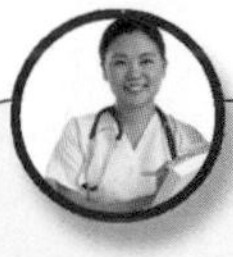

▶ *Take* NOTE!

Good food sources of folic acid include dark green vegetables, such as broccoli, romaine lettuce, and spinach; baked beans; black-eyed peas; citrus fruits; peanuts; and liver.

Fish and shellfish are an important part of a healthy diet because they contain high-quality protein, are low in saturated fat, and contain omega-3 fatty acids. However, nearly all fish and shellfish contain traces of mercury and some contain higher levels of mercury that may harm a developing fetus if ingested by pregnant women in large amounts. With this in mind, the FDA and the Environmental Protection Agency (EPA) are advising women who may become pregnant, pregnant women, and nursing mothers to do the following:

- Avoid eating shark, swordfish, king mackerel, and tilefish.
- Eat up to 12 ounces (two average meals) weekly of these fish:
  - Shrimp, canned light tuna, salmon
  - Pollock and catfish
- Check local advisories about the safety of fish caught by family and friends in local lakes, rivers, and coastal areas (Hibbeln et al., 2007)

EVIDENCE-BASED PRACTICE 11.1
Effects of Zinc Supplementation in Pregnancy on Maternal, Fetal, Neonatal, and Infant Outcomes

● **Study**

It has been suggested that low serum zinc levels may be associated with suboptimal outcomes of pregnancy such as prolonged labor, atonic postpartum hemorrhage, pregnancy-induced hypertension, preterm labor, and post-term pregnancies, although many of these associations have not yet been established.

Many women of childbearing age may have mild to moderate zinc deficiency. Low zinc levels may cause preterm birth or may prolong labor. It is also possible that zinc deficiency may affect infant growth.

A review of 17 trials, involving over 9,000 women and their babies, found that although zinc supplementation has a small effect on reducing preterm births, it does not help to prevent low-birthweight babies. Finding ways to improve women's overall nutritional status, particularly in low-income areas, will do more to improve the health of mothers and babies than giving pregnant women zinc supplements.

▲ **Findings**

The 14% relative reduction in preterm birth for zinc compared with placebo was primarily in the group of studies involving women of low income, and this has some relevance in areas of high perinatal mortality. There was no convincing evidence that zinc supplementation during pregnancy results in other important benefits. Since the preterm association could well reflect poor nutrition, studies to address ways of improving the overall nutritional status of populations in impoverished areas, rather than focusing on micronutrient and/or zinc supplementation in isolation, should be a priority.

■ **Nursing Implications**

Nurses can dispel any myths associated with the use of zinc as a preventive measure for preterm births, since research doesn't seem to validate this. Encouraging better nutrition, increasing water consumption, and taking rest periods throughout the day are all associated with longevity of pregnancy. At this point, the exact triggering mechanism for preterm labor is not known.

Mahomed, K., Bhutta, Z., & Middleton, P. (2007). Zinc supplementation for improving pregnancy and infant outcome. *Cochrane Database of Systematic Reviews,* Issue 2. Art. No.: CD000230. DOI: 10.1002/14651858.CD000230.pub3.

Maternal Weight Gain

The amount of weight that a woman gains during pregnancy is not as important as what she eats. A woman can lose extra weight after a pregnancy, but she can never make up for a poor nutritional status during the pregnancy. Currently, the American College of Obstetricians & Gynecologists (2005) recommends a 25- to 35-pound weight gain during pregnancy. Table 11.6 summarizes the distribution of weight gain during pregnancy.

The best way to assess whether a pregnant woman is consuming enough calories is to follow her pattern of weight gain. If she is gaining in a steady, gradual manner, then she is taking in enough calories. However, consuming an adequate amount of calories doesn't guarantee that her nutrients are sufficient. It is critical to evaluate both the quantity and the quality of the foods eaten.

The IOM has issued recommendations for weight gain during pregnancy based on prepregnancy body mass index (BMI; Box 11.3). A woman who is underweight before pregnancy or who has a low maternal weight gain pattern should be monitored carefully because she is at risk of giving birth to a low-birthweight infant (<2,500 g or 5.5 pounds). Frequently these women simply need advice on what to eat to add weight. Encourage the woman to eat snacks that are high in calories such as nuts, peanut butter, milkshakes, cheese, fruit, yogurt, and ice cream. Any woman who has a prepregnancy BMI of less than 19.8 is considered to be high risk and should be referred to a nutritionist. These women are encouraged to gain 28 to 40 pounds during the pregnancy (IOM, 2006a).

Conversely, women who start a pregnancy while overweight (BMI >25 to 29) run the risk of having a high-

TABLE 11.6   NORMAL DISTRIBUTION OF WEIGHT GAIN DURING PREGNANCY

Component	Weight
Fetus	7.5–8.5 pounds
Blood	4 pounds
Uterus	2 pounds
Breasts	1 pound
Placenta and umbilical cord	1.5 pounds
Fat and protein stores	7.5 pounds
Tissue fluids	2.7 pounds
Amniotic fluid	1.8 pounds
Approximate total weight gain	29 pounds

Sources: ACOG, 2005; Blackburn, 2007; Dudek, 2006.

BOX 11.3 Body Mass Index

Body Mass Index (BMI) provides an accurate estimate of total body fat and is considered a good method to assess overweight and obesity in people. BMI is a weight-to-height ratio calculation that can be determined by dividing a woman's weight in kilograms by her height in meters squared. BMI can also be calculated by weight in pounds divided by the height in inches squared, multiplied by 704.5.

The Centers for Disease Control and Prevention (CDC) categorizes BMI as follows:
• Underweight: less than 18.5
• Healthy weight: 18.5 to 24.9
• Overweight: 25 to 29.9
• Obese: 30 or higher (CDC, 2007)

Use this example to calculate BMI:
Mary is 5-foot-5 tall and weighs 150 pounds.
1. Convert weight into kilograms 150 divided by 2.2 lb/kg = 68.18 kg.
2. Convert height into meters:
   a. 5-foot-5 = 65 inches times 2.54 cm/in = 165.1 cm
   b. 165.1 cm/100 cm = 1.65 m
3. Then square the height in meters: 1.65 times 1.65 = 2.72
4. Calculate BMI 68.18 divided by 2.72 = 25

birthweight infant, with resulting cephalopelvic disproportion and, potentially, a surgical birth. Dieting during pregnancy is never recommended, even for women who are obese. Severe restriction of caloric intake is associated with a decrease in birthweight. Because of the expansion of maternal blood volume and the development of fetal and placental tissues, some weight gain is essential for a healthy pregnancy. Women who gain more than the recommended weight during pregnancy and who fail to lose this weight 6 months after giving birth are at much higher risk of being obese nearly a decade later (ACOG, 2005). Women who are overweight when beginning a pregnancy should gain no more than 15 to 25 pounds during the pregnancy, depending on their nutritional status and degree of obesity (ACOG, 2005).

All pregnant women should aim for a steady rate of weight gain throughout pregnancy. During the first trimester, for women whose prepregnant weight is within the normal weight range, weight gain should be about 3.5 to 5 pounds. For underweight women, weight gain should be at least 5 pounds. For overweight women, weight gain should be about 2 pounds. Much of the weight gained during the first trimester is caused by growth of the uterus and expansion of the blood volume.

During the second and third trimesters, the following pattern is recommended. For women whose prepregnant weight is within the normal weight range, weight

gain should be about 1 pound per week. For underweight women, weight gain should be slightly more than 1 pound per week. For overweight women, weight gain should be about two thirds of a pound per week (Blackburn, 2007).

Nutrition Promotion

Through education, nurses can play an important role in ensuring adequate nutrition for pregnant women. During the initial prenatal visit, health care providers conduct a thorough assessment of a woman's typical dietary practices and address any conditions that may cause inadequate nutrition, such as nausea and vomiting or lack of access to adequate food. Assess and reinforce dietary information at every prenatal visit to promote good nutrition. A normal pregnancy and a well-balanced diet generally provide most of the recommended nutrients except iron and folate, both of which must be supplemented in the form of prenatal vitamins.

The Food Guide Pyramid, developed in 1992 and revised in 2005 by the U.S. Department of Agriculture, is the typical tool used for nutritional education and is recognized by the general population as the gold standard for healthy eating patterns (Dudek, 2006). Use this well-known tool as a basis for dietary instruction and tailor it to meet each woman's individual needs (Teaching Guidelines 11.1).

Special Nutritional Considerations

Many factors play an important role in shaping a person's food habits, and these factors must be taken into account

TEACHING GUIDELINES 11.1

Teaching to Promote Optimal Nutrition During Pregnancy

• Follow the Food Guide Pyramid and select a variety of foods from each group.
• Gain weight in a gradual and steady manner as follows:
  a. Normal-weight woman—25 to 35 pounds
  b. Underweight woman—28 to 40 pounds
  c. Overweight woman—15 to 25 pounds
  d. Obese woman—15 pounds
• Take your prenatal vitamin/mineral supplementation daily.
• Avoid weight-reduction diets during pregnancy.
• Do not skip meals; eat three meals with one or two snacks daily.
• Limit the intake of sodas and caffeine-rich drinks.
• Avoid the use of diuretics during pregnancy.
• Do not restrict the use of salt unless instructed to do so by your health care provider.
• Engage in reasonable physical activity daily.

if nutritional counseling is to be realistic and appropriate. Nurses need to be aware of these factors to ensure individualized teaching and care.

Cultural Variations and Restrictions

Food is important to every cultural group. It is often part of celebrations and rituals. When working with women from various cultures, the nurse needs to adapt American nutritional guidelines to meet their nutritional needs within their cultural framework. Food choices and variations for different cultures might include the following:

- Bread, cereal, rice and pasta group:
  - Bolello
  - Couscous
  - Hau juan
  - Flaxseed
- Vegetable group:
  - Agave
  - Bok choy
  - Jicama
  - Okra
  - Water chestnuts
- Protein group:
  - Bean paste
  - Blood sausage
  - Legumes
  - Shellfish
- Fruit group:
  - Catabopy
  - Kumquats
  - Plantain
  - Yucca fruit
  - Zapate
- Milk and dairy:
  - Buttermilk
  - Buffalo milk
  - Soybean milk

Lactose Intolerance

The best source of calcium is milk and dairy products, but for women with lactose intolerance, adaptations are necessary. Women with lactose intolerance lack an enzyme (lactase) needed for the breakdown of lactose into its component simple sugars, glucose, and galactose. Without adequate lactase, lactose passes through the small intestine undigested and causes abdominal discomfort, gas, and diarrhea. Lactose intolerance is especially common among women of African, Asian, and Middle Eastern descent (Dudek, 2006).

Additional or substitute sources of calcium may be necessary. These may include peanuts, almonds, sunflower seeds, broccoli, salmon, kale, and molasses (Escott-Stump, 2007). In addition, encourage the woman to drink lactose-free dairy products or calcium-enriched orange juice or soy milk.

Vegetarians

Vegetarian diets are becoming increasing prevalent in the United States. People choose a vegetarian diet for various reasons, including environmental, animal rights, philosophical, religious, and health beliefs (Hughes & Brown, 2006). Vegetarians choose not to eat meat, chicken, and fish. Their diets consist mostly of plant-based foods, such as legumes, vegetables, whole grains, nuts, and seeds. Vegetarians fall into groups defined by the types of foods they eat. Lacto-ovo-vegetarians omit red meat, fish, and poultry but eat eggs, milk, and dairy products, in addition to plant-based foods. Lacto-vegetarians consume milk and dairy products along with plant-based foods; they omit eggs, meat, fish, and poultry. Vegans eliminate all foods from animals, including milk, eggs, and cheese, and eat only plant-based foods (Dudek, 2006).

The concern with any form of vegetarianism, especially during pregnancy, is that the diet may be inadequate in nutrients. Other risks of vegetarian eating patterns during pregnancy may include low gestational weight gain, iron-deficiency anemia, compromised protein utilization, and decreased mineral absorption (Dudek, 2006). A diet can become so restrictive that a woman is not gaining weight or is consistently not eating enough from one or more of the food groups. Generally, the more restrictive the diet, the greater the chance of nutrient deficiencies.

Well-balanced vegetarian diets that include dairy products provide adequate caloric and nutrient intake and do not require special supplementation; however, vegan diets do not include any meat, eggs, or dairy products. Pregnant vegetarians must pay special attention to their intake of protein, iron, calcium, and vitamin B12. Suggestions include:

- For protein: substitute soy foods, beans, lentils, nuts, grains, and seeds.
- For iron: eat a variety of meat alternatives, along with vitamin C-rich foods.
- For calcium: substitute soy, calcium-fortified orange juice, and tofu.
- For vitamin B12: eat fortified soy foods and a B12 supplement.

The woman may also take a multivitamin prenatal supplement (Hughes & Brown, 2006).

Pica

Many women experience unusual food cravings during their pregnancy. Having cravings during pregnancy is perfectly normal. Sometimes, however, women crave substances that have no nutritional value and can even be dangerous to themselves and their fetus. **Pica** is the compulsive ingestion of nonfood substances. Pica is derived from the Latin term for magpie, a bird that is known to consume a variety of nonfood substances. Unlike the bird, however, pregnant women who develop a pica habit typically have one or two specific cravings.

The exact cause of pica is not known. Many theories have been advanced to explain it, but none has been proven scientifically. The incidence of pica is difficult to determine, since it is underreported. It is more common in the United States among African-American women compared to other ethnicities, but the practice of pica is not limited to any one geographic area, race, creed, or culture. In the United States, pica is also common in women from rural areas and women with a family history of it (Mikkelsen, Andersen, & Olsen, 2007)

The three main substances consumed by women with pica are soil or clay (geophagia), ice (pagophagia), and laundry starch (amylophagia). Nutritional implications include:

- Soil: replaces nutritive sources and causes iron-deficiency anemia
- Clay: produces constipation; can contain toxic substances and cause parasitic infection
- Ice: can cause iron-deficiency anemia, tooth fractures, freezer burn injuries
- Laundry starch: replaces iron-rich foods, leads to iron deficiencies, and replaces protein metabolism, thus depriving the fetus of amino acids needed for proper development (Blackburn, 2007)

Clinical manifestations of anemia often precede the identification of pica because it is rarely addressed by the health care provider and the woman does not usually volunteer such information (Cunningham et al., 2005). Secrecy surrounding this habit makes research and diagnosis difficult because some women fail to view their behavior as anything unusual, harmful, or worth reporting. Because of the clinical implications, pica should be discussed with all pregnant women as a preventive measure. The topic can be part of a general discussion of cravings, and the nurse should stress the harmful effects outlined above.

Suspect pica when the woman exhibits anemia although her dietary intake is appropriate. Ask about her usual dietary intake, and include questions about the ingestion of nonfood substances. Consider the potential negative outcomes for the pregnant woman and her fetus, and take appropriate action.

Psychosocial Adaptations During Pregnancy
WATCH & LEARN

Pregnancy is a unique time in a woman's life. It is a time of dramatic alterations in her body and her appearance, as well as a time of change in her social status. All these changes occur simultaneously. Concurrent with the physiologic changes within her body systems are psychosocial changes within the mother and family members as they face significant role and lifestyle changes.

Maternal Emotional Responses

Motherhood, perhaps more than any role in society, has acquired a special significance for women. Women are taught they should find fulfillment and satisfaction in the role of the "ever-bountiful, ever-giving, self-sacrificing mother" (Thies & Travers, 2006). With such high expectations, many pregnant women experience various emotions throughout their pregnancy. The woman's approach to these emotions is influenced by her emotional makeup, her sociologic and cultural background, her acceptance or rejection of the pregnancy, whether the pregnancy was planned, if the father is known, and her support network (Alexander et al., 2007).

Despite the wide-ranging emotions associated with the pregnancy, many women experience similar responses. These responses commonly include ambivalence, introversion, acceptance, mood swings, and changes in body image.

Ambivalence

The realization of a pregnancy can lead to fluctuating responses, possibly at the opposite ends of the spectrum. For example, regardless of whether the pregnancy was planned, the woman may feel proud and excited at her achievement while at the same time fearful and anxious of the implications. The reactions are influenced by several factors, including the way the woman was raised, her current family situation, the quality of the relationship with the expectant father, and her hopes for the future. Some women express concern over the timing of the pregnancy, wishing that goals and life objectives had been met before becoming pregnant. Other women may question how a newborn or infant will affect their career or their relationships with friends and family. These feelings can cause conflict and confusion about the pregnancy.

Ambivalence, or having conflicting feelings at the same time, is a universal feeling and is considered normal when preparing for a lifestyle change and new role. Pregnant women commonly experience ambivalence during the first trimester. Usually ambivalence evolves into acceptance by the second trimester, when fetal movement is felt. The woman's personality, her ability to adapt to changing circumstances, and the reactions of her partner will affect her adjustment to being pregnant and her acceptance of impending motherhood.

Introversion

Introversion, or focusing on oneself, is common during the early part of pregnancy. The woman may withdraw and become increasingly preoccupied with herself and her fetus. As a result, her participation with the outside world may be less, and she will appear passive to her family and friends.

This introspective behavior is a normal psychological adaptation to motherhood for most women. Introversion seems to heighten during the first and third trimesters, when the woman's focus is on behaviors that will ensure a safe and health pregnancy outcome. Couples need to be aware of this behavior and should be informed about measures to maintain and support the focus on the family.

Acceptance

During the second trimester, the physical changes of the growing fetus with an enlarging abdomen and fetal movement bring reality and validity to the pregnancy. There are many tangible signs that someone separate from herself is present. The pregnant woman feels fetal movement and may hear the heartbeat. She may see the fetal image on an ultrasound screen and feel distinct parts, recognizing independent sleep and wake patterns. She becomes able to identify the fetus as a separate individual and accepts this.

Many women will verbalize positive feelings about the pregnancy and will conceptualize the fetus. The woman may accept her new body image and talk about the new life within. Generating a discussion about the woman's feelings and offering support and validation at prenatal visits are important.

Mood Swings

Emotional lability is characteristic throughout most pregnancies. One moment a woman can feel great joy, and within a short time she can feel shock and disbelief. Frequently, pregnant women will start to cry without any apparent cause. Some women feel as though they are riding an "emotional roller-coaster." These extremes in emotion can make it difficult for partners and family members to communicate with the pregnant woman without placing blame on themselves for their mood changes. Clear explanations about how common mood swings are during pregnancy are essential.

Change in Body Image

The way in which pregnancy affects a woman's body image varies greatly from person to person. Some women feel as if they have never been more beautiful, whereas others spend their pregnancy feeling overweight and uncomfortable. For some women pregnancy is a relief from worrying about weight, whereas for others it only exacerbates their fears of weight gain. Changes in body image are normal but can be very stressful for the pregnant woman. Offering a thorough explanation and initiating discussion of the expected bodily changes may help the family to cope with them.

Maternal Role Tasks

Reva Rubin (1984) identified maternal tasks that a woman must accomplish to incorporate the maternal role into her personality. Accomplishing these tasks helps the expectant mother to develop her self-concept as a mother and

---

BOX 11.4 **Maternal Role Tasks**

- **Ensuring safe passage throughout pregnancy and birth**
  - Primary focus of the woman's attention
  - First trimester: woman focuses on herself, not on the fetus
  - Second trimester: woman develops attachment of great value to her fetus
  - Third trimester: woman has concern for herself and her fetus as a unit
  - Participation in positive self-care activities related to diet, exercise, and overall well-being
- **Seeking acceptance of infant by others**
  - First trimester: acceptance of pregnancy by herself and others
  - Second trimester: family needs to relate to the fetus as member
  - Third trimester: unconditional acceptance without rejection
- **Seeking acceptance of self in maternal role to infant ("binding in")**
  - First trimester: mother accepts idea of pregnancy, but not of infant
  - Second trimester: with sensation of fetal movement (quickening), mother acknowledges fetus as a separate entity within her
  - Third trimester: mother longs to hold infant and becomes tired of being pregnant
- **Learning to give of oneself**
  - First trimester: identifies what must be given up to assume new role
  - Second trimester: identifies with infant, learns how to delay own desires
  - Third trimester: questions her ability to become a good mother to infant (Rubin, 1984)

---

to form a mutually gratifying relationship with her infant. These tasks are listed in Box 11.4.

Pregnancy and Sexuality

The way a pregnant woman feels and experiences her body during pregnancy can affect her sexuality. The woman's changing shape, emotional status, fetal activity, changes in breast size, pressure on the bladder, and other discomforts of pregnancy result in increased physical and emotional demands. These can produce stress on the sexual relationship between the pregnant woman and her partner. As the changes of pregnancy ensue, many partners become confused, anxious, and fearful of how the relationship may be affected.

Sexual desire of pregnant women may change throughout the pregnancy. During the first trimester, the woman may be less interested in sex because of fatigue, nausea, and fear of disturbing the early embryonic development. During the second trimester, her interest may increase because of the stability of the pregnancy. During the third trimester, her enlarging size may produce discomfort during sexual activity (Frieden & Chan, 2007).

A woman's sexual health is intimately linked to her own self-image. Sexual positions to increase comfort as the pregnancy progresses as well as alternative noncoital modes of sexual expression, such as cuddling, caressing, and holding, should be discussed. Giving permission to talk about and then normalizing sexuality can help enhance the sexual experience during pregnancy and, ultimately, the couple's relationship. If avenues of communication are open regarding sexuality during pregnancy, any fears and myths the couple may have can be dispelled.

Pregnancy and the Partner

Nursing care related to childbirth has expanded from a narrow emphasis on the physical health needs of the mother and infant to a broader focus on family-related, social and emotional needs. One prominent feature of this family-centered approach is the recent movement toward promoting the mother–infant bond. To achieve a truly family-centered practice, nursing must make a comparable commitment to understanding and meeting the needs of the partner in the emerging family. Recent studies suggest that the partner's potential contribution to the infant's overall development has been misperceived or devalued and that the partner's ability and willingness to assume a more active role in the infant's care may have been underestimated.

Reactions to pregnancy and to the psychological and physical changes by the woman's partner vary greatly. Some enjoy the role of being the nurturer, whereas others experience alienation and may seek comfort or companionship elsewhere. Some expectant fathers may view pregnancy as proof of their masculinity and assume the dominant role, whereas others see their role as minimal, leaving the pregnancy up to the woman entirely. Each expectant partner reacts uniquely.

Emotionally and psychologically, expectant partners may undergo less visible changes than women, but most of these changes remain unexpressed and unappreciated (Thies & Travers, 2006). Expectant partners also experience a multitude of adjustments and concerns. Physically, they may gain weight around the middle and experience nausea and other GI disturbances—what is termed couvade syndrome, a sympathetic response to their partner's pregnancy. They also experience ambivalence during early pregnancy, with extremes of emotions (e.g., pride and joy versus an overwhelming sense of impending responsibility).

During the second trimester of pregnancy, partners go through acceptance of their role of breadwinner, caretaker, and support person. They come to accept the reality of the fetus when movement is felt, and they experience confusion when dealing with the woman's mood swings and introspection. During the third trimester, the expectant partner prepares for the reality of this new role and negotiates what the role will be during the labor and birthing process. Many express concern about being the primary support person during labor and birth and worry how they will react when faced with their loved one in pain. Expectant partners share many of the same anxieties as their pregnant partners. However, it is uncommon for them to reveal these anxieties to the pregnant partner or health care professionals. Often, how the expectant partner responds during the third trimester depends on the state of the marriage or partnership. When the marriage or partnership is struggling, the impending increase in responsibility toward the end of pregnancy acts to drive the expectant partner further away. Often it manifests as working late, staying out late with friends, or beginning new or superficial relationships. In the stable marriage or partnership, the expectant partner who may have been struggling to find his or her place in the pregnancy now finds concrete tasks to do—for example, painting the nursery, assembling the car seat, attending Lamaze classes, and so on.

Pregnancy and Siblings

A sibling's reaction to pregnancy is age-dependent. Some children might express excitement and anticipation, whereas others might have negative reactions. A young toddler might regress in toilet training or ask to drink from a bottle again. An older school-aged child may ignore the new addition to the family and engage in outside activities to avoid the new member. The introduction of an infant into the family is often the beginning of sibling rivalry, which results from the child's fear of change in the security of the relationship with his or her parents (Thies & Travers, 2006). Preparation of the siblings for the anticipated birth is imperative and must be designed according to the age and life experiences of the sibling at home. Constant reinforcement of love and caring will help to reduce the older child's fear of change and worry about being replaced by the new family member.

If possible, parents should include siblings in preparation for the birth of the new baby to help them feel as if they have an important role to play (Fig. 11.6). Parents must also continue to focus on the older sibling after the birth to reduce regressive or aggressive behavior toward the newborn.

■■■ Key Concepts

- Pregnancy is a normal life event that involves considerable physical, psychosocial, emotional, and relationship adjustments.
- The signs and symptoms of pregnancy have been grouped into those that are subjective (presumptive)

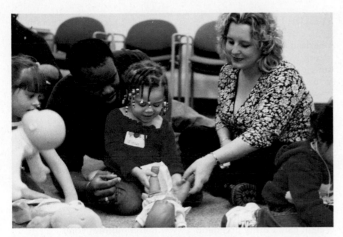

FIGURE 11.6 Parents preparing sibling for the birth of a new baby.

and experienced by the woman herself, those that are objective (probable) and observed by the health care professional, and those that are the positive, beyond-the-shadow-of-a-doubt signs.

- Physiologically, almost every system of a woman's body changes during pregnancy with startling rapidity to accommodate the needs of the growing fetus. A majority of the changes are influenced by hormonal changes.

- The placenta is a unique kind of endocrine gland; it has a feature possessed by no other endocrine organ—the ability to form protein and steroid hormones.

- Occurring in conjunction with the physiologic changes in the woman's body systems are psychosocial changes occurring within the mother and family members as they face significant role and lifestyle changes.

- Commonly experienced emotional responses to pregnancy in the woman include ambivalence, introversion, acceptance, mood swings, and changes in body image.

- Reactions of expectant partners to pregnancy and to the physical and psychological changes in the woman vary greatly.

- A sibling's reaction to pregnancy is age dependent. The introduction of a new infant to the family is often the beginning of sibling rivalry, which results from the established child's fear of change in security of their relationships with their parents. Therefore, preparation of the siblings for the anticipated birth is imperative.

REFERENCES

Alexander, L. L., et al. (2007). *New dimensions in women's health* (4th ed.). Sudbury, MA: Jones and Bartlett Publishers.

American College of Obstetricians and Gynecologists (ACOG). (2005). Body mass index. Provider advice, and target gestational weight gain. *Obstetrics & Gynecology, 105*(3), 633–638.

Arenson, J., & Drake, P. (2007). *Maternal and newborn health.* Sudbury, MA: Jones and Bartlett Publishers.

Blackburn, S. T. (2007). *Maternal, fetal, and neonatal physiology: A clinical perspective* (3rd ed.). St. Louis, MO: Saunders Elsevier.

Centers for Disease Control and Prevention (CDC). (2007). BMI for adults: Body mass index calculator. Available at: http://www.cdc.gov/nccdphp/dnpa/bmi/calc-bmi.htm

Cunningham, F., et al. (2005). *William's obstetrics* (22nd ed.). New York: McGraw-Hill.

Dudek, S. G. (2006). *Nutrition essentials for nursing practice* (5th ed.). Philadelphia: Lippincott Williams & Wilkins.

Escott-Stump, S. (2007). *Nutrition and diagnosis-related care* (6th ed.). Philadelphia: Lippincott Williams & Wilkins.

Fitzgerald, M. P., & Graziano, S. (2007). Anatomic and functional changes in the lower urinary tract during pregnancy. *Urologic Clinics of North America, 34*(1), 7–12.

Frieden, F. J., & Chan, Y. (2007). Antepartum care. In R. E. Rakel & E. T. Bope (Eds.), *Conn's current therapy* (Section 16; pp. 1169–1175). Philadelphia: Saunders Elsevier.

Graham, H. (2007). Breast health and pregnancy. *British Journal of Midwifery, 15*(3), 137–140.

Hackley, B., Kriebs, J. M., & Rousseau, M. E. (2007). *Primary care of women: A guide for midwives and women's health providers.* Sudbury, MA: Jones and Bartlett Publishers.

Hibbeln, J. R., Davis, J. M., Steer, C., Emmett, P., Rogers, I., Williams, C., & Golding, J. (2007). Benefits may outweigh risks of maternal seafood consumption in pregnancy. *Lancet, 369*(9561), 578–585.

Hughes, J. V., & Brown, J. (2006). A meat-free pregnancy. *Vegetarian Times,* April (340), 23–25.

Institute of Medicine (IOM). (2006a). *Nutrition during pregnancy. Part I: Weight gain. Part II: Nutrient supplements.* National Academy of Sciences. Washington, DC: National Academy Press.

Institute of Medicine (IOM). (2006b). *Dietary reference intakes for calcium, phosphorus, magnesium, vitamin D and fluoride.* Washington, DC: National Academy Press.

Institute of Medicine (IOM). (2006c). *Dietary reference intakes for thiamine, riboflavin, niacin, vitamin B6, vitamin B 12, pantothenic acid, biotin, and choline.* Washington, DC: National Academy Press.

Institute of Medicine (IOM). (2006d). *Dietary reference intakes for vitamin C, vitamin E, selenium, and carotenoids.* Washington, DC: National Academy Press.

Institute of Medicine (IOM). (2006e). *Dietary reference intakes for vitamin A, vitamin K, arsenic, boron, chromium, copper, iodine, manganese, molybdenum, nickel, silicon, vanadium, and zinc.* Washington, DC: National Academy Press.

Institute of Medicine (IOM). (2006f). *Dietary reference intakes for energy, carbohydrates, fiber, protein and amino acids.* Washington, DC: National Academy Press.

Jeyabalan, A., & Lain, K. Y. (2007). Anatomic and functional changes in the upper urinary tract during pregnancy. *Urologic Clinics of North America, 34*(1), 1–6.

Ko, C. W. (2006). Risk factors for gallstone-related hospitalization during pregnancy and the postpartum. *American Journal of Gastroenterology, 101*(10), 2263–2268.

Lane, C. A. (2007). Nausea and vomiting in pregnancy: A tailored approach to treatment. *Clinical Obstetrics & Gynecology, 50*(1), 100–111.

Levano, K. J., Cunningham, F. G., Alexander, J. M., et al. (2007). *Williams' manual of obstetrics: Pregnancy complications* (22nd ed.). New York: McGraw-Hill.

Likes, R. L., & Rittenhouse, E. (2007). Pregnancy diagnosis. *eMedicine.* Available at: http://www.emedicine.com/med/topic3277.htm

Martin, S. R., & Foley, M. R. (2006). Intensive care in obstetrics: An evidence-based review. *American Journal of Obstetrics & Gynecology, 195*(3), 673–689.

Mashburn, J. (2006). Etiology, diagnosis, and management of vaginitis. *Journal of Midwifery & Women's Health, 51*(6), 423–430.

National Academy of Sciences. (2007). *Dietary reference intakes for energy, carbohydrates, fiber, fat, protein and amino acids (macronutrients).* Washington, DC: National Academies Press, pp. 5–64.

Ochedalski, T., Subburaju, S., Wynn, P. C., & Aguilera, G. (2007). Interaction between estrogen and oxytocin on hypothalamic-pituitary-adrenal axis activity. *Journal of Neuroendocrinology, 19*(3), 189–197.

Osman, H., Rubeiz, N., Tamim, H., & Nassar, A. H. (2007). Risk factors for the development of striae gravidarum. *American Journal of Obstetrics & Gynecology, 196*(1), 62–65.

Poppe, K., Velkeniers, B., & Glinoer, D. (2007). Thyroid disease and female reproduction. *Clinical Endocrinology, 66*(3), 309–321.

Pretorius, C., Jagatt, A., & Lamont, R. F. (2007). The relationship between periodontal disease, bacterial vaginosis, and preterm birth. *Journal of Perinatal Medicine, 35*(2), 93–99.

Rubin, R. (1984). *Maternal identity and the maternal experience.* New York: Springer.

Thies, K. M., & Travers, J. F. (2006). *Handbook of human development for health care professionals.* Sudbury, MA: Jones and Bartlett Publishers.

Torgersen, K. L., & Curran, C. A. (2006). A systematic approach to the physiologic adaptations of pregnancy. *Critical Care Nursing Quarterly, 29*(1), 2–19.

Tunzi, M., & Gray, G. R. (2007). Common skin conditions during pregnancy. *American Family Physician, 75*(2), 211–218.

United States Department of Agriculture (USDA). (2005). *Dietary guidelines for Americans 2005.* Center for Nutrition Policy and Promotion. Available: http://www.mypyramid.gov/

Walsh, D. (2007). *Evidence-based care for normal labor and birth: A guide for midwives.* London: Taylor & Francis, Inc.

WEBSITES

American College of Nurse Midwives: 202-347-5445, www.acnm.org

American College of Obstetricians and Gynecologists: www.acog.com

Association of Women's Health: Obstetrics & Neonatal Nurses: www.awhonn.org

Dietary Guidelines for Americans: http://www.nal.usda.gov/fnic/dga

International Childbirth Education Association: www.icea.org

March of Dimes: www.modimes.org

Mayo Clinic Pregnancy Center: www.mayoclinic.org

National Center for Education in Maternal and Child Health: www.ncemch.org

Nutrition during pregnancy and breastfeeding: www.nal.usda.gov/fnic/pubs/topics/pregnancy/precom.html

Vegan diet during pregnancy: www.vrg.org/nutrition/veganpregnancy.htm

Weight gain during pregnancy: www.marchofdimes.com/pnhec/159_153.asp

CHAPTER WORKSHEET

MULTIPLE CHOICE QUESTIONS

1. What factors would change during a pregnancy if the hormone progesterone were reduced or withdrawn?

   a. The woman's gums would become red and swollen and would bleed easily.

   b. The uterus would contract more and peristalsis would increase.

   c. Morning sickness would increase and would be prolonged.

   d. It would inhibit the secretion of prolactin by the pituitary gland.

2. Which of the following is a presumptive sign or symptom of pregnancy?

   a. Restlessness

   b. Elevated mood

   c. Urinary frequency

   d. Low backache

3. When obtaining a blood test for pregnancy, which hormone would the nurse expect the test to measure?

   a. hCG

   b. hPL

   c. FSH

   d. LH

4. During pregnancy, which of the following should the expectant mother reduce or avoid?

   a. Raw meat or uncooked shellfish

   b. Fresh, washed fruits and vegetables

   c. Whole grains

   d. Protein and iron from meat sources

5. A feeling expressed by most women upon learning they are pregnant is:

   a. Acceptance

   b. Depression

   c. Jealousy

   d. Ambivalence

6. Reva Rubin identified four major tasks that the pregnant woman undertakes to form a mutually gratifying relationship with her infant. What is "binding in"?

   a. Ensuring safe passage through pregnancy, labor, and birth

   b. Seeking acceptance of this infant by others

   c. Seeking acceptance of self as mother to the infant

   d. Learning to give of oneself on behalf of the infant

CRITICAL THINKING EXERCISES

1. When interviewing a woman at her first prenatal visit, the nurse asks about her feelings. The woman replies, "I'm frightened and confused. I don't know whether I want to be pregnant or not. Being pregnant means changing our whole life, and now having somebody to care for all the time. I'm not sure I would be a good mother. Plus I'm a bit afraid of all the changes that would happen to my body. Is this normal? Am I okay?"

   a. How should the nurse answer this question?

   b. What specific information is needed to support the client during this pregnancy?

2. Sally, age 23, is 9 weeks pregnant. At her clinic visit she says, "I'm so tired I can barely make it home from work. Then once I'm home, I don't have the energy to make dinner." She says she is so sick in the morning that she is frequently late to work and spends much of the day in the bathroom. Sally's current lab work is within normal limits.

   a. What explanation can the nurse offer Sally about her discomforts?

   b. What interventions can the nurse offer to Sally?

3. Bringing a new infant into the family affects the siblings. What strategies can a nurse discuss when a mother asks how to deal with this?

STUDY ACTIVITIES

1. Go to your local health department's maternity clinic and interview several women regarding their feelings and the bodily changes that have taken place since they became pregnant. Based on your findings, place them into appropriate trimesters of their pregnancy.

2. Search the Internet for information about the psychological changes that occur during pregnancy. Share your websites with your clinical group.

3. During pregnancy, the plasma volume increases by 50% but the RBC volume increases by only 25% to 33%. This disproportion is manifested as

   _____.

4. When a pregnant woman in her third trimester lies on her back and experiences dizziness and lightheadedness, the underlying cause of this is

   _____.

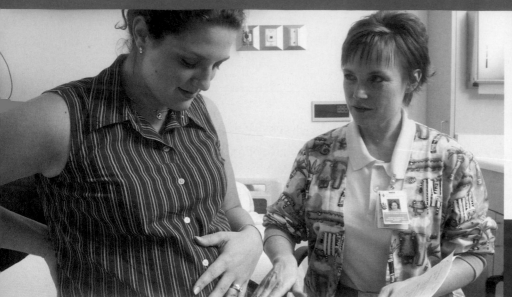

CHAPTER 12

NURSING MANAGEMENT DURING PREGNANCY

KEY TERMS

alpha–fetoprotein
amniocentesis
biophysical profile
chorionic villus
   sampling (CVS)

gravida
high–risk pregnancy
linea nigra
natural childbirth

para
perinatal education
preconception care

LEARNING OBJECTIVES

Upon completion of the chapter, the learner will be able to:

1. Define the key terms used in this chapter.
2. Identify the information typically collected at the initial prenatal visit.
3. Explain the assessments completed at follow-up prenatal visits.
4. Describe the tests used to assess maternal and fetal well-being, including nursing management for each.
5. Outline appropriate nursing management to promote maternal self-care and to minimize the common discomforts of pregnancy.
6. List the key components of perinatal education.

Linda and her husband, Rob, are eager to start a family within the next year. They are stable in their careers and financially secure. They decide to check out a new nurse-midwife practice associated with the local hospital, and they go for a preconception appointment. They leave their appointment overwhelmed with all the information they were given about having a healthy pregnancy.

Wow

The secret of human touch is simple: showing a sincere liking and interest in people. Nurses need to use touch often.

P̲regnancy is a time of many physiologic and psychological changes that can positively or negatively affect the woman, her fetus, and her family. Misconceptions, inadequate information, and unanswered questions about pregnancy, birth, and parenthood are common. The ultimate goal of any pregnancy is the birth of a healthy newborn, and nurses play a major role in helping the pregnant woman and her partner achieve this goal. Ongoing assessment and education are essential.

This chapter describes the nursing management required during pregnancy. It begins with a brief discussion of preconception care and then describes the assessment of the woman at the first prenatal visit and on follow-up visits. The chapter discusses tests commonly used to assess maternal and fetal well-being, including specific nursing management related to each test. The chapter also identifies important strategies to minimize the common discomforts of pregnancy and promote self-care. Lastly, the chapter discusses perinatal education, including childbirth education, birthing options, care provider options, preparation for breastfeeding or bottle feeding, and final preparation for labor and birth.

Preconception Care

Ideally, couples thinking about having a child should schedule a visit with their health care provider for preconception counseling to ensure that they are in the best possible state of health before pregnancy. **Preconception care** is the promotion of the health and well-being of a woman and her partner before pregnancy. The goal of preconception care is to identify any areas such as health problems, lifestyle habits, or social concerns that might unfavorably affect pregnancy (Dunlop, Jack, & Frey, 2007).

Risk Factors for Adverse Pregnancy Outcomes

Preconception care is just as important as prenatal care to reduce adverse pregnancy outcomes such as maternal and infant mortality, preterm births, and low-birthweight infants. Adverse pregnancy outcomes constitute a major public health challenge: 12% of infants are born premature; 8% are born with low birthweight; 3% have major birth defects; and 32% of women suffer pregnancy complications (Centers for Disease Control & Prevention [CDC], 2007b).

Risk factors for these adverse pregnancy outcomes are prevalent among women of reproductive age, as demonstrated by the following statistics:

- 12% of women smoke during pregnancy, contributing to fetal addiction to nicotine.
- 13% consume alcohol during pregnancy, leading to fetal alcohol spectrum disorder.
- 70% of women do not take folic acid supplements, increasing the risk of neural tube defects in the newborn.

Taking folic acid reduces the incidence of neural tube defects by two thirds.
- 32% of women starting a pregnancy are obese, which may increase their risk of developing hypertension, diabetes, and thromboembolic disease and may increase the need for cesarean birth.
- 3% take prescription or over-the-counter drugs that are known teratogens (substances harmful to the developing fetus).
- 5% of women have preexisting medical conditions that can negatively affect pregnancy if unmanaged (CDC, 2007b).

All of the factors above pose risks to pregnancy and could be addressed with early interventions if the woman sought preconception health care. Specific recognized risk factors for adverse pregnancy outcomes that fall into one or more of the above categories are listed in Box 12.1.

The period of greatest environmental sensitivity and consequent risk for the developing embryo is between days 17 and 56 after conception. The first prenatal visit, which is usually a month or later after a missed menstrual period, may occur too late to affect reproductive outcomes associated with abnormal organogenesis secondary to poor lifestyle choices. In some cases, such as with unplanned pregnancies, women may delay seeking health care, denying that they are pregnant. Thus, commonly used prevention practices may begin too late to avert the morbidity and mortality associated with congenital anomalies and low birthweight (Atrash et al., 2006). Therefore, it is best that the woman and her partner seek preconception care.

W̲hat is the purpose of couples like Linda and Rob going for preconception counseling? What are the goals of preconception care for this couple?

BOX 12.1 Risk Factors for Adverse Pregnancy Outcomes

- Taking retinoic acid (Accutane) to clear cystic acne
- Alcohol use
- Anti-epileptic drugs
- Autoimmune disorders
- Diabetes (preconception)
- Folic acid deficiency
- HIV/AIDS
- Maternal phenylketonuria (PKU)
- Rubella seronegativity
- Obesity
- STI
- Smoking (CDC, 2006)
- Underweight

Sources: CDC (2008); NIH (2008); March of Dimes (2008).

Nursing Management

Preconception care involves obtaining a complete health history and physical examination of the woman and her partner. Key areas include:

- Immunization status of the woman
- Underlying medical conditions, such as cardiovascular and respiratory problems or genetic disorders
- Reproductive health data, such as pelvic examinations, use of contraceptives, and sexually transmitted infections (STIs)
- Sexuality and sexual practices, such as safer-sex practices and body image issues
- Nutrition history and present status
- Lifestyle practices, including occupation and recreational activities
- Psychosocial issues such as levels of stress, exposure to abuse and violence
- Medication and drug use, including use of tobacco, alcohol, over-the-counter and prescription medications, and illicit drugs
- Support system, including family, friends, and community (Fig. 12.1 gives a sample preconception screening tool)

This information provides a foundation for planning health-promotion activities and education. For example, to have a positive impact on the pregnancy:

- Ensure that the woman's immunizations are up to date.
- Take a thorough history of both partners to identify any medical or genetic conditions that need treatment or a referral to specialists.
- Identify history of STIs and high-risk sexual practices so they can be modified.
- Complete a dietary history combined with nutritional counseling.
- Gather information regarding exercise and lifestyle practices to encourage daily exercise for well-being and weight maintenance.
- Stress the importance of taking folic acid to prevent neural tube defects.
- Urge the woman to achieve optimal weight before a pregnancy.
- Identify work environment and any needed changes to promote health.
- Address substance use issues, including smoking and drugs.
- Identify victims of violence and assist them to get help.
- Manage chronic conditions such as diabetes and asthma.
- Educate the couple about environmental hazards, including metals and herbs.
- Offer genetic counseling to identify carriers.
- Suggest the availability of support systems, if needed (Graham, 2006).

Nurses can act as advocates and educators, creating healthy, supportive communities for women and their partners in the childbearing phases of their lives. It is important to enter into a collaborative partnership with the woman and her partner, enabling them to examine their own health and its influence on the health of their future baby. Provide information to allow the woman and her partner to make an informed decision about having a baby, but keep in mind that this decision rests solely with the couple.

▶ *Take* NOTE!

"Preconception care should be integrated into the women's health care continuum to achieve high levels of lifetime wellness for all women" (Dunlop, Jack, & Frey, 2007).

*L*inda and Rob decide to change several aspects of their lifestyle and nutritional habits before conceiving a baby, based on advice from the nurse-midwife. They both want to lose weight, stop smoking, and increase their intake of fruits and vegetables. How will these lifestyle and dietary changes benefit Linda's future pregnancy? What other areas might need to be brought up to date to prepare for a future pregnancy?

The First Prenatal Visit

Once a pregnancy is suspected and, in some cases, tentatively confirmed by a home pregnancy test, the woman should seek prenatal care to promote a healthy outcome. Although the most opportune window (preconception) for improving pregnancy outcomes may be missed, appropriate nursing management starting at conception and continuing throughout the pregnancy can have a positive impact on the health of pregnant women and their unborn children.

The assessment process begins at this initial prenatal visit and continues throughout the pregnancy. The initial visit is an ideal time to screen for factors that might place the woman and her fetus at risk for problems such as preterm delivery. The initial visit also is an optimal time to begin educating the client about changes that will affect her life.

Counseling and education of the pregnant woman and her partner are critical to ensure healthy outcomes for mother and her infant. Pregnant women and their partners frequently have questions, misinformation, or misconceptions about what to eat, weight gain, physical discomforts, drug and alcohol use, sexuality, and the birthing process. The nurse needs to allow time to answer questions and provide anticipatory guidance during the pregnancy and to make appropriate community referrals to meet the needs of these clients. To address these issues and foster the

PRECONCEPTION SCREENING AND COUNSELING CHECKLIST

NAME	BIRTHPLACE	AGE

DATE: / /   ARE YOU PLANNING TO GET PREGNANT IN THE NEXT SIX MONTHS? ___ Y ___N

IF YOUR ANSWER TO A QUESTION IS YES, PUT A CHECK MARK ON THE LINE IN FRONT OF THE QUESTION. FILL IN OTHER INFORMATION THAT APPLIES TO YOU.

DIET AND EXERCISE

What do you consider a healthy weight for you?_____
___Do you eat three meals a day?
___Do you follow a special diet (vegetarian, diabetic, other)?
___Which do you drink (__ coffee __ tea __ cola __ milk __ water __ soda/pop
other_____)?
___Do you eat raw or undercooked food (meat, other)?
___Do you take folic acid?
___Do you take other vitamins daily (__ multivitamin __ vitamin A __ other)?
___Do you take dietary supplements (__ black cohosh __ pennyroyal __ other)?
___Do you have current/past problems withh eating disorders?
___Do you exercise? Type/frequency:_____
Notes:

LIFESTYLE

___Do you smoke cigarettes or use other tobacco products?
   How many cigarettes/packs a day?_____
___Are you exposed to second-hand smoke?
___Do you drink alcohol?
   What kind?_____How often?_____How much?_____
___Do you use recreational drugs (cocaine, heroin, ecstasy, meth/ice, other)?
   List:_____
___Do you see a dentist regularly?
   What kind of work do you do?_____
___Do you work or live near possible hazards (chemicals, x-ray or other radiation,
   lead)? List:_____
___Do you use saunas or hot tubs?
Notes:

MEDICATION /DRUGS

___Are you taking prescribed drugs (Accutane, valproic acid, blood thinners)? List
   them_____
___Are you taking non-prescribed drugs?
   List them:_____
___Are you using birth control pills?
___Do you get injectable contraceptives or shots for birth control?
___Do you use any herbal remedies or alternative medicine?
   List:_____
NOTES:

MEDICAL/FAMILY HISTORY

Do you have or have you ever had:
___Epilepsy?
___Diabetes?
___Asthma?
___High blood pressure?
___Heart disease?
___Anemia?
___Kidney or bladder disorders?
___Thyroid disease?
___Chickenpox?
___Hepatitis C?
___Digestive problems?
___Depression or other mental health problem?
___Surgeries?
___Lupus?
___Scleroderma?
___Other conditions?
Have you ever been vaccinated for:
___Measles, mumps, rubella?
___Hepatitis B?
___Chickenpox?
NOTES:

WOMEN'S HEALTH

___Do you have any problems with your menstrual cycle?
___How many times have you been pregnant?
   What was/ were the outcomes(s)?_____
___Did you have difficulty getting pregnant last time?
___I lave you been treated for infertility?
   Have you had surgery on your uterus, cervix, ovaries, or tubes?
___Did you mother take the hormone DES during pregnancy?
   Have you ever had HPV, genital warts or chlamydia?
___Have you ever been treated for a sexually transmitted infection (genital herpes,
   gonorrhea, syphilis, HIV/AIDS, other)? List:_____
NOTES:

GENETICS

Does your family have a history of	Or	Your partner's family
___Hemophilia?		___
___Other bleeding disorders?		___
___Tay-Sachs disease?		___
___Blood diseases (sickle cell, thalassemia, other)?		___
___Muscular dystrophy?		___
___Down syndrome/mental retardation?		___
___Cystic fibrosis?		___
___Birth defects (spine/heart/kidney)?		___

Your ethnic background is:_____
Your partner's ethnic background is: _____
NOTES:

HOME ENVIRONMENT

___Do you feel emotionally supported at home?
___Do you have help from relatives or friends if needed?
___Do you feel you have serious money/financial worries?
___Are you in a stable relationship?
___Do you feel safe at home?
___Does anyone threaten or physically hurt you?
___Do you have pets (cats, rodents, exotic animals)? List:_____
___Do have any contact with soil, cat litter, or sandboxes?

Baby preparation (if planning pregnancy):
___Do you have a place for a baby to sleep?
___Do you need any baby items?
NOTES:

OTHER

IS THERE ANYTHING ELSE YOU'D LIKE ME TO KNOW?

ARE THERE ANY QUESTIONS YOU'D LIKE TO ASK ME?

FIGURE 12.1 Sample preconception screening tool. (Used with permission. Copyright March of Dimes.)

overall well-being of pregnant women and their fetuses, specific National Health Goals have been established (see the Healthy People 2010 box).

Comprehensive Health History

During the initial visit, a comprehensive health history is obtained, including age, menstrual history, prior obstetric history, past medical and surgical history, family history, genetic screening, medication or drug use, and history of exposure to infections (STIs) (Frieden & Chan, 2007). Often, using a prenatal history form (Fig. 12.2) is the best way to document the data collected.

The initial health history typically includes questions about three major areas: the reason for seeking care; the client's past medical, surgical, and personal history, including that of the family and her partner; and the client's reproductive history. During the history-taking process, the nurse and client establish the foundation of a trusting relationship and jointly develop a plan of care for the pregnancy. Tailor this plan to the client's lifestyle as much as possible and focus primarily on education for overall wellness during the pregnancy. The ultimate goal is early detection and prevention of any problems that occur during the pregnancy (Frieden & Chan, 2007).

HEALTHY PEOPLE 2010

Objective	Nursing Implications
Increase the proportion of pregnant women who receive early and adequate prenatal care: • Increase the number of women receiving maternal prenatal care beginning in the first trimester of pregnancy from a baseline of 83% to 90% of live births. • Increase the number of women receiving early and adequate prenatal care from a baseline of 74% to 90% of live births.	Will contribute to reduced rates of perinatal illness, disability, and death by helping to identify possible risk factors and implementing measures to lessen these factors that contribute to poor outcomes
Increase the proportion of pregnant women who attend a series of prepared childbirth classes.	Will contribute to a more pleasant birthing experience because women will be prepared for what they will face; also help in reducing pain and anxiety
Increase abstinence from alcohol, cigarettes, and illicit drugs among pregnant women.	Will help to reduce the wide-ranging effects, such as spontaneous abortion, low birthweight, and preterm birth, associated with prenatal substance use

Source: U.S. Department of Health & Human Services, 2000.

Reason for Seeking Care

The woman commonly comes for prenatal care based on the suspicion that she is pregnant. She may report that she has missed her menstrual period or has had a positive result on a home pregnancy test. Ask the woman for the date of her last menstrual period (LMP). Also ask about any presumptive or probable signs of pregnancy that she might be experiencing. Typically a urine or blood test to check for evidence of human chorionic gonadotropin (hCG) is done to confirm the pregnancy.

Past History

Ask about the woman's past medical and surgical history. This information is important because conditions that the woman experienced in the past (e.g., urinary tract infections) may recur or be exacerbated during pregnancy. Also, chronic illnesses, such as diabetes or heart disease, can increase the risk for complications during pregnancy for the woman and her fetus. Ask about any history of allergies to medications, foods, or environmental substances. Ask about any mental health problems, such as depression or anxiety. Gather similar information about the woman's family and her partner.

The woman's personal history also is important. Ask about her occupation, possible exposure to teratogens, exercise and activity level, recreational patterns (including the use of substances such as alcohol, tobacco, and drugs), use of alternative and complementary therapies, sleep patterns, nutritional habits, and general lifestyle. Each of these may have an impact on the outcome of the pregnancy. For example, if the woman smokes during pregnancy, nicotine in the cigarettes causes vasoconstriction in the mother, leading to reduced placental perfusion. As a result, the newborn may be small for gestational age. The newborn will also go through nicotine withdrawal soon after birth. In addition, no safe level of alcohol ingestion in pregnancy has been determined. Many fetuses exposed to heavy alcohol levels during pregnancy develop fetal alcohol syndrome, a collection of deformities and disabilities.

Reproductive History

The woman's reproductive history includes a menstrual, obstetric, and gynecologic history. Typically, this history begins with a description of the woman's menstrual cycle, including her age at menarche, number of days in her cycle, typical flow characteristics, and any discomfort experienced. The use of contraception also is important, including when the woman last used any contraception.

Ask the woman the date of her LMP to determine the estimated or expected date of birth (EDB) or delivery (EDD). Several methods may be used to estimate the date of birth. Nagele's rule can be used to establish the EDD or EDB. Using this rule, subtract 3 months and then add 7 days to the first day of the LMP. Then correct the year by adding 1 to it. This date has a margin of error of plus or minus 2 weeks. For instance, if a woman reports that her LMP was Oct. 14, 2007, you would subtract 3 months

(text continues on page 295)

Health History Summary
Maternal/Newborn Record System

Page 1 of 2

Patient's name _____

ID. No. _____

_____

_____

Demographic data

Date of birth _____ Age _____ Language ☐ _____ ☐ English ☐ N/A

☐ None

Interpreter ☐ _____

Religion ☐ _____ Race/ethnicity _____

Marital status S M SEP D W   Name of baby's father _____

Allergy/sensitivity

☐ None ☐ Latex

☐ Other _____

Primary/referring physician

Education	Occupation	Full	Part	Self	Unemp	Work Tel No	Home Tel No
Patient		☐	☐	☐	☐		
Father of baby		☐	☐	☐	☐		

Menstrual history

	Menarche yrs	Interval days	Length days	Abnormalities ☐ None	

Certain ☐ Yes ☐ No

LMP ___/___/___ Normal ☐ Yes ☐ No

Positive pregnancy test ___/___/___

☐ Blood
☐ Urine

EDD

By dates ___/___/___

By ultrasound ___/___/___

Date of ultrasound ___/___/___

Pregnancy history	Gravida	Full term	Premature	Spontaneous Ab	Induced Ab	Ectopic	Multiple births	Live

No	Month/year	Infant sex	Weight at birth	Wks gest	Hours in labor	Type of delivery	Anesthesia	Comments/complications
1								
2								
3								
4								
5								
6								
7								

Medical history

Check and detail positive findings below. Use reference numbers.

Obstetric

Patient

1. Anemia _____ ☐
2. Fetal/neonatal death or anomaly _____ ☐
3. Gestational diabetes _____ ☐
4. Hemorrhage _____ ☐
5. Hyperemesis _____ ☐
6. Incompetent cervix _____ ☐
7. Intrauterine growth retardation _____ ☐
8. Isoimmunization _____ ☐
9. Polyhydramnios _____ ☐
10. Postpartum depression _____ ☐
11. Pregnancy-induced hypertension _____ ☐
12. Preterm labor or birth _____ ☐
13. PROM-chorioamnionitis _____ ☐
14. Rhogam given _____ ☐
15. RH neg _____ ☐

Gynecologic

16. Contraceptive use _____ ☐
17. Abnormal PAP _____ ☐
18. Fibroids _____ ☐
19. Gyn· surgery _____ ☐

Gynecologic (cont'd.)

Patient

20. Infertility _____ ☐
21. In utero exposure to DES _____ ☐
22. Uterine/cervical anomaly _____ ☐

Sexually transmitted diseases

23. Chlamydia _____ ☐
24. Gonorrhea _____ ☐
25. Herpes (HSV) _____ ☐
26. Syphilis _____ ☐

Vaginal/genital infections

27. Trichomonas _____ ☐
28. Condylomata _____ ☐
29. Candidiasis _____ ☐

Other infections

30. Toxoplasmosis _____ ☐
31. Group B streptococcus _____ ☐
32. Rubella or immunization _____ ☐
33. Varicella or immunization _____ ☐
34. Cytomegalovirus (CMV) _____ ☐
35. AIDS (HIV) _____ ☐
36. Hepatitis (type _____) _____ ☐ or immunization (type _____)

FIGURE 12.2 Sample prenatal history form. (Used with permission. Copyright Briggs Corporation, 2001.)

Health History Summary
Maternal/newborn record system

Page 2 of 2

Patient's name _____

ID. No. _____

_____

_____

Cardiovascular — Patient / Family
37. Myocardial infarction ____ ☐ ☐
38. Heart disease ____ ☐ ☐
39. Rheumatic fever ____ ☐
40. Valve disease ____ ☐
41. Chronic hypertension ____ ☐ ☐
42. Disease of the aorta ____ ☐ ☐
43. Varicosities Thrombophlebitis ____ ☐ ☐
44. Previous pulmonary embolism ____ ☐
45. Blood disorders ____ ☐ ☐
46. Anemia/ hemoglobinopathy ____ ☐ ☐
47. Blood transfusions ____ ☐
48. Other ____ ☐

Pulmonary
49. Asthma ____ ☐
50. Tuberculosis ____ ☐ ☐
51. Chronic obstructive pulmonary disease ____ ☐ ☐

Endocrine
52. Diabetes ____ ☐ ☐
53. Thyroid dysfunction ____ ☐ ☐
54. Maternal PKU ____ ☐
55. Endocrinopathy ____ ☐ ☐
56. Gastrointestinal ____ ☐
57. Liver disease ____ ☐

Check and detail positive findings below. Use reference numbers.

Renal disease — Patient / Family
58. Cystitis ____ ☐
59. Pyelonephritis ____ ☐
60. Asymptomatic bacteriuria ____ ☐
61. Chronic renal disease ____ ☐ ☐
62. Autoimmune disease ____ ☐ ☐
63. Cancer ____ ☐ ☐

Neurologic disease
64. Cerebrovascular accident ____ ☐ ☐
65. Seizure disorder ____ ☐ ☐
66. Migraine headaches ____ ☐ ☐
67. Degenerative disease ____ ☐ ☐
68. Other ____ ☐

Psychological/surgical
69. Psychiatric disease Mental lillness ____ ☐ ☐
70. Physical abuse or neglect ____ ☐ ☐
71. Emotional abuse or neglect ____ ☐ ☐
72. Addiction (drug, alcohol, nicotine) ____ ☐ ☐
73. Major accidents ____ ☐
74. Surgery ____ ☐
75. Anesthetic complications ____ ☐
76. Non-surgical hospitalization ____ ☐
77. Other ____ ☐
78. **No known disease/problems** ____ ☐

Genetic history — Patient / Father of baby / Family
79. Age 35 or older (female) 50 or older (male) ____ ☐ ☐ ☐
80. Cerebral palsy ____ ☐ ☐ ☐
81. Cleft lip/palate ____ ☐ ☐ ☐
82. Congenital anomalies ____ ☐ ☐ ☐
83. Congenital heart disease ____ ☐ ☐ ☐
84. Consanguinity ____ ☐ ☐ ☐
85. Cystic fibrosis ____ ☐ ☐ ☐
86. Down's syndrome ____ ☐ ☐ ☐
87. Hemophilia ____ ☐ ☐ ☐
88. Huntington's chorea ____ ☐ ☐ ☐

89. Mental retardation ____ ☐ ☐ ☐
90. Muscular dystrophy ____ ☐ ☐ ☐
91. Neural tube defect ____ ☐ ☐ ☐
92. Sickle cell disease or trait ____ ☐ ☐ ☐
93. Tay-sachs disease ____ ☐ ☐ ☐
94. Test for fragile X ____ ☐ ☐ ☐
95. Thalassemia A or B ____ ☐ ☐ ☐
96. Other ____ ☐ ☐ ☐
97. Other ____ ☐ ☐ ☐
98. Other ____ ☐ ☐ ☐

Historical risk status   ☐ **No risk factors noted**

☐ **At risk (identify)**

Signature

FIGURE **12.2** (continued)

(July) and add 7 days (21), then add 1 year (2008). The woman's EDD or EDB is July 21, 2008.

Because of the normal variations in women's menstrual cycles, differences in the normal length of gestation between ethnic groups, and errors in dating methods, there is no such thing as an exact due date. In general, a birth 2 weeks before or 2 weeks after the EDD or EDB is considered normal. Nagele's rule is less accurate if the woman's menstrual cycles are irregular, if the woman conceives while breastfeeding or before her regular menstrual cycle is established, if she is ovulating although she is amenorrheic, or after she discontinues oral contraceptives (Hackley, Kriebs, & Rousseau, 2007).

A gestational or birth calculator or wheel can also be used to calculate the due date (Fig. 12.3). Some practitioners use ultrasound to more accurately determine the gestational age and date the pregnancy.

Typically, an obstetric history provides information about the woman's past pregnancies, including any problems encountered during the pregnancy, labor, delivery, and afterward. Such information can provide clues to problems that might develop in the current pregnancy. Some common terms used to describe and document an obstetric history include:

- Gravid: the state of being pregnant
- **Gravida**: a pregnant woman; gravida I (primigravida) during the first pregnancy, gravida II (secundigravida) during the second pregnancy, and so on

- **Para**: The number of pregnancies that a woman has, regardless of whether the newborn is born alive or dead. Thus, a primipara is a woman who has given birth once after a pregnancy of at least 20 weeks, commonly referred to as a "primip" in clinical practice. A multipara is a woman who has had two or more pregnancies resulting in viable offspring, commonly referred to as a "multip." Nullipara (para 0) is a woman who has not produced a viable offspring.

Other systems may be used to document a woman's obstetric history. These systems often break down the category of para more specifically (Box 12.2).

Information about the woman's gynecologic history is important. Ask about any reproductive tract surgeries the woman has undergone. For example, surgery on the uterus may affect its ability to contract effectively during labor. A history of tubal pregnancy increases the woman's risk for another tubal pregnancy. Also ask about safe-sex practices and any history of STIs.

Physical Examination

The next step in the assessment process is the physical examination, which detects any physical problems that may affect the pregnancy outcome. The initial physical examination provides the baseline for evaluating changes during future visits.

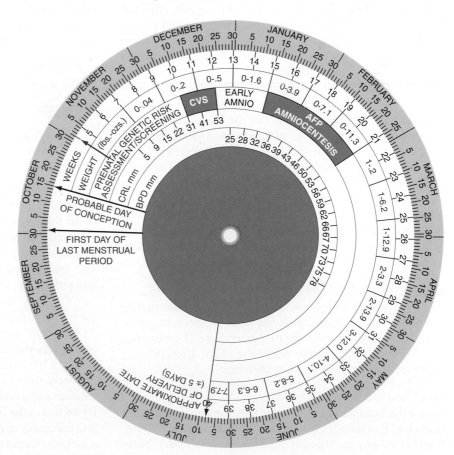

FIGURE 12.3 EDB using a birth wheel. The first day of the woman's last normal menstrual period was October 1. Using the birth wheel, her EDB would be approximately July 8 of the following year. (Used with permission. Copyright March of Dimes, 2007.)

BOX 12.2 Obstetric History Terms

GTPAL or TPAL

G = gravida, T = term births, P = preterm births, A = abortions, L = living children

    G—the current pregnancy

    T—the number of pregnancies ending >37 weeks' gestation, at term

    P—the number of preterm pregnancies ending >20 weeks or viability but before completion of 37 weeks

    A—the number of pregnancies ending before 20 weeks or viability

    L—the number of children currently living

Consider this example:

Mary Johnson is pregnant for the fourth time. She had one abortion at 8 weeks' gestation. She has a daughter who was born at 40 weeks' gestation and a son born at 34 weeks. Mary's obstetric history would be documented as follows:

Using the gravida/para method: gravida 4, para 2

Using the TPAL method: 1112 (T = 1 [daughter born at 40 weeks]; P = 1 [son born at 34 weeks], A = 1 [abortion at 8 weeks]; L = 2 [two living children])

Preparation

Instruct the client to undress and put on a gown. Also ask her to empty her bladder and, in doing so, to collect a urine specimen. Typically this specimen is a clean-catch urine specimen that is sent to the laboratory for a urinalysis to detect a possible urinary tract infection.

Begin the physical examination by obtaining vital signs, including blood pressure, respiratory rate, temperature, and pulse. Also measure the client's height and weight. Abnormalities such as an elevated blood pressure may suggest pregestational hypertension, requiring further evaluation. Abnormalities in pulse rate and respiration require further investigation for possible cardiac or respiratory disease. If the woman weighs less than 100 pounds or more than 200 pounds or there has been a sudden weight gain, report these findings to the primary care provider; medical treatment or nutritional counseling may be necessary.

Head-to-Toe Assessment

A complete head-to-toe assessment is usually performed by the health care professional. Every body system is assessed. Some of the major areas are discussed here. Throughout the assessment, be sure to drape the client appropriately to ensure privacy and prevent chilling.

Head and Neck

Assess the head and neck area for any previous injuries and sequelae. Evaluate for any limitations in range of motion. Palpate for any enlarged lymph nodes or swelling. Note any edema of the nasal mucosa or hypertrophy of gingival tissue in the mouth; these are typical responses to increased estrogen levels in pregnancy. Palpate the thyroid gland for enlargement. Slight enlargement is normal, but marked enlargement may indicate hyperthyroidism, requiring further investigation.

Chest

Auscultate heart sounds, noting any abnormalities. A soft systolic murmur caused by the increase in blood volume may be noted. Anticipate an increase in heart rate by 10 to 15 beats per minute (starting between 14 and 20 weeks of pregnancy) secondary to increases in cardiac output and blood volume. The body adapts to the increase in blood volume with peripheral dilatation to maintain blood pressure. Progesterone causes peripheral dilatation.

Auscultate the chest for breath sounds, which should be clear. Also note symmetry of chest movement and thoracic breathing patterns. Estrogen promotes relaxation of the ligaments and joints of the ribs, with a resulting increase in the anteroposterior chest diameter. Expect a slight increase in respiratory rate to accommodate the increase in tidal volume and oxygen consumption.

Inspect and palpate the breasts. Increases in estrogen and progesterone and blood supply make the breasts feel full and more nodular, with increased sensitivity to touch. Blood vessels become more visible and there is an increase in breast size. Striae gravidarum (stretch marks) may be visible in women with large breasts. Darker pigmentation of the nipple and areola is present, along with enlargement of Montgomery's glands.

 ▶ **Take** NOTE!

Use this opportunity to reinforce and teach breast self-examination.

Abdomen

The appearance of the abdomen depends on the number of weeks of gestation. The abdomen enlarges progressively as the fetus grows. Palpate the abdomen, which should be rounded and nontender. A decrease in muscle tone may be noted due to the influence of progesterone. Inspection also may reveal striae gravidarum (stretch marks) and linea nigra, depending on the duration of the pregnancy.

Typically, the height of the fundus is measured when the uterus arises out of the pelvis to evaluate fetal growth. At 12 weeks' gestation the fundus can be palpated at the symphysis pubis. At 16 weeks' gestation the fundus is midway between the symphysis and the umbilicus. At 20 weeks the fundus can be palpated at the umbilicus and measures approximately 20 cm from the symphysis pubis. By 36 weeks the fundus is just below the ensiform cartilage and measures approximately 36 cm. The uterus maintains a globular/ovoid shape throughout pregnancy (Frieden & Chan, 2007).

Extremities

Inspect and palpate both legs for dependent edema, pulses, and varicose veins. If edema is present in early pregnancy, further evaluation may be needed to rule out gestational hypertension. Ask the woman if she has any pain in her calf that increases when she ambulates. This might indicate a deep vein thrombosis (DVT). High levels of estrogen during pregnancy place women at higher risk for DVT.

Pelvic Examination

The pelvic examination provides information about the internal and external reproductive organs. In addition, it aids in assessing some of the presumptive and probable signs of pregnancy and allows for determination of pelvic adequacy. During the pelvic examination, remain in the examining room to assist the health care provider with any specimen collection, fixation, and labeling. Also provide comfort and emotional support for the woman, who might be anxious. Throughout the examination, explain what is happening and why, and answer any questions as necessary.

External Genitalia

After the client is placed in the lithotomy position and draped appropriately, the external genitalia are inspected visually. They should be free from lesions, discharge, hematomas, varicosities, and inflammation upon inspection. A culture for STIs may be collected at this time.

Internal Genitalia

Next, the internal genitalia are examined via a speculum. The cervix should be smooth, long, thick, and closed. Because of increased pelvic congestion, the cervix will be softened (Goodell's sign), the uterine isthmus will be softened (Hegar's sign), and there will be a bluish coloration of the cervix and vaginal mucosa (Chadwick's sign).

The uterus typically is pear-shaped and mobile, with a smooth surface. It will undergo cell hypertrophy and hyper-plasia so that it enlarges throughout the pregnancy to accommodate the growing fetus.

During the pelvic examination, a Papanicolaou (Pap) smear may be obtained. Additional cultures, such as for gonorrhea and chlamydia screening and group B streptococcus screening, also may be obtained. Ensure that all specimens obtained are labeled correctly and sent to the laboratory for evaluation. A rectal examination is done last to assess for lesions, masses, prolapse, or hemorrhoids.

Once the examination of the internal genitalia is completed and the speculum is removed, a bimanual examination is performed to estimate the size of the uterus to confirm dates and to palpate the ovaries. The ovaries should be small and nontender, without masses. At the conclusion of the bimanual examination, the health care professional reinserts the index finger into the vagina and the middle finger into the rectum to assess the strength and regularity of the posterior vaginal wall.

Pelvic Size, Shape, and Measurements

The size and shape of the women's pelvis can affect her ability to deliver vaginally. Pelvic shape is typically classified as one of four types: gynecoid, android, anthropoid, and platypelloid. Refer to Chapter 13 for an in-depth discussion of pelvic size and shape.

Taking internal pelvic measurements determines the actual diameters of the inlet and outlet through which the fetus will pass. This is extremely important if the woman has never given birth vaginally. Taking pelvic measurements is unnecessary for the woman who has given birth vaginally before (unless she has experienced some type of trauma to the area) because vaginal delivery demonstrates that the pelvis is adequate for the passage of the fetus.

Three measurements are assessed: diagonal conjugate, true conjugate, and ischial tuberosity (Fig. 12.4). The diagonal conjugate is the distance between the anterior surface of the sacral prominence and the anterior surface

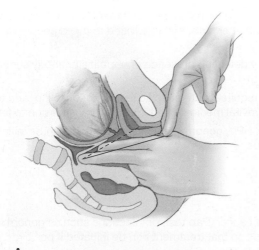

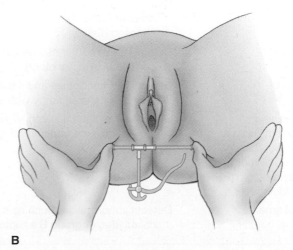

A   **B**

FIGURE 12.4 Pelvic measurements. (**A**) Diagonal conjugate (solid line) and true conjugate (dotted line). (**B**) Ischial tuberosity diameter.

of the inferior margin of the symphysis pubis (Frieden & Chan, 2007). This measurement, usually 12.5 cm or greater, represents the anteroposterior diameter of the pelvic inlet. The diagonal conjugate is the most useful measurement for estimating pelvic size because a misfit with the fetal head occurs if it is too small.

The true conjugate, also called the obstetric conjugate, is the measurement from the anterior surface of the sacral prominence to the posterior surface of the inferior margin of the symphysis pubis. This diameter cannot be measured directly; rather, it is estimated by subtracting 1 to 2 cm from the diagonal conjugate measurement. The average true conjugate diameter is at least 11.5 cm (Cunningham et al., 2005). This measurement is important because it is the smallest front-to-back diameter through which the fetal head must pass when moving through the pelvic inlet.

The ischial tuberosity diameter is the transverse diameter of the pelvic outlet. This measurement is made outside the pelvis at the lowest aspect of the ischial tuberosities. A diameter of 10.5 cm or more is considered adequate for passage of the fetal head (Blackburn, 2007).

Laboratory Tests

A series of tests are generally ordered during the initial visit so that baseline data can be obtained, allowing for early detection and prompt intervention if any problems occur. Tests that are generally conducted for all pregnant women include urinalysis and blood studies. The urine is analyzed for albumin, glucose, ketones, and bacteria casts. Blood studies usually include a complete blood count (hemoglobin, hematocrit, red and white blood cell counts, and platelets), blood typing and Rh factor, a rubella titer, hepatitis B surface antibody antigen, HIV, VDRL, and RPR tests, and cervical smears to detect STIs (Common Laboratory and Diagnostic Tests 12.1). In addition, most offices and clinics have ultrasound equipment available to validate an intrauterine pregnancy and assess early fetal growth.

The need for additional laboratory studies is determined by a woman's history, physical examination findings, current health status, and risk factors identified in the initial interview. Additional tests can be offered, but ultimately the woman and her partner make the decision about undergoing them. Educate the client and her partner about the tests, including the rationale. In addition, support the client and her partner in their decision-making process, regardless of whether you agree with the couple's decision. The couple's decisions about their health care are based on the ethical principle of autonomy, which allows an individual the right to make decisions about his or her own body.

COMMON LABORATORY AND DIAGNOSTIC TESTS 12.1

Test	Explanation
Complete blood cell count (CBC)	Evaluates hemoglobin (12–14 g) and hematocrit (42% +/– 5) levels and red blood cell count (4.2–5.4 million/mm^3) to detect presence of anemia; identifies WBC (5,000–10,000/mm^3), which if elevated may indicate an infection; determines platelet count (150,000–450,000 cubic mL) to assess clotting ability
Blood typing	Determines woman's blood type and Rh status to rule out any blood incompatibility issues early; Rh-negative mother would likely receive RhoGAM (at 28 weeks) if she is Rh sensitive via indirect Coombs test
Rubella titer	Detects antibodies for the virus that causes German measles; if titer is 1:8 or less, the woman is not immune, requires immunization after birth, and is advised to avoid people with undiagnosed rashes
Hepatitis B	Determines if mother has hepatitis B by detecting presence of hepatitis antibody surface antigen (HbsAg) in her blood
HIV testing	Detects HIV antibodies and if positive requires more specific testing, counseling, and treatment during pregnancy with antiretroviral medications to prevent transmission to fetus
STI screening: Venereal Disease Research Laboratory (VDRL) or rapid plasma reagin (RPR) serologic tests	Detects STIs (such as syphilis, herpes, HPV, gonorrhea) so that treatment can be initiated early to prevent transmission to fetus
Cervical smears	Detects abnormalities such as cervical cancer (Pap test) or infections such as gonorrhea, chlamydia, or group B streptococcus so that treatment can be initiated if positive

Sources: Skidmore-Roth 2004; Spratto and Woods, 2004

Remember Linda and Rob, the couple who want to start a family? Ten months after the preconception appointment, Linda calls to make a first prenatal appointment. What key areas will be addressed at this first prenatal visit? What interventions might be suggested for Linda to implement in order to ensure a healthy newborn?

Follow-Up Visits

Continuous prenatal care is important for a successful pregnancy outcome. The recommended follow-up visit schedule for a healthy pregnant woman is as follows:

- Every 4 weeks up to 28 weeks (7 months)
- Every 2 weeks from 29 to 36 weeks
- Every week from 37 weeks to birth

At each subsequent prenatal visit the following assessments are completed:

- Weight and blood pressure, which are compared to baseline values
- Urine testing for protein, glucose, ketones, and nitrites
- Fundal height measurement to assess fetal growth
- Assessment for quickening/fetal movement to determine fetal well-being
- Assessment of fetal heart rate (should be 110 to 160 bpm)

At each follow-up visit, answer questions, provide anticipatory guidance and education, review nutritional guidelines, and evaluate the client for compliance with prenatal vitamin therapy. Throughout the pregnancy, encourage the woman's partner to participate if possible.

Fundal Height Measurement

Fundal height is the distance (in cm) measured with a tape measure from the top of the pubic bone to the top of the uterus (fundus) with the client lying on her back with her knees slightly flexed (Fig. 12.5). Measurement in this

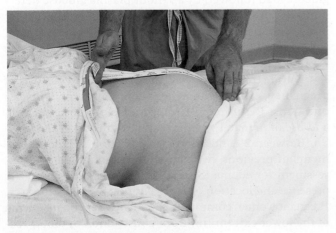

FIGURE 12.5 Fundal height measurement.

way is termed the McDonald's method. Fundal height typically increases as the pregnancy progresses; it reflects fetal growth and provides a gross estimate of the duration of the pregnancy.

Between 12 and 14 weeks' gestation, the fundus can be palpated above the symphysis pubis. The fundus reaches the level of the umbilicus at approximately 20 weeks and measures 20 cm. Fundal measurement should approximately equal the number of weeks of gestation until week 36. For example, a fundal height of 24 cm suggests a fetus at 24 weeks' gestation. After 36 weeks, the fundal height then drops due to lightening and may no longer correspond with the week of gestation.

It is expected that the fundal height will increase progressively throughout the pregnancy, reflecting fetal growth. However, if the growth curve flattens or stays stable, it may indicate the presence of intrauterine growth restriction (IUGR). If the fundal height measurement is greater than 4 cm from the estimated gestational age, further evaluation is warranted if a multifetal gestation has not been diagnosed or hydramnios has not been ruled out (Dillon, 2007).

Fetal Movement Determination

Fetal movement is usually perceived by the client between 16 and 20 weeks' gestation. Perceived fetal movement is most often related to trunk and limb motion and rollovers, or flips (Arenson & Drake, 2007). Fetal movement is a gross indicator of fetal well-being. Decreased fetal movement may indicate asphyxia and IUGR. If compromised, the fetus decreases its oxygen requirements by decreasing activity (Mangesi & Hofmeyr, 2007). A decrease in fetal movement may be related to other factors as well, such as maternal use of central nervous system depressants, fetal sleep cycles, hydrocephalus, bilateral renal agenesis, and bilateral hip dislocation (Arenson & Drake, 2007).

Two suggested techniques for determining fetal movement, also called fetal movement counts, are the Cardiff technique and the Sadovsky technique (Box 12.3). Fetal movement is a noninvasive method of screening and can be easily taught to all pregnant women. Both techniques require client participation.

Instruct the client about how to count fetal movements, the reasons for doing so, and the significance of decreased fetal movements. Urge the client to perform the counts in a relaxed environment and a comfortable position, such as semi-Fowler's or side-lying. Provide the client with detailed information concerning fetal movement counts and stress the need for consistency in monitoring (at approximately the same time each day) and the importance of informing the health care provider promptly of any reduced movements. Providing clients with "fetal kick count" charts to record movement helps promote compliance. There is no established number of fetal movements that indicates fetal well-being, but instruct the

BOX 12.3 **Techniques for Fetal Movement Counts**

Maternal perception of fetal movements or counting fetal movements is an inexpensive, noninvasive method of assessing fetal well-being. Several different techniques, two of which are described below, can be used. Scientific evidence has not shown that one technique is better than another. However, the amount of time required for the client to complete the count varies. Additionally, because counts are highly subjective on the mother's part, consistency is essential when performing fetal movement counts. Fetal movement counts should be done at approximately the same time each day, and further testing should be initiated within 12 hours of a client's perception of decreased activity (Mangesti & Hofmeyr, 2007).

Cardiff Technique
The woman lies or sits and concentrates on fetal movements until she records 10 movements. She must record the length of time during which the 10 movements occurred. She is instructed to notify her health care provider if she doesn't feel at least 10 movements within 1 hour. Further follow-up testing is indicated.

Sadovsky Technique
The woman lies down on her left side for 1 hour after meals and concentrates on fetal movement. Four movements should be felt within 1 hour. If four movements have not been felt within 1 hour, then the woman should monitor movement for a second hour. If after 2 hours four movements haven't been felt, the client should contact her health care provider.

Nursing Procedure 12.1

MEASURING FETAL HEART RATE

Purpose: To assess fetal well-being

1. Assist the woman onto the examining table and have her lie down.
2. Cover her with a sheet to ensure privacy, and then expose her abdomen.
3. Palpate the abdomen to determine the fetal lie, position, and presentation.
4. Locate the back of the fetus (the ideal position to hear the heart rate).
5. Apply lubricant gel to abdomen in the area where the back has been located.
6. Turn on the handheld Doppler device and place it on the spot over the fetal back.
7. Listen for the sound of the amplified heart rate, moving the device slightly from side to side as necessary to obtain the loudest sound. Assess the woman's pulse rate and compare it to the amplified sound. If the rates appear the same, reposition the Doppler device.
8. Once the fetal heart rate has been identified, count the number of beats in 1 minute and record the results.
9. Remove the Doppler device and wipe off any remaining gel from the woman's abdomen and the device.
10. Record the heart rate on the woman's medical record.
11. Provide information to the woman regarding fetal well-being based on findings.

woman to report a count of less than three fetal movements within an hour. Further investigation with a nonstress test or biophysical profile is usually warranted (Mangesi & Hofmeyr, 2007).

Fetal Heart Rate Measurement

Fetal heart rate measurement is integral to fetal surveillance throughout the pregnancy. Auscultating the fetal heart rate with a handheld Doppler at each prenatal visit helps confirm that the intrauterine environment is still supportive to the growing fetus. The purpose of assessing fetal heart rate is to determine rate and rhythm. Nursing Procedure 12.1 lists the steps in measuring fetal heart rate.

Follow-Up Visit Intervals and Assessments

Up to 28 weeks' gestation, follow-up visits involve assessment of the client's blood pressure and weight. The urine is tested for protein and glucose. Fundal height and fetal heart rate are assessed at every office visit. Between weeks 24 and 28, a blood glucose level is obtained using a 50-g glucose load followed by a 1-hour plasma glucose determination. If the result is more than 140 mg/dL, further testing, such as a 3-hour 100-g glucose tolerance test, is warranted to determine whether gestational diabetes is present.

During this time, review the common discomforts of pregnancy, evaluate any client complaints, and answer questions. Reinforce the importance of good nutrition and use of prenatal vitamins, along with daily exercise.

Between 29 and 36 weeks' gestation, all the assessments of previous visits are completed, along with assessment for edema. Special attention is focused on the presence and location of edema during the last trimester. Pregnant women commonly experience dependent edema of the lower extremities from constriction of blood vessels secondary to the heavy gravid uterus. Periorbital edema around the eyes, edema of the hands, and pretibial edema are abnormal and could be signs of gestational hypertension. Inspecting and palpating both extremities, listening for complaints of tight rings on fingers, and observing for swelling around the eyes are important assessments. Abnormal findings in any of these areas need to be reported.

If the mother is Rh negative, her antibody titer is re-evaluated. RhoGAM is given if indicated. The client also is evaluated for risk of preterm labor. At each visit, ask if she is experiencing any common signs or symptoms of preterm labor (e.g., uterine contractions, dull backache, feeling of pressure in the pelvic area or thighs, increased vaginal discharge, menstrual-like cramps, vaginal bleeding). A pelvic examination is performed to assess the cervix for position, consistency, length, and dilation. If the woman has had a previous preterm birth, she is at risk for another and close monitoring is warranted.

Counsel the woman about choosing a health care provider for the newborn, if she has not selected one yet. Along with completion of a breast assessment, discuss the choice of breastfeeding versus bottle-feeding. Reinforce the importance of daily fetal movement monitoring as an indicator of fetal well-being. Re-evaluate hemoglobin and hematocrit levels to assess for anemia.

Between 37 and 40 weeks' gestation, the same assessments are done as for the previous weeks. In addition, screening for group B streptococcus, gonorrhea, and chlamydia is done. Fetal presentation and position (via Leopold's maneuvers) are assessed. Review the signs and symptoms of labor and forward a copy of the prenatal record to the hospital labor department for future reference. Review the client's desire for family planning after birth as well as her decision to breastfeed or bottle-feed. Remind the client that an infant car seat is required by law and must be used to drive the newborn home from the hospital or birthing center.

Teaching About the Danger Signs of Pregnancy

It is important to educate the client about danger signs during pregnancy that require further evaluation. Explain that she should contact her health care provider immediately if she experiences any of the following:

- During the first trimester: spotting or bleeding (miscarriage), painful urination (infection), severe persistent vomiting (hyperemesis gravidarum), fever higher than 100°F (infection), and lower abdominal pain with dizziness and accompanied by shoulder pain (ruptured ectopic pregnancy)
- During the second trimester: regular uterine contractions (preterm labor); pain in calf, often increased with foot flexion (blood clot in deep vein); sudden gush or leakage of fluid from vagina (premature rupture of

membranes); and absence of fetal movement for more than 24 hours (possible fetal distress or demise)
- During the third trimester: sudden weight gain; periorbital or facial edema, severe upper abdominal pain, or headache with visual changes (pregnancy-induced hypertension); and a decrease in fetal daily movement for more than 24 hours (possible demise). Any of the previous warning signs and symptoms can also be present in this last trimester (March of Dimes, 2008c).

One of the warning signs that should be emphasized is early contractions, which can lead to preterm birth. All pregnant women need to be able to recognize early signs of contractions to prevent preterm labor, which is a major public health problem in the United States. Approximately 12% of all live births—or one out of eight babies—is born too soon (March of Dimes, 2008c). These preterm infants (born at less than 37 weeks' gestation) can suffer lifelong health consequences such as mental retardation, chronic lung disease, cerebral palsy, seizure disorders, and blindness, among other problems (March of Dimes, 2008c). Preterm labor can happen to any pregnant women at any time. In many cases it can be stopped with medications if it is recognized early, before significant cervical dilation has taken place. If the woman experiences menstrual-like cramps occurring every 10 minutes accompanied by a low, dull backache, she should stop what she is doing and lie down on her left side for 1 hour and drink two or three glasses of water. If the symptoms worsen or don't subside after 1 hour, she should contact her health care provider.

Assessment of Fetal Well-Being

During the antepartum period, several tests are performed routinely to monitor fetal well-being and to detect possible problems. When a high-risk pregnancy is identified, additional antepartum testing can be initiated to promote positive maternal, fetal, and neonatal outcomes. **High-risk pregnancies** include those that are complicated by maternal or fetal conditions (coincidental with or unique to pregnancy) that jeopardize the health status of the mother and put the fetus at risk for uteroplacental insufficiency, hypoxia, and death (Gilbert, 2007). However, additional antepartum fetal testing should take place only when the results obtained will guide future care, whether it is reassurance, more frequent testing, admission to the hospital, or the need for immediate delivery (Gilbert, 2007).

Ultrasonography

Since its introduction in the late 1950s, ultrasonography has become a very useful diagnostic tool in obstetrics. Real-time scanners can produce a continuous picture of the fetus on a monitor screen. A transducer that emits high-frequency sound waves is placed on the mother's abdomen and moved to visualize the fetus (Fig. 12.6). The fetal

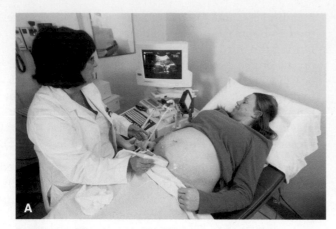 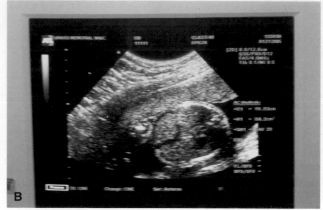

FIGURE 12.6 Ultrasound. (**A**) Ultrasound device being applied to client's abdomen. (**B**) View of monitor.

heartbeat and any malformations in the fetus can be assessed and measurements can be made accurately from the picture on the monitor screen.

Ultrasound, which is noninvasive, is considered a safe, accurate, and cost-effective tool. It provides important information about fetal activity, growth, and gestational age, assesses fetal well-being, and determines the need for invasive intrauterine tests (Valley & Fly, 2006).

There are no hard-and-fast rules as to the number of ultrasounds a woman should have during her pregnancy. An ultrasound usually is performed in the first trimester to confirm pregnancy, exclude ectopic or molar pregnancies, and confirm cardiac pulsation. A second scan may be performed at about 18 to 20 weeks to look for congenital malformations, exclude multifetal pregnancies, and verify dates and growth. A third scan may be done at around 34 weeks to evaluate fetal size, assess fetal growth, and verify placental position (Valley & Fly, 2006). An ultrasound is used to confirm placental location during amniocentesis and to provide visualization during chorionic villus sampling. An ultrasound is also ordered whenever an abnormality is suspected based on clinical grounds.

Nursing management during the ultrasound focuses on educating the woman about the ultrasound test and reassuring her that she will not experience any sensation from the sound waves during the test. No special client preparation is needed before performing the ultrasound, although in early pregnancy the woman may need to have a full bladder. Inform her that she may experience some discomfort from the pressure on the full bladder during the scan, but it will last only a short time. Tell the client that the conducting gel used on the abdomen during the scan may feel cold initially.

Doppler Flow Studies

Doppler flow studies can be used to measure the velocity of blood flow via ultrasound. Doppler flow studies can detect fetal compromise in high-risk pregnancies. The test is noninvasive and has no contraindications. The color im-

ages produced help to identify abnormalities in diastolic flow within the umbilical vessels. The velocity of the fetal red blood cells can be determined by measuring the change in the frequency of the sound wave reflected off the cells. Thus, Doppler flow studies can detect the movement of red blood cells in vessels (Gilbert, 2007). In pregnancies complicated by hypertension or IUGR, diastolic blood flow may be absent or even reversed (Gilbert, 2007). Doppler flow studies also can be used to evaluate the blood flow through other fetal blood vessels, such as the aorta and those in the brain. Research continues to determine the indications for Doppler flow studies to improve pregnancy outcomes. Nursing management of the woman undergoing Doppler flow studies is similar to that described for an ultrasound.

Alpha–Fetoprotein Analysis

Alpha-fetoprotein (AFP) is a substance produced by the fetal liver between weeks 13 and 20 of gestation. About 30 years ago, elevated levels of maternal serum AFP or amniotic fluid AFP were first linked to the occurrence of fetal neural tube defects. This biomarker screening test is now recommended for all pregnant women (Alexander et al., 2007; ACOG, 2007a).

AFP is present in amniotic fluid in low concentrations between 10 and 14 weeks of gestation and can be detected in maternal serum beginning approximately at 12 to 14 weeks of gestation (Gilbert, 2007). If there is a developmental defect, such as failure of the neural tube to close, more AFP escapes into amniotic fluid from the fetus. AFP then enters the maternal circulation by crossing the placenta, and the level in maternal serum can be measured. The optimal time for AFP screening is 16 to 18 weeks of gestation (ACOG, 2007a). Correct information about gestational dating, maternal weight, race, number of fetuses, and insulin dependency is necessary to ensure the accuracy of this screening test. If incorrect maternal information is submitted or the blood specimen is not drawn during the appropriate time frame, false-positive results may occur, increasing the woman's anxiety. Subsequently, further testing might be ordered based on an inaccurate interpretation, resulting in additional financial and emotional costs to the woman.

A variety of situations can lead to elevation of maternal serum AFP, including open neural tube defect, underestimation of gestational age, the presence of multiple fetuses, gastrointestinal defects, low birthweight, oligohydramnios, and decreased maternal weight (Frieden & Chan, 2007). Lower-than-expected maternal serum AFP levels are seen when fetal gestational age is overestimated or in cases of fetal death, hydatidiform mole, increased maternal weight, maternal type I diabetes, and fetal trisomy 21 (Down syndrome) or trisomy 18 (Edward's syndrome) (Gilbert, 2007).

Measurement of maternal serum AFP is minimally invasive, requiring only a venipuncture for a blood sample. It detects approximately 80% of all open neural tube defects and open abdominal wall defects in early pregnancy (Dashe et al., 2006). AFP has now been combined with other biomarker screening tests to determine the risk of neural tube defects and Down syndrome.

Nursing management for AFP testing consists of preparing the woman for this screening test by gathering accurate information about the date of her LMP, weight, race, and gestational dating. Accurately determining the window of 16 to 18 weeks' gestation will help to ensure that the test results are correct. Also explain that the test involves obtaining a blood specimen.

Marker Screening Tests

Two additional blood screening tests may be used to determine the risk of open neural tube defects and Down syndrome: the triple-marker screen and the addition of a fourth marker, inhibin A, which is used to enhance the accuracy of screening for Down syndrome in women younger than 35 years of age. Low inhibin A levels indicate the possibility of Down syndrome (Frieden & Chan, 2007). These tests combine three or four procedures to enhance the ability to make a diagnosis. These biomarkers are merely screening tests and identify women who need further definitive procedures (i.e., amniocentesis and genetic counseling) to make a diagnosis of neural tube defects (anencephaly, spina bifida, and encephalocele) or Down syndrome in the fetus. Most screening tests are performed between 15 to 22 weeks of gestation (16 to 18 weeks is ideal) (Blackburn, 2007).

The triple-marker screening or triple screening test is performed at 16 to 18 weeks of gestation. It uses the levels of three maternal serum markers (AFP, unconjugated estriol, and hCG), in combination with maternal age, to calculate risk (Frieden & Chan, 2007). With this screening, low maternal serum AFP and unconjugated estriol levels and a high hCG level suggests the possibility of Down syndrome. Elevated levels of maternal serum AFP are associated with open neural tube defects, ventral wall defects, some renal abnormalities, multiple gestation, certain skin disorders, fetal demise, and placental abnormality. The addition of the other two markers enhances the detection rate, from 25% using AFP alone to approximately 69% using all three (Frieden & Chan, 2007).

The screening test using four maternal markers (i.e., quadruple-marker screening) is also used to screen for Down syndrome. It uses maternal age at term and the concentration of four biomarkers in maternal serum: AFP, unconjugated estriol, hCG, and inhibin A. This test is done at 14 to 22 weeks of pregnancy and is reported to detect 85% of trisomy 21 cases; the triple screen was reported to detect only 69% (Hackley, Kriebs, & Rousseau, 2007). AFP and inhibin A levels are decreased in infants with trisomy 21 (Down syndrome).

Nursing management related to marker screening tests consists primarily of providing education about the tests. Prenatal screening has become standard in prenatal care. However, for many couples it remains confusing, emotionally charged, and filled with uncertain risks. Offer a thorough explanation of the test, reinforcing the information given by the health care professional. Provide couples with a description of the risks and benefits of performing these screens, emphasizing that these tests are for screening purposes only. Remind the couple that a definitive diagnosis is not made without further tests such as an amniocentesis. Answer any questions about these prenatal screening tests and respect the couple's decision if they choose not to have them done. Many couples may choose not to know because they would not consider having an abortion regardless of the test results.

Nuchal Translucency Screening

Nuchal translucency screening (ultrasound) is also done in the first trimester between 11 and 14 weeks. This allows for earlier detection and diagnosis of some fetal chromosomal and structural abnormalities. Ultrasound is used to identify an increase in nuchal translucency, which is due to the subcutaneous accumulation of fluid behind the fetal neck. Increased nuchal translucency is associated with chromosomal abnormalities such as trisomy 21, 18, and 13. Infants with trisomies tend to have more collagen and elastic connective tissue, allowing for accumulation (Caughey et al., 2007).

Amniocentesis

Amniocentesis involves a transabdominal puncture of the amniotic sac to obtain a sample of amniotic fluid for analysis. The fluid contains fetal cells that are examined to detect chromosomal abnormalities and several hereditary metabolic defects in the fetus before birth. In addition, amniocentesis is used to confirm a fetal abnormality when other screening tests detect a possible problem.

Amniocentesis is performed in the second trimester, usually between weeks 16 and 18. It can be done as early as week 14 or as late as week 20 (Singh & Singh, 2007). Over 40 different chromosomal abnormalities, inborn errors of metabolism, and neural tube defects can be diagnosed with amniocentesis. It can replace a genetic probability with a diagnostic certainty, allowing the woman and her partner to make an informed decision about the option of therapeutic abortion.

Amniocentesis can be performed in any of the three trimesters of pregnancy. An early amniocentesis (performed between weeks 11 and 14) is done to detect genetic anomalies. However, early amniocentesis has been associated with a high risk of spontaneous miscarriage and postprocedural amniotic fluid leakage compared with transabdominal chorionic villus screening (Singh & Singh, 2007). ACOG (2004) has issued a position statement on first-trimester screening methods, recommending chorionic villus sampling and nuchal translucency to detect Down syndrome rather than amniocentesis because of the increased risks associated with the early procedure. However, early screening and diagnosis can provide the couple with time to make decisions about the pregnancy outcome.

In the second trimester the procedure is performed between 15 and 20 weeks to detect chromosomal abnormalities, evaluate the fetal condition when the woman is sensitized to the Rh-positive blood, diagnose intrauterine infections, and investigate amniotic fluid AFP when the maternal serum AFP level is elevated (Gilbert, 2007).

In the third trimester amniocentesis is most commonly indicated to determine fetal lung maturity after the 35th week of gestation via analysis of lecithin-to-sphingomyelin ratios (L/S ratio) and to evaluate the fetal condition with Rh isoimmunization. Table 12.1 lists amniotic fluid analysis findings and their implications.

The second trimester is the most common time to have an amniocentesis for any prenatal diagnosis since it carries such high risk if done earlier. By week 14 to 16 of gestation, there is sufficient amniotic fluid for sampling yet enough time for a safe abortion, if desired. Amniocentesis is offered to women who are 35 years of age or older, women who have a child with a neural tube defect, and women with elevated maternal serum AFP levels. It also

TABLE 12.1   **AMNIOTIC FLUID ANALYSIS AND IMPLICATIONS**

Test Component	Normal Findings	Fetal Implications of Abnormal Findings
Color	Clear with white flecks of vernix caseosa in a mature fetus	Blood of maternal origin is usually harmless. "Port wine" fluid may indicate abruptio placentae. Fetal blood may indicate damage to the fetal, placental, or umbilical cord vessels.
Bilirubin	Absent at term	High levels indicate hemolytic disease of the neonate in isoimmunized pregnancy.
Meconium	Absent (except in breech presentation)	Presence indicates fetal hypotension or distress.
Creatinine	More than 2 mg/dL in a mature fetus	Decrease may indicate immature fetus (less than 37 weeks).
Lecithin–sphingomyelin ratio (L/S ratio)	More than 2 generally indicates fetal pulmonary maturity.	A ratio of less than 2 indicates pulmonary immaturity and subsequent respiratory distress syndrome.
Phosphatidylglycerol	Present	Absence indicates pulmonary immaturity.
Glucose	Less than 45 mg/dL	Excessive increases at term or near term indicate hypertrophied fetal pancreas and subsequent neonatal hypoglycemia.
Alpha-fetoprotein	Variable, depending on gestation age and laboratory technique; highest concentration (about 18.5 µg/mL) occurs at 13 to 14 weeks	Inappropriate increases indicate neural tube defects such as spina bifida or anencephaly, impending fetal death, congenital nephrosis, or contamination of fetal blood.
Bacteria	Absent	Presence indicates chorioamnionitis.
Chromosomes	Normal karyotype	Abnormal karyotype may indicate fetal sex and chromosome disorders.
Acetylcholinesterase	Absent	Presence may indicate neural tube defects, exomphalos, or other serious malformations.

Sources: Blackburn, 2007; Dillon, 2007; Frieden & Chang, 2007.

may be used to detect chromosomal aberrations when a parent has a chromosomal abnormality or is a carrier for a metabolic disease (Cunningham et al., 2005).

Procedure

Amniocentesis is performed after an ultrasound examination identifies an adequate pocket of amniotic fluid free of fetal parts, the umbilical cord, or the placenta (Fig. 12.7). The health care provider inserts a long pudendal or spinal needle, a 22-gauge, 5-inch needle, into the amniotic cavity and aspirates amniotic fluid, which is placed in an amber or foil-covered test tube to protect it from light. When the desired amount of fluid has been withdrawn, the needle is removed and slight pressure is applied to the site. If there is no evidence of bleeding, a sterile bandage is applied to the needle site. The specimens are then sent to the laboratory immediately for the cytologist to evaluate.

Examining a sample of fetal cells directly produces a definitive diagnosis rather than a "best guess" diagnosis based on indirect screening tests. It is an invaluable diagnostic tool, but the risks include spontaneous abortion (1 in 200), maternal or fetal infection, fetal-maternal hemorrhage, leakage of amniotic fluid, and maternal discomfort after the procedure. The test results may take up to 3 weeks.

Nursing Management

When preparing the woman for an amniocentesis, explain the procedure and encourage her to empty her bladder just before the procedure to avoid the risk of bladder puncture.

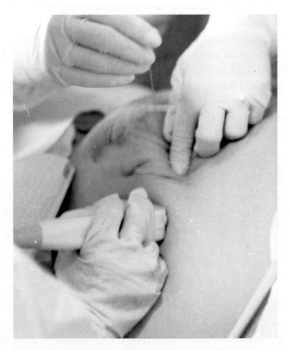

FIGURE 12.7 Technique for amniocentesis: Inserting needle.

Inform her that a 20-minute electronic fetal monitoring strip usually is obtained to evaluate fetal well-being and obtain a baseline to compare after the procedure is completed. Obtain and record maternal vital signs.

After the procedure, assist the woman to a position of comfort and administer RhoGAM intramuscularly if the woman is Rh negative to prevent potential sensitization to fetal blood. Assess maternal vital signs and fetal heart rate every 15 minutes for an hour after the procedure. Observe the puncture site for bleeding or drainage. Instruct the client to rest after returning home and remind her to report fever, leaking amniotic fluid, vaginal bleeding, or uterine contractions or any changes in fetal activity (increased or decreased) to the health care provider.

When the test results come back, be available to offer support, especially if a fetal abnormality is found. Also prepare the woman and her partner for the need for genetic counseling. Trained genetic counselors can provide accurate medical information and help couples to interpret the results of the amniocentesis so they can make the decisions that are right for them as a family.

Chorionic Villus Sampling

Chorionic villus sampling (CVS) is a procedure for obtaining a sample of the chorionic villi for prenatal evaluation of chromosomal disorders, enzyme deficiencies, and fetal gender determination and to identify sex-linked disorders such as hemophilia, sickle cell anemia, and Tay-Sachs disease (Blackburn, 2007). Chorionic villi are finger-like projections that cover the embryo and anchor it to the uterine lining before the placenta is developed. Because they are of embryonic origin, sampling provides information about the developing fetus. CVS can be used to detect numerous genetic disorders, with the exception of neural tube defects (Jenkins et al., 2007).

There has been an impetus to develop earlier prenatal diagnostic procedures so that couples can make an early decision to terminate the pregnancy if an anomaly is confirmed. Early prenatal diagnosis by CVS was proposed as an alternative to routine amniocentesis, which carries fewer risks if done later in the pregnancy. In addition, results of CVS testing are available sooner than those of amniocentesis, usually within 48 hours.

Procedure

CVS is generally performed 10 to 13 weeks after the LMP. Earlier, chorionic villi may not be sufficiently developed for adequate tissue sampling and the risk of limb defects is increased (Kenner & Lott, 2007). First, an ultrasound is done to confirm gestational age and viability. Then, under continuous ultrasound guidance, CVS is performed using either a transcervical or transabdominal approach. With the transcervical approach, the woman is placed in the lithotomy position and a sterile catheter is introduced through the cervix and inserted in the placenta, where a sample of chorionic villi is aspirated. This approach requires the client to have a full bladder to push the uterus and placenta into a position that is more accessible to the catheter. A full bladder also helps in better visualization of the structures. With the transabdominal approach, an 18-gauge spinal needle is inserted through the abdominal wall into the placental tissue and a sample of chorionic villi is aspirated. Regardless of the approach used, the sample is sent to the cytogenetics laboratory for analysis.

Potential complications of CVS include mild vaginal bleeding and cramping, spontaneous abortion, limb abnormalities, rupture of membranes, infection, chorioamnionitis, and fetal-maternal hemorrhage (Blackburn, 2007). The pregnancy loss rate is approximately 1.3%, which is somewhat higher than with traditional amniocentesis (Walling, 2007). In addition, women who are Rh negative should receive immune globulin (RhoGAM) to avoid isoimmunization (Gilbert, 2007).

Nursing Management

Explain to the woman that the procedure will last about 15 minutes. An ultrasound will be done first to locate the embryo, and a baseline set of vital signs will be taken before starting. Make sure she is informed of the risks related to the procedure, including their incidence.

If a transabdominal CVS procedure is planned, advise her to fill her bladder by drinking increased amounts of water. Inform her that a needle will be inserted through her abdominal wall and samples will be collected. Once the samples are collected, the needle will be withdrawn and the samples will be sent to the genetics laboratory for evaluation.

For transcervical CVS, inform the women that a speculum will be placed into the vagina under ultrasound guidance. Then the vagina is cleaned and a small catheter is inserted through the cervix. The samples obtained through the catheter are then sent to the laboratory.

After either procedure, assist the woman to a position of comfort and clean any excess lubricant or secretions from the area. Instruct her about signs to watch for and report, such as fever, cramping, and vaginal bleeding. Urge her not to engage in any strenuous activity for the next 48 hours. Assess the fetal heart rate for changes and administer RhoGAM to an unsensitized Rh-negative woman after the procedure.

Percutaneous Umbilical Blood Sampling

Percutaneous umbilical blood sampling (PUBS) permits the collection of a blood specimen directly from the fetal circulation (Fig. 12.8). This test allows for rapid chromo-

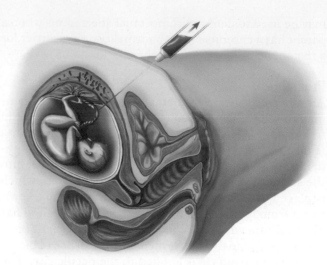

FIGURE 12.8 Collecting blood sample for PUBS.

somal analysis to achieve a timely diagnosis. It is done specifically for women at risk for genetic anomalies and those with potential blood disorders, such as blood incompatibility or hemoglobinopathies.

Procedure

Under continuous ultrasound guidance, a fine needle is inserted through the mother's abdomen and uterine wall into an umbilical cord vessel. Specimens can be evaluated for coagulation studies, blood group typing, complete blood count, karyotyping, and blood gas analysis (Singh & Singh, 2008). Fetal infection, Rh incompatibility, and fetal acid–base status can be determined. The blood sample is usually drawn late in the second trimester to assist in medical management, but PUBS can be done anytime after 16 weeks of gestation.

Although the information gained from this procedure is valuable and can be life-saving for many fetuses, PUBS is not without risks. Potential complications include leakage of blood from the puncture site, cord laceration, cord hematomas, transient fetal bradycardia, infection, thromboembolism in the umbilical cord, preterm labor, infection, and premature rupture of membranes (Blackburn, 2007).

Nursing Management

Explain the procedure thoroughly to the woman. Position her properly on the examination table and help clean the area for needle insertion. Monitor vital signs and fetal heart rate throughout the procedure. At the conclusion of the procedure, closely monitor the mother and fetus for changes. Assess fetal heart rate continuously and perform external fetal monitoring for up to 2 hours before the woman is discharged from the outpatient area. A repeat ultrasound is usually done within an hour after the procedure to rule out bleeding or hematoma formation.

Prior to discharge, instruct the woman to report signs of infection, an increase in contractions, or a change in fetal activity level from normal. Reinforce the need to count fetal movements, and review the technique so she can assess them when she is discharged home.

Nonstress Test

The nonstress test (NST) is an indirect measurement of uteroplacental function. Unlike the fetal movement counting done by the mother alone, this procedure requires specialized equipment and trained personnel. The basis for the nonstress test is that the normal fetus produces characteristic fetal heart rate patterns in response to fetal movements. In the healthy fetus there is an acceleration of the fetal heart rate with fetal movement. Currently, an NST is recommended twice weekly (after 28 weeks of gestation) for clients with diabetes and other high-risk conditions, such as IUGR, preeclampsia, postterm pregnancy, renal disease, and multifetal pregnancies (Cunningham et al., 2005).

NST is a noninvasive test that requires no initiation of contractions. It is quick to perform and there are no known side effects. However, it is not as sensitive to fetal oxygen reserves as the contraction stress test, and there is a high false-positive rate (Gilbert, 2007).

Procedure

Before the procedure the client eats a meal to stimulate fetal activity. Then she is placed in the left lateral recumbent position to avoid supine hypotension syndrome. An external electronic fetal monitoring device is applied to her abdomen. The device consists of two belts, each with a sensor. One of the sensors records uterine activity; the second sensor records fetal heart rate. The client is handed an "event marker" with a button that she pushes every time she perceives fetal movement. When the button is pushed, the fetal monitor strip is marked to identify that fetal movement has occurred. The procedure usually lasts 20 to 30 minutes.

Nursing Management

Prior to the NST, explain the testing procedure and have the woman empty her bladder. Position her in a semi-Fowler's position and apply the two external monitor belts. Document the date and time the test is started, patient information, the reason for the test, and the maternal vital signs. Obtain a baseline fetal monitor strip over 15 to 30 minutes.

During the test, observe for signs of fetal activity with a concurrent acceleration of the fetal heart rate. Interpret the NST as reactive or nonreactive. A "reactive" NST includes at least two fetal heart rate accelerations from the baseline of at least 15 bpm for at least 15 seconds within the 20-minute recording period. If the test does not meet these criteria after 40 minutes, it is considered nonreactive. A "nonreactive" NST is characterized by the absence of two fetal heart rate accelerations using the 15-by-15 criterion in a 20-minute time frame. A nonreactive test has been correlated with a higher incidence of fetal distress during labor, fetal mortality, and IUGR. Additional testing, such as a contraction stress test or biophysical profile, should be considered (Frieden & Chan, 2007).

After the NST procedure, assist the woman off the table, provide her with fluids, and allow her to use the restroom. Typically the results are discussed with the woman at this time by the health care provider. Provide teaching about signs and symptoms to report. If serial NSTs are being done, schedule the next testing session.

Contraction Stress Test

Because blood flow to the uterus and placenta is slowed during uterine contractions, the contraction stress test (CST), formerly called the oxytocin-challenge test, is a diagnostic procedure performed to determine the fetal heart rate response under stress, such as during contractions. The goal of the test is to achieve three uterine contractions in a 10-minute period. This can occur spontaneously with the aid of nipple stimulation, which causes the release of endogenous oxytocin, or through the use of an oxytocin infusion. Its use has been indicated in pregnancies in which placental insufficiency is suspected—preeclampsia, IUGR, diabetes mellitus, postterm pregnancy, a previous stillbirth—or when an irregularity of the fetal heart rate has been observed. However, the CST has given way to the biophysical profile and has limited use today (Blackburn, 2007).

Biophysical Profile

A **biophysical profile** uses a real-time ultrasound to allow assessment of various parameters of fetal well-being: fetal tone, breathing, motion, and amniotic fluid volume. These four parameters, together with the NST, constitute the biophysical profile. Each parameter is controlled by a different structure in the fetal brain: fetal tone by the cortex; fetal movements by the cortex and motor nuclei; fetal breathing movements by the centers close to the fourth ventricle; and the NST by the posterior hypothalamus and medulla. The amniotic fluid is the result of fetal urine volume. Not all facilities perform an NST unless other parameters of the profile are abnormal (Gilbert, 2007). The biophysical profile is based on the concept that a fetus that experiences hypoxia loses certain behavioral parameters in the reverse order in which they were acquired during fetal development (normal order of development: tone at 8 weeks; movement at 9 weeks; breathing at 20 weeks; and fetal heart rate reactivity at 24 weeks).

Scoring and Interpretation

The biophysical profile is a scored test with five components, each worth 2 points if present. A total score of 10 is possible if the NST is used. Thirty minutes are allotted for testing, although fewer than 10 minutes are usually needed. The following criteria must be met to obtain a score of 2; anything less is scored as 0 (Gilbert, 2007):

- Body movements: three or more discrete limb or trunk movements
- Fetal tone: one or more instances of full extension and flexion of a limb or trunk
- Fetal breathing: one or more fetal breathing movements of more than 30 seconds
- Amniotic fluid volume: one or more pockets of fluid measuring 2 cm
- NST: normal NST = 2 points; abnormal NST = 0 points

Interpretation of the biophysical profile score can be complicated, depending on several fetal and maternal variables. Because it is indicated as a result of a non-reassuring finding from previous fetal surveillance tests, this test can be used to quantify the interpretation, and intervention can be initiated if appropriate. One of the important factors is the amniotic fluid volume, taken in conjunction with the results of the NST. Amniotic fluid is largely composed of fetal urine. As placental function decreases, perfusion of fetal organs, such as kidneys, decreases, and this can lead to a reduction of amniotic fluid. If oligohydramnios or decreased amniotic fluid is present, the potential exists for antepartum or intrapartum fetal compromise (Gearhart & Sehdev, 2007).

Overall, a score of 8 to 10 is considered normal if the amniotic fluid volume is adequate. A score of 6 or below is suspicious, possibly indicating a compromised fetus; further investigation of fetal well-being is needed.

Because the biophysical profile is an ultrasonographic assessment of fetal behavior, it requires more extensive equipment and more highly trained personnel than other testing modalities. The cost is much greater than with less sophisticated tests. It permits conservative therapy and prevents premature or unnecessary intervention. There are fewer false-positive results than with the NST alone or CST (Gearhart & Sehdev, 2007).

Nursing Management

Nursing management focuses primarily on offering the client support and answering her questions. Expect to complete the NST before scheduling the biophysical profile, and explain why further testing might be needed. Tell the woman that the ultrasound will be done in the diagnostic imaging department.

Nursing Management for the Common Discomforts of Pregnancy

Most women experience common discomforts during pregnancy and ask a nurse's advice about ways to minimize them. However, other women will not bring up their concerns unless asked. Therefore, the nurse needs to address the common discomforts that occur in each trimester at each prenatal visit and provide realistic measures to help the client deal with them (Teaching Guidelines 12.1). Nursing Care Plan 12.1 applies the nursing process to the care of a woman experiencing some discomforts of pregnancy.

First-Trimester Discomforts

During the first 3 months of pregnancy, the woman's body is undergoing numerous changes. Some women experience many discomforts, but others have few. These discomforts are caused by the changes taking place within the body and pass as the pregnancy progresses.

Urinary Frequency or Incontinence

Urinary frequency or incontinence is common in the first trimester because the growing uterus compresses the bladder. This also is a common complaint during the third trimester, especially when the fetal head settles into the pelvis. However, the discomfort tends to improve in the second trimester, when the uterus becomes an abdominal organ and moves away from the bladder region.

After infection and gestational diabetes have been ruled out as causative factors of increased urinary frequency, suggest that the woman decrease her fluid intake 2 to 3 hours before bedtime and limit her intake of caffeinated beverages. Increased voiding is normal, but encourage the client to report any pain or burning during urination. Also explain that increased urinary frequency may subside as she enters her second trimester, only to recur in the third trimester. Teach the client to perform Kegel exercises throughout the day to help strengthen perineal muscle tone, thereby enhancing urinary control and decreasing the possibility of incontinence.

Fatigue

Fatigue plagues all pregnant women, primarily in the first and third trimesters (the highest energy levels typically occur during the second trimester), even if they get their normal amount of sleep at night. First-trimester fatigue most often is related to the many physical changes (e.g., increased oxygen consumption, increased levels of progesterone and relaxin, increased metabolic demands) and psychosocial changes (e.g., mood swings, multiple role demands) of pregnancy. Third-trimester fatigue can be caused by sleep disturbances from increased weight (many women cannot find a comfortable sleeping position due to the enlarging abdomen), physical discomforts such as heartburn, and insomnia due to mood swings, multiple role anxiety, and a decrease in exercise (Trupin, 2006).

Once anemia, infection, and blood dyscrasias have been ruled out as contributing to the client's fatigue, advise

TEACHING GUIDELINES 12.1

Teaching to Manage the Discomforts of Pregnancy

Urinary Frequency or Incontinence

- Try Kegel exercises to increase control over leakage.
- Empty your bladder when you first feel a full sensation.
- Avoid caffeinated drinks, which stimulate voiding.
- Reduce your fluid intake after dinner to reduce nighttime urination.

Fatigue

- Attempt to get a full night's sleep, without interruptions.
- Eat a healthy balanced diet.
- Schedule a nap in the early afternoon daily.
- When you are feeling tired, rest.

Nausea and Vomiting

- Avoid an empty stomach at all times.
- Munch on dry crackers/toast in bed before arising.
- Eat several small meals throughout the day.
- Drink fluids between meals rather than with meals.
- Avoid greasy, fried foods or ones with a strong odor, such as cabbage or Brussels sprouts.

Backache

- Avoid standing or sitting in one position for long periods.
- Apply heating pad (low setting) to the small of your back.
- Support your lower back with pillows when sitting.
- Stand with your shoulders back to maintain correct posture.

Leg Cramps

- Elevate legs above heart level frequently throughout the day.
- If you get a cramp, straighten both legs and flex your feet toward your body.
- Ask your health care provider about taking additional calcium supplements, which may reduce leg spasms.

Varicosities

- Walk daily to improve circulation to extremities.
- Elevate both legs above heart level while resting.
- Avoid standing in one position for long periods of time.
- Don't wear constrictive stockings and socks.
- Don't cross the legs when sitting for long periods.
- Wear support stockings to promote better circulation.

Hemorrhoids

- Establish a regular time for daily bowel elimination.
- Prevent straining by drinking plenty of fluids and eating fiber-rich foods and exercising daily.
- Use warm sitz baths and cool witch hazel compresses for comfort.

Constipation

- Increase your intake of foods high in fiber and drink at least eight 8-ounce glasses of fluid daily.
- Exercise each day (brisk walking) to promote movement through the intestine.
- Reduce the amount of cheese consumed.

Heartburn/Indigestion

- Avoid spicy or greasy foods and eat small frequent meals.
- Sleep on several pillows so that your head is elevated.
- Stop smoking and avoid caffeinated drinks to reduce stimulation.
- Avoid lying down for at least 2 hours after meals.
- Try drinking sips of water to reduce burning sensation.
- Take antacids sparingly if burning sensation is severe.

Braxton Hicks Contractions

- Keep in mind that these contractions are a normal sensation.
- Try changing your position or engaging in mild exercise to help reduce the sensation.
- Drink more fluids if possible.

---

her to arrange work, childcare, and other demands in her life to permit additional rest periods. Work with the client to devise a realistic schedule for rest. Using pillows for support in the side-lying position relieves pressure on major blood vessels that supply oxygen and nutrients to the fetus when resting (Fig. 12.9). Also recommend the use of relaxation techniques, providing instructions as necessary, and suggest she increase her daily exercise level.

Nausea and Vomiting

Nausea and vomiting are common discomforts during the first trimester: at least 50% of women experience nausea during pregnancy (Hackley, Kriebs, & Rousseau, 2007). The physiologic changes that cause nausea and vomiting are unknown, but research suggests that unusually high levels of estrogen, progesterone, and hCG and a vitamin B6 deficiency may be contributing factors. Symp-

Nursing Care Plan 12.1

OVERVIEW OF THE WOMAN EXPERIENCING COMMON DISCOMFORTS OF PREGNANCY

Alicia, a 32-year-old, G1 P0, at 10 weeks' gestation, comes to the clinic for a visit. During the interview she tells you, "I'm running to the bathroom to urinate it seems like all the time, and I'm so nauseous that I'm having trouble eating." She denies any burning or pain on urination. Vital signs are within acceptable limits.

NURSING DIAGNOSIS: Impaired urinary elimination related to frequency secondary to physiologic changes of pregnancy

Outcome Identification and Evaluation

Client will report a decrease in urinary complaints, as evidenced by a decrease in the number of times she uses the bathroom to void, reports that she feels her bladder is empty after voiding, and use of Kegel exercises.

Interventions: Promoting Normal Urinary Elimination Patterns

- Assess client's usual bladder elimination patterns to establish a baseline for comparison.
- Obtain a urine specimen for analysis to rule out infection or glucosuria.
- Review with client the physiologic basis for the increased frequency during pregnancy; inform client that frequency should abate during the second trimester and that it most likely will return during her third trimester. This will promote understanding of the problem.
- Encourage the client to empty her bladder when first feeling a sensation of fullness to minimize risk of urinary retention.
- Suggest client avoid caffeinated drinks, which can stimulate the need to void.
- Encourage client to drink adequate amounts of fluid throughout the day; however, have client reduce her fluid intake before bedtime to reduce nighttime urination.
- Urge client to keep perineal area clean and dry to prevent irritation and excoriation from any leakage.
- Instruct client in Kegel exercises to increase perineal muscle tone and control over leakage.
- Teach client about the signs and symptoms of urinary tract infection and urge her to report them should they occur to ensure early detection and prompt intervention.

NURSING DIAGNOSIS: Imbalanced nutrition, less than body requirements, related to nausea and vomiting

Outcome Identification and Evaluation

Client will ingest adequate amounts of nutrients for maternal and fetal well-being as evidenced by acceptable weight gain pattern and statements indicating an increase in food intake with a decrease in the number of episodes of nausea and vomiting.

Interventions: Promoting Adequate Nutrition

- Obtain weight and compare to baseline to determine effects of nausea and vomiting on nutritional intake.
- Review client's typical dietary intake over 24 hours to determine nutritional intake and patterns so that suggestions can be individualized.
- Encourage client to eat five or six small frequent meals throughout the day to prevent her stomach from becoming empty.
- Suggest that she munch on dry crackers, toast, cereal, or cheese or drink a small amount of lemonade before arising to minimize nausea.
- Encourage client to arise slowly from bed in the morning and avoid sudden movements to reduce stimulation of the vomiting center.
- Advise client to drink fluids between meals rather than with meals to avoid overdistention of the abdomen and subsequent increase in abdominal pressure.
- Encourage her to increase her intake of foods high in vitamin B6 such as meat, poultry, bananas, fish, green leafy vegetables, peanuts, raisins, walnuts, and whole grains, as tolerated, to ensure adequate nutrient intake.
- Advise the client to avoid greasy, fried, or highly spiced foods and to avoid strong odors, including foods such as cabbage, to minimize gastrointestinal upset.
- Encourage the client to avoid wearing tight or restricting clothes to minimize pressure on the expanding abdomen.
- Arrange for consultation with nutritionist as necessary to assist with diet planning.

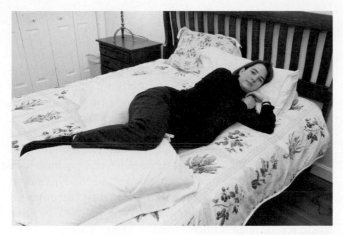

FIGURE 12.9   Using pillows for support in the side-lying position.

toms generally last until the second trimester and are generally associated with a positive pregnancy outcome (Cunningham et al., 2005).

To help alleviate nausea and vomiting, advise the woman to eat small, frequent meals (five or six a day) to prevent her stomach from becoming completely empty. Other helpful suggestions include eating dry crackers, Cheerios, lemonade, or cheese before getting out of bed in the morning and increasing her intake of foods high in vitamin B6, such as meat, poultry, bananas, fish, green leafy vegetables, peanuts, raisins, walnuts, and whole grains, or making sure she is receiving enough vitamin B6 by taking her prescribed prenatal vitamins. Other helpful tips to deal with nausea and vomiting include:

• Get out of bed in the morning very slowly.
• Avoid sudden movements.
• Open a window to remove odors of food being cooked.
• Limit intake of fluids or soups during meals (drink them between meals).
• Avoid fried foods and foods cooked with grease, oils, or fatty meats, for they tend to upset the stomach.
• Avoid highly seasoned foods such as those cooked with garlic, onions, peppers, and chili.
• Drink a small amount of caffeine-free carbonated beverage (ginger ale) if nauseated.
• Avoid strong smells.
• Avoid wearing tight or restricting clothes, which might place increased pressure on the expanding abdomen.
• Avoid stress (Lane, 2007).

Breast Tenderness

Due to increased estrogen and progesterone levels, which cause the fat layer of breasts to thicken and the number of milk ducts and glands to increase during the first trimester, many women experience breast tenderness. Offering a thorough explanation to the woman about the reasons for the breast discomfort is important. Wearing a larger bra with good support can help alleviate this discomfort.

Advise her to wear a supportive bra, even while sleeping. As her breasts increase in size, advise her to change her bra size to ensure adequate support.

Constipation

Increasing levels of progesterone during pregnancy lead to decreased contractility of the gastrointestinal tract, slowed movement of substances through the colon, and a resulting increase in water absorption. All of these factors lead to constipation. Lack of exercise or too little fiber or fluids in the diet can also promote constipation. In addition, the large bowel is mechanically compressed by the enlarging uterus, adding to this discomfort. The iron and calcium in prenatal vitamins can also contribute to constipation during the first and third trimesters.

Explain how pregnancy exacerbates the symptoms of constipation and offer the following suggestions:

• Eat fresh or dried fruit daily.
• Eat more raw fruits and vegetables, including their skins.
• Eat whole-grain cereals and breads such as raisin bran or bran flakes.
• Participate in physical activity every day.
• Eat meals at regular intervals.
• Establish a time of day to defecate, and elevate your feet on a stool to avoid straining.
• Drink six to eight glasses of water daily.
• Decrease your intake of refined carbohydrates.
• Drink warm fluids on arising to stimulate bowel motility.
• Decrease your consumption of sugary sodas.
• Avoid eating large amounts of cheese.

If the suggestions above are ineffective, suggest that the woman use a bulk-forming laxative such as Metamucil.

Nasal Stuffiness, Bleeding Gums, Epistaxis

Increased levels of estrogen cause edema of the mucous membranes of the nasal and oral cavities. Advise the woman to drink extra water for hydration of the mucous membranes or to use a cool mist humidifier in her bedroom at night. If she needs to blow her nose to relieve nasal stuffiness, advise her to blow gently, one nostril at a time. Advise her to avoid the use of nasal decongestants and sprays.

If a nosebleed occurs, advise the woman to loosen the clothing around her neck, sit with her head tilted forward, pinch her nostrils with her thumb and forefinger for 10 to 15 minutes, and apply an ice pack to the bridge of her nose.

If the woman has bleeding gums, encourage her to practice good oral hygiene by using a soft toothbrush and flossing daily. Warm saline mouthwashes can relieve discomfort. If the gum problem persists, instruct her to see her dentist.

Cravings

Desires for certain foods and beverages are likely to begin during the first trimester but do not appear to reflect any physiologic need. Foods with a high sodium or sugar content often are the ones craved. At times, some women crave non-food substances such as clay, cornstarch, laundry detergent, baking soda, soap, paint chips, dirt, ice, or wax. This craving for non-food substances, termed pica, may indicate a severe dietary deficiency of minerals or vitamins, or it may have cultural roots (Lynch, 2007). Pica is discussed in Chapter 11.

Leukorrhea

Increased vaginal discharge begins during the first trimester and continues throughout pregnancy. The physiologic changes behind leukorrhea arise from the high levels of estrogen, which cause increased vascularity and hypertrophy of cervical glands as well as vaginal cells (Cunningham et al., 2005). The result is progressive vaginal secretions throughout pregnancy.

Advise the woman to keep the perineal area clean and dry, washing the area with mild soap and water during her daily shower. Also recommend that she avoid wearing pantyhose and other tight-fitting nylon clothes that prevent air from circulating to the genital area. Encourage the use of cotton underwear and suggest wearing a nightgown rather than pajamas to allow for increased airflow. Also instruct the woman to avoid douching and tampon use.

Second-Trimester Discomforts

A sense of well-being typically characterizes the second trimester for most women. By this time, the fatigue, nausea, and vomiting have subsided and the uncomfortable changes of the third trimester are a few months away. Not every woman experiences the same discomforts during this time, so nursing assessments and interventions must be individualized.

Backache

Backache, experienced by many women during the second trimester, is due to a shift in the center of gravity caused by the enlarging uterus. Muscle strain results. In addition, a high level of circulating progesterone softens cartilage and loosens joints, thus increasing discomfort. Upper back pain also can be caused by increased breast size (ACOG, 2007b).

After exploring other reasons that might cause backache, such as uterine contractions, urinary tract infection, ulcers, or musculoskeletal back disorders, the following instructions may be helpful:

- Maintain correct posture, with head up and shoulders back.
- Wear low-heeled shoes with good arch support.
- When standing for long periods, place one foot on a stool or box.
- Use good body mechanics when lifting objects.
- When sitting, use foot supports and pillows behind the back.

- Try pelvic tilt or rocking exercises to strengthen the back (ACOG, 2007b).

The pelvic tilt or pelvic rock is used to alleviate pressure on the lower back during pregnancy by stretching the lower back muscles. It can be done sitting, standing, or on all fours. To do it on all fours, the hands are positioned directly under the shoulders and the knees under the hips. The back should be in a neutral position with the head and neck aligned with the straight back. The woman then presses up with the lower back and holds this position for a few seconds, then relaxes to a neutral position. This action of pressing upward is repeated frequently throughout the day to prevent a sore back (ACOG, 2007b). See Evidence-Based Practice 12.1.

Leg Cramps

Leg cramps occur primarily in the second and third trimesters and could be related to the pressure of the gravid uterus on pelvic nerves and blood vessels (Arenson & Drake, 2007). Diet can also be a contributing factor if the woman is not consuming enough of certain minerals, such as calcium and magnesium. The sudden stretching of leg muscles may also play a role in causing leg cramps (Trupin, 2006).

Encourage the woman to gently stretch the muscle by dorsiflexing the foot up toward the body. Wrapping a warm, moist towel around the leg muscle can also help the muscle to relax. Advise the client to avoid stretching her legs, pointing her toes, and walking excessively. Stress the importance of wearing low-heeled shoes and support hose and arising slowly from a sitting position. If the leg cramps are due to deficiencies in minerals, the condition can be remedied by eating more foods rich in these nutrients. Also instruct the woman on calf-stretching exercises: have her stand 3 feet from the wall and lean toward it, resting her lower arms against it, while keeping her heels on the floor. This may help reduce cramping if it is done before going to bed.

Elevating the legs throughout the day will help relieve pressure and minimize strain. Wearing support hose and avoiding curling the toes may help to relieve leg discomfort. Also instruct the client to avoid standing in one spot for a prolonged period or crossing her legs. If she must stand for prolonged periods, suggest that she change her position at least every 2 hours by walking or sitting to reduce the risk of leg cramps. Encourage her to drink eight 8-ounce glasses of fluid throughout the day to ensure adequate hydration.

Varicosities of the Vulva and Legs

Varicosities of the vulva and legs are associated with the increased venous stasis caused by the pressure of the gravid uterus on pelvic vessels and the vasodilation resulting from increased progesterone levels. Progesterone relaxes the vein walls, making it difficult for blood to return to the heart from the extremities; pooling can result. Genetic predispo-

EVIDENCE-BASED PRACTICE 12.1
Interventions for Preventing and Treating Pelvic and Back Pain in Pregnancy

● **Study**

More than two thirds of pregnant women experience back pain and almost one fifth experience pelvic pain. The pain increases with advancing pregnancy and interferes with work, daily activities, and sleep. Many women experience back or pelvic pain during pregnancy. This pain generally increases as pregnancy advances and it interferes with daily activities (like carrying, cleaning, sitting, and walking), can prevent women from going to work, and sometimes disturbs sleep. Suggestions to help manage the pain are varied and include special pregnancy exercises, frequent rest, hot and cold compresses, a supportive belt, massage, acupuncture, chiropractic, aromatherapy, relaxation, herbs, yoga, and Reiki. Sometimes drugs like acetaminophen have also been suggested. No studies were found dealing with the prevention of back and pelvic pain.

For treatment, the review of trials found eight studies, involving 1,305 participants, that examined the effects of various pregnancy-specific exercises, physiotherapy programs, acupuncture, and using special pillows added to usual prenatal care. They were compared to usual pregnancy care or other treatments. The quality of the studies was not the best, and so the findings should be treated with caution.

▲ **Findings**

The review found that specifically tailored strengthening exercises, sitting pelvic tilt exercise programs, and water gymnastics all reported beneficial effects. In addition, acupuncture seemed more effective than physiotherapy. Adverse effects, when reported, appeared minor and transient. More research is needed on this widespread problem of pregnancy.

■ **Nursing Implications**

Nurses can apply these findings to help pregnant women cope with and actively participate in their therapy to relieve their pelvic and back discomfort. The nurse should offer a thorough explanation of the reasons for the discomfort and then proceed to outline the effective therapies. In addition, the nurse can provide instruction and demonstrate how to go through each exercise.

Source: Pennick, V. E., & Young, G. (2007). Interventions for preventing and treating pelvic and back pain in pregnancy. *Cochrane Database of Systematic Reviews* 2007, Issue 2. Art. No.: CD001139. DOI: 10.1002/14651858.CD001139.pub2.

sition, inactivity, obesity, and poor muscle tone are contributing factors.

Encourage the client to wear support hose and teach her how to apply them properly. Advise her to elevate her legs above her heart while lying on her back for 10 minutes before she gets out of bed in the morning, thus promoting venous return before she applies the hose. Instruct the client to avoid crossing her legs and avoid wearing knee-high stockings. They cause constriction of leg vessels and muscles and contribute to venous stasis. Also encourage the client to elevate both legs above the level of the heart for 5 to 10 minutes at least twice a day (Fig. 12.10); to wear low-heeled shoes; and to avoid long periods of standing or sitting, frequently changing her position. If the client has vulvar varicosities, suggest she apply ice packs to the area when she is lying down. See Evidence-Based Practice 12.2.

Hemorrhoids

Hemorrhoids are varicosities of the rectum and may be external (outside the anal sphincter) or internal (above the sphincter) (ACOG, 2007d). They occur as a result of progesterone-induced vasodilation and from pressure of the enlarged uterus on the lower intestine and rectum. Hemorrhoids are more common in women with constipation, poor fluid intake or poor dietary habits, smokers, or those with a previous history of hemorrhoids (Arenson & Drake, 2007).

Instruct the client in measures to prevent constipation, including increasing fiber intake and drinking at least 2 liters of fluid per day. Recommend the use of topical anesthetics (e.g., Preparation H, Anusol, witch hazel compresses) to reduce pain, itching, and swelling, if permitted by the health care provider. Teach the client about local comfort measures such as warm sitz baths, witch hazel compresses, or cold compresses. To minimize her risk of straining while defecating, suggest that she elevate her feet on a stool. Also encourage her to avoid prolonged sitting or standing (ACOG, 2007d).

Flatulence With Bloating

The physiologic changes that result in constipation (reduced gastrointestinal motility and dilation secondary to progesterone's influence) may also result in increased flatulence. As the enlarging uterus compresses the bowel, it delays the passage of food through the intestines, thus allowing more time for gas to be formed by bacteria in

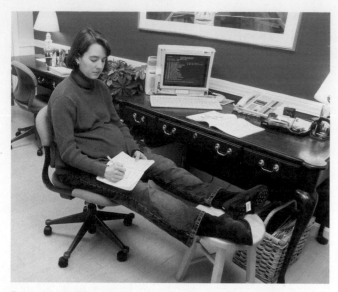

FIGURE 12.10 Woman elevating her legs while working.

the colon. The woman usually reports increased passage of rectal gas, abdominal bloating, or belching. Instruct the woman to avoid gas-forming foods, such as beans, cabbage, and onions, as well as foods that have a high content of white sugar. Adding more fiber to the diet, increasing fluid intake, and increasing physical exercise are also helpful in reducing flatus. In addition, reducing the swallowing of air when chewing gum or smoking will reduce gas build-up. Reducing the intake of carbonated beverages and cheese and eating mints can also help reduce flatulence during pregnancy (Trupin, 2006).

Third-Trimester Discomforts

As women enter their third trimester, many experience a return of the first-trimester discomforts of fatigue, urinary frequency, leukorrhea, and constipation. These discomforts are secondary to the ever-enlarging uterus compressing adjacent structures, increasing hormone

---

EVIDENCE-BASED PRACTICE 12.2
Interventions for Varicose Veins and Leg Edema in Pregnancy

● **Study**

Pregnancy is presumed to be a major contributory factor in the increased incidence of varicose veins in women, which can in turn lead to venous insufficiency and leg edema. The most common symptom of varicose veins and edema is substantial pain, as well as night cramps, numbness, and tingling; also, the legs may feel heavy and achy and the veins may be unsightly.

Varicose veins, sometimes called varicosity, occur when a valve in the blood vessel walls weakens and the blood stagnates. This leads to problems with the circulation in the veins and to edema or swelling. The vein then becomes distended and its walls stretch and sag, allowing the vein to swell into a tiny balloon near the surface of the skin. The veins in the legs are most commonly affected as they are working against gravity, but the vulva (vaginal opening) or rectum, resulting in hemorrhoids (piles), can be affected too.

Treatment of varicose veins is usually divided into three main groups: surgery, pharmacological, and non-pharmacological treatments. Treatment for leg edema mostly involves symptom reduction rather than cure and uses pharmacological and non-pharmacological approaches.

The review identified three trials involving 159 women. Although the drug rutoside seemed to be effective in reducing symptoms, the study was too small to be able to say this with real confidence. Similarly, with compression stockings and reflexology, there were insufficient data to be able to assess benefits and harms, but they looked promising. More research is needed.

▲ **Findings**

Rutoside appears to relieve the symptoms of varicose veins in late pregnancy. However, this finding is based on one small study (69 women), and there are not enough data presented in the study to assess its safety in pregnancy. It therefore cannot be routinely recommended. Reflexology appears to improve symptoms for women with leg edema, but again this is based on one small study (43 women). External compression stockings do not appear to have any advantages in reducing edema.

■ **Nursing Implications**

Nurses can use this evidence to instruct women about varicose veins and outline the various therapies available to treat them. It is not clear that any of the therapies are totally successful in relieving the discomfort associated with varicose veins, based on this analysis, but comfort therapies can be covered to help with the discomfort. Maintaining an ideal weight gain throughout the pregnancy will also help reduce the risk of varicose vein formation.

Source: Bamigboye, A. A., & Smyth, R. (2007). Interventions for varicose veins and leg edema in pregnancy. *Cochrane Database of Systematic Reviews* 2007, Issue 1. Art. No.: CD001066. DOI: 10.1002/14651858.CD001066.pub2.

levels, and the metabolic demands of the fetus. In addition to these discomforts, many women experience shortness of breath, heartburn and indigestion, swelling, and Braxton Hicks contractions.

Shortness of Breath and Dyspnea

The increasing growth of the uterus prevents complete lung expansion late in pregnancy. As the uterus enlarges upward, the expansion of the diaphragm is limited. Dyspnea can occur when the woman lies on her back and the pressure of the gravid uterus against the vena cava reduces venous return to the heart (Arenson & Drake, 2007).

Explain to the woman that dyspnea is normal and will improve when the fetus drops into the pelvis (lightening). Instruct her to adjust her body position to allow for maximum expansion of the chest and to avoid large meals, which increase abdominal pressure. Raising the head of the bed on blocks or placing pillows behind her back is helpful too. In addition, stress that lying on her side will displace the uterus off the vena cava and improve her breathing. Advise the woman to avoid exercise that precipitates dyspnea, to rest after exercise, and to avoid overheating in warm climates. If she still smokes, encourage her to stop.

Heartburn and Indigestion

Heartburn and indigestion result when high progesterone levels cause relaxation of the cardiac sphincter, allowing food and digestive juices to flow backward from the stomach into the esophagus. Irritation of the esophageal lining occurs, causing the burning sensation known as heartburn. It occurs in up to 70% of women at some point during pregnancy, with an increased frequency seen in the third trimester (Blackburn, 2007). The pain may radiate to the neck and throat. It worsens when the woman lies down, bends over after eating, or wears tight clothes. Indigestion (vague abdominal discomfort after meals) results from eating too much or too fast; from eating when tense, tired, or emotionally upset; from eating food that is too fatty or spicy; and from eating heavy food or food that has been badly cooked or processed (Trupin, 2006). In addition, the stomach is displaced upward and compressed by the large uterus in the third trimester, thus limiting the stomach's capacity to empty quickly. Food sits, causing heartburn and indigestion.

Review the client's usual dietary intake and suggest that she limit or avoid gas-producing or fatty foods and large meals. Encourage the client to maintain proper posture and remain in the sitting position for 1 to 3 hours after eating to prevent reflux of gastric acids into the esophagus by gravity. Urge the client to eat slowly, chewing her food thoroughly to prevent excessive swallowing of air, which can lead to increased gastric pressure. Instruct the client to avoid highly spiced foods, chocolate, coffee, alcohol, sodas, and spearmint or peppermint. These items stimulate the release of gastric digestive acids, which may cause reflux into the esophagus. Avoid late-night or large meals and gum chewing.

Dependent Edema

Swelling is the result of increased capillary permeability caused by elevated hormone levels and increased blood volume. Sodium and water are retained and thirst increases. Edema occurs most often in dependent areas such as the legs and feet throughout the day due to gravity; it improves after a night's sleep. Warm weather or prolonged standing or sitting may increase edema. Generalized edema, appearing in the face, hands, and feet, can signal preeclampsia if accompanied by dizziness, blurred vision, headaches, upper quadrant pain, or nausea (Trupin, 2006). This edema should be reported to the health care provider.

Appropriate suggestions to minimize dependent edema include:

- Elevate your feet and legs above the level of the heart.
- Wear support hose when standing or sitting for long periods.
- Change position frequently throughout the day.
- Walk at a sensible pace to help contract leg muscles to promote venous return.
- When taking a long car ride, stop to walk around every 2 hours.
- When standing, rock from the ball of the foot to the toes to stimulate circulation.
- Lie on your left side to keep the gravid uterus off the vena cava to return blood to the heart.
- Avoid foods high in sodium, such as lunch meats, potato chips, and bacon.
- Avoid wearing knee-high stockings.
- Drink six to eight glasses of water daily to replace fluids lost through perspiration.
- Avoid high intake of sugar and fats, because they cause water retention.

Braxton Hicks Contractions

Braxton Hicks contractions are irregular, painless contractions that occur without cervical dilation. Typically they intensify in the third trimester in preparation for labor. In reality, they have been present since early in the pregnancy but may have gone unnoticed. They are thought to increase the tone of uterine muscles for labor purposes (ACOG, 2007e).

Reassure the client that these contractions are normal. Instruct the client in how to differentiate between Braxton Hicks and labor contractions. Explain that true labor contractions usually grow longer, stronger, and closer together and occur at regular intervals. Walking usually strengthens true labor contractions, whereas Braxton Hicks contractions tend to decrease in intensity and taper off. Advise the client to keep herself well hydrated and to rest in a side-lying position to help relieve the discomfort. Suggest that she use breathing techniques such as Lamaze techniques to ease the discomfort.

▶ *Consider* THIS!

One has to wonder sometimes why women go through what they do. During my first pregnancy I was sick for the first 2 months. I would experience waves of nausea from the moment I got out of bed until midmorning. Needless to say, I wasn't the happiest camper around. After the third month, my life seemed to settle down and I was beginning to think that being pregnant wasn't too bad after all. For the moment, I was fooled. Then, during my last 2 months, another wave of discomfort struck—heartburn and constipation—a double whammy! I now feared eating anything that might trigger acid indigestion and also might remain in my body too long. I literally had to become the "fiber queen" to combat these two challenges. Needless to say, my "suffering" was well worth our bright-eyed baby girl in the end.

Thoughts: Despite the various discomforts associated with pregnancy, most women wouldn't change their end result. Do most women experience these discomforts? What suggestions could be made to reduce them?

Nursing Management to Promote Self-Care

Pregnancy is considered a time of health, not illness. Health promotion and maintenance activities are key to promoting an optimal outcome for the woman and her fetus.

Pregnant women commonly have many questions about the changes occurring during pregnancy, how these changes affect their usual routine, such as working, traveling, exercising, or engaging in sexual activity, how the changes influence their typical self-care activities, such as bathing, perineal care, or dental care, and whether these changes are signs of a problem.

▶ *Take* NOTE!

Women may have heard stories about or been told by others what to do and what not to do during pregnancy, leading to many misconceptions and much misinformation.

Nurses can play a major role in providing anticipatory guidance and teaching to foster the woman's responsibility for self-care, helping to clarify misconceptions and correct any misinformation. Educating the client to identify threats to safety posed by her lifestyle or environment and proposing ways to modify them to avoid a negative

outcome are important. Counseling should also include healthy ways to prepare food, advice to avoid medications unless they are prescribed for her, and advice on identifying teratogens within her environment or at work and how to reduce her risk from exposure. The pregnant client can better care for herself and the fetus if her concerns are anticipated and identified by the nurse and are incorporated into teaching sessions at each prenatal visit.

Personal Hygiene

Hygiene is a necessity for the maintenance of good health. Cleansing the skin removes dirt, bacteria, sweat, dead skin cells, and body secretions. Counsel women to wash their hands frequently throughout the day to lower the bacterial count on their hands and under their fingernails. During pregnancy a woman's sebaceous (sweat) glands become more active under the influence of hormones, and sweating is more profuse. This increase may make it necessary to use a stronger deodorant and shower more frequently. The cervical and vaginal glands also produce more secretions during pregnancy. Frequent showering helps to keep the area dry and promotes better hygiene. Encourage the use of cotton underwear to allow greater air circulation. Taking a tub bath in early pregnancy is permitted, but closer to term, when the woman's center of gravity shifts, it is safer to shower to prevent the risk of slipping.

Hot Tubs and Saunas

Caution pregnant women to avoid using hot tubs, saunas, whirlpools, and tanning beds during pregnancy. The heat may cause fetal tachycardia as well as raise the maternal temperature. Exposure to bacteria in hot tubs that have not been cleaned sufficiently is another reason to avoid them during pregnancy.

Perineal Care

The glands in the cervical and vaginal areas become more active during pregnancy secondary to hormonal influences. This increase in activity will produce more vaginal secretions, especially in the last trimester. Advise pregnant women to shower frequently and wear all-cotton underwear to minimize the effects of these secretions. Caution pregnant women not to douche, because douching can increase the risk of infection, and not to wear panty liners, which block air circulation and promote moisture. Explain that they should also avoid perfumed soaps, lotions, perineal sprays, and harsh laundry detergents to help prevent irritation and potential infection.

Dental Care

Research has established that the elevated levels of estrogen and progesterone during pregnancy cause women to be more sensitive to the effects of bacterial dental plaque, which can cause gingivitis, an oral infection characterized by swollen and bleeding gums (Hackley, Kriebs, & Rousseau, 2007). Brushing and flossing teeth twice daily will help reduce bacteria in the mouth. Advise the woman to visit her dentist early in the pregnancy to address any dental caries and have a thorough cleaning to prevent possible infection later in the pregnancy. Advise her to avoid exposure to x-rays by informing the hygienist of the pregnancy. If x-rays are necessary, the abdomen should be shielded with a lead apron.

Researchers are exploring a link between prematurity and periodontitis, an oral infection that spreads beyond the gum tissues to invade the supporting structures of the teeth. Periodontitis is characterized by bleeding gums, loss of tooth attachment, loss of supporting bone, and bad breath due to pus formation. Unfortunately, because this infection is chronic and often painless, women frequently don't realize they have it. Additional guidelines that the nurse should stress regarding maintaining dental health include:

- Seek professional dental care during the first trimester for assessment and care.
- Obtain treatment for dental pain and infection promptly during pregnancy.
- Brush twice daily for 2 minutes, especially before bed, with fluoridated toothpaste and rinse well. Use a soft-bristled toothbrush and be sure to brush at the gum line to remove food debris and plaque to keep gums healthy.
- Eat healthy foods, especially those high in vitamins A, C, and D and calcium.
- Avoid sugary snacks.
- Chew sugar-free gum for 10 minutes after a meal if brushing isn't possible.
- After vomiting, rinse your mouth immediately with baking soda ($\frac{1}{4}$ teaspoon) and warm water (1 cup) to neutralize the acid (Hackley, Kriebs, & Rousseau, 2007).

Breast Care

Since the breasts enlarge significantly and become heavier throughout pregnancy, stress the need to wear a firm, supportive bra with wide straps to balance the weight of the breasts. Instruct the woman to anticipate buying a larger-sized bra about halfway through her pregnancy because of the increasing size of the breasts. Advise her to avoid using soap on the nipple area because it can be very drying. Encourage her to rinse the nipple area with plain water while bathing to keep it clean. The Montgomery glands secrete a lubricating substance that keeps the nipples moist and discourages growth of bacteria, so there is no need to use alcohol or other antiseptics on the nipples.

If the mother has chosen to breastfeed, nipple preparation is unnecessary unless her nipples are inverted and do not become erect when stimulated. Breast shells can be worn during the last 2 months to address this issue (Alexander et al., 2007).

Around week 16 of pregnancy, colostrum secretion begins, which the woman may notice as moisture in her bra. Advise the woman to place breast pads or a cotton cloth in her bra and change them frequently to prevent build-up, which may lead to excoriation.

Clothing

Many contemporary clothes are loose-fitting and layered, so the woman may not need to buy an entirely new wardrobe to accommodate her pregnancy. Some pregnant women may continue to wear tight clothes. Point out that loose clothing will be more comfortable for the client and her expanding waistline.

Advise pregnant women to avoid wearing constricting clothes and girdles that compress the growing abdomen. Urge the woman to avoid knee-high hose, which might impede lower-extremity circulation and increase the risk of developing deep vein thrombosis. Low-heeled shoes will minimize pelvic tilt and possible backache. Wearing layered clothing may be more comfortable, especially toward term, when the woman may feel overheated.

Exercise

Exercise is well tolerated by a healthy woman during pregnancy. It promotes a feeling of well-being, improves circulation, helps reduce constipation, bloating, and swelling, increases energy level, improves posture, helps sleep, promotes relaxation and rest, and relieves the lower back discomfort that often arises as the pregnancy progresses (ACOG, 2007h). However, the duration and difficulty of exercise should be modified throughout pregnancy because of a decrease in performance efficiency with gestational age. Some women continue to push themselves to maintain their prior level of exercise, but most find that as their shape changes and their abdominal area enlarges, they must modify their exercise routines. Modification also helps to reduce the risk of injury caused by laxity of the joints and connective tissue due to the hormonal effects (ACOG, 2007h).

Exercise during pregnancy is contraindicated in women with preterm labor, poor weight gain, anemia, facial and hand edema, pain, hypertension, threatened abortion, dizziness, shortness of breath, incompetent cervix, multiple gestation, decreased fetal activity, cardiac disease, and palpitations (Trupin, 2006).

ACOG has stated that healthy pregnant women can perform the same activity recommended for the general population: 30 minutes or more of moderate exercise every day (ACOG, 2007h; Fig. 12.11). It is believed that pregnancy is a unique time for behavior modification and that healthy behaviors maintained or adopted during

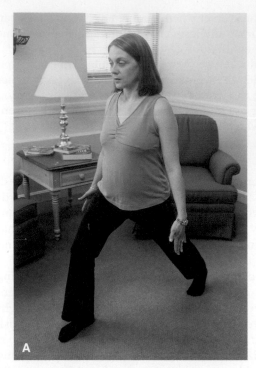

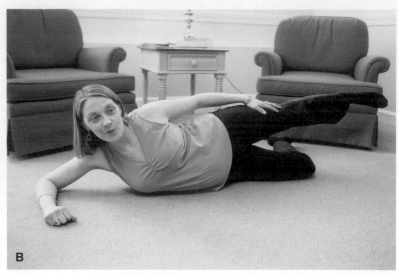

FIGURE 12.11 Exercising during pregnancy.

pregnancy may improve the woman's health for the rest of her life. The excess weight gained in pregnancy, which some women never lose, is a major public health problem (Trupin, 2006). Exercise helps the woman avoid gaining excess weight during pregnancy.

Exercise during pregnancy helps return a woman's body to good health after the baby is born. The long-term benefits of exercise that begin in early pregnancy include improved posture, weight control, and improved muscle tone; exercise also aids in the prevention of osteoporosis after menopause and assists in keeping the birthweight of the fetus within the normal range (Perkins et al., 2007). Teaching Guidelines 12.2 highlights recommendations for exercise during pregnancy.

Sleep and Rest

Getting enough sleep helps a person feel better and promotes optimal performance levels during the day. The body releases its greatest concentration of growth hormone during sleep, helping the body to repair damaged tissue and grow. Also, with the increased metabolic demands during pregnancy, fatigue is a constant challenge to many pregnant women, especially during the first and third trimesters.

The following tips can help promote adequate sleep:

• Stay on a regular schedule by going to bed and waking up at the same times.
• Eat regular meals at regular times to keep external body cues consistent.

• Take time to unwind and relax before bedtime.
• Establish a bedtime routine or pattern and follow it.
• Create a proper sleep environment by reducing the light and lowering the room temperature.

TEACHING GUIDELINES 12.2

Teaching to Promote Exercise During Pregnancy

• Consume liquids before, during, and after exercising.
• Exercise three or four times each week, not sporadically.
• Engage in brisk walking, swimming, biking, or low-impact aerobics; these are considered ideal activities.
• Avoid getting overheated during exercise.
• Reduce the intensity of workouts in late pregnancy.
• Avoid jerky, bouncy, or high-impact movements.
• Avoid lying flat (supine) after the fourth month because of hypotensive effect.
• Use pelvic tilt and pelvic rocking to relieve backache.
• Start with 5 to 10 minutes of stretching exercises.
• Rise slowly following an exercise session to avoid dizziness.
• Avoid activities such as skiing, surfing, scuba diving, and ice hockey.
• Never exercise to the point of exhaustion.

Sources: ACOG (2007b); AAFP (2008); APA (2008).

• Go to bed when you feel tired; if sleep doesn't occur, read a book until you are sleepy.
• Reduce caffeine intake later in the day.
• Limit fluid intake after dinner to minimize trips to the bathroom.
• Exercise daily to improve circulation and well-being.
• Use a modified Sims position to improve circulation in the lower extremities.
• Avoid lying on your back after the fourth month, which may compromise circulation to the uterus.
• Avoid sharply bending your knees, which promotes venous stasis below the knees.
• Keep anxieties and worries out of the bedroom. Set aside a specific area in the home or time of day for them.

Sexual Activity and Sexuality

Pregnancy is characterized by intense biological, psychological, and social changes. These changes have direct and indirect, conscious and unconscious effects on a woman's sexuality. The woman experiences dramatic alterations in her physiology, her appearance, and her body, as well as her relationships. A woman's sexual responses during pregnancy vary widely. Common symptoms such as fatigue, nausea, vomiting, breast soreness, and urinary frequency may reduce her desire for sexual intimacy. However, many women report enhanced sexual desire due to increasing levels of estrogen.

> ▶ **Take** NOTE!
>
> *Fluctuations in sexual desire are normal and a highly individualized response throughout pregnancy.*

The physical and emotional adjustments of pregnancy can cause changes in body image, fatigue, mood swings, and sexual activity. The woman's changing shape, emotional status, fetal activity, changes in breast size, pressure on the bladder, and other common discomforts of pregnancy result in increased physical and emotional demands. These can produce stress on the sexual relationship of the pregnant woman and her partner. However, most women adjust well to the alterations and experience a satisfying sexual relationship (ACOG, 2007c).

Often pregnant women ask whether sexual intercourse is allowed during pregnancy or whether there are specific times when they should refrain from having sex. This is a good opportunity to educate clients about sexual behavior during pregnancy and also to ask about their expectations and individual experience related to sexuality and possible changes. It is also a good time for nurses to address the impact of the changes associated with pregnancy on sexual desire and behavior. For example, some women experience increased sexual desire while others experience less. Couples may enjoy sexual activity more because there is no fear of pregnancy and no need to disrupt spontaneity by using birth control. An increase in pelvic congestion and lubrication secondary to estrogen influence may heighten orgasm for many women. Some women have a decrease in desire because of a negative body image, fear of harming the fetus by engaging in intercourse, and fatigue, nausea, and vomiting (Trupin, 2006). A couple may need assistance to adjust to the various changes brought about by pregnancy.

Reassure the women and her partner that sexual activity is permissible during pregnancy unless there is a history of any of the following:

• Vaginal bleeding
• Placenta previa
• Risk of preterm labor
• Multiple gestation
• Incompetent cervix
• Premature rupture of membranes
• Presence of infection (Trupin, 2006)

Inform the couple that the fetus will not be injured by intercourse. Suggest that alternative positions may be more comfortable (e.g., woman on top, side-lying), especially during the later stages of pregnancy.

Many women feel a particular need for closeness during pregnancy, and the woman should communicate this need to her partner (Thies & Travers, 2006). Emphasize to the couple that closeness and cuddling need not culminate in intercourse, and that other forms of sexual expression, such as mutual masturbation, foot massage, holding hands, kissing, and hugging can be very satisfying (Thies & Travers, 2006).

Women will experience a myriad of symptoms, feelings, and physical sensations during their pregnancy. Having a satisfying sexual relationship during pregnancy is certainly possible, but it requires honest communication between partners to determine what works best for them, and a good relationship with their health care provider to ensure safety (March of Dimes, 2007a).

Employment

For the most part, women can continue working until delivery if they have no complications during their pregnancy and the workplace does not present any special hazards (ACOG, 2007a). Hazardous occupations include health care workers, daycare providers, laboratory technicians, chemists, painters, hairstylists, veterinary workers, and carpenters (ACOG, 2007a). Jobs requiring strenuous work such as heavy lifting, climbing, carrying heavy objects, and standing for prolonged periods place a pregnant woman at risk if modifications are not instituted.

Assess for environmental and occupational factors that place a pregnant women and her fetus at risk for injury. Interview the woman about her employment environment. Ask about possible exposure to teratogens (substances with the potential to alter the fetus permanently in form or function) and the physical demands of employment: Is she exposed to temperature extremes? Does she need to stand for prolonged periods in a fixed position? A description of the work environment is important in providing anticipatory guidance to the woman. Stress the importance of taking rest periods throughout the day, because constant physically intensive workloads increase the likelihood of low birthweight and preterm labor and birth (Cunningham et al., 2005).

Due to the numerous physiologic and psychosocial changes that women experience during their pregnancies, the employer may need to make special accommodations to reduce the pregnant woman's risk of hazardous exposures and heavy workloads. The employer may need to provide adequate coverage so that the woman can take rest breaks; remove the woman from any areas where she might be exposed to toxic substances; and avoid work assignments that require heavy lifting, hard physical labor, continuous standing, or constant moving. Some recommendations for working while pregnant are given in Teaching Guidelines 12.3.

Travel

Pregnancy does not curtail a woman's ability to travel in a car or in a plane. However, women should follow a few safety guidelines to minimize risk to themselves and their fetuses. According to ACOG, pregnant women can travel safely throughout their pregnancy, although the second trimester is perhaps the best time to travel because there is the least chance of complications (ACOG, 2007f). Pregnant women considering international travel should evaluate the problems that could occur during the journey as well as the quality of medical care available at the destination.

▶ **Take** NOTE!

In general, pregnant women with serious underlying illnesses should not travel to developing countries (CDC, 2007c).

Advise pregnant women to be aware of the potential for injuries and trauma related to traveling, and teach women ways to prevent these from occurring. Teaching Guidelines 12.4 offers tips for safe travel on planes and to foreign areas.

When traveling by car, the major risk is a car accident. The impact and momentum can lead to traumatic separation of the placenta from the wall of the uterus. Shock and massive hemorrhage might result (Trupin, 2006). Tips that nurses can offer to promote safety during ground travel include:

- Always wear a three-point seat belt, no matter how short the trip, to prevent ejection or serious injury from collision.
- Apply a nonpadded shoulder strap properly; it should cross between the breasts and over the upper abdomen, above the uterus (Fig. 12.12).
- If no seat belts are available (buses or vans), ride in the back seat of the vehicle.
- Use a lap belt that crosses over the pelvis below the uterus.
- Deactivate the airbag if possible. If you can't, move the seat as far back from the dashboard as possible to minimize impact on the abdomen.
- Avoid using a cellular phone while driving to prevent distraction.
- Avoid driving when very fatigued in the first and third trimesters.
- Avoid late-night driving, when visibility might be compromised.
- Direct a tilting steering wheel away from the abdomen (Hackley, Kriebs, & Rousseau, 2007).

Immunizations and Medications

Ideally, clients should receive all childhood immunizations before conception to protect the fetus from any risk of congenital anomalies. If the client comes for a preconception visit, discuss immunizations such as measles, mumps, and rubella (MMR), hepatitis B, and diphtheria/tetanus (every 10 years); administer them at this time if needed.

TEACHING GUIDELINES 12.3

Teaching for the Pregnant Working Woman

- Plan to take two 10- to 15-minute breaks within an 8-hour workday.
- Be sure there is a place available for you to rest, preferably in the side-lying position, with a restroom readily available.
- Avoid jobs that require strenuous workloads; if this is not possible, then request a modification of work duties (lighter tasks) to reduce your workload.
- Change your position from standing to sitting or vice versa at least every 2 hours.
- Ensure that you are allowed time off without penalty, if necessary, to ensure a healthy outcome for you and your fetus.
- Make sure the work environment is free of toxic substances.
- Ensure the work environment is smoke-free so passive smoking isn't a concern.
- Minimize heavy lifting if associated with bending.

TEACHING GUIDELINES 12.4

Teaching to Promote Safe Travel on Planes and in Foreign Countries

- Bring along a copy of the prenatal record if your travel will be prolonged in case there is a medical emergency away from home.
- When traveling abroad, carry a foreign dictionary that includes words or phrases for the most common pregnancy emergencies.
- Travel with at least one companion at all times for personal safety.
- Check with your health care provider before receiving any immunizations necessary for foreign travel; some may be harmful to the fetus.
- When in a foreign country, avoid fresh fruit, vegetables, and local water.
- Avoid any milk that is not pasteurized.
- Eat only meat that is well cooked to avoid exposure to toxoplasmosis.
- Request an aisle seat and walk about the airplane every 2 hours.
- While sitting on long flights, practice calf-tensing exercises to improve circulation to the lower extremities.
- Be aware of typical problems encountered by pregnant travelers, such as fatigue, heartburn, indigestion, constipation, vaginal discharge, leg cramps, urinary frequency, and hemorrhoids.
- Always wear support hose while flying to prevent the development of blood clots.
- Drink plenty of water to keep well hydrated throughout the flight.

Sources: ACOG (2007f), APA (2008).

The risk to a developing fetus from vaccination of the mother during pregnancy is primarily theoretical. Routine immunizations are not usually indicated during pregnancy. However, no evidence exists of risk from vaccinating pregnant women with inactivated virus or bacterial vaccines or toxoids. A number of other vaccines have not been adequately studied, and thus theoretical risks of vaccination must be weighed against the risks of the disease to mother and fetus (Hackley, Kriebs, & Rousseau, 2007).

▶ *Take NOTE!*

Advise pregnant women to avoid live virus vaccines (MMR and varicella) and to avoid becoming pregnant within 1 month of having received one of these vaccines because of the theoretical risk of transmission to the fetus (CDC, 2007a).

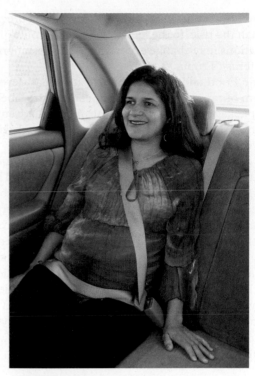

FIGURE **12.12** Proper application of a seat belt during pregnancy.

CDC guidelines for vaccine administration are highlighted in Box 12.4.

It is best for pregnant women not to take any medications. At the very least, encourage them to discuss with the health care provider their current medications and any herbal remedies they take so that they can learn about any potential risks should they continue to take them during pregnancy. Generally, if the woman is taking medicine for seizures, high blood pressure, asthma, or depression,

BOX 12.4 **CDC Guidelines for Vaccine Administration During Pregnancy**

Vaccines That Should be Considered If Otherwise Indicated
- Hepatitis B
- Influenza (inactivated)
- Tetanus/diphtheria
- Meningococcal
- Rabies

Vaccines Contraindicated During Pregnancy
- Influenza (live, attenuated vaccine)
- Measles
- Mumps
- Rubella
- Varicella

Sources: CDC (2007a); March of Dimes (2008); Future Medicine (2007).

the benefits of continuing the medicine during pregnancy outweigh the risks to the fetus. The safety profile of some medications may change according to the gestational age of the fetus (Trupin, 2006).

The Food and Drug Administration has developed a system of ranking drugs that appears on the labels and in the package inserts. These risk categories are summarized in Box 12.5. Always advise women to check with the health care provider for guidance.

A common concern of many pregnant women involves the use of over-the-counter medications and herbal agents. Many women consider these products benign simply because they are available without a prescription (Cragan et al., 2006). While herbal medications are commonly thought of as "natural" alternatives to other medicines, they can be just as potent as some prescription medications. A major concern about herbal medicine is the lack of consistent potency in the active ingredients in any given batch of product, making it difficult to know the exact strength by reading the label. Also, many herbs contain chemicals that cross the placenta and may cause harm to the fetus.

BOX 12.5 FDA Pregnancy Risk Classification of Drugs

- Category A: These drugs have been tested and found safe during pregnancy. Examples: folic acid, vitamin B6, and thyroid medicine.
- Category B: These drugs have been used frequently during pregnancy and do not appear to cause major birth defects or other fetal problems. Examples: antibiotics, acetaminophen (Tylenol), aspartame (artificial sweetener), famotidine (Pepcid), prednisone (cortisone), insulin, and ibuprofen.
- Category C: These drugs are more likely to cause problems and safety studies have not been completed. Examples: prochlorperazine (Compazine), fluconazole (Diflucan), ciprofloxacin (Cipro), and some antidepressants.
- Category D: These drugs have clear health risks for the fetus. Examples: alcohol, lithium (treats bipolar disorders), phenytoin (Dilantin); all chemotherapeutic agents used to treat cancer.
- Category X: These drugs have been shown to cause birth defects and should never be taken during pregnancy. Examples: Accutane (treats cystic acne), androgens (treat endometriosis), Coumadin (prevents blood clots), antithyroid medications for overactive thyroid; radiation therapy (cancer treatment), Tegison or Soriatane (treats psoriasis), streptomycin (treats tuberculosis); thalidomide (treats insomnia), diethylstilbestrol (DES) (treats menstrual disorders), and organic mercury from contaminated food.

Sources: Trupin (2006); USDHHS (2007).

Nurses are often asked about the safety of over-the-counter medicines and herbal agents. Unfortunately, many drugs have not been evaluated in controlled studies, and it is difficult to make general recommendations for these products. Therefore, encourage pregnant women to check with their health care provider before taking anything. Questions about the use of over-the-counter and herbal products are part of the initial prenatal interview.

Nursing Management to Prepare the Woman and Her Partner for Labor, Birth, and Parenthood

Childbirth today is a very different experience from childbirth in previous generations. In the past, women were literally "put to sleep" with anesthetics, and they woke up with a baby. Most women never remembered the details and had a passive role in childbirth as the physician delivered the newborn. In the 1950s, consumers began to insist on taking a more active role in their health care, and couples desired to be together during the extraordinary event of childbirth. Beginning in the 1970s, the father or significant other support person remained with the mother throughout labor and birth (Lleras, 2007).

Childbirth education began because women demanded to become more involved in their birthing experience rather than simply turning control over to a health care provider. Nurses played a pivotal role in bringing about this change by providing information and supporting clients and their families, fostering a more active role in preparing for the upcoming birth.

Traditional childbirth education classes focused on developing and practicing techniques for use in managing pain and facilitating the progress of labor. Recently, the focus of this education has broadened: it now encompasses not only preparation for childbirth, but also preparation for breastfeeding, infant care, transition to new parenting roles, relationship skills, family health promotion, and sexuality (Risica & Phipps, 2007). The term used to describe this broad range of topics is **perinatal education**. Subjects commonly addressed in perinatal education include:

- Anatomy and physiology of reproduction
- Fetal growth and development
- Prenatal maternal exercise
- Physiologic and emotional changes during pregnancy
- Sex during pregnancy
- Infant growth and development
- Nutrition and healthy eating habits during pregnancy
- Teratogens and their impact on the fetus
- Signs and symptoms of labor
- Preparation for labor and birth (for parents, siblings, and other family members)
- Options for birth
- Infant nutrition, including preparation for breastfeeding
- Infant care, including safety, CPR, and first aid
- Family planning (March of Dimes, 2007b)

Childbirth Education Classes

Childbirth education classes teach pregnant women and their support person about pregnancy, birth, and parenting. The classes are offered in local communities or online and are usually taught by certified childbirth educators.

Most childbirth classes support the concept of **natural childbirth** (a birth without pain-relieving medications) so that the woman can be in control throughout the experience as much as possible. The classes differ in their approach to specific comfort techniques and breathing patterns. The three most common childbirth methods are the Lamaze (psychoprophylactic) method, the Bradley (partner-coached childbirth) method, and the Dick-Read (natural childbirth) method.

Lamaze Method

Lamaze is a psychoprophylactic ("mind prevention") method of preparing for labor and birth that promotes the use of specific breathing and relaxation techniques. Dr. Fernand Lamaze, a French obstetrician, popularized this method of childbirth preparation in the 1960s. Lamaze believed that conquering fear through knowledge and support was important. He also believed women needed to alter the perception of suffering during childbirth. This perception change would come about by learning conditioned reflexes that, instead of signaling pain, would signal the work of producing a child, and thus would carry the woman through labor awake, aware, and in control of her own body (Leonard, 2007). Lamaze felt strongly that all women have the right to deliver their babies with minimal or no medication while maintaining their dignity, minimizing their pain, maximizing their self-esteem, and enjoying the miracle of birth.

Lamaze classes include information on toning exercises, relaxation exercises and techniques, and breathing methods for labor. The breathing techniques are used in labor to enhance relaxation and to reduce the woman's perception of pain. The goal is for women to become aware of their own comfortable rate of breathing in order to maintain relaxation and adequate oxygenation of the fetus. Breathing techniques are an effective attention-focusing strategy to reduce pain.

Paced breathing involves breathing techniques used to decrease stress responses and therefore decrease pain. This type of breathing implies self-regulation by the woman. The woman starts off by taking a cleansing breath at the onset and end of each contraction. This cleansing breath symbolizes freeing her mind from worries and concerns. This breath enhances oxygenation and puts the woman in a relaxed state.

Slow-paced breathing is associated with relaxation and should be half the normal breathing rate (six to nine breaths per minute). This type of breathing is the most relaxed pattern and is recommended throughout labor.

Abdominal or chest breathing may be used. It is generally best to breathe in through the nose and breathe out either through the nose or mouth, whichever is more comfortable for the woman.

Modified-paced breathing can be used for increased work or stress during labor to increase alertness or focus attention or when slow-paced breathing is no longer effective in keeping the woman relaxed. The woman's respiratory rate increases, but it does not exceed twice her normal rate. Modified-paced breathing is a quiet upper chest breath that is increased or decreased according to the intensity of the contraction. The inhalation and the exhalation are equal. This breathing technique should be practiced during pregnancy for optimal use during labor.

Patterned-paced breathing is similar to modified-paced breathing but with a rhythmic pattern. It uses a variety of patterns, with an emphasis on the exhalation breath at regular intervals. Different patterns can be used, such as 4/1, 6/1, 4/1. A 4/1 rhythm is four upper chest breaths followed by an exhalation (a sighing out of air, like blowing out a candle). Random patterns can be chosen for use as long as the basic principles of rate and relaxation are met.

Couples practice these breathing patterns typically during the last few months of the pregnancy until they feel comfortable using them. Focal points (visual fixation on a designated object), effleurage (light abdominal massage), massage, and imagery (journey of the mind to a relaxing place) are also added to aid in relaxation. From the nurse's perspective, encourage the woman to breathe at a level of comfort that allows her to cope. Always remain quiet during the woman's periods of imagery and focal point visualization to avoid breaking her concentration.

Bradley Method (Partner-Coached)

The Bradley method uses various exercises and slow, controlled abdominal breathing to accomplish relaxation. Dr. Robert Bradley, a Denver-based obstetrician, advocated a completely unmedicated labor and birth experience. The Bradley method emphasizes the pleasurable sensations of childbirth, teaching women to concentrate on these sensations while "turning on" to their own bodies (Leonard, 2007). In 1965, he wrote *Husband-Coached Childbirth*, which advocated the active participation of the husband as labor coach.

A woman is conditioned to work in harmony with her body using breath control and deep abdominopelvic breathing to promote general body relaxation during labor. This method stresses that childbirth is a joyful, natural process and emphasizes the partner's involvement during pregnancy, labor, birth, and the early newborn period. Thus, the training techniques are directed toward the coach, not the mother. The coach is educated in massage/comfort techniques to use on the mother throughout the labor and birth process.

Dick–Read Method

In 1944 Grantly Dick-Read, a British obstetrician, wrote *Childbirth Without Fear.* He believed that the attitude of a woman toward her birthing process had a considerable influence on the ease of her labor, and he believed that fear is the primary pain-producing agent in an otherwise normal labor. He felt that fear builds a state of tension, creating an antagonistic effect on the laboring muscles of the uterus, which results in pain. Pain causes more fear, which further increases the tension, and the vicious cycle of "fear–tension–pain" is established (Leonard, 2007). Dick-Read sought to interrupt the circular pattern of fear, tension, and pain during the labor and birthing process. He promoted the belief that the degree of fear could be diminished with increased understanding of the normal physiologic response to labor (Alexander et al., 2007).

Dick-Read believed that prenatal instruction was essential for pain relief and that emotional factors during labor interfered with the normal labor progression. The woman achieves relaxation and reduces pain by arming herself with the knowledge of normal childbirth and using abdominal breathing during contractions.

Nursing Management and Childbirth Education

Childbirth education is less about methods than about mastery. The overall aim of any of the methods is to promote an internal locus of control that will enable each woman to yield her body to the process of birth. As the woman gains success and tangible benefits from the exercises she is taught, she begins to reframe her beliefs and gains practical knowledge, and the impetus will be there for her to engage in the conscious use of the techniques (Fig. 12.13). Nurses play a key role in supporting and encouraging each couple's use of the techniques taught in childbirth education classes.

Every woman's labor is unique, and it is important for nurses not to generalize or stereotype women. The most effective support a nurse can offer couples using prepared childbirth methods is encouragement and presence. These nursing measures must be adapted to each individual throughout the labor process. Offering encouraging phrases such as "great job" or "you can do it" helps to reinforce their efforts and at the same time empowers them to continue. Using eye-to-eye contact to engage the woman's total attention is important if she appears overwhelmed or appears to lose control during the transition phase of labor.

Nurses play a significant role in enhancing the couple's relationship by respecting the involvement of the partner and demonstrating concern for his needs throughout labor. Offering to stay with the woman to give him a break periodically allows him to meet his needs while at the same time still actively participating. Offer anticipatory guidance to the couple and assist during critical times in labor. Demonstrate many of the coping techniques to the partner and praise their successful use, which increases self-esteem. Focus on their strengths and the positive elements of the labor experience. Congratulating the couple for a job well done is paramount.

Throughout the labor experience, demonstrate personal warmth and project a friendly attitude. Frequently, a nurse's touch may help to prevent a crisis by reassuring the mother that she is doing fine.

Options for Birth Settings and Care Providers

From the moment a woman discovers she is pregnant, numerous decisions await her—where the infant will be born, what birth setting is best, and who will assist with the birth. The great majority of women are well and healthy and can consider the full range of birth settings—hospital, birth center, or home setting—and care providers. They should be given information about each to ensure the most informed decision.

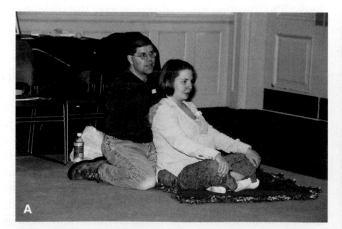
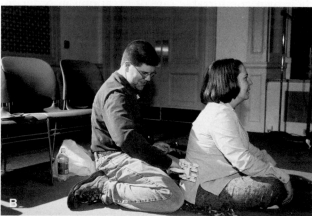

FIGURE 12.13 A couple practicing the techniques taught in a childbirth education class.

Birth Settings

Hospitals are the most common site for birth in the United States. If the woman has a serious medical condition or is at high risk for developing one, she will probably need to plan to give birth in a hospital setting under the care of an obstetrician. Giving birth in a hospital is advantageous for several reasons. Hospitals are best equipped to diagnose and treat women and newborns with complications; trained personnel are available if necessary; and no transportation is needed if a complication should arise during labor or birth. Disadvantages include the high-tech atmosphere; strict policies and restrictions that might limit who can be with the woman; and the medical model of care.

Within the hospital setting, however, choices do exist regarding birth environments. The conventional delivery room resembles an operating room, where the health care professional delivers the newborn from the woman, who is positioned in stirrups. The woman is then transferred to the recovery area on a stretcher and then again to the postpartum unit. The birthing suite is the other option within the hospital setting. In the birthing suite, the woman and her partner remain in one place for labor, birth, and recovery. The birthing suite is a private room decorated to look as homelike as possible. For example, the bed converts to allow for various birthing positions, and there may be a rocking chair or an easy chair for the woman's partner. Despite the homey atmosphere, the room is still equipped with emergency resuscitative obstetric equipment and electronic fetal monitors in case they are needed quickly (Fig. 12.14A). Such settings provide a more personal childbirth experience in a less formal and intimidating atmosphere compared to the traditional delivery room.

A freestanding birth center (Fig. 12.14B) can be a good choice for a woman who wants more personalized care than in a hospital but does not feel comfortable with a home birth. In contrast to the institutional environment in hospitals, most freestanding birth centers have a homelike atmosphere, and many are, in fact, located in converted homes. Some are located on hospital property and are affiliated with them. Birth centers are designed to provide maternity care to women judged to be at low risk for obstetric complications. Women are allowed and encouraged to give birth in the position most comfortable for them. Care in birth centers is often provided by midwives and is more relaxed, with no routine intravenous lines, fetal monitoring, and restrictive protocols. A disadvantage of the birth center is the need to transport the woman to a hospital quickly if an emergency arises, because emergency equipment is not readily available. In a research study comparing homelike to conventional institutional settings, the author concluded that there appeared to be some benefits from homelike settings for childbirth, although increased support from caregivers may be more important (Walsh, 2007).

Most women who choose a home birth believe that birth is a natural process that requires little medical intervention (Mayor, 2007). Home births can be safe if there are qualified, experienced attendants and an emergency transfer system in place in case of serious complications. Many women choose the home setting out of a strong desire to control their child's birth and to give birth surrounded by family members. Most home birth caregivers are midwives who have provided continuous care to the woman throughout the pregnancy. Disadvantages include the need to transport the woman to the hospital during or after labor if a problem arises, and the limited pain management available in the home setting.

Care Providers

While most women in the United States still receive pregnancy care from an obstetrician, an increasing number are choosing a midwife for their care. The difference is a matter of degrees. Obstetricians must finish a 4-year residency in obstetrics and gynecology in addition to medical school. Certified nurse-midwives complete 1 to 2 years of graduate work in midwifery following nursing school. Obstetricians can handle high-risk pregnancies and delivery emergencies; can administer or order pain-relief

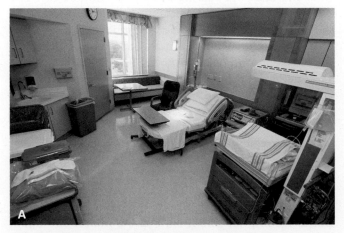
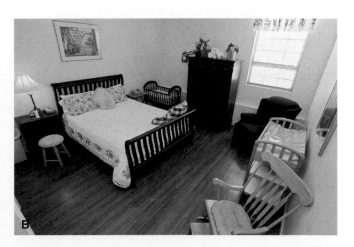

FIGURE 12.14 (**A**) Birthing suite. (**B**) Birthing center.

drugs; and are assisted by a support staff in the hospital setting. Midwives work in hospitals, birthing centers, and home settings to deliver care. They believe in the normalcy of birth and tolerate wide variations of what is considered normal during labor, which leads to fewer interventions applied during the childbirth process (Knowlton, 2007). They are not able to handle high-risk births and some birth emergencies.

In addition to the woman's primary health care professional, some women hire a doula to be with them during the childbearing process. Doula is a Greek word that means "woman's servant." A doula is a laywoman trained to provide women and their families with encouragement, emotional and physical support, and information through late pregnancy, labor, birth, and postpartum. Doulas provide the woman with continuous support throughout labor but do not perform any clinical procedures.

Preparation for Breastfeeding or Bottle-Feeding

Pregnant women are faced with a decision about which method of feeding to choose. Educate the pregnant client about the advantages and disadvantages of each method, allowing the woman and her partner to make an informed decision about the best method for their situation. Providing the client and her partner with this information will increase the likelihood of a successful experience regardless of the method of feeding chosen.

Breastfeeding

Substantial scientific evidence exists documenting the health benefits of breastfeeding for newborns. Human milk provides an ideal balance of nutrients for newborns (ACOG, 2006). Breastfeeding is advantageous for the following reasons:

- Human milk is digestible and economical and requires no preparation.
- Bonding between mother and child is promoted.
- Cost is less than purchasing formula.
- Ovulation is suppressed (however, this is not a reliable birth control method).
- The risk of ovarian cancer and the incidence of premenopausal breast cancer are reduced for the woman.
- Extra calories are used, which promotes weight loss gradually without dieting.
- Oxytocin is released to promote more rapid uterine involution with less bleeding.
- Sucking helps to develop the muscles in the infant's jaw.
- Absorption of lactose and minerals in the newborn is improved.
- The immunologic properties of breast milk help prevent infections in the baby.
- The composition of breast milk adapts to meet the infant's changing needs.

- Constipation in the baby is not a problem with adequate intake.
- Food allergies are less likely to develop in the breast-fed baby.
- The incidence of otitis media and upper respiratory infections in the infant is reduced.
- Breastfed babies are less likely to be overfed, thus reducing the risk of adult obesity.
- Breastfed newborns are less prone to vomiting (ACOG, 2006).

One could say that lactation and breastfeeding are so natural that they should just happen on their own accord, but this is not the case. Learning to breastfeed takes practice, requires support from the partner, and requires dedication and patience on the part of the mother; it may be necessary to work closely with a lactation consultant to be successful and comfortable in doing it.

Breastfeeding also has disadvantages. These include breast discomfort, sore nipples, mastitis, engorgement, milk stasis, vaginal dryness, and decreased libido (Blackburn, 2007). Some mothers feel it is inconvenient or embarrassing, limits other activities, limits partner involvement, increases their dependency by being tied to the infant all the time, and restricts their use of alcohol or drugs. Nurses can help mothers to cope with their fear of dependency and feelings of obligation by emphasizing the positive aspects of breastfeeding and encouraging bonding experiences.

Nipple preparation is not necessary during the prenatal period unless the nipples are inverted and do not become erect when stimulated. Assess for this by placing the forefinger and thumb above and below the areola and compressing behind the nipple. If it flattens or inverts, advise the client to wear breast shields during the last 2 months of pregnancy. Breast shields exert a continuous pressure around the areola, pushing the nipple through a central opening in the inner shield (ACOG, 2006). The shields are worn inside the bra. Initially the shields are worn for 1 hour, and then the woman progressively increases the wearing time up to 8 hours daily. The client maintains this schedule until after delivery, and then she wears the shield 24 hours a day until the infant latches on easily (ACOG, 2006). In addition, suggest that the woman wear a supportive nursing bra 24 hours a day.

Encourage the woman to attend a breastfeeding support group (e.g., La Leche League), provide her with sources of information about infant feeding, and suggest that she read a good reference book about lactation. All of these activities will help in her decision-making process and will be invaluable to her should she choose to breastfeed her newborn.

Bottle Feeding

Bottle-feeding an infant isn't just a matter of "open, pour, and feed." Parents need information on types of formulas, preparation and storage of formula, equipment, and feeding positions. It is recommended that normal full-term infants receive conventional cow's milk-based formula; the physician should direct this choice. If the infant has a reaction (diarrhea, vomiting, abdominal pain, excessive gas) to the first formula, another formula should be tried. Sometimes a soy-based formula is substituted. In terms of preparation of formula and its use, the following guidelines should be stressed:

- Obtain adequate equipment (six 4-ounce bottles, eight 8-ounce bottles, and nipples).
- Consistency is important. Stay with a nipple that is comfortable to the infant.
- Frequently assess nipples for any loose pieces of rubber at the opening.
- Correct formula preparation is critical to the health and development of the infant. Formula is available in three forms: ready-to-feed, concentrate, and powder.
- Read the formula label thoroughly before mixing.
- Correct formula dilution is important to avoid fluid imbalances. For ready-to-use, use as is without dilution. For concentrated formulas, dilute with equal parts of water. For powdered formulas, mix one scoop of powder with 2 ounces of water.
- If the water supply is safe, sterilization is not necessary.
- Bottles and nipples should be washed in hot, sudsy water using a bottle brush.
- Formula should be served at room temperature.
- If the water supply is questionable, water should be boiled for 5 minutes before use.
- Formula should not be heated in a microwave oven, because it is heated unevenly.
- Formula can be prepared 24 hours ahead of time and stored in the refrigerator.

Teach the woman and other caretakers to feed the infant in a semi-upright position using the cradle hold in the arms. This position allows for face-to-face contact between the infant and caretaker. Advise the caretaker to hold the bottle so that the nipple is kept full of formula to prevent excessive air swallowing. Instruct the caretaker to feed the infant every 3 to 4 hours and adapt the feeding times to the infant's needs. Frequent burping of the infant (every ounce) helps prevent gas from building up in the stomach. Caution the caretaker not to prop the bottle; propping the bottle can cause choking (Lawson, 2007).

Bottle-feeding should mirror breastfeeding as closely as possible. While nutrition is important, so are the emotional and interactive components of feeding. Encourage the caretaker to cuddle the infant closely and position the infant so that his or her head is in a comfortable position. Also encourage communication with the infant during feedings.

> ▶ *Take* NOTE!
>
> *Warn the caretaker about the danger of putting the infant to bed with a bottle; this can lead to "baby bottle tooth decay" because sugars in the formula stay in contact with the infant's developing teeth for prolonged periods.*

Final Preparation for Labor and Birth

The nurse has played a supportive/education role for the couple throughout the pregnancy and now needs to assist in preparing them for their "big event" by making sure they have made informed decisions and completed the following checklist:

- Attended childbirth preparation classes and practiced breathing techniques
- Selected a birth setting and made arrangements there
- Know what to expect during labor and birth
- Toured the birthing facility
- Packed a suitcase to take to the birthing facility when labor starts
- Made arrangements to have siblings and/or pets taken care of during labor
- Have been instructed on signs and symptoms of labor and what to do
- Know what to do if membranes rupture prior to going into labor
- Know how to reach their health care professional when labor starts
- Communicated their needs and desires concerning pain management
- Discussed the possibility of a cesarean birth if complications occur
- Discussed possible names for the newborn
- Selected a feeding method (bottle or breast) with which they feel comfortable
- Made a decision regarding circumcision if they have a boy
- Purchased an infant safety seat in which to bring their newborn home
- Decided on a pediatrician
- Have items needed to prepare for the newborn's homecoming:
  - Infant clothes in several sizes
  - Nursing bras
  - Infant crib with spaces between the slats that are 2⅜ inches or less apart
  - Diapers (cloth or disposable)
  - Feeding supplies (bottles and nipples if bottle-feeding)
  - Infant thermometer
- Selected a family planning method to use after the birth

At each prenatal visit the nurse has had the opportunity to discuss and reinforce the importance of being prepared for the birth of the child with the parents. It is now up to the parents to use the nurse's guidance and put it into action to be ready for their upcoming "big event."

■■■ Key Concepts

- Preconception care is the promotion of the health and well-being of a woman and her partner before pregnancy. The goal of preconception care is to identify any areas such as health problems, lifestyle habits, or social concerns that might unfavorably affect pregnancy.

- A thorough history and physical examination is performed on the initial prenatal visit.

- A primary aspect of nursing management during the antepartum period is counseling and educating the pregnant women and her partner to promote healthy outcomes for all involved.

- Nagele's rule can be used to establish the estimated date of birth. Using this rule, subtract 3 months, add 7 days to the first day of the last normal menstrual period, then correct the year by adding 1 to it. This date is within plus or minus 2 weeks (margin of error).

- Pelvic shape is typically classified as one of four types: gynecoid, android, anthropoid, and platypelloid. The gynecoid type is the typical female pelvis and offers the best shape for a vaginal delivery.

- Continuous prenatal care is important for a successful outcome. The recommended schedule is every 4 weeks up to 28 weeks (7 months); every 2 weeks from 29 to 36 weeks; and every week from 37 weeks to birth.

- The height of the fundus is measured when the uterus arises out of the pelvis to evaluate fetal growth.

- The fundus reaches the level of the umbilicus at approximately 20 weeks and measures 20 cm. Fundal measurement should approximately equal the number of weeks of gestation until week 36.

- At each visit the woman is asked whether she is having any common signs or symptoms of preterm labor, which might include uterine contractions, dull backache, pressure in the pelvic area or thighs, increased vaginal discharge, menstrual-like cramps, and vaginal bleeding.

- Prenatal screening has become standard in prenatal care to detect neural tube defects and genetic abnormalities.

- The nurse should address common discomforts that occur in each trimester matter-of-factly at all prenatal visits and should provide realistic measures to help the client deal with them effectively.

- The pregnant client can better care for herself and the fetus if her concerns are anticipated by the nurse and incorporated into guidance sessions at each prenatal visit.

- Iron and folic acid need to be supplemented because their increased requirements during pregnancy are usually too great to be met through diet alone.

- The American College of Obstetricians and Gynecologists recommends a 25- to 35-pound weight gain during pregnancy.

- For a pregnant woman to meet recommended dietary reference intakes (DRIs), it is important for her to eat according to the USDA's Food Guide Pyramid.

- Throughout pregnancy, a well-balanced diet is critical for a healthy baby.

- Perinatal education has broadened its focus to include preparation for pregnancy and family adaptation to the new parenting roles. Childbirth education began because of increasing pressure from consumers who wanted to become more involved in their birthing experience.

- Three common childbirth education methods are Lamaze (psychoprophylactic), Bradley (partner-coached childbirth), and Dick-Read (natural childbirth).

- The great majority of women in the United States are well and healthy and can consider the full range of birth settings: hospital, birth center, or home setting.

- All pregnant women need to be able to recognize early signs of contractions to prevent preterm labor.

REFERENCES

Alexander, L. L., LaRosa, J. H., Bader, H., & Garfield, S. (2007). *New dimensions in women's health* (4th ed.). Sudbury, MA: Jones and Bartlett Publishers.

American Academy of Family Physicians (AAFP). (2008). Pregnancy and exercise: What you can do for a healthy pregnancy. Available at: http://familydoctor.org/online/famdocen/home/women/pregnancy/basics/305.html

American College of Obstetricians and Gynecologists (ACOG). (2004). *ACOG issues position on first-trimester screening methods.* ACOG News Release. Available at: http://acog.org/from_home/publications/press_releases/nr06-30-04.cfm

American College of Obstetricians and Gynecologists (ACOG). (2006). *Breastfeeding your baby.* Available at: http://www.acog.org/publications/patient_education/bp029.cfm

American College of Obstetricians and Gynecologists (ACOG). (2007a). *Planning for your pregnancy and birth* (4th ed.). Washington, DC: Author.

American College of Obstetricians and Gynecologists (ACOG). (2007b). *Easing back pain during pregnancy.* Available at: http://www.acog.org/publications/patient_education/bp115.cfm

American College of Obstetricians and Gynecologists (ACOG). (2007c). *Sexuality and sexual problems.* Available at: http://www.acog.org/publications/patient_education/bp072.cfm

American College of Obstetricians and Gynecologists (ACOG). (2007d). *Problems of the digestive system.* Available at: http://www.acog.org/publications/patient_education/bp120.cfm

American College of Obstetricians and Gynecologists (ACOG). (2007e). *How to tell when labor begins.* Available at: http://www.acog.org/publications/patient_education/bp004.cfm

American College of Obstetricians and Gynecologists (ACOG). (2007f). *Air travel during pregnancy* (ACOG Committee Opinion No. 264). Washington, DC: Author.

American College of Obstetricians and Gynecologists (ACOG). (2007g). *Neural tube defects* (ACOG Practice Bulletin No. 44). Available at http://www.guideline.gov/summary/summary.aspx?ss=15&doc_id=3994&nbr=3131

American College of Obstetricians and Gynecologists (ACOG). (2007h). *Exercise during pregnancy.* Available at: http://www.acog.org/publications/patient_education/bp119.cfm

American Pregnancy Association (APA). (2008). Effect of exercise on pregnancy. Available at: http://www.americanpregnancy.org/pregnancy/health/effectsofexerciseonpreg.html

American Pregnancy Association (APA). (2008). Pregnancy and travel. Available at: http://www.americanpregnancy.org/pregnancyhealth/travel.html

Arenson, J., & Drake, P. (2007). *Maternal and newborn nursing.* Sudbury, MA: Jones and Bartlett Publishers.

Atrash, H. K., Johnson, K., Adams, M., Cordero, J. F., & Howse, J. (2006). Preconception care for improved perinatal outcomes: The time to act. *Maternal & Child Health, 10*(5), Supplement: S3–11.

Blackburn, S. T. (2007). *Maternal, fetal, and neonatal physiology: A clinical perspective* (3rd ed.). St. Louis, MO: Saunders Elsevier.

Caughey, A. B., Musci, T. J., Belluomini, J., Main, D., Otto, C., & Goldberg, J. (2007). Nuchal translucency screening: How do women actually utilize the results? *Prenatal Diagnosis, 27*(2), 119–123.

Centers for Disease Control and Prevention (CDC). (2006). *Recommendations to improve preconception health and health care—United States.* Atlanta, GA: CDC.

Centers for Disease Control and Prevention (CDC). (2007a). *Guidelines for vaccinating pregnant women.* Recommendations of the Advisory Committee on Immunization Practices (ACIP). Atlanta, GA: CDC.

Centers for Disease Control and Prevention (CDC). (2007b). *Preconception health and care.* Available at: http://www.cdc.gov/ncbddd/preconception/default.htm

Centers for Disease Control and Prevention (CDC). (2007c). *Pregnancy, breast-feeding and travel: Factors affecting the decision to travel.* Traveler's Health. Available at: http://www.cdc.gov/travel/pregnant.htm

Centers for Disease Control and Prevention (CDC). (2008). Having a healthy pregnancy. Available at: http://www.cdc.gov/ncbdd/bd.abc.htm

Cragan, J. D., Friedman, J. M., Holmes, L. B., Uhl, K., Green, N. S., & Riley, L. (2006). Ensuring the safe and effective use of medications during pregnancy: Planning and prevention through preconception care. *Maternal & Child Health Journal,* Supplement, Vol. 10, 129–135.

Cunningham, F., et al. (2005). *William's obstetrics* (22nd ed.). New York: McGraw-Hill.

Dashe, J. S., Twickler, D. M., Santos-Ramos, R. McIntire, D. D., & Ramus, R. M. (2006). Alpha-fetoprotein detection of neural tube defects and the impact of standard of ultrasound. *American Journal of Obstetrics & Gynecology, 195*(6), 1623–1628.

Dillon, P. M. (2007). *Nursing health assessment: A critical thinking, case studies approach.* Philadelphia: F. A. Davis Company.

Dunlop, A. L., Jack, B., & Frey, K. (2007). National recommendations for preconception care: The essential role of the family physician. *Journal of the American Board of Family Medicine, 20*(1), 81–84.

Frieden, F. J., & Chan, Y. (2007). Antepartum care. In R. E. Rakel & E. T. Bope (Eds.), *Conn's current therapy 2007* (Section 16; pp. 1169–1174), Philadelphia: Saunders Elsevier.

Future Medicine. (2007). Vaccination during pregnancy. Available at: http://futuremedicine.com/doi/abs/10.2217/17455057.3.2.227

Gearhart, P. A., & Sehdev, H. M. (2007). Biophysical profile. *eMedicine.* Available at: http://emedicine.com/radio/topic758.htm

Gilbert, E. S. (2007). *Manual of high-risk pregnancy and delivery* (4th ed.). St. Louis, MO: Mosby.

Graham, L. (2006). CDC releases guidelines on improving preconception health care. *American Family Physician, 74*(11), 1967–1970.

Hackley, B., Kriebs, J. M., & Rousseau, M. E. (2007). *Primary care of women: A guide for midwives and women's health practitioners.* Sudbury, MA: Jones and Bartlett Publishers.

Jenkins, T. M., Caughey, A. B., Hopkins, L. M., & Norton, M. E. (2007). Chorionic villus sampling compared with amniocentesis and the difference in the rate of pregnancy loss. *Obstetrics & Gynecology, 109*(1), 204–206.

Kenner, C., & Lott, J. W. (2007). *Comprehensive neonatal care: An interdisciplinary approach* (4th ed.). St. Louis, MO: Saunders Elsevier.

Knowlton, L. (2007). Labor of love: Nurse midwife Ruth Watson Lubic. *American Journal of Nursing, 107*(4), 86–87.

Lane, C. A. (2007). Nausea and vomiting in pregnancy: A tailored approach treatment. *Clinical Obstetrics & Gynecology, 50*(1), 100–111.

Lawson, M. (2007). Contemporary aspects of infant feeding. *Pediatric Nursing, 19*(2), 39–44.

Leonard, P. (2007). Childbirth education: A handbook for nurses. *Nursing Spectrum.* Available at: http://nsweb.nursingspectrum.com/ce/m350a.htm

Lleras, D. (2007). The childbirth experience: An obstetrical nurse's experience. *International Journal of Childbirth Education, 22*(1), 19–21.

Lynch, S. W. (2007). Greater expectations. *Alternative Medicine Magazine,* March (95), 64–71.

Mangesi, L., & Hofmeyr, G. (2007). Fetal movement counting for assessment of fetal well-being. *Cochrane Database of Systematic Reviews.* (Cochrane Database Syst Rev) 2007(1). Cochrane AN: CD004909.

March of Dimes. (2007a). The joy of sex during pregnancy. Available at: http://www.marchofdimes.com/printableArticles/159_516.asp?printable=true

March of Dimes. (2007b). Childbirth educational classes. Available at: http://www.marchofdimes.com/pnhec/159_12929.asp

March of Dimes. (2007c). Prematurity: The answers can't come soon enough. Available at: http://www.marchofdimes.com/prematurity

March of Dimes. (2008). Before pregnancy: Preconception. Available at: http://www.marchofdimes.com/pnhec/173.asp

March of Dimes. (2008). Vaccination during pregnancy. Available at: http://www.marchofdimes.com/pnhec/159_16189.asp

Mayor, S. (2007). NICE recommends women should choose where to give birth after discussing the risks. *British Medical Journal, 334*(7295), 654–660.

Mikkelsen, T. B., Andersen, A. N., & Olsen, S. F. (2007). Pica in pregnancy in a privileged population: Myth or reality? *Obstetrical & Gynecological Survey, 62*(2), 94–95.

National Institutes of Health (NIH). (2008). High-risk pregnancy. Available at: http://www.nichd.nih.gov/healthtopics/high_risk_pregnancy.cfm

Perkins, C., Pivarnik, J. M., Paneth, N., & Stein, A. D. (2007). Physical activity and fetal growth during pregnancy. *Obstetrics & Gynecology, 109*(1), 81–87.

Risica, P. M., & Phipps, M. G. (2007). Educational preferences in a prenatal clinic population. *International Journal of Childbirth Education, 21*(4), 4–7.

Singh, D., & Singh, J. R. (2008). Prenatal diagnosis for congenital malformations and genetic disorders. *eMedicine.* Available at: http://www.emedicine.com/oph/topic485.htm

Thies, K. M., & Travers, J. F. (2006). *Handbook of human development for health care professionals.* Sudbury, MA: Jones and Bartlett Publishers.

Trupin, S. R. (2006). Common pregnancy complaints and questions. *eMedicine.* Available at: http://emedicine.com/med/topic3238.htm

U.S. Department of Health and Human Services. (2000). *Healthy People 2010.* Washington, DC: US Department of Health and Human Services.

U.S. Department of Health and Human Services (USDHHS). (2007). Pregnancy and medicines. Available at: http://www.4women.gov/faq/pregmed.htm

Valley, V. T., & Fly, C. A. (2006). Pelvic ultrasonography. *eMedicine.* Available at: http://www.emedicine.com/emerg/topic622.htm

Walling, A. D. (2007). Pregnancy loss after amniocentesis and CVS. *American Family Physician, 75*(2), 258–259.

Walsh, D. J. (2007). A birth center's encounters with discourses of childbirth: how resistance led to innovation. *Sociology of Health & Illness, 29*(2), 216–232.

WEBSITES

American Academy of Husband-Coached Childbirth: www.bradleybirth.com

American College of Nurse Midwives: (202) 347-5445, www.acnm.org

American College of Obstetricians and Gynecologists (ACOG): www.acog.com

Association of Women's Health, Obstetrics & Neonatal Nurses: www.awhonn.org

Doulas of North America (DONA): (206) 324-5440, www.dona.com

International Childbirth Education Association: www.icea.org

International Lactation Consultation Association (ILCA): www.ilca.org

La Leche League International: (800) 525-3243, www.lalacheleague.org

Lamaze International: (800) 368-4404, www.lamaze-childbirth.com

March of Dimes: www.modimes.com

Mayo Clinic Pregnancy Center: www.mayoclinic.org

National Center for Education in Maternal and Child Health: www.ncemch.org

Prepared Childbirth Education: www.childbirtheducation.org

Special Supplemental Nutrition Program for Women, Infants, and Children (WIC): www.usda.gov/fns/wic.html

CHAPTER WORKSHEET

MULTIPLE CHOICE QUESTIONS

1. Which of the following biophysical profile findings indicate poor oxygenation to the fetus?

   a. Two pockets of amniotic fluid

   b. Well-flexed arms and legs

   c. Nonreactive fetal heart rate

   d. Fetal breathing movements noted

2. The nurse teaches the pregnant client how to perform Kegel exercises as a way to accomplish which of the following?

   a. Prevent perineal lacerations

   b. Stimulate postdates labor

   c. Increase pelvic muscle tone

   d. Lose pregnancy weight quickly

3. During a clinic visit, a pregnant client at 30 weeks' gestation tells the nurse, "I've had some mild cramps that are pretty irregular. What does this mean?" The cramps are probably:

   a. the beginning of labor in the very early stages

   b. an ominous finding indicating that the client is about to have a miscarriage

   c. related to overhydration in the client

   d. Braxton Hicks contractions, which occur throughout pregnancy

4. The nurse teaches a pregnant woman about exercise and activity, including activities not recommended during pregnancy. The nurse determines that the teaching was effective when the pregnant woman states that which of the following activities is not recommended during pregnancy?

   a. Swimming

   b. Walking

   c. Scuba diving

   d. Bike riding

5. A pregnant client's last normal menstrual period was on August 10. Using Nagele's rule, the nurse calculates that her estimated date of birth (EDB) will be which of the following?

   a. June 23

   b. July 10

   c. July 30

   d. May 17

CRITICAL THINKING EXERCISES

1. Mary Jones comes to the Women's Health Center, where you work as a nurse. She is in her first trimester of pregnancy and tells you her main complaints are nausea and fatigue, to the point that she wants to sleep most of the time and eats one meal daily. She appears pale and tired. Her mucous membranes are pale. She reports that she gets 8 to 9 hours of sleep each night but still can't seem to stay awake and alert at work. She tells you she knows that she is not eating as she should, but she isn't hungry. Her hemoglobin and hematocrit are low.

   a. What subjective and objective data do you have to make your assessment?

   b. What is your impression of this woman?

   c. What nursing interventions would be appropriate for this client?

   d. How will you evaluate the effectiveness of your interventions?

2. Monica, a 16-year-old African-American high school student, is here for her first prenatal visit. Her last normal menstrual period was 2 months ago, and she states she has been "sick ever since." She is 5 feet, 6 inches tall and weighs 110 pounds. In completing her dietary assessment, the nurse asks about her intake of milk and dairy products. Monica reports that she doesn't like "that stuff" and doesn't want to put on too much weight because it "might ruin my figure."

   a. In addition to the routine obstetric assessments, which additional ones might be warranted for this teenager?

   b. What dietary instruction should be provided to this teenager based on her history?

   c. What follow-up monitoring should be included in subsequent prenatal visits?

3. Maria, a 27-year-old Hispanic woman in her last trimester of pregnancy (34 weeks), complains to the clinic nurse that she is constipated and feels miserable most of the time. She reports that she has started taking laxatives, but mostly they don't help her. When questioned about her dietary habits, she replies that she eats beans and rice and drinks tea with most meals. She says she has tried to limit her fluid intake so she doesn't have to go to the bathroom so much because she doesn't

want to miss any of her daytime soap operas on television.

a. What additional information would the nurse need to assess her complaint?

b. What interventions would be appropriate for Maria?

c. What adaptations will Maria need to make to alleviate her constipation?

STUDY ACTIVITIES

1. Visit a freestanding birth center and compare it to a traditional hospital setting in terms of restrictions, type of pain management available, and costs.

2. Arrange to shadow a nurse-midwife for a day to see her role in working with the childbearing family.

3. Select two of the websites supplied at the end of this chapter and note their target audience, the validity of information offered, and their appeal to expectant couples. Present your findings.

4. Request permission to attend a childbirth education class in your local area and help a woman without a partner practice the paced breathing exercises. Present the information you learned and think about how you can apply it while taking care of a woman during labor.

5. A laywoman with a specialized education and experience in assisting women during labor is a

_____.

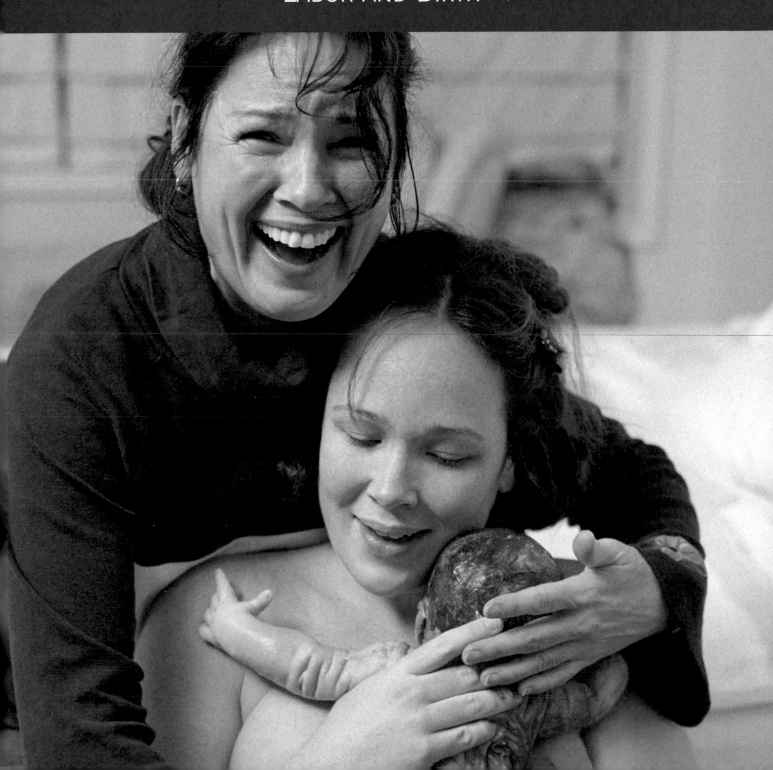

UNIT FOUR

LABOR AND BIRTH

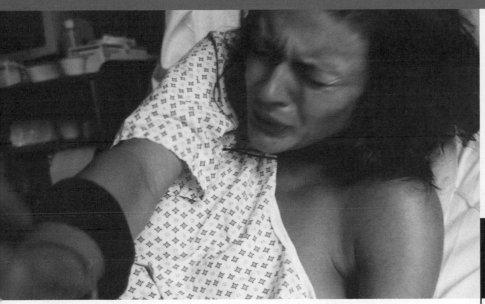

CHAPTER 13

LABOR AND BIRTH PROCESS

KEY TERMS

attitude	engagement	molding
dilation	frequency	position
doula	intensity	presentation
duration	lie	station
effacement	lightening	

LEARNING OBJECTIVES

Upon completion of the chapter, the learner will be able to:

1. Outline premonitory signs of labor.
2. Compare and contrast true versus false labor.
3. Categorize the critical factors affecting labor and birth.
4. Analyze the cardinal movements of labor.
5. Identify the maternal and fetal responses to labor and birth.
6. Classify the stages of labor and the critical events in each stage.
7. Explain the normal physiologic/psychological changes occurring during all four stages of labor.
8. Formulate the concept of pain as it relates to the woman in labor.

Kathy and Chuck have been eagerly awaiting the birth of their first child for what seems to them an eternity. When Kathy finally feels contractions in her abdomen, she and Chuck rush to the birthing center. After the OB nurse completes a complete history and physical assessment, she informs Kathy and her husband that she must have experienced "false labor" and that they should return home until she starts true labor.

Wow

Intense physical and emotional support promotes a positive and memorable birthing experience.

The process of labor and birth involves more than the birth of a newborn. Numerous physiologic and psychological events occur that ultimately result in the birth of a newborn and the creation or expansion of the family.

This chapter describes labor and birth as a process. It addresses initiation of labor, the premonitory signs of labor, including true and false labor, critical factors affecting labor and birth, maternal and fetal response to the laboring process, and the four stages of labor. The chapter also identifies critical factors related to each stage of labor: the "10 P's" of labor.

Initiation of Labor

Labor is a complex, multifaceted interaction between the mother and fetus. It is a series of processes by which the fetus is expelled from the uterus. It is difficult to determine exactly why labor begins and what initiates it. Although several theories have been proposed to explain the onset and maintenance of labor, none of these has been proved scientifically. It is widely believed that labor is influenced by a combination of factors, including uterine stretch, progesterone withdrawal, increased oxytocin sensitivity, and increased release of prostaglandins.

One theory suggests that labor is initiated by a change in the estrogen-to-progesterone ratio. During the last trimester of pregnancy, estrogen levels increase and progesterone levels decrease. This change leads to an increase in the number of myometrium gap junctions. Gap junctions are proteins that connect cell membranes and facilitate coordination of uterine contractions and myometrial stretching (Gilbert, 2007).

Although physiologic evidence for the role of oxytocin in the initiation of labor is inconclusive, the number of oxytocin receptors in the uterus increases at the end of pregnancy. This creates an increased sensitivity to oxytocin. Estrogen, the levels of which are also rising, increases myometrial sensitivity to oxytocin. With the increasing levels of oxytocin in the maternal blood in conjunction with fetal production, initiation of uterine contractions can occur. Oxytocin also aids in stimulating prostaglandin synthesis through receptors in the decidua. Prostaglandins lead to additional contractions, cervical softening, gap junction induction, and myometrial sensitization, thereby leading to a progressive cervical **dilation** (the opening or enlargement of the external cervical os) (Blackburn, 2007).

Prostaglandins are produced in the decidua and fetal membranes and have a central role in the initiation of labor. Prostaglandin levels increase late during pregnancy secondary to elevated estrogen levels. Prostaglandins stimulate smooth muscle contraction of the uterus. An increase in prostaglandins leads to myometrial contractions and a reduction in cervical resistance. Subsequently, the cervix softens, thins out, and dilates during labor.

Premonitory Signs of Labor

Before the onset of labor, a pregnant woman's body undergoes several changes in preparation for the birth of the newborn. The changes that occur often lead to characteristic signs and symptoms that suggest that labor is near. These premonitory signs and symptoms can vary, and not every woman experiences every one of them.

Cervical Changes

Before labor begins, cervical softening and possible cervical dilation with descent of the presenting part into the pelvis occurs. These changes can occur 1 month to 1 hour before actual labor begins.

As labor approaches, the cervix changes from an elongated structure to a shortened, thinned segment. Cervical collagen fibers undergo enzymatic rearrangement into smaller, more flexible fibers that facilitate water absorption, leading to a softer, more stretchable cervix. These changes occur secondary to the effects of prostaglandins and pressure from Braxton Hicks contractions (Blackburn, 2007).

Lightening

Lightening occurs when the fetal presenting part begins to descend into the maternal pelvis. The uterus lowers and moves into a more anterior position. The shape of the abdomen changes as a result of the change in the uterus. With this descent, the woman usually notes that her breathing is much easier. However, she may complain of increased pelvic pressure, cramping, and low back pain. She may notice an increase in vaginal discharge and more frequent urination. Also, edema of the lower extremities may occur as a result of the increased stasis of pooling blood. In primiparas, lightening can occur 2 weeks or more before labor begins; among multiparas it may not occur until labor (Walsh, 2007).

Increased Energy Level

Some women report a sudden increase in energy before labor. This is sometimes referred to as nesting, because many women will focus this energy toward childbirth preparation by cleaning, cooking, preparing the nursery, and spending extra time with other children in the household. The increased energy level usually occurs 24 to 48 hours before the onset of labor. It is thought to be the result of an increase in epinephrine release caused by a decrease in progesterone (Cheng & Caughey, 2007).

Bloody Show

At the onset of labor, the mucous plug that fills the cervical canal during pregnancy is expelled as a result of cervical softening and increased pressure of the presenting part. These ruptured cervical capillaries release a small amount of blood that mixes with mucus, resulting in the pink-tinged secretions known as bloody show.

Braxton Hicks Contractions

Braxton Hicks contractions, which the woman may have been experiencing throughout the pregnancy, may become stronger and more frequent. Braxton Hicks contractions are typically felt as a tightening or pulling sensation of the top of the uterus. They occur primarily in the abdomen and groin and gradually spread downward before relaxing. In contrast, true labor contractions are more commonly felt in the lower back. These contractions aid in moving the cervix from a posterior position to an anterior position. They also help in ripening and softening the cervix. However, the contractions are irregular and can be decreased by walking, voiding, eating, increasing fluid intake, or changing position.

Braxton Hicks contractions usually last about 30 seconds but can persist for as long as 2 minutes. As birth draws near and the uterus becomes more sensitive to oxytocin, the frequency and intensity of these contractions increase. However, if the contractions last longer than 30 seconds and occur more often than four to six times an hour, advise the woman to contact her health care provider so that she can be evaluated for possible preterm labor, especially if she is less than 38 weeks pregnant.

▶ *Take* NOTE!

An infant born between 34 and 36 completed weeks of gestation is identified as "late preterm" and experiences many of the same health issues as other preterm birth infants (AWHONN, 2007).

Spontaneous Rupture of Membranes

One in four women will experience spontaneous rupture of the membranes before the onset of labor (Institute of Medicine, 2007). The rupture of membranes can result in either a sudden gush or a steady leakage of amniotic fluid. Although much of the amniotic fluid is lost when the rupture occurs, a continuous supply is produced to ensure protection of the fetus until birth.

After the amniotic sac has ruptured, the barrier to infection is gone and an ascending infection is possible. In addition, there is a danger of cord prolapse if engagement has not occurred with the sudden release of fluid and pressure with rupture. Due to the possibility of these complications, advise women to notify their health care provider and go in for an evaluation.

▶ *Consider* THIS!

I always pictured myself a dignified woman and behaved in ways to demonstrate that, for that was the way I was raised. My mother and grandmother always stressed that you should look good, dress well, and do nothing to embarrass yourself in public. I did a fairly good job of living up to their expectations until I become pregnant. I recall I was overdue according to my dates and was miserable in the summer heat. I decided to go to the store for some ice cream. As I waddled down the grocery aisles, all of a sudden my water broke and came pouring down my legs all over the floor. Not wanting to make a spectacle of myself and remembering what my mother always said about being dignified at all times in public, I quickly reached up onto the grocery shelf and "accidentally" knocked off a large jar of pickles right where my puddle was. As I walked hurriedly away from that mess without my ice cream, I heard on the store loudspeaker, "Clean-up on aisle 13!"

Thoughts: We tend to live by what we are taught, and in this case, this woman needed to save face from her ruptured membranes. Many women experience ruptured membranes before the onset of labor, so it is not out of the ordinary for this to happen in public. What risks can occur when membranes do rupture? What action should this woman take now to minimize these risks? How will the nurse validate this woman's ruptured membranes?

True Versus False Labor

False labor is a condition occurring during the latter weeks of some pregnancies in which irregular uterine contractions are felt, but the cervix is not affected. In contrast, true labor is characterized by contractions occurring at regular intervals that increase in frequency, duration, and intensity. True labor contractions bring about progressive cervical dilation and effacement. Table 13.1 summarizes the differences between true and false labor. False labor, prodromal labor, and Braxton Hicks contractions are all names for contractions that do not contribute in a measurable way toward the goal of birth.

Many women fear being sent home from the hospital with "false labor." All women feel anxious when they feel contractions, but they should be informed that labor could be a long process, especially if it is their first pregnancy. Encourage the woman to think of false labor or "pre-labor signs" as positive, as they are part of the entire labor continuum. With first pregnancies, the cervix can take up to 20 hours to dilate completely (Cunningham et al., 2005).

TABLE 13.1 DIFFERENCES BETWEEN TRUE AND FALSE LABOR

Parameters	True Labor	False Labor
Contraction timing	Regular, becoming closer together, usually 4–6 minutes apart, lasting 30–60 seconds	Irregular, not occurring close together
Contraction strength	Become stronger with time, vaginal pressure is usually felt	Frequently weak, not getting stronger with time or alternating (a strong one followed by weaker ones)
Contraction discomfort	Starts in the back and radiates around toward the front of the abdomen	Usually felt in the front of the abdomen
Any change in activity	Contractions continue no matter what positional change is made	Contractions may stop or slow down with walking or making a position change
Stay or go?	Stay home until contractions are 5 minutes apart, last 45–60 seconds, and are strong enough so that a conversation during one is not possible—then go to the hospital or birthing center.	Drink fluids and walk around to see if there is any change in the intensity of the contractions; if the contractions diminish in intensity after either or both—stay home.

Sources: Arenson & Drake, 2007; Blackburn, 2007; Cunningham et al., 2005.

Remember Kathy and Chuck, the anxious couple who came to the hospital too early? Kathy felt sure she was in labor and is now confused. What explanations and anticipatory guidance should be offered to this couple? What term would describe her earlier contractions?

Factors Affecting the Labor Process

In many references, the critical factors that affect the process of labor and birth are outlined as the "five P's":

1. Passageway (birth canal)
2. Passenger (fetus and placenta)
3. Powers (contractions)
4. Position (maternal)
5. Psychological response

These critical factors are commonly accepted and discussed by health care professionals. However, five additional "P's" can also affect the labor process:

1. Philosophy (low-tech, high-touch)
2. Partners (support caregivers)
3. Patience (natural timing)
4. Patient preparation (childbirth knowledge base)
5. Pain control (comfort measures)

These five additional "P's" are helpful in planning care for the laboring family. These patient-focused factors are an attempt to foster labor that can be managed through the use of high touch, patience, support, knowledge, and pain management.

Passageway

The birth passageway is the route through which the fetus must travel to be born vaginally. The passageway consists of the maternal pelvis and soft tissues. Of the two, however, the maternal bony pelvis is more important because it is relatively unyielding (except for the coccyx). Typically the pelvis is assessed and measured during the first trimester, often at the first visit to the health care provider, to identify any abnormalities that might hinder a successful vaginal birth. As the pregnancy progresses, the hormones relaxin and estrogen cause the connective tissues to become more relaxed and elastic and cause the joints to become more flexible to prepare the mother's pelvis for birth. Additionally, the soft tissues usually yield to the forces of labor.

Bony Pelvis

The maternal bony pelvis can be divided into the true and false portions. The false (or greater) pelvis is composed of the upper flared parts of the two iliac bones with their concavities and the wings of the base of the sacrum. The false pelvis is divided from the true pelvis by an imaginary line drawn from the sacral prominence at the back to the superior aspect of the symphysis pubis at the front of the pelvis. This imaginary line is called the linea terminalis. The false pelvis lies above this imaginary line; the true pelvis lies below it (Fig. 13.1). The true pelvis is the bony passageway through which the fetus must travel. It is made up of three planes: the inlet, the mid-pelvis (cavity), and the outlet.

Pelvic Inlet

The pelvic inlet allows entrance to the true pelvis. It is bounded by the sacral prominence in the back, the ilium on the sides, and the superior aspect of the symphysis pubis in

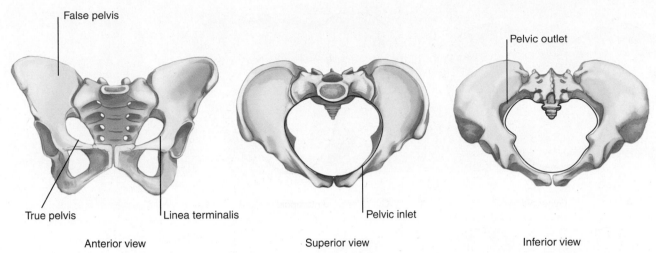

FIGURE **13.1** The bony pelvis.

the front (Edmonds, 2007). The pelvic inlet is wider in the transverse aspect (sideways) than it is from front to back.

Mid-Pelvis

The mid-pelvis (cavity) occupies the space between the inlet and outlet. It is through this snug, curved space that the fetus must travel to reach the outside. As the fetus passes through this small area, its chest is compressed, causing lung fluid and mucus to be expelled. This expulsion removes the space-occupying fluid so that air can enter the lungs with the newborn's first breath.

Pelvic Outlet

The pelvic outlet is bound by the ischial tuberosities, the lower rim of the symphysis pubis, and the tip of the coccyx. In comparison with the pelvic inlet, the outlet is wider from front to back. For the fetus to pass through the pelvis, the outlet must be large enough.

To ensure the adequacy of the pelvic outlet for vaginal birth, the following pelvic measurements are assessed:

- Diagonal conjugate of the inlet (distance between the anterior surface of the sacral prominence and the anterior surface of the inferior margin of the symphysis pubis)
- Transverse or ischial tuberosity diameter of the outlet (distance at the medial and lowest aspect of the ischial tuberosities, at the level of the anus; a known hand span or clenched-fist measurement is generally used to obtain this measurement)
- True or obstetric conjugate (distance estimated from the measurement of the diagonal conjugate; 1.5 cm is subtracted from the diagonal conjugate measurement)

For more information about pelvic measurements, see Chapter 12.

If the diagonal conjugate measures at least 11.5 cm and the true or obstetric conjugate measures 10 cm or more (1.5 cm less than the diagonal conjugate, or about 10 cm), then the pelvis is large enough for a vaginal birth of what would be considered a normal-size newborn.

Pelvic Shape

In addition to size, the shape of a woman's pelvis is a determining factor for a vaginal birth. The pelvis is divided into four main shapes: gynecoid, anthropoid, android, and platypelloid (Fig. 13.2).

The gynecoid pelvis is considered the true female pelvis, occurring in about 50% of all women; it is less common in men (Leonard, 2007). Vaginal birth is most favorable with this type of pelvis because the inlet is round and the outlet is roomy. This shape offers the optimal diameters in all three planes of the pelvis. This type of pelvis allows early and complete fetal internal rotation during labor.

The anthropoid pelvis is common in men and occurs in 20% to 30% of women (Billington & Stevenson, 2007). The pelvic inlet is oval and the sacrum is long, producing a deep pelvis (wider front to back [anterior to posterior] than side to side [transverse]). Vaginal birth is more favorable with this pelvic shape compared to the android or platypelloid shape (Frieden & Chan, 2007).

The android pelvis is considered the male-shaped pelvis and is characterized by a funnel shape. It occurs in approximately 20% of women (Cunningham et al., 2005). The pelvic inlet is heart-shaped and the posterior segments are reduced in all pelvic planes. Descent of the fetal head into the pelvis is slow, and failure of the fetus to rotate is common. The prognosis for labor is poor, subsequently leading to cesarean birth.

The platypelloid or flat pelvis is the least common type of pelvic structure among men and women, with an approximate incidence of 5% (Billington & Stevenson, 2007). The pelvic cavity is shallow but widens at the pelvic outlet, making it difficult for the fetus to descend through

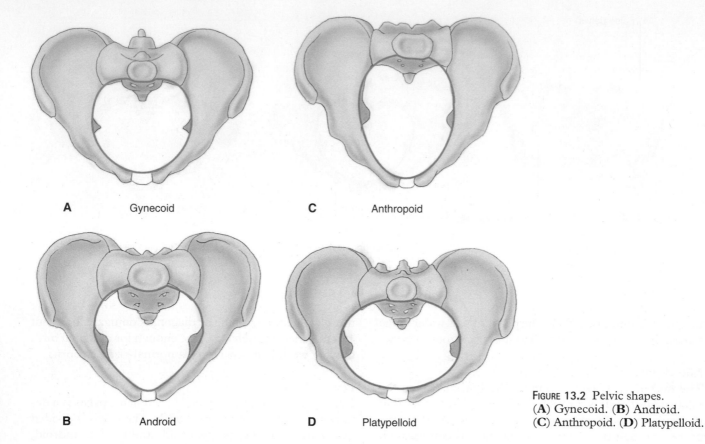

A Gynecoid

C Anthropoid

B Android

D Platypelloid

FIGURE 13.2 Pelvic shapes.
(**A**) Gynecoid. (**B**) Android.
(**C**) Anthropoid. (**D**) Platypelloid.

the mid-pelvis. It is not favorable for a vaginal birth unless the fetal head can pass through the inlet. Women with this type of pelvis usually require cesarean birth.

An important principle is that most pelves are not purely defined but occur in nature as mixed types. Many women have a combination of these four basic pelvis types, with no two pelves being exactly the same. Regardless of the shape, the newborn will be born if size and positioning remain compatible. The narrowest part of the fetus attempts to align itself with the narrowest pelvic dimension (e.g., biparietal to interspinous diameters, which means the fetus generally tends to rotate to the most ample portion of the pelvis).

Soft Tissues

The soft tissues of the passageway consist of the cervix, the pelvic floor muscles, and the vagina. Through **effacement**, the cervix effaces (thins) and dilates (opens) to allow the presenting fetal part to descend into the vagina.

▶ *Take* NOTE!

Cervical effacement and dilation is similar to pulling a turtleneck sweater over your head.

The pelvic floor muscles help the fetus to rotate anteriorly as it passes through the birth canal. The soft tissues of the vagina expand to accommodate the fetus during birth.

Passenger

The fetus (with placenta) is the passenger. The fetal head (size and presence of molding), fetal attitude (degree of body flexion), fetal lie (relationship of body parts), fetal presentation (first body part), fetal position (relationship to maternal pelvis), fetal station, and fetal engagement are all important factors that have an impact on the ultimate outcome in the birthing process.

Fetal Head

The fetal head is the largest and least compressible fetal structure, making it an important factor in relation to labor and birth. Considerable variation in the size and diameter of the fetal skull is often seen.

Compared with an adult, the fetal head is large in proportion to the rest of the body, usually about one quarter of the body surface area (Kenner & Lott, 2007). The bones that make up the face and cranial base are fused and essentially fixed. However, the bones that make up the rest of the cranium (two frontal bones, two parietal bones, and the occipital bone) are not fused; rather, they are soft and pliable, with gaps between the plates of bone. These gaps, which are membranous spaces between the cranial bones, are called sutures, and the intersections of these sutures are called fontanelles. Sutures are important because they allow the cranial bones to overlap in order for the head to adjust in shape (elongate) when pressure is exerted on it by uterine contractions or the maternal bony pelvis. Some diameters shorten whereas others lengthen as the head is molded during the labor and birthing process. This malleability of the fetal skull may decrease fetal skull dimensions by 0.5 to 1 cm (Blackburn, 2007). After birth, the sutures close as the bones grow and the brain reaches its full growth.

The changed (elongated) shape of the fetal skull at birth as a result of overlapping of the cranial bones is known as **molding**. Along with molding, fluid can also collect in the scalp (caput succedaneum) or blood can collect beneath the scalp (cephalohematoma), further distorting the shape and appearance of the fetal head. Caput succedaneum can be described as edema of the scalp at the presenting part. This swelling crosses suture lines and disappears within 3 to 4 days. Cephalhematoma is a collection of blood between the periosteum and the bone. It does not cross suture lines and is generally reabsorbed over the next 4 to 6 weeks (Arenson & Drake, 2007).

▶ **Take** NOTE!

Parents may become concerned about the distortion of their newborn's head. However, reassurance that the oblong shape is only temporary is usually all that is needed to reduce their anxiety.

Sutures also play a role in helping to identify the position of the fetal head during a vaginal examination. Figure 13.3 shows a fetal skull. The coronal sutures are located between the frontal and parietal bones and extend transversely on both sides of the anterior fontanelles. The frontal suture is located between the two frontal bones. The lambdoidal sutures are located between the occipital bone and the two parietals, extending transversely on either side of the posterior fontanelles. The sagittal suture is located between the parietal bones and divides the skull into the right and left halves. During a pelvic examination, palpation of these sutures by the examiner reveals the position of the fetal head and the degree of rotation that has occurred.

The anterior and posterior fontanelles are also useful in helping to identify the position of the fetal head, and they allow for molding. In addition, the fontanelles are important when evaluating the newborn. The anterior

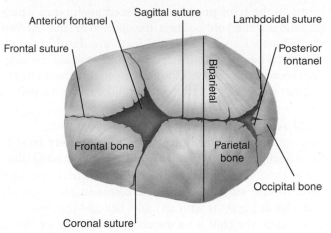

FIGURE 13.3 Fetal skull.

fontanelle is the famous "soft spot" of the newborn's head. It is diamond-shaped and measures about 2 to 3 cm. It remains open for 12 to 18 months after birth to allow for growth of the brain (Edmonds, 2007). The posterior fontanelle corresponds to the anterior one but is located at the back of the fetal head; it is triangular. This one closes within 8 to 12 weeks after birth and measures, on average, 0.5 to 1 cm at its widest diameter (Kenner & Lott, 2007).

The diameter of the fetal skull is an important consideration during the labor and birth process. Fetal skull diameters are measured between the various landmarks of the skull. Diameters include occipitofrontal, occipitomental, suboccipitobregmatic, and biparietal (Fig. 13.4). The two most important diameters that can affect the birth process are the suboccipitobregmatic (approximately 9.5 cm at term) and the biparietal (approximately 9.25 cm at term) diameters. The suboccipitobregmatic diameter, measured from the base of the occiput to the center of the anterior fontanelle, identifies the smallest anteroposterior diameter of the fetal skull. The biparietal diameter measures the largest transverse diameter of the fetal skull: the distance between the two parietal bones. In a cephalic (headfirst) presentation, which occurs in 95% of all term

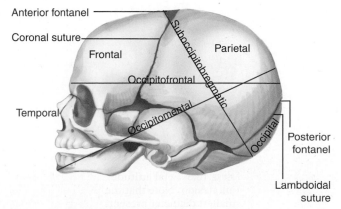

FIGURE 13.4 Fetal skull diameters.

births, if the fetus presents in a flexed position in which the chin is resting on the chest, the optimal or smallest fetal skull dimensions for a vaginal birth are demonstrated. If the fetal head is not fully flexed at birth, the anteroposterior diameter increases. This increase in dimension might prevent the fetal skull from entering the maternal pelvis.

Fetal Attitude

Fetal attitude is another important consideration related to the passenger. Fetal **attitude** refers to the posturing (flexion or extension) of the joints and the relationship of fetal parts to one another. The most common fetal attitude when labor begins is with all joints flexed—the fetal back is rounded, the chin is on the chest, the thighs are flexed on the abdomen, and the legs are flexed at the knees (Fig. 13.5). This normal fetal position is most favorable for vaginal birth, presenting the smallest fetal skull diameters to the pelvis.

When the fetus presents to the pelvis with abnormal attitudes (no flexion or extension), the diameter can increase the diameter of the presenting part as it passes through the pelvis, increasing the difficulty of birth. An attitude of extension tends to present larger fetal skull diameters, which may make birth difficult.

Fetal Lie

Fetal **lie** refers to the relationship of the long axis (spine) of the fetus to the long axis (spine) of the mother. There are two primary lies: longitudinal (which is the most common) and transverse (Fig. 13.6).

A longitudinal lie occurs when the long axis of the fetus is parallel to that of the mother (fetal spine to maternal spine side-by-side). A transverse lie occurs when the long axis of the fetus is perpendicular to the long axis of the mother (fetus spine lies across the maternal abdomen and crosses her spine). A fetus in a transverse lie position cannot be delivered vaginally (Billington & Stevenson, 2007).

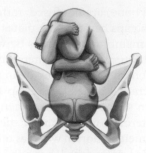

A. Longitudinal lie

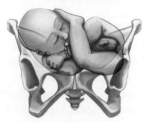

B. Transverse lie
FIGURE 13.6 Fetal lie.

Fetal Presentation

Fetal **presentation** refers to the body part of the fetus that enters the pelvic inlet first (the "presenting part"). This is the fetal part that lies over the inlet of the pelvis or the cervical os. Knowing which fetal part is coming first at birth is critical for planning and initiating appropriate interventions.

The three main fetal presentations are cephalic (head first), breech (pelvis first), and shoulder (scapula first). The majority of term newborns (95%) enter this world in a cephalic presentation; breech presentation accounts for 3% of term births, shoulder presentations for approximately 2% (Edmonds, 2007).

In a cephalic presentation, the presenting part is usually the occiput portion of the fetal head (Fig. 13.7). This presentation is also referred to as a vertex presentation. Variations in a vertex presentation include the military, brow, and face presentations.

Breech presentation occurs when the fetal buttocks or feet enter the maternal pelvis first and the fetal skull enters last. This abnormal presentation poses several challenges at birth. Primarily, the largest part of the fetus (skull) is born last and may become "hung up" or stuck in the pelvis. In addition, the umbilical cord can become compressed between the fetal skull and the maternal pelvis after the fetal chest is born because the head is the last to exit. Moreover, unlike the hard fetal skull, the buttocks are soft and are not as effective as a cervical dilator during labor compared with a cephalic presentation. Finally, there is the possibility of trauma to the head as a result of the lack of opportunity for molding.

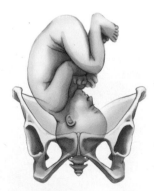

FIGURE 13.5 Fetal attitude: Full flexion. Note that the smallest diameter presents to the pelvis.

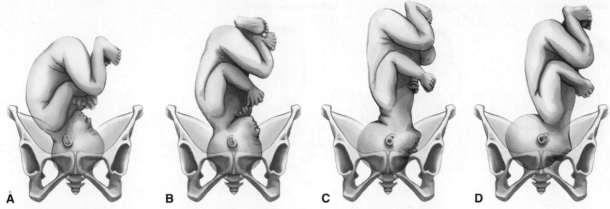

FIGURE **13.7** Fetal presentation: cephalic presentations. (**A**) Vertex. (**B**) Military. (**C**) Brow. (**D**) Face.

The types of breech presentations are determined by the positioning of the fetal legs (Fig. 13.8). In a frank breech (50% to 70%), the buttocks present first with both legs extended up toward the face. In a full or complete breech (5% to 10%), the fetus sits crossed-legged above the cervix. In a footling or incomplete breech (10% to 30%), one or both legs are presenting. Breech presentations are associated with prematurity, placenta previa, multiparity, uterine abnormalities (fibroids), and some congenital anomalies such as hydrocephaly (Fischer, 2007). A frank breech can result in a vaginal birth, but complete, footling, and incomplete breech presentations generally necessitate a cesarean birth.

A shoulder presentation occurs when the fetal shoulders present first, with the head tucked inside. Odds of a shoulder presentation are one in 1,000 (Cunningham et al., 2005). The fetus is in a transverse lie with the shoulder as the presenting part. Conditions associated with shoulder presentation include placenta previa, multiple gestation, or fetal anomalies. A cesarean birth is typically necessary (Edmonds, 2007).

Fetal Position

Fetal **position** describes the relationship of a given point on the presenting part of the fetus to a designated point of the maternal pelvis (Walsh, 2007). The landmark fetal presenting parts include the occipital bone (O), which designates a vertex presentation; the chin (mentum [M]), which designates a face presentation; the buttocks (sacrum [S]), which designate a breech presentation; and the scapula (acromion process [A]), which designates a shoulder presentation.

In addition, the maternal pelvis is divided into four quadrants: right anterior, left anterior, right posterior, and left posterior. These quadrants designate whether the presenting part is directed toward the front, back, left, or right side of the pelvis. Fetal position is determined first by identifying the presenting part and then the maternal quadrant the presenting part is facing (Fig. 13.9). Position is indicated by a three-letter abbreviation as follows:

• The first letter defines whether the presenting part is tilted toward the left (L) or the right (R) side of the maternal pelvis.

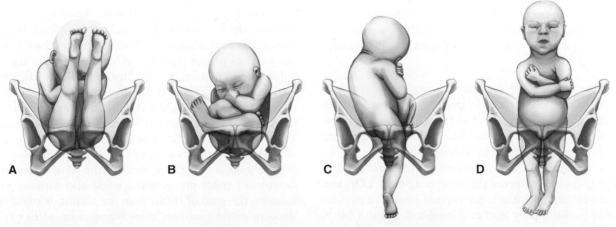

FIGURE **13.8** Breech presentations. (**A**) Frank breech. (**B**) Complete breech. (**C**) Single footling breech. (**D**) Double footling breech.

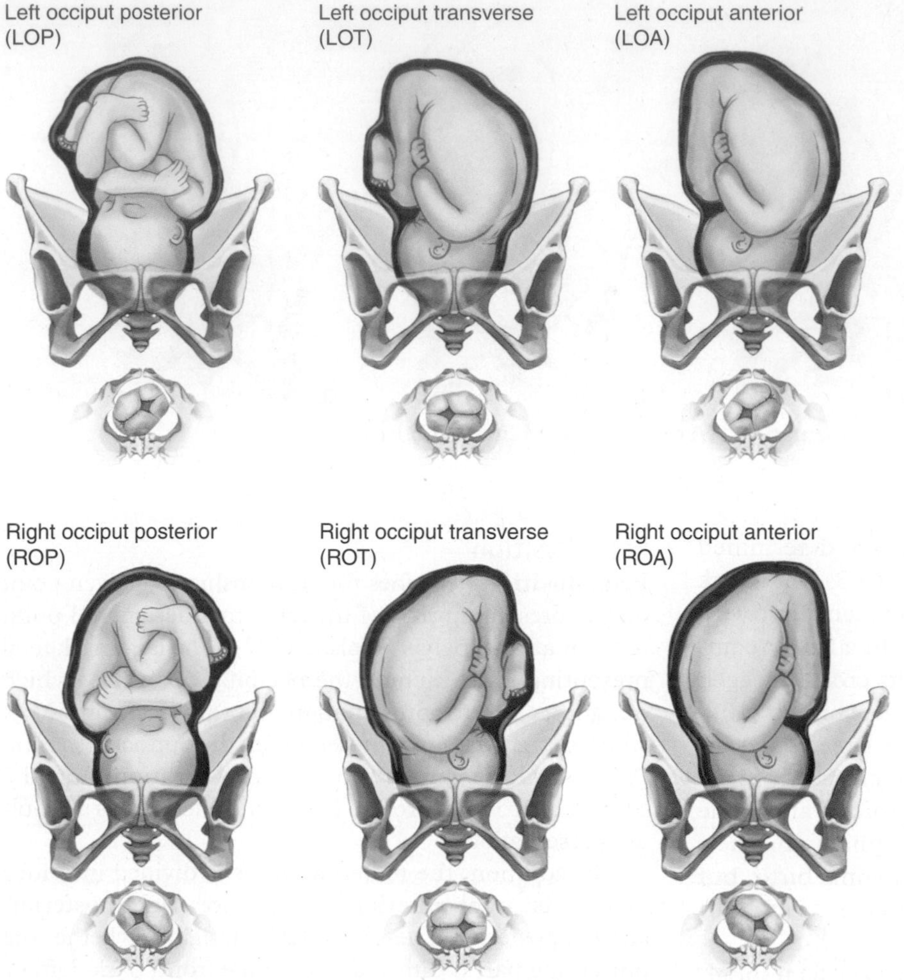

Left occiput posterior
(LOP)

Left occiput transverse
(LOT)

Left occiput anterior
(LOA)

Right occiput posterior
(ROP)

Right occiput transverse
(ROT)

Right occiput anterior
(ROA)

FIGURE 13.9 Examples of fetal positions in a vertex presentation. The lie is longitudinal for each illustration. The attitude is one of flexion. Notice that the view of the top illustration is seen when facing the pregnant woman. The bottom view is that seen with the woman in a dorsal recumbent position.

- The second letter represents the particular presenting part of the fetus: O for occiput, S for sacrum (buttocks), M for mentum (chin), A for acromion process, and D for dorsal (refers to the fetal back) when denoting the fetal position in shoulder presentations (Cheng & Caughey, 2007).
- The third letter defines the location of the presenting part in relation to the anterior (A) portion of the maternal pelvis or the posterior (P) portion of the maternal pelvis. If the presenting part is directed to the side of the maternal pelvis, the fetal presentation is designated as transverse (T).

For example, if the occiput is facing the left anterior quadrant of the pelvis, then the position is termed left occipitoanterior and is recorded as LOA. LOA is the most common (and most favorable) fetal position for birthing today, followed by right occipitoanterior (ROA).

The positioning of the fetus allows the fetal head to contour to the diameters of the maternal pelvis. LOA and ROA are optimal positions for vaginal birth. An occiput posterior position may lead to a long and difficult birth, and other positions may or may not be compatible with vaginal birth.

Fetal Station

Station refers to the relationship of the presenting part to the level of the maternal pelvic ischial spines. Fetal station is measured in centimeters and is referred to as a minus or plus, depending on its location above or below the ischial spines. Typically, the ischial spines are the narrowest part of the pelvis and are the natural measuring point for the birth progress.

Zero (0) station is designated when the presenting part is at the level of the maternal ischial spines. When the presenting part is above the ischial spines, the distance is recorded as minus stations. When the presenting part is below the ischial spines, the distance is recorded as plus stations. For instance, if the presenting part is above the ischial spines by 1 cm, it is documented as being a −1 station; if the presenting part is below the ischial spines by 1 cm, it is documented as being a +1 station. An easy way to understand this concept is to think in terms of meeting the goal, which is the birth. If the fetus is descending downward (past the ischial spines) and moving toward meeting the goal of birth, then the station is positive and the centimeter numbers grow bigger from +1 to +4. If the fetus is not descending past the ischial spines, then the station is negative and the centimeter numbers grow bigger from −1 to −4. The farther away the presenting part from the outside, the larger the negative number (-4 cm). The closer the presenting part of the fetus is to the outside, the larger the positive number (+4 cm). Figure 13.10 shows stations of presenting part.

Fetal Engagement

Engagement signifies the entrance of the largest diameter of the fetal presenting part (usually the fetal head) into the smallest diameter of the maternal pelvis (Blackburn, 2007). The fetus is said to be "engaged" in the pelvis when the presenting part reaches 0 station. Engagement is determined by pelvic examination.

The largest diameter of the fetal head is the biparietal diameter. It extends from one parietal prominence to the other. It is an important factor in the navigation through the maternal pelvis. Engagement typically occurs in primigravidas 2 weeks before term, whereas multiparas may experience engagement several weeks before the onset of labor or not until labor begins.

> ▶ *Take NOTE!*
>
> *The term* floating *is used when engagement has not occurred, because the presenting part is freely movable above the pelvic inlet.*

Cardinal Movements of Labor

The fetus goes through many positional changes as it travels through the passageway. These positional changes are known as the cardinal movements of labor. They are deliberate, specific, and very precise movements that allow the smallest diameter of the fetal head to pass through a corresponding diameter of the mother's pelvic structure. Although cardinal movements are conceptualized as separate and sequential, the movements are typically concurrent (Fig. 13.11).

Engagement

Engagement occurs when the greatest transverse diameter of the head in vertex (biparietal diameter) passes through the pelvic inlet (usually 0 station). The head usually enters the pelvis with the sagittal suture aligned in the transverse diameter.

Descent

Descent is the downward movement of the fetal head until it is within the pelvic inlet. Descent occurs intermittently with contractions and is brought about by one or more of the following forces:

• Pressure of the amniotic fluid
• Direct pressure of the fundus on the fetus' buttocks or head (depending on which part is located in the top of the uterus)
• Contractions of the abdominal muscles (second stage)
• Extension and straightening of the fetal body

Descent occurs throughout labor, ending with birth. During this time, the mother experiences discomfort, but she is unable to isolate this particular fetal movement from her overall discomfort.

Flexion

Flexion occurs as the vertex meets resistance from the cervix, the walls of the pelvis, or the pelvic floor. As a result, the chin is brought into contact with the fetal thorax and the presenting diameter is changed from occipitofrontal to suboccipitobregmatic (9.5 cm), which achieves the smallest fetal skull diameter presenting to the maternal pelvic dimensions.

Internal Rotation

After engagement, as the head descends, the lower portion of the head (usually the occiput) meets resistance from one side of the pelvic floor. As a result, the head rotates about 45 degrees anteriorly to the midline under the symphysis. This movement is known as internal rotation. Internal rotation brings the anteroposterior diameter of the head in line with the anteroposterior diameter of the pelvic outlet. It aligns the long axis of the fetal head with the long axis of the maternal pelvis. The widest portion of the maternal pelvis is the anteroposterior diameter, and thus the fetus must rotate to accommodate the pelvis.

Extension

With further descent and full flexion of the head, the nucha (the base of the occiput) becomes impinged under

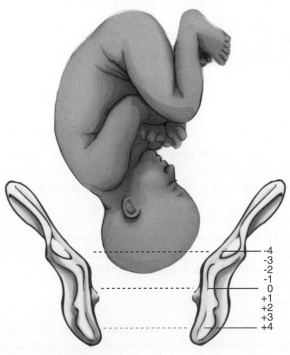

FIGURE 13.10 Fetal stations.

-4
-3
-2
-1
0
+1
+2
+3
+4

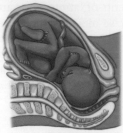

Engagement, Descent, Flexion

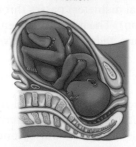

Internal Rotation

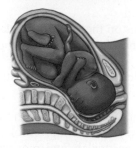

Extension Beginning (rotation complete)

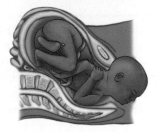

Extension Complete

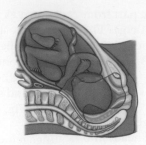

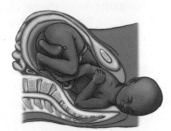

External Rotation restitution)

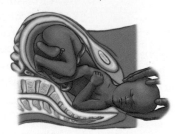

External Rotation (shoulder rotation)

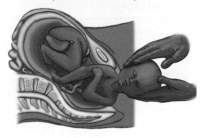

Expulsion

FIGURE 13.11 Cardinal movements of labor.

the symphysis. Resistance from the pelvic floor causes the fetal head to extend so that it can pass under the pubic arch. Extension occurs after internal rotation is complete. The head emerges through extension under the symphysis pubis along with the shoulders. The anterior fontanel, brow, nose, mouth, and chin are born successively.

External Rotation (Restitution)

After the head is born and is free of resistance, it untwists, causing the occiput to move about 45 degrees back to its original left or right position (restitution). The sagittal suture has now resumed its normal right-angle relationship to the transverse (bisacromial) diameter of the shoulders (i.e., the head realigns with the position of the back in the birth canal). External rotation of the fetal head allows the shoulders to rotate internally to fit the maternal pelvis.

Expulsion

Expulsion of the rest of the body occurs more smoothly after the birth of the head and the anterior and posterior shoulders (Cheng & Caughey, 2007).

Powers

The primary stimulus powering labor is uterine contractions. Contractions cause complete dilation and effacement of the cervix during the first stage of labor. The secondary powers in labor involve the use of intra-abdominal pressure (voluntary muscle contractions) exerted by the woman as she pushes and bears down during the second stage of labor.

Uterine Contractions

Uterine contractions are involuntary and therefore cannot be controlled by the woman experiencing them, regardless of whether they are spontaneous or induced. Uterine contractions are rhythmic and intermittent, with a period of relaxation between contractions. This pause allows the woman and the uterine muscles to rest. In addition, this pause restores blood flow to the uterus and placenta, which is temporarily reduced during each uterine contraction.

Uterine contractions are responsible for thinning and dilating the cervix, and they thrust the presenting part toward the lower uterine segment. With each uterine contraction, the upper segment of the uterus becomes shorter and thicker, whereas the lower passive segment and the cervix become longer, thinner, and more distended. The division between the contractile upper portion (fundus) of the uterus and the lower portion is described as the physiologic retraction ring. Longitudinal traction on the cervix by the fundus as it contracts and retracts leads to cervical effacement and dilation. Uterine contractions cause the upper uterine segment to shorten, making the cervix paper-thin when it becomes fully effaced.

The cervical canal reduces in length from 2 cm to a paper-thin entity and is described in terms of percentages from 0 to 100%. In primigravidas, effacement typically starts before the onset of labor and usually begins before dilation; in multiparas, however, neither effacement nor dilation may start until labor ensues. On clinical examination the following may be assessed:

- Cervical canal 2 cm in length would be described as 0% effaced.
- Cervical canal 1 cm in length would be described as 50% effaced.

- Cervical canal 0 cm in length would be described as 100% effaced.

Dilation is dependent on the pressure of the presenting part and the contraction and retraction of the uterus. The diameter of the cervical os increases from less than 1 cm to approximately 10 cm to allow for birth. When the cervix is fully dilated, it is no longer palpable on vaginal examination. Descriptions may include the following:

- External cervical os closed: 0 cm dilated
- External cervical os half open: 5 cm dilated
- External cervical os fully open: 10 cm dilated

During early labor, uterine contractions are described as mild, they last about 30 seconds, and they occur about every 5 to 7 minutes. As labor progresses, contractions last longer (60 seconds), occur more frequently (2 to 3 minutes apart), and are described as being moderate to high in intensity.

Each contraction has three phases: increment (build-up of the contraction), acme (peak or highest intensity), and decrement (descent or relaxation of the uterine muscle fibers; Fig. 13.12).

Uterine contractions are monitored and assessed according to three parameters: frequency, duration, and intensity.

1. **Frequency** refers to how often the contractions occur and is measured from the increment of one contraction to the increment of the next contraction.
2. **Duration** refers to how long a contraction lasts and is measured from the beginning of the increment to the end of the decrement for the same contraction.
3. **Intensity** refers to the strength of the contraction determined by manual palpation or measured by an internal intrauterine catheter (IUPC). The catheter is positioned in the uterine cavity through the cervix after the membranes have ruptured. It reports intensity by measuring the pressure of the amniotic fluid inside the uterus in millimeters of mercury (Edmonds, 2007).

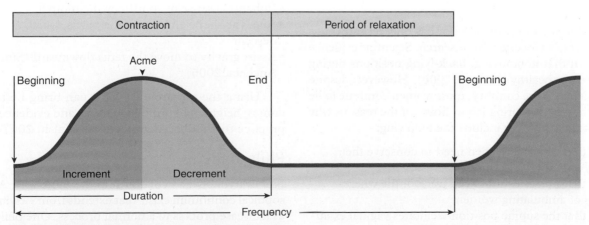

FIGURE **13.12** The three phases of a uterine contraction.

Intra-Abdominal Pressure

Increased intra-abdominal pressure (voluntary muscle contractions) compresses the uterus and adds to the power of the expulsion forces of the uterine contractions (Blackburn, 2007). Coordination of these forces in unison promotes birth of the fetus and expulsion of the fetal membranes and placenta from the uterus. Interference with these forces (such as when a woman is highly sedated or extremely anxious) can compromise the effectiveness of these powers.

Psychological Response

Childbearing can be one of the most life-altering experiences for a woman. The experience of childbirth goes beyond the physiologic aspects: it influences her self-confidence, self-esteem, and view of life, relationships, and children. Her state of mind (psyche) throughout the entire process is critical to bring about a positive outcome for her and her family. Factors promoting a positive birth experience include:

- Clear information about procedures
- Support; not being alone
- Sense of mastery, self-confidence
- Trust in staff caring for her
- Positive reaction to the pregnancy
- Personal control over breathing
- Preparation for the childbirth experience

Having a strong sense of self and meaningful support from others can often help women manage labor well. Feeling safe and secure typically promotes a sense of control and ability to withstand the challenges of the childbearing experience. Anxiety and fear, however, decrease a woman's ability to cope with the discomfort of labor. Maternal catecholamines secreted in response to anxiety and fear can inhibit uterine blood flow and placental perfusion. In contrast, relaxation can augment the natural process of labor (Leonard, 2007). Preparing mentally for childbirth is important so that the woman can work with, rather than against, the natural forces of labor.

Position (Maternal)

Maternal positioning during labor has only recently been the subject of well-controlled research. Scientific evidence has shown that nonmoving, back-lying positions during labor are not healthy (Hanson 2006). However, despite this evidence to the contrary, most women continue to lie flat on their backs during labor. Some of the reasons why this practice continues include the following:

- Belief that laboring women need to conserve their energy and not tire themselves
- Belief that nurses cannot keep track of the whereabouts of ambulating women
- Belief that the supine position facilitates vaginal examinations and external belt adjustment

- Belief that a bed is "where one is supposed to be" in a hospital setting
- Belief that the position is more convenient for the delivering health professional
- Belief that laboring women are "connected to things" that impede movement (Hanson, 2006)

Although many labor and birthing facilities claim that all women are allowed to adopt any position of comfort during their laboring experience, the great majority of women spend their time on their backs during labor and birth.

▶ **Take** NOTE!

If the only furniture provided is a bed, this is what the woman will use. Furnishing rooms with comfortable chairs, beanbags, and other birth props allows a woman to choose from a variety of positions and to be free to move during labor.

Changing positions and moving around during labor and birth offer several benefits. Maternal position can influence pelvic size and contours. Changing position and walking affect the pelvis joints, which may facilitate fetal descent and rotation. Squatting enlarges the pelvic outlet by approximately 25%, whereas a kneeling position removes pressure on the maternal vena cava and helps to rotate the fetus in the posterior position (Terry et al., 2006). The use of any upright or lateral position, compared with supine or lithotomy positions, may:

- Reduce the length of the first stage of labor
- Reduce the duration of the second stage of labor
- Reduce the number of assisted deliveries (vacuum and forceps)
- Reduce episiotomies and perineal tears
- Contribute to fewer abnormal fetal heart rate patterns
- Increase comfort/reduce requests for pain medication
- Enhance a sense of control by the mother
- Alter the shape and size of the pelvis, which assists in descent
- Assist gravity to move the fetus downward (Simkin & Ancheta, 2006)

Using the research available can bring better outcomes, heightened professionalism, and evidence-based practice to childbearing practices (Walsh, 2007).

Philosophy

Not everyone views childbirth in the same way. A philosophical continuum exists that extends from viewing labor as a disease process to a normal process. One philosophy assumes that women cannot manage the birth experience

EVIDENCE-BASED PRACTICE 13.1
Continuous Support for Women During Childbirth

● Study

Historically, women have been attended and supported by other women during labor. However, in recent decades in hospitals worldwide, continuous support during labor has become the exception rather than the rule. Concerns about the consequent dehumanization of the birth experiences have led to calls for a return to continuous support by women for women during labor.

This review of studies included 16 trials, from 11 countries, involving over 13,000 women in a wide range of settings and circumstances. The primary outcome was to assess the effects, on mothers and their babies, of continuous, one-to-one intrapartum support compared with usual care. The secondary outcome was to determine whether the effects of continuous support are influenced by (1) routine practices and policies in the birth environment that may affect a woman's autonomy, freedom of movement, and ability to cope with labor; (2) whether the caregiver is a member of the staff of the institution; and (3) whether the continuous support begins early or later in labor.

▲ Findings

Women who received continuous labor support were more likely to give birth "spontaneously" (vaginally, without vacuum or forceps). They were less likely to use pain medications, were more likely to be satisfied with their experience, and had slightly shorter labors. In general, labor support appeared to be more effective when it was provided by women who were not part of the hospital staff. It also appeared to be more effective when it started early in labor. No adverse effects were identified.

■ Nursing Implications

Knowing the results of this evidence-based study, all nurses should strive to be a real "presence" for all of their laboring couples. Based on the findings, continuous nursing support promotes positive birthing outcomes and fewer technical/surgical interventions. Both maternal and fetal well-being is preserved when nurses are present and involved during the childbirth experience.

Hodnett, E. D., Gates, S., Hofmeyr, G. J., & Sakala, C. (2007). Continuous support for women during childbirth. *Cochrane Database of Systematic Reviews* 2007, 3. Art. No.: CD003766. DOI: 10.1002/14651858.CD003766.pub2.

adequately and therefore need constant expert monitoring and management. The other philosophy assumes that women are capable, reasoning individuals who can actively participate in their birth experience.

The health care system in the United States today appears to be leaning toward the former philosophy, applying technological interventions to most mothers who enter the hospital system. Giving birth in a hospital in the 21st century for many women has become "intervention intensive"—designed to start, continue, and end labor through medical management rather than allowing the normal process of birth to unfold. Advances in medical care have improved the safety for women with high-risk pregnancies. However, the routine use of intravenous therapy, electronic fetal monitoring, augmentation, and epidural anesthesia has not necessarily improved birth outcomes for all women (Leonard, 2007). Perhaps a middle-of-the-road philosophy for intervening when circumstances dictate, along with weighing the risks and benefits before doing so, may be appropriate.

During the 1970s, family-centered maternity care was developed in response to the consumer reaction to the depersonalization of birth. The hope was to shift the philosophy from "technologization" to personalization to humanize childbirth. The term "family-centered birthing" is more appropriate today to denote the low-tech, high-touch approach requested by many childbearing women, who view childbirth as a normal process.

Certified nurse midwives (CNMs) are champions of family-centered birthing, and their participation in the childbirth process is associated with fewer unnecessary interventions when compared to obstetricians. CNMs subscribe to a normal birth process where the woman uses her own instincts and bodily signs during labor. In short, midwives empower women within the birthing environment (Russell, 2007; Steppe, 2007).

No matter what philosophy is held, it is ideal if everyone involved in the particular birth process—from the health care provider to the mother—shares the same philosophy toward the birth process.

Partners

Women desire support and attentive care during labor and birth. Caregivers can convey emotional support by offering their continued presence and words of encouragement. Throughout the world, few women are left to labor totally alone: emotional, physical, or spiritual support during labor is the norm for most cultures (Ballen & Fulcher, 2006). A caring partner can use massage, light touch, acupressure, hand-holding, stroking, and relaxation, can help the woman communicate her wishes to the staff, and can provide a continuous, reassuring presence, all of which bring some degree of comfort to the laboring woman (Ballen & Fulcher, 2006). Although the presence of the baby's father at the birth provides special emotional support, a partner can be anyone who is present to support the woman throughout the experience.

Worldwide, women usually support other women in childbirth. Hodnett et al. (2003) reported that the continuous presence of a trained female support person (**doula**) reduced the need for medication for pain relief, the use of vacuum or forceps delivery, and the need for cesarean births. Continuous support was also associated with a slight reduction in the length of labor. The doula, who is an experienced labor companion, provides the woman and her partner with emotional and physical support and information throughout the entire labor and birth experience.

A similar study in the United States found that nursing care decreases the likelihood of negative evaluations of the childbirth experience, feelings of tenseness during labor, and finding labor worse than expected. Also reported were less perineal trauma, reduced difficulty in mothering, and reduced likelihood of early cessation of breastfeeding (Ballen & Fulcher, 2006).

Given the many benefits of intrapartum support, laboring women should always have the option to receive partner support, whether from nurses, doulas, significant others, or family. Whoever the support partner is, he or she should provide the mother with continuous presence and hands-on comfort and encouragement.

Patience

The birth process takes time. If more time were allowed for women to labor naturally without intervention, the cesarean birth rate would most likely be reduced (Simkin & Ancheta, 2006). The literature suggests that delaying interventions can give a woman enough time to progress in labor and reduce the need for surgical intervention (American College of Obstetricians and Gynecologists [ACOG], 2007). *Healthy People 2010* has two goals related to cesarean births in the United States:

1. Reduce the rate of cesarean births among low-risk (full-term, singleton, vertex presentation) women having their first child to 15% of live births, from a baseline of 18%.
2. Reduce the rate of cesarean births among women who have had a prior cesarean birth to 63% of live births, from a baseline of 72% (USDHHS, 2000).

We are a long way from achieving these goals, since the current cesarean birth rate in the United States—30%—is the highest since these data first became available from birth certificates in 1989. Cesarean birth is associated with increased morbidity and mortality for both mother and infant, as well as increased inpatient length of stay and health care costs (CDC, 2007).

It is difficult to predict how a labor will progress and therefore equally difficult to determine how long a woman's labor will last. There is no way to estimate the likely strength and frequency of uterine contractions, the extent to which the cervix will soften and dilate, and how much the fetal head will mold to fit the birth canal. We cannot know beforehand whether the complex fetal rotations needed for an efficient labor will take place properly. All of these factors are unknowns when a woman starts labor.

There is a trend in health care, however, to attempt to manipulate the process of labor through medical means such as artificial rupture of membranes and augmentation of labor with oxytocin (Walsh, 2007). The labor induction rate has increased dramatically in the United States since the 1980s (Gulmezoglu, Crowther, & Middleton, 2007).

Approximately one in five women are induced or have labor augmented with uterine-stimulating drugs or artificial rupture of membranes to accelerate their progress (Bricker & Luckas, 2007). An amniotomy (artificial rupture of the fetal membranes) may be performed to augment or induce labor when the membranes have not ruptured spontaneously. Doing so allows the fetal head to have more direct contact with the cervix to dilate it. This procedure is performed with the fetal head at −2 station or lower, with the cervix dilated to at least 3 cm. Synthetic oxytocin (Pitocin) is also used to induce or augment labor by stimulating uterine contractions. It is administered piggybacked into the primary intravenous line with an infusion pump titrated to uterine activity.

There is compelling evidence that elective induction of labor significantly increases the risk of cesarean birth, especially for nulliparous women (Simkin & Ancheta, 2006). The belief is that many cesarean births could be avoided if women were allowed to labor longer and if the natural labor process were allowed to complete the job. The longer wait (using the intervention of patience) usually results in less intervention.

The ACOG attributes the dramatic increase in inductions in part to pressure from women, convenience for physicians, and liability concerns. They recommend a "cautious approach" regarding elective induction until clinical trials can validate a more liberal use of labor inductions (ACOG, 2002). There are medical indications for inducing labor, such as spontaneous rupture of membranes and when labor does not start; a pregnancy more than 42 weeks' gestation; maternal hypertension, diabetes, or lung disease; and a uterine infection (ACOG, 2006).

When the laboring woman feels the urge to bear down, pushing begins. Most women respond extremely well to messages from their body without being directed by the nurse. A more natural, undirected approach allows the woman to wait and bear down when she feels the urge to push. Having patience and letting nature take its course will reduce the incidence of physiologic stress in the mother, resulting in less trauma to her perineal tissue.

Patient Preparation

Basic prenatal education can help women manage their labor process and feel in control of their birthing experience. The literature indicates that if a woman is prepared before the labor and birth experience, the labor is more likely to remain normal or natural (without the need for medical intervention) (Gagnon, 2006). An increasing body of evidence also indicates that the well-prepared woman, with good labor support, is less likely to need analgesia or anesthesia and is unlikely to require cesarean birth (Risica & Phipps, 2006).

Prenatal education teaches the woman about the childbirth experience and increases her sense of control. She is then able to work as an active participant during the labor and birth experience (Brodsky, 2006). The research also suggests that prenatal preparation may affect intrapartum and postpartum psychosocial outcomes. For example, prenatal education covering parenting communication classes had a significant effect on postpartum anxiety and postpartum adjustment. Prenatal education should be viewed as an opportunity to strengthen families by providing anticipatory guidance and improve family members' life skills. In short, prenatal education helps to promote healthy families during the transition to parenthood and beyond (Polomeno, 2006).

▶ *Take NOTE!*

Learning about labor and birth allows women and couples to express their needs and preferences, enhances their confidence, and improves communication between themselves and the staff.

Pain Management

Labor and birth, although a normal physiologic process, can produce significant pain. Pain during labor is a nearly universal experience. Controlling the pain without harm to the fetus or labor process is the major focus of pain management during childbirth.

Pain is a subjective experience involving a complex interaction of physiologic, spiritual, psychosocial, cultural, and environmental influences (Smith et al., 2006). Cultural values and learned behaviors influence perception and response to pain, as do anxiety and fear, both of which tend to heighten the sense of pain (Walsh, 2007). The challenge for care providers is to find the right combination of pain management methods to keep the pain manageable while minimizing the negative effect on the fetus, the normal physiology of labor, maternal–infant bonding, breastfeeding, and a woman's perception of the labor itself (Wood, 2007). Chapter 14 presents a full discussion of pain management during labor and birth.

Physiologic Responses to Labor

Labor is the physiologic process by which the uterus expels the fetus and placenta from the body. During pregnancy, progesterone secreted from the placenta suppresses the spontaneous contractions of a typical uterus, keeping the fetus within the uterus. In addition, the cervix remains firm and noncompliant. At term, however, changes occur in the cervix that make it softer. In addition, uterine contractions become more frequent and regular, signaling the onset of labor.

The labor process involves a series of rhythmic, involuntary, usually quite uncomfortable uterine muscle contractions. They bring about a shortening that causes effacement and dilation of the cervix and a bursting of the fetal membranes. Then, accompanied by both reflex and voluntary contractions of the abdominal muscles (pushing), the uterine contractions result in the birth of the baby (Blackburn, 2007). During labor, the mother and fetus make several physiologic adaptations.

Maternal Responses

As the woman progresses through childbirth, numerous physiologic responses occur that assist her to adapt to the laboring process. The labor process stresses several of the woman's body systems, which react through numerous compensatory mechanisms. Maternal physiologic responses include:

- Heart rate increases by 10 to 20 bpm.
- Cardiac output increases by 10% to 15% during the first stage of labor and by 30% to 50% during the second stage of labor.
- Blood pressure increases by 10 to 30 mm Hg during uterine contractions in all labor stages.
- The white blood cell count increases to 25,000 to 30,000 cells/mm^3, perhaps as a result of tissue trauma.
- Respiratory rate increases and more oxygen is consumed related to the increase in metabolism.
- Gastric motility and food absorption decrease, which may increase the risk of nausea and vomiting during the transition stage of labor.
- Gastric emptying and gastric pH decrease, increasing the risk of vomiting with aspiration.
- Temperature rises slightly, possibly due to an increase in muscle activity.
- Muscular aches/cramps occur as a result of the stressed musculoskeletal system.
- Basal metabolic rate increases and blood glucose levels decrease because of the stress of labor (Blackburn, 2007; Cheng & Caughey, 2007).

A woman's ability to adapt to the stress of labor is influenced by her psychological and physical state. Among the many factors that affect her coping ability are:

- Previous birth experiences and their outcomes
- Current pregnancy experience (planned versus unplanned, discomforts experienced, age, risk status of pregnancy, chronic illness, weight gain)
- Cultural considerations (values and beliefs about health status)
- Support system (presence and support of a valued partner during labor)
- Childbirth preparation (attended childbirth classes and has practiced paced breathing techniques)
- Exercise during pregnancy
- Expectations of the birthing experience
- Anxiety level
- Fear of labor and loss of control
- Fatigue and weariness (Edmonds, 2007)

Fetal Responses

Although the focus during labor may be on assessing the mother's adaptations, several physiologic adaptations occur in the fetus as well. The fetus is experiencing labor along with the mother. If the fetus is healthy, the stress of labor usually has no adverse effects. The nurse needs to be alert to any abnormalities in the fetus' adaptation to labor. Fetal responses to labor include:

- Periodic fetal heart rate accelerations and slight decelerations related to fetal movement, fundal pressure, and uterine contractions
- Decrease in circulation and perfusion to the fetus secondary to uterine contractions (a healthy fetus is able to compensate for this drop)
- Increase in arterial carbon dioxide pressure (PCO_2)
- Decrease in fetal breathing movements throughout labor
- Decrease in fetal oxygen pressure with a decrease in the partial pressure of oxygen (PO_2) (Kenner & Lott, 2007)

▶ *Take* NOTE!

Respiratory changes during labor help to prepare the fetus for extrauterine respiration immediately after birth.

Stages of Labor

Labor is typically divided into four stages: dilation, expulsive, placental, and restorative. Table 13.2 summarizes the major events of each stage.

The first stage is the longest: it begins with the first true contraction and ends with full dilation (opening) of the cervix. Because this stage lasts so long, it is divided into three phases, each corresponding to the progressive dilation of the cervix.

Stage two of labor, or the expulsive stage, begins when the cervix is completely dilated and ends with the birth of the newborn. The expulsive stage can last from minutes to hours.

The third stage, or the placental stage, starts after the newborn is born and ends with the separation and birth of the placenta. Continued uterine contractions typically cause the placenta to be expelled within 5 to 30 minutes.

The fourth stage, or the restorative stage, lasts from 1 to 4 hours after birth. This period is when the mother's body begins to stabilize after the hard work of labor and the loss of the products of conception. The fourth stage is often not recognized as a true stage of labor, but it is a critical period for maternal physiologic transition as well as new family attachment (Arenson & Drake, 2007).

First Stage

During the first stage of labor, the fundamental change underlying the process is progressive dilation of the cervix. Cervical dilation is gauged subjectively by vaginal examination and is expressed in centimeters. The first stage ends when the cervix is dilated to 10 cm in diameter and is large enough to permit the passage of a fetal head of average size. The fetal membranes, or bag of waters, usually rupture during the first stage, but they may have burst earlier or may even remain intact until birth. For the primigravida, the first stage of labor lasts about 12 hours. However, this time can vary widely: for the multiparous woman, it is usually only half that.

During the first stage of labor, women usually perceive the visceral pain of diffuse abdominal cramping and uterine contractions. Pain during the first stage of labor is primarily a result of the dilation of the cervix and lower uterine segment, and the distention (stretching) of these structures during contractions. The first stage is divided into three phases: latent or early phase, active phase, and transition phase.

Latent or Early Phase

The latent or early phase gives rise to the familiar signs and symptoms of labor. This phase begins with the start of regular contractions and ends when rapid cervical dilation begins. Cervical effacement occurs during this phase, and the cervix dilates from 0 to 3 cm.

Contractions usually occur every 5 to 10 minutes, last 30 to 45 seconds, and are described as mild by palpation. Effacement of the cervix is from 0% to 40%. Most women are very talkative during this period, perceiving their contractions to be similar to menstrual cramps. Women may remain at home during this phase, contacting their health care professional about the onset of labor.

For the nulliparous woman, the latent phase typically lasts about 9 hours; in the multiparous woman, it lasts about 6 hours (Cheng & Caughey, 2007). During this phase, women are apprehensive but excited about the start of their labor after their long gestational period.

TABLE 13.2 STAGES AND PHASES OF LABOR

	First Stage	Second Stage	Third Stage	Fourth Stage
Description	From 0–10 cm dilation; consists of three phases	From complete dilation (10 cm) to birth of the newborn; lasts up to 1 hour	Separation and delivery of the placenta	1–4 hours after the birth of the newborn; time of maternal physiologic adjustment
Phases	**Latent phase** (0–3 cm dilation) – Cervical dilation from 0 to 3 cm – Cervical effacement from 0% to 40% – Nullipara, lasts up to 9 hours; multipara, lasts up to 5–6 hours – Contraction frequency every 5–10 minutes – Contraction duration 30–45 seconds – Contraction intensity mild to palpation **Active phase** (4–7 cm dilation) – Cervical dilation from 4 to 7 cm – Cervical effacement from 40% to 80% – Nullipara, lasts up to 6 hours; multipara, lasts up to 4 hours – Contraction frequency every 2–5 minutes – Contraction duration 45–60 seconds – Contraction intensity moderate to palpation **Transition phase** (8–10 cm dilation) – Cervical dilation from 8 to 10 cm – Cervical effacement from 80% to 100% – Nullipara lasts up to 1 hour; multipara, lasts up to 30 minutes – Contraction frequency every 1–2 minutes – Contraction duration 60–90 seconds – Contraction intensity strong by palpation	**Pelvic phase** (period of fetal descent) **Perineal phase** (period of active pushing) – Nullipara, lasts up to 1 hour; multipara, lasts up to 30 minutes – Contraction frequency every 2–3 minutes or less – Contraction duration 60–90 seconds – Contraction intensity strong by palpation – Strong urge to push during the later perineal phase	**Placental separation:** detaching from uterine wall **Placental expulsion:** coming outside the vaginal opening	

Think back to the couple who were sent home from the hospital birthing center. Three days later Kathy awoke with a wet sensation and intense discomfort in her back, spreading around to her abdomen. She decided to go for a walk, but her contractions didn't diminish; instead, they continued to occur every few minutes and grew stronger in intensity. She and Chuck decided to go back to the hospital birthing center. Was there a difference in the location of Kathy's discomfort this time? What changes will the admission nurse find in Kathy if this is true labor?

Active Phase

Cervical dilation begins to occur more rapidly during the active phase. The cervix usually dilates from 4 to 7 cm, with 40% to 80% effacement taking place. This phase can last up to 6 hours for the nulliparous woman and 4.5 hours for the multiparous woman (Simkin & Ancheta, 2006). The fetus descends farther in the pelvis. Contractions become more frequent (every 2 to 5 minutes) and increase in duration (45 to 60 seconds). The woman's discomfort intensifies (moderate to strong by palpation). She becomes more intense and inwardly focused, absorbed in the serious work of her labor. She limits interactions with those in the room. If she and her partner have attended childbirth education classes, she will begin to use the relaxation and paced breathing techniques that they learned to cope with the contractions. The typical dilation rate for the nulliparous woman is 1.2 cm/hour; for the multiparous woman, it is 1.5 cm/hour (Cunningham et al., 2005).

Transition Phase

The transition phase is the last phase of the first stage of labor. During this phase, dilation slows, progressing from 8 to 10 cm, with effacement from 80% to 100%. The transition phase is the most difficult and, fortunately, the shortest phase for the woman, lasting approximately 1 hour in the first birth and perhaps 15 to 30 minutes in successive births (Walsh, 2007). During transition, the contractions are stronger (hard by palpation), more painful, and more frequent (every 1 to 2 minutes), and they last longer (60 to 90 seconds). The average rate of fetal descent is 1 cm/hour in nulliparous women and 2 cm/hour in multiparous women. Pressure on the rectum is great, and there is a strong desire to contract the abdominal muscles and push.

Other maternal features during the transitional phase include nausea and vomiting, trembling extremities, backache, increased apprehension and irritability, restless movement, increased bloody show from the vagina, inability to relax, diaphoresis, feelings of loss of control, and being overwhelmed (the woman may say, "I can't take it any more"). This phase should not last longer than 3 hours for nulliparas and 1 hour for multiparas (Cunningham et al., 2005).

In assessing Kathy, the nurse finds she is 4 cm dilated and 50% effaced with ruptured membranes. In what stage and phase of labor would this assessment finding place Kathy?

Second Stage

The second stage of labor begins with complete cervical dilation (10 cm) and effacement and ends with the birth of the newborn. Although the previous stage of labor primarily involved the thinning and opening of the cervix, this stage involves moving the fetus through the birth canal and out of the body. The cardinal movements of labor occur during the early phase of passive descent in the second stage of labor.

Contractions occur every 2 to 3 minutes, last 60 to 90 seconds, and are described as strong by palpation. The average length of the second stage of labor in a nullipara is approximately 1 hour and less than half that time for the multipara. During this expulsive stage, the mother usually feels more in control and less irritable and agitated. She is focused on the work of pushing. Traditionally, women have been taught to hold their breath to the count of 10, inhale again, push again, and repeat the process several times during a contraction. This sustained, strenuous style of pushing has been shown to lead to hemodynamic changes in the mother and interfere with oxygen exchange between the mother and the fetus. In addition, it is associated with pelvic floor damage: the longer the push, the more damage to the pelvic floor (Hanson, 2006). The newest protocol from the Association of Women's Health and Newborn Nursing (AWHONN) recommends an open-glottis method in which air is released during pushing to prevent the buildup of intrathoracic pressure. Doing so also supports mother's involuntary bearing-down efforts (Roberts, Gonzalez, & Sampselle, 2007).

During the second stage of labor, pushing can either follow the mother's spontaneous urge or be directed by the caregiver. Much debate still exists between spontaneous and directed pushing during the second stage of labor. Although directed pushing is common practice in hospitals, there is evidence to suggest that directed pushing should be avoided. Research seems to support spontaneous pushing—when the woman is allowed to follow her own instincts (Hanson, 2006). Evidence is mounting that the management of the second stage, particularly pushing, is a modifiable risk factor in long-term perinatal outcomes. Valsalva (holding breath) bearing down and supine maternal positions are linked to negative maternal–fetal hemodynamics and outcomes. The adoption of a physiologic, woman-directed approach to bearing down is advocated (Roberts, Gonzalez, & Sampselle, 2007).

Evidence-based practice focuses on a physiologic approach to the second stage of labor. Behaviors demonstrated by laboring women during this time include pushing at the onset of the urge to bear down; using their own pattern and technique of bearing down in response to sensations they experience; using open-glottis bearing down with contractions; pushing with variations in strength and duration; pushing down with progressive intensity; and using multiple positions to increase progress and comfort. This approach is in stark contrast to management by arbitrary time limits and the directed bearing-down efforts seen in practice today (Hanson, 2006).

Laboring down (promotion of passive descent) is an alternative strategy for second-stage management in women with epidurals. Using this approach, the fetus descends and is born without coached maternal pushing.

The second stage of labor has two phases (pelvic and perineal) related to the existence and quality of the maternal urge to push and to obstetric conditions related to fetal descent. The early phase of the second stage is called the pelvic phase, because it is during this phase that the fetal head is negotiating the pelvis, rotating, and advancing in descent. The later phase is called the perineal phase, because at this point the fetal head is lower in the pelvis and is distending the perineum. The occurrence of a strong urge to push characterizes the later phase of the second stage and has also been called the phase of active pushing (Roberts, Gonzalez, & Sampselle, 2007).

The later perineal phase occurs when the mother feels a tremendous urge to push as the fetal head is lowered and is distending the perineum. The perineum bulges and there is an increase in bloody show. The fetal head becomes apparent at the vaginal opening but disappears between contractions. When the top of the head no longer regresses between contractions, it is said to have crowned. The fetus rotates as it maneuvers out. The second stage commonly lasts up to 3 hours in a first labor and up to an hour in subsequent ones (Fig. 13.13).

Third Stage

The third stage of labor begins with the birth of the newborn and ends with the separation and birth of the placenta. It consists of two phases: placental separation and placental expulsion.

Placental Separation

After the infant is born, the uterus continues to contract strongly and can now retract, decreasing markedly in size. These contractions cause the placenta to pull away from the uterine wall. The following signs of separation indicate that the placenta is ready to deliver:

- The uterus rises upward.
- The umbilical cord lengthens.
- A sudden trickle of blood is released from the vaginal opening.
- The uterus changes its shape to globular.

Spontaneous birth of the placenta occurs in one of two ways: the fetal side (shiny gray side) presenting first (called Schultz's mechanism or more commonly called "shiny Schultz's") or the maternal side (red raw side) presenting first (termed Duncan's mechanism or "dirty Duncan").

Placental Expulsion

After separation of the placenta from the uterine wall, continued uterine contractions cause the placenta to be expelled within 2 to 30 minutes unless there is gentle external traction to assist. After the placenta is expelled, the uterus is massaged briefly by the attending physician or midwife until it is firm so that uterine blood vessels constrict, minimizing the possibility of hemorrhage. Normal blood loss is approximately 500 mL for a vaginal birth and 1,000 mL for a cesarean birth (Arenson & Drake, 2007).

If the placenta does not spontaneously deliver, the health care professional assists with its removal by manual extraction. On expulsion, the placenta is inspected for its intactness by the health care professional and the nurse to make sure all sections are present. If any piece is still attached to the uterine wall, it places the woman at risk for postpartum hemorrhage because it becomes a space-occupying object that interferes with the ability of the uterus to contract fully and effectively.

Fourth Stage

The fourth stage begins with completion of the expulsion of the placenta and membranes and ends with the initial physiologic adjustment and stabilization of the mother (1 to 4 hours after birth). This stage initiates the postpartum period. The mother usually feels a sense of peace and excitement, is wide awake, and is very talkative initially. The attachment process begins with her inspecting her newborn and desiring to cuddle and breastfeed him or her. The mother's fundus should be firm and well contracted. Typically it is located at the midline between the umbilicus and the symphysis, but it then slowly rises to the level of the umbilicus during the first hour after birth (Walsh, 2007). If the uterus becomes boggy, it is massaged to keep it firm. The lochia (vaginal discharge) is red, mixed with small clots, and of moderate flow. If the woman has had an episiotomy during the second stage of labor, it should be intact, with the edges approximated and clean and no redness or edema present.

The focus during this stage is to monitor the mother closely to prevent hemorrhage, bladder distention, and venous thrombosis. Usually the mother is thirsty and hungry during this time and may request food and drink. Her bladder is hypotonic and thus she has limited sensation to acknowledge a full bladder or to void. Vital signs, the amount and consistency of the vaginal discharge (lochia), and the uterine fundus are usually monitored every 15 minutes for at least 1 hour. The woman will be

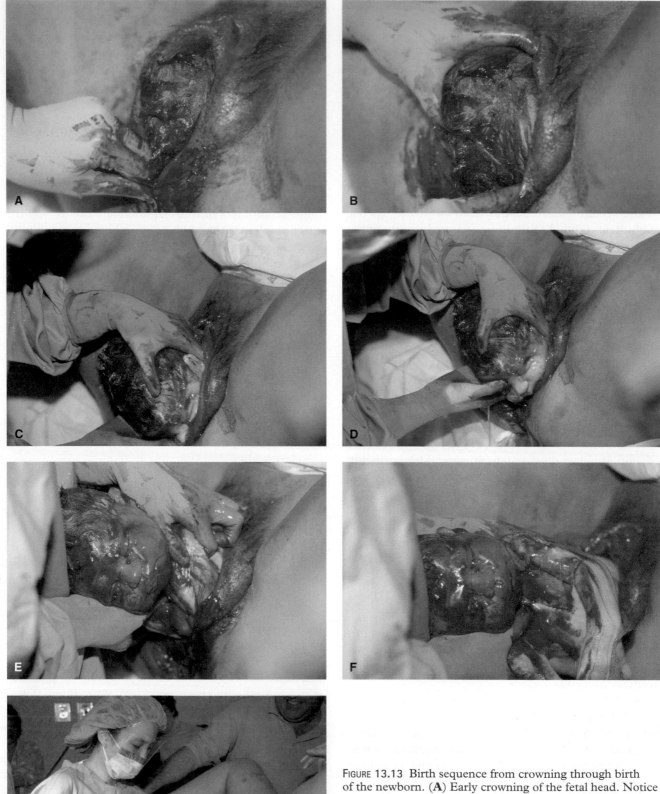

FIGURE 13.13 Birth sequence from crowning through birth of the newborn. (**A**) Early crowning of the fetal head. Notice the bulging of the perineum. (**B**) Late crowning. Notice that the fetal head is appearing face down. This is the normal OA position. (**C**) As the head extends, you can see that the occiput is to the mother's right side—ROA position. (**D**) The cardinal movement of extension. (**E**) The shoulders are born. Notice how the head has turned to line up with the shoulders—the cardinal movement of external rotation. (**F**) The body easily follows the shoulders. (**G**) The newborn is held for the first time! (© B. Proud.)

feeling cramp-like discomfort during this time due to the contracting uterus.

■■■ Key Concepts

■ Labor is a complex, multifaceted interaction between the mother and fetus. Thus, it is difficult to determine exactly why labor begins and what initiates it.

■ Before the onset of labor, a pregnant woman's body undergoes several changes in preparation for the birth of the newborn, often leading to characteristic signs and symptoms that suggest that labor is near. These changes include cervical changes, lightening, increased energy level, bloody show, Braxton Hicks contractions, and spontaneous rupture of membranes.

■ False labor is a condition seen during the latter weeks of some pregnancies in which irregular uterine contractions are felt, but the cervix is not affected.

■ The critical factors in labor and birth are designated as the 10 P's: passageway (birth canal), passenger (fetus and placenta), powers (contractions), psychological response, maternal position, philosophy (low tech, high touch), partners (support caregivers), patience (natural timing), patient preparation (childbirth knowledge base), and pain control (comfort measures).

■ The size and shape of a woman's pelvis are determining factors for a vaginal birth. The female pelvis is classified according to four main groups: anthropoid, android, gynecoid, and platypelloid.

■ The labor process is comprised of a series of rhythmic, involuntary, usually quite uncomfortable uterine muscle contractions that bring about a shortening (effacement) and opening (dilation) of the cervix, and a bursting of the fetal membranes. Important parameters of uterine contractions are frequency, duration, and intensity.

■ The diameters of the fetal skull vary considerably, with some diameters shortening and others lengthening as the head is molded during the labor and birth process.

■ Pain during labor is a nearly universal experience for childbearing women. Having a strong sense of self and meaningful support from others can often help women manage labor well and reduce their sensation of pain.

■ Preparing mentally for childbirth is important for women to enable them to work with the natural forces of labor and not against them.

■ As the woman experiences and progresses through childbirth, numerous physiologic responses occur that assist her adaptation to the laboring process.

■ Labor is typically divided into four stages that are unequal in length.

■ During the first stage, the fundamental change underlying the process is progressive dilation of the cervix. It is further divided into three phases: latent phase, active phase, and transition.

■ The second stage of labor is from complete cervical dilation (10 cm) and effacement through the birth of the infant.

■ The third stage is that of separation and birth of the placenta. It consists of two phases: placental separation and placental expulsion.

■ The fourth stage begins after the birth of the placenta and membranes and ends with the initial physiologic adjustment and stabilization of the mother (1–4 hours).

REFERENCES

American College of Obstetricians and Gynecologists (ACOG). (2002). *ACOG news release commentary—Nonmedical indications help fuel rise in induction rate*. [Released June 30, 2002.] Washington, DC: ACOG.

American College of Obstetricians and Gynecologists (ACOG). (2006). *Planning your pregnancy and birth*. Washington, DC: ACOG.

American College of Obstetricians and Gynecologists (ACOG). (2007). *Evaluation of cesarean birth*. Washington, DC: ACOG.

Arenson, J., & Drake, P. (2007) *Maternal and newborn health*. Sudbury, MA: Jones and Bartlett Publishers.

Association of Women's Health, Obstetric and Neonatal Nurses (AWHONN). (2007). The late preterm infant assessment guide. *AWHONN News*, Spring 2007, p. 11.

Ballen, L. E., & Fulcher, A. J. (2006). Nurses and doulas: Complementary roles to provide optimal maternity care. *Journal of Obstetrics, Gynecologic & Neonatal Nursing, 35*(2), 304–311.

Billington, M., & Stevenson, M. (2007). *Critical care in childbirth for midwives*. Malden, MA: Blackwell Publishers.

Blackburn, S. T. (2007). *Maternal, fetal and neonatal physiology: A clinical perspective* (3rd ed.). St. Louis, MO: Saunders Elsevier.

Bricker, L., & Luckas, M. (2007). Amniotomy alone for induction of labor updated. *Cochrane Database of Systematic Reviews, 2*. Art No.: CD002862. DOI: 1002/14651858.CD002862.

Brodsky, P. L. (2006). Childbirth: A journey through time. *International Journal of Childbirth Education, 21*(3), 10–15.

Centers for Disease Control and Prevention (CDC). (2007). Quick-Stats: Percentage of all live births by cesarean delivery—National Vital Statistics, United States. *MMWR, 56*(15), 373.

Cheng, Y. W., & Caughey, A. B. (2007). Normal labor and delivery. *eMedicine*. Available at: http://www.emedicine.com/MED/topic3239.htm

Cunningham, G., Gant, N. F., Leveno, K. J., Gilstrap, L. C., Hauth, J. C., & Wenstrom, K. D. (2005). *Williams' obstetrics* (22nd ed.). New York: McGraw-Hill.

Edmonds, K. (2007). *Dewhurst's textbook of obstetrics and gynecology* (7th ed.). Oxford, UK: Blackwell Publishers Limited.

Fischer, R. (2007). Breech presentation. *eMedicine*. Available at www.emedicine.com/med/topic3272.htm

Gagnon, A. J. (2006). Individual or group antenatal education for childbirth/parenthood. *Cochrane Library* 2006(4), CD002869.

Gulmezoglu, A. M., Crowther, C. A., & Middleton, P. (2007). Induction of labor for improving birth outcomes for women at or beyond term. *Cochrane Database of Systematic Reviews 2007, 4*. Art. No. CD004945. DIO: 10.1002/14651858.CD004945.pub2.

Gilbert, E. S. (2007). *Manual of high-risk pregnancy and birth*. St. Louis: Mosby.

Hanson, L. (2006). Pushing for change. *Journal of Perinatal & Neonatal Nursing, 20*(4), 282–284.

Hodnett, E. D., Gates, S., Hofmeyr, G. J., & Sakala, C. (2003). Continuous support for women during childbirth. *Cochrane Database of Systematic Reviews, 3*. Art. No. CD003766 DOI: 10.1002/14651858.CD003766.

Institute of Medicine (IOM). (2007). *Preterm birth: Causes, consequences, and prevention*. Washington, DC: National Academies Press.

Kenner, C., & Lott, J. W. (2007). *Comprehensive neonatal care: An interdisciplinary approach* (4th ed.). St. Louis: Saunders Elsevier.

Leonard, P. (2007). Childbirth education: A handbook for nurses. *Nursing Spectrum*. Available at: http://nsweb.nursingspectrum.com/ ce/m350b.htm.

Polomeno, V. (2006). Relationship or content? Which is more important in perinatal education? *International Journal of Childbirth Education, 22*(1), 4–16.

Risica, P. M., & Phipps, M. G. (2006). Educational preferences in a prenatal clinic. *International Journal of Childbirth Education, 21*(4), 4–7.

Roberts, J. M., Gonzalez, C. B., & Sampselle, C. (2007). Why do supportive birth attendants become directive of maternal bearing-down efforts in second-stage labor? *Journal of Midwifery & Women's Health, 52*(2), 134–141.

Russell, K. E. (2007). Mad, bad or different? Midwives and normal birth in obstetric-led units. *British Journal of Midwifery, 15*(3), 128–131.

Simkin, P., & Ancheta, R. S. (2006). *The labor progress handbook* (2nd ed.). Malden, MA: Blackwell Publishers.

Smith, C. A., Collins, C. T., Cyna, A. M., & Crowther, C. A. (2006). Complementary and alternative therapies for pain management in labor. *Cochrane Library,* 2006(4), CD003521: 2009358378.

Steppe, B. (2007). In honor of the midwife. *International Journal of Childbirth Education, 22*(1), 39–40.

Terry, R. R., Westcott, J., O'Shea, L., & Kelly, F. (2006). Postpartum outcomes in supine delivery by physicians vs. nonsupine delivery by midwives. *Journal of the American Osteopathic Association, 106*(4), 199–205.

U.S. Department of Health and Human Services (USDHHS). (2000). *Healthy people 2010.* Washington, DC: Author.

Walsh, D. (2007). *Evidence-based care for normal labor and birth.* Andover, UK: Taylor & Francis, Inc.

Wood, S. (2007). Coping with labor pain. *March of Dimes.* Available at: http://www.marchofdimes.com/printableArticles/240_12936.asp

WEBSITES

Academy for Guided Imagery, Inc.: www.interactiveimagery.com/

American College of Obstetricians and Gynecologists: www.acog.org

American College of Nurse Midwives: www.midwife.org

American Public Health Association: www.apha.org

Association of Labor Assistants and Childbirth Educators: www.alace.org

Association of Women's Health, Obstetric and Neonatal Nurses (AWHONN): www.awhonn.org

Birthworks: www.birthworks.org

Childbirth Organization: www.childbirth.org

Diversity Rx: www.diversityrx.org

Doulas of North America: www.dona.org

Evidence-Based Nursing: www.evidencebasednursing.com

HypnoBirthing Institute: www.hypnobirthing.com

International Childbirth Education Association: www.icea.org

Lamaze International: www.lamaze-childbirth.com

National Association of Childbearing Centers: www.birthcenters.org

CHAPTER WORKSHEET

MULTIPLE CHOICE QUESTIONS

1. When determining the frequency of contractions, the nurse would measure which of the following?

   a. Start of one contraction to the start of the next contraction

   b. Beginning of one contraction to the end of the same contraction

   c. Peak of one contraction to the peak of the next contraction

   d. End of one contraction to the beginning of the next contraction

2. Which fetal lie is most conducive to a spontaneous vaginal birth?

   a. Transverse

   b. Longitudinal

   c. Perpendicular

   d. Oblique

3. Which of the following observations would suggest that placental separation is occurring?

   a. Uterus stops contracting altogether.

   b. Umbilical cord pulsations stop.

   c. Uterine shape changes to globular.

   d. Maternal blood pressure drops.

4. As the nurse is explaining the difference between true versus false labor to her childbirth class, she states that the major difference between them is:

   a. Discomfort level is greater with false labor.

   b. Progressive cervical changes occur in true labor.

   c. There is a feeling of nausea with false labor.

   d. There is more fetal movement with true labor.

5. The shortest but most intense phase of labor is the:

   a. Latent phase

   b. Active phase

   c. Transition phase

   d. Placental expulsion phase

6. A laboring woman is admitted to the labor and birth suite at 6 cm dilation. She would be in which phase of the first stage of labor?

   a. Latent

   b. Active

   c. Transition

   d. Early

7. Which assessment would indicate that a women is in true labor?

   a. Membranes are ruptured and fluid is clear

   b. Presenting part is engaged and not floating

   c. Cervix is 4 cm dilated, 90% effaced

   d. Contractions last 30 seconds, every 5 to 10 minutes

CRITICAL THINKING EXERCISES

1. Cindy, a 20-year-old primipara, calls the birthing center where you work as a nurse and reports she thinks she is in labor because she feels labor pains. Her due date is this week. The midwives have been giving her prenatal care throughout this pregnancy.

   a. What additional information do you need to respond appropriately?

   b. What suggestions/recommendations would you make to her?

   c. What instructions need to be given to guide her decision making?

   d. What other premonitory signs of labor might the nurse ask about?

   e. What manifestations would be found if Cindy is experiencing true labor?

2. You are assigned to lead a community education class for women in their third trimester of pregnancy to prepare them for their upcoming birth. Prepare an outline of topics that should be addressed.

STUDY ACTIVITIES

1. During clinical post-conference, share with the other nursing students how the critical forces of labor influenced the length of labor and the birthing process for a laboring woman assigned to you.

2. The cardinal movements of labor include which of the following? Select all that apply.

   a. Extension and rotation

   b. Descent and engagement

   c. Presentation and position

   d. Attitude and lie

   e. Flexion and expulsion

3. Interview a woman on the mother–baby unit who has given birth within the past few hours. Ask her to describe her experience and examine psychological factors that may have influenced her laboring process.

4. On the following illustration, identify the parameters of uterine contractions by marking an "X" where the nurse would measure the duration of the contraction.

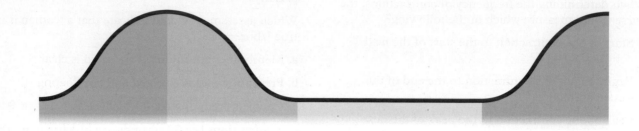

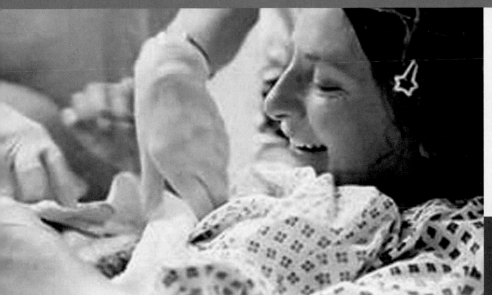

CHAPTER 14

NURSING MANAGEMENT DURING LABOR AND BIRTH

KEY TERMS

accelerations
artifact
baseline fetal heart rate
baseline variability
crowning

deceleration
electronic fetal
   monitoring
episiotomy
Leopold's maneuvers

neuraxial analgesia/
   anesthesia
periodic baseline changes

LEARNING OBJECTIVES

Upon completion of the chapter, the learner will be able to:

1. Define the key terms related to the labor and birth process.
2. Discuss the measures used to evaluate maternal status during labor and birth.
3. Explain the advantages and disadvantages of external and internal fetal monitoring, including the appropriate use for each.
4. Choose appropriate nursing interventions to address nonreassuring fetal heart rate patterns.
5. Outline the nurse's role in fetal assessment.
6. Explain the various comfort-promotion and pain-relief strategies used during labor and birth.
7. Summarize the assessment data collected on admission to the perinatal unit.
8. Discuss the ongoing assessments involved in each stage of labor and birth.
9. Explain the nurse's role throughout the labor and birth process.

Sheila is admitted in active labor (5 cm dilated) to the labor and birth suite at term. This is her second pregnancy and she is prepared to avoid pain medications this time so she can be more involved with the birthing process. She has been using modified-paced breathing with success thus far.

Wow

Wise nurses are not always silent, but they know when to be during the miracle of birth.

The laboring and birthing process is a life-changing event for many women. Nurses need to be respectful, available, encouraging, supportive, and professional in dealing with all women. Nursing management for labor and birth involves assessment, comfort measures, emotional support, information and instruction, advocacy, and support for the partner (Sauls, 2007).

The health of mothers and their infants is of critical importance, both as a reflection of the current health status of a large segment of our population and as a predictor of the health of the next generation. *Healthy People 2010* (USDHHS, 2000) addresses maternal health in two objectives: reducing maternal deaths and reducing maternal illness and complications due to pregnancy. In addition, another objective addresses increasing the proportion of pregnant women who attend prepared childbirth classes. (See Chapters 12 and 22 for more information on these objectives.)

This chapter provides information about nursing management during labor and birth. First, the essentials for in-depth assessment of maternal and fetal status during labor and birth are discussed. This is followed by a thorough description of the major methods of promoting comfort and providing pain management. The chapter concludes by putting all the information together with a discussion of the nursing care specific to each stage of labor, including the necessary data to be obtained with the admission assessment, methods to evaluate labor progress during the first stage of labor, and key nursing measures that focus on maternal and fetal assessments and pain relief for all stages of labor.

Maternal Assessment During Labor and Birth

During labor and birth, various techniques are used to assess maternal status. These techniques provide an ongoing source of data to determine the woman's response and her progress in labor. Assess maternal vital signs, including temperature, blood pressure, pulse, respiration, and pain, which are primary components of the physical examination and ongoing assessment. Also review the prenatal record to identify risk factors that may contribute to a decrease in uteroplacental circulation during labor. If there is no vaginal bleeding on admission, a vaginal examination is performed to assess cervical dilation, after which it is monitored periodically as necessary to identify progress. Evaluate maternal pain and the effectiveness of pain-management strategies at regular intervals during labor and birth.

Vaginal Examination

Although not all nurses perform vaginal examinations on laboring women in all practice settings, most nurses working in community hospitals do so because physicians are not routinely present in labor and birth suites. Since most newborns in the United States are born in community hospitals, nurses are performing vaginal examinations (American Hospital Association, 2007). Vaginal examinations are also performed by midwives and physicians.

▶ *Take* NOTE!

A vaginal examination is an assessment skill that takes time and experience to develop; only by doing it frequently in clinical practice can the practitioner's skill level improve.

The purpose of performing a vaginal examination is to assess the amount of cervical dilation, the percentage of cervical effacement, and the fetal membrane status and to gather information on presentation, position, station, degree of fetal head flexion, and presence of fetal skull swelling or molding (Fig. 14.1). Prepare the woman by informing her about the procedure, what information will be obtained from it, how she can assist with the procedure, how it will be performed, and who will be performing it.

The woman is typically on her back during the vaginal examination. The vaginal examination is performed gently, with concern for the woman's comfort. If it is the initial vaginal examination to check for membrane status, water is used as a lubricant. If the membranes have already ruptured, an antiseptic solution is used to prevent an ascending infection. After donning sterile gloves, the examiner inserts his or her index and middle fingers into the vaginal introitus. Next, the cervix is palpated to assess dilation, effacement, and position (e.g., posterior or an-

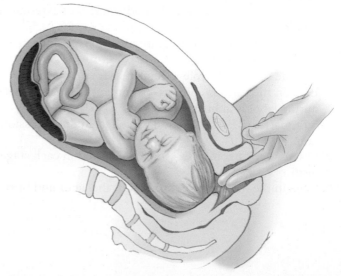

FIGURE 14.1 Vaginal examination to determine cervical dilation and effacement.

terior). If the cervix is open to any degree, the presenting fetal part, fetal position, station, and presence of molding can be assessed. In addition, the membranes can be evaluated and described as intact, bulging, or ruptured.

At the conclusion of the vaginal examination, the findings are discussed with the woman and her partner to bring them up to date about labor progress. In addition, the findings are documented either electronically or in writing and reported to the primary health care professional in charge of the case.

Cervical Dilation and Effacement

The amount of cervical dilation and the degree of cervical effacement are key areas assessed during the vaginal examination as the cervix is palpated with the gloved index finger. Although this finding is somewhat subjective, experienced examiners typically come up with similar findings. The width of the cervical opening determines dilation, and the length of the cervix assesses effacement. The information yielded by this examination serves as a basis for determining which stage of labor the woman is in and what her ongoing care should be.

Fetal Descent and Presenting Part

In addition to cervical dilation and effacement findings, the vaginal examination can also determine fetal descent (station) and presenting part. During the vaginal examination, the gloved index finger is used to palpate the fetal skull (if vertex presentation) through the opened cervix or the buttocks in the case of a breech presentation. Station is assessed in relation to the maternal ischial spines and the presenting fetal part. These spines are not sharp protrusions but rather blunted prominences at the midpelvis. The ischial spines serve as landmarks and have been designated as zero station. If the presenting part is palpated higher than the maternal ischial spines, a negative number is assigned; if the presenting fetal part is felt below the maternal ischial spines, a plus number is assigned, denoting how many centimeters below zero station.

Progressive fetal descent (−5 to +4) is the expected norm during labor—moving downward from the negative stations to zero station to the positive stations in a timely manner. If progressive fetal descent does not occur, a disproportion between the maternal pelvis and the fetus might exist and needs to be investigated.

Rupture of Membranes

The integrity of the membranes can be determined during the vaginal examination. Typically, if intact, the membranes will be felt as a soft bulge that is more prominent during a contraction. If the membranes have ruptured, the woman may have reported a sudden gush of fluid. Membrane rupture also may occur as a slow trickle of fluid. When membranes rupture, the priority focus should be on assessing fetal heart rate (FHR) first to identify a deceleration, which might indicate cord compression secondary to cord prolapse. If the membranes are ruptured

when the woman comes to the hospital, it is important to ascertain when it occurred. Prolonged ruptured membranes increase the risk of infection as a result of ascending vaginal organisms for both mother and fetus. Signs of intrauterine infection to be alert for include maternal fever, fetal and maternal tachycardia, foul odor of vaginal discharge, and an increase in white blood cell count.

To confirm that membranes have ruptured, a sample of fluid is taken from the vagina and tested with Nitrazine paper to determine the fluid's pH. Vaginal fluid is acidic, whereas amniotic fluid is alkaline and turns Nitrazine paper blue. Sometimes, however, false-positive results may occur, especially in women experiencing a large amount of bloody show, because blood is alkaline. The membranes are most likely intact if the Nitrazine test tape remains yellow to olive green, with pH between 5 and 6. The membranes are probably ruptured if the Nitrazine test tape turns a blue-green to deep blue, with pH ranging from 6.5 to 7.5 (Frieden & Chan, 2007).

If the Nitrazine test is inconclusive, an additional test, called the fern test, can be used to confirm rupture of membranes. With this test, a sample of fluid is obtained, applied to a microscope slide, and allowed to dry. Using a microscope, the slide is examined for a characteristic fern pattern that indicates the presence of amniotic fluid.

Assessing Uterine Contractions

The primary power of labor is uterine contractions, which are involuntary. Uterine contractions increase intrauterine pressure, causing tension on the cervix. This tension leads to cervical dilation and thinning, which in turn eventually forces the fetus through the birth canal. Normal uterine contractions have a contraction (systole) and a relaxation (diastole) phase. The contraction resembles a wave, moving downward to the cervix and upward to the fundus of the uterus. Each contraction starts with a building up (increment), gradually reaching an acme (peak intensity), and then a letting down (decrement). Each contraction is followed by an interval of rest, which ends when the next contraction begins. At the acme (peak) of the contraction, the entire uterus is contracting, with the greatest intensity in the fundal area. The relaxation phase follows and occurs simultaneously throughout the uterus.

Uterine contractions during labor are monitored by palpation and by electronic monitoring. Assessment of the contractions includes frequency, duration, intensity, and uterine resting tone (see Chapter 13 for a more detailed discussion).

Uterine contractions with an intensity of 30 mm Hg or greater initiate cervical dilation. During active labor, the intensity usually reaches 50 to 80 mm Hg. Resting tone is normally between 5 and 10 mm Hg in early labor and between 12 and 18 mm Hg in active labor (Gilbert, 2007).

To palpate the fundus for contraction intensity, place the pads of your fingers on the fundus and describe how

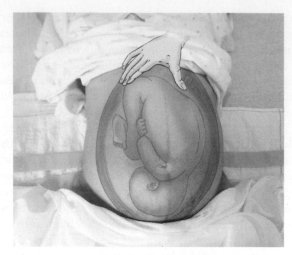

FIGURE 14.2 Nurse palpating the woman's fundus during a contraction.

it feels: like the tip of the nose (mild), like the chin (moderate), or like the forehead (strong). Palpation of intensity is a subjective judgment of the indentability of the uterine wall; a descriptive term is assigned (mild, moderate, or strong) (Fig. 14.2).

> ▶ **Take** NOTE!
>
> *Frequent clinical experience is needed to gain accuracy in assessing the intensity of uterine contractions.*

The second method used to assess the intensity of uterine contractions is electronic monitoring, either external or internal. Both methods provide an accurate measurement of the actual intensity of uterine contractions. Although the external fetal monitor is sometimes used to estimate the intensity of uterine contractions, it is not as accurate an assessment tool.

For woman at risk for preterm birth, home uterine activity monitoring can be used to screen for prelabor uterine contractility so that escalating contractility can be identified, allowing earlier intervention to prevent preterm birth. The home uterine activity monitor consists of a pressure sensor attached to a belt that is held against the abdomen and a recording/storage device that is carried on a belt or hung from the shoulder. Uterine activity is typically recorded by the woman for one hour twice daily, while she is performing routine activities. The stored data are transmitted via telephone to a perinatal nurse, and a receiving device prints out the data. The woman is contacted if there are any problems.

Although in theory identifying early contractions to initiate interventions to arrest the labor sounds reasonable, research shows that uterine activity monitoring in asymptomatic high-risk women is inadequate for predicting preterm birth (Herbst & Nilsson, 2006). This practice continues even though numerous randomized trials have found no relationship between monitoring and actual reduction of preterm labor. In more recent research findings, cervical length is predictive of preterm birth in all populations studied. A cervical length less than 25 mm warrants intervention to improve the health outcomes of pregnant women and their infants (Grimes-Dennis & Berghella, 2007).

Performing Leopold's Maneuvers

Leopold's maneuvers are a method for determining the presentation, position, and lie of the fetus through the use of four specific steps. This method involves inspection and palpation of the maternal abdomen as a screening assessment for malpresentation. A longitudinal lie is expected, and the presentation can be cephalic, breech, or shoulder. Each maneuver answers a question:

• What fetal part (head or buttocks) is located in the fundus (top of the uterus)?
• On which maternal side is the fetal back located? (Fetal heart tones are best auscultated through the back of the fetus.)
• What is the presenting part?
• Is the fetal head flexed and engaged in the pelvis?

Leopold's maneuvers are described in Nursing Procedure 14.1.

Fetal Assessment During Labor and Birth

A fetal assessment identifies well-being or signs that indicate compromise. The character of the amniotic fluid is assessed, but the fetal assessment focuses primarily on determining the FHR pattern. Fetal scalp sampling, fetal pulse oximetry, and fetal stimulation are additional assessments performed as necessary in the case of questionable FHR patterns.

Analysis of Amniotic Fluid

Amniotic fluid should be clear when the membranes rupture, either spontaneously or artificially through an amniotomy (a disposable plastic hook [Amnihook] is used to perforate the amniotic sac). Cloudy or foul-smelling amniotic fluid indicates infection. Green fluid may indicate that the fetus has passed meconium secondary to transient hypoxia; however, it is considered a normal occurrence if the fetus is in a breech presentation. If it is determined that meconium-stained amniotic fluid is due to fetal hypoxia, the maternity and pediatric teams work together to prevent meconium aspiration syndrome. This would necessitate suctioning after the head is born before the infant takes a breath and perhaps direct tracheal suctioning

Nursing Procedure 14.1

PERFORMING LEOPOLD'S MANEUVERS

Purpose: To Determine Fetal Presentation, Position, and Lie

1. Place the woman in the supine position and stand beside her.
2. Perform the first maneuver to determine presentation.
   a. Facing the woman's head, place both hands on the abdomen to determine fetal position in the uterine fundus.
   b. Feel for the buttocks, which will feel soft and irregular (indicates vertex presentation); feel for the head, which will feel hard, smooth, and round (indicates a breech presentation).

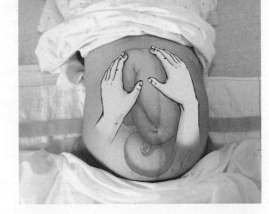

3. Complete the second maneuver to determine position.
   a. While still facing the woman, move hands down the lateral sides of the abdomen to palpate on which side the back is located (feels hard and smooth).
   b. Continue to palpate to determine on which side the limbs are located (irregular nodules with kicking and movement).

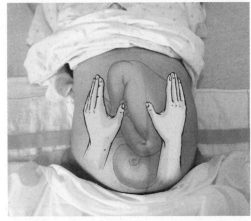

4. Perform the third maneuver to confirm presentation.
   a. Move hands down the sides of the abdomen to grasp the lower uterine segment and palpate the area just above the symphysis pubis.
   b. Place thumb and fingers of one hand apart and grasp the presenting part by bringing fingers together.
   c. Feel for the presenting part. If the presenting part is the head, it will be round, firm, and ballottable; if it is the buttocks, it will feel soft and irregular.

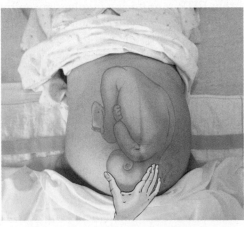

(continued)

5. Perform the fourth maneuver to determine attitude.
   a. Turn to face the client's feet and use the tips of the first three fingers of each hand to palpate the abdomen.
   b. Move fingers toward each other while applying downward pressure in the direction of the symphysis pubis. If you palpate a hard area on the side opposite the fetal back, the fetus is in flexion, because you have palpated the chin. If the hard area is on the same side as the back, the fetus is in extension, because the area palpated is the occiput.

Also, note how your hands move. If the hands move together easily, the fetal head is not descended into the woman's pelvic inlet. If the hands do not move together and stop because of resistance, the fetal head is engaged into the woman's pelvic inlet (Dillon, 2007).

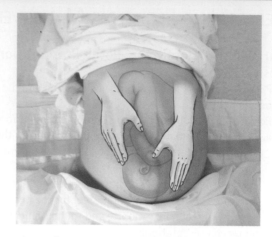

---

after birth if the Apgar score is low. In some cases an amnioinfusion (introduction of warmed, sterile normal saline or Ringer's lactate solution into the uterus) is used to dilute moderate to heavy meconium released in utero to assist in preventing meconium aspiration syndrome.

Analysis of the FHR

Analysis of the FHR is one of the primary evaluation tools used to determine fetal oxygen status indirectly. FHR assessment can be done intermittently using a fetoscope (a modified stethoscope attached to a headpiece) or a Doppler (ultrasound) device, or continuously with an electronic fetal monitor applied externally or internally.

Intermittent FHR Monitoring

Intermittent FHR monitoring involves auscultation via a fetoscope or a hand-held Doppler device that uses ultrasound waves that bounce off the fetal heart, producing echoes or clicks that reflect the rate of the fetal heart (Fig. 14.3). Traditionally, a fetoscope was used to assess fetal heart rate, but the Doppler device has been found to have a greater sensitivity than the fetoscope (Edmonds, 2007); thus, at present it is more commonly used.

▶ **Take** *NOTE!*

Doppler devices are relatively low in cost and are not used only in hospitals. They are used in home births and birthing centers, and pregnant women can also purchase them to help reduce anxiety between clinical examinations if they had a previous problem during pregnancy (Walsh, 2007).

Intermittent FHR monitoring allows the woman to be mobile in the first stage of labor. She is free to move around and change position at will since she is not attached to a stationary electronic fetal monitor. However, intermittent monitoring does not provide a continuous FHR recording and does not document how the fetus responds to the stress of labor (unless listening is done during the contraction). The best way to assess fetal well-being would be to start listening to the FHR at the end of the contraction (not after one) so that late decelerations could be detected. However, the pressure of the device during a contraction is uncomfortable and can distract the woman from using her paced-breathing patterns.

Intermittent FHR auscultation can be used to detect FHR baseline and rhythm and changes from baseline. However, it cannot detect variability and types of decelerations, as electronic fetal monitoring can (Murray, 2007).

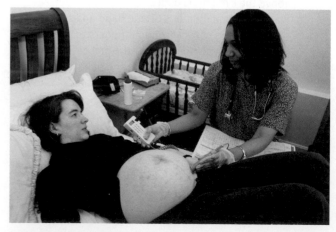

FIGURE 14.3 Auscultating fetal heart rate.

During intermittent auscultation to establish a baseline, the FHR is assessed for a full minute after a contraction. From then on, unless there is a problem, listening for 30 seconds and multiplying the value by two is sufficient. If the woman experiences a change in condition during labor, auscultation assessments should be more frequent. Changes in condition include ruptured membranes or the onset of bleeding. In addition, more frequent assessments occur after periods of ambulation, a vaginal examination, admin-

istration of pain medications, or other clinically important events (Hale, 2007).

The FHR is heard most clearly at the fetal back. In a cephalic presentation, the FHR is best heard in the lower quadrant of the maternal abdomen. In a breech presentation, it is heard at or above the level of the maternal umbilicus (Fig. 14.4). As labor progresses, the FHR location will change accordingly as the fetus descends into the maternal pelvis for the birthing process. To ensure that

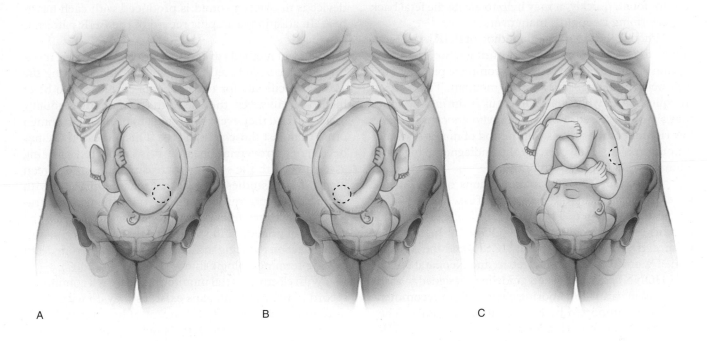

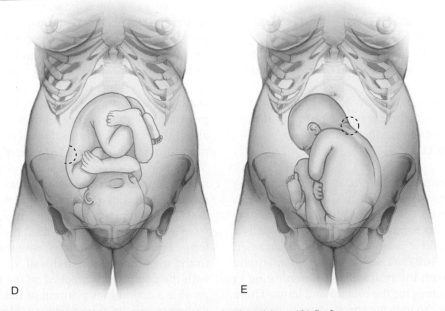

FIGURE 14.4 Locations for auscultating fetal heart rate based on fetal position. (**A**) Left occiput anterior (LOA). (**B**) Right occiput anterior (ROA). (**C**) Left occiput posterior (LOP). (**D**) Right occiput posterior (ROP). (**E**) Left sacral anterior (LSA).

the maternal heart rate is not confused with the FHR, palpate the client's radial pulse simultaneously while the FHR is being auscultated through the abdomen.

The procedure for using a fetoscope or Doppler device to assess FHR is similar (see Nursing Procedure 12.1 in Chapter 12). The main difference is that a small amount of water-soluble gel is applied to the woman's abdomen or ultrasound device before auscultation with the Doppler device to promote sound wave transmission. This gel is not needed when a fetoscope is used. Usually the FHR is best heard in the woman's lower abdominal quadrants; if it is not found quickly, it may help to locate the fetal back by performing Leopold's maneuvers.

Although the intermittent method of FHR assessment allows the client to move about during labor, the information obtained fails to provide a complete picture of the well-being of the fetus moment to moment. This leads to the question of what the fetal status is during the times that are not assessed. For women who are considered at low risk for complications, this period of non-assessment is not a problem. However, for the undiagnosed high-risk woman, it might prove ominous.

National professional organizations have provided general guidelines for the frequency of assessments based on existing evidence. The American College of Obstetricians and Gynecologists (ACOG), the Institute for Clinical Systems Improvement (ICSI), and the Association of Women's Health, Obstetric, and Neonatal Nurses (AWHONN) have published guidelines designed to assist clinicians in caring for laboring clients. Their recommendations are supported by large controlled studies. They recommend the following guidelines for assessing FHR:

- Initial 10- to 20-minute continuous FHR assessment on entry into labor/birth area
- Completion of a prenatal and labor risk assessment on all clients
- Intermittent auscultation every 30 minutes during active labor for a low-risk woman and every 15 minutes for a high-risk woman
- During the second stage of labor, every 15 minutes for the low-risk woman and every 5 minutes for the high-risk woman and during the pushing stage (ACOG, 2005; AWHONN, 2006; ICSI, 2007).

In several randomized controlled studies comparing intermittent auscultation with electronic monitoring in both low- and high-risk clients, no difference in intrapartum fetal death was found. However, in each study a nurse–client ratio of 1:1 was consistently maintained during labor (ICSI, 2007). This suggests that adequate staffing is essential with intermittent FHR monitoring to ensure optimal outcomes for the mother and fetus. There is insufficient evidence to indicate specific situations where continuous electronic fetal monitoring might result in better outcomes when compared to intermittent assess-ment. However, in pregnancies involving an increased risk of perinatal death, cerebral palsy, or neonatal encephalopathy and when oxytocin is used for induction or augmentation, it is recommended that continuous electronic fetal monitoring be used rather than intermittent fetal auscultation (Society of Obstetricians and Gynecologists of Canada, 2006).

Continuous Electronic Fetal Monitoring

Electronic fetal monitoring uses a machine to produce a continuous tracing of the FHR. When the monitoring device is in place, a sound is produced with each heartbeat. In addition, a graphic record of the FHR pattern is produced.

Current methods of continuous electronic fetal monitoring were introduced in the United States during the 1960s, specifically for use in clients considered to be at high risk. However, the use of these methods gradually increased and they eventually came to be used for women other than just those at high risk. This increased use has become controversial because it is suspected of being associated with the steadily increasing rates of cesarean births. Many studies suggest that when compared with standardized intermittent auscultation, the use of intrapartum electronic fetal monitoring seems to increase the number of preterm and surgical births but has no significant effect on reducing the incidence of intrapartum death or long-term neurologic injury (Lockwood, 2007).

With electronic fetal monitoring, there is a continuous record of the FHR: no gaps exist, as they do with intermittent auscultation. The concept of hearing and evaluating every beat of the fetus's heart to allow for early intervention seems logical. On the downside, however, using continuous monitoring can limit maternal movement and encourages the woman to lie in the supine position, which reduces placental perfusion. Despite the criticisms, electronic fetal monitoring remains an accurate method for determining fetal health status by providing a moment-to-moment printout of FHR status.

Various groups within the medical community have criticized the use of continuous fetal monitoring for all pregnant clients, whether high risk or low risk. Concerns about the efficiency and safety of routine electronic fetal monitoring in labor have led expert panels in the United States to recommend that such monitoring be limited to high-risk pregnancies. However, its use in low-risk pregnancies continues globally (Gagnon, Meier, & Waghorn, 2007). This remains an important research issue.

Continuous electronic fetal monitoring can be performed externally (indirectly), with the equipment attached to the maternal abdominal wall, or internally (directly), with the equipment attached to the fetus. Both methods provide a continuous printout of the FHR, but they differ in their specificity. The efficacy of electronic fetal monitoring depends on the accurate interpretation of the tracings, not necessarily which method (external vs. internal) is used.

Continuous External Monitoring

In external or indirect monitoring, two ultrasound transducers, each of which is attached to a belt, are applied around the woman's abdomen. They are similar to the hand-held Doppler device. One transducer, called a tocotransducer, detects changes in uterine pressure and converts the pressure registered into an electronic signal that is recorded on graph paper (Murray, 2007). The tocotransducer is placed over the uterine fundus in the area of greatest contractility to monitor uterine contractions. The other ultrasound transducer records the baseline FHR, long-term variability, accelerations, and decelerations. It is positioned on the maternal abdomen in the midline between the umbilicus and the symphysis pubis. The diaphragm of the ultrasound transducer is moved to either side of the abdomen to obtain a stronger sound and is then attached to the second elastic belt. This transducer converts the fetal heart movements into beeping sounds and records them on graph paper (Fig. 14.5).

Good continuous data are provided on the FHR. External monitoring can be used while the membranes are still intact and the cervix is not yet dilated. It is noninvasive and can detect relative changes in abdominal pressure between uterine resting tone and contractions. External monitoring also measures the approximate duration and frequency of contractions, providing a permanent record of FHR (Murray, 2007).

However, external monitoring can restrict the mother's movements. It also cannot detect short-term variability. Signal disruptions can occur due to maternal obesity, fetal malpresentation, and fetal movement, as well as by artifact. **Artifact** describes irregular variations or absence of FHR on the fetal monitor record that result from mechanical limitations of the monitor or electrical interference. For instance, the monitor may pick up transmissions from CB radios used by truck drivers on nearby roads and translate them into a signal. Additionally, gaps in the monitor strip can occur periodically without explanation.

Continuous Internal Monitoring

Continuous internal monitoring is usually indicated for women or fetuses considered to be at high risk. Possible conditions might include multiple gestation, decreased fetal movement, abnormal FHR on auscultation, intrauterine growth restriction (IUGR), maternal fever, preeclampsia, dysfunctional labor, preterm birth, or medical conditions such as diabetes or hypertension. It involves the placement of a spiral electrode into the fetal presenting part, usually the head, to assess FHR and a pressure transducer placed internally within the uterus to record uterine contractions (Fig. 14.6). The fetal spiral electrode is considered the most accurate method of detecting fetal heart characteristics and patterns because it involves receiving a signal directly from the fetus (Murray, 2007). Trained labor and birth nurses can place the spiral electrode on the fetal head when the membranes rupture in some health care facilities, but they do not place the intrauterine pressure catheter in the uterus. Internal monitoring does not have to include both an intrauterine pressure catheter and a scalp electrode. A fetal scalp electrode can be used to monitor the fetal heartbeat without monitoring the maternal intrauterine pressure.

Both the FHR and the duration and interval of uterine contractions are recorded on the graph paper. This method permits evaluation of baseline heart rate and changes in rate and pattern.

Four specific criteria must be met for this type of monitoring to be used:

• Ruptured membranes
• Cervical dilation of at least 2 cm

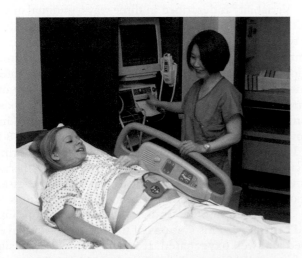

FIGURE 14.5 Continuous external electronic fetal monitoring device applied to the woman in labor.

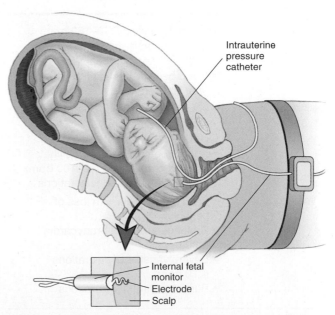

FIGURE 14.6 Continuous internal electronic fetal monitoring.

- Presenting fetal part low enough to allow placement of the scalp electrode
- Skilled practitioner available to insert spiral electrode (ICSI, 2007)

Compared to external monitoring, continuous internal monitoring can accurately detect both short-term (moment-to-moment) changes and long-term variability (fluctuations within the baseline) and FHR dysrhythmias. In addition, maternal position changes and movement do not interfere with the quality of the tracing.

Determining FHR Patterns

Assessment parameters of the FHR are classified as baseline rate, baseline variability (long-term and short-term), and periodic changes in the rate (accelerations and decelerations). The nurse must be able to interpret the various FHR parameters to determine if the pattern is reassuring (indicating fetal well-being) or nonreassuring (indicating fetal problems) to care for the woman effectively during labor and birth. Table 14.1 summarizes these patterns.

Baseline FHR

Baseline fetal heart rate refers to the average FHR that occurs during a 10-minute segment that excludes periodic or episodic rate changes, such as tachycardia or bradycardia. It is assessed when the woman has no contractions and the fetus is not experiencing episodic FHR changes. The normal baseline FHR ranges between 110 and 160 beats per minute (bpm) (National Institute of Child Health and Human Development [NICHD], 2006). The normal baseline FHR can be obtained by auscultation, ultrasound, or Doppler, or by a continuous internal direct fetal electrode.

TABLE 14.1 INTERPRETING FHR PATTERNS

Reassuring FHR signs	• Normal baseline (110–160 bpm) • Moderate bradycardia (100–110 bpm); good variability • Good beat-to-beat variability and fetal accelerations
Nonreassuring signs	• Fetal tachycardia (>160 bpm) • Moderate bradycardia (100–110 bpm); lost variability • Absent beat-to-beat variability • Marked bradycardia (90–100 bpm) • Moderate variable decelerations
Ominous signs	• Fetal tachycardia with loss of variability • Prolonged marked bradycardia (<90 bpm) • Severe variable decelerations (<70 bpm) • Persistent late decelerations

Sources: Hale, 2007; Lockwood, 2007; Murray, 2007, NICHD, 2006.

Fetal bradycardia occurs when the FHR is below 110 bpm and lasts 10 minutes or longer (NICHD, 2006). It can be the initial response of a healthy fetus to asphyxia. Causes of fetal bradycardia might include fetal hypoxia, prolonged maternal hypoglycemia, fetal acidosis, administration of drugs to the mother, hypothermia, maternal hypotension, prolonged umbilical cord compression, and fetal congenital heart block (Arenson & Drake, 2007). Bradycardia may be benign if it is an isolated event, but it is considered an ominous sign when accompanied by a decrease in long-term variability and late decelerations.

Fetal tachycardia is a baseline FHR greater than 160 bpm that lasts for 10 minutes or longer (NICHD, 2006). It can represent an early compensatory response to asphyxia. Other causes of fetal tachycardia include fetal hypoxia, maternal fever, maternal dehydration, amnionitis, drugs (e.g., cocaine, amphetamines, nicotine), maternal hyperthyroidism, maternal anxiety, fetal anemia, prematurity, fetal heart failure, and fetal arrhythmias. Fetal tachycardia is considered an ominous sign if it is accompanied by a decrease in variability and late decelerations (Hale, 2007).

Baseline Variability

Baseline variability is defined as normal physiologic variations in the time intervals that elapse between each fetal heartbeat observed along the baseline in the absence of contractions, decelerations, and accelerations (Menihan & Kopel, 2008). It represents the interplay between the parasympathetic and sympathetic nervous systems. The constant interplay (push-and-pull effect) on the FHR from the parasympathetic and sympathetic systems produces a moment-to-moment change in the FHR. Because variability is in essence the combined result of autonomic nervous system branch function, its presence implies that the both branches are working and receiving adequate oxygen (Hale, 2007). Thus, variability is one of the most important characteristics of the FHR.

Variability is described in three ways: minimal or absent, moderate, and marked. Minimal or absent variability typically is caused by uteroplacental insufficiency, cord compression, maternal hypotension, uterine hyperstimulation, abruptio placentae, or a fetal dysrhythmia. Interventions to improve uteroplacental blood flow and perfusion through the umbilical cord include lateral positioning of the mother, increasing the IV fluid rate to improve maternal circulation, administering oxygen at 8 to 10 L/min by mask, considering internal fetal monitoring, documenting findings and reporting to the health care provider. Preparation for a surgical birth may be necessary if no changes occur after attempting the interventions.

Moderate viability indicates that the autonomic and central nervous systems of the fetus are well developed and well oxygenated. It is considered a good sign of fetal well-being and correlates with the absence of significant metabolic acidosis (Fig. 14.7).

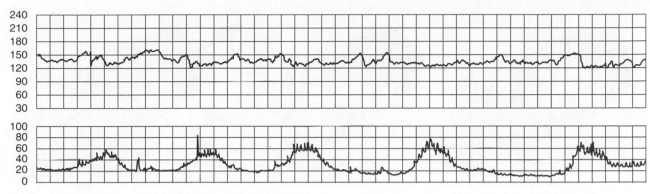

FIGURE 14.7 Long-term variability (average or moderate).

Marked variability occurs when there are more than 25 beats of fluctuation in the FHR baseline. Causes of this include cord prolapse or compression, maternal hypotension, uterine hyperstimulation, and abruptio placentae. Interventions include determining the cause if possible, lateral positioning, increasing IV fluid rate, administering oxygen at 8 to 10 L/min by mask, discontinuing oxytocin infusion, observing for changes in tracing, considering internal fetal monitoring, communicating an abnormal pattern to the health care provider, and preparing for a surgical birth if no change in pattern is noted (Menihan & Kopel, 2008).

FHR variability is an important clinical indicator that is predictive of fetal acid–base balance and cerebral tissue perfusion (Bakker et al., 2007). As the central nervous system is desensitized by hypoxia and acidosis, FHR decreases until a smooth baseline pattern appears. Loss of variability may be associated with a poor outcome. Some causes of decreased variability include fetal hypoxia/acidosis, drugs that depress the central nervous system, congenital abnormalities, fetal sleep, prematurity, and fetal tachycardia (Walsh, 2007).

> ▶ *Take* NOTE!
>
> *External electronic fetal monitoring cannot assess short-term variability. Therefore, if external monitoring shows a baseline that is smoothing out, use of an internal spiral electrode should be considered to gain a more accurate picture of the fetal health status.*

Periodic Baseline Changes

Periodic baseline changes are temporary, recurrent changes made in response to a stimulus such as a contraction. The FHR can demonstrate patterns of acceleration or deceleration in response to most stimuli. Fetal **accel-erations** are transitory increases in the FHR above the baseline associated with sympathetic nervous stimulation. They are visually apparent, with elevations of FHR of more than 15 bpm above the baseline, and their duration is less than 2 minutes (NICHD, 2006). They are generally considered reassuring and require no interventions. Accelerations denote fetal movement and fetal well-being and are the basis for nonstress testing.

A **deceleration** is a transient fall in FHR caused by stimulation of the parasympathetic nervous system. Decelerations are described by their shape and association to a uterine contraction. They are classified as early, late, variable, and prolonged (Fig. 14.8).

Early decelerations are characterized by a gradual decrease in the FHR in which the nadir (lowest point) occurs at the peak of the contraction. They rarely decrease more than 30 to 40 bpm below the baseline. Typically, the onset, nadir, and recovery of the deceleration occur at the same time as the onset, peak and recovery of the contraction. They are most often seen during the active stage of any normal labor, during pushing, crowning, or vacuum extraction. They are thought to be a result of fetal head compression that results in a reflex vagal response with a resultant slowing of the FHR during uterine contractions. Early decelerations are not indicative of fetal distress and do not require intervention.

Late decelerations are transitory decreases in FHR that occur after a contraction begins. The FHR does not return to baseline levels until well after the contraction has ended. Delayed timing of the deceleration occurs, with the nadir of the uterine contraction. Late decelerations are associated with uteroplacental insufficiency, which occurs when blood flow within the intervillous space is decreased to the extent that fetal hypoxia exists (Bakker et al., 2007). Conditions that may decrease uteroplacental perfusion with resultant decelerations include maternal hypotension, gestational hypertension, placental aging secondary to diabetes and postmaturity, hyperstimulation via oxytocin infusion, maternal smoking, anemia, and

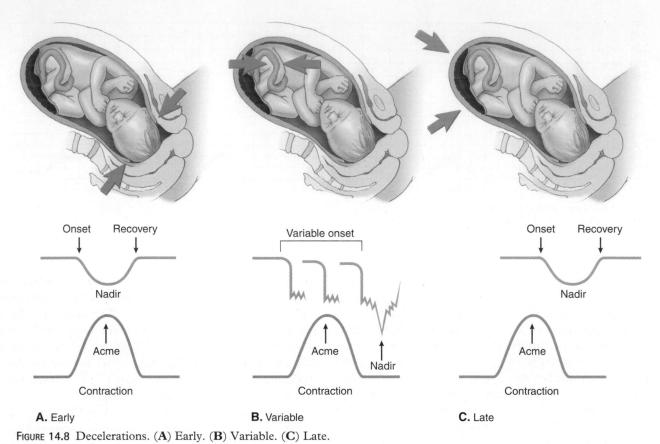

A. Early   **B.** Variable   **C.** Late

FIGURE 14.8 Decelerations. (**A**) Early. (**B**) Variable. (**C**) Late.

cardiac disease. They imply some degree of fetal hypoxia. Repetitive late decelerations and late decelerations with decreasing baseline variability are nonreassuring signs. Box 14.1 highlights interventions for decelerations.

Variable decelerations present as visually apparent abrupt decreases in FHR below baseline and have an unpredictable shape on the FHR baseline, possibly demonstrating no consistent relationship to uterine contractions. The shape of variable decelerations may be U, V, or W, or they may not resemble other patterns (Hale, 2007). Variable decelerations usually occur abruptly with quick deceleration. They are the most common deceleration pattern found in the laboring woman and are usually transient and correctable (Murray, 2007). Variable decelerations are associated with cord compression. However, they become a nonreassuring sign when the FHR decreases to less than 60 bpm, persists at that level for at least 60 seconds, and is repetitive (ICSI, 2007). The pattern of variable deceleration consistently related to the contractions with a slow return to FHR baseline is also nonreassuring.

Prolonged decelerations are abrupt FHR declines of at least 15 bpm that last longer than 2 minutes but less than 10 minutes (NICHD, 2006). The rate usually drops to less than 90 bpm. Many factors are associated with this pattern, including prolonged cord compression, abruptio placentae, cord prolapse, supine maternal position, vaginal examination, fetal blood sampling, maternal seizures, regional anesthesia, or uterine rupture (Murray, 2007). Prolonged decelerations can be remedied by identifying the underlying cause and correcting it.

Combinations of FHR patterns obtained by electronic fetal monitoring during labor are not infrequent. Nonreassuring patterns are more significant if they are mixed and persist for long periods. Other nonreassuring patterns include prolonged late decelerations, absent or minimal variability, bradycardia or tachycardia, and prolonged variable decelerations lower than 60 bpm. The likelihood of fetal compromise is increased if various nonreassuring patterns coexist, particularly those associated with decreased baseline variability or abnormal contraction patterns (ICSI, 2007).

Other Fetal Assessment Methods

In situations suggesting the possibility of fetal compromise, such as inconclusive or nonreassuring FHR patterns, further ancillary testing such as fetal scalp sampling, fetal pulse oximetry, and fetal stimulation may be used to validate the FHR findings and assist in planning interventions.

BOX 14.1 Interventions for Nonreassuring Decelerations

If a patient develops a nonreassuring deceleration pattern such as late or variable decelerations:

- Notify the health care provider about the pattern and obtain further orders, making sure to document all interventions and their effects on the FHR pattern.
- Reduce or discontinue oxytocin as dictated by the facility's protocol, if it is being administered.
- Provide reassurance that interventions are being done to effect a pattern change.

Additional interventions specific for a late deceleration FHR pattern would include:

- Turning the client on her left side to increase placental perfusion
- Administering oxygen by mask to increase fetal oxygenation
- Increasing the IV fluid rate to improve intravascular volume
- Assessing client for any underlying contributing causes
- Providing reassurance that interventions are to effect pattern change

Specific interventions for a variable deceleration FHR pattern would include:

- Changing the client's position to relieve compression on the cord
- Providing reassurance that interventions are to effect pattern change
- Giving oxygen and IV fluids as ordered

▶ *Take NOTE!*

During the past decade, the use of fetal scalp sampling has decreased, being replaced by less invasive techniques that yield similar information.

Fetal Oxygen Saturation Monitoring (Fetal Pulse Oximetry)

Fetal pulse oximetry measures fetal oxygen saturation directly and in real time. It is used with electronic fetal monitoring as an adjunct method of assessment when the FHR pattern is nonreassuring or inconclusive. Normal oxygen saturation of a healthy fetus is 30% to 70% (Miller, 2007). If the fetal oxygen saturation is reassuring (a trend of more than 30% between contractions), unnecessary cesarean births, invasive procedures such as fetal blood sampling, and operative vaginal births can be minimized (Peek, Condous, & Nanan, 2007). Any reduction in un-

necessary interventions during labor and birth has the potential to improve maternal and fetal outcomes and reduce costs.

Adequate maintenance of fetal oxygenation is necessary for fetal well-being. Fetal oxygen saturation monitoring is used for a singleton term fetus in a vertex presentation, at a −2 station or below, and with a nonreassuring FHR pattern. In addition, the fetal membranes must be ruptured and the cervix dilated at least 2 cm (Gilbert, 2007). A soft sensor is introduced through the dilated cervix and placed on the cheek, forehead, or temple of the fetus. It is held in place by the uterine wall. The sensor then is attached to a special adaptor on the fetal monitor that provides a real-time recording that is displayed on the uterine activity panel of the tracing. It is a noninvasive, safe, and accurate method for assessing fetal oxygenation.

The fetal pulse oximetry traces along the contraction portion of the monitoring strip, so it is easy to see how the saturation changes with the contraction. This adjunct test can help support decisions to allow labor to continue or to intervene surgically. Observing the trend of oxygen saturation on the tracing and documenting the values on the labor flow sheet or other medical record forms is crucial. The physician or midwife must be notified if the fetal oxygen saturation becomes nonreassuring (less than 30% between contractions) in conjunction with a nonreassuring FHR pattern. Ongoing communication is needed between the nurse and the primary care provider to enhance the maternal–fetus status.

Fetal Stimulation

An indirect method used to evaluate fetal oxygenation and acid–base balance to identify fetal hypoxia is fetal scalp stimulation and vibroacoustic stimulation. If the fetus does not have adequate oxygen reserves, carbon dioxide builds up, leading to acidemia and hypoxemia. These metabolic states are reflected in nonreassuring FHR patterns as well as fetal inactivity. Fetal stimulation is performed to promote fetal movement with the hope that FHR accelerations will accompany the movement.

Fetal movement can be stimulated with a vibroacoustic stimulator (artificial larynx) applied to the woman's lower abdomen and turned on for a few seconds to produce sound and vibration or by tactile stimulation via pelvic examination and stimulation of the fetal scalp with the gloved fingers. A well-oxygenated fetus will respond when stimulated (tactile or by noise) by moving in conjunction with an acceleration of 15 bpm above the baseline heart rate that lasts at least 15 seconds. This FHR acceleration reflects a pH of more than 7 and a fetus with an intact central nervous system. Fetal scalp stimulation is not done if the fetus is preterm, or if the woman has an intrauterine infection, a diagnosis of placenta previa (which could lead to hemorrhage), or a fever (which increases the risk of an ascending infection) (Gilbert, 2007).

Promoting Comfort and Providing Pain Management During Labor

Pain during labor is a universal experience, although the intensity of the pain may vary. Although labor and childbirth are viewed as natural processes, both can produce significant pain and discomfort. The physical causes of pain during labor include cervical stretching, hypoxia of the uterine muscle due to a decrease in perfusion during contractions, pressure on the urethra, bladder, and rectum, and distention of the muscles of the pelvic floor (Leonard, 2007). A woman's pain perception can be influenced by her previous experiences with pain, fatigue, pain anticipation, positive or negative support system, labor and birth environment, cultural expectations, and level of emotional stress and anxiety (Albers, 2007).

The techniques used to manage the pain of labor vary according to geography and culture. For example, some Appalachian women believe that placing a hatchet or knife under the bed of a laboring woman may help "cut the pain of childbirth," and a woman from this background may wish to do so in the hospital setting (Bowers, 2007). Asian, Latino, and Orthodox Jewish women may request that their own mothers, not their husbands, attend their births; husbands do not actively participate in the birthing process. Cherokee, Hmong, and Japanese women will often remain quiet during labor and birth and not complain of pain because outwardly expressing pain is not appropriate in their cultures. Never interpret their quietness as freedom from pain (Bowers, 2007).

Culturally diverse childbearing families present to the labor and birth suites with the same needs and desires of all families. Give them the same respect and sense of welcome shown to all families. Make sure they have a high-quality birth experience: uphold their religious, ethnic, and cultural values and integrate them into care.

Today, women have many safe nonpharmacologic and pharmacologic choices for the management of pain during labor and birth, which may be used separately or in combination with one another.

Nurses are in an ideal position to provide childbearing women with balanced, clear, concise information about effective nonpharmacologic and pharmacologic measures to relieve pain. Pain management standards issued by JCAHO mandate that pain be assessed in all clients admitted to a health care facility. Thus, it is important for nurses to be knowledgeable about the most recent scientific research on labor pain-relief modalities, to make sure that accurate and unbiased information about effective pain-relief measures is available to laboring women, to be sure that the woman determines what is an acceptable labor pain level for her, and to allow the woman the choice of pain-relief method.

Nonpharmacologic Measures

Nonpharmacologic measures may include continuous labor support, hydrotherapy, ambulation and position changes, acupuncture and acupressure, attention focusing and imagery, therapeutic touch and massage, breathing techniques, and effleurage. Most of these methods are based on the "gate control" theory of pain, which proposes that local physical stimulation can interfere with pain stimuli by closing a hypothetical gate in the spinal cord, thus blocking pain signals from reaching the brain (Arenson & Drake, 2007). It has long been a standard of care for labor nurses to first provide or encourage a variety of nonpharmacologic measures before moving to the pharmacologic interventions.

Nonpharmacologic measures are usually simple, safe, and inexpensive to use. Many of these measures are taught in childbirth classes, and women should be encouraged to try a variety of methods prior to the real labor. Many of the measures need to be practiced for best results and coordinated with the partner/coach. The nurse provides support and encouragement for the woman and her partner using nonpharmacologic methods. Although women can't consciously direct the labor contractions, they can control how they respond to them, thereby enhancing their feelings of control.

Continuous Labor Support

Continuous labor support involves offering a sustained presence to the laboring woman by providing emotional support, comfort measures, advocacy, information and advice, and support for the partner (Gagnon, Meier, & Waghorn, 2007). A woman's family, a midwife, a nurse, a doula, or anyone else close to the woman can provide this continuous presence. A support person can assist the woman to ambulate, reposition herself, and use breathing techniques. A support person can also aid with the use of acupressure, massage, music therapy, or therapeutic touch. During the natural course of childbirth, a laboring woman's functional ability is limited secondary to pain, and she often has trouble making decisions. The support person can help make them based on his or her knowledge of the woman's birth plan and personal wishes.

Research has validated the value of continuous labor support versus intermittent support in terms of lower operative deliveries, cesarean births, and requests for pain medication (Armstrong & Feldman, 2007).

▶ ***Take*** NOTE!

The human presence is of immeasurable value to make the laboring woman feel secure.

Hydrotherapy

Hydrotherapy is a nonpharmacologic measure in which the woman immerses herself in warm water for relaxation and relief of discomfort. When the woman enters the warm water, the warmth and buoyancy help to release muscle tension and can impart a sense of well-being (Koenig, 2007). Warm water provides soothing stimulation of nerves in the skin, promoting vasodilatation, reversal of sympathetic nervous response, and a reduction in catecholamines (Blackburn, 2007). Contractions are usually less painful in warm water because the warmth and buoyancy of the water have a relaxing effect.

There are a wide range of hydrotherapy options available, from ordinary bathtubs to whirlpool baths and showers, combined with low lighting and music. Many hospitals provide showers and whirlpool baths for laboring women for pain relief. However, hydrotherapy is more commonly practiced in birthing centers managed by midwives. The recommendation for initiating hydrotherapy is that the woman be in active labor (more than 5 cm dilated) to prevent the slowing of labor contractions secondary to muscular relaxation. The woman's membranes can be intact or ruptured. Women are encouraged to stay in the bath or shower as long as they feel they are comfortable. The water temperature should not exceed body temperature, and the bath time typically is limited to 1 to 2 hours (Koenig, 2007).

Hydrotherapy is an effective pain-management option for many women. Women who are experiencing a healthy pregnancy can be offered this option, but the potential benefits or risks to the woman are still not known (Fink, Irwin, & Mitchell, 2007).

Ambulation and Position Changes

Ambulation and position changes during labor are another extremely useful comfort measure. Historically, women adopted a variety of positions during labor, rarely using the recumbent position until recently. The medical profession has favored recumbent positions during labor, but without evidence to demonstrate their appropriateness (Sleutel, Schultz, & Wyble, 2007).

Changing position frequently (every 30 minutes or so)—sitting, walking, kneeling, standing, lying down, getting on hands and knees, and using a birthing ball—helps relieve pain (Fig. 14.9). Position changes also may help to speed labor by adding the benefits of gravity and changing the shape of the pelvis. Research has found that the position that the woman assumes and the frequency of position changes have a profound effect on uterine activity and efficiency. Allowing the woman to obtain a position of comfort frequently facilitates a favorable fetal rotation by altering the alignment of the presenting part with the pelvis. As the mother continues to change position based on comfort, the optimal presentation is afforded (Gilbert, 2007). Supine and sitting positions should be avoided, since they may interfere with labor progress and can cause compression of the vena cava and decrease blood return to the heart.

Swaying from side to side, rocking, or other rhythmic movements may also be comforting. If labor is progressing slowly, ambulating may speed it up again. Upright positions such as walking, kneeling forward, or doing the lunge on the birthing ball give most women a greater sense of control and active movement than just lying down. Table 14.2 highlights some of the more common positions that can be used during labor and birth.

Acupuncture and Acupressure

Acupuncture and acupressure can be used to relieve pain during labor. Although controlled research studies of these methods are limited, there is adequate evidence that both are useful in relieving pain associated with labor and birth. However, both methods require a trained, certified clinician, and such a person is not available in many birth facilities (Hantoushzadeh, Alhusseini, & Lebaschi, 2007).

Acupuncture involves stimulating key trigger points with needles. This form of Chinese medicine has been practiced for approximately 3,000 years. Classical Chinese teaching holds that throughout the body there are meridians or channels of energy (*qi*) that when in balance regulate body functions. Pain reflects an imbalance or obstruction of the flow of energy. The purpose of acupuncture is to restore *qi*, thus diminishing pain (Koenig, 2007). Stimulating the trigger points causes the release of endorphins, reducing the perception of pain.

Acupressure involves the application of a firm finger or massage at the same trigger points to reduce the pain sensation. The amount of pressure is important. The intensity of the pressure is determined by the needs of the woman. Holding and squeezing the hand of a woman in labor may trigger the point most commonly used for both techniques. Some acupressure points are found along the spine, neck, shoulder, toes, and soles of the feet (Armstrong & Feldman, 2007). A Cochrane Collaboration review found that acupuncture may indeed reduce labor pain, but the number of women studied has been small (Smith et al., 2006).

Attention Focusing and Imagery

Attention focusing and imagery uses many of the senses and the mind to focus on stimuli. The woman can focus on tactile stimuli such as touch, massage, or stroking. She may focus on auditory stimuli such as music, humming, or verbal encouragement. Visual stimuli might be any object in the room, or the woman can imagine the beach, a mountaintop, a happy memory, or even the contractions of the uterine muscle pulling the cervix open and the fetus pressing downward to open the cervix. Some women focus on a particular mental activity such as a song, a chant, counting backwards, or a Bible verse. Breathing, relaxation, positive thinking, and positive visualization work well for mothers in labor. The use of these techniques keeps the sensory input perceived during the contraction from reaching the pain center in the cortex of the brain (Armstrong & Feldman, 2007).

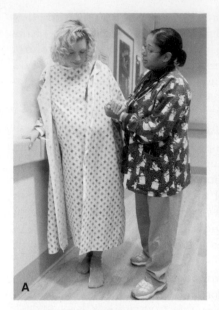
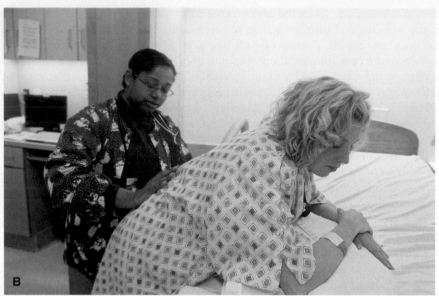
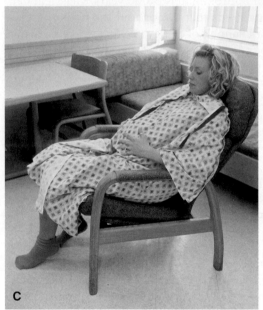
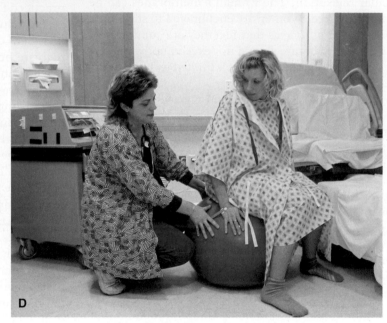

FIGURE 14.9 Various positions for use during labor. (**A**) Ambulation. (**B**) Leaning forward. (**C**) Sitting in a chair. (**D**) Using a birthing ball.

Therapeutic Touch and Massage

Therapeutic touch and massage use the sense of touch to promote relaxation and pain relief. Massage works as a form of pain relief by increasing the production of endorphins in the body. Endorphins reduce the transmission of signals between nerve cells and thus lower the perception of pain (Blackburn, 2007). In addition, touching and massage distract the woman from discomfort.

Therapeutic touch is based on the premises that the body contains energy fields that lead to either good or ill health and that the hands can be used to redirect the energy fields that lead to pain (Arenson & Drake, 2007). To be done correctly, this technique must be learned and practiced. Some women prefer a light touch, while others find a firmer touch more soothing. Massage of the neck, shoulders, back, thighs, feet, and hands can be very comforting. The use of firm counterpressure in the lower back or sacrum is especially helpful for back pain during contractions (Fig. 14.10). Contraindications for massage include skin rashes, varicose veins, bruises, or infections (Leonard, 2007).

Effleurage is a light, stroking, superficial touch of the abdomen, in rhythm with breathing during contractions. It is used as a relaxation and distraction technique from discomfort. The external fetal monitor belts may interfere with the ability to accomplish this.

TABLE 14.2 **COMMON POSITIONS FOR USE DURING LABOR AND BIRTH**

Standing	• Takes advantage of gravity during and between contractions • Makes contractions feel less painful and be more productive • Helps fetus line up with angle of maternal pelvis • Helps to increase urge to push in second stage of labor
Walking	• Has the same advantages as standing • Causes changes in the pelvic joints, helping the fetus move through the birth canal
Standing and leaning forward on partner, bed, birthing ball	• Has the same advantages as standing • Is a good position for a backrub • May feel more restful than standing • Can be used with electronic fetal monitor
Slow dancing (standing with woman's arms around partner's neck, head resting on his chest or shoulder, with his hands rubbing woman's lower back; sway to music and breathe in rhythm if it helps)	• Has the same advantages as walking • Back pressure helps relieve back pain • Rhythm and music help woman relax and provide comfort
The lunge (standing facing a straight chair with one foot on the seat with knee and foot to the side; bending raised knee and hip, and lunging sideways repeatedly during a contraction, holding each lunge for 5 seconds; partner holds chair and helps with balance)	• Widens one side of the pelvis (the side toward lunge) • Encourages rotation of baby • Can also be done in a kneeling position
Sitting upright	• Helps promote rest • Has more gravity advantage than lying down • Can be used with electronic fetal monitor
Semi-sitting (setting the head of the bed at a 45-degree angle with pillows used for support)	• Has the same advantages as sitting upright • Is an easy position if on a bed
Sitting on toilet or commode	• Has the same advantages as sitting upright • May help relax the perineum for effective bearing down
Rocking in a chair	• Has the same advantages as sitting upright • May help speed labor (rocking movement)
Sitting, leaning forward with support	• Has the same advantages as sitting upright • Is a good position for a backrub
On all fours, on hands and knees	• Helps relieve backache • Assists rotation of baby in posterior position • Allows for pelvic rocking and body movement • Relieves pressure on hemorrhoids • Allows for vaginal examinations • Is sometimes preferred as a pushing position by women with back labor
Kneeling, leaning forward with support on a chair seat, the raised head of the bed, or on a birthing ball	• Has the same advantages as all-fours position • Puts less strain on wrists and hands
Side-lying	• Is a very good position for resting and convenient for many kinds of medical interventions • Helps lower elevated blood pressure • May promote progress of labor when alternated with walking • Is useful to slow a very rapid second stage • Takes pressure off hemorrhoids • Facilitates relaxation between contractions

(continued)

TABLE 14.2   COMMON POSITIONS FOR USE DURING LABOR AND BIRTH (continued)

Squatting	• May relieve backache • Takes advantage of gravity • Requires less bearing-down effort • Widens pelvic outlet • May help fetus turn and move down in a difficult birth • Helps if the woman feels no urge to push • Allows freedom to shift weight for comfort • Offers an advantage when pushing, since upper trunk presses on the top of the uterus
Supported squat (leaning back against partner, who supports woman under the arms and takes the entire woman's weight; standing up between contractions)	• Requires great strength in partner • Lengthens trunk, allowing more room for fetus to maneuver into position • Lets gravity help
Dangle (partner sitting high on bed or counter with feet supported on chairs or footrests and thighs spread; woman leaning back between partner's legs, placing flexed arms over partner's thighs; partner gripping sides with his thighs; woman lowering herself and allowing partner to support her full weight; standing up between contractions)	• Has the same advantages of a supported squat • Requires less physical strength from the partner

Sources: Albers, 2007; Armstrong & Feldman, 2007; Koenig, 2007; Walsh, 2007.

EVIDENCE-BASED PRACTICE 14.1
The Effects of Complementary and Alternative Therapies for Pain Management in Labor on Maternal and Perinatal Morbidity

● Study

The pain of labor can be intense, with tension, anxiety, and fear making it worse. Many women would like to labor without using drugs and turn to alternatives to manage pain. These alternative methods include acupuncture, mind-body techniques, massage, reflexology, herbal medicines or homoeopathy, hypnosis, and music. This review examined currently available evidence supporting the use of alternative and complementary therapies for pain management in labor. Fourteen trials were included in the review, with data reporting on 1,537 women using different modalities of pain management; 1,448 women were included in the meta-analysis.

▲ Findings

Acupuncture and hypnosis may help relieve labor pain. There is insufficient evidence about the benefits of music, massage, relaxation, white noise, acupressure, and aromatherapy, and no evidence about the effectiveness of massage or other complementary therapies. In summary, acupuncture and hypnosis may be beneficial for the management of pain during labor; however, the number of women studied has been small. Few other complementary therapies have been subjected to proper scientific study.

■ Nursing Implications

Although this study didn't offer conclusive evidence that alternative therapies for pain management work better than pharmacologic or invasive methods, they should not be discounted. Many women wish to avoid artificial means to control the discomfort of labor. The nurse should be supportive and open-minded about a woman's efforts to meet her pain management goals.

Smith, C. A., Collins, C. T., Cyna, A. M., & Crowther, C. A. (2006). Complementary and alternative therapies for pain management in labor. *Cochrane Database of Systematic Reviews* 2006, Issue 4. Art. No.: CD003521. DOI: 10.1002/14651858.CD003521.pub2.

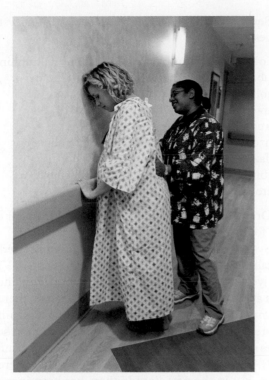

FIGURE **14.10** Nurse massaging the client's back during a contraction while she ambulates during labor.

Breathing Techniques

Breathing techniques are effective in producing relaxation and pain relief through the use of distraction. If the woman is concentrating on slow-paced rhythmic breathing, she isn't likely to fully focus on contraction pain. Breathing techniques are often taught in childbirth education classes (see Chapter 12 for additional information).

Breathing techniques use controlled breathing to reduce the pain experienced through a stimulus–response conditioning. The woman selects a focal point within her environment to stare at during the first sign of a contraction. This focus creates a visual stimulus that goes directly to her brain. The woman takes a deep cleansing breath, which is followed by rhythmic breathing. Verbal commands from her partner supply an ongoing auditory stimulus to her brain. Effleurage can be combined with the breathing to provide a tactile stimulus, all blocking pain sensations to her brain.

Benefits of practicing patterned breathing include:

- Breathing becomes an automatic response to pain.
- Breathing increases relaxation and can be used for deal with life's everyday stresses.
- The steady rhythm of breathing is calming during labor.
- Breathing provides a sense of well-being and a measure of control.
- Breathing brings purpose to each contraction, making them more productive.
- Breathing provides more oxygen for the mother and fetus (American Pregnancy Association, 2007).

Many couples learn patterned-paced breathing during their childbirth education classes. Three levels may be taught, each beginning and ending with a cleansing breath. In the first pattern, also known as slow-paced breathing, the woman inhales slowly through her nose and exhales through pursed lips. The breathing rate is typically 6 to 9 bpm. In the second pattern, also called shallow or modified-paced breathing, the woman inhales and exhales through her mouth at a rate of 4 breaths every 5 seconds. The rate can be accelerated to 2 breaths per second to assist her to relax. The third pattern, pattern paced breathing, is similar to modified-paced breathing except that the breathing is punctuated every few breaths by a forceful exhalation through pursed lips. All breaths are kept equal and rhythmic and can increase as contractions increase in intensity (Lyon, 2007).

Many childbirth educators do not recommend specific breathing techniques or try to teach parents to breathe the "right" way during labor and birth. Couples are encouraged to find breathing styles that enhance their relaxation and use them. There are numerous benefits to controlled and rhythmic breathing in childbirth (outlined above), and many women choose these techniques to manage their discomfort during labor.

Pharmacologic Measures

With varying degrees of success, generations of women have sought ways to relieve the pain of childbirth. Pharmacologic pain relief during labor includes systemic analgesia and regional or local anesthesia. Women have seen dramatic changes in pharmacologic pain management options over the years. Methods have evolved from biting down on a stick to a more complex pharmacologic approach such as epidural/intrathecal analgesia. Systemic analgesia and regional analgesia/anesthesia have become less common, while newer neuraxial analgesia/anesthesia techniques involving minimal motor blockade have become more popular. **Neuraxial analgesia/anesthesia** is the administration of analgesic (opioids) or anesthetic (medication capable of producing a loss of sensation in an area of the body) agents, either continuously or intermittently, into the epidural or intrathecal space to relieve pain. Low-dose and ultra-low-dose epidural analgesia, spinal analgesia, and combined spinal-epidural analgesia have replaced the traditional epidural for labor (Kuczkowski, 2007). This shift in pain management allows a woman to be an active participant in labor.

▶ *Take* NOTE!

Regardless of which approach is used during labor, the woman has the right to choose the methods of pain control that will best suit her and meet her needs.

▶ *Consider* THIS!

When I was expecting my first child, I was determined to put my best foot forward and do everything right. I was an experienced OB nurse, and in my mind doing everything right was expected behavior. I was already 2 weeks past my calculated due date and I was becoming increasingly worried. That particular day I went to work with a backache but felt no contractions.

I managed to finish my shift but felt completely wiped out. As I walked to my car outside the hospital, my water broke and I felt the warm fluid run down my legs. I went back inside to be admitted for this much-awaited event.

Although I had helped thousands of women go through their childbirth experience, I was now the one in the bed and not standing alongside it. My husband and I had practiced our breathing techniques to cope with the discomfort of labor, but this "discomfort" in my mind was more than I could tolerate. So despite my best intentions of doing everything right, within an hour I begged for a painkiller to ease the pain. While the medication took the edge off my pain, I still felt every contraction and truly now appreciate the meaning of the word "labor." Although I wanted to use natural childbirth without any medication, I know that I was a full participant in my son's birthing experience, and that is what "doing everything right" was for me!

Thoughts: Doing what is right varies for each individual, and as nurses we need to support whatever that is. Having a positive outcome from the childbirth experience is the goal; the means it takes to achieve it is less important. How can nurses support women in making their personal choices to achieve a healthy outcome? Are any women "failures" if they ask for pain medication to tolerate labor? How can nurses help women overcome this stigma of being a "wimp"?

Systemic Analgesia

Systemic analgesia involves the use of one or more drugs administered orally, intramuscularly, or intravenously; they become distributed throughout the body via the circulatory system. Depending on which administration method is used, the therapeutic effect of pain relief can occur within minutes and last for several hours. The most important complication associated with the use of this class of drugs is respiratory depression. Therefore, women given these drugs require careful monitoring. Opioids given close to the time of birth can cause central nervous system depression in the newborn, necessitating the administration of naloxone (Narcan) to reverse the depressant effects of the opioids.

Several drug categories may be used for systemic analgesia:

- Opioids, such as butorphanol (Stadol), nalbuphine (Nubain), meperidine (Demerol), or fentanyl (Sublimaze)
- Ataractics, such as hydroxyzine (Vistaril) or promethazine (Phenergan)
- Benzodiazepines, such as diazepam (Valium) or midazolam (Versed)
- Barbiturates, such as secobarbital (Seconal) or pentobarbital (Nembutal)

Drug Guide 14.1 highlights some of the major drugs used for systemic analgesia.

Systemic analgesics are typically administered parenterally, usually through an existing intravenous (IV) line. Nearly all medications given during labor cross the placenta and have a depressant effect on the fetus; therefore, it is important for the woman to receive the least amount of systemic medication that relieves her discomfort so that it does not cause any harm to the fetus (Cheng & Caughey, 2007). Historically opioids have been administered by nurses, but in the past decade there has been increasing use of client-controlled intravenous analgesia (patient-controlled analgesia [PCA]). With this system, the woman is given a button connected to a computerized pump on the IV line. When the woman desires analgesia, she presses the button and the pump delivers a preset amount of medication. This system provides the woman with a sense of control over her own pain management and active participation in the childbirth process.

Opioids

Opioids are morphine-like medications that are most effective for the relief of moderate to severe pain. Opioids typically are administered IV. Of all of the synthetic opioids (butorphanol [Stadol], nalbuphine [Nubain], fentanyl [Sublimaze], and meperidine [Demerol]), meperidine is the most commonly used opioid for the management of pain during labor. Opioids are associated with newborn respiratory depression, decreased alertness, inhibited sucking, and a delay in effective feeding (Bagwell, 2007).

Opioids decrease the transmission of pain impulses by binding to receptor site pathways that transmit the pain signals to the brain. The effect is increased tolerance to pain and respiratory depression related to a decrease in sensitivity to carbon dioxide (Skidmore-Roth, 2007).

All opioids are considered good analgesics. However, respiratory depression can occur in the mother and fetus depending on the dose given. They may also cause a decrease in FHR variability identified on the fetal monitor strip. This FHR pattern change is usually transient. Other systemic side effects include nausea, vomiting, pruritus, delayed gastric emptying, drowsiness, hypoventilation, and newborn depression. To reduce the incidence of new-

DRUG GUIDE 14.1   COMMON AGENTS USED FOR SYSTEMIC ANALGESIA

Type	Drug	Comments
Opioids	Morphine 2–5 mg IV	May be given IV, intrathecally, or epidurally Rapidly crosses the placenta Can cause maternal and neonatal CNS depression Decreases uterine contractions
	Meperidine (Demerol) 25–50 mg IV	May be given IV or epidurally with maximal fetal uptake 2–3 hours after administration Can cause CNS depression Decreases fetal variability
	Butorphanol (Stadol) 1 mg IV q3–4h	Is given IV Is rapidly transferred across the placenta Causes neonatal respiratory depression
	Nalbuphine (Nubain) 10 mg IV	Is given IV Causes less maternal nausea and vomiting Causes decreased FHR variability, fetal bradycardia and respiratory depression
	Fentanyl (Sublimaze) 25–50 mcg IV	Is given IV or epidurally Can cause maternal hypotension, maternal and fetal respiratory depression Rapidly crosses placenta
Ataractics	Hydroxyzine (Vistaril) 50 mg IM	Does not relieve pain but reduces anxiety and potentiates opioid analgesic effects Is used to decrease nausea and vomiting
	Promethazine (Phenergan) 25 mg IV	Is used for antiemetic effect when combined with opioids Causes sedation and reduces apprehension May contribute to maternal hypotension and neonatal depression
Benzodiazepines	Diazepam (Valium) 2–5 mg IV	Is given to enhance pain relief of opioid and cause sedation May be used to stop eclamptic seizures Decreases nausea and vomiting Can cause newborn depression; therefore, lowest possible dose should be used
	Midazolam (Versed) 1–5 mg IV	Is not used for analgesic but amnesia effect Is used as adjunct for anesthesia Is excreted in breast milk
Barbiturates	Secobarbital (Seconal) 100 mg PO/IM	Causes sedation Is used in very early labor to alter a dysfunctional pattern
	Pentobarbital (Nembutal) 100 mg PO/IM	Is not used for pain relief in active labor Crosses placenta and is secreted in breast milk

Sources: Cheng & Caughey, 2007; Edmonds, 2007; Evron & Ezri, 2007; Skidmore-Roth, 2007; Wood, 2007.

born depression, birth should occur within 1 hour or after 4 hours of administration to prevent the fetus from receiving the peak concentration (Cheng & Caughey, 2007).

Opioid antagonists such as naloxone (Narcan) are given to reverse the effects of the central nervous system depression, including respiratory depression, caused by opioids. Opioid antagonists also are used to reverse the side effects of neuraxial opioids, such as pruritus, urinary retention, nausea, and vomiting, without significantly decreasing analgesia (Skidmore-Roth, 2007). Consult a current drug guide for more specifics on these drug categories.

Ataractics

The ataractic group of medications is used in combination with an opioid to decrease nausea and vomiting and lessen anxiety. These adjunct drugs potentiate the effectiveness of the opioid so that a lesser dose can be given. They may also be used to increase sedation. Promethazine (Phenergan) can be given IV, but hydroxyzine (Vistaril) must be given by mouth or by intramuscular injection into a large muscle mass. Neither drug affects the progress of labor, but either may cause a decrease in FHR variability and possible newborn depression (Albers, 2007).

Benzodiazepines

Benzodiazepines are used for minor tranquilizing and sedative effects. Diazepam (Valium) also is given IV to stop seizures due to pregnancy-induced hypertension. However, it is not used during labor itself. It can be administered to calm a woman who is out of control, thereby enabling her to relax enough so that she can participate effectively during her labor process rather than fighting against it. Lorazepam (Ativan) can also be used for its tranquilizing effect, but increased sedation is experienced with this medication (Skidmore-Roth, 2007). Midazolam (Versed), also given IV, produces good amnesia but no analgesia. It is most commonly used as an adjunct for anesthesia. Diazepam and midazolam cause central nervous system depression for both the woman and the newborn.

Barbiturates

The barbiturate drug group is used only in early labor or in a prolonged latent phase that produces enough discomfort that the woman cannot sleep. Barbiturates are given orally or intramuscularly to produce a light sleep to alter a dysfunctional labor pattern or to calm a very anxious woman in early labor. The goal in giving a barbiturate is to promote therapeutic rest for a few hours to enhance the woman's ability to cope with active labor. These drugs cross the placenta and cause central nervous system depression in the newborn (Skidmore-Roth, 2007).

Regional Analgesia/Anesthesia

Regional analgesia/anesthesia provides pain relief without loss of consciousness. It involves the use of local anesthetic agents, with or without added opioids, to bring about pain relief or numbness through the drug's effects on the spinal cord and nerve roots. Obstetric regional analgesia generally refers to a partial or complete loss of pain sensation below the T8 to T10 level of the spinal cord (Edmonds, 2007).

The routes for regional pain relief include epidural block, combined spinal–epidural block, local infiltration, pudendal block, and intrathecal (spinal) analgesia/anesthesia. Local and pudendal routes are used during birth for episiotomies; epidural and intrathecal routes are used for pain relief during active labor and birth. The major advantage of regional pain-management techniques is that the woman can participate in the birthing process and still have good pain control.

Epidural Block

Approximately 60% of laboring women in the United States receive an epidural block for pain relief during labor. In urban areas, many hospitals approach 90% use of epidurals (Kuczkowski, 2007).

An epidural block involves the injection of a drug into the epidural space, which is located outside the dura mater between the dura and the spinal canal. The epidural space is typically entered through the third and fourth lumbar vertebrae with a needle, and a catheter is threaded into the epidural space. The needle is removed and the catheter is left in place to allow for continuous infusion or intermittent injections of medicine (Fig. 14.11). An epidural block provides analgesia and anesthesia and can be used for both vaginal and cesarean births. It has evolved from a regional block producing total loss of sensation to analgesia with minimal blockade. The effectiveness of epidural analgesia depends on the technique and medications used. It is usually started after labor is well established, typically when cervical dilation is greater than 5 cm.

Theoretically, epidural local anesthetics could block all labor pain if used in large volumes and high concentrations. However, pain relief is balanced against other goals such as walking during the first stage of labor, pushing effectively in the second stage, and minimizing maternal and fetal side effects.

An epidural is contraindicated for women with a previous history of spinal surgery or spinal abnormalities, coagulation defects, infections, and hypovolemia. It also is contraindicated for the woman who is receiving anticoagulation therapy.

Complications include nausea and vomiting, hypotension, fever, pruritus, intravascular injection, and respiratory depression. Effects on the fetus during labor include fetal distress secondary to maternal hypotension (Bagwell, 2007). Ensuring that the woman avoids a supine position after an epidural catheter has been placed will help to minimize hypotension.

Changes in epidural drugs and techniques have been made to optimize pain control while minimizing side effects. Today most women receive a continuous lumbar epidural infusion of a local anesthetic, typically a drug whose name ends in "caine," and an opioid. To decrease motor blockade, bupivacaine (Sensorcaine) and ropivacaine (Naropin) have replaced lidocaine (Xylocaine), and drug concentrations have been lowered (Kuczkowski, 2007).

The addition of opioids, such as fentanyl or morphine, to the local anesthetic helps decrease the amount of motor block obtained. Continuous infusion pumps are used to administer the epidural analgesia, allowing the woman to be in control and administer a bolus dose on demand (Smiley & Stephenson, 2007).

Combined Spinal–Epidural Analgesia

Another epidural technique is combined spinal–epidural (CSE) analgesia. This technique involves inserting the epidural needle into the epidural space and subsequently inserting a small-gauge spinal needle through the epidural needle into the subarachnoid space. An opioid, without a local anesthetic, is injected into this space. The spinal needle is then removed and an epidural catheter is inserted for later use.

CSE is advantageous because of its rapid onset of pain relief (within 3 to 5 minutes) that can last up to 3 hours. It also allows the woman's motor function to remain active.

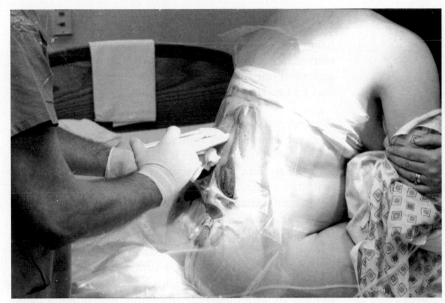

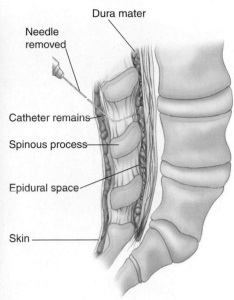

Dura mater

Needle removed

Catheter remains

Spinous process

Epidural space

Skin

A   **B**

FIGURE **14.11** Epidural catheter insertion. (**A**) A needle is inserted into the epidural space. (**B**) A catheter is threaded into the epidural space; the needle is then removed. The catheter allows medication to be administered intermittently or continuously to relieve pain during labor and childbirth.

Her ability to bear down during the second stage of labor is preserved because the pushing reflex is not lost, and her motor power remains intact. The CSE technique provides greater flexibility and reliability for labor than either spinal or epidural analgesia alone (Kuczkowski, 2007). When compared with traditional epidural or spinal analgesia, which often keeps the woman lying in bed, CSE allows her to ambulate ("walking epidural") (Kuczkowski, 2007). Ambulating during labor provides several benefits: it may help control pain better, shorten the first stage of labor, increase the intensity of the contractions, and decrease the possibility of an operative vaginal or cesarean birth.

Although women can walk with CSE, they often choose not to because of sedation and fatigue. Often health care providers don't encourage or assist women to ambulate for fear of injury (Ros et al., 2007). Currently, anesthesiologists are performing walking epidurals using continuous infusion techniques as well as CSE and patient-controlled epidural analgesia (Smiley & Stephenson, 2007).

Complications include maternal hypotension, intravascular injection, accidental intrathecal blockade, postdural puncture headache, inadequate or failed block, and pruritus. Hypotension and associated FHR changes are managed with maternal positioning (semi-Fowler's position), intravenous hydration, and supplemental oxygen (Kuczkowski, 2007).

Patient-Controlled Epidural Analgesia

Patient-controlled epidural analgesia (PCEA) involves the use of an indwelling epidural catheter with an infusion of medication and a programmed pump that allows the woman to control the dosing. This method allows the woman to have a sense of control over her pain and reach her own individually acceptable analgesia level. When compared with the traditional epidural analgesia, PCEA provides equivalent analgesia with lower anesthetic use, lower rates of supplementation, and higher client satisfaction (Smiley & Stephenson, 2007).

With PCEA, the woman uses a hand-held device connected to an analgesic agent that is attached to an epidural catheter. When she pushes the button, a bolus dose of agent is administered via the catheter to reduce her pain. This method allows her to manage her pain at will without having to ask a staff member to provide pain relief.

Local Infiltration

Local infiltration involves the injection of a local anesthetic, such as lidocaine, into the superficial perineal nerves to numb the perineal area. This technique is done by the physician or midwife just before performing an episiotomy (surgical incision into the perineum to facilitate birth) or before suturing a laceration. Local infiltration does not alter the pain of uterine contractions, but it does numb the immediate area of the episiotomy or laceration. Local infiltration does not cause side effects for the woman or her newborn.

Pudendal Nerve Block

A pudendal nerve block refers to the injection of a local anesthetic agent (e.g., bupivacaine, ropivacaine) into the

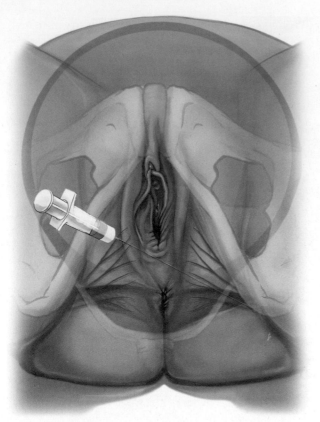

FIGURE 14.12 Pudendal nerve block.

pudendal nerves near each ischial spine. It provides pain relief in the lower vagina, vulva, and perineum (Fig. 14.12).

A pudendal block is used for the second stage of labor, an episiotomy, or an operative vaginal birth with outlet forceps or vacuum extractor. It must be administered about 15 minutes before it would be needed to ensure its full effect. A transvaginal approach is generally used to inject an anesthetic agent at or near the pudendal nerve branch. Neither maternal nor fetal complications are common.

Spinal (Intrathecal) Analgesia/Anesthesia

The spinal (intrathecal) pain-management technique involves injection of an anesthetic "caine" agent, with or without opioids, into the subarachnoid space to provide pain relief during labor or cesarean birth. The contraindications are similar to those for the epidural block. Adverse reactions for the woman include hypotension and spinal headache.

The subarachnoid injection of opioids alone, a technique termed intrathecal narcotics, has been gaining popularity since it was introduced in the 1980s. A narcotic is injected into the subarachnoid space, providing rapid pain relief while still maintaining motor function and sensation (Edmonds, 2007). An intrathecal narcotic is given during the active phase (more than 5 cm dilation) of labor. Compared with epidural blocks, intrathecal narcotics are easy to administer, provide rapid-onset pain relief, are less

likely to cause newborn respiratory depression, and do not cause motor blockade (Edmonds, 2007). Although pain relief is rapid with this technique, it is limited by the narcotic's duration of action, which may be only a few hours and not last through the labor. Additional pain measures may be needed to sustain pain management.

General Anesthesia

General anesthesia is typically reserved for emergency cesarean births when there is not enough time to provide spinal or epidural anesthesia or if the woman has a contraindication to the use of regional anesthesia. It can be started quickly and causes a rapid loss of consciousness. General anesthesia can be administered by IV injection, inhalation of anesthetic agents, or both. Commonly, thiopental, a short-acting barbiturate, is given IV to produce unconsciousness. This is followed by administration of a muscle relaxant. After the woman is intubated, nitrous oxide and oxygen are administered. A volatile halogenated agent may also be administered to produce amnesia (Cheng & Caughey, 2007).

All anesthetic agents cross the placenta and affect the fetus. The primary complication with general anesthesia is fetal depression, along with uterine relaxation and potential maternal vomiting and aspiration.

Although the anesthesiologist or nurse anesthetist administers the various general anesthesia agents, the nurse needs to be knowledgeable about the pharmacologic aspects of the drugs used and must be aware of airway management. Ensure that the woman is NPO and has a patent IV. In addition, administer a non-particulate (clear) oral antacid (e.g., Bicitra or sodium citrate) or a proton pump inhibitor (Protonix) as ordered to reduce gastric acidity. Assist with placement of a wedge under the woman's right hip to displace the gravid uterus and prevent vena cava compression in the supine position. Once the newborn has been removed from the uterus, assist the perinatal team in providing supportive care.

Nursing Care During Labor and Birth

WATCH & LEARN

Childbirth, a physiologic process that is fundamental to all human existence, is one of the most significant cultural, psychological, spiritual, and behavioral events in a woman's life. Although the act of giving birth is a universal phenomenon, it is a unique experience for each woman. Continuous evaluation and appropriate intervention for women during labor are key to promoting a positive outcome for the family.

The nurse's role in childbirth is to ensure a safe environment for the mother and her newborn. Nurses begin evaluating the mother and fetus during the admission procedures at the health care agency and continue to do so throughout labor. It is critical to provide anticipatory guidance and explain each procedure (fetal monitoring, intravenous therapy, medications given, and expected reactions) and what will happen next. This will prepare the woman for the upcoming physical and emotional challenges, thereby helping to reduce her anxiety. Acknowledging her support systems (family or partner) helps allay their fears and concerns, thereby assisting them in carrying out their supportive role. Knowing how and when to evaluate a woman during the various stages of labor is essential for all labor and birth nurses to ensure a positive maternal experience and a healthy newborn.

A major focus of care for the woman during labor and birth is assisting her with maintaining control over her pain, emotions, and actions while being an active participant. Nurses can help and support women to be actively involved in their childbirth experience by allowing time for discussion, offering companionship, listening to worries and concerns, paying attention to the woman's emotional needs, and offering information to help her understand what is happening in each stage of labor.

Nursing Care During the First Stage of Labor

Depending on how far advanced the woman's labor is when she arrives at the facility, the nurse will determine assessment parameters of maternal–fetal status and plan care accordingly. The nurse will provide high-touch, low-tech supportive nursing care during the first stage of labor when admitting the woman and orienting her to the labor and birth suite. Nursing care during this stage will include taking an admission history (reviewing the prenatal record); checking the results of routine laboratory tests and any special tests such as chorionic villi sampling, amniocentesis, genetic studies, and biophysical profile done during pregnancy; asking the woman about her childbirth preparation (birth plan, classes taken, coping skills); and completing a physical assessment of the woman to establish a baseline of values for future comparison.

Key nursing interventions include:

- Identifying the estimated date of birth from the client and the prenatal chart
- Validating the client's prenatal history to determine fetal risk status
- Determining fundal height to validate dates and fetal growth
- Performing Leopold's maneuvers to determine fetal position, lie, and presentation
- Checking FHR
- Performing a vaginal examination (as appropriate) to evaluate effacement and dilation progress
- Instructing the client and her partner about monitoring techniques and equipment
- Assessing fetal response and FHR to contractions and recovery time

- Interpreting fetal monitoring strips
- Checking FHR baseline for accelerations, variability, and decelerations
- Repositioning the client to obtain an optimal FHR pattern
- Recognizing FHR problems and initiating corrective measures
- Checking amniotic fluid for meconium staining, odor, and amount
- Comforting client throughout testing period and labor
- Supporting client's decisions regarding intervention or avoidance of intervention
- Assessing client's support system and coping status frequently

In addition to these interventions to promote optimal outcomes for the mother and fetus, the nurse must document care accurately and in a timely fashion. Accurate and timely documentation helps to decrease professional liability exposure and minimize the risk of preventable injuries to women and infants during labor and birth (Walsh, 2007). Guidelines for recording care include documenting:

- All care rendered, to prove that standards were met
- Conversations with all providers, including notification times
- Nursing interventions before and after notifying provider
- Use of the chain of command and response at each level
- All flow sheets and forms, to validate care given
- All education given to client and response to it
- Facts, not personal opinions
- Initial nursing assessment, all encounters, and discharge plan
- All telephone conversations (Hamilton & Wright, 2007)

This standard of documentation is needed to prevent or defend against litigation, which is prevalent in the childbirth arena.

Assessing the Woman upon Admission

The nurse usually first comes in contact with the woman either by phone or in person. It is important to ascertain whether the woman is in true or false labor and whether she should be admitted or sent home. Upon admission to the labor and birth suite, the highest priorities include assessing FHR, assessing cervical dilation/effacement, and determining whether membranes have ruptured or are intact. These assessment data will guide the critical thinking in planning care for the patient.

If the initial contact is by phone, establish a therapeutic relationship with the woman. Speaking in a calm, caring tone facilitates this. When completing a phone assessment, include questions about the following:

- Estimated date of birth, to determine if term or preterm
- Fetal movement (frequency in the past few days)

- Other premonitory signs of labor experienced
- Parity, gravida, and previous childbirth experiences
- Time from start of labor to birth in previous labors
- Characteristics of contractions, including frequency, duration, and intensity
- Appearance of any vaginal bloody show
- Membrane status (ruptured or intact)
- Presence of supportive adult in household or if she is alone

When speaking with the woman over the telephone, review the signs and symptoms that denote true versus false labor, and suggest various positions she can assume to provide comfort and increase placental perfusion. Also suggest walking, massage, and taking a warm shower to promote relaxation. Outline what foods and fluids are appropriate for oral intake in early labor. Throughout the phone call, listen to the woman's concerns and answer any questions clearly.

Reducing the risk of liability exposure and avoiding preventable injuries to mothers and fetuses during labor and birth can be accomplished by adhering to two basic tenets of clinical practice: (1) use applicable evidence and/or published standards and guidelines as the foundation of care, and (2) whenever a clinical choice is presented, chose client safety (Collins, 2006). With these two tenets in mind, advise the woman on the phone to contact her health care provider for further instructions or to come to the facility to be evaluated, since ruling out true labor and possible maternal–fetal complications cannot be done accurately over the phone.

Additional nursing responsibilities associated with a phone assessment include:

- Consulting the woman's prenatal record for parity status, estimated date of birth, and untoward events
- Calling the health care provider to inform him or her of the woman's status
- Preparing for admission to the perinatal unit to ensure adequate staff assignment
- Notifying the admissions office of a pending admission

If the nurse's first encounter with the woman is in person, an assessment is completed to determine whether she should be admitted to the perinatal unit or sent home until her labor advances. Entering a facility is often an intimidating and stressful event for women since it is an unfamiliar environment. Giving birth for the first time is a pivotal event in the lives of most women. Therefore, demonstrate respect when addressing the client; listen carefully and express interest and concern. Nurses must value and respect women and promote their self-worth and sense of control by allowing them to participate in making decisions (Hackley, Kriebs, & Rousseau, 2007).

An admission assessment includes maternal health history, physical assessment, fetal assessment, laboratory studies, and assessment of psychological status. Usually the facility has a form that can be used throughout labor and birth to document assessment findings (Fig. 14.13).

Maternal Health History

A maternal health history should include typical biographical data such as the woman's name and age and the name of the delivering health care provider. Other information that is collected includes the prenatal record data, including the estimated date of birth, a history of the current pregnancy, and the results of any laboratory and diagnostic tests, such as blood type, Rh status, and group B streptococcal status; past pregnancy and obstetric history; past health history and family history; prenatal education; list of medications; risk factors such as diabetes, hypertension, and use of tobacco, alcohol, or illicit drugs; reason for admission, such as labor, cesarean birth, or observation for a complication; history of potential domestic violence; history of previous preterm births; allergies; time of last food ingestion; method chosen for infant feeding; name of birth attendant and pediatrician; and pain management plan.

Ascertaining this information is important so that an individualized plan of care can be developed for the woman. If, for example, the woman's due date is still 2 months away, it is important to establish this information so interventions can be initiated to arrest the labor immediately or notify the intensive perinatal team to be available. In addition, if the woman is a diabetic, it is critical to monitor her glucose levels during labor, to prepare for a surgical birth if dystocia of labor occurs, and to alert the newborn nursery of potential hypoglycemia in the newborn after birth. By collecting important information about each woman they care for, nurses can help improve the outcomes for all concerned.

Be sure to observe the woman's emotions, support system, verbal interaction, body language and posture, perceptual acuity, and energy level. Also note her cultural background and language spoken. This psychosocial information provides cues about the woman's emotional state, culture, and communication systems. For example, if the woman arrives at the labor and birth suite extremely anxious, alone, and unable to communicate in English, how can the nurse meet her needs and plan her care appropriately? It is only by assessing each woman physically and psychosocially that the nurse can make astute decisions regarding proper care. In this case, an interpreter would be needed to assist in the communication process between the staff and the woman to initiate proper care.

It is important to acknowledge and try to understand the cultural differences in women with cultural backgrounds different from that of the nurse. Attitudes toward childbirth are heavily influenced by the culture in which the woman has been raised. As a result, within every society, specific attitudes and values shape the woman's childbearing behaviors. Be aware of what these are. When carrying out a cultural assessment during the admission

ADMISSION ASSESSMENT OBSTETRICS

▲ PATIENT IDENTIFICATION ▲

ADMISSION DATA

Date		Time		Via		
				☐ Ambulatory ☐ Wheelchair ☐ Stretcher		

Grav.	Term	Pre-term	Ab.	Living	EDC	LMP	GA

Prev. adm. date _____ Reason _____

Obstetrician _____ Pediatrician _____

Ht. _____ Wt. _____ Wt. gain _____

Allergies (meds/food) ☐ None _____ ☐ Hx latex sensitivity

BP _____ T _____ P _____ R _____

FHR _____ Vag exam _____

Reason for Admission

☐ Labor / SROM   ☐ Induction _____

☐ Primary C/S _____   ☐ Repeat C/S

☐ Observation _____

☐ OB / Medical complication _____

Onset of labor: ☐ Not in labor

Date _____ Time _____

Membranes: ☐ Intact

☐ Ruptured / Date _____ Time _____

☐ Clear   ☐ Meconium   ☐ Bloody   ☐ Foul

Vaginal bleeding: ☐ None

☐ Normal show   ☐ _____

Current Pregnancy Labs   ☐ NPC

☐ POL   ☐ PPROM   ☐ Cerclage

☐ PIH   ☐ Chr. HTN   ☐ Other _____

☐ Diabetes _____ Diet _____

☐ Insulin _____

☐ Amniocentesis _____ Results _____

Bld type / RH ____ Date Rhogam ____

Antibody screen ☐ Neg ☐ Pos

Rubella ☐ Non-immune ☐ Immune

Diabetic screen ☐ Normal ☐ Abnormal

Recent exposure to chick pox ☐

Current meds: _____

	Pos	Neg	Tested
Hepatitis B	☐	☐	☐ No
HIV	☐	☐	☐ No
Group B strep	☐	☐	☐ No
GC	☐	☐	☐ No
Chlamydia	☐	☐	☐ No
RPR	☐	☐	☐ No

Previous OB History

☐ POL   ☐ Multiple gestation

☐ Prev C/S type _____ Reason _____

☐ PIH   ☐ Chronic HTN   ☐ Diabetes _____

☐ Stillbirth/demise   ☐ Neodeath   ☐ Anomalies

☐ Precipitous labor (<3 H)   ☐ Macrosomia

☐ PP Hemorrhage

☐ Hx Transfusion reaction   ☐ Yes   ☐ No

☐ Other _____

Latest risk assessment   ☐ None

1. _____   3. _____

2. _____   4. _____

Date _____

Signature _____ Time _____

NEUROLOGICAL

☐ WNL

Variance: ☐ HA

☐ Scotoma / visual changes

Reflexes   ☐ < 2 +   ☐ > 2 +

☐ Clonus ____ bts

☐ Numbness   ☐ Tingling

☐ Hx Seizures

☐ _____

RESPIRATORY

☐ WNL

Variance: ☐ Hx Asthma ☐ URI

Respirations: ☐ < 12 ☐ > 24

Effort: ☐ SOB

☐ Shallow ☐ Labored

Auscultation:

☐ Diminished ☐ Crackles

☐ Wheezes ☐ Rhonchi   No Yes

	No	Yes
Cough for greater than 2 weeks?	☐	☐
Is the cough productive?	☐	☐
Blood in the sputum?	☐	☐
Experiencing any fever or night sweats?	☐	☐
Ever had TB in the past?	☐	☐
Recent exposure to TB?	☐	☐
Weight loss in last 3 weeks?	☐	☐

If the patient answers yes to any three of the above questions implement policy and procedure # 5725-0704.

GASTROINTESTINAL

☐ WNL

Variance: ☐ Heartburn

☐ Epigastric pain   Nausea

☐ Vomiting ☐ Diarrhea

☐ Constipation ☐ Pain

☐ Wt. Gain < 2lbs / month**

☐ Recent change in appetite of < 50% of usual intake for > 5 days

☐ _____

INTEGUMENTARY

☐ WNL

Variance: ☐ Rash ☐ Lacerations

☐ Abrasion ☐ Swelling

☐ Uticaria ☐ Bruising

☐ Diaphoretic/hot

☐ Clammy/cold

☐ Scars

☐ _____

FETAL ASSESSMENT

☐ WNL

Variance:

☐ NRFS

FHR ☐ < 110   ☐ > 160

LTV ☐ Absent ☐ Minimal

☐ Increased

STV Absent

Decelerations: _____

☐ Decreased fetal movement

☐ IUGR

☐ _____

Tobacco use	☐ Denies	☐ Yes	Amt _____
Alcohol use	☐ Denies	☐ Yes	Amt _____
Drug use	☐ Denies	☐ Yes	Amt type _____
Primary language	☐ English	☐ Spanish	

CARDIOVASCULAR

☐ WNL

Variance:

☐ MVP

Heart rate: ☐ < 60   ☐ > 100

B/P: Systolic: ☐ < 90 ☐ > 140

Diastolic: ☐ < 50 ☐ > 90

☐ Edema _____

☐ Chest pain / palpitations

☐ _____

MUSCULOSKELETAL

☐ WNL

Variance:

☐ Numbness ☐ Tingling

☐ Paralysis ☐ Deformity

☐ Scoliosis

☐ _____

GENITOURINARY

☐ WNL

Variance: ☐ Albumin _____

Output: ☐ < 30 cc/Hr.

☐ UTI ☐ Rx ☐ Frequency

☐ Dysuria ☐ Hematuria

☐ CVA Tenderness

☐ Hx STD

☐ Vag. discharge _____

☐ Rash ☐ Blisters

☐ Warts ☐ Lesions

☐ _____

EARS, NOSE, THROAT, AND EYES

☐ WNL

Variance:

☐ Sore throat   ☐ Eyeglasses

☐ Runny nose   ☐ Contact lenses

☐ Nasal congestion

☐ _____

PSYCHOSOCIAL

☐ WNL

Variance: ☐ Hx depression

☐ Yes   ☐ No

☐ Emotional behavioral care

Affect: ☐ Flat ☐ Anxious

☐ Uncooperative ☐ Combative

Living will   ☐ Yes   ☐ No

☐ On chart

Healthcare surrogate ☐ Yes ☐ No

☐ On chart

Are you being hurt, hit, frightened by anyone at home or in your life? ☐ Yes ☐ No

Religious preference _____

☐ _____

PAIN ASSESSMENT

1. Do you have any ongoing pain problems?   ☐ No ☐ Yes

2. Do you have any pain now?   ☐ No ☐ Yes

3. If any of the above questions are answered yes, the patient has a positive pain screening.

4. *Patient to be given pain management education material. Complete pain / symptom assessment on flowsheet.*

5. Please proceed to complete pain assessment.

FIGURE 14.13 Sample documentation form used for admission to the perinatal unit. (Used with permission. Briggs Corporation, 2001.)

Questions for Providing Culturally Competent Care During Labor and Birth

- Where were you born? How long have you lived in the Untied States?
- What languages do you speak and read?
- Who are your major support people?
- What are your religious practices?
- How do you view childbearing?
- Are there any special precautions or restrictions that are important?
- Is birth considered a private or a social experience?
- How would you like to manage your labor discomfort?
- Who will provide your labor support?

Sources: Bowers (2007); D'Avanzo (2008); Giger & Davidhizar (2007).

process, ask questions (Box 14.2) to help plan culturally competent care during labor and birth.

Physical Examination

The physical examination typically includes a generalized assessment of the woman's body systems, including hydration status, vital signs, auscultation of heart and lung sounds, and measurement of height and weight. The physical examination also includes the following assessments:

- Fundal height measurement
- Uterine activity, including contraction frequency, duration, and intensity
- Status of membranes (intact or ruptured)
- Cervical dilatation and degree of effacement
- Fetal status, including heart rate, position, and station
- Pain level

These assessment parameters form a baseline against which the nurse can compare all future values throughout labor. The findings should be similar to those of the woman's prepregnancy and pregnancy findings, with the exception of her pulse rate, which might be elevated secondary to her anxious state with beginning labor.

Laboratory Studies

On admission, laboratory studies typically are done to establish a baseline. Although the exact tests may vary among facilities, they usually include a urinalysis via clean-catch urine specimen and complete blood count (CBC). Blood typing and Rh factor analysis may be necessary if the results of these are unknown or unavailable. In addition, if the following test results are not included in the maternal prenatal history, it may be necessary to perform them at this time. They include syphilis screening, hepatitis B (HbsAg) screening, group B streptococcus, HIV testing

(if woman gives consent), and possible drug screening if the history is positive.

Group B streptococcus (GBS) is a gram-positive organism that is present in 10% to 30% of all healthy women (Kenner & Lott, 2007). These women are asymptomatic carriers but can cause GBS disease of the newborn through vertical transmission. The mortality rate of infected newborns varies according to time of onset (early or late). Risk factors for GBS include maternal intrapartum fever, prolonged ruptured membranes, previous birth of an infected newborn, and GBS bacteriuria in the present pregnancy.

In 2002 ACOG and the American Academy of Pediatrics (AAP) issued guidelines that advised universal screening of pregnant women at 35 to 37 weeks' gestation for GBS and intrapartum antibiotic therapy for GBS carriers (Reingold et al., 2007). Maternal infections associated with GBS include acute chorioamnionitis, endometritis, and urinary tract infection. Neonatal clinical manifestations include pneumonia and sepsis. Identified GBS carriers receive IV antibiotic prophylaxis (penicillin G or ampicillin) at the onset of labor or ruptured membranes.

If her HIV status is not documented, the woman being admitted to the labor and birth suite should have rapid HIV testing done. To reduce perinatal transmission, HIV-positive women are given zidovudine (2 mg/kg IV over an hour, and then a maintenance infusion of 1 mg/kg per hour until birth) or a single 200-mg oral dose of nevirapine at the onset of labor; the newborn is given 2 mg/kg orally between 48 and 72 hours of life (Kenner & Lott, 2007). To further reduce the risk of perinatal transmission, ACOG and the U.S. Public Health Service recommend that HIV-infected women with plasma viral loads of more than 1,000 copies per milliliter be counseled regarding the benefits of elective cesarean birth (Jamieson et al., 2007). Additional interventions to reduce the transmission risk would include avoiding use of scalp electrode for fetal monitoring or doing a scalp blood sampling for fetal pH, delaying amniotomy, and avoiding invasive procedures such as forceps or vacuum-assisted devices. The nurse stresses the importance of all interventions and the goal to reduce transmission of HIV to the newborn.

Continuing Assessment During the First Stage of Labor

After the admission assessment is complete, assessment continues for changes that would indicate that labor is progressing as expected. Assess the woman's knowledge, experience, and expectations of labor. Typically, blood pressure, pulse, and respirations are assessed every hour during the latent phase of labor unless the clinical situation dictates that vital signs be taken more frequently. During the active and transition phases, they are assessed every 30 minutes. The temperature is taken every 4 hours throughout the first stage of labor unless the clinical situation dictates more frequent measurement (maternal fever).

Vaginal examinations are performed periodically to track labor progress. This assessment information is shared with the woman to reinforce that she is making progress toward the goal of birth. Uterine contractions are monitored for frequency, duration, and intensity every 30 to 60 minutes during the latent phase, every 15 to 30 minutes during the active phase, and every 15 minutes during transition. Note the changes in the character of the contractions as labor progresses, and inform the woman of her progress. Continually determine the woman's level of pain and her ability to cope and use relaxation techniques effectively.

When the fetal membranes rupture, spontaneously or artificially, assess the FHR and check the amniotic fluid for color, odor, and amount. Assess the FHR intermittently or continuously via electronic monitoring. During the latent phase of labor, assess the FHR every 30 to 60 minutes; in the active phase, assess FHR at least every 15 to 30 minutes. Also, be sure to assess the FHR before ambulation, prior to any procedure, and prior to administering analgesia or anesthesia to the mother. Table 14.3 summarizes assessments for the first stage of labor.

*R*emember Sheila from the chapter-opening scenario? What is the nurse's role with Sheila in active labor? What additional comfort measures can the labor nurse offer Sheila?

Nursing Interventions

Nursing interventions during the admission process should include:

- Asking about the client's expectations of the birthing process
- Providing information about labor, birth, pain-management options, and relaxation techniques
- Presenting information about fetal monitoring equipment and the procedures needed
- Monitoring FHR and identifying patterns that need further intervention
- Monitoring the mother's vital signs to obtain a baseline for later comparison
- Reassuring the client that her labor progress will be monitored closely and nursing care will focus on ensuring fetal and maternal well-being throughout

As the woman progresses through the first stage of labor, nursing interventions include:

- Encouraging the woman's partner to participate
- Keeping the woman and her partner up to date on the progress of the labor
- Orienting the woman and her partner to the labor and birth unit and explaining all of the birthing procedures
- Providing clear fluids (e.g., ice chips) as needed or requested
- Maintaining the woman's parenteral fluid intake at the prescribed rate if she has an IV

TABLE 14.3 SUMMARY OF ASSESSMENTS DURING THE FIRST STAGE OF LABOR

Assessments*	Latent Phase (0–3 cm)	Active Phase (4–7 cm)	Transition (8–10 cm)
Vital signs (BP, pulse, respirations)	Every 30–60 min	Every 30 min	Every 15–30 min
Temperature	Every 4 hours	Every 4 hours	Every 4 hours
Contractions (frequency, duration, intensity)	Every 30–60 min by palpation or continuously if EFM	Every 15–30 min by palpation or continuously if EFM	Every 15 min by palpation or continuously if EFM
Fetal heart rate	Every hour by Doppler or continuously by EFM	Every 30 min by Doppler or continuously by EFM	Every 15–30 min by Doppler or continuously by EFM
Vaginal examination	Initially on admission to determine phase and as needed based on maternal cues to document labor progression	As needed to monitor labor progression	As needed to monitor labor progression
Behavior/psychosocial	With every client encounter: talkative, excited, anxious	With every client encounter: self-absorbed in labor; intense and quiet now	With every client encounter: discouraged, irritable, feels out of control, declining coping ability

*The frequency of assessments is dictated by the health status of the woman and fetus and can be altered if either one of their conditions changes.
EFM, electronic fetal monitoring.

• Initiating or encouraging comfort measures, such as backrubs, cool cloths to the forehead, frequent position changes, ambulation, showers, slow dancing, leaning over a birth ball, side-lying, or counterpressure on lower back (Teaching Guidelines 14.1)
• Encouraging the partner's involvement with breathing techniques
• Assisting the woman and her partner to focus on breathing techniques
• Informing the woman that the discomfort will be intermittent and of limited duration; urging her to rest between contractions to preserve her strength; and encouraging her to use distracting activities to lessen the focus on contractions
• Changing bed linens and gown as needed
• Keeping the perineal area clean and dry

TEACHING GUIDELINES 14.1

Positioning During the First Stage of Labor

• Walking with support from your partner (adds the force of gravity to contractions to promote fetal descent)
• Slow-dancing position with your partner holding you (adds the force of gravity to contractions and promotes support from and active participation of your partner)
• Side-lying with pillows between the knees for comfort (offers a restful position and improves oxygen flow to the uterus)
• Semi-sitting in bed or on a couch leaning against the partner (reduces back pain because fetus falls forward, away from the sacrum)
• Sitting in a chair with one foot on the floor and one on the chair (changes pelvic shape)
• Leaning forward by straddling a chair, a table, or a bed or kneeling over a birth ball (reduces back pain, adds the force of gravity to promote descent; possible pain relief if partner can apply sacral pressure)
• Sitting in a rocking chair or on a birth ball and shifting weight back and forth (provides comfort because rocking motion is soothing; uses the force of gravity to help fetal descent)
• Lunge by rocking weight back and forth with foot up on chair during contraction (uses force of gravity by being upright; enhances rotation of fetus through rocking)
• Open knee–chest position (helps to relieve back discomfort) (Armstrong & Feldman, 2007)

• Supporting the woman's decisions about pain management
• Monitoring maternal vital signs frequently and reporting any abnormal values
• Ensuring that the woman takes deep cleansing breaths before and after each contraction to enhance gas exchange and oxygen to the fetus
• Educating the woman and her partner about the need for rest and helping them plan strategies to conserve strength
• Monitoring FHR for baseline, accelerations, variability, and decelerations
• Checking on bladder status and encouraging voiding at least every 2 hours to make room for birth
• Repositioning the woman as needed to obtain optimal heart rate pattern
• Communicating requests from the woman to appropriate personnel
• Respecting the woman's sense of privacy by covering her when appropriate
• Offering human presence by being present with the woman, not leaving her alone for long periods
• Being patient with the natural labor pattern to allow time for change
• Reporting any deviations from normal to the health care professional so that interventions can be initiated early to be effective (Sauls, 2007)

See Nursing Care Plan 14.1.

Remember Sheila, who was admitted in active labor? She has progressed to the transition phase (8 cm dilated) and is becoming increasingly more uncomfortable. She is using a patterned-paced breathing pattern now but thrashing around in the hospital bed.

Nursing Management During the Second Stage of Labor

Nursing care during the second stage of labor focuses on supporting the woman and her partner in making active decisions about her care and labor management, implementing strategies to prolong the early passive phase of fetal descent, supporting involuntary bearing-down efforts, providing instruction and assistance, and using maternal positions that can enhance descent and reduce pain (Sleutel, Schultz, & Wyble, 2007). Research suggests that strong pushing during the second stage may be accompanied by a significant decline in fetal pH and may cause maternal muscle and nerve damage if done too early (Sauls, 2007). Shortening the phase of active pushing and lengthening the early phase of passive descent can be achieved by encouraging the woman not to push until she has a strong desire to do so and until the descent and rotation of the fetal head are well advanced. Effective

Nursing Care Plan 14.1

OVERVIEW OF THE WOMAN IN THE ACTIVE PHASE OF THE FIRST STAGE OF LABOR

Candice, a 23-year-old gravida 1, para 0 (G1,P0) is admitted to the labor and birth suite at 39 weeks' gestation having contractions of moderate intensity every 5 to 6 minutes. A vaginal examination reveals her cervix is 80% effaced and 5 cm dilated. The presenting part (vertex) is at 0 station and her membranes ruptured spontaneously 4 hours ago at home. She is admitted and an IV is started for hydration and vascular access. An external fetal monitor is applied. FHR is 140 bpm and regular. Her partner is present at her bedside. Candice is now in the active phase of the first stage of labor, and her assessment findings are as follows: cervix dilated 7 cm, 80% effaced; moderate to strong contractions occurring regularly, every 3 to 5 minutes, lasting 45 to 60 seconds; at 0 station on pelvic examination; FHR auscultated loudest below umbilicus at 140 bpm; vaginal show—pink or bloody vaginal mucus; currently apprehensive, inwardly focused, with increased dependency; voicing concern about ability to cope with pain; limited ability to follow directions.

NURSING DIAGNOSIS: Anxiety related to labor and birth process and fear of the unknown related to client's first experience

Outcome Identification and Evaluation

Client will remain calm and in control as evidenced by ability to make decisions and use positive coping strategies.

Interventions: Promoting Positive Coping Strategies

- Provide instruction regarding the labor process to allay anxiety.
- Reorient the woman to the physical environment and equipment as necessary to keep her informed of events.
- Encourage verbalization of feelings and concerns to reduce anxiety.
- Listen attentively to woman and partner to demonstrate interest and concern.
- Inform woman and partner of standard procedures/processes to ensure adequate understanding of events and procedures.
- Frequently update woman of progress and labor status to provide positive reinforcement for actions.
- Reinforce relaxation techniques and provide instruction if needed to aid in coping.
- Encourage participation of the partner in the coaching role; role-model to facilitate partner participation in labor process to provide support and encouragement to the client.
- Provide a presence and remain with woman as much as possible to provide comfort and support.

NURSING DIAGNOSIS: Pain related to effects of contractions and cervical dilatation and events of labor

Outcome Identification and Evaluation

Client will maintain a tolerable level of pain and discomfort as evidenced by statements of pain relief, pain rating of 2 or less on pain rating scale, and absence of adverse effects in client and fetus from analgesia or anesthesia.

Interventions: Providing Pain Relief

- Monitor vital signs, observe for signs of pain, and have client rate pain on a scale of 0 to 10 to provide baseline for comparison.
- Encourage client to void every 1 to 2 hours to decrease pressure from a full bladder.
- Assist woman to change positions frequently to increase comfort and promote labor progress.
- Encourage use of distraction to reduce focus on contraction pain.
- Suggest pelvic rocking, massage, or back counterpressure to reduce pain.
- Assist with use of relaxation and breathing techniques to promote relaxation.
- Use touch appropriately (backrub) when desired by the woman to promote comfort.
- Integrate use of nonpharmacologic measures for pain relief, such as warm water, birthing ball, or other techniques to facilitate pain relief.
- Administer pharmacologic agents as ordered when requested to control pain.
- Provide reassurance and encouragement between contractions to foster self-esteem and continued participation in labor process.

(continued)

Nursing Care Plan 14.1 (continued)

NURSING DIAGNOSIS: Risk of infection related to vaginal examinations following rupture of membranes

Outcome Identification and Evaluation
Client will remain free of infection as evidenced by absence of signs and symptoms of infection, vital signs and FHR within acceptable parameters, lab test results within normal limits, and clear amniotic fluid without odor.

Interventions: Preventing Infection
- Monitor vital signs (every 1 to 2 hours after ROM) and FHR frequently as per protocol to allow for early detection of problems; report fetal tachycardia (early sign of maternal infection) to ensure prompt treatment.
- Provide frequent perineal care and pad changes to maintain good perineal hygiene.
- Change linens and woman's gown as needed to maintain cleanliness.
- Ensure that vaginal examinations are performed only when needed to prevent introducing pathogens into the vaginal vault.
- Monitor lab test results such as white blood cell count to assess for elevations indicating infection.
- Use aseptic technique for all invasive procedures to prevent infection transmission.
- Carry out good handwashing techniques before and after procedures and use standard precautions as appropriate to minimize risk of infection transmission.
- Document amniotic fluid characteristics—color, odor—to establish baseline for comparison.

---

pushing can be achieved by assisting the woman to assume a more upright or squatting position (Hanson, 2006).

Perineal lacerations or tears can occur during the second stage when the fetal head emerges through the vaginal introitus. The extent of the laceration is defined by depth: a first-degree laceration extends through the skin; a second-degree laceration extends through the muscles of the perineal body; a third-degree laceration continues through the anal sphincter muscle; and a fourth-degree laceration also involves the anterior rectal wall. Special attention needs to be paid to third- and fourth-degree lacerations to prevent fecal incontinence (Lowder et al., 2007). The primary care provider should repair any lacerations during the third stage of labor.

An **episiotomy** is an incision made in the perineum to enlarge the vaginal outlet and theoretically to shorten the second stage of labor. Alternative measures such as warm compresses and continual massage with oil have been successful in stretching the perineal area to prevent cutting it. Certified nurse midwives (CNMs) can cut and repair episiotomies, but they frequently use alternative measures if possible.

▶ *Take* NOTE!

Further research needs to be done to validate the efficacy of natural measures versus the episiotomy.

The midline episiotomy is the most commonly used one in the United States because it can be easily repaired and causes the least amount of pain (Albers & Borders, 2007). Figure 14.14 shows episiotomy locations.

Assessment
Assessment is continuous during the second stage of labor. Hospital policies dictate the specific type and timing of assessments, as well as the way in which they are documented. Assessment involves identifying the signs typical of the second stage of labor, including:

- Increase in apprehension or irritability
- Spontaneous rupture of membranes
- Sudden appearance of sweat on upper lip
- Increase in blood-tinged show
- Low grunting sounds from the woman
- Complaints of rectal and perineal pressure
- Beginning of involuntary bearing-down efforts

Other ongoing assessments include the contraction frequency, duration, and intensity; maternal vital signs every 5 to 15 minutes; fetal response to labor as indicated by FHR monitor strips; amniotic fluid for color, odor, and amount when membranes are ruptured; and the woman and her partner's coping status (Table 14.4).

Assessment also focuses on determining the progress of labor. Associated signs include bulging of the perineum, labial separation, advancing and retreating of the newborn's head during and between bearing-down efforts,

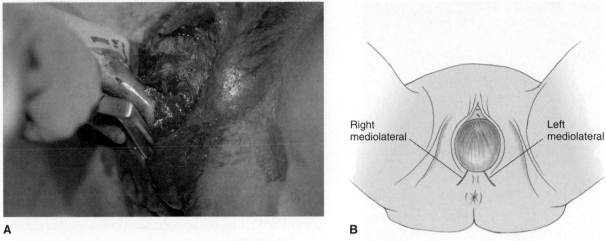

FIGURE 14.14 Location of an episiotomy. (**A**) Midline episiotomy. (**B**) Right and left mediolateral episiotomies.

and **crowning** (fetal head is visible at vaginal opening; Fig. 14.15).

A vaginal examination is completed to determine if it is appropriate for the woman to push. Pushing is appropriate if the cervix has fully dilated to 10 cm and the woman feels the urge to do so.

Nursing Interventions

Nursing interventions during this stage focus on motivating the woman, encouraging her to put all her efforts to pushing this newborn to the outside world, and giving her feedback on her progress. If the woman is pushing and not making progress, suggest that she keep her eyes open

TABLE 14.4 SUMMARY OF ASSESSMENTS DURING THE SECOND, THIRD, AND FOURTH STAGES OF LABOR

Assessments*	Second Stage of Labor (Birth of Neonate)	Third Stage of Labor (Placenta Expulsion)	Fourth Stage of Labor (Recovery)
Vital signs (BP, pulse, respirations)	Every 5–15 min	Every 15 min	Every 15 min
Fetal heart rate	Every 5–15 min by Doppler or continuously by EFM	Apgar scoring at 1 and 5 min	Newborn—complete head-to-toe assessment; vital signs every 15 min until stable
Contractions/uterus	Palpate every one	Observe for placental separation	Palpating for firmness and position every 15 min for first hour
Bearing down/pushing	Assist with every effort	None	None
Vaginal discharge	Observe for signs of descent—bulging of perineum, crowning	Assess bleeding after expulsion	Assess every 15 min with fundus firmness
Behavior/psychosocial	Observe every 15 min: cooperative, focus is on work of pushing newborn out	Observe every 15 min: often feelings of relief after hearing newborn crying; calmer	Observe every 15 min: usually excited, talkative, awake; needs to hold newborn, be close, and inspect body

*The frequency of assessments is dictated by the health status of the woman and fetus and can be altered if either one of their conditions changes.
EFM, electronic fetal monitoring.

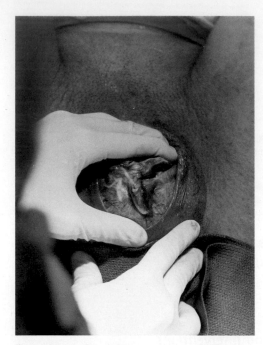

FIGURE **14.15** Crowning.

during the contractions and look toward where the infant is coming out. Changing positions every 20 to 30 minutes will also help in making progress. Positioning a mirror so the woman can visualize the birthing process and how successful her pushing efforts are can help motivate her.

During the second stage of labor, an ideal position would be one that opens the pelvic outlet as wide as possible, provides a smooth pathway for the fetus to descend through the birth canal, takes advantage of gravity to assist the fetus to descend, and gives the mother a sense of being safe and in control of the labor process (Hanson, 2006). Some suggestions for positions in the second stage include:

- Lithotomy with feet up in stirrups: most convenient position for caregivers
- Semi-sitting with pillows underneath knees, arms, and back
- Lateral/side-lying with curved back and upper leg supported by partner
- Sitting on birthing stool: opens pelvis, enhances the pull of gravity, and helps with pushing
- Squatting/supported squatting: gives the woman a sense of control
- Kneeling with hands on bed and knees comfortably apart

Other important nursing interventions during the second stage include:

- Providing continuous comfort measures such as mouth care, position changes, changing bed linen and underpads, and providing a quiet, focused environment
- Instructing the woman on the following bearing-down positions and techniques:

- Pushing only when she feels an urge to do so
- Using abdominal muscles when bearing down
- Using short pushes of 6 to 7 seconds
- Focusing attention on the perineal area to visualize the newborn
- Relaxing and conserving energy between contractions
- Pushing several times with each contraction
- Pushing with an open glottis and slight exhalation (Roberts, Gonzalez, & Sampselle, 2007)
- Continuing to monitor contraction and FHR patterns to identify problems
- Providing brief, explicit directions throughout this stage
- Continuing to provide psychosocial support by reassuring and coaching
- Facilitating the upright position to encourage the fetus to descend
- Continuing to assess blood pressure, pulse, respirations, uterine contractions, bearing-down efforts, FHR, coping status of the client and her partner
- Providing pain management if needed
- Providing a continuous nursing presence
- Offering praise for the client's efforts
- Preparing for and assisting with delivery by:
  - Notifying the health care provider of the estimated time frame for birth
  - Preparing the delivery bed and positioning client
  - Preparing the perineal area according to the facility's protocol
  - Offering a mirror and adjusting it so the woman can watch the birth
  - Explaining all procedures and equipment to the client and her partner
  - Setting up delivery instruments needed while maintaining sterility
  - Receiving newborn and transporting him or her to a warming environment, or covering the newborn with a warmed blanket on the woman's abdomen
  - Providing initial care and assessment of the newborn (see the Birth section that follows)

Sheila is completely dilated now and experiencing the urge to push. How can the nurse help Sheila with her pushing efforts? What additional interventions can the labor nurse offer Sheila now?

Birth

The second stage of labor ends with the birth of the newborn. The maternal position for birth varies from the standard lithotomy position to side-lying to squatting to standing or kneeling, depending on the birthing location, the woman's preference, and standard protocols. Once the woman is positioned for birth, cleanse the vulva and perineal areas. The primary health care provider then takes charge after donning protective eyewear, masks, gowns, and gloves and performing hand hygiene.

Once the fetal head has emerged, the primary care provider explores the fetal neck to see if the umbilical cord is wrapped around it. If it is, the cord is slipped over the head to facilitate delivery. As soon as the head emerges, the health care provider suctions the newborn's mouth first (because the newborn is an obligate nose breather) and then the nares with a bulb syringe to prevent aspiration of mucus, amniotic fluid, or meconium (Fig. 14.16). The umbilical cord is double-clamped and cut between the clamps. With the first cries of the newborn, the second stage of labor ends.

In addition to encouraging Sheila to rest between pushing and offering praise for her efforts, what is the nurse's role during the birthing process?

Immediate Care of the Newborn

Once the infant is born, place him or her under the radiant warmer, dry him or her, assess him or her, wrap him or her in warmed blankets, and place him or her on the woman's abdomen for warmth and closeness. In some health care facilities, the newborn is placed on the woman's abdomen immediately after birth and covered with a warmed blanket. In either scenario, the stability of the newborn dictates the location of aftercare. The nurse can also assist the mother with breastfeeding her newborn for the first time.

Assessment of the newborn begins at the moment of birth and continues until the newborn is discharged. Drying the newborn and providing warmth to prevent heat loss by evaporation is essential to help support thermoregulation and provide stimulation. Placing the newborn under a radiant heat source and putting on a stockinet cap will further reduce heat loss after drying.

Assess the newborn by assigning an Apgar score at 1 and 5 minutes. The Apgar score assesses five parameters—heart rate (absent, slow, or fast), respiratory effort (absent, weak cry, or good strong yell), muscle tone (limp, or lively and active), response to irritation stimulus, and color—that evaluate a newborn's cardiorespiratory adaptation after birth. The parameters are arranged from the most important (heart rate) to the least important (color). The newborn is assigned a score of 0 to 2 in each of the five parameters. The purpose of the Apgar assessment is to evaluate the physiologic status of the newborn; see Chapter 18 for additional information on Apgar scoring.

Secure two identification bands on the newborn's wrist and ankle that match the band on the mother's wrist to ensure the newborn's identity. This identification process is completed in the birthing suite before anyone leaves the room. Some health care agencies also take an early photo of the newborn for identification in the event of abduction (Healthcare Risk Management, 2007).

Other types of newborn security systems can also be used to prevent abduction. Some systems have sensors that are attached to the newborn's identification bracelet or cord clamp. An alarm is set off if the bracelet or clamp activates receivers near exits. Others have an alarm that is activated when the sensor is removed from the newborn (Fig. 14.17). Even with the use of electronic sensors, the parents, nursing staff, and security personnel are responsible for prevention strategies and ensuring the safety and protection of all newborns (Healthcare Risk Management, 2007).

Sheila gave birth to a healthy 7-pound, 7-ounce baby girl. She is eager to hold and nurse her newborn. What is the initial care of the newborn? How can the nurse meet the needs of both the newborn and Sheila, who is exhausted but eager to bond with her newborn?

Nursing Management During the Third Stage of Labor

During the third stage of labor, strong uterine contractions continue at regular intervals under the continuing influence of oxytocin. The uterine muscle fibers shorten, or retract, with each contraction, leading to a gradual decrease in the

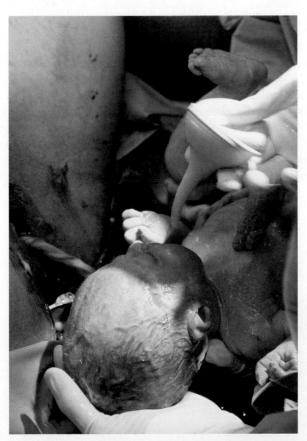

FIGURE 14.16 Suctioning the newborn immediately after birth.

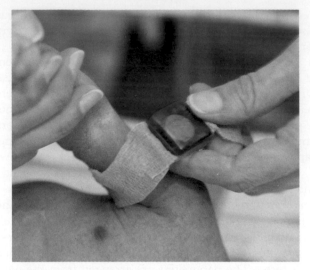

FIGURE 14.17 An example of a security sensor applied to a newborn's arm.

size of the uterus, which helps shear the placenta away from its attachment site. The third stage is complete when the placenta is delivered. Nursing care during the third stage of labor primarily focuses on immediate newborn care and assessment and being available to assist with the delivery of the placenta and inspecting it for intactness.

Three hormones play important roles in the third stage. During this stage the woman experiences peak levels of oxytocin and endorphins, while the high adrenaline levels that occurred during the second stage of labor to aid with pushing begin falling. The hormone oxytocin causes uterine contractions and helps the woman to enact instinctive mothering behaviors such as holding the newborn close to her body and cuddling the baby.

Skin-to-skin contact immediately after birth and the newborn's first attempt at breastfeeding further augment maternal oxytocin levels, strengthening the uterine contractions that will help the placenta to separate and the uterus to contract to prevent hemorrhage. Endorphins,

the body's natural opiates, produce an altered state of consciousness and aid in blocking out pain. In addition, the drop in adrenaline level from the second stage, which had kept the mother and baby alert at first contact, causes most women to shiver and feel cold shortly after giving birth.

> ▶ *Take* NOTE!
>
> *A crucial role for nurses during this time is to protect the natural hormonal process by ensuring unhurried and uninterrupted contact between mother and newborn after birth, providing warmed blankets to prevent shivering, and allowing skin-to-skin contact and breastfeeding.*

Assessment

Assessment during the third stage of labor includes:

• Monitoring placental separation by looking for the following signs:
  • Firmly contracting uterus
  • Change in uterine shape from discoid to globular ovoid
  • Sudden gush of dark blood from vaginal opening
  • Lengthening of umbilical cord protruding from vagina
• Examining placenta and fetal membranes for intactness the second time (the health care provider assesses the placenta for intactness the first time) (Fig. 14.18)
• Assessing for any perineal trauma, such as the following, before allowing the birth attendant to leave:
  • Firm fundus with bright-red blood trickling: laceration
  • Boggy fundus with red blood flowing: uterine atony
  • Boggy fundus with dark blood and clots: retained placenta

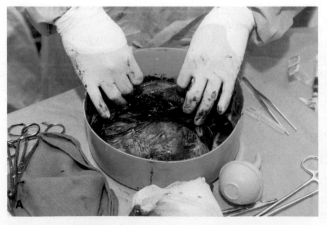
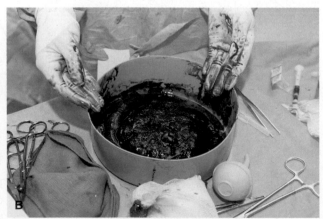

FIGURE 14.18 Placenta. (**A**) Fetal side. (**B**) Maternal side.

- Inspecting the perineum for condition of episiotomy, if performed
- Assessing for perineal lacerations and ensuring repair by birth attendant

Nursing Interventions

Interventions during the third stage of labor include:

- Describing the process of placental separation to the couple
- Instructing the woman to push when signs of separation are apparent
- Administering an oxytocic if ordered and indicated after placental expulsion
- Providing support and information about episiotomy and/or laceration
- Cleaning and assisting client into a comfortable position after birth, making sure to lift both legs out of stirrups (if used) simultaneously to prevent strain
- Repositioning the birthing bed to serve as a recovery bed if applicable
- Assisting with transfer to the recovery area if applicable
- Providing warmth by replacing warmed blankets over the woman
- Applying an ice pack to the perineal area to provide comfort to episiotomy if indicated
- Explaining what assessments will be carried out over the next hour and offering positive reinforcement for actions
- Ascertaining any needs
- Monitoring maternal physical status by assessing:
  - Vaginal bleeding: amount, consistency, and color
  - Vital signs: blood pressure, pulse, and respirations taken every 15 minutes
  - Uterine fundus, which should be firm, in the midline, and at the level of the umbilicus
- Recording all birthing statistics and securing primary caregiver's signature
- Documenting birthing event in the birth book (official record of the facility that outlines every birth event), detailing any deviations

Nursing Management During the Fourth Stage of Labor

The fourth stage of labor begins after the placenta is expelled and lasts up to 4 hours after birth, during which time recovery takes place. This recovery period may take place in the same room where the woman gave birth, in a separate recovery area, or in her postpartum room. During this stage, the woman's body is beginning to undergo the many physiologic and psychological changes that occur after birth. The focus of nursing management during the fourth stage of labor involves frequent close observation for hemorrhage, provision of comfort measures, and promotion of family attachment.

Assessment

Assessments during the fourth stage center on the woman's vital signs, status of the uterine fundus and perineal area, comfort level, lochia amount, and bladder status. During the first hour after birth, vital signs are taken every 15 minutes, then every 30 minutes for the next hour if needed. The woman's blood pressure should remain stable and within normal range after giving birth. A decrease may indicate uterine hemorrhage; an elevation might suggest preeclampsia.

The pulse usually is typically slower (60 to 70 bpm) than during labor. This may be associated with a decrease in blood volume following placental separation. An elevated pulse rate may be an early sign of blood loss. The blood pressure usually returns to its prepregnancy level and therefore is not a reliable early indicator of shock. Fever is indicative of dehydration (less than 100.4°F or 38°C) or infection (above 101°F), which may involve the genitourinary tract. Respiratory rate is usually between 16 and 24 breaths per minute and regular. Respirations should be unlabored unless there is an underlying preexisting respiratory condition.

Assess fundal height, position, and firmness every 15 minutes during the first hour following birth. The fundus needs to remain firm to prevent excessive postpartum bleeding. The fundus should be firm (feels like the size and consistency of a grapefruit), located in the midline and below the umbilicus. If it is not firm (boggy), gently massage it until it is firm (see Nursing Procedure 22.1 for more information). Once firmness is obtained, stop massaging.

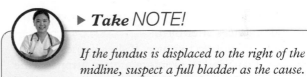

▶ **Take** NOTE!

If the fundus is displaced to the right of the midline, suspect a full bladder as the cause.

The vagina and perineal areas are quite stretched and edematous following a vaginal birth. Assess the perineum, including the episiotomy if present, for possible hematoma formation. Suspect a hematoma if the woman reports excruciating pain or cannot void or if a mass is noted in the perineal area. Also assess for hemorrhoids, which can cause discomfort.

Assess the woman's comfort level frequently to determine the need for analgesia. Ask the woman to rate her pain on a scale of 1 to 10; it should be less than 3. If it is higher, further evaluation is needed to make sure there aren't any deviations contributing to her discomfort.

Assess vaginal discharge (lochia) every 15 minutes for the first hour and every 30 minutes for the next hour. Palpate the fundus at the same time to ascertain its firmness and help to estimate the amount of vaginal discharge. In addition, palpate the bladder for fullness, since many women receiving an epidural block experience limited sensation in the bladder region. Voiding should produce large amounts of urine (diuresis) each time. Palpation of the woman's bladder after each voiding helps to ensure complete emptying. A full bladder will displace the uterus to either side of the midline and potentiate uterine hemorrhage secondary to bogginess.

Nursing Interventions

Nursing interventions during the fourth stage might include:

- Providing support and information to the woman regarding episiotomy repair and related pain-relief and self-care measures
- Applying an ice pack to the perineum to promote comfort and reduce swelling
- Assisting with hygiene and perineal care; teaching the woman how to use the perineal bottle after each pad change and voiding; helping the woman into a new gown
- Monitoring for return of sensation and ability to void (if regional anesthesia was used)
- Encouraging the woman to void by ambulating to bathroom, listening to running water, or pouring warm water over the perineal area with the peribottle
- Monitoring vital signs and fundal and lochia status every 15 minutes and documenting them
- Promoting comfort by offering analgesia for afterpains and warm blankets to reduce chilling
- Offering fluids and nourishment if desired
- Encouraging parent–infant attachment by providing privacy for the family
- Being knowledgeable about and sensitive to typical cultural practices after birth
- Assisting the mother to nurse, if she chooses, during the recovery period to promote uterine firmness (the release of oxytocin from the posterior pituitary gland stimulates uterine contractions)
- Teaching the woman how to assess her fundus for firmness periodically and to massage it if it is boggy
- Describing the lochia flow and normal parameters to observe for postpartum
- Teaching safety techniques to prevent newborn abduction
- Demonstrating the use of the portable sitz bath as a comfort measure for her perineum if she had a laceration or an episiotomy repair
- Explain comfort/hygiene measures and when to use them
- Assisting with ambulation when getting out of bed for the first time
- Providing information about the routine on the mother–baby unit or nursery for her stay
- Observing for signs of early parent–infant attachment: fingertip touch to palm touch to enfolding of the infant (Leonard, 2007)

■■■ Key Concepts

- A nurse provides physical and emotional support during the labor and birth process to assist a woman to achieve her goals.
- When a woman is admitted to the labor and birth area, the admitting nurse must assess and evaluate the risk status of the pregnancy and initiate appropriate interventions to provide optimal care for the client.
- Completing an admission assessment includes taking a maternal health history; performing physical assessment on the woman and fetus, including her emotional and psychosocial status; and obtaining the necessary laboratory studies.
- The nurse's role in fetal assessment for labor and birth includes determining fetal well-being and interpreting signs and symptoms of possible compromise. Determining the fetal heart rate (FHR) pattern and assessing amniotic fluid characteristics are key.
- FHR can be assessed intermittently or continuously. Although the intermittent method allows the client to move about during labor, the information obtained intermittently does not provide a complete picture of fetal well-being from moment to moment.
- Assessment parameters of the FHR are classified as baseline rate, baseline variability (long-term and short-term), and periodic changes in the rate (accelerations and decelerations).
- The nurse monitoring the laboring client needs to be knowledgeable about which parameters are reassuring, nonreassuring, and ominous so that appropriate interventions can be instituted.
- For a nonreassuring FHR pattern, the nurse should notify the health care provider about the pattern and obtain further orders, making sure to document all interventions and their effects on the FHR pattern.
- In addition to interpreting assessment findings and initiating appropriate inventions for the laboring client, accurate and timely documentation must be carried out continuously.
- Today's women have many safe nonpharmacologic and pharmacologic choices for the management of pain during childbirth. They may be used individually or in combination to complement one another.
- Nursing management for the woman during labor and birth includes comfort measures, emotional support, information and instruction, advocacy, and support for the partner.
- Nursing care during the first stage of labor includes taking an admission history (reviewing the prenatal record), checking the results of routine laboratory work and special tests done during pregnancy, asking the woman about her childbirth preparation (birth plan, classes taken, coping skills), and completing a physical assessment of the woman to establish a baseline of values for future comparison.

- Nursing care during the second stage of labor focuses on supporting the woman and her partner in making decisions about her care and labor management, implementing strategies to prolong the early passive phase of fetal descent, supporting involuntary bearing-down efforts, providing instruction and assistance, and encouraging the use of maternal positions that can enhance descent and reduce the pain.

- Nursing care during the third stage of labor primarily focuses on immediate newborn care and assessment and being available to assist with the delivery of the placenta and inspecting it for intactness.

- The focus of nursing management during the fourth stage of labor involves frequently observing the mother for hemorrhage, providing comfort measures, and promoting family attachment.

REFERENCES

Albers, L. L. (2007). The evidence for physiologic management of the active phase of the first stage of labor. *Journal of Midwifery & Women's Health, 52*(3), 207–215.

Albers, L. L., & Borders, N. (2007). Minimizing genital tract trauma and related pain following spontaneous vaginal birth. *Journal of Midwifery & Women's Health, 52*(3), 246–253.

American College of Obstetricians and Gynecologists (ACOG). (2005). *Fetal heart rate patterns: Monitoring, interpretation, and management* (Practice Bulletin Number 62). Washington, DC: Author.

American Hospital Association (AHA). (2007). *Hospital statistics.* Chicago: Author.

American Pregnancy Association. (2007). *Patterned breathing during labor.* Available at: http://www.americanpregnancy.org/labornbirth/patternedbreathing.htm.

Arenson, J., & Drake, P. (2007). *Maternal and newborn health.* Sudbury, MA: Jones and Bartlett Publishers.

Armstrong, P., & Feldman, S. (2007). *A wise birth: Bringing together the best of natural childbirth and modern medicine.* London, UK: Pinter and Martin Limited.

Association of Women's Health, Obstetric and Neonatal Nurses (AWHONN). (2006). *Fetal assessment* (Clinical Position Statement). Washington, DC: Author.

Bagwell, G. A. (2007). Resuscitation and stabilization of the newborn and infant. In C. Kenner & J. W. Lott (Eds.), *Comprehensive neonatal care: An interdisciplinary approach* (Chapter 38, pp. 666–676). St. Louis, MO: Saunders Elsevier.

Bakker, P. C., Kurver, P. H., Kuik, D. J., & Van Grijn, H. P. (2007). Elevated uterine activity increases the risk of fetal acidosis at birth. *American Journal of Obstetrics and Gynecology, 196*(4), 313–319.

Blackburn, S. T. (2007) *Maternal, fetal, and neonatal physiology: A clinical perspective* (3rd ed.). St. Louis, MO: Saunders Elsevier.

Bowers, P. (2007). Cultural perspectives in childbearing. *Nursing Spectrum.* Available at: http://www.nurse.com/ce/course.html?CCID=3245.

Cheng, Y. W., & Caughey, A. B. (2007). Normal labor and delivery. *eMedicine.* Available at: http://www.emedicine.com/med/topic3239.htm

Collins, D. (2006). Legally speaking: Risk management in obstetrics and gynecology. *Contemporary OB/GYN, 51*(11), 38–42.

D'Avanzo, C. E. (2008). *Cultural health assessment* (4th ed.). St. Louis: Mosby Elsevier.

Dillon, P. M. (2007). *Nursing health assessment: A critical thinking, case studies approach* (2nd ed.). Philadelphia: F. A. Davis Company.

Edmonds, K. (2007). *Dewhurst's textbook of obstetrics and gynecology* (7th ed.). Oxford, UK: Blackwell Publishers Limited

Evron, S., & Ezri, T. (2007). Options for systemic labor analgesia. *Current Opinions in Anesthesiology, 20*(3), 181–185.

Fink, J. L., Irwin, G., & Mitchell, R. (2007). Clinical tips. *RN, 70*(2), 44–45.

Frieden, F. J., & Chan, Y. (2007). Antepartum care. In R. E. Rakel & E. T. Bope (Eds.), *Conn's current therapy 2007* (Section 16, pp. 1168–1175). Philadelphia: Saunders Elsevier.

Gagnon, A. J., Meier, K. M., & Waghorn, K. (2007). Continuity of nursing care and its link to cesarean birth rate. *Birth: Issues in Perinatal Care, 34*(1), 26–31.

Giger, J. N., & Davidhizar, R. E. (2007). *Transcultural nursing* (5th ed.). St. Louis: Mosby.

Gilbert, E. S. (2007). *Manual of high risk pregnancy and delivery* (4th ed.). St. Louis, MO: Mosby.

Grimes-Dennis, J., & Berghella, V. (2007). Cervical length and prediction of preterm delivery. *Current Opinion in Obstetrics & Gynecology, 19*(2), 191–195.

Hackley, B., Kriebs, J. M., & Rousseau, M. E. (2007) *Primary care of women: A guide for midwives and women's health providers.* Sudbury, MA: Jones and Bartlett Publishers.

Hale, R. (2007). Monitoring fetal and maternal wellbeing. *British Journal of Midwifery, 15*(2), 107–110.

Hamilton, E., & Wright, E. (2007). Labor pains: Unraveling the complexity of OB decision making. *Critical Care Nursing Quarterly, 29*(4), 342–353.

Hanson, L. (2006). Pushing for change. *Journal of Perinatal & Neonatal Nursing, 20*(4), 282–285.

Hantoushzadeh, S., Alhusseini, N., & Lebaschi, A. H. (2007). The effects of acupuncture during labor on nulliparous women: A randomized controlled trial. *Australian & New Zealand Journal of Obstetrics & Gynecology, 47*(1), 26–30.

Healthcare Risk Management. (2007). Infant abduction raises questions about health care security and vigilance. *Healthcare Risk Management, 29*(5), 49–52.

Herbst, A., & Nilsson, C. (2006). Diagnosis of early preterm labor. *British Journal of Obstetrics & Gynecology,* Supplement 2, 113, 60–67.

Institute for Clinical Systems Improvement (ICSI). (2007). *ICSI Health Care Guidelines: Management of labor* (2nd ed.). Available at: http://www.icsi.org/labor/labor__management_of__full_version__2.html.

Jamieson, D. J., Read, J. S., Kourtis, A., et al. (2007). Cesarean delivery for HIV-infected women: Recommendations and controversies. *American Journal of Obstetrics and Gynecology, 197*(3 Suppl), S96–100.

Kenner, C., & Lott, J. W. (2007). *Comprehensive neonatal care: An interdisciplinary approach* (4th ed.). St. Louis, MO: Saunders Elsevier.

Koenig, D. (2007). Special delivery. *Natural Health, 37*(4), 51–58.

Kuczkowski, K. M. (2007). Labor pain and its management with the combined spinal-epidural analgesia: What does an obstetrician need to know? *Archives of Gynecology & Obstetrics, 275*(3), 183–185.

Leonard, P. (2007). Childbirth education: A handbook for nurses. *Nursing Spectrum.* Available at: http://nsweb/nursingspectrum.com/ce/m350c.htm.

Lockwood, C. (2007). Intrapartum EFM: How can we better identify the at-risk fetus? *Contemporary OB/GYN, 52*(1), 15–16.

Lowder, J. L., Burrows, L. J., Krohn, M. A., & Weber, A. M. (2007). Risk factors for primary and subsequent anal sphincter lacerations: A comparison of cohorts by parity and prior mode of delivery. *American Journal of Obstetrics & Gynecology, 196*(4), 344–349.

Lyon, E. (2007). *Big book of birth.* New York: Penguin Group (USA).

Menihan, C. A., & Kopel, E. (2008). *Electronic fetal monitoring: Concepts and applications* (2nd ed.). Philadelphia: Lippincott Williams & Wilkins.

Miller, K. E. (2007). Maternal oxygen affects nonreassuring FHR patterns. *American Family Physician, 75*(1), 111–114.

Moses, S. (2007). Fetal scalp blood sampling. *Family Practice Notebook.* Available at: http://www.fpnotebook.com/OB76.htm.

Murray, M. L. (2007). *Antepartal and intrapartal fetal monitoring* (3rd ed.). New York: Springer Publishing Company, Inc.

National Institute of Child Health and Human Development (NICHD). (2006). *NICHD terminology for fetal heart rate characteristics.* Available at: http://www.nichd.nih.gov/search.cfm?search_string=electronic+fetal+monitoring.

Peek, M. J., Condous, G. S., & Nanan, R. K. (2007). Fetal pulse oximetry and cesarean delivery. *New England Journal of Medicine, 356*(13), 1337–1340.

Reingold, A., Gershman, K., Petit, S., et al. (2007). Perinatal group B streptococcal disease after universal screening recommendations. *Journal of the American Medical Association, 298*(12), 1390–1392.

Roberts, J. M., Gonzalez, C. B., & Sampselle, C. (2007). Why do supportive birth attendants become directive of maternal bearing-down efforts in second-stage labor? *Journal of Midwifery & Women's Health, 52*(2), 134–141.

Ros, A., Felberbaum, R., Jahnke, I., Diedrich, K., Schmucker, P., & Huppe, M. (2007). Epidural anesthesia for labor: Does it influence the mode of delivery? *Archives of Gynecology & Obstetrics, 275*(4), 269–274.

Sauls, D. (2007). Nurses' attitudes toward provision of care and related health outcomes. *Nursing Research, 56*(2), 117–123.

Skidmore-Roth, L. (2007). *Mosby's 2007 nursing drug reference* (20th ed.). St. Louis, MO: Mosby Elsevier.

Sleutel, M., Schultz, S., & Wyble, K. (2007). Nurses' views of factors that help and hinder their intrapartum care. *Journal of Obstetric, Gynecologic & Neonatal Nursing, 36*(3), 203–211.

Smiley, R. M., & Stephenson, L. (2007). Patient-controlled analgesia for labor. *International Anesthesiology Clinics, 45*(1), 83–98.

Smith, C. A., Collins, C. T., Cyna, A. M., & Crowther, C. A. (2006). Complementary and alternative therapies for pain management in labor. *Cochrane Library.* 2006(4), CD003521; 2009358378.

Society of Obstetricians and Gynecologists of Canada (SOGC). (2006). Fetal health surveillance in labor (SOGC Clinical Practice Guidelines). *Journal of Obstetrics and Gynecology in Canada.* Available at: http://www.sogc.org/.

U.S. Department of Health and Human Services (USDHHS). (2000). *Healthy people 2010: Understanding and improving health* (2nd ed.). Chapter 16: Maternal, Infant, and Child Health. (DHHS Publication 017-001-00550-9). Washington, DC: Author.

Walsh, D. (2007). *Evidence-based care for normal labor and birth.* Andover, UK: Taylor & Francis, Inc.

Wood, S. (2007). Coping with labor pain. *March of Dimes.* Available at: http://www.marchofdimes.com/pnhec/240_12936.asp.

WEBSITES

Academy for Guided Imagery, Inc.: www.interactiveimagery.com

American College of Obstetricians and Gynecologists: www.acog.org

American Public Health Association: www.apha.org

Association of Labor Assistants and Childbirth Educators: www.alace.org

Association of Women's Health, Obstetric and Neonatal Nurses (AWHONN): www.awhonn.org

Birthworks: www.birthworks.org

Evidence-Based Nursing: www.evidencebasednursing.com

Child Find: www.childfind.org

Department of Health and Human Services: www.4women.gov

Diversity Rx: www.diversityrx.org

Doulas of North America: www.dona.org

Ethnomed: http://ethnomed.org

HypnoBirthing Institute: www.hypnobirthing.com

International Childbirth Education Association: www.icea.org

Lamaze International: www.lamaze-childbirth.com

National Center for Missing and Exploited Children: www.missingkids.com

Transcultural Health Links: www.iun.edu/~libemb/trannurs/trannurs.htm

CHAPTER WORKSHEET

MULTIPLE CHOICE QUESTIONS

1. When a client in labor is fully dilated, which instruction would be most effective to assist her in encouraging effective pushing?

   a. Hold your breath and push through entire contraction.

   b. Use chest-breathing with the contraction.

   c. Pant and blow during each contraction.

   d. Push for 6 to 7 seconds several times during each contraction.

2. During the fourth stage of labor, the nurse palpates the uterus on the right side and sees a saturated perineal pad. What is the nurse's first action?

   a. Massage the uterus vigorously.

   b. Have the client void and reassess her.

   c. Notify the primary care provider.

   d. Document as a normal finding.

3. When managing a client's pain during labor, nurses should:

   a. Make sure the agents given don't prolong labor.

   b. Know that all pain-relief measures are similar.

   c. Support the client's decisions and requests.

   d. Not recommend nonpharmacologic methods.

4. When caring for a client during the active phase of labor without continuous electronic fetal monitoring, the nurse would intermittently assess FHR every:

   a. 15 minutes

   b. 5 minutes

   c. 30 minutes

   d. 60 minutes

5. The nurse notes the presence of transient fetal accelerations on the fetal monitoring strip. Which intervention would be most appropriate?

   a. Reposition the client on the left side.

   b. Begin 100% oxygen via face mask.

   c. Document this reassuring pattern.

   d. Call the health care provider immediately.

CRITICAL THINKING EXERCISES

1. Carrie, a 20-year-old primigravida at term, comes to the birthing center in active labor (dilation 5 cm and 80% effaced, −1 station) with ruptured membranes. She states she wants an "all-natural" birth without medication. Her partner is with her and appears anxious but supportive. On the admission assessment, Carrie's prenatal history is unremarkable; vital signs are within normal limits; FHR via Doppler ranges between 140 and 144 bpm and is regular.

   a. Based on your assessment data and the woman's request not to have medication, what nonpharmacologic interventions could you offer her?

   b. What positions might be suggested to facilitate fetal descent?

2. Several hours later, Carrie complains of nausea and turns to her partner and angrily tells him to not touch her and to go away.

   a. What assessment needs to be done to determine what is happening?

   b. What explanation can you offer Carrie's partner regarding her change in behavior?

STUDY ACTIVITIES

1. Share experiences within a post-clinical conference group regarding the pain management interventions of the patients to which you were assigned. Compare and evaluate the effectiveness of different methods used, maternal behavior observed, and neonatal outcome in terms of Apgar scores.

2. On the fetal heart monitor, the nurse notices an elevation of the fetal baseline with the onset of contractions. This elevation would describe _____.

3. Compare and contrast a local birthing center to a community hospital's birthing suite in terms of the pain-management techniques and fetal monitoring used.

4. Select a childbirth website for expectant parents and critique the information provided in terms of its educational level and amount of advertising.

UNIT FIVE

POSTPARTUM PERIOD

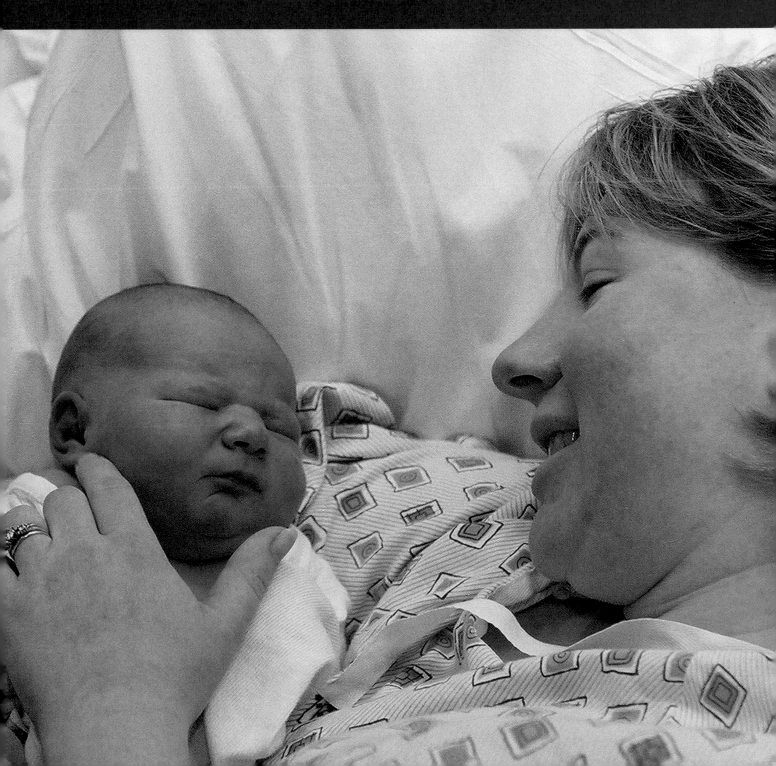

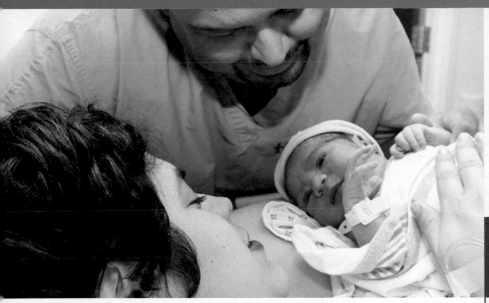

CHAPTER 15

POSTPARTUM ADAPTATIONS

KEY TERMS

engorgement
engrossment
involution
lactation

letting-go phase
lochia
puerperium

taking-hold phase
taking-in phase
uterine atony

LEARNING OBJECTIVES

Upon completion of the chapter, the learner will be able to:

1. Define the key terms used in this chapter.
2. Explain the systemic physiologic changes occurring in the woman after childbirth.
3. Identify the phases of maternal role adjustment as described by Reva Rubin.
4. Analyze the psychological adaptations occurring in the mother's partner after childbirth.

Betsy had been home only 3 days when she called the OB unit where she had given birth and asked to speak to the lactation consultant. She reported pain in both breasts. Her nipples were tender due to frequent breastfeeding and she described her breasts as heavy, hard, and swollen.

Wow

A new mother's expectations are seen through rose-colored glasses, and at times her fantasy is better than the reality.

The postpartum period is a critical transitional time for a woman, her newborn, and her family on physiologic and psychological levels. The **puerperium** period begins after the delivery of the placenta and lasts approximately 6 weeks. During this period the woman's body begins to return to its prepregnant state, and these changes generally resolve by the sixth week after giving birth. However, the postpartum period can also be defined to include the changes in all aspects of the mother's life that occur during the first year after a child is born. Some believe that the postpartum adjustment period lasts well into the first year, making the fourth phase of labor the longest. Keeping this in mind, the true postpartum period may last between 9 and 12 months as the mother works to lose the weight she gained while pregnant, adjusts psychologically to the changes in her life, and takes on the new role of mother.

This chapter describes the major physiologic and psychological changes that occur in a woman after childbirth. Various systemic adaptations take place throughout the woman's body. In addition, the mother and the family adjust to the new addition psychologically. The birth of a child changes the family structure and the roles of the family members. The adaptations are dynamic and continue to evolve as physical changes occur and new roles emerge.

Maternal Physiologic Adaptations

During pregnancy, the woman's entire body changed to accommodate the needs of the growing fetus. After birth, the woman's body once again undergoes significant changes in all body systems to return her body to its prepregnant state.

Reproductive System Adaptations

The reproductive system goes through tremendous adaptations to return to the prepregnancy state. All organs and tissues of the reproductive system are involved. The female reproductive system is unique in its capacity to remodel throughout the woman's reproductive life. The events after birth, with the shedding of the placenta and subsequent uterine involution, involve substantial tissue destruction and subsequent repair and remodeling. For example, the woman's menstrual cycle, interrupted during pregnancy, will begin to return several weeks after childbirth. The uterus, which has undergone tremendous expansion during pregnancy to accommodate progressive fetal growth, will return to its prepregnant size over several weeks. The mother's breasts have grown to prepare for lactation and do not return to their prepregnant size as the uterus does.

Uterus

The uterus returns to its normal size through a gradual process of **involution**, which involves retrogressive changes that return it to its nonpregnant size and condition. Involution involves three retrogressive processes:

1. Contraction of muscle fibers to reduce those previously stretched during pregnancy
2. Catabolism, which reduces enlarged, individual myometrial cells
3. Regeneration of uterine epithelium from the lower layer of the decidua after the upper layers have been sloughed off and shed during lochial discharge (Blackburn, 2007)

The uterus, which weighs approximately 1,000 g (2.2 lb) soon after birth, undergoes physiologic involution as it returns to its nonpregnant state. Approximately 1 week after birth, the uterus shrinks in size by 50% and weighs about 500 g (1 lb); at the end of 6 weeks, it weighs approximately 60 g (2 oz), about the weight before the pregnancy (Arenson & Drake, 2007; Blackburn, 2007; Fig. 15.1). During the first few days after birth, the uterus typically descends from the level of the umbilicus at a rate of 1 cm (1 fingerbreadth) per day. By 3 days, the fundus lies 2 to 3 fingerbreadths below the umbilicus (or slightly higher in multiparous women). By the end of 10 days, the fundus usually cannot be palpated because it has descended into the true pelvis.

If these retrogressive changes do not occur as a result of retained placental fragments or infection, subinvolution results. Subinvolution is generally responsive to early diagnosis and treatment. Factors that facilitate uterine involution include complete expulsion of amniotic membranes and placenta at birth, a complication-free labor and birth process, breastfeeding, and early ambulation.

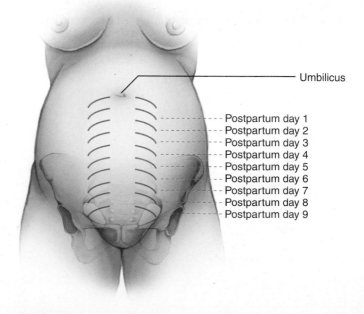

Umbilicus

Postpartum day 1
Postpartum day 2
Postpartum day 3
Postpartum day 4
Postpartum day 5
Postpartum day 6
Postpartum day 7
Postpartum day 8
Postpartum day 9

FIGURE 15.1 Uterine involution.

Factors that inhibit involution include a prolonged labor and difficult birth, incomplete expulsion of amniotic membranes and placenta, uterine infection, overdistention of uterine muscles (such as by multiple gestation, hydramnios, or a large singleton fetus), a full bladder (which displaces the uterus and interferes with contractions), anesthesia (which relaxes uterine muscles), and close childbirth spacing (frequent and repeated distention decreases tone and causes muscular relaxation).

Lochia

Lochia is the vaginal discharge that occurs after birth. It results from involution, during which the superficial layer of the decidua basalis becomes necrotic and is sloughed off. Immediately after childbirth, lochia is bright red and consists mainly of blood, fibrinous products, decidual cells, and red and white blood cells. The lochia from the uterus is alkaline but becomes acidic as it passes through the vagina. It is roughly equal to the amount occurring during a heavy menstrual period. The average amount of lochial discharge is 240 to 270 mL (8 to 9 oz) (Nash, 2007).

Women who have had cesarean births tend to have less flow because the uterine debris is removed manually along with delivery of the placenta. Lochia is present in most women for at least 3 weeks after childbirth, but it persists in some women for as long as 6 weeks.

Lochia passes through three stages: lochia rubra, lochia serosa, and lochia alba:

- Lochia rubra is a deep-red mixture of mucus, tissue debris, and blood that occurs for the first 3 to 4 days after birth. As uterine bleeding subsides, it becomes paler and more serous.
- Lochia serosa is the second stage. It is pinkish brown and is expelled 3 to 10 days postpartum. Lochia serosa primarily contains leukocytes, decidual tissue, red blood cells, and serous fluid.
- Lochia alba is the final stage. The discharge is creamy white or light brown and consists of leukocytes, decidual tissue, and reduced fluid content. It occurs from days 10 to 14 but can last 3 to 6 weeks postpartum in some women and still be considered normal.

Lochia at any stage should have a fleshy smell; an offensive odor usually indicates an infection, such as endometritis.

> ▶ **Take** NOTE!
>
> A danger sign is the reappearance of bright-red blood after lochia rubra has stopped. Reevaluation by the health care professional is essential if this occurs.

Afterpains

Part of the involution process involves uterine contractions. Subsequently, many women are frequently bothered by painful uterine contractions termed afterpains. All women experience afterpains, but they are more acute in multiparous women secondary to repeated stretching of the uterine muscles. This repeated stretching reduces muscle tone, allowing for alternate uterine contraction and relaxation. The uterus of a primiparous woman tends to remain contracted after giving birth unless she is breastfeeding; had a prolonged, difficult labor and birth; or had an overdistended uterus secondary to multiple gestation, hydramnios, or retained blood clots or placental fragments.

> ▶ **Take** NOTE!
>
> Afterpains are usually stronger during breastfeeding because oxytocin released by the sucking reflex strengthens the contractions. Mild analgesics can reduce this discomfort.

Cervix

The cervix typically returns to its prepregnant state by week 6 of the postpartum period. The cervix gradually closes but never regains its prepregnant appearance. Immediately after childbirth, the cervix is shapeless and edematous and is easily distensible for several days. The cervical os gradually closes and returns to normal by 2 weeks, whereas the external os widens and never appears the same after childbirth. The external cervical os is no longer shaped like a circle, but instead appears as a jagged slit-like opening, often described as a "fish mouth" (Fig. 15.2).

Vagina

Shortly after birth, the vaginal mucosa is edematous and thin, with few rugae. As ovarian function returns and estrogen production resumes, the mucosa thickens and rugae return in approximately 3 weeks. The vagina gapes at the

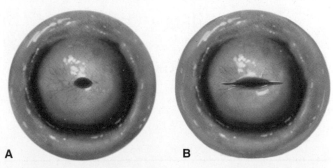

FIGURE 15.2 Appearance of the cervical os. (**A**) Before the first pregnancy. (**B**) After pregnancy.

opening and is generally lax. The vagina returns to its approximate prepregnant size by 6 to 8 weeks postpartum but will always remain a bit larger than it had been before pregnancy.

Normal mucus production and thickening of the vaginal mucosa usually return with ovulation (Edmonds, 2007). Ovulation can return as early as a month after childbirth in women who are not breastfeeding, with a mean time frame of 3 months. The mean time to ovulation in breastfeeding women is approximately 6 months, but this can vary greatly depending on breast-feeding patterns (Walsh, 2007). Localized dryness and coital discomfort (dyspareunia) usually plague most women until menstruation returns. Water-soluble lubricants can reduce discomfort during intercourse. Box 15.1 lists some commonly available water-soluble lubricants.

Perineum

The perineum is often edematous and bruised for the first day or two after birth. If the birth involved an episiotomy or laceration, complete healing may take as long as 4 to 6 months in the absence of complications at the site, such as hematoma or infection (Blackburn, 2007). Perineal lacerations may extend into the anus and cause considerable discomfort for the mother when she is attempting to defecate or ambulate. The presence of swollen hemorrhoids may also heighten discomfort. Local comfort measures such as ice packs, pouring warm water over the area via a peribottle, witch hazel pads, anesthetic sprays, and sitz baths can relieve pain. See Evidence-Based Practice 15.1.

Supportive tissues of the pelvic floor are stretched during the childbirth process, and restoring their tone may take up to 6 months. Pelvic relaxation can occur in any woman experiencing a vaginal birth. Nurses should

---

BOX 15.1 **Water-Soluble Lubricants**

- Astroglide
- Aqua Lube Personal
- Devine No. 9
- Emerita
- Eros
- ID Glide sensual lubricant
- JO water-based lubricant
- K-Y personal lubricant
- Life Styles personal lubricant
- Liquid Silk
- Nature's Dew
- Pre-Seed Intimate
- Replens
- Slippery Stuff

---

encourage all women to practice Kegel exercises to improve pelvic floor tone, strengthen the perineal muscles, and promote healing.

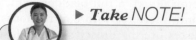

▶ *Take* NOTE!

Failure to maintain and restore perineal muscular tone leads to urinary incontinence later in life for many women.

Cardiovascular System Adaptations

The cardiovascular system undergoes dramatic changes after birth. During pregnancy, the heart is displaced slightly upward and to the left. This reverses as the uterus undergoes involution. Cardiac output remains high for the first few days postpartum and then gradually declines to nonpregnant values within 3 months of birth.

Blood volume, which increased substantially during pregnancy, drops rapidly after birth and returns to normal within 4 weeks postpartum (Arenson & Drake, 2007). The decrease in both cardiac output and blood volume reflects the birth-related blood loss (an average of 500 mL with a vaginal birth and 1,000 mL with a cesarean birth). Blood plasma volume is further reduced through diuresis, which occurs during the early postpartum period (Cheng & Caughey, 2007). Despite the decrease in blood volume, the hematocrit level remains relatively stable and may even increase, reflecting the predominant loss of plasma. Thus, an acute decrease in hematocrit is not an expected finding and may indicate hemorrhage.

Pulse and Blood Pressure

The increase in cardiac output during pregnancy begins to diminish after birth. This decrease in cardiac output is reflected in bradycardia (50 to 70 bpm) for the first 2 weeks postpartum. This slowing of the heart rate is related to the increased blood that flows back to the heart and to the central circulation after it is no longer perfusing the placenta. This increase in central circulation brings about an increased stroke volume and allows a slower heart rate to provide ample maternal circulation. Gradually, cardiac output returns to prepregnant levels by 3 months after childbirth (Blackburn, 2007).

Tachycardia (heart rate above 100 bpm) in the postpartum woman warrants further investigation. It may indicate hypovolemia, dehydration, or hemorrhage. However, because of the increased blood volume during pregnancy, a considerable loss may be well tolerated and not cause a compensatory cardiovascular response such as tachycardia. In most instances of postpartum hemorrhage, blood pressure and cardiac output remain increased because of the compensatory increase in heart rate. Thus, a decrease

EVIDENCE-BASED PRACTICE 15.1
Rectal Analgesia for Pain From Perineal Trauma Following Childbirth

● Study
Perineal pain from a tear and/or surgical cut (episiotomy) is a common problem following vaginal birth. Strategies to reduce perineal trauma and the appropriate repair of any perineal damage sustained are important for avoiding and alleviating pain. Numerous pain-relief treatments are used in clinical practice, such as local anesthetics, oral analgesics, therapeutic ultrasound, antiseptics, and nonpharmacologic applications such as ice packs and baths. This review assesses the evidence for using rectal analgesia for pain relief following perineal trauma caused by childbirth.

▲ Findings
This review of trials found that NSAID rectal suppositories are associated with less pain up to 24 hours after birth, and less additional analgesia is required. More research is required to assess the longer-term outcomes, maternal satisfaction, and effects, if any, on breast milk, mother–baby bonding, and sexual functioning.

■ Nursing Implications
According to the study, NSAID rectal suppositories were helpful in relieving postpartum pain. Nurses can offer this intervention to their patients and explain the evidence-based practice behind it.

Hedayati, H., Parsons, J., & Crowther, C. A. (2003). Rectal analgesia for pain from perineal trauma following childbirth. *Cochrane Database of Systematic Reviews* 2003, Issue 3. Art. No.: CD003931. DOI: 10.1002/14651858.CD003931.

---

in blood pressure and cardiac output are not expected changes during the postpartum period. Early identification is essential to ensure prompt intervention.

Blood pressure values should be similar to those obtained during the labor process. In some women there may be a slight transient increase lasting for about a week after childbirth (Edmonds, 2007). A significant increase accompanied by headache might indicate preeclampsia and requires further investigation. A decreased blood pressure may suggest orthostatic hypotension or uterine hemorrhage.

Coagulation
Clotting factors that increased during pregnancy tend to remain elevated during the early postpartum period. Giving birth stimulates this hypercoagulability state further. As a result, these coagulation factors remain elevated for 2 to 3 weeks postpartum (Hackley, Kriebs, & Rousseau, 2007). This hypercoagulable state, combined with vessel damage during birth and immobility, places the woman at risk for thromboembolism (blood clots) in the lower extremities and the lungs.

Blood Cellular Components
Red blood cell production ceases early in the puerperium, causing mean hemoglobin and hematocrit levels to decrease slightly in the first 24 hours. Over the next 2 weeks, both levels rise slowly. The white blood count, which increases in labor, remains elevated for first 4 to 6 days after birth but then falls to 6,000 to 10,000/mm³. This white blood cell elevation can complicate a diagnosis of infection in the immediate postpartum period.

Urinary System Adaptations

Pregnancy and birth can have profound effects on the urinary system. During pregnancy, the glomerular filtration rate and renal plasma flow increase significantly. Both usually return to normal by 6 weeks after birth.

Many women have difficulty feeling the sensation to void after giving birth if they received an anesthetic block during labor (which inhibits neural functioning of the bladder) or if they received oxytocin to induce or augment their labor (antidiuretic effect). These women will be at risk for incomplete emptying, bladder distention, difficulty voiding, and urinary retention. In addition, urination may be impeded by:

- Perineal lacerations
- Generalized swelling and bruising of the perineum and tissues surrounding the urinary meatus
- Hematomas
- Decreased bladder tone as a result of regional anesthesia
- Diminished sensation of bladder pressure as a result of swelling, poor bladder tone, and numbing effects of regional anesthesia used during labor (Nash, 2007)

Difficulty voiding can lead to urinary retention, bladder distention, and ultimately urinary tract infection (UTI). Urinary retention and bladder distention can cause displacement of the uterus from the midline to the right and can inhibit the uterus from contracting properly, which increases the risk of postpartum hemorrhage. Urinary retention is a major cause of **uterine atony**, which allows excessive bleeding. Frequent voiding of small amounts (less than 150 mL) suggests urinary retention with overflow, and catheterization may be necessary to empty the bladder to restore tone.

Postpartum diuresis occurs as a result of several mechanisms: the large amounts of intravenous fluids given during labor, a decreasing antidiuretic effect of oxytocin as its level declines, the buildup and retention of extra fluids during pregnancy, and a decreasing production of aldosterone—the hormone that decreases sodium retention and increases urine production (Blackburn, 2007). All these factors contribute to rapid filling of the bladder within 12 hours of birth. Diuresis begins within 12 hours after childbirth and continues throughout the first week postpartum. Normal function returns within a month after birth (Edmonds, 2007).

▶ *Consider* THIS!

Have you ever felt like a real idiot by not being able to complete a simple task in life? I had a beautiful baby boy after only 6 hours of labor. My epidural worked well and I actually felt very little discomfort throughout my labor. Because it was in the middle of the night when they brought me to my postpartum room, I felt a few hours of sleep would be all I needed to be back to normal. During an assessment early the next morning, the nurse found my uterus had shifted to the right from my midline, and I was instructed to empty my bladder. I didn't understand why the nurse was concerned about where my uterus was located and, besides, I didn't feel any sensation of a full bladder. But I did get up anyway and tried to comply. Despite all the nurse's tricks of running the faucet for sound effects, in addition to having warm water poured over my thighs via the peri-bottle, I was unable to urinate. How could I not accomplish one of life's simplest tasks?

Thoughts: Women who receive regional anesthesia frequently experience reduced sensation to their perineal area and do not feel a full bladder. The nursing assessment revealed a displaced uterus secondary to a full bladder. What additional "tricks" can be used to assist this woman to void? What explanation should be offered to her regarding why she is having difficulty urinating?

Gastrointestinal System Adaptations

The GI system quickly returns to normal because the gravid uterus is no longer filling the abdominal cavity and producing pressure on the abdominal organs. Progesterone levels, which caused relaxation of smooth muscle during pregnancy and diminished bowel tone, also are declining.

Regardless of the type of delivery, most women experience decreased bowel tone and sluggish bowels for several days after birth. Decreased peristalsis occurs in response to analgesics, surgery, diminished intraabdominal pressure, low-fiber diet and insufficient fluid intake,

and diminished muscle tone. In addition, women with an episiotomy, perineal laceration, or hemorrhoids may fear pain or damage to the perineum with their first bowel movement and may attempt to delay it. Subsequently, constipation is a common problem during the postpartum period. A stool softener can be prescribed for this reason.

Most women are hungry and thirsty after childbirth, commonly related to NPO restrictions and the energy expended during labor. Their appetite returns to normal immediately after giving birth.

▶ *Take* NOTE!

Anticipate the woman's need to replenish her body with food and fluids, and provide both soon after she gives birth.

Musculoskeletal System Adaptations

The effects of pregnancy on the muscles and joints vary widely. During pregnancy, the hormones relaxin, estrogen, and progesterone relax the joints. After birth, levels of these hormones decline, resulting in a return of all joints to their prepregnant state, with the exception of the woman's feet. Parous women will note a permanent increase in their shoe size (Hackley, Kriebs, & Rousseau, 2007).

Woman commonly experience fatigue and activity intolerance and have a distorted body image for weeks after birth secondary to declining relaxin and progesterone levels, which cause hip and joint pain that interferes with ambulation and exercise. Good body mechanics and correct position are important during this time to prevent low back pain and injury to the joints. Within 6 to 8 weeks after delivery, joints are completely stabilized and return to normal.

During pregnancy, stretching of the abdominal wall muscles occurs to accommodate the enlarging uterus. This stretching leads to a loss in muscle tone and possibly separation of the longitudinal muscles (rectus abdominis muscles) of the abdomen. Separation of the rectus abdominis muscles, called diastasis recti, is more common in women who have poor abdominal muscle tone before pregnancy. After birth, muscle tone is diminished and the abdominal muscles are soft and flabby. Specific exercises are necessary to help the woman regain muscle tone. Fortunately, diastasis responds well to exercise, and abdominal muscle tone can be improved (see Chapter 16 for more information about exercises to improve muscle tone).

▶ *Take* NOTE!

If rectus muscle tone is not regained through exercise, support may not be adequate during future pregnancies.

Integumentary System Adaptations

Another system that experiences lasting effects of pregnancy is the integumentary system. As estrogen and progesterone levels decrease, the darkened pigmentation on the abdomen (linea nigra), face (melasma), and nipples gradually fades. Some women experience hair loss during pregnancy and the postpartum periods. Approximately 90% of hairs are growing at any one time, with the other 10% entering a resting phase. Because of the high estrogen levels present during pregnancy, an increased number of hairs go into the resting phase, which is part of the normal hair loss cycle. The most common period for hair loss is within 3 months after birth, when estrogen returns to normal levels and more hairs are allowed to fall out. This hair loss is temporary, and regrowth generally returns to normal levels in 6 to 12 months (Lyon, 2007).

Striae gravidarum (stretch marks) that developed during pregnancy on the breasts, abdomen, and hips gradually fade to silvery lines. However, these lines do not disappear completely. Although many products on the market claim to make stretch marks disappear, their effectiveness is highly questionable.

The profuse diaphoresis (sweating) that is common during the early postpartum period is one of the most noticeable adaptations in the integumentary system. Many women will wake up drenched with perspiration during the puerperium. This postpartal diaphoresis is a mechanism to reduce the amount of fluids retained during pregnancy and restore prepregnant body fluid levels. It can be profuse at times. It is common, especially at night during the first week after birth. Reassure the client that this is normal and encourage her to change her gown to prevent chilling.

Respiratory System Adaptations

Respirations usually remain within the normal adult range of 16 to 24 breaths per minute. As the abdominal organs resume their nonpregnant position, the diaphragm returns to its usual position. Anatomic changes in the thoracic cavity and rib cage caused by increasing uterine growth resolve quickly. As a result, discomforts such as shortness of breath and rib aches are relieved. Tidal volume, minute volume, vital capacity, and functional residual capacity return to prepregnant values, typically within 1 to 3 weeks of birth (Blackburn, 2007).

Endocrine System Adaptations

The endocrine system undergoes several changes rapidly after birth. Levels of circulating estrogen and progesterone drop quickly with delivery of the placenta. Decreased estrogen levels are associated with breast engorgement and with the diuresis of excess extracellular fluid accumulated during pregnancy (Edmonds, 2007). Estrogen is at its lowest level a week after birth. For the woman who is not breastfeeding, estrogen levels begin to increase by 2 weeks after birth. For the breastfeeding woman, estrogen levels remain low until breastfeeding frequency decreases.

Other placental hormones (hCG, hPL, progesterone) decline rapidly after birth. hCG levels are nonexistent at the end of the first postpartum week and hPL is undetectable within 1 day after birth (Blackburn, 2007). Progesterone levels are undetectable by 3 days after childbirth, and production is reestablished with the first menses. Prolactin levels decline within 2 weeks for the woman who is not breastfeeding and remain elevated for the lactating woman (Blackburn, 2007).

Think back to Betsy, the woman experiencing painful changes in her breasts. What is Betsy describing to the lactation consultant? Why has the condition of her breasts changed compared to when she was in the hospital?

Lactation

Lactation is the secretion of milk by the breasts. It is thought to be brought about by the interaction of progesterone, estrogen, prolactin, and oxytocin. Breast milk typically appears 3 days after childbirth.

During pregnancy, the breasts increase in size and functional ability in preparation for breastfeeding. Within the first month of gestation, the ducts of the mammary glands grow branches, forming more lobules and alveoli. These structural changes make the breasts larger, more tender, and heavy. Each breast gains nearly 1 lb in weight by term, the glandular cells fill with secretions, blood vessels increase in number, and there are increased amounts of connective tissue and fat cells (Blackburn, 2007).

Prolactin from the anterior pituitary gland, secreted in increasing levels throughout pregnancy, triggers the synthesis and secretion of milk after the woman gives birth. During pregnancy, prolactin, estrogen, and progesterone cause synthesis and secretion of colostrum, which contains protein and carbohydrate but no milk fat. It is only after birth takes place, when the high levels of estrogen and progesterone are abruptly withdrawn, that prolactin is able to stimulate the glandular cells to secrete milk instead of colostrum. This takes place within 2 to 3 days after giving birth. Oxytocin acts so that milk can be ejected from the alveoli to the nipple. Therefore, sucking by the newborn will release milk. Prolactin levels increase in response to nipple stimulation during feedings. Prolactin and oxytocin result in milk production if stimulated by sucking (Walsh, 2007) (Fig. 15.3). If the stimulus (sucking) is not present, as with a woman who is not breastfeeding, breast engorgement and milk production will subside within 2 to 3 days postpartum.

Typically, during the first 2 days after birth, the breasts are soft and nontender. The woman also may report a tingling sensation in both breasts. After this time, breast changes depend on whether the mother is breastfeeding or taking measures to prevent lactation.

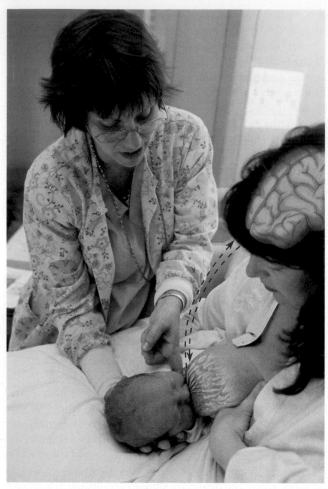

FIGURE 15.3 Physiology of lactation.

Engorgement is the process of swelling of the breast tissue as a result of an increase in blood and lymph supply as a precursor to lactation (Bainbridge, 2007). Breasts increase in vascularity and swell in response to prolactin 2 to 4 days after birth. If engorged, the breasts will be hard and tender to touch. They are temporarily full, tender, and very uncomfortable until the milk supply is ready. Frequent emptying of the breasts helps to minimize discomfort and resolve engorgement. Standing in a warm shower or applying warm compresses immediately before feedings will help to soften the breasts and nipples in order to allow the newborn to latch on easier. These measures will also enhance the letdown reflex. Between feedings, applying cold compresses to the breasts helps to reduce swelling. To maintain milk supply, the breasts need to be stimulated by a nursing infant, a breast pump, or manual expression of the milk (Fig. 15.4).

Remember Betsy, with the breast discomfort? The lactation consultant explained that she was experiencing normal breast engorgement and offered several suggestions to help her. What relief measures might they be? What reassurance can be given to Betsy at this time?

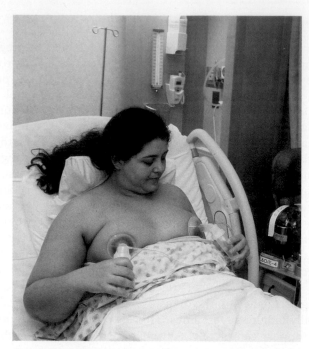

FIGURE 15.4 Mother using breast pumps to stimulate milk production.

If the woman is not breastfeeding, relief measures include wearing a tight, supportive bra 24 hours daily, applying ice to her breasts for approximately 15 to 20 minutes every other hour, and not stimulating the breasts by squeezing or manually expressing milk from the nipples. In addition, avoiding exposing the breasts to warmth (e.g., a hot shower) will help relieve breast engorgement. In women who are not breastfeeding, engorgement typically subsides within 2 to 3 days with these measures.

Ovulation and Return of Menstruation

Changing hormone levels constantly interact with one another to produce bodily changes. Four major hormones are influential during the postpartum period: estrogen, progesterone, prolactin, and oxytocin. Estrogen is the major female hormone during pregnancy, but levels drop profoundly at birth and reach their lowest level a week into the postpartum period. Progesterone quiets the uterus to prevent a preterm birth during pregnancy, and its increasing levels during pregnancy prevent lactation from starting before birth takes place. As with estrogen, progesterone levels decrease dramatically after birth and are undetectable 72 hours after birth. Progesterone levels are reestablished with the first menstrual cycle (Blackburn, 2007).

During the postpartum period, oxytocin stimulates the uterus to contract during the breastfeeding session and for as long as 20 minutes after each feeding. Oxytocin also acts on the breast by eliciting the milk letdown reflex during breastfeeding. Prolactin is also associated with the breastfeeding process by stimulating milk production. In women who breastfeed, prolactin levels remain elevated into the sixth week after birth (Nash, 2007). The levels of the hormone increase and decrease in proportion to nipple stimulation. Prolactin levels decrease in nonlactating women, reaching prepregnant levels by the third postpartum week (Edmonds, 2007). High levels of prolactin have been found to delay ovulation by inhibiting ovarian response to FSH (Edmonds, 2007).

The timing of first menses and ovulation after birth differs between women who are and are not breastfeeding. For nonlactating women, menstruation usually resumes 7 to 9 weeks after giving birth, with the first cycle being anovulatory (Walsh, 2007). The return of menses in the lactating woman depends on breastfeeding frequency and duration. It can return anytime from 2 to 18 months after childbirth, depending on whether the woman is exclusively breastfeeding or supplementing with formula. The first postpartum menstrual period may be heavier than prepregnant ones and is frequently anovulatory (Hackley, Kriebs, & Rousseau, 2007).

> ▶ *Take* NOTE!
>
> *Ovulation may occur before menstruation; therefore, breastfeeding is not a reliable method of contraception. Other methods of family planning must be used to control fertility (Alexander et al., 2007).*

Betsy tries several of the measures the lactation consultant suggested to relieve her breast discomfort but is still having heaviness and pain. She feels discouraged and tells the nurse she is thinking of reducing her breastfeeding and using formula to feed her newborn. Is that a good choice? Why or why not? What interventions will help Betsy get through this difficult time?

Psychological Adaptations

Mothers' and fathers' experiences of pregnancy are necessarily different, and this difference continues after childbirth as they both adjust to their new parenting roles. Parenting involves caring for infants physically and emotionally to foster the growth and development of responsible, caring adults. During the early months of parenthood, mothers experience more life changes and get more satisfaction from their new roles than fathers. However, fathers interact with their newborns much like mothers (Thorpe, 2007). Early parent–infant contact after birth improves attachment behaviors. Other members of the newborn's family, such as siblings and grandparents, also

experience changes related to the birth of the newborn. Chapter 16 describes these changes.

Maternal Psychological Adaptations

Postpartum depression affects the transition to the maternal role for many mothers. Between 50% and 80% of new mothers suffer from the short-lived postpartum mood disorder termed "baby blues." In addition, each year in the United States, up to 28% of new mothers or more than 400,000 new mothers suffer debilitating postpartum depression, a prevalence that continues unabated (AWHONN, 2007). Postpartum depression can lead to alienation from loved ones, daily dysfunction secondary to overwhelming sorrow and disorientation, and, at its most extreme, personal terror resulting in dangerous thoughts and violent actions. For additional information, see Chapter 22.

The woman experiences a variety of responses as she adjusts to a new family member, postpartum discomforts, changes in her body image, and the reality of change in her life. In the early 1960s, Reva Rubin identified three phases that a mother goes through to adjust to her new maternal role. Rubin's maternal role framework can be used to monitor the client's progress as she "tries on" her new role as a mother. Absence of these processes or inability to progress through the phases satisfactorily may impede the appropriate development of the maternal role (Rubin, 1984). Although Rubin's maternal role development theories are of value, some of her observations regarding the length of each phase may not be completely relevant for the contemporary woman of the 21st century. Today, many women know their infant's gender, have "seen" their fetus in utero through four-dimensional ultrasound, and have a working knowledge of childbirth and child care. They are less passive than in years past and progress through the phases of attaining the maternal role at a much faster pace than Rubin would have imagined. Still, Rubin's framework is timeless for assessing and monitoring expected role behaviors when planning care and appropriate interventions.

Taking-In Phase

The **taking-in phase** is the time immediately after birth when the client needs sleep, depends on others to meet her needs, and relives the events surrounding the birth process. This phase is characterized by dependent behavior. During the first 24 to 48 hours after giving birth, mothers often assume a very passive role in meeting their own basic needs for food, fluids, and rest, allowing the nurse to make decisions for them concerning activities and care. They spend time recounting their labor experience to anyone who will listen. Such actions help the mother integrate the birth experience into reality—that is, the pregnancy is over and the newborn is now a unique individual, separate from herself. When interacting with the newborn, new mothers spend time claiming the newborn and touching him or her, commonly identifying specific features in the newborn, such as "he has my nose" or "his fingers are long like his father's" (Fig. 15.5).

▶ **Take** NOTE!

The taking-in phase typically lasts 1 to 2 days and may be the only phase observed by nurses in the hospital setting because of the shortened postpartum stays that are the norm today.

Taking-Hold Phase

The **taking-hold phase**, the second phase of maternal adaptation, is characterized by dependent and independent maternal behavior. This phase typically starts on the second to third day postpartum and may last several weeks.

As the client regains control over her bodily functions during the next few days, she will be taking hold and becoming preoccupied with the present. She will be particularly concerned about her health, the infant's condition, and her ability to care for him or her. She demonstrates increased autonomy and mastery of her own body's functioning, and a desire to take charge with support and help from others. She will show independence by caring for herself and learning to care for her newborn, but she still requires assurance that she is doing well as a mother. She expresses a strong interest in caring for the infant by herself.

Letting-Go Phase

In the **letting-go phase**, the third phase of maternal adaptation, the woman reestablishes relationships with other people. She adapts to parenthood through her new role as a mother. She assumes the responsibility and care for the newborn with a bit more confidence now (Arenson & Drake, 2007). The focus of this phase is to move forward by assuming the parental role and to separate herself from the symbiotic relationship that she and her newborn had during pregnancy. She establishes a lifestyle that includes the infant. The mother relinquishes the fantasy infant and accepts the real one.

Partner Psychological Adaptations

For partners, whether they are husbands, significant others, boyfriends, same-sex life partners, or just friends, becoming a parent or just sharing the childbirth experience can be a perplexing time as well as a time of great change. This transition is influenced by many factors, including participation in childbirth, relationships with significant others, competence in child care, the family role organization, the individual's cultural background, and the method of infant feeding.

▶ **Take** NOTE!

Most research findings stress the importance of early contact between the father or significant other and the newborn, as well as participation in infant care activities, to foster the relationship (Thorpe, 2007).

Infants have a powerful effect on their fathers and others, who become intensely involved with them (Fig. 15.6). The father's or significant other's developing bond with the newborn—a time of intense absorption, preoccupation, and interest—is called engrossment.

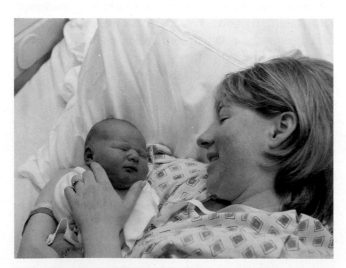

FIGURE 15.5 Mother bonding with newborn during the taking-in phase.

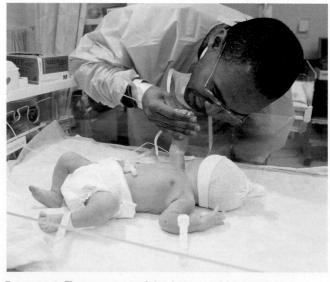

FIGURE 15.6 Engrossment of the father and his newborn.

Engrossment

Engrossment is characterized by seven behaviors:

1. Visual awareness of the newborn—the father or partner perceives the newborn as attractive, pretty, or beautiful
2. Tactile awareness of the newborn—the father or partner has a desire to touch or hold the newborn and considers this activity to be pleasurable
3. Perception of the newborn as perfect—the father or partner does not "see" any imperfections
4. Strong attraction to the newborn—the father or partner focuses all attention on the newborn when he is in the room
5. Awareness of distinct features of the newborn—the father or partner can distinguish his newborn from others in the nursery
6. Extreme elation—the father or partner feels a "high" after the birth of his child
7. Increased sense of self-esteem—the father or partner feels proud, "bigger," more mature, and older after the birth of his child (Sears & Sears, 2006)

Frequently, fathers or partners are portrayed as well-meaning but bumbling when caring for newborns. However, they have their own unique way of relating to their newborns and can become as nurturing as mothers. A father or partner's nurturing responses may be less automatic and slower to unfold than a mother's, but they are capable of a strong bonding attachment to their newborns (Sears & Sears, 2006). Encouraging fathers or partners to express their feelings by seeing, touching, and holding their son or daughter and by cuddling, talking to, and feeding him or her will help to cement this new relationship. Reinforcement of this engrossing behavior helps fathers or partners to make a positive attachment during this critical period.

Three-Stage Role Development Process

Similar to mothers, fathers or partners also go through a predictable three-stage process during the first 3 weeks as they too "try on" their roles as parents. The three stages are expectations, reality, and transition to mastery (Sears & Sears, 2006).

Stage 1: Expectations

New fathers or partners pass through stage 1 (expectations) with preconceptions about what home life will be like with a newborn. Many men may be unaware of the dramatic changes that can occur when this newborn comes home to live with them. For some, it is an eye-opening experience.

Stage 2: Reality

Stage 2 (reality) occurs when fathers or partners realize that their expectations in stage 1 are not realistic. Their feelings change from elation to sadness, ambivalence, jealousy, and frustration. Many wish to be more involved in the newborn's care and yet do not feel prepared to do so. Some find parenting fun but at the same time do not feel fully prepared to take on that role.

Stage 3: Transition to Mastery

In stage 3 (transition to mastery), the father or partner makes a conscious decision to take control and be at the center of his newborn's life regardless of his preparedness. This adjustment period is similar to that of the mother's letting-go phase, when she incorporates the newest member into the family.

■■■ Key Concepts

- The puerperium period refers to the first 6 weeks after delivery. During this period, the mother experiences many physiologic and psychological adaptations to return her to the prepregnant state.
- Involution involves three processes: contraction of muscle fibers to reduce stretched ones, catabolism (which reduces enlarged, individual cells), and regeneration of uterine epithelium from the lower layer of the decidua after the upper layers have been sloughed off and shed in lochia.
- Lochia passes through three stages: lochia rubra, lochia serosa, and lochia alba during the postpartal period.
- Maternal blood plasma volume decreases rapidly after birth and returns to normal within 4 weeks postpartum.
- Reva Rubin (1984) identified three phases the mother goes through to adjust to her new maternal role. The phases of maternal postpartum adjustment are taking in, taking hold, and letting go.
- The transition to fatherhood is influenced by many factors, including participation in childbirth, relationships with significant others, competence in child care, the family role organization, the father's cultural background, and the method of infant feeding.
- Like mothers, men go through a predictable three-stage process during the first 3 weeks as they too "try on" their roles as fathers or partners. The three stages include expectations, reality, and transition to mastery.

REFERENCES

Alexander, L. L., LaRosa, J. H., Bader, H., & Garfield, S. (2007). *New dimensions in women's health* (4th ed.). Sudbury, MA: Jones and Bartlett Publishers.

Arenson, J., & Drake, P. (2007). *Maternal and newborn health.* Sudbury, MA: Jones and Bartlett Publishers.

AWHONN. (2007). Conquering postpartum depression. *Nursing for Women's Health, 11*(4), 422–423.

Bainbridge, J. (2007). Dealing with breast and nipple soreness when breastfeeding. *British Journal of Midwifery, 13*(9), 552–556.

Blackburn, S. T. (2007). *Maternal, fetal, and neonatal physiology* (3rd ed.). Philadelphia: Saunders Elsevier.

Cheng, Y. W., & Caughey, A. B. (2007) Normal labor and delivery. *eMedicine*. Available at: http://www.emedicine.com/MED/topic3239.htm.

Edmonds, K. (2007). *Dewhurst's textbook of obstetrics and gynecology* (7th ed.). Oxford, UK: Blackwell Publishing Limited.

Hackley, B., Kriebs, J. M., & Rousseau, M. E. (2007). *Primary care of women: A guide for midwives and women's health providers*. Sudbury, MA: Jones & Bartlett Publishers.

Lyon, E. (2007). *Big book of birth*. New York: Penguin Group (USA).

Nash, L. R. (2007). Postpartum care. In R. E. Rachel & E. T. Bope (Eds.), *Conn's current therapy 2007* (Section 16, pp. 1190–1193). Philadelphia: Saunders Elsevier.

Rubin, R. (1984). *Maternal identity and the maternal experience*. New York: Springer.

Sears, R. W., & Sears, J. M. (2006). *Fathers' first steps: 25 things every dad should know*. Boston, MA: Harvard Common Press.

Thorpe, K. (2007). Child health nurses supporting parents. *Australian Nursing Journal, 14*(8), 32–35.

Walsh, D. (2007). *Evidence-based care for normal labor and birth: A guide for midwives*. Andover, UK: Taylor & Francis, Inc.

WEBSITES

American College of Nurse-Midwives: www.midwife.org
Association for Perinatal Psychology and Health: www.birthpsychology.com
Association of Maternal & Child Health Programs: www.amchpl.org
Center for Postpartum Health: www.postpartumhealth.com
Depression after Delivery: www.depressionafterdelivery.com
Home-Based Working Moms: www.hbwm.com
International Lactation Consultants Association: www.ilca.org
La Leche League: www.lalecheleague.org
Midwifery Today, Inc.: www.midwiferytoday.com
National Center for Fathering: www.fathers.com
National Parenting Center: www.tnpc.com
National Women's Health Information Center: www.4women.gov
Parenthood Web: www.parenthoodweb.com
Parenting Q & A: www.parenting-qa.com
Parents Anonymous, Inc.: www.parentsanonymous.org
Parents Helping Parents: www.php.com
Postpartum Support International: www.chss.iup.edu/postpartum/

CHAPTER WORKSHEET

MULTIPLE CHOICE QUESTIONS

1. Postpartal breast engorgement occurs 48 to 72 hours after giving birth. What physiologic change influences breast engorgement?

   a. An increase in blood and lymph supply to the breasts

   b. A decrease in estrogen and progesterone levels

   c. Colostrum production increases dramatically

   d. Fluid retention in the breasts due to the intravenous fluids given during labor

2. In the taking-in maternal role phase described by Rubin (1984), the nurse would expect the woman's behavior to be characterized as which of the following?

   a. Gaining self-confidence

   b. Adjusting to her new relationships

   c. Being passive and dependent

   d. Resuming control over her life

3. The nurse is explaining to a postpartal woman that the afterpains she is experiencing can be the result of which of the following?

   a. Manipulation of the uterus during labor

   b. A large infant weighing more than 8 lb

   c. Pregnancies that were too closely spaced

   d. Contractions of the uterus after birth

4. The nurse would expect a postpartal woman to demonstrate lochia in which sequence?

   a. Rubra, alba, scrosa

   b. Rubra, serosa, alba

   c. Serosa, alba, rubra

   d. Alba, rubra, serosa

5. The nurse is assessing Ms. Smith, who gave birth to her first child 5 days ago. What findings by the nurse would be expected?

   a. Cream-colored lochia; uterus above the umbilicus

   b. Bright-red lochia with clots; uterus 2 fingerbreadths below umbilicus

   c. Light pink or brown lochia; uterus 4 to 5 fingerbreadths below umbilicus

   d. Yellow, mucousy lochia; uterus at the level of the umbilicus

6. Prioritize the postpartum mother's needs 4 hours after giving birth by placing a number 1, 2, 3, or 4 in the blank before each need.

   _____ Learn how to hold and cuddle the infant

   _____ Watch a baby bath demonstration given by the nurse

   _____ Sleep and rest without being disturbed for a few hours

   _____ Interaction time with the infant to facilitate bonding

CRITICAL THINKING EXERCISES

1. A new nurse assigned to the postpartum mother–baby unit makes a comment to the oncoming shift that Ms. Griffin, a 25-year-old primipara, seems lazy and shows no initiative in taking care of herself or her baby. The nurse reported that Ms. Griffin talks excessively about her labor and birth experience and seems preoccupied with herself and her needs, not her newborn's care. She wonders if something is wrong with this mother because she seems so self-centered and has to be directed to do everything.

   a. Is there something "wrong" with Ms. Griffin's behavior? Why or why not?

   b. What maternal role phase is being described by the new nurse?

   c. What role can the nurse play to support the mother through this phase?

2. Mrs. Lenhart, a primipara, gave birth to a healthy baby boy yesterday. Her husband John seemed elated at the birth, calling his friends and family on his cell phone minutes after the birth. He passed out cigars and praised his wife for her efforts. Today, when the nurse walked into their room, Mr. Lenhart seemed very anxious around his new son and called for the nurse whenever the baby cried or needed a diaper change. He seemed standoffish when asked to hold his son, and he spent time talking to other fathers in the waiting room, leaving his wife alone in the room.

   a. Would you consider Mr. Lenhart's paternal behavior to be normal at this time?

   b. What might Mr. Lenhart be feeling at this time?

   c. How can the nurse help this new father adjust to his new role?

STUDY ACTIVITIES

1. Find an Internet resource that discusses general postpartum care for new mothers who might have questions after discharge. Evaluate the website's information as to how credible, accurate, and current it is.

2. Prepare a teaching plan for new mothers, outlining the various physiologic changes that will take place after discharge.

3. The term that describes the return of the uterus to its prepregnant state is _____.

4. A deviated fundus to the right side of the abdomen would indicate a _____.

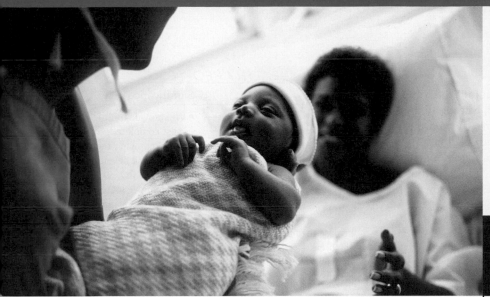

CHAPTER 16

NURSING MANAGEMENT DURING THE POSTPARTUM PERIOD

KEY TERMS

attachment
bonding
en face position

Kegel exercises
mastitis
peribottle

postpartum blues
sitz bath

LEARNING OBJECTIVES

Upon completion of the chapter, the learner will be able to:

1. Define the key terms.
2. List the parameters that need to be assessed during the postpartum period.
3. Compare the bonding and attachment process.
4. Identify behaviors that enhance or inhibit the attachment process.
5. Outline nursing management for the woman and her family during the postpartum period.
6. Discuss the role of the nurse in promoting successful breast-feeding.
7. List areas of health education needed for discharge planning, home care, and follow-up.

Raina is a 24-year-old Muslim primipara who has just been admitted to the postpartum unit. Her husband sits at the bedside but doesn't seem to give her any physical or emotional support after her lengthy labor and difficult birth.

WoW *Parenting is an intimate, interactive, continuous, lifelong process.*

419

The postpartum period is a time of major adjustments and adaptations not just for the mother, but for all members of the family. It is during this time that parenting starts and a relationship with the newborn begins. A positive, loving relationship between parents and their newborn promotes the emotional well-being of all. This relationship endures and has profound effects on the child's growth and development.

> ▶ **Take** NOTE!
>
> *Parenting is a skill that is often learned by trial and error, with varying degrees of success. Successful parenting, a continuous and complex interactive process, requires the parents to learn new skills and to integrate the new member into the family.*

HEALTHY PEOPLE 2010

Objective	Significance
Increase the proportion of mothers who breast-feed their babies.	• Will provide infants with the most complete form of nutrition, improving their health, growth and development, and immunity
Increase the number of mothers who breast-feed during early postpartum from a baseline of 64% to 75%.	• Will improve maternal health via breast-feeding's beneficial effects
Increase the number of mothers who breast-feed at 6 months from a baseline of 29% to 50%.	• Will increase the rate of breast-feeding, particularly among low-income and certain racial and ethnic populations who are less likely to begin breast-feeding in the hospital or to sustain it through the infant's first year
Increase the number of mothers who breast-feed at 1 year from a baseline of 16% to 25%.	

Once the infant is born, each system in the mother's body takes several weeks to return to its nonpregnant state. The physiologic changes in women during the postpartum period are dramatic. Nurses should be aware of these changes and should be able to make observations and assessments to validate normal occurrences and detect any deviations.

In addition to physical assessment and care of the woman in the postpartum period, strong social support is vital to help her integrate the baby into the family. In today's mobile society, extended families may live far away and may be unable to help care for the new family. As a result, many new parents turn to health care professionals for information as well as physical and emotional support during this adjustment period. Nurses can be an invaluable resource by serving as mentors, teaching about self-care measures and baby care basics, and providing emotional support. Nurses can "mother" the new mother by offering physical care, emotional support, and information and practical help. The nurse's support and care through this critical time can increase the new parents' confidence, giving them a sense of accomplishment in their parenting skills.

One important intervention during the postpartum period is promotion of breast-feeding. *Healthy People 2010* includes breast-feeding as a goal for maternal, infant, and child health.

As in all nursing care, nurses should provide culturally competent care during the postpartum period. The nurse should engage in ongoing cultural self-assessment and overcome any stereotypes that perpetuate prejudice or discrimination against any cultural group (Bowers, 2007). Providing culturally competent nursing care during the postpartum period requires time, open-mindedness, and patience. To promote positive outcomes, the nurse should be sensitive to the woman's and family's culture, religion, and ethnic influences (see "Providing Optimal Cultural Care" in the Nursing Interventions section).

Remember the couple introduced at the beginning of the chapter? When the postpartum nurse comes to examine Raina, her husband quickly leaves the room and returns a short time later after the examination is complete. How do you interpret his behavior toward his wife? What might you communicate to this couple?

This chapter describes the nursing management of the woman and her family during the postpartum period. It outlines physical assessment parameters for new mothers and newborns. It also focuses on bonding and attachment behaviors; nurses need to be aware of these behaviors so they can perform appropriate interventions. Steps to address physiologic needs such as comfort, self-care, nutrition, and contraception are described. Ways to help the woman and her family adapt to the birth of the newborn are also discussed (Fig. 16.1).

Nursing management during the postpartum period focuses on assessing the woman's ability to adapt to the physiologic and psychological changes occurring at this time (see Chap. 15 for a detailed discussion of these adaptations). Family members are also assessed to determine how well they are making the transition to this new stage. Based on assessment findings, the nurse plans and implements care to address the family's needs. Because of today's shortened lengths of stay, the nurse may be able to focus only on priority needs and may need to arrange for follow-up in the home to ensure that all the family's needs are met.

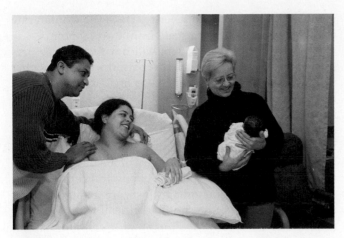

FIGURE **16.1** Parents and grandmother interacting with the newborn.

Assessment

Comprehensive nursing assessment begins within an hour after the woman gives birth and continues through discharge.

▶ **Take** NOTE!

Nurses need a firm grasp of normal findings so that they can recognize abnormal findings and intervene appropriately.

This assessment includes vital signs and physical and psychosocial assessments. Although the exact protocol may vary among facilities, postpartum assessment typically is performed as follows:

• During the first hour: every 15 minutes
• During the second hour: every 30 minutes
• During the first 24 hours: every 4 hours
• After 24 hours: every 8 hours (Simpkin & James, 2006)

During each assessment, keep in mind risk factors that may lead to complications, such as infection or hemorrhage, during the recovery period (Box 16.1). Early identification is critical to ensure prompt intervention.

As with any assessment, always review the woman's medical record for information about her pregnancy, labor, and birth. Note any preexisting conditions, any complications that occurred during pregnancy, labor, birth, and immediately afterward, and any treatments provided.

Postpartum assessment of the mother typically includes vital signs, pain level, and a systematic head-to-toe review of body systems. The acronym BUBBLE-EE—breasts, uterus, bladder, bowels, lochia, episiotomy/perineum, extremities, and emotional status—can be used as a guide for this head-to-toe review (Blackburn, 2007).

BOX 16.1 **Factors Increasing the Woman's Risk for Postpartum Complications**

Risk Factors for Postpartum Infection
• Operative procedure (forceps, cesarean birth, vacuum extraction)
• History of diabetes, including gestational-onset diabetes
• Prolonged labor (more than 24 hours)
• Use of indwelling urinary catheter
• Anemia (hemoglobin less than 10.5 mg/dL)
• Multiple vaginal examinations during labor
• Prolonged rupture of membranes (more than 24 hours)
• Manual extraction of placenta
• Compromised immune system (HIV positive)

Risk Factors for Postpartum Hemorrhage
• Precipitous labor (less than 3 hours)
• Uterine atony
• Placenta previa or abruptio placentae
• Labor induction or augmentation
• Operative procedures (vacuum extraction, forceps, cesarean birth)
• Retained placental fragments
• Prolonged third stage of labor (more than 30 minutes)
• Multiparity, more than three births closely spaced
• Uterine overdistention (large infant, twins, hydramnios)

While assessing the woman and her family during the postpartum period, be alert for danger signs (Box 16.2). Notify the primary health care provider immediately if any are noted.

Postpartum assessment also includes assessing the parents and other family members, such as siblings and grandparents, for attachment and bonding with the newborn.

BOX 16.2 **Postpartum Danger Signs**

• Fever more than 38°C (100.4°F)
• Foul-smelling lochia or an unexpected change in color or amount
• Visual changes, such as blurred vision or spots, or headaches
• Calf pain with dorsiflexion of the foot
• Swelling, redness, or discharge at the episiotomy site
• Dysuria, burning, or incomplete emptying of the bladder
• Shortness of breath or difficulty breathing
• Depression or extreme mood swings

Vital Signs

Obtain vital signs and compare them with the previous values, noting and reporting any deviations. Vital sign changes can be an early indicator of complications.

Temperature

Use a consistent measurement technique (oral, axillary, or tympanic) to get the most accurate readings. Typically, the new mother's temperature during the first 24 hours postpartum is within the normal range. Some women experience a slight fever, up to 38°C (100.4°F), during the first 24 hours. This elevation may be the result of dehydration because of fluid loss during labor. Temperature should be normal after 24 hours with replacement of fluids lost during labor and birth (Arenson & Drake, 2007). A temperature above 38°C (100.4°F) at any time or an abnormal temperature after the first 24 hours may indicate infection and must be reported. Abnormal temperature readings warrant continued monitoring until an infection can be ruled out through cultures or blood studies.

Pulse

Because of the changes in blood volume and cardiac output after delivery, relative bradycardia may be noted. The woman's pulse rate may range from 50 to 70 bpm. Pulse usually stabilizes to prepregnancy levels within 10 days (Blackburn, 2007).

Tachycardia in the postpartum woman can suggest anxiety, excitement, fatigue, pain, excessive blood loss, infection, or underlying cardiac problems. Further investigation is warranted to rule out complications.

Respirations

Respiratory rates in the postpartum woman should be within the normal range of 16 to 20 breaths per minute. Any change in respiratory rate out of the normal range might indicate pulmonary edema, atelectasis, or pulmonary embolism and must be reported. Lungs should be clear on auscultation.

Blood Pressure

Assess the woman's blood pressure and compare it with her usual range. Report any deviation from this range. Elevations in blood pressure from baseline might suggest pregnancy-induced hypertension; decreases may suggest dehydration or excessive blood loss.

Blood pressure also may vary based on the woman's position, so assess blood pressure with the woman in the same position every time. Be alert for orthostatic hypotension, which can occur when the woman moves rapidly from a lying or sitting position to a standing one.

Pain

Pain, the fifth vital sign, is assessed along with the other four parameters. Question the woman about the type of pain and its location and severity. Have the woman rate the pain using a numeric scale from 0 to 10 points.

Many postpartum orders will have the nurse premedicate the woman routinely for afterbirth pains rather than wait for her to experience them first. The goal of pain management is to have the woman's pain scale rating maintained between 0 to 2 points at all times, especially after breast-feeding. This can be accomplished by assessing the woman's pain level frequently and preventing pain by administering analgesics. If the woman has severe pain in the perineal region despite use of physical comfort measures, check for a hematoma by inspecting and palpating the area. If one is found, notify the health care provider immediately.

Breasts

Inspect the breasts for size, contour, asymmetry, engorgement, or erythema. Check the nipples for cracks, redness, fissures, or bleeding, and note whether they are erect, flat, or inverted. Flat or inverted nipples can make breast-feeding challenging for both mother and infant. Cracked, blistered, fissured, bruised, or bleeding nipples in the breast-feeding woman are generally indications that the baby is improperly positioned on the breast. Palpate the breasts lightly to ascertain if they are soft, filling, or engorged, and document your findings. For women who are not breast-feeding, use a gentle, light touch to avoid breast stimulation, which would exacerbate engorgement. As milk is starting to come in, the breasts become firmer; this is charted as "filling." Engorged breasts are hard, tender, and taut. Ask the woman if she is having any nipple discomfort. Palpate the breasts for any nodules, masses, or areas of warmth, which may indicate a plugged duct that may progress to **mastitis** if not treated promptly. Any discharge from the nipple should be described and documented if it is not colostrum (creamy yellow) or foremilk (bluish white).

Uterus

Assess the fundus (top portion of the uterus) to determine the degree of uterine involution. If possible, have the woman empty her bladder before assessing the fundus. If the patient has had a cesarean birth and has a PCA pump, instruct her to self-medicate prior to fundal assessment to decrease her discomfort. Using a two-handed approach with the woman in the supine position and the bed in a flat position or as low as possible, palpate the abdomen gently, feeling for the top of the uterus while the other hand is placed on the lower segment of the uterus to stabilize it (Fig. 16.2).

The fundus should be midline and should feel firm. A boggy or relaxed uterus is a sign of uterine atony. This can be the result of bladder distention, which displaces the uterus upward and to the right, or retained placental fragments. Either situation predisposes the woman to hemorrhage.

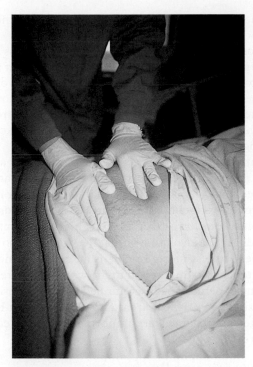

FIGURE 16.2 Palpating the fundus.

Once the fundus is located, place your index finger on the fundus and count the number of fingerbreadths between the fundus and the umbilicus (1 fingerbreadth is approximately equal to 1 cm). One to 2 hours after birth, the fundus typically is between the umbilicus and the symphysis pubis. Approximately 6 to 12 hours after birth, the fundus usually is at the level of the umbilicus.

Normally, the fundus progresses downward at a rate of one fingerbreadth (or 1 cm) per day after childbirth (Cunningham et al., 2005). On the first postpartum day, the top of the fundus is located 1 cm below the umbilicus and is recorded as U-1. Similarly, on the second postpartum day, the fundus would be 2 cm below the umbilicus and should be recorded as U-2, and so on. If the fundus is not firm, gently massage the uterus using a circular motion until it becomes firm.

Bladder

Considerable diuresis—as much as 3,000 mL—may follow for several days after childbirth, decreasing by the third day (Blackburn, 2007). However, many postpartum women do not sense the need to void even if their bladder is full. Women who received regional anesthesia during labor are at risk for bladder distention and for difficulty voiding until sensation returns within several hours after birth.

Assess for voiding problems by asking the woman the following questions:

• Have you (passed your water, urinated, gone to the bathroom) yet?
• Have you noticed any burning or discomfort with urination?
• Do you have any difficulty passing your urine?
• Do you feel that your bladder is empty when you finish urinating?
• Do you have any signs of infection such as urgency, frequency, or pain?
• Are you able to control the flow of urine by squeezing your muscles?
• Have you noticed any leakage of urine when you cough, laugh, or sneeze?

Assess the bladder for distention and adequate emptying after efforts to void. Palpate the area over the symphysis pubis. If empty, the bladder is not palpable. Palpation of a rounded mass suggests bladder distention. Also percuss the area: a full bladder is dull to percussion. If the bladder is full, lochia drainage will be more than normal because the uterus cannot contract to suppress the bleeding.

> ▶ **Take** NOTE!
>
> *Note the location and condition of the fundus; a full bladder tends to displace the uterus up and to the right.*

After the woman voids, palpate and percuss the area again to determine adequate emptying of the bladder. If the bladder remains distended, the woman may be retaining urine in her bladder, and measures to initiate voiding should be instituted. Be alert for signs of infection, including infrequent or insufficient voiding (less than 200 mL), discomfort, burning, urgency, or foul-smelling urine (Simpkin & James, 2006). Document urine output.

Bowels

Spontaneous bowel movements may not occur for 2 to 3 days after giving birth because of a decrease in muscle tone in the intestines during labor. Normal patterns of bowel elimination usually return within 8 to 14 days after birth (Blackburn, 2007).

Inspect the woman's abdomen for distention, auscultate for bowel sounds in all four quadrants, and palpate for tenderness. The abdomen typically is soft, nontender, and nondistended. Bowel sounds are present in all four quadrants. Ask the woman if she has had a bowel movement or has passed gas since giving birth, because constipation is a common problem during the postpartum period and most women do not offer this information unless asked about it. Normal assessment findings are active bowel sounds, passing gas, and a nondistended abdomen.

Lochia

Assess lochia in terms of amount, color, odor, and change with activity and time. To assess how much a woman is bleeding, ask her how many perineal pads she has used in the past 1 to 2 hours and how much drainage was on each pad. For example, did she saturate the pad completely, or was only half of the pad covered with drainage? Ask about the color of the drainage, odor, and the presence of any clots. Lochia has a definite musky scent, with an odor similar to that of menstrual flow without any large clots. Foul-smelling lochia suggests an infection, and large clots suggest poor uterine involution, necessitating additional intervention.

To determine the amount of lochia, observe the amount of lochia saturation on the perineal pad and relate it to time (Fig. 16.3). Lochia flow will increase when the woman gets out of bed (lochia pools in the vagina and the uterus while she is lying down) and when she breastfeeds (oxytocin release causes uterine contractions). A woman who saturates a perineal pad within 30 to 60 minutes is bleeding much more than one who saturates a pad in 2 hours. Typically, the amount of lochia is described as follows:

- Scant: a 1- to 2-inch lochia stain on the perineal pad or approximately a 10-mL loss
- Light or small: an approximately 4-inch stain or a 10- to 25-mL loss
- Moderate: a 4- to 6-inch stain with an estimated loss of 25 to 50 mL
- Large or heavy: a pad is saturated within 1 hour after changing it (Nash, 2007)

The total volume of lochia is approximately 240 to 270 mL (8 to 9 oz), and the amount decreases daily (Blackburn, 2007). Check under the woman to make sure there isn't additional blood hidden and not absorbed on her perineal pad.

Report any abnormal findings, such as heavy, bright-red lochia with large tissue fragments or a foul odor. If excessive bleeding occurs, the first step would be to massage the boggy fundus until it is firm to reduce the flow of blood. Document all findings.

Women who had a cesarean birth will have less lochia discharge than those who had a vaginal birth, but stages and color changes remain the same. Although the woman's abdomen will be tender after surgery, the nurse must palpate the fundus and assess the lochia to make sure they are within the normal range and that there is no excessive bleeding.

Anticipatory guidance to give the woman at discharge should include information about lochia and the expected changes. Urge the woman to notify her health care provider if lochia rubra returns after the serosa and alba transitions have taken place. This is abnormal and may indicate subinvolution or that the woman is too active and needs to rest more. Lochia is an excellent medium for bacterial growth. Explain to the woman that frequent changing of perineal pads, continued use of her peribottle for rinsing her perineal area, and handwashing before and after pad changes are important infection control measures.

Episiotomy and Perineum

To assess the episiotomy and perineal area, position the woman on her side with her top leg flexed upward at the knee and drawn up toward her waist. If necessary, use a penlight to provide adequate lighting during the assessment. Wearing gloves and standing at the woman's side with her back to you, gently lift the upper buttock to expose the perineum and anus (Fig. 16.4). Inspect the episiotomy for irritation, ecchymosis, tenderness, or hematomas. Assess for hemorrhoids and their condition.

During the early postpartum period, the perineal tissue surrounding the episiotomy is typically edematous and slightly bruised. The normal episiotomy site should not have redness, discharge, or edema. The majority of healing takes place within the first 2 weeks, but it may take 4 to 6 months for the episiotomy to heal completely (Blackburn, 2007).

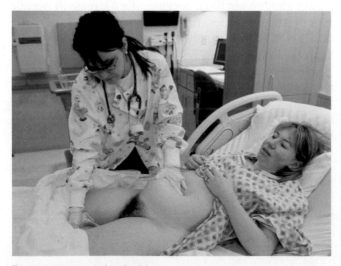

FIGURE 16.3 Assessing lochia.

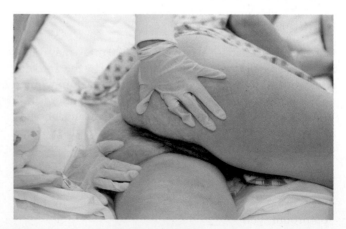

FIGURE 16.4 Inspecting the perineum.

Lacerations to the perineal area sustained during the birthing process that were identified and repaired also need to be assessed to determine their healing status. Lacerations are classified based on their severity and tissue involvement:

- First-degree laceration—involves only skin and superficial structures above muscle
- Second-degree laceration—extends through perineal muscles
- Third-degree laceration—extends through the anal sphincter muscle
- Fourth-degree laceration—continues through anterior rectal wall

Assess the episiotomy and any lacerations at least every 8 hours to detect hematomas or signs of infection. Large areas of swollen, bluish skin with complaints of severe pain in the perineal area indicate pelvic or vulvar hematomas. Redness, swelling, increasing discomfort, or purulent drainage may indicate infection. Both findings need to be reported immediately.

A white line the length of the episiotomy is a sign of infection, as is swelling or discharge. Severe, intractable pain, perineal discoloration, and ecchymosis indicate a perineal hematoma, a potentially dangerous condition. Report any unusual findings. Ice can be applied to relieve discomfort and reduce edema; sitz baths also can promote comfort and perineal healing (see "Promoting Comfort" in the Nursing Interventions section).

Extremities

During pregnancy, the state of hypercoagulability protects the mother against excessive blood loss during childbirth and placental separation. However, this hypercoagulable state can increase the risk of thromboembolic disorders during pregnancy and postpartum. Three factors predispose women to thromboembolic disorders during pregnancy: stasis (compression of the large veins because of the gravid uterus), altered coagulation (state of pregnancy), and localized vascular damage (may occur during birthing process). All of these increase the risk of clot formation.

> ▶ **Take** NOTE!
>
> *Pulmonary embolism occurs in 1 in 2,000 pregnancies and is a major cause of maternal mortality (Moses, 2007).*

Pulmonary emboli typically result from dislodged deep vein thrombi in the lower extremities. Risk factors associated with thromboembolic conditions include:

- Anemia
- Diabetes mellitus
- Cigarette smoking
- Obesity
- Preeclampsia secondary to exaggeration of hypercoagulable state
- Hypertension
- Varicose veins
- Pregnancy
- Oral contraceptive use
- Cesarean birth
- Previous thromboembolic disease
- Multiparity
- Inactivity
- Advanced maternal age (Hackley, Kriebs, & Rousseau, 2007)

Because of the subtle presentation of thromboembolic disorders, the physical examination may not be enough to detect them. The woman may report lower extremity tightness or aching when ambulating that is relieved with rest and elevation of the leg. Edema in the affected leg (typically the left), along with warmth and tenderness, may also be noted. A duplex ultrasound (two-dimensional ultrasound and Doppler ultrasound that compresses the vein to assess for changes in venous flow) in conjunction with the physical findings frequently is needed for a conclusive diagnosis (Kuntz, Cheesman, & Powers, 2006).

Women with an increased risk for this condition during the postpartum period should wear antiembolism stockings or use sequential compression devices to reduce their risk of thrombophlebitis. Encouraging the client to ambulate after childbirth reduces the incidence of thrombophlebitis.

Emotional Status

Assess the woman's emotional status by observing how she interacts with her family, her level of independence, energy levels, eye contact with her infant (within a cultural context), posture and comfort level while holding the newborn, and sleep and rest patterns. Be alert for mood swings, irritability, or crying episodes.

Remember Raina and her "quiet" husband, the Muslim couple? The postpartum nurse informs Raina that her doctor, Nancy Schultz, has been called away for emergency surgery and won't be available the rest of the day. The nurse explains that Dr. Robert Nappo will be making rounds for her. Raina and her husband become upset. Why? Is culturally competent care being provided to this couple?

Bonding and Attachment

Nurses can be instrumental in promoting attachment by assessing attachment behaviors (positive and negative) and intervening appropriately if needed. Nurses must be able to identify any family discord that might interfere with the attachment process. Remember, however, that mothers from different cultures may behave differently from what is expected in your own culture. For example, Native American mothers tend to handle their newborns less often and use cradle boards to carry them. Native American mothers and many Asian-American mothers delay breast-feeding until their milk comes in, because colostrum is considered harmful for the newborn (Bowers, 2007). Don't assume that different behavior is wrong.

Meeting the newborn for the first time after birth can be an exhilarating experience for parents. Although the mother has spent many hours dreaming of her unborn and how he or she will look, it is not until after birth that they meet face to face. They both need to get to know one another and to develop feelings for one another.

Bonding is the close emotional attraction to a newborn by the parents that develops during the first 30 to 60 minutes after birth. It is unidirectional, from parent to infant. It is thought that optimal bonding of the parents to a newborn requires a period of close contact within the first few minutes to a few hours after birth (Mercer, 2006). The mother initiates bonding when she caresses her infant and exhibits certain behaviors typical of a mother tending her child. The infant's responses to this, such as body and eye movements, are a necessary part of the process. During this initial period, the infant is in a quiet, alert state, looking directly at the holder.

> ▶ **Take** NOTE!
>
> *The length of time necessary for bonding depends on the health of the infant and mother, as well as the circumstances surrounding the labor and birth (Fowles & Horowitz, 2006).*

Attachment is the development of strong affection between an infant and a significant other (mother, father, sibling, and caretaker) (Grossman, Grossman, & Waters, 2006). This tie between two people is psychological rather than biological, and it does not occur overnight. The process of attachment follows a progressive or developmental course that changes over time. Attachment is an individualized and multifactorial process that differs based on the health of the infant, the mother, environmental circumstances, and the quality of care the infant receives (Wilson et al., 2007). It occurs through mutually satisfying experiences. Maternal attachment begins during pregnancy as the result of fetal movement and maternal fantasies about the infant and continues through the birth and postpartum periods. Attachment behaviors include seeking, staying close to, and exchanging gratifying experiences with the infant (Grossman, Grossman,

& Waters, 2006). In a high-risk pregnancy, the attachment process may be complicated by premature birth (lack of time to develop a relationship with the unborn baby) and by parental stress due to the fetal and/or maternal vulnerability.

Bonding is a vital component of the attachment process and is necessary in establishing parent–infant attachment and a healthy, loving relationship. During this early period of acquaintance, mothers touch their infants in a very characteristic manner. Mothers visually and physically "explore" their infants, initially using their fingertips on the infant's face and extremities and progressing to massaging and stroking the infant with their fingers. This is followed by palm contact on the trunk. Eventually, mothers draw their infant toward them and hold the infant. Mothers also interact with their infants through eye-to-eye contact in the *en face* position (Mercer, 2006) (Fig. 16.5).

Generally, research on attachment has found that the process is similar for fathers as for mothers, but the pace may be different. Like mothers, fathers manifest attachment behaviors during pregnancy; indeed, Grossman et al. (2006) found that the best predictor of early postnatal attachment for fathers is fetal attachment. Becoming a father requires a man to build on the experiences he has had throughout childhood and adolescence. Fathers develop an emotional tie with their infants in a variety of ways. They seek and maintain closeness with the infant and can recognize characteristics of the infant. They feel a sense of responsibility for the infant's growth and development (Wilson et al., 2007).

Attachment is a process; it does not occur instantaneously, even though many parents believe in a romanticized version of attachment, which happens right after birth. A delay in the attachment process can occur if a mother's physical and emotional states are adversely affected by exhaustion, pain, the absence of a support system, anesthesia, or an unwanted outcome (Feldman, 2007).

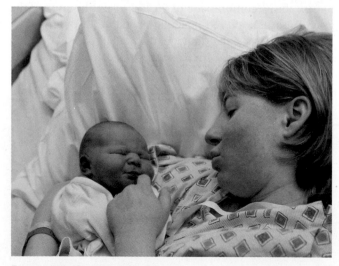

FIGURE **16.5** *En face* position.

> ▶ *Take* NOTE!
>
> *Many midwives teach fathers to massage their partners, which has been proven to have a positive effect on the pregnancy, labor, bonding and attachment, and perhaps on family dynamics (Whitehouse, 2006).*

The developmental task for the infant is learning to differentiate between trust and mistrust. If the mother or caretaker is consistently responsive to the infant's care, meeting the baby's physical and psychological needs, the infant will likely learn to trust the caretaker, view the world as a safe place, and grow up to be secure, self-reliant, trusting, cooperative, and helpful. However, if the infant's needs are not met, the child is more likely to face developmental delays, neglect, and child abuse (Logsdon, Wisner, & Pinto-Foltz, 2006).

"Becoming" a parent may take 4 to 6 months. The transition to parenthood, according to Mercer (2006), involves four stages:

1. Commitment, attachment, and preparation for an infant during pregnancy
2. Acquaintance with and increasing attachment to the infant, learning how to care for the infant, and physical restoration during the first weeks after birth
3. Moving toward a new normal routine in the first 4 months after birth
4. Achievement of a parenthood role around 4 months

The stages overlap, and the timing of each is affected by variables such as the environment, family dynamics, and the partners (Mercer, 2006).

Factors Affecting Attachment

Attachment behaviors are influenced by three major factors:

1. Parents' background (includes the care that the parents received when growing up, cultural practices, relationship within the family, experience with previous pregnancies and planning and course of events during pregnancy, postpartum depression)
2. Infant (includes the infant's temperament and health at birth)
3. Care practices (the behaviors of physicians, midwives, nurses, and hospital personnel, care and support during labor, first day of life in separation of mother and infant, and rules of the hospital or birthing center) (Grossman, Grossman, & Waters 2006)

Attachment occurs more readily with the infant whose temperament, health, appearance, and gender fit the par-

ent's expectations. If the infant does not meet these expectations, attachment can be delayed (Wilson et al., 2007).

Factors associated with the health care facility or birthing unit can also hinder attachment. These include:

- Separation of infant and parents immediately after birth and for long periods during the day
- Policies that discourage unwrapping and exploring the infant
- Intensive care environment, restrictive visiting policies
- Staff indifference or lack of support for parent's caretaking attempts and abilities

Critical Attributes of Attachment

The terms "bonding" and "attachment" are often used interchangeably, even though they involve different time frames and interactions. Attachment stages include proximity, reciprocity, and commitment.

Proximity refers to the physical and psychological experience of the parents being close to their infant. This attribute has three dimensions:

1. Contact—The sensory experiences of touching, holding, and gazing at the infant are part of proximity-seeking behavior.
2. Emotional state—The emotional state emerges from the affective experience of the new parents toward their infant and their parental role.
3. Individualization—Parents are aware of the need to differentiate the infant's needs from themselves and to recognize and respond to them appropriately, making the attachment process also, in some way, one of detachment.

Reciprocity is the process by which the infant's abilities and behaviors elicit parental response. Reciprocity is described by two dimensions: complementary behavior and sensitivity. Complementary behavior involves taking turns and stopping when the other is not interested or becomes tired. An infant can coo and stare at the parent to elicit a similar parental response to complement his or her behavior. Parents who are sensitive and responsive to their infant's cues will promote their development and growth. Parents who become skilled at recognizing the ways their infant communicates will respond appropriately by smiling, vocalizing, touching, and kissing.

Commitment refers to the enduring nature of the relationship. The components of this are twofold: centrality and parent role exploration. In centrality, parents place the infant at the center of their lives. They acknowledge and accept their responsibility to promote the infant's safety, growth, and development. Parent role exploration is the parents' ability to find their own way and integrate the parental identity into themselves (Grossman, Grossman, & Waters, 2006).

TABLE 16.1 POSITIVE AND NEGATIVE ATTACHMENT BEHAVIORS

	Positive Behaviors	Negative Behaviors
Infant	Smiles; is alert; demonstrates strong grasp reflex to hold parent's finger; sucks well, feeds easily; enjoys being held close; makes eye-to-eye contact; follows parent's face; appears facially appealing; is consolable when crying	Feeds poorly, regurgitates often; cries for long periods, colicky and inconsolable; shows flat affect, rarely smiles even when prompted; resists holding and closeness; sleeps with eyes closed most of time; stiffens body when held; is unresponsive to parents; doesn't pay attention to parents' faces
Parent	Makes direct eye contact; assumes *en face* position when holding infant; claims infant as family member, pointing out common features; expresses pride in infant; assigns meaning to infant's actions; smiles and gazes at infant; touches infant, progressing from fingertips to holding; names infant; requests to be close to infant as much as allowed; speaks positively about infant	Expresses disappointment or displeasure in infant; fails to "explore" infant visually or physically; fails to claim infant as part of family; avoids caring for infant; finds excuses not to hold infant close; has negative self-concept; appears uninterested in having infant in room; frequently asks to have infant taken back to nursery to be cared for; assigns negative attributes to infant and calls infant inappropriate, negative names (e.g., frog, monkey, tadpole)

Sources: Grossman, Grossman, & Waters, 2007; Nash, 2007; Oppenheim & Goldsmith, 2007.

Positive and Negative Attachment Behaviors

Positive bonding behaviors include maintaining close physical contact, making eye-to-eye contact, speaking in soft, high-pitched tones, and touching and exploring the infant. Table 16.1 highlights typical positive and negative behaviors of attachment.

Nursing Interventions

In terms of postpartum hospital stays today, "less is more." If the woman had a vaginal delivery, she may be discharged within 48 hours. If she had a cesarean birth, she may remain hospitalized from 72 to 96 hours. This shortened stay leaves little time for nurses to prepare the woman and her family for the many changes that will occur when she returns home. Nurses need to use this limited time to address the following topics: pain and discomfort, immunizations, nutrition, activity and exercise, lactation, discharge teaching, sexuality and contraception, and follow-up (see Nursing Care Plan 16.1).

▶ *Take NOTE!*

Always adhere to standard precautions when providing direct care to reduce the risk of disease transmission.

Providing Optimal Cultural Care

As the face of America is becoming more diverse, nurses must be prepared to care for childbearing families from various cultures. In many cultures, women and their families are cared for and nurtured by their community for weeks and even months after the birth of a new family member. Box 16.3 highlights some of the major cultural variants during the postpartum period.

Nurses need to remember that childbearing practices and beliefs vary in different cultures. To provide appropriate nursing care, the nurse should determine the patient's preferences before intervening. Cultural practices may include dietary restrictions, certain clothes, taboos, activities for maintaining mental health, and the use of silence, prayer, or meditation. Restoring health may involve taking folk medicines or conferring with a tribal healer (Srivastava, 2007).

Raina and her husband are upset at the thought of having a male doctor care for her because Muslim women are very modest and prefer having a same-sex care provider. What should the nurse do in this situation?

Promoting Comfort

The postpartum woman may have discomfort and pain from a variety of sources, such as an episiotomy, perineal lacerations, an edematous perineum, inflamed hemorrhoids, engorged breasts, afterbirth pains secondary to uterine contractions in breast-feeding and multiparous mothers, and sore nipples if breast-feeding. Nonpharmacologic and pharmacologic measures can be used to decrease pain and discomfort.

Applications of Cold and Heat

Commonly, an ice pack is the first measure used after a vaginal birth to relieve perineal discomfort from edema, an

Nursing Care Plan 16.1

OVERVIEW OF THE POSTPARTUM WOMAN

Belinda, a 26-year-old G2P2, is a patient on the mother–baby unit after giving birth to a term 8-lb, 12-oz baby boy yesterday. The night nurse reports that she has an episiotomy, complains of a pain rating of 7 points on a scale of 1 to 10, is having difficulty breast-feeding, and had heavy lochia most of the night. The nurse also reports that the patient seems focused on her own needs and not on her infant. Assessment this morning reveals the following:

B: Breasts are soft with colostrum leaking; nipples cracked
U: Uterus is one fingerbreadth below the umbilicus; deviated to right
B: Bladder is palpable; patient states she hasn't been up to void yet
B: Bowels have not moved; bowel sounds present; passing flatus
L: Lochia is moderate; peripad soaked from night accumulation
E: Episiotomy site intact; swollen, bruised; hemorrhoids present
—
E: Extremities; no edema over tibia, no warmth or tenderness in calf
E: Emotional status is "distressed" as a result of discomfort and fatigue

NURSING DIAGNOSIS: Impaired tissue integrity related to episiotomy

Outcome Identification and Evaluation
The woman remains free of infection, without any signs and symptoms of infection, and exhibits evidence of progressive healing as demonstrated by clean, dry, intact episiotomy site.

Interventions: Promoting Tissue Integrity
- Monitor episiotomy site for redness, edema, and signs of infection.
- Assess vital signs at least every 4 hours *to identify changes suggesting infection.*
- Apply ice pack to episiotomy site *to reduce swelling.*
- Instruct patient on use of sitz bath *to promote healing, hygiene, and comfort.*
- Encourage frequent perineal care and peripad changes *to prevent infection.*
- Recommend ambulation *to improve circulation and promote healing.*
- Instruct patient on positioning *to relieve pressure on perineal area.*
- Demonstrate use of anesthetic sprays *to numb perineal area.*

NURSING DIAGNOSIS: Pain related to episiotomy, sore nipples, and hemorrhoids

Outcome Identification and Evaluation
The woman experiences a decrease in pain, reporting that her pain has diminished to a tolerable level, rating it as 2 points or less.

Interventions: Providing Pain Relief
- Thoroughly inspect perineum *to rule out hematoma as cause of pain.*
- Administer analgesic medication as ordered as needed *to promote comfort.*
- Carry out comfort measures to episiotomy as outlined earlier *to reduce pain.*
- Explain discomforts and reassure the client that they are time-limited to assist in coping with pain.
- Apply Tucks pads to swollen hemorrhoids *to induce shrinkage and reduce pain.*
- Suggest frequent use of sitz bath *to reduce hemorrhoid pain.*
- Administer stool softener and laxative *to prevent straining with first bowel movement.*
- Observe positioning and latching-on technique while breast-feeding. Offer suggestions based on observations to correct positioning/latching on *to minimize trauma to the breast.*
- Suggest air-drying of nipples after breast-feeding and use of plain water *to prevent nipple cracking.*
- Teach relaxation techniques when breast-feeding *to reduce anxiety and discomfort.*

(continued)

Nursing Care Plan 16.1 (continued)

NURSING DIAGNOSIS: Risk for ineffective coping related to mood alteration and pain

Outcome Identification and Evaluation
The woman copes with mood alterations, as evidenced by positive statements about newborn and participation in newborn care.

Interventions: Promoting Effective Coping

- Provide a supportive, nurturing environment and encourage the mother to vent her feelings and frustrations to relieve anxiety.
- Provide opportunities for the mother to rest and sleep *to combat fatigue.*
- Encourage the mother to eat a well-balanced diet *to increase her energy level.*
- Provide reassurance and explanations that mood alterations are common after birth secondary to waning hormones after pregnancy *to increase the mother's knowledge.*
- Allow the mother relief from newborn care *to afford opportunity for self-care.*
- Discuss with partner expected behavior from mother and how additional support and help are needed during this stressful time *to promote partner's participation in care.*
- Make appropriate community referrals for mother–infant support *to ensure continuity of care.*
- Encourage frequent skin-to-skin contact and closeness between mother and infant *to facilitate bonding and attachment behaviors.*
- Encourage client to participate in infant care and provide instructions as needed *to foster a sense of independence and self-esteem.*
- Offer praise and reinforcement of positive mother–infant interactions *to enhance self-confidence in care.*

---

episiotomy, or laceration. It is applied during the fourth stage of labor and can be used for the first 24 hours to reduce perineal edema and to prevent hematoma formation, thus reducing pain and promoting healing. Ice packs are wrapped in a disposable covering or clean washcloth and are applied to the perineal area. Usually the ice pack is applied for 20 minutes and removed for 10 minutes. Many commercially prepared ice packs are available, but a latex glove filled with crushed ice and covered can also be used if the mother is not allergic to latex. Ensure that the ice pack is changed frequently to promote good hygiene and to allow for periodic assessments.

The **peribottle** is a plastic squeeze bottle filled with warm tap water that is sprayed over the perineal area after each voiding and before applying a new perineal pad. Usually the peribottle is introduced to the woman when she is assisted to the bathroom to freshen up and void for the first time—in most instances, once vital signs are stable after the first hour. Provide the woman with instructions on how and when to use the peribottle. Reinforce this practice each time she changes her pad, voids, or defecates, making sure that she understands to direct the flow of water from front to back. The woman can take the peribottle home and use it over the next several weeks until her lochia discharge stops. The peribottle can be used by women who had either vaginal or cesarean births to provide comfort and hygiene to the perineal area.

After the first 24 hours, a **sitz bath** with warm water may be prescribed and substituted for the ice pack to

reduce local swelling and promote comfort for an episiotomy, perineal trauma, or inflamed hemorrhoids. The change from cold to warm therapy enhances vascular circulation and healing (Steen, Briggs, & King, 2006). Before using a sitz bath, the woman should cleanse the perineum with a peribottle or take a shower using mild soap.

Most health care agencies use plastic disposable sitz baths that women can take home. The plastic sitz bath consists of a basin that fits on the commode; a bag filled with warm water is hung on a hook and connected via a tube onto the front of the basin (Fig. 16.6). Teaching Guidelines 16.1 highlights the steps in using a sitz bath.

Advise the woman to use the sitz bath several times daily to provide hygiene and comfort to the perineal area. Encourage her to continue this measure after discharge.

Some facilities have hygienic sitz baths called Suri-Gators in the bathroom that spray an antiseptic, water, or both onto the perineum. The woman sits on the toilet with legs apart so that the nozzle spray reaches her perineal area.

Keep in mind that tremendous hemodynamic changes are taking place within the mother during this early postpartum period, and her safety must be a priority. Fatigue, blood loss, the effects of medications, and lack of food may cause her to feel weak when she stands up. Assisting the woman to the bathroom to instruct her on how to use the peribottle and sitz bath is necessary to ensure her safety. Many women become lightheaded or dizzy when they get out of bed and need direct physical assistance. Staying in the woman's room, ensuring that the emer-

BOX 16.3 Cultural Influences During the Postpartum Period

African-American
- Mother may share care of the infant with extended family members.
- Experiences of older women within the family influence infant care.
- Mothers may protect their newborns from strangers for several weeks.
- Mothers may not bathe their newborns for the first week. Oils are applied to skin and hair to prevent dryness and cradle cap.
- Silver dollars may be taped over the infant's umbilicus in an attempt to flatten the slightly protruding umbilical stump.
- Sleeping with parents is a common practice (Bowers, 2007).

Amish
- Women consider childbearing their primary role in society.
- They generally oppose birth control.
- Pregnancy and childbirth are considered a private matter; they may conceal it from public knowledge.
- Women typically do not respond favorably when hurried to complete a self-care task. Nurses need to take cues from women indicating their readiness to complete morning self-care activities (Bowers, 2007).

Appalachian
- Infant colic is treated by passing the newborn through a leather horse's collar or administering weak catnip tea.
- An asafetida bag (a gum resin with a strong odor) is tied around the infant's neck to ward off disease.
- Women may avoid eye contact with nurses and health care providers.
- Women typically avoid asking questions even though they do not understand directions.
- The grandmother may rear the infant for the mother (Armstrong & Feldman, 2007).

Filipino-American
- Grandparents often assist in the care of their grandchildren.
- Breast-feeding is encouraged, and some mothers breast-feed their children for up to 2 years.
- Women have difficulty discussing birth control and sexual matters.
- Strong religious beliefs prevail and bedside prayer is common.
- Families are very close-knit and numerous visitors can be expected to the hospital after childbirth (Srivastava, 2007).

Japanese-American
- Cleanliness and protection from cold are essential components of newborn care. Nurses should give the daily bath to the infant.

- Newborns routinely are not taken outside the home because it is believed that they should not be exposed to outside or cold air. Infants should be kept in a quiet, clean, warm place for the first month of life.
- Breast-feeding is the primary method of feeding.
- Many women stay in their parents' home for 1 to 2 months after birth.
- Bathing the infant can be the center of family activity at home (Bowers, 2007).

Mexican-American
- The newborn's grandmother lives with the mother for several weeks after birth to help with housekeeping and child care.
- Most women will breast-feed more than 1 year. The infant is carried in a *rebozo* (shawl) that allows easy access for breast-feeding.
- Women may avoid eye contact and may not feel comfortable being touched by a stranger. Nurses need to respect this feeling.
- Some women may bring religious icons to the hospital and may want to display them in their room (Srivastava, 2007).

Muslim
- Modesty is a primary concern; nurses need to protect the client's modesty.
- Muslims are not permitted to eat pork; check all food items before serving.
- Muslims prefer a same-sex health care provider; male–female touching is prohibited except in an emergency situation.
- A Muslim woman stays in the house for 40 days after birth, being cared for by the female members of her family.
- Most women will breast-feed, but religious events call for periods of fasting, which may increase the risk of dehydration or malnutrition.
- Women are exempt from obligatory five-times-daily prayers as long as lochia is present.
- Extended family is likely to be present throughout much of the woman's hospital stay. They will need an empty room to perform their prayers without having to leave the hospital (Cassar, 2006).

Native American
- Women are secretive about pregnancies and do not reveal them early.
- Touching is not a typical female behavior and eye contact is brief.
- They resent being hurried and need time for sitting and talking.
- Most mothers breast-feed and practice birth control (Srivastava, 2007).

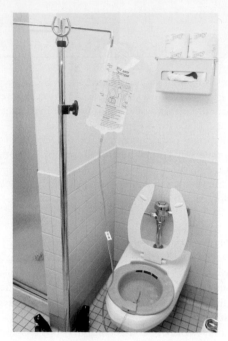

FIGURE 16.6 Sitz bath set-up.

TEACHING GUIDELINES 16.1

Using a Sitz Bath

1. Close clamp on tubing before filling bag with water to prevent leakage.
2. Fill sitz bath basin and plastic bag with warm water (comfortable to touch).
3. Place the filled basin on the toilet with the seat raised and the overflow opening facing toward the back of the toilet.
4. Hang the filled plastic bag on a hook close to the toilet or an IV pole.
5. Attach the tubing to the opening on the basin.
6. Sit on the basin positioned on the toilet seat and release the clamp to allow warm water to irrigate the perineum.
7. Remain sitting on the basin for approximately 15 to 20 minutes.
8. Stand up and pat the perineum area dry. Apply a clean peripad.
9. Tip the basin to remove any remaining water and flush the toilet.
10. Wash the basin with warm water and soap and dry it in the sink.
11. Store basin and tubing in a clean, dry area until the next use.
12. Wash hands with soap and water.

---

gency call light is readily available, and being available if needed during this early period will ensure safety and prevent accidents and falls.

Topical Preparations

Several treatments may be applied topically for temporary relief of pain and discomfort. One such treatment is a local anesthetic spray such as Dermoplast or Americaine. These agents numb the perineal area and are used after cleansing the area with water via the peribottle and/or a sitz bath.

For hemorrhoid discomfort, cool witch hazel pads, such as Tucks Pads, can be used. The pads are placed at the rectal area, between the hemorrhoids and the perineal pad. These pads cool the area, help relieve swelling, and minimize itching.

Analgesics

Analgesics such as acetaminophen (Tylenol) and oral nonsteroidal anti-inflammatory drugs (NSAIDs) such as ibuprofen (Motrin) are prescribed to relieve mild postpartum discomfort. For moderate to severe pain, a narcotic analgesic such as codeine or oxycodone in conjunction with aspirin or acetaminophen may be prescribed. Instruct the woman about adverse effects of any medication prescribed. Common adverse effects of oral analgesics include dizziness, lightheadedness, nausea and vomiting, constipation, and sedation (Skidmore-Roth, 2007).

Also inform the woman that the drugs are secreted in breast milk. Nearly all medications that the mother takes are passed into her breast milk; however, the mild analgesics (e.g., acetaminophen or ibuprofen) are considered relatively safe for breast-feeding mothers (Tomasulo, 2007). Administering a mild analgesic approximately an hour before breast-feeding will usually relieve afterpains and/or perineal discomfort.

Assisting With Elimination

The bladder is edematous, hypotonic, and congested immediately postpartum. Consequently, bladder distention, incomplete emptying, and inability to void are common. A full bladder interferes with uterine contraction and may lead to hemorrhage, because it will displace the uterus out of the midline. Encourage the woman to void. Often, assisting her to assume the normal voiding position on the commode facilitates this. If the woman has difficulty voiding, pouring warm water over the perineal area, hearing the sound of running tap water, blowing bubbles through a straw, taking a warm shower, drinking fluids, or placing her hand in a basin of warm water may stimulate voiding. If these actions do not stimulate urination within 4 to 6 hours after giving birth, catheterization may be needed. Palpate the bladder for distention and ask the woman if she is voiding in small amounts (less than 100 mL) frequently (retention with overflow). If catheterization is necessary, use sterile technique to reduce the risk of infection.

EVIDENCE-BASED PRACTICE 16.1
Topically Applied Anesthetics for Treating Perineal Pain After Childbirth

● Study

The perineum (the area between the vagina and rectum) may be traumatized during childbirth following a tear or a surgical cut (episiotomy). Perineal trauma after childbirth affects millions of women around the world each year. The degree of perineal pain and discomfort associated with perineal trauma is often underestimated. Pain often interferes with basic daily activities such as walking, sitting, and passing urine and also detracts from the experience of motherhood. Local anesthetics are easy to use and inexpensive, but their effectiveness needs to be assessed. A study was performed to assess the effects of topically applied anesthetics to relieve perineal pain after childbirth while the mother was still in the hospital and after discharge. This review of trials found eight studies using a variety of anesthetics.

▲ Findings

Data were insufficient to show that the topical anesthetics helped relieve perineal pain, and long-term effects were not assessed. More research is required to assess the effectiveness of topical anesthetics on pain, longer-term outcomes, women's relationships, and quality of life, as well as the effectiveness of different topical anesthetics.

■ Nursing Implications

Although this study could not validate topical anesthetics' effectiveness in relieving perineal pain, they do provide relief to many postpartum women. The nurse should assess each woman individually and offer other comfort alternatives such as warm sitz baths, ice packs, and ambulation. Further research will be needed to offer proof that topical anesthetics are an effective pain relief measure.

Hedayati, H., Parsons, J., & Crowther, C. A. (2006). Topically applied anesthetics for treating perineal pain after childbirth. *Cochrane Database of Systematic Reviews* 2006, Issue 2. Art. No.: CD004223. DOI: 10.1002/14651858.CD004223.pub2.

Decreased bowel motility during labor, high iron content in prenatal vitamins, postpartum fluid loss, and the adverse effects of pain medications and/or anesthesia may predispose the postpartum woman to constipation. In addition, the woman may fear that bowel movements will cause pain or injury, especially if she had an episiotomy or a laceration that was repaired with sutures.

Usually a stool softener, such as docusate (Colace), with or without a laxative might be helpful if the client has difficulty with bowel elimination. Other measures, such as ambulating and increasing fluid and fiber intake, may also help. Nutritional instruction might include increasing fruits and vegetables in the diet; drinking plenty of fluids (8 to 12 cups) to keep the stool soft; drinking small amounts of prune juice and/or hot liquids to stimulate peristalsis; eating high-fiber foods such as bran cereals, whole grains, dried fruits, fresh fruits, and raw vegetables; and walking daily.

Promoting Activity, Rest, and Exercise

The postpartum period is an ideal time for nurses to promote the importance of physical fitness, help women incorporate exercise into their lifestyle, and encourage them to overcome barriers to exercise. The lifestyle changes that occur postpartum may affect a woman's health for decades. Early ambulation is encouraged to reduce the risk of thromboembolism and to improve strengthening.

Many changes occur postpartum, and caring for a newborn alters the woman's eating and sleeping habits, work schedules, and time allocation. Postpartum fatigue is common during the early days after childbirth, and it may continue for weeks or months (Runquist, 2007). It affects the mother's relationships with significant others and her ability to fulfill household and child care responsibilities. Be sure that the mother recognizes her need for rest and sleep and is realistic about her expectations. Some suggestions include the following:

- Nap when the infant is sleeping, because getting uninterrupted sleep at night is difficult.
- Reduce participation in outside activities and limit the number of visitors.
- Determine the infant's sleep–wake cycles and attempt to increase wakeful periods during the day so the baby sleeps for longer periods at night.
- Eat a balanced diet to promote healing and to increase energy levels.
- Share household tasks to conserve your energy.
- Ask the father or other family members to provide infant care during the night periodically so that you can get an uninterrupted night of sleep.
- Review your family's daily routine and see if you can "cluster" activities to conserve energy and promote rest.

The demands of parenthood may reduce or prevent exercise in even the most committed person. A targeted exercise program and proper body mechanics can help new mothers deal with the physical challenges of motherhood. Emphasize the benefits of a regular exercise program, which include:

- Helps the woman to lose pregnancy weight
- Increases energy level so the woman can cope with her new responsibilities

• Speeds the return to prepregnant size and shape
• Provides an outlet for stress (Druxman & Petersen, 2006)

More than one third of American women are overweight (CDC, Office of Women's Health, 2007). Although the average gestational weight gain is small (approximately 25 to 35 lb), excess weight gain and failure to lose weight after pregnancy are important predictors of long-term obesity. Breast-feeding and exercise may help to control weight in the long term (AAP, 2005).

> ▶ *Take* NOTE!
>
> *Women who have not returned to their prepregnant weight by 6 months are likely to retain the extra weight (Hackley, Kriebs, & Rousseau, 2007). Encourage women to lose their pregnancy weight by 6 months postpartum, and refer those who don't to community weight-loss programs.*

The postpartum woman may face some obstacles to exercising, including physical changes (ligament laxity), competing demands (newborn care), lack of information about weight retention (inactivity equates to weight gain), and stress incontinence (leaking of urine during activity).

A healthy woman with an uncomplicated vaginal birth can resume exercise in the immediate postpartum period. Advise the woman to start slowly and increase the level of exercise over a period of several weeks as tolerated. Jogging strollers may be an option for some women, allowing them to exercise with their newborns. Also, exercise videos and home exercise equipment allow mothers to work out while the newborn naps.

Exercising after giving birth promotes feelings of well-being and restores muscle tone lost during pregnancy. Routine exercise should be resumed gradually, beginning with Kegel exercises on the first postpartum day and, by the second week, progressing to abdominal, buttock, and thigh-toning exercises (Druxman & Petersen, 2006). Walking is an excellent form of early exercise as long as the woman avoids jarring and bouncing movements, because joints do not stabilize until 6 to 8 weeks postpartum. Exercising too much too soon can cause the woman to bleed more and her lochia may return to bright red.

Recommended exercises for the first few weeks postpartum include abdominal breathing, head lifts, modified sit-ups, double knee roll, and pelvic tilt (Teaching Guidelines 16.2). The number of exercises and their duration is gradually increased as the woman gains strength.

Remember that cultures have different attitudes toward exercise. Some cultures (e.g., Haitian, Arab-

TEACHING GUIDELINES 16.2

Exercising

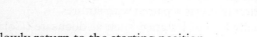

Abdominal Breathing

1. While lying on a flat surface (floor or bed), take a deep breath through your nose and expand your abdominal muscles (they will rise up from your midsection).
2. Slowly exhale and tighten your abdominal muscles for 3 to 5 seconds.
3. Repeat this several times.

Head Lift

1. Lie on a flat surface with knees flexed and feet flat on the surface.
2. Lift your head off the flat surface, tuck it onto your chest, and hold for 3 to 5 seconds.
3. Relax your head and return to the starting position.
4. Repeat this several times.

Modified Sit-Ups

1. Lie on a flat surface and raise your head and shoulders 6 to 8 inches so that your outstretched hands reach your knees.
2. Keep your waist on the flat surface.

3. Slowly return to the starting position.
4. Repeat, increasing in frequency as your comfort level allows.

Double Knee Roll

1. Lie on a flat surface with your knees bent.
2. While keeping your shoulders flat, slowly roll your knees to your right side to touch the flat surface (floor or bed).
3. Roll your knees back over your body to the left side until they touch the opposite side of the flat surface.
4. Return to the starting position on your back and rest.
5. Repeat this exercise several times.

Pelvic Tilt

1. Lie on your back on a flat surface with your knees bent and your arms at your side.
2. Slowly contract your abdominal muscles while lifting your pelvis up toward the ceiling.
3. Hold for 3 to 5 seconds and slowly return to your starting position.
4. Repeat several times..

American, and Mexican) expect new mothers to observe a specific period of bed rest or activity restriction; thus, it would be inappropriate to recommend active exercise during the early postpartum period (Bowers, 2007).

Preventing Stress Incontinence

Fifty percent of all parous women develop some degree of pelvic prolapse in their lifetime that is associated with stress incontinence (Thomason & DeLancey, 2007). The more vaginal deliveries a woman has had, the more likely she is to have stress incontinence. Stress incontinence can occur with any activity that causes an increase in intra-abdominal pressure. Postpartum women might consider low-impact activities such as walking, biking, swimming, or low-impact aerobics so they can resume physical activity while strengthening the pelvic floor.

Suggestions to prevent stress incontinence are:

- Start a regular program of Kegel exercises after childbirth.
- Lose weight if necessary; obesity is associated with stress incontinence.
- Avoid smoking; limit intake of alcohol and caffeinated beverages, which irritate the bladder.

Kegel exercises help to strengthen the pelvic floor muscles if done properly and regularly (Lemarck, 2007). Kegel exercises were originally developed by Dr. Arnold Kegel as a method of controlling incontinence in women after childbirth. The principle behind these exercises is that strengthening the muscles of the pelvic floor improves urethral sphincter function.

While providing postpartum care, instruct women on primary prevention of stress incontinence by discussing the value and purpose of Kegel exercises. Approach the subject sensitively, avoiding the term "incontinent." The terms "leakage," "loss of urine," or "bladder control issues" are more acceptable to most women.

> ▶ **Take** NOTE!
>
> *When properly performed, Kegel exercises have been effective in preventing or improving urinary continence (Lemack, 2007).*

Women can perform Kegel exercises, doing ten 5-second contractions, whenever they change diapers, talk on the phone, or watch TV. Teach the woman to perform Kegel exercises properly; help her to identify the correct muscles by trying to stop and start the flow of urine when sitting on the toilet (Teaching Guidelines 16.3). Kegel exercises can be done without anyone knowing.

Assisting With Self-Care Measures

Demonstrate and discuss with the woman ways to prevent infection during the postpartum period. Because she

TEACHING GUIDELINES 16.3

Performing Kegel Exercises

1. Identify the correct pelvic floor muscles by contracting them to stop the flow of urine while sitting on the toilet.
2. Repeat this contraction several times to become familiar with it.
3. Start the exercises by emptying the bladder.
4. Tighten the pelvic floor muscles and hold for 10 seconds.
5. Relax the muscle completely for 10 seconds.
6. Perform 10 exercises at least three times daily. Progressively increase the number that you perform.
7. Perform the exercises in different positions, such as standing, lying, and sitting.
8. Keep breathing during the exercises.
9. Don't contract your abdominal, thigh, leg, or buttocks muscles during these exercises.
10. Relax while doing Kegel exercises and concentrate on isolating the right muscles.
11. Attempt to tighten your pelvic muscles before sneezing, jumping, or laughing.
12. Remember that you can perform Kegel exercises anywhere without anyone noticing.

may experience lochia drainage for as long as a month after childbirth, describe practices to promote well-being and healing. These measures include:

- Frequently change perineal pads, applying and removing them from front to back to prevent spreading contamination from the rectal area to the genital area.
- Avoid using tampons after giving birth to decrease the risk of infection.
- Shower once or twice daily using a mild soap. Avoid using soap on nipples.
- Use a sitz bath after every bowel movement to cleanse the rectal area and relieve enlarged hemorrhoids.
- Use the peribottle filled with warm water after urinating and before applying a new perineal pad.
- Avoid tub baths for 4 to 6 weeks, until joints and balance are restored, to prevent falls.
- Wash your hands before changing perineal pads, after disposing of soiled pads, and after voiding (Brown, 2006).

To reduce the risk of infection at the episiotomy site, reinforce proper perineal care with the client, showing her how to rinse her perineum with the peribottle after she voids or defecates. Stress the importance of always patting gently from front to back and washing her hands thoroughly before and after perineal care. For hemorrhoids, have the client apply witch hazel-soaked pads

(Tucks Pads), ice packs to relieve swelling, or hemorrhoidal cream or ointment if ordered.

Ensuring Safety

One of the safety concerns during the postpartum period is orthostatic hypotension. When the woman moves from a lying or sitting position to a standing one rapidly, her blood pressure can suddenly drop, causing her pulse rate to increase. She may become dizzy and faint. Be aware of this problem and initiate the following safeguards:

- Check blood pressure first before ambulating the client.
- Elevate the head of the bed for a few minutes before ambulating the client.
- Have the client sit on the side of the bed for a few moments before getting up.
- Help the client to stand up, and stay with her.
- Ambulate alongside the client and provide support if needed.
- Frequently ask the client how her head feels.
- Stay close by to assist if she feels lightheaded.

Additional topics to address concern infant safety. Instruct the woman to place the newborn back in the crib on his or her back if she is feeling sleepy. If the woman falls asleep while holding the infant, she might drop him or her. Also, instruct mothers to keep the door to their room closed when their infant is in their room with them. They should check the identification of anyone who enters their room or who wants to take the infant out of the room. This will prevent infant abduction.

Counseling About Sexuality and Contraception

Sexuality is an important part of every woman's life. Women want to get back to "normal" as soon as possible after giving birth, but the couple's sexual relationship cannot be isolated from the psychological and psychosocial adjustments that both partners are going through.

Postpartum women may hesitate to resume sexual relations for a number of reasons. Many postpartum women have fatigue, weakness, vaginal bleeding, perineal discomfort, hemorrhoids, sore breasts, decreased vaginal lubrication resulting from low estrogen levels, and dyspareunia. Fatigue, the physical demands made by the infant, and the stress of new roles and responsibilities may stress the emotional reserves of couples. New parents may not get much privacy or rest, both of which are necessary for sexual pleasure (Pastore, Owens, & Raymond, 2007).

Men may feel they now have a secondary role within the family, and they may not understand their partner's daily routine. These issues, combined with the woman's increased investment in the mothering role, can strain the couple's sexual relationship.

Although couples are reluctant to ask, they often want to know when they can safely resume sexual intercourse after childbirth. Typically, sexual intercourse can be resumed once bright-red bleeding has stopped and the perineum is healed from an episiotomy or lacerations. This is usually by the third to the sixth week postpartum. However, there is not a set, prescribed time to resume sexual intercourse after childbirth. Each couple must set their own time frame when they feel it is appropriate to resume sexual intercourse.

When counseling the couple about sexuality, determine what knowledge and concerns the couple have about their sexual relationship. Inform the couple that fluctuations in sexual interest are normal. Also inform the couple about what to expect when resuming sexual intercourse and how to prevent discomfort. Precoital vaginal lubrication may be impaired during the postpartum period, especially in women who are breast-feeding. Use of water-based gel lubricants (KY jelly, Astroglide) can help. Pelvic floor exercises, in addition to preventing stress incontinence, can also enhance sensation.

Contraceptive options should be included in the discussions with the couple so that they can make an informed decision before resuming sexual activity. Many couples are overwhelmed with the amount of new information given to them during their brief hospitalization, so many are not ready for a lengthy discussion about contraceptives. Presenting a brief overview of the options, along with literature, may be appropriate. It may be suitable to ask them to think about contraceptive needs and preferences and advise them to use a barrier method (condom with spermicidal gel or foam) until they choose another form of contraceptive. This advice is especially important if the follow-up appointment will not occur for 4 to 6 weeks after childbirth, as many couples will resume sexual activity before this time. Some postpartum women ovulate before their menstrual period returns and thus need contraceptive protection to prevent another pregnancy.

Open and effective communication is necessary for effective contraceptive counseling so that information is clearly understood. Provide clear, consistent information appropriate to the woman and her partner's language, culture, and educational level. This will help them select the best contraceptive method (Engin-Ustun et al., 2007).

Promoting Nutrition

The postpartum period can be a stressful one for myriad reasons, such as fatigue, the physical stress of pregnancy and birth, and the nonstop work required to take care of the newborn and to meet the needs of other family members. As a result, the new mother may ignore her own nutrition needs. Whether she is breast-feeding or bottle-feeding, encourage the new mother to take good care of herself and eat a healthy diet so that the nutrients lost during pregnancy can be replaced and she can return to a healthy weight. In general, nutrition recommendations for the postpartum woman include the following:

- Eat a wide variety of foods with high nutrient density.
- Eat meals that require little or no preparation.

- Avoid high-fat fast foods.
- Drink plenty of fluids daily—at least 2,500 mL (approximately 84 oz).
- Avoid fad weight-reduction diets and harmful substances such as alcohol, tobacco, and drugs.
- Avoid excessive intake of fat, salt, sugar, and caffeine.
- Eat the recommended daily servings from each food group (Box 16.4).

The breast-feeding mother's nutritional needs are higher than they were during pregnancy. The mother's diet and nutritional status influence the quantity and quality of breast milk. To meet the needs for milk production, the woman's nutritional needs increase as follows:

- Calories: +500 cal/day for the first and second 6 months of lactation
- Protein: +20 g/day, adding an extra 2 cups of skim milk
- Calcium: +400 mg daily—consumption of four or more servings of milk
- Fluid: +2 to 3 quarts of fluids daily (milk, juice or water); no sodas

Certain foods (usually gaseous or strong-flavored ones) eaten by the mother may affect the flavor of the breast milk or cause gastrointestinal problems for the infant. Not all infants are affected by the same foods. If the particular food item seems to cause a problem, urge the mother to eliminate that food for a few days to see if the problem disappears.

BOX 16.4 **Nutritional Recommendations for Nutrition During the Postpartum Period**

Recommendations for the Lactating Woman From the Food Guide Pyramid
- Fruits: 4 servings
- Vegetables: 4 servings
- Milk: 4 to 5 servings
- Bread, cereal, pasta: 12 or more servings
- Meat, poultry, fish, eggs: 7 servings
- Fats, oils, and sweets: 5 servings (Dudek, 2006)

General Dietary Guidelines for Americans from the Food Guide Pyramid (for the Non-lactating Woman)
- Fruits: 2 to 4 servings
- Vegetables: 3 to 5 servings
- Milk: 2 to 3 servings
- Breads, grains, and cereals: 6 to 11 servings
- Meat, poultry, fish, eggs: 2 to 3 servings
- Fats, oils, and sweets: use sparingly (USDA & USDHHS, 2005)

▶ *Take NOTE!*

During the woman's brief stay in the health care facility, she may demonstrate a healthy appetite and eat well. Nutritional problems usually start at home when the mother needs to make her own food selections and prepare her own meals. This is a crucial area to address during follow-up.

Supporting the Woman's Choice of Feeding Method

While there is considerable evidence that breast-feeding has numerous health benefits, many mothers choose to feed their infants formula for the first year of life. Nurses must be able to deliver sound, evidence-based information to help the new mother choose the best way to feed her infant and must support her in her decision (Lawson, 2007).

Many factors affect a woman's choice of feeding method, such as culture, employment demands, support from significant others and family, and knowledge base. Although breast-feeding is encouraged, be sure that couples have the information they need to make an informed decision. Whether a couple chooses to breast-feed or bottle-feed the newborn, support and respect their choice.

Certain women should not breast-feed. Drugs such as antithyroid drugs, antineoplastic drugs, alcohol, or street drugs (amphetamines, cocaine, PCP, marijuana) enter the breast milk and would harm the infant, so women taking these substances should not breast-feed. To prevent HIV transmission to the newborn, women who are HIV positive should not breast-feed. Other contraindications to breast-feeding include a newborn with an inborn error of metabolism such as galactosemia or PKU, a current pregnancy, or a serious mental health disorder that would prevent the mother from remembering to feed the infant consistently.

Providing Assistance With Breast-Feeding and Bottle-Feeding

First-time mothers often have many questions about feeding, and even women who have had experience with feeding may have questions. Regardless of whether the postpartum woman is breast-feeding or bottle-feeding her newborn, she can benefit from instruction.

Providing Assistance with Breast-Feeding

WATCH&LEARN

The American Academy of Pediatrics (AAP, 2005) recommends breast-feeding for all full-term newborns. Exclusive breast-feeding is sufficient to support optimal growth and development for approximately the first 6 months of life. Breast-feeding should be continued for at least the first year of life and beyond for as long as mutually desired by mother and child. Educating a mother about breast-feeding will increase the likelihood of a successful breast-feeding experience.

At birth, all newborns should be quickly dried, assessed, and, if stable, placed immediately in uninterrupted skin-to-skin contact (kangaroo care) with their mother. This is good practice whether the mother is going to breast-feed or bottle-feed her infant. Kangaroo care provides the newborn with optimal physiologic stability, warmth, and opportunities for the first feed (Kenner & Lott, 2007).

The benefits of breast-feeding are clear (see Chap. 18). To promote breast-feeding, the Baby-Friendly Hospital Initiative, an international program of the World Health Organization and the United Nations Children's Fund, was started in 1991. As part of this program, the hospital or birth center should take the following 10 steps to provide "an optimal environment for the promotion, protection, and support of breast-feeding":

1. Have a written breast-feeding policy that is communicated to all staff.
2. Educate all staff to implement this written policy.
3. Inform all women about the benefits and management of breast-feeding.
4. Show all mothers how to initiate breast-feeding within 30 minutes of birth.
5. Give no food or drink other than breast milk to all newborns.
6. Demonstrate to all mothers how to initiate and maintain breast-feeding.
7. Encourage breast-feeding on demand.
8. Allow no pacifiers to be given to breast-feeding infants.
9. Establish breast-feeding support groups and refer mothers to them.
10. Practice rooming-in 24 hours daily (UNICEF, 2007).

The nurse is responsible for encouraging breast-feeding when appropriate. For the woman who chooses to breast-feed her infant, the nurse or lactation consultant will need to spend time instructing her how to do so successfully. Many women have the impression that breast-feeding is simple. Although it is a natural process, women may experience some difficulty in breast-feeding their newborns. Nurses can assist mothers in smoothing out this transition. Assist and provide one-to-one instruction to breast-feeding mothers, especially first-time breast-feeding mothers, to ensure correct technique. Suggestions are highlighted in Teaching Guidelines 16.4.

▶ **Take** NOTE!

Some newborns "latch on and catch on" right away, and others take more time and patience. Inform new mothers about this to reduce their frustration and uncertainty about their ability to breast-feed.

Tell mothers that they need to believe in themselves and their ability to accomplish this task. They should not panic if breast-feeding does not go smoothly at first; it takes time and practice. Additional suggestions to help mothers relax and feel more comfortable breast-feeding, especially when they return home, include the following:

- Select a quiet corner or room where you won't be disturbed.
- Use a rocking chair to soothe both you and your infant.
- Take long, slow deep breaths to relax before nursing.
- Drink while breast-feeding to replenish body fluids.
- Listen to soothing music while breast-feeding.
- Cuddle and caress the infant while feeding.
- Set out extra cloth diapers within reach to use as burping cloths.
- Allow sufficient time to enjoy each other in an unhurried atmosphere.
- Involve other family members in all aspects of the infant's care from the start.

Providing Assistance With Bottle-Feeding

If the mother or couple has chosen to bottle-feed their newborn, the nurse should respect and support their decision. Discuss with the parents what type of formula they will use. Commercial formulas are classified as cow's milk-based (Enfamil, Similac), soy protein-based (Isomil, Prosobee, Nursoy), or specialized or therapeutic formulas for infants with protein allergies (Nutramigen, Pregestimil, Alimentum). Commercial formulas can also be purchased in various forms: powdered (must be mixed with water), condensed liquid (must be diluted with equal amounts of water), ready to use (poured directly into bottles), and prepackaged (ready to use in disposable bottles).

Newborns need about 108 cal/kg or approximately 650 cal/day (Dudek, 2006). Therefore, explain to parents that a newborn will need to 2 to 4 ounces to feel satisfied at each feeding. Until about age 4 months, most bottle-fed infants need six feedings a day. After this time, the number of feedings declines to accommodate other foods in the diet, such as fruits, cereals, and vegetables (Escott-Stump, 2007). For more information on newborn nutrition and bottle feeding, see Chapter 18.

When teaching the mother about bottle-feeding, provide the following guidelines:

- Make feeding a relaxing time, a time to provide both food and comfort to your newborn.
- Use the feeding period to promote bonding by smiling, singing, making eye contact, and talking to the infant.
- Always hold the newborn when feeding. Never prop the bottle.
- Use a comfortable position when feeding the newborn. Place the newborn in your dominant arm, which is supported by a pillow. Or have the newborn in a semi-upright position supported in the crook of your arm (this position reduces choking and the flow of milk into the middle ear).

TEACHING GUIDELINES 16.4

Breast-Feeding Suggestions

- Explain that breast-feeding is a learned skill for both parties.
- Offer a thorough explanation about the procedure.
- Instruct the mother to wash her hands before starting.
- Inform her that her afterpains will increase during breast-feeding.
- Make sure the mother is comfortable (pain-free) and not hungry.
- Tell the mother to start the feeding with an awake and alert infant showing hunger signs.
- Assist the mother to position herself correctly for comfort.
- Urge the mother to relax to encourage the let-down reflex.
- Guide the mother's hand to form a "C" to access the nipple.
- Have the mother lightly tickle the infant's upper lip with her nipple to stimulate the infant to open the mouth wide.
- Help her to latch on by bringing the infant rapidly to the breast with a wide-open mouth.
- Show her how to check that the newborn's mouth position is correct, and tell her to listen for a sucking noise.
- Demonstrate correct removal from the breast, using her finger to break the suction.
- Instruct the mother on how to burp the infant between breasts.
- Show her different positions, such as cradle and football holds and side-lying positions (see Chap. 18).
- Reinforce and praise the mother for her efforts.
- Allow ample time to answer questions and address concerns.
- Refer the mother to support groups and community resources.

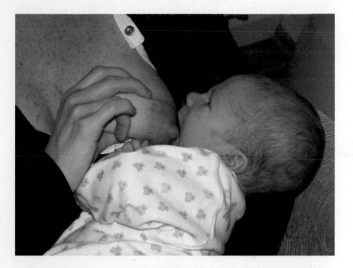

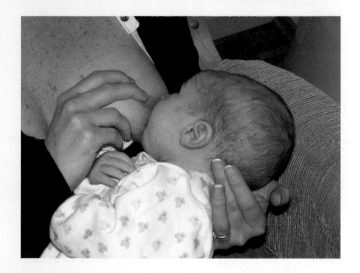

- Tilt the bottle so that the nipple and the neck of the bottle are always filled with formula. This prevents the infant from taking in too much air.
- Stimulate the sucking reflex by touching the nipple to the infant's lips.
- Refrigerate any powdered formula that has been combined with tap water.
- Discard any formula not taken; do not keep it for future feedings.
- Burp the infant frequently, and place the baby on his or her back or side for sleeping.
- Use only iron-fortified infant formula for first year (Lawson, 2007).

Teaching About Breast Care

Regardless of whether or not the mother is breast-feeding her newborn, urge her to wear a very supportive, snug bra 24 hours a day to support enlarged breasts and promote comfort. A woman who is breast-feeding should wear a supportive bra throughout the lactation period. A woman who is not nursing should wear it until engorgement ceases, and then should wear a less restrictive one. The bra should fit snugly while still allowing the mother to breathe without restriction. All new mothers should use plain water to clean their breasts, especially the nipple area; soap is drying and should be avoided.

Assessing the Breasts

Instruct the mother how to examine her breasts daily. Daily assessment includes the milk supply (breasts will feel full as they are filling), the condition of the nipples (red, bruised, fissured, or bleeding), and the success of breast-feeding. The fullness of the breasts may progress to engorgement in the breast-feeding mother if feedings are delayed or breast-feeding is ineffective. Palpating both breasts will help identify whether the breasts are soft, filling, or engorged. A similar assessment of the breasts should be completed on the nonlactating mother to identify any problems, such as engorgement or mastitis.

Alleviating Breast Engorgement

Breast engorgement usually occurs during the first week postpartum. It is a common response of the breasts to the sudden change in hormones and the presence of an increased amount of milk. Reassure the woman that this condition is temporary and usually resolves within 72 hours.

Alleviating Breast Engorgement in the Breastfeeding Woman

If the mother is breast-feeding, encourage frequent feedings, at least every 2 to 3 hours, using manual expression just before feeding to soften the breast so the newborn can latch on more effectively. Advise the mother to allow the newborn to feed on the first breast until it softens before switching to the other side. See Chapter 18 for more information on alleviating breast engorgement and other common breast-feeding concerns.

Alleviating Breast Engorgement and Suppressing Lactation in the Bottle-Feeding Woman

If the woman is bottle-feeding, explain that breast engorgement is a self-limiting phenomenon that disappears as increasing estrogen levels suppress milk formation (i.e., lactation suppression). Encourage the woman to use ice packs, to wear a snug, supportive bra 24 hours a day, and to take mild analgesics such as acetaminophen. Encourage her to avoid any stimulation to the breasts that might foster milk production, such as warm showers or pumping or massaging the breasts. Medication is no longer given to hasten lactation suppression. Teaching Guidelines 16.5 provides tips on lactation suppression.

Promoting Family Adjustment and Well-Being

The postpartum period involves extraordinary physiologic, psychological, and sociocultural changes in the life of a woman and her family. Adapting to the role of a parent is not an easy process. The postpartum period is a "getting-to-know-you" time when parents begin to integrate the newborn into their lives as they reconcile the fantasy child with the real one. This can be a very challenging

TEACHING GUIDELINES 16.5

Suppressing Lactation

1. Wear a supportive, snugly fitting bra 24 hours daily, but not one that binds the breasts too tightly or interferes with your breathing.
2. Suppression may take 5 to 7 days to accomplish.
3. Take mild analgesics to reduce breast discomfort.
4. Let shower water flow over your back rather than your breasts.
5. Avoid any breast stimulation in the form of sucking or massage.
6. Drink to quench your thirst. Restricting your fluid intake will not dry up your milk.
7. Reduce your salt intake to decrease fluid retention.
8. Use ice packs or cool compresses (e.g., cool cabbage leaves) inside the bra to decrease local pain and swelling; change them every 30 minutes (Arenson & Drake, 2007).

period for families. Nurses play a major role in assisting families to adapt to the changes, promoting a smooth transition into parenthood. Appropriate and timely interventions can help parents adjust to the role changes and promote attachment to the newborn.

For couples who already have children, the addition of a new member may bring role conflict and challenges. The nurse should provide anticipatory guidance about siblings' responses to the new baby, increased emotional tension, child development, and meeting the multiple needs of the expanding family. Although the multiparous woman has had experience with newborns, do not assume that her knowledge is current and accurate, especially if some time has elapsed since her previous child was born. Reinforcing information is important for all families.

Promoting Parental Roles

Parents' roles develop and grow when they interact with their newborn (see Chap. 15 for information on maternal and paternal adaptation). The pleasure they derive from this interaction stimulates and reinforces this behavior. With repeated, continued contact with the newborn, parents learn to recognize cues and understand the newborn's behavior. This positive interaction contributes to family harmony.

Nurses need to know the stages parents go through as they make their new parenting roles fit into their life experience. Assess the parents for attachment behaviors (normal and deviant), adjustment to the new parental role, family member adjustment, social support system, and educational needs. To promote parental role adaptation and parent–newborn attachment, include the following nursing interventions:

- Provide as much opportunity as possible for parents to interact with their newborn. Encourage exploration, holding, and providing care.
- Model behaviors by holding the newborn close and speaking positively.
- Always refer to the newborn by name in front of the parents.
- Speak directly to the newborn in a calm voice.
- Encourage both parents to pick up and hold the newborn.
- Point out the newborn's response to parental stimulation.
- Point out the positive physical features of the newborn.
- Involve both parents in the newborn's care and praise them for their efforts.
- Evaluate the family's strengths and weaknesses and readiness for parenting.
- Assess for risk factors such as lack of social support and the presence of stressors.
- Observe the effect of culture on the family interaction to determine whether it is appropriate.
- Monitor parental attachment behaviors to determine whether alterations require referral. Positive behaviors include holding the newborn closely or in an *en face* position, talking to or admiring the newborn, or demonstrating closeness. Negative behaviors include avoiding contact with the newborn, calling it names, or showing a lack of interest in caring for the newborn (see Table 16.1).
- Monitor the parents' coping behaviors to determine alterations that need intervention. Positive coping behaviors include positive conversations between the partners, both parents wanting to be involved with newborn care, and lack of arguments between the parents. Negative behaviors include not visiting, limited conversations or periods of silence, and heated arguments or conflict.
- Identify the support systems available to the new family and encourage them to ask for help. Ask direct questions about home or community support. Make referrals to community resources to meet the family's needs.
- Arrange for community home visits in high-risk families to provide positive reinforcement of parenting skills and nurturing behaviors with the newborn.
- Provide anticipatory guidance about the following before discharge to reduce the new parents' frustration:
  - Newborn sleep–wake cycles (they may be reversed)
  - Variations in newborn appearance
  - Infant developmental milestones (growth spurts)
  - How to interpret crying cues (hunger, wet, discomfort)
  - Techniques to quiet a crying infant (car ride)
  - Sensory enrichment/stimulation (colorful mobile)
  - Signs and symptoms of illness and how to assess for fever
  - Important phone numbers, follow-up care, and needed immunizations

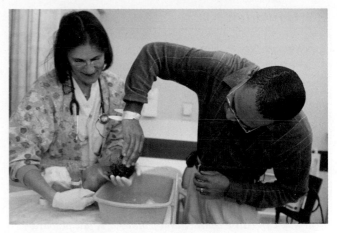

FIGURE 16.7 Father participating in newborn care.

- Physical and emotional changes associated with the postpartum period
- Need to integrate siblings into care of the newborn; stress that sibling rivalry is normal and offer ways to reduce it
- Ways to make time together for the couple
- Appropriate community referral resources

In addition, nurses can help fathers to feel more competent in assuming their parental role by teaching and providing information (Fig. 16.7). Education can dispel any unrealistic expectations they may have, helping them to cope more successfully with the demands of fatherhood and thereby fostering a nurturing family relationship.

Explaining Sibling Roles

It can be overwhelming to a young child to have another family member introduced into his or her small, stable world. Although most parents try to prepare siblings for the arrival of their new little brother or sister, many young children experience stress. They may view the new infant as competition, or fear that they will be replaced in the parents' affection. All siblings need extra attention from their parents and reassurance that they are loved and important.

▶ **Consider** THIS!

Katie and Molly have been excited about having a new baby sister since they were told about their mother's pregnancy. The 6-year-old twins are eagerly looking out the front window, waiting for their parents to bring their new sister, Jessica, home. The girls are big enough to help their mother care for their new sibling, and for the past few months they have been fixing up the new nursery and selecting baby clothes. They practiced diapering their dolls—their mother was specific about not using any powder or lotion on Jessica's bottom—and

(continued)

▶ *Consider* THIS! *(continued)*

holding them correctly to feed them bottles. Finally, their mother arrives home from the hospital with Jessica in her arms!

The girls notice that their mother is very protective of Jessica and watches them carefully when they care for her. They fight over the opportunity to hold her or feed her. What is special to both of them is the time they spend alone with their parents. Although a new family member has been added, the twins still feel special and loved by their parents.

Thoughts: Bringing a new baby into an established family can cause conflict and jealousy. What preparation did the older siblings have before Jessica arrived? Why is it important for parents to spend time with each sibling separately?

Many parents need reassurance that sibling rivalry is normal. Suggest the following to help parents minimize sibling rivalry:

- Expect and tolerate some regression (thumb sucking, bedwetting).
- Explain childbirth in an appropriate way for the child's age.
- Encourage discussion about the new infant during relaxed family times.
- Encourage the sibling(s) to participate in decisions, such as the baby's name and toys to buy.
- Take the sibling on the tour of the maternity suite.
- Buy a T-shirt that says "I'm the [big brother or big sister]."
- Spend "special time" with the child.
- Read with the child. Some suggested title include *Things to Do with A New Baby* (Ormerod, 1984); *Betsy's Baby Brother* (Wolde, 1975); *The Berenstain Bears' New Baby* (Berenstain, 1974); and *Mommy's Lap* (Horowitz & Sorensen, 1993).
- Plan time for each child throughout the day.
- Role-play safe handling of a newborn, using a doll. Give the preschooler or school-age child a doll to care for.
- Encourage older children to verbalize emotions about the newborn.
- Purchase a gift that the child can give to the newborn.
- Purchase a gift that can be given to the child by the newborn.
- Arrange for the child to come to the hospital to see the newborn (Fig. 16.8).
- Move the sibling from his or her crib to a youth bed months in advance of the birth of the newborn.
- Encourage grandparents to pay attention to the older child when visiting (Rector, 2007).

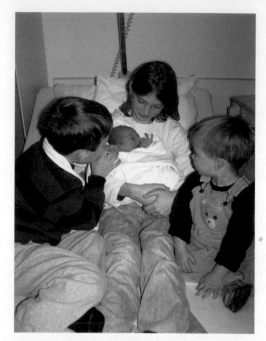

FIGURE 16.8 Sibling visitation.

Discussing Grandparents' Role

Grandparents can be a source of support and comfort to the postpartum family if effective communication skills are used and roles are defined. The grandparents' role and involvement will depend on how close they live to the family, their willingness to become involved, and cultural expectations of their role. Just as parents and siblings go through developmental changes, so too do grandparents. These changes can have a positive or negative effect on the relationship.

Newborn care, feeding, and childrearing practices have changed since the grandparents raised the parents. New parents may lack parenting skills but nonetheless want their parents' support without criticism. A grandparent's "take-charge approach" may not be welcome by new parents who are testing their own parenting roles, and family conflict may ensue. However, many grandparents respect their adult children's wishes for autonomy and remain "resource people" for them when requested.

▶ *Take* NOTE!

Grandparents' involvement can enrich the lives of the entire family if accepted in the right context and dose by the family.

Nurses can assist in the grandparents' role transition by assessing their communication skills, role expectations, and support skills during the prenatal period. Find out whether the grandparents are included in the couple's social support network and whether their support is wanted or helpful. If they are, and it is, then encourage the grandparents to learn about the parenting, feeding, and childrearing skills their children have learned in childbirth classes. This information is commonly found in "grandparenting" classes, which introduce new parenting concepts and bring the grandparents up to date on childbirth practices today.

Teaching About Postpartum Blues

The postpartum period is typically a happy yet stressful time, because the birth of an infant is accompanied by enormous physical, social, and emotional changes. The postpartum woman may report feelings of emotional lability, such as crying one minute and laughing the next. **Postpartum blues** are transient emotional disturbances beginning in the first week after childbirth and are characterized by anxiety, irritability, insomnia, crying, loss of appetite, and sadness (Fooladi, 2006). These symptoms typically begin 3 to 4 days after childbirth and resolve by day 10 (Bennett, 2007). These mood swings may be confusing to new mothers but usually are self-limiting.

Postpartum blues are thought to affect up to 75% of all new mothers; this condition is the mildest form of emotional disturbance associated with childbearing (March of Dimes, 2007). The mother maintains contact with reality consistently and symptoms tend to resolve spontaneously without therapy within 1 to 2 weeks.

> ▶ **Take** NOTE!
>
> *Postpartum blues have been regarded as brief, benign, and without clinical significance, but several studies have proposed a link between blues and subsequent depression in the 6 months following childbirth (Vaughn, 2006).*

Postpartum blues requires no formal treatment other than support and reassurance because it does not usually interfere with the woman's ability to function and care for her infant. Further evaluation is necessary, however, if symptoms persist more than 2 weeks (Ey, 2007). Nurses can ease a mother's distress by encouraging her to vent her feelings and by demonstrating patience and understanding with her and her family. Suggest that getting outside help with housework and infant care might help her to feel less overwhelmed until the blues ease. Provide telephone numbers she can call when she feels down during the day. Making women aware of this disorder while they are pregnant will increase their knowledge about this mood disturbance, which may lessen their embarrassment and increase their willingness to ask for and accept help if it does occur.

The postpartum woman also is at risk for postpartum depression and postpartum psychosis; these conditions are discussed in Chapter 22.

Preparing for Discharge

The AAP and the American College of Obstetricians and Gynecologists (ACOG) state that the length of stay in the health care facility should be individualized for each mother and baby. A shortened hospital stay may be indicated if the following criteria are met:

- Mother is afebrile and vital signs are within normal range.
- Lochia is appropriate amount and color for stage of recovery.
- Hemoglobin and hematocrit values are within normal range.
- Uterine fundus is firm; urinary output is adequate.
- ABO blood groups and RhD status are known and, if indicated, anti-D immunoglobulin has been administered.
- Surgical wounds are healing and no signs of infection are present.
- Mother is able to ambulate without difficulty.
- Food and fluids are taken without difficulty.
- Self-care and infant care are understood and demonstrated.
- Family or other support system is available to care for both.
- Mother is aware of possible complications (AAP & ACOG, 2007).

Providing Immunizations

Prior to discharge, check the immunity status for rubella for all mothers and give a subcutaneous injection of rubella vaccine if they are not serologically immune (titer less than 1:10). Be sure that the client signs a consent form to receive the vaccine. Nursing mothers can be vaccinated because the live, attenuated rubella virus is not communicable. Inform all mothers receiving immunization about adverse effects (rash, joint symptoms, and a low-grade fever 5 to 21 days later) and the need to avoid pregnancy for at least 28 days after being vaccinated because of the risk of teratogenic effects (CDC, 2007).

If the client is Rh negative, check the Rh status of the newborn. Verify that the woman is Rh negative and has not been sensitized, that the Coombs' test is negative, and that the newborn is Rh positive. Mothers who are Rh negative and have given birth to an infant who is Rh positive should receive an injection of Rh immunoglobulin within 72 hours after birth to prevent a sensitization reaction in the Rh-negative woman who received Rh-positive blood cells during the birthing process. The usual protocol for the Rh-negative woman is to receive two doses of Rh immunoglobulin (RhoGAM), one at 28 weeks' gestation and the second dose within 72 hours after childbirth. A signed consent form is needed after a thorough explanation is provided about the procedure, including its purpose, possible adverse effects, and effect on future pregnancies.

Ensuring Follow-Up Care

New mothers and their families need to be attended to over an extended period of time by nurses knowledgeable about mother care, infant feeding (breast-feeding and bottle-feeding), infant care, and nutrition. Although continuous nursing care stops on discharge from the hospital or birthing center, extended episodic nursing care needs to be provided at home. Some of the challenges faced by the current families after discharge are described in Box 16.5.

Many new mothers are reluctant to "cut the cord" after their brief stay in the health care facility and need expanded community services. Women who are discharged too early from the hospital run the risk of uterine subinvolution, discomfort at an episiotomy or cesarean site, infection, fatigue, and maladjustment to their new role. Postpartum nursing care should include a range of family-focused care, including telephone calls, outpatient clinics, and home visits. Typically, public health nurses, community and home health nurses, and the health care provider's office staff will provide postpartum care after hospital discharge.

Providing Telephone Follow-Up

Telephone follow-up typically occurs during the first week after discharge to check on how things are going at home. Calls can be made by perinatal nurses within the agency as part of follow-up care or by the local health department nurses. A disadvantage to a phone call assessment is that the nurse cannot see the client and thus must rely on the mother or the family's observations. The experienced nurse needs to be able to recognize distress and give appropriate advice and referral information if needed.

BOX 16.5 Challenges Facing Families After Discharge

- Lack of role models for breast-feeding and infant care
- Lack of support from the new mother's own mother if she did not breast-feed
- Increased mobility of society, which means that extended family may live far away and cannot help care for the newborn and support the new family
- Feelings of isolation and limited community ties for women who work full time
- Shortened hospital stays: parents may be overwhelmed by all the information they are given in the brief hospital stay
- Prenatal classes usually focus on the birth itself rather than on skills needed to care for themselves and the newborn during the postpartum period
- Limited access to education and support systems for families from diverse cultures

---

Source: Nash, 2007.

Providing Outpatient Follow-Up

For mothers with established health care providers such as private pediatricians and obstetricians, visits to the office are arranged soon after discharge. For the woman with an uncomplicated vaginal birth, an office visit is usually scheduled for 4 to 6 weeks after childbirth. A woman who had a cesarean birth frequently is seen within 2 weeks after hospital discharge. Hospital discharge orders will specify when these visits should be made. Newborn examinations and further diagnostic laboratory studies are scheduled within the first week.

▶ **Take** NOTE!

Infants discharged before they are 48 hours old should be seen by a pediatrician or health care provider by the time they are 96 hours old; those discharged after they are 48 hours old should be seen by the time they are 120 hours old (Langan, 2006).

Outpatient clinics are available in many communities. If family members run into a problem, the local clinic is available to provide assessment and treatment. Clinic visits can replace or supplement home visits. Although these clinics are open during daytime hours only and the staff members are unfamiliar with the family, they can be a valuable resource for the new family with a problem or concern.

Providing Home Visit Follow-Up

Home visits are usually made within the first week after discharge to assess the mother and newborn. During the home visit, the nurse assesses for and manages common physical and psychosocial problems. In addition, the home nurse can help the new parents adjust to the change in their lives. The postpartum home visit usually includes the following:

- Maternal assessment: general well-being, vital signs, breast health and care, abdominal and musculoskeletal status, voiding status, fundus and lochia status, psychological and coping status, family relationships, proper feeding technique, environmental safety check, newborn care knowledge and health teaching needed (Fig. 16.9 shows sample assessment forms)
- Infant assessment: physical examination, general appearance, vital signs, home safety check, child development status, any education needed to improve parents' skills

The home care nurse must be prepared to support and educate the woman and her family in the following areas:

- Breast-feeding or bottle-feeding technique and procedures

(text continues on page 448)

Maternal Assessment
Maternal/Newborn Record System

Page 1 of 2

PATIENT IDENTIFICATION

Record No. _____

Name _____

Home address _____

STREET

CITY   STATE   ZIP

Date __MO__ /__DAY__ /__YR__ Time begin: _____ Date of delivery __MO__ / __DAY__ / __YR__

Time end: _____

Medication allergy ☐ None Identify_____
Significant health history ☐ None Identify_____

PHYSICAL

TEMP.	PULSE	RESP.	BP /

Breasts ☐ Nursing ☐ Non-nursing
Color ☐ Normal ☐ Reddened
Condition ☐ Soft ☐ Firm ☐ Engorged ☐ Blocked ducts
Secretion ☐ Colostrum ☐ Milk ☐ Other _____
Support bra ☐ No ☐ Yes, fit ☐ Appropriate
     ☐ Inappropriate
Nipples (If nursing) ☐ Erect ☐ Flat ☐ Inverted
   Condition ☐ Intact ☐ Bruised ☐ Blistered
     ☐ Fissured ☐ Bleeding ☐ Scabbed
   Care ☐ Water only ☐ Soap ☐ Air dry
     ☐ Topical agent (type/frequency) _____

     ☐ Other _____
Self-exam ☐ Accurate ☐ Inaccurate/instructed

Abdomen
Diastasis recti ☐ Absent ☐ Present_____cm
     ☐ Exercise taught
Incision ☐ None
   Type ☐ Transverse ☐ Vertical ☐ Umbilical
   Closure ☐ Staples ☐ Sutures ☐ Steri-strips
   Condition ☐ Approximated ☐ Open _____ cm
     ☐ Redness _____
     ☐ Swelling _____
     ☐ Discharge _____
     ☐ Other _____

Reproductive Tract
Uterus ☐ Firm ☐ Firm with massage ☐ Boggy
   Height _____ ☐ Midline ☐ Displaced L R
   ☐ Non tender ☐ Tender ☐ With touch ☐ Constant
Lochia ☐ Rubra ☐ Serosa ☐ Alba
   ☐ Clots (describe) _____
   ☐ Fleshy odor ☐ Foul odor
   Pads Type _____ Number/day _____

     Saturation % ├───┼───┼───┼───┤
           0   25   50   75   100

Perineum ☐ Intact ☐ Laceration
   ☐ Episiotormy Type _____ Extension _____
   Condition ☐ Redness _____
     ☐ Edema _____
     ☐ Eccymosis _____
     ☐ Discharge _____
     ☐ Approximation _____
   Care ☐ Front-to-back cleansing ☐ Peri-bottle
     ☐ Soap/water
     ☐ Ice ☐ Sitz bath ☐ Warm ☐ Cool
     ☐ Topical agent (type/frequency) _____

     ☐ Other _____

Elimination
Urinary tract
   Voiding pattern ☐ Normal ☐ Incontinence
     ☐ Bladder distention ☐ Catheter (type) _____
   Signs of infection ☐ None/reviewed ☐ Urgency ☐ Frequency
     ☐ Dysuria ☐ CVA tenderness L R
Gastrointestinal tract
   Bowel pattern ☐ Normal ☐ No BM
     ☐ Constipation ☐ Diarrhea
     ☐ Meds/treatments (type, frequency, effect) _____

   Hemorrhoids ☐ No ☐ Yes (describe) _____
     ☐ Meds/treatments (type, frequency, effect) _____

Lower Extremities
Edema ☐ None ☐ Pedal ☐ Ankle ☐ Pretibial ☐ Thigh
   ☐ Pitting (describe) _____
Signs of thrombophlebitis ☐ None

	L	R		L	R
Homan's sign	☐	☐	Redness	☐	☐
Pain	☐	☐	Warmth	☐	☐
Swelling	☐	☐			

Pain

	No	Yes Managed	Yes Problematic
Abdominal incision	☐	☐	☐
Back	☐	☐	☐
Breasts	☐	☐	☐
Headache	☐	☐	☐
Hemorrhoid	☐	☐	☐
Nipple	☐	☐	☐
Perineum	☐	☐	☐
Uterine cramping	☐	☐	☐
Other _____	☐	☐	☐

Analgesic ☐ No
   ☐ Yes (type/dose/frequency) _____

Reportable danger signs ☐ Aware ☐ Unaware/instructed

TESTS ☐ None
   ☐ Urinalysis
   ☐ CBC
   ☐ _____

IDENTIFIED NEEDS

_____
_____
_____
_____
_____
_____
_____
_____

Signature _____

A

FIGURE 16.9 Sample postpartum home visit assessment form. (**A**) Maternal assessment. *(continued)*

Maternal Assessment
Maternal/Newborn Record System

Page 2 of 2

PATIENT IDENTIFICATION

Record No. _____

Name _____

Home address _____
STREET

CITY _____ STATE _____ ZIP

ACTIVITIES OF DAILY LIVING - 24 HOUR HISTORY

Date __MO__ / __DAY__ / __YR__

Nutrition

Appetite	☐ Good	☐ Fair	☐ Poor
Usual pattern	☐ Yes	☐ No	_____
Special diet	☐ No	☐ Yes	_____
Food intolerance/allergy	☐ No	☐ Yes	_____
Vitamin/mineral supplement	☐ No	☐ Yes	_____

Fluid intake (type/amount) _____

BREAKFAST	LUNCH	DINNER	SNACKS
_____	_____	_____	_____
_____	_____	_____	_____
_____	_____	_____	_____

General Hygiene ☐ Adequate   ☐ Inadequate (describe)

Sleep/Activity

Amount of Activity	Activities	Exercise
Night, uninterrupted _____ hrs	Limitations ☐ None Identify _____	☐ None

Amount of Activity

Night, uninterrupted _____ hrs

Naps ☐ No ☐ Yes _____ hrs

Fatigue ☐ None ☐ Minimal ☐ Moderate ☐ Exhausted

Activities

Limitations ☐ None Identify _____

	Appropriate	Inappropriate/instructed
☐ Self-care	☐ Infant care	
Stair climbing	☐	☐
Lifting	☐	☐
Household tasks	☐	☐
Outside home	☐	☐
Other _____		

Exercise

☐ None

	Accurate	Inaccurate/instructed
Kegel	☐	☐
Postpartum	☐	☐
Other _____		

PSYCHOLOGICAL

Review of Labor and Birth

Missing pieces	☐ No	☐ Yes
Unmet expectations	☐ No	☐ Yes
Unresolved feelings	☐ No	☐ Yes

Pertinent data _____

Postpartum Timetable (Key on reverse side)
☐ Taking in ☐ Taking hold ☐ Letting go

Emotional Status ☐ Happy ☐ Ambivalent ☐ Anxious
☐ Sad ☐ Other _____

Postpartum-depression (Key on reverse side)
☐ 0 ☐ 1 ☐ 2 ☐ 3 ☐ 4
☐ Signs/Symptoms Reviewed

General Comments (body image, role changes, concerns) _____
_____
_____

SEXUALITY

	Aware	Unaware/instructed
Relationship with partner		
Adjustment	☐	☐
Expressions of affection	☐	☐
Resuming Intercourse		
Timing (lack of lochia, comfort)	☐	☐
Vaginal dryness	☐	☐
Milk ejection (if lactating)	☐	☐
Position variation	☐	☐
Libidinal changes	☐	☐
Return of Menses	☐	☐

Contraceptive Method

☐ None   ☐ Undecided/aware of options
☐ Natural family planning
☐ Cervical cap
☐ Condom
☐ Diaphragm
☐ Hormones ☐ Pill ☐ Injection ☐ Implant
☐ IUD
☐ Spermicide
☐ Sterilization ☐ Female ☐ Male
☐ Other _____

Accurate use ☐ Yes ☐ No/instructed

IDENTIFIED NEEDS

_____
_____
_____

Signature _____

FIGURE 16.9 (continued)

Maternal Assessment
Maternal/Newborn Record System

Date MO / DAY / YR   Time begin: _____   Date of Birth MO / DAY / YR
Time end: _____

Significant history ☐ None   Identify_____

PHYSICAL

Temp _____ Pulse (rate/rhythm) _____ Resp _____
Weight _____ Birth weight _____ % Change _____
Length_____ Head _____ Chest _____

HEAD/NECK

	Level	Bulging	Depressed
1. Fontanels			
Anterior	☐	☐	☐
Posterior	☐	☐	☐

Sutures   ☐ Open   ☐ Closed   ☐ Overriding
2. Variations   ☐ Molding   ☐ Caput   ☐ Cephalhematoma

	NORMAL	ABNORMAL	DETAIL VARIATIONS/ABNORMAL FINDINGS
3. Face (symmetry)	☐	☐	
4. Eyes (symmetry, conjunctiva, sciera, eyelids, PERL)	☐	☐	
5. Ears (shape, position, auditory response)	☐	☐	
6. Nose (patency)	☐	☐	
7. Mouth (lip, mucous membranes, tongue, palate)	☐	☐	

Chest

8. Neck (ROM, symmetry)	☐	☐	
9. Appearance (shape, breasts, nipples)	☐	☐	
10. Breath sounds	☐	☐	
11. Clavicles	☐	☐	

Cardiovascular

12. Heart sounds	☐	☐	
13. Brachial/femoral pulses (compare strength, equality)	☐	☐	

Abdomen

14. Appearance (shape, size)	☐	☐	
15. Cord (condition)	☐	☐	
16. Liver (less than or equal to 3 cm ↓ ®costal margin)	☐	☐	

Genitalia

17. Female (labia, introitus, discharge	☐	☐	
18. Male (meatus, scrotum, testes)	☐	☐	
19. Circumcision ☐ No ☐ Yes	☐	☐	

Musculoskeletal

20. Muscle tone	☐	☐	
21. Extremities (symmetry, digits, ROM)	☐	☐	
22. Hips (symmetry, ROM)	☐	☐	
23. Spine (alignment, integrity)	☐	☐	

Neurologic

24. Reflexes (presence, symmetry)			
Moro	☐	☐	
Grasp	☐	☐	
Babinski	☐	☐	
25. Cry (presence, quality)	☐	☐	

PHYSICAL (CONT'D)
Skin

Turgor   ☐ Good   ☐ Poor
Condition ☐ Smooth   ☐ Dry, cracked   ☐ Peeling
Color   ☐ Pink   ☐ Ruddy   ☐ Cyanotic   ☐ Pale
☐ Jaundice (note levels)
  ☐ Head (3 mg/dl)
  ☐ Head and upper chest (6 mg/dl)
  ☐ Head and entire chest (9 mg/dl)
  ☐ Head, chest and abdomen to umbilicus (12 mg/dl)
  ☐ Head, chest and entire abdomen (15 mg/dl)
  ☐ Head, chest, abdomen, legs and feet (18 mg/dl)

Variations (Rashes, lesions, birthmarks). _____

NUTRITION
Feeding

Reflexes ☐ Root   ☐ Suck   ☐ Swallow
Hunger cues identified   ☐ Yes   ☐ No/instructed

BREAST	FORMULA
Frequency___times in _____ hours	Type _____
Time per breast_____ min _____min	Amount _____ oz.
Positioning ☐ Correct	Frequency _____
☐ Incorrect_____	Preparation ☐ Correct
Latch ☐ Correct	☐ Incorrect_____
☐ Incorrect_____	
Appropriate audible swallows	☐ Correct
☐ Yes ☐ No_____	☐ _____

Satiation demonstrated   ☐ Yes
  ☐ No (describe) _____
Regurgitation ☐ No ☐ Yes (describe)_____
Pacifier use ☐ No ☐ Yes (type/pattern)_____

Stool (number/day, color, consistency)_____
Urine (number/day, color)_____

BEHAVIOR
Sleep/Activity Pattern (24 hours)

Sleep (16–20 hrs)   ☐ Yes ☐ No (describe)_____

Awake-alert (2–3 hrs)   ☐ Yes ☐ No (describe)_____

Awake-crying (2–4 hrs)   ☐ Yes ☐ No (describe)_____

Consolability (Key on reverse)   ☐ 0 ☐ 1 ☐ 2 ☐ 3 ☐ 4

TESTS   ☐ None   Time
☐ Metabolic screen kit no. _____   _____
☐ Bilirubin   _____
☐ Hematocrit   _____
☐ _____   _____
☐ _____   _____

INENTIFIED NEEDS _____

_____

_____

_____

Signature _____

B

FIGURE **16.9** (continued) (**B**) Newborn assessment. (Used with permission: Copyright Briggs Corporation. Professional Nurse Associates.)

- Appropriate parenting behavior and problem solving
- Maternal/newborn physical, psychosocial, and culture–environmental needs
- Emotional needs of the new family
- Warning signs of problems and how to prevent or eliminate them
- Sexuality issues, including contraceptive use
- Immunization needs for both mother and infant
- Family dynamics for smooth transition
- Links to health care providers and community resources

■■■ Key Concepts

■ The transitional adjustment period between birth and parenthood includes education about baby care basics, the role of the new family, emotional support, breast-feeding or bottle-feeding support, and maternal mentoring.

■ Sensitivity to how childbearing practices and beliefs vary for multicultural families and how best to provide appropriate nursing care to meet their needs are important during the postpartum period.

■ A thorough postpartum assessment is key to preventing complications as is frequent handwashing by the nurse, especially between handling mothers and infants.

■ The postpartum assessment using the acronym BUBBLE-EE (breasts, uterus, bowel, bladder, lochia, episiotomy/perineum, extremities, and emotions) is a helpful guide in performing a systematic head-to-toe postpartum assessment.

■ Lochia is assessed according to its amount, color, and change with activity and time. It proceeds from lochia rubra to serosa to alba.

■ Because of shortened agency stays, nurses must use this brief time with the client to address areas of comfort, elimination, activity, rest and exercise, self-care, sexuality and contraception, nutrition, family adaptation, discharge, and follow-up.

■ The AAP advocates breast-feeding for all full-term newborns, maintaining that, ideally, breast milk should be the sole nutrient for the first 6 months and continued with foods until 12 months of life or longer.

■ Successful parenting is a continuous and complex interactive process that requires the acquisition of new skills and the integration of the new member into the existing family unit.

■ Bonding is a vital component of the attachment process and is necessary in establishing parent–infant attachment and a healthy, loving relationship; attachment behaviors include seeking and maintaining close proximity to, and exchanging gratifying experiences with, the infant.

■ Nurses can be instrumental in facilitating attachment by first understanding attachment behaviors (positive and negative) of newborns and parents, and intervening appropriately to promote and enhance attachment.

■ New mothers and their families need to be attended to over an extended period of time by nurses knowledgeable about mother care, newborn feeding (breastfeeding and bottle-feeding), newborn care, and nutrition.

REFERENCES

American Academy of Pediatrics (AAP) & American College of Obstetricians & Gynecologists (ACOG). (2007). *Pediatric clinical practice guidelines and policies* (7th ed.). Washington, DC: American Academy of Pediatrics.

American Academy of Pediatrics (AAP). (2005). Policy Statement: Breastfeeding and the use of human milk. *Pediatrics, 115*(2), 496–507.

Arenson, J., & Drake, P. (2007). *Maternal and newborn health.* Sudbury, MA: Jones and Bartlett Publishers.

Armstrong, P., & Feldman, S. (2007). *A wise birth: Bringing together the best of natural childbirth and modern medicine.* London: Pinter & Martin Limited.

Bennett, S. S. (2007). *Postpartum depression for dummies.* Indianapolis: John Wiley & Sons, Inc.

Blackburn, S. T. (2007). *Maternal, fetal, and neonatal physiology* (3rd ed.). Philadelphia: Saunders Elsevier.

Bowers, P. (2007). *Cultural perspectives in childbearing.* Available at: http://www.nurse.com/ce/course.html?CCID=3245.

Brown, S. H. E. (2006). Tender Beginnings program: An educational continuum for the maternity patient. *Journal of Perinatal & Neonatal Nursing, 20*(3), 210–219.

Cassar, L. (2006). Cultural expectations of Muslims and Orthodox Jews in regard to pregnancy and the postpartum period: A study in comparison and contrast. *International Journal of Childbirth Education, 21*(2), 27–30.

Center for Disease Control and Prevention, Office of Women's Health. (2007). *Overweight and obesity among U.S. adults.* Available at: www.cdc.gov/od/spotlight/nwhw/pubs/overwght.htm.

Centers for Disease Control and Prevention (CDC). (2007). *Adult immunizations.* Available at: http://www.cdc.gov/nip/publications/VIS/vis-mmr.pdf.

Cunningham, F. G., Gant, N. F., Leveno, K. J., Gilstrap, L. C., Hauth, J. C., & Wenstrom, K. D. (2005). *Williams' obstetrics* (22nd ed.). New York: Lippincott Williams & Wilkins.

Druxman, L., & Peterson, C. (2006). Postpartum exercise. *IDEA Fitness Journal, 3*(10), 34–37.

Dudek, S. G. (2006). *Nutrition essentials for nursing practice* (5th ed.). Philadelphia: Lippincott Williams & Wilkins.

Engin-Ustun, Y., Ustun, Y., Cetin, F., Meydanli, M., Kafkasli, A., & Sezgin, B. (2007). Effect of postpartum counseling on postpartum contraceptive use. *Archives of Gynecology & Obstetrics, 275*(6), 429–432.

Escott-Stump, S. (2007). *Nutrition and diagnosis-related care* (6th ed.). Philadelphia: Lippincott Williams & Wilkins.

Ey, J. L. (2007). Postpartum depression. *Clinical Pediatrics, 46*(3), 290–291.

Feldman, R. (2007). Parent-infant synchrony and the construct of shared timing; physiologic precursors, developmental outcomes, and risk conditions. *Journal of Child Psychology & Psychiatry, 48*(3/4), 329–354.

Fooladi, M. M. (2006). Therapeutic tears and postpartum blues. *Holistic Nursing Practice, 20*(4), 204–211.

Fowles, E. R., & Horowitz, A. (2006). Clinical assessment of mothering during infancy. *JOGNN, 35*(5), 662–670.

Grossman, K. E., Grossman, K., & Waters, E. (2006). *Attachment from infancy to adulthood.* New York: Guilford Publications, Inc.

Hackley, B., Kriebs, J. M., & Rousseau, M. E. (2007). *Primary care of women: A guide for midwives and women's health providers.* Sudbury, MA: Jones and Bartlett Publishers.

Insel, P., Ross, D., & Turner, E. (2007). *Nutrition* (3rd ed.) Sudbury, MA: Jones and Bartlett.

Kenner, C., & Lott, J. W. (2007). *Comprehensive neonatal care: An interdisciplinary approach* (4th ed.). St. Louis: Saunders Elsevier.

Kersey-Matusiak, G., Gerace, L. M., Bowers, P., & Salimbene, S. (2007). Cultural competence for the global nurse. *Nursing Spectrum.* Available at: http://www.nurse.com/ce/course.html?CCID=3687.

Kuntz, J. G., Cheesman, J. D., & Powers, R. D. (2006). Acute thrombotic disorders. *American Journal of Emergency Medicine, 24*(4), 460–467.

Langan, R. C. (2006). Discharge procedures for healthy newborns. *American Family Physician, 73*(5), 849–853.

Lawson, M. (2007). Contemporary aspects in infant feeding. *Pediatric Nursing, 19*(2), 39–44.

Lemack, G. E. (2007). Incontinence: Helping women stay in control. *Cortlandt Forum, 20*(1), 53–54.

Logsdon, M. C., Wisner, K. L., & Pinto-Foltz, M. D. (2006). The impact of postpartum depression on mothering. *JOGNN, 35*(5), 652–658.

March of Dimes. (2007). *The postpartum blues.* Available at: http://www.marchofdimes.com/pnhec/188_15754.asp.

Mercer, R. T. (2006). Nursing support of the process of becoming a mother. *JOGNN, 35*(5), 649–651.

Moses, S. (2007). Pulmonary embolism in pregnancy. *Family Practice Notebook.* Available at: http://www.fpnotebook.com/ LUN117.htm.

Nash, L. R. (2007). Postpartum care. In R. E. Rakel & E. T. Bope (Eds.), *Conn's current therapy 2007* (Section 16, pp. 1190–1193). Philadelphia: Saunders Elsevier.

Oppenheim, D., & Goldsmith, D. F. (2007). *Attachment theory in clinical work with children: Bridging the gap between research and practice.* New York: Guilford Publications, Inc.

Pastore, L., Owens, A., & Raymond, C. (2007). Postpartum sexuality concerns among first-time parents from one U.S. academic hospital. *Journal of Sexual Medicine, 4*(1), 115–123.

Rector, L. (2007). *Supporting siblings and their families during intensive baby care.* Baltimore: Paul H. Brookes Publishing.

Runquist, J. (2007). Persevering through postpartum fatigue. *JOGNN, 36*(1), 28–37.

Simpkin, K. R., & James, D. C. (2006). Postpartum care. *Nursing Spectrum.* Available at: http://www.nurse.com/ce/syllabus.html?CCID=3455.

Skidmore-Roth, L. (2007). *Mosby's 2007 nursing drug reference* (20th ed.). St. Louis: Mosby Elsevier.

Srivastava, R. (2007). *The healthcare professional's guide to clinical cultural competence.* Philadelphia: Elsevier Health Sciences.

Steen, M., Briggs, M., & King, D. (2006). Alleviating postnatal perineal trauma: To cool or not to cool? *British Journal of Midwifery, 14*(5), 304–308.

Thomason, A., & DeLancey, J. (2007). Urinary incontinence symptoms during and after pregnancy in continent and incontinent primiparas. *International Urogynecology Journal & Pelvic Floor Dysfunction, 18*(2), 147–151.

Tomasulo, P. (2007). LactMed-New NLM Database on drugs and lactation. *Medical Reference Services Quarterly, 26*(1), 51–58.

United States Department of Agriculture (USDA), United States Department of Health and Human Services (USDHHS). (2005). *Healthy eating pyramid.* Center for Nutrition Policy and Promotion. Available at: www.cnpp.usda.gov/pyramid-update/index.html.

United States Department of Health and Human Resources (USDHHS), Public Health Department. (2000). *Healthy people 2010.* Available at: www.healthypeople.gov/document/HTML/Volume2/16MICH.htm.

United Nations International Children's Emergency Fund (UNICEF). (2007). *The Baby-Friendly Hospital Initiative.* Available at: http://www.unicef.org/programme/breastfeeding/baby.htm#10.

Vaughn, J. E. (2006). Behavioral health. When it's not postpartum blues: Recognizing postpartum depression. *Case Management, 12*(3), 8–9.

Whitehouse, K. (2006). That loving touch. *Practicing Midwife, 9*(3), 22–25.

Wilson, C. L., Rholes, W. S., Simpson, J. A., & Tran, S. (2007). Labor, delivery, and early parenthood: An attachment theory perspective. *Personality and Social Psychology Bulletin, 33*(4), 505–518.

WEBSITES

American College of Nurse-Midwives: www.midwife.org

Association for Perinatal Psychology and Health: www.birthpsychology.com

Association of Maternal & Child Health Programs: www.amchpl.org

Baby-Friendly USA: www.babyfriendlyusa.org

Center for Postpartum Health, www.postpartumhealth.com

Depression after Delivery: www.depressionafterdelivery.com

Home-Based Working Moms: www.hbwm.com

International Lactation Consultants Association: www.ilca.org

La Leche League International: www.lalecheleague.org

Midwifery Today, Inc.: www.midwiferytoday.com

National Alliance for Breast-feeding Advocacy: www.naba-breast-feeding.org

National Center for Fathering: www.fathers.com

National Parenting Center: www.tnpc.com

National Women's Health Information Center: www.4women.gov

Parenthood Web: www.parenthoodweb.com

Parenting Q & A: www.parenting-qa.com

Parents Anonymous, Inc.: www.parentsanonymous.org

Parents Helping Parents: www.php.com

CHAPTER WORKSHEET

MULTIPLE CHOICE QUESTIONS

1. When assessing a postpartum woman, which of the following would lead the nurse to suspect postpartum blues?

   a. Panic attacks and suicidal thoughts

   b. Anger toward self and infant

   c. Periodic crying and insomnia

   d. Obsessive thoughts and hallucinations

2. Which of these activities would best help the postpartum nurse to provide culturally sensitive care for the childbearing family?

   a. Taking a transcultural course

   b. Caring for only families of his or her cultural origin

   c. Teaching Western beliefs to culturally diverse families

   d. Educating himself or herself about diverse cultural practices

3. Which of the following suggestions would be most appropriate to include in the teaching plan for a postpartum woman who needs to lose weight?

   a. Increase fluid intake and acid-producing foods in her diet.

   b. Avoid empty-calorie foods and increase exercise.

   c. Start a high-protein diet and restrict fluids.

   d. Eat no snacks or carbohydrates.

4. After teaching a group of breast-feeding women about nutritional needs, the nurse determines that the teaching was successful when the women state that they need to increase their intake of which nutrients?

   a. Carbohydrates and fiber

   b. Fats and vitamins

   c. Calories and protein

   d. Iron-rich foods and minerals

5. Which of the following would lead the nurse to suspect that a postpartum woman was developing a complication?

   a. Fatigue and irritability

   b. Perineal discomfort and pink discharge

   c. Pulse rate of 60 bpm

   d. Swollen, tender, hot area on breast

6. Which of the following would the nurse assess as indicating positive bonding between the parents and their newborn?

   a. Holding the infant close to the body

   b. Having visitors hold the infant

   c. Buying expensive infant clothes

   d. Requesting that the nurses care for the infant

7. Which activity would the nurse include in the teaching plan for parents with a newborn and an older child to reduce sibling rivalry when the newborn is brought home?

   a. Punishing the older child for bedwetting behavior

   b. Sending the sibling to the grandparents' house

   c. Planning a special time daily for the older sibling

   d. Allowing the sibling to share a room with the infant

8. The major purpose of the first postpartum homecare visit is to:

   a. Identify complications that require interventions

   b. Obtain a blood specimen for PKU testing

   c. Complete the official birth certificate

   d. Support the new parents in their parenting roles

CRITICAL THINKING EXERCISES

1. As a nurse working on a postpartum unit, you enter the room of Ms. Jones, a 22-year-old primipara, and find her chatting on the phone while her newborn is crying loudly in the bassinette, which has been pushed into the bathroom. You pick up and comfort the newborn. While holding the baby, you ask the client if she was aware her newborn was crying. She replies, "That's about all that monkey does since she was born!" You hand the newborn to her and she places the newborn on the bed away from her and continues her phone conversation.

   a. What is your nursing assessment of this encounter?

   b. What nursing interventions would be appropriate?

   c. What specific discharge interventions may be needed?

2. Jennifer Adamson, a 34-year-old single primipara, left the hospital after a 36-hour stay with her newborn son. She lives alone in a one-bedroom walk-up apartment. As the postpartum home health nurse visiting her 2 days later, you find the following:

- Tearful client pacing the floor holding her crying son
- Home cluttered and in disarray
- Fundus firm and displaced to right of midline
- Moderate lochia rubra; episiotomy site clean, dry, and intact
- Vital signs within normal range; pain rating less than 3 points on scale of 1 to 10
- Breasts engorged slightly; supportive bra on
- Newborn assessment within normal limits
- Distended bladder upon palpation; reporting urinary frequency

a. Which of these assessment findings warrants further investigation?

b. What interventions are appropriate at this time, and why?

c. What health teaching is needed before you leave this home?

3. The nurse walks into the room of Lisa Drew, a 24-year-old primigravida. She asks the nurse to hand her the bottle sitting on the bedside table, stating, "I'm going to finish it off because my baby only ate half of it 3 hours ago when I fed him."

a. What response by the nurse would be appropriate at this time?

b. What action should the nurse take?

c. What health teaching is needed for Lisa prior to discharge?

STUDY ACTIVITIES

1. Identify three questions that a nurse would ask a postpartum woman to assess for postpartum blues.

2. Find a website that offers advice to new parents about breast-feeding. Critique the site, the author's credentials, and the accuracy of the content.

3. Outline instructions you would give to a new mother on how to use her peribottle.

4. Breast tissue swelling secondary to vascular congestion after childbirth and preceding lactation describes _____.

5. Listen to the postpartum story of one of your assigned patients and share it with your peers in class or as part of online discussion.

UNIT SIX

THE NEWBORN

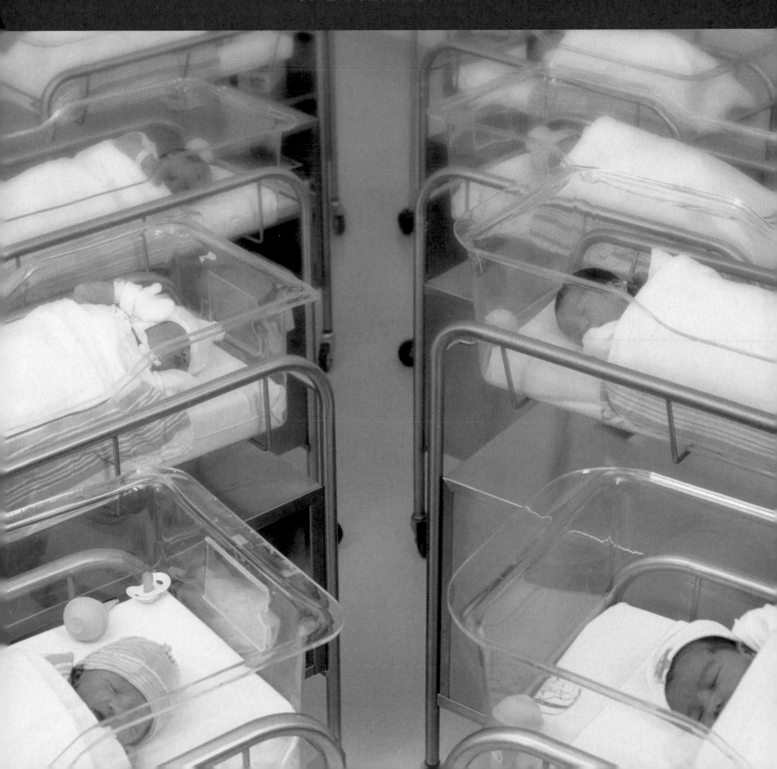

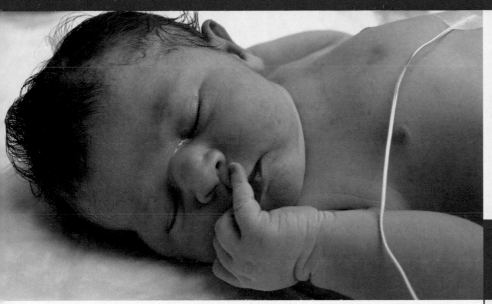

NEWBORN ADAPTATION

KEY TERMS

cold stress
jaundice
meconium
neonatal period

neurobehavioral response
neutral thermal
   environment (NTE)

periodic breathing
reflex
thermoregulation

LEARNING OBJECTIVES

Upon completion of the chapter, the learner will be able to:

1. Define the key terms used in this chapter.
2. Identify the major changes in body systems that occur as the newborn adapts to extrauterine life.
3. List the primary challenges faced by the newborn during the adaptation to extrauterine life.
4. Explain the three behavioral patterns of newborn behavioral adaptation.
5. Discuss the five typical behavioral responses of the newborn.

The Healthy Start home care nurse reviewed the patient's file in her car before she got out: 18-year-old primipara, 1 week postpartum with a term newborn girl weighing 7 pounds. The new mother, Maria, greeted the nurse at the door and let her inside the house. After performing a postpartum assessment on Maria and an assessment of her newborn daughter, the nurse asked Maria if she had any questions or concerns. Maria's eyes welled up with tears: she is worried that her daughter can't see.

Wow

Newborns can't always be judged by their outer wrapping; rather, we should focus on the awesome gift inside.

When a child is born, the exhaustion and stress of labor are over for the parents, but now the newborn must begin the work of physiologically and behaviorally adapting to the new environment. The first 24 hours of life can be the most precarious (Blackburn, 2007).

The **neonatal period** is defined as the first 28 days of life. After birth, the newborn is exposed to a whole new world of sounds, colors, smells, and sensations. The newborn, previously confined to the warm, dark, wet intrauterine environment, is now thrust into an environment that is much brighter and cooler. As the newborn adapts to life after birth, numerous physiologic changes occur (Table 17.1).

Awareness of the adaptations that are occurring forms the foundation for providing support to the newborn during this crucial time. Physiologic and behavioral changes occur quickly during this transition period. Being aware of any deviations from the norm is crucial to ensure early identification and prompt intervention.

This chapter describes the physiologic changes of the newborn's major body systems. It also discusses the behavioral adaptations, including behavioral patterns and the newborn's behavioral responses, that occur during this transition period.

Physiologic Adaptations

The mechanics of birth require a change in the newborn for survival outside the uterus. Immediately, respiratory gas exchange, along with circulatory modifications, must occur to sustain extrauterine life. During this time, as newborns strive to attain homeostasis, they also experience complex changes in major organ systems. Although the transition usually takes place within the first 6 to 10 hours of life, many adaptations take weeks to attain full maturity.

Cardiovascular System Adaptations

During fetal life, the heart relies on certain unique structures that assist it in providing adequate perfusion of vital body parts. The umbilical vein carries oxygenated blood from the placenta to the fetus. The ductus venosus allows the majority of the umbilical vein blood to bypass the liver and merge with blood moving through the vena cava, bringing it to the heart sooner. The foramen ovale allows more than half the blood entering the right atrium to cross immediately to the left atrium, thereby passing the pulmonary circulation. The ductus arteriosus connects the pulmonary artery to the aorta, which allows bypassing of the pulmonary circuit. Only a small portion of blood passes through the pulmonary circuit for the main purpose of perfusion of the structure, rather than for oxygenation. The fetus depends on the placenta to provide oxygen and nutrients and to remove waste products.

At birth, the circulatory system must switch from fetal to newborn circulation and from placental to pulmonary gas exchange. The physical forces of the contractions of labor and birth, mild asphyxia, increased intracranial pressure as a result of cord compression and uterine contractions, as well as cold stress immediately experienced after birth lead to an increased release in catecholamines that is critical for the changes involved in the transition to

TABLE 17.1 ANATOMIC AND PHYSIOLOGIC COMPARISON OF THE FETUS AND NEWBORN

Comparison	Fetus	Newborn
Respiratory system	Fluid-filled, high-pressure system causes blood to be shunted from the lungs through the ductus arteriosus to the rest of the body.	Air-filled, low-pressure system encourages blood flow through the lungs for gas exchange; increased oxygen content of blood in the lungs contributes to the closing of the ductus arteriosus (becomes a ligament).
Site of gas exchange	Placenta	Lungs
Circulation through the heart	Pressures in the right atrium are greater than in the left, encouraging blood flow through the foreman ovale.	Pressures in the left atrium are greater than in the right, causing the foreman ovale to close.
Hepatic portal circulation	Ductus venosus bypasses; maternal liver performs filtering functions	Ductus venosus closes (becomes a ligament); hepatic portal circulation begins.
Thermoregulation	Body temperature is maintained by maternal body temperature and the warmth of the intrauterine environment.	Body temperature is maintained through a flexed posture and brown fat.

Source: Klossner, N. J., & Hatfield, N. (2006). *Introductory maternity and pediatric nursing.* Philadelphia: Lippincott Williams & Wilkins.

extrauterine life. The increased levels of epinephrine and norepinephrine stimulate increased cardiac output and contractility, surfactant release, and promotion of pulmonary fluid clearance (Kenner & Lott, 2007).

Fetal Structures

Changes in circulation occur immediately at birth as the fetus separates from the placenta (Fig. 17.1). When the umbilical cord is clamped, the first breath is taken and the lungs begin to function. As a result, systemic vascular resistance increases and blood return to the heart via the inferior vena cava decreases. Concurrently with these changes, there is a rapid decrease in pulmonary vascular resistance and an increase in pulmonary blood flow (Blackburn, 2007). The foramen ovale functionally closes with a decrease in pulmonary vascular resistance, which leads to a decrease in right-sided heart pressures. An increase in systemic pressure, after clamping of the cord, leads to an increase in left-sided heart pressures. Ductus arteriosus, ductus venosus, and umbilical vessels that were vital during fetal life are no longer needed. Over a period of months these fetal vessels form nonfunctional ligaments.

Before birth, the foramen ovale allowed most of the oxygenated blood entering the right atrium from the inferior vena cava to pass into the left atrium of the heart. With the newborn's first breath, air pushes into the lungs, triggering an increase in pulmonary blood flow and pulmonary venous return to the left side of the heart. As a result, the pressure in the left atrium becomes higher than in the right atrium. The increased left atrial pressure causes the foramen ovale to close, thus allowing the output from the right ventricle to flow entirely to the lungs. With closure of this fetal shunt, oxygenated blood is now separated from nonoxygenated blood. The subsequent increase in tissue oxygenation further promotes the increase in systemic blood pressure and continuing blood flow to the lungs. The foramen ovale normally closes functionally at birth when left atrial pressure increases and right atrial pressure decreases. Permanent anatomic closure, though, really occurs throughout the next several weeks.

During fetal life, the ductus arteriosus, located between the aorta and the pulmonary artery, protected the lungs against circulatory overload by shunting blood (right to left) into the descending aorta, bypassing the pulmonary circulation. Its patency during fetal life is promoted by continual production of prostaglandin E2 (PGE2) by the ductus arteriosus (T. W. Hansen, 2007). The ductus arteriosus becomes functionally closed within the first few hours after birth. Oxygen is the most important factor in controlling its closure. Closure depends on the high oxygen content of the aortic blood resulting from aeration of the lungs at birth. At birth, pulmonary vascular resistance decreases, allowing pulmonary blood flow to increase and oxygen exchange to occur in the lungs. It occurs secondary to an increase in PO_2 coincident with the first breath and umbilical cord occlusion when it is clamped.

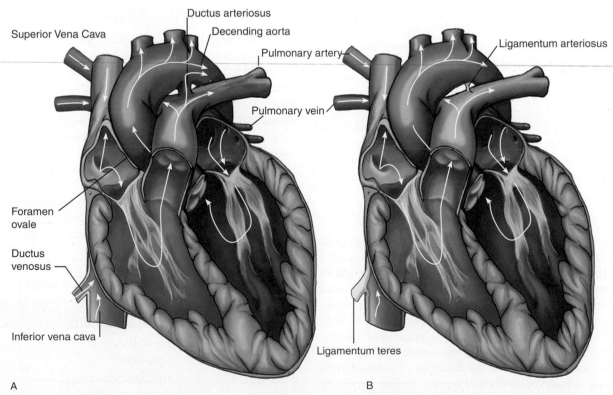

FIGURE **17.1** Cardiovascular adaptations of the newborn. Note the changes in oxygenation between (**A**) prenatal circulation and (**B**) postnatal (pulmonary) circulation.

The ductus venosus shunted blood from the left umbilical vein to the inferior vena cava during intrauterine life. It closes within a few days after birth, because this shunting is no longer needed as a result of activation of the liver. The activated liver now takes over the functions of the placenta (which was expelled at birth). The ductus venosus becomes a ligament in extrauterine life.

The two umbilical arteries and one umbilical vein begin to constrict at birth, because with placental expulsion, blood flow ceases. In addition, peripheral circulation increases. Thus, the vessels are no longer needed and they too become ligaments.

Heart Rate

During the first few minutes after birth, the newborn's heart rate is approximately 120 to 180 bpm. Thereafter, it begins to decrease to an average of 120 to 130 bpm (Arenson & Drake, 2007). The newborn is highly dependent on heart rate for maintenance of cardiac output and blood pressure. Although the blood pressure is not taken routinely in the healthy term newborn, it is usually highest after birth and reaches a plateau within a week after birth.

> ▶ **Take** NOTE!
>
> *Transient functional cardiac murmurs may be heard during the neonatal period as a result of the changing dynamics of the cardiovascular system at birth (Wheeler & McCaffrey, 2007).*

The fluctuations in both the heart rate and blood pressure tend to follow the changes in the newborn's behavioral state. An increase in activity, such as wakefulness, movement, or crying, corresponds to an increase in heart rate and blood pressure. In contrast, the compromised newborn demonstrates markedly less physiologic variability overall. Tachycardia may be found with volume depletion, cardiorespiratory disease, drug withdrawal, and hyperthyroidism. Bradycardia is often associated with apnea and is often seen with hypoxia.

Blood Volume

The blood volume of the newborn depends on the amount of blood transferred from the placenta at birth. It is usually estimated to be 80 to 85 mL/kg of body weight in the term infant (Blackburn, 2007). However, the volume may vary as much as 25% to 40%, depending on when clamping of the umbilical cord occurs. Early (before 30 to 40 seconds) or late (after 3 minutes) clamping of the umbilical cord changes circulatory dynamics during transition. Recent studies show the benefits of delayed cord clamping as improving the newborn's cardiopulmonary adaptation, preventing childhood anemia without increasing hypervolemia-related risks, increasing blood pressure, improving oxygen transport, and increasing red blood

cell flow. Although a tailored approach is required in the case of cord clamping, the balance of available data suggests that delayed cord clamping should be the method of choice (Levy & Blickstein, 2006; Mercer et al., 2007). Further research is needed to explain the relationship among oxygen transport, red blood cell volume, and initiation of breathing, thereby indicating whether early or delayed cord clamping is beneficial.

Blood Components

Fetal red blood cells are large, but few in number. After birth, the red cell count gradually increases as the cell size decreases, because they live in an environment with much higher PO_2. A newborn's red cells have a life span of 80 to 100 days, compared to 120 days in adults.

Hemoglobin initially declines as a result of a decrease in neonatal red cell mass (physiologic anemia of infancy). Leukocytosis (elevated white blood cells) is present as a result of birth trauma soon after birth. The newborn's platelet count and aggregation ability are the same as adults.

The newborn's hematologic values are affected by the site of the blood sample (capillary blood has higher levels of hemoglobin and hematocrit compared with venous blood), placental transfusion (delayed cord clamping and normal shift of plasma to extravascular spaces, which causes higher levels of hemoglobin and hematocrit), and gestational age (increased age is associated with increased numbers of red cells and hemoglobin) (Blackburn, 2007). Table 17.2 lists normal newborn blood values.

Respiratory System Adaptations

The first breath of life is a gasp that generates an increase in transpulmonary pressure and results in diaphragmatic descent. Hypercapnia, hypoxia, and acidosis resulting from normal labor become stimuli for initiating respirations. Inspiration of air and expansion of the lungs allow for an increase in tidal volume (amount of air brought into the lungs). Surfactant is a surface tension-reducing lipoprotein found in the newborn's lungs that prevents alveolar collapse at the end of expiration and loss of lung volume. It lines the alveoli to enhance aeration of gas-free lungs, thus reducing surface tension and lowering the pressure required to open the alveoli. Normal lung function is dependent upon surfactant, which permits a decrease in

TABLE 17.2 **NORMAL NEWBORN BLOOD VALUES**

Lab Data	Normal Range
Hemoglobin	17–20 g/dL
Hematocrit	52%–63%
Platelets	100,000–300,000/μL
Red blood cells	5.1–5.8 (1,000,000/μL)
White blood cells	10–30,000/mm³

surface tension at end-expiration (to prevent atelectasis) and an increase in surface tension during lung expansion (to facilitate elastic recoil on inspiration). Surfactant provides the lung stability needed for gas exchange. The newborn's first breath, in conjunction with surfactant, overcomes the surface forces to permit aeration of the lungs. The chest wall of the newborn is floppy because of the high cartilage content and poorly developed musculature. Thus, accessory muscles to help in breathing are ineffective.

One of the most crucial adaptations that the newborn makes at birth is adjusting from a fluid-filled intrauterine environment to a gaseous extrauterine environment. During fetal life, the lungs are expanded with an ultrafiltrate of the amniotic fluid. During and after birth, this fluid must be removed and replaced with air. Passage through the birth canal allows intermittent compression of the thorax, which helps eliminate the fluid in the lungs. Pulmonary capillaries and the lymphatics remove the remaining fluid.

If fluid is removed too slowly or incompletely (e.g., with decreased thoracic squeezing during birth or diminished respiratory effort), transient tachypnea (respiratory rate above 60 bpm) of the newborn occurs. Examples of situations involving decreased thoracic compression and diminished respiratory effort include cesarean birth and sedation in newborns (Kenner & Lott, 2007).

> ▶ **Take** NOTE!
>
> *A baby born by cesarean delivery does not have the same benefit of the birth canal squeeze as does the newborn born by vaginal delivery. Closely observe the respirations of the newborn after cesarean delivery.*

Lungs

Before the newborn's lungs can maintain respiratory function, the following events must occur:

- Initiation of respiratory movement
- Expansion of the lungs
- Establishment of functional residual capacity (ability to retain some air in the lungs on expiration)
- Increased pulmonary blood flow
- Redistribution of cardiac output (McLenan, 2007)

Initial breathing is probably the result of a reflex triggered by pressure changes, noise, light, chilling, compression of the fetal chest during delivery, and high carbon dioxide and low oxygen concentrations of the newborn's blood. Many theories address the initiation of respiration in the newborn, but most are based on speculation from observations rather than on empirical research (Wheeler & McCaffrey, 2007). Research continues to search for answers to these questions.

Respirations

After respirations are established in the newborn, they are shallow and irregular, ranging from 30 to 60 breaths per minute, with short periods of apnea (less than 15 seconds). The newborn's respiratory rate varies according to his or her activity; the more active the newborn, the higher the respiratory rate, on average. Signs of respiratory distress to observe for include cyanosis, tachypnea, expiratory grunting, sternal retractions, and nasal flaring. Respirations should not be labored, and the chest movements should be symmetric. In some cases, **periodic breathing** may occur, which is the cessation of breathing that lasts 5 to 10 seconds without changes in color or heart rate (Arenson & Drake, 2007). Periodic breathing may be observed in newborns within the first few days of life and requires close monitoring.

> ▶ **Take** NOTE!
>
> *Apneic periods lasting more than 15 seconds with cyanosis and heart rate changes require further evaluation (Kenner & Lott, 2007).*

Body Temperature Regulation

Newborns are dependent on their environment for the maintenance of body temperature, much more so immediately after birth than later in life. One of the most important elements in a newborn's survival is obtaining a stable body temperature to promote an optimal transition to extrauterine life. On average, a newborn's temperature ranges from 36.5° to 37.5°C (97.9° to 99.7°F).

Thermoregulation is the process of maintaining the balance between heat loss and heat production. It is a critical physiologic function that is closely related to the transition and survival of the newborn. An appropriate thermal environment is essential for maintaining a normal body temperature. Compared with adults, newborns tolerate a narrower range of environmental temperatures and are extremely vulnerable to both under- and overheating. Nurses play a key role in providing an appropriate environment to help newborns maintain thermal stability.

> ▶ **Consider** THIS!
>
> *When I look down at my little miracle of life in my arms, I can't help but beam with pride at this great accomplishment. She seems so vulnerable and defenseless, and yet is equipped with everything she needs to survive at birth. When the nurse brought my daughter in for the first time after birth, I wanted to see and feel every part of her. Much to my dismay, she was*

(continued)

▶ *Consider* THIS! *(continued)*

wrapped up like a mummy in a blanket and she had a pink knit cap on her head. I asked the nurse why all the babies had to look like they were bound for the North Pole with all these layers on. Wasn't she aware it was summertime and probably at least 80 degrees outside?

The nurse explained that newborns lose body heat easily and need to be kept warm until their temperature stabilizes. Even though I wanted to get up close and personal with my baby, I decided to keep the pink polar bear outfit on her.

Thoughts: Newborns may be born with "everything they need to survive" on the outside, but they still experience temperature instability and lose heat through radiation, evaporation, convection, and conduction. Because the newborn's head is the largest body part, a great deal of heat can be lost if a cap is not kept on the head. What guidance can be given to this mother before discharge to stabilize her daughter's temperature while at home? What simple examples can be used to demonstrate your point?

Heat Loss

Newborns have several characteristics that predispose them to heat loss:

- Thin skin with blood vessels close to the surface
- Lack of shivering ability to produce heat involuntarily
- Limited stores of metabolic substrates (glucose, glycogen, fat)
- Limited use of voluntary muscle activity or movement to produce heat
- Large body surface area relative to body weight
- Lack of subcutaneous fat, which provides insulation
- Little ability to conserve heat by changing posture (fetal position)
- No ability to adjust their own clothing or blankets to achieve warmth
- Inability to communicate that they are too cold or too warm

Every newborn struggles to maintain body temperature from the moment of birth, when the newborn's wet body is exposed to the much cooler environment of the birthing room. The amniotic fluid covering the newborn cools as it evaporates rapidly in the low humidity and air-conditioning of the room. The newborn's temperature may decrease 3 to 5 degrees within minutes after leaving the warmth of the mother's uterus (99.6°F) (Mercer et al., 2007).

The transfer of heat depends on the temperature of the environment, air speed, and water vapor pressure or humidity. Heat exchange between the environment and the newborn involves the same mechanisms as those with any physical object and its environment. These mechanisms are conduction, convection, evaporation, and radiation. Prevention of heat loss is a key nursing intervention (Fig. 17.2).

Conduction

Conduction involves the transfer of heat from one object to another when the two objects are in direct contact with each other. Conduction refers to heat fluctuation between the newborn's body surface when in contact with other solid surfaces, such as a cold mattress, scale, or circumcision restraining board. Heat loss by conduction can also occur when touching a newborn with cold hands or when the newborn has direct contact with a colder object such as a metal scale. Using a warmed cloth diaper or blanket to cover any cold surface touching a newborn directly helps to prevent heat loss through conduction.

Convection

Convection involves the flow of heat from the body surface to cooler surrounding air or to air circulating over a body surface. An example of convection-related heat loss would be a cool breeze that flows over the newborn. To prevent heat loss by this mechanism, keep the newborn out of direct cool drafts (open doors, windows, fans, air conditioners) in the environment, work inside an isolette as much as possible and minimize opening portholes that allow cold air to flow inside, and warm any oxygen or humidified air that comes in contact with the newborn. Using clothing and blankets in isolettes is an effective means of reducing the newborn's exposed surface area and providing external insulation. Also, transporting the newborn to the nursery in a warmed isolette, rather than carrying him or her, helps to maintain warmth and reduce exposure to the cool air.

Evaporation

Evaporation involves the loss of heat when a liquid is converted to a vapor. Evaporative loss may be insensible (such as from skin and respiration) or sensible (such as from sweating). Insensible loss occurs, but the individual isn't aware of it. Sensible loss is objective and can be noticed. It depends on air speed and the absolute humidity of the air. For example, when the baby is born, the body is covered with amniotic fluid. The fluid evaporates into the air, leading to heat loss. Heat loss via evaporation also occurs when bathing a newborn. Drying newborns immediately after birth with warmed blankets and placing a cap on their head will help to prevent heat loss through evaporation. In addition, drying the newborn after bathing will help prevent heat loss through evaporation. Promptly changing wet linens, clothes, or diapers will also reduce heat loss and prevent chilling.

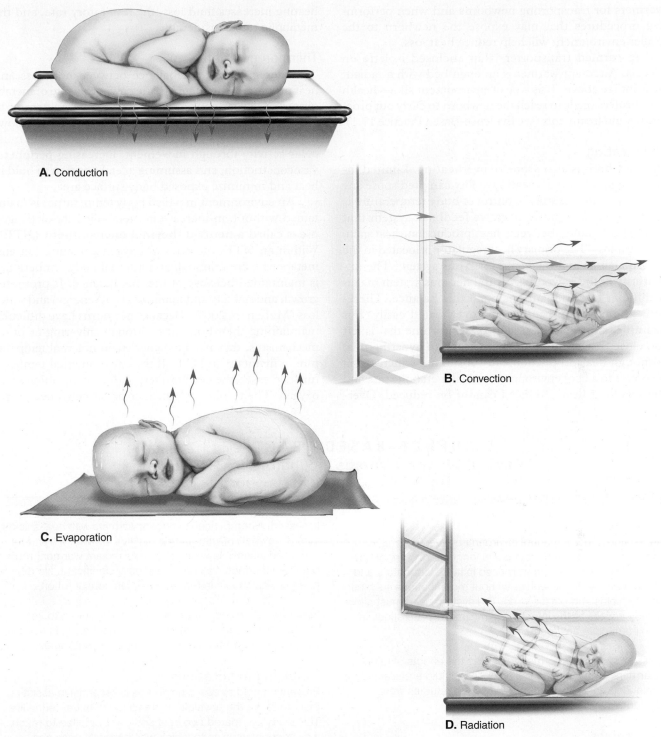

FIGURE 17.2 The four mechanisms of heat loss in the newborn. (**A**) Conduction.
(**B**) Convection. (**C**) Evaporation. (**D**) Radiation.

Radiation

Radiation involves loss of body heat to cooler, solid surfaces in close proximity but not in direct contact with the newborn. The amount of heat loss depends on the size of the cold surface area, the surface temperature of the body, as well as the temperature of the receiving surface area. For example, when a newborn is placed in a single-wall isolette next to a cold window, heat loss from radiation occurs. Newborns will become cold even though they are in a heated isolette. To reduce heat loss by radiation, keep cribs and isolettes away from outside walls, cold windows, and air conditioners. Also, using radiant warmers for transporting newborns and when performing procedures that may expose the newborn to the cooler environment will help reduce heat loss.

A warmed transporter is an enclosed isolette on wheels. A radiant warmer is an open bed with a radiant heat source above. This type of environment allows health care professionals to reach the newborn to carry out procedures and treatments (see Evidence-Based Practice 17.1).

Overheating

The newborn is also prone to overheating. Limited insulation and limited sweating ability can predispose any newborn to overheating. Control of body temperature is achieved via a complex negative feedback system that creates a balance between heat production, heat gain, and heat loss. The primary heat regulator is located in the hypothalamus and the central nervous system. The immaturity of the newborn's central nervous system makes it difficult to create and maintain this balance. Therefore, the newborn can become overheated easily. For example, an isolette that is too warm or one that is left too close to a sunny window may lead to hyperthermia. Although heat production can substantially increase in response to a cool environment, basal metabolic rate and the resultant heat produced cannot be reduced. Over-

heating increases fluid loss, the respiratory rate, and the metabolic rate considerably.

Thermoregulation

Thermoregulation, the balance between heat loss and heat production, is related to the newborn's rate of metabolism and oxygen consumption. The newborn attempts to conserve heat and increase heat production in the following ways: increasing the metabolic rate, increasing muscular activity through movement, increasing peripheral vasoconstriction, and assuming a fetal position to hold in heat and minimize exposed body surface area.

An environment in which body temperature is maintained without an increase in metabolic rate or oxygen use is called a **neutral thermal environment (NTE)**. Within an NTE, the rates of oxygen consumption and metabolism are minimal, and internal body temperature is maintained because of thermal balance. It promotes growth and stability and minimizes heat (energy) and water loss (McLenan, 2007). Because newborns have difficulty maintaining their body heat through shivering or other mechanisms, they need a higher environmental temperature to maintain an NTE. If the environmental temperature decreases, the newborn responds by consuming more oxygen. The respiratory rate increases (tachypnea) in re-

EVIDENCE-BASED PRACTICE 17.1
Radiant Warmers Versus Incubators for Regulating Body Temperature in Newborns

● Study

Providing a thermoneutral environment is an essential component of the immediate and longer-term care of newborn. The methods currently used include incubators and open-care systems, with or without modifications such as heat shields and plastic wrap. The system used must allow ready access to the infant while minimizing alterations in the immediate environment.

This study was performed to assess the effects of radiant warmers versus incubators on neonatal fluid and electrolyte balance, morbidity, and mortality. Eight studies were included in this review.

▲ Findings

Compared with incubators, radiant warmers caused a statistically significant increase in insensible water loss and a trend toward increased oxygen consumption that was not statistically significant. Due to small numbers, effects on important clinical outcomes could not be adequately

assessed. A comparison of radiant warmers with heat shields versus incubators without heat shields showed a trend for increased insensible water loss in the radiant warmer group, but the difference was not statistically significant. No difference was shown in terms of oxygen consumption.

Further randomized controlled trials are required to assess the effects of radiant warmers versus incubators in neonatal care on important short- and long-term outcomes.

■ Nursing Implications

Preventing cold stress in newborns is essential in assisting them to make the physiologic transition to extrauterine life. This study compared two heat sources but failed to reach a clear consensus as to which was better. Nurses can apply these results in caring for newborns by making sure that fluid intake is sufficient to make up for insensible water loss when the baby is under either heat source. In addition, they can assist in future research about heat sources that support thermoregulation in the newborn.

Flenady, V. J., & Woodgate, P. G. (2007). Radiant warmers versus incubators for regulating body temperature in newborn infants. *Cochrane Database of Systematic Reviews,* 00075320-100000000-00251, Issue 4, 2007.

sponse to the increased need for oxygen. As a result, the newborn's metabolic rate increases.

The newborn's primary method of heat production is through nonshivering thermogenesis, a process in which brown fat (adipose tissue) is oxidized in response to cold exposure. Brown fat is a special kind of highly vascular fat found only in newborns. The brown coloring is derived from the fat's rich supply of blood vessels and nerve endings. These fat deposits, which are capable of intense metabolic activity—and thus generate a great deal of heat—are found between the scapulae, at the nape of the neck, in the mediastinum, and in areas surrounding the kidneys and adrenal glands. Brown fat makes up about 2% to 6% of body weight in the full-term newborn (Blackburn, 2007). When the newborn experiences a cold environment, the release of norepinephrine increases, which in turn stimulates brown fat metabolism by the breakdown of triglycerides. Cardiac output increases, increasing blood flow through the brown fat tissue. Subsequently, this blood becomes warmed as a result of the increased metabolic activity of the brown fat.

Newborns can experience heat loss through all four mechanisms, ultimately resulting in cold stress. **Cold stress** is excessive heat loss that requires a newborn to use compensatory mechanisms (such as nonshivering thermogenesis and tachypnea) to maintain core body temperature (Cinar & Filiz, 2006). The consequences of cold stress can be quite severe. As the body temperature decreases, the newborn becomes less active, lethargic, hypotonic, and weaker. All newborns are at risk for cold stress, particularly within the first 12 hours of life. However, preterm newborns are at the greatest risk for cold stress and experience more profound effects than full-term newborns because they have less fat stores, poorer vasomotor responses, and less insulation to cope with a hypothermic event.

Cold stress in the newborn can lead to the following problems if not reversed: depleted brown fat stores, increased oxygen needs, respiratory distress, increased glucose consumption leading to hypoglycemia, metabolic acidosis, jaundice, hypoxia, and decreased surfactant production (McLenan, 2007).

> ▶ **Take** NOTE!
>
> *Nurses must be aware of the thermoregulatory needs of the newborn and must ensure that these needs are met to provide the newborn with the best start possible.*

To minimize the effects of cold stress and maintain an NTE, the following interventions are helpful:

- Prewarming blankets and hats to reduce heat loss through conduction
- Keeping the infant transporter (warmed isolette) fully charged and heated at all times
- Drying the newborn completely after birth to prevent heat loss from evaporation
- Encouraging skin-to-skin contact with the mother if the newborn is stable
- Promoting early breastfeeding to provide fuels for nonshivering thermogenesis
- Using heated and humidified oxygen
- Always using radiant warmers and double-wall isolettes to prevent heat loss from radiation
- Deferring bathing until the newborn is medically stable, and using a radiant heat source while bathing (Fig. 17.3)
- Avoiding the placement of a skin temperature probe over a bony area or one with brown fat, because it does not give an accurate assessment of the whole body temperature (most temperature probes are placed over the liver when the newborn is supine or side-lying)

Hepatic System Function

At birth, the newborn's liver assumes the functions that the placenta handled during fetal life. These functions include

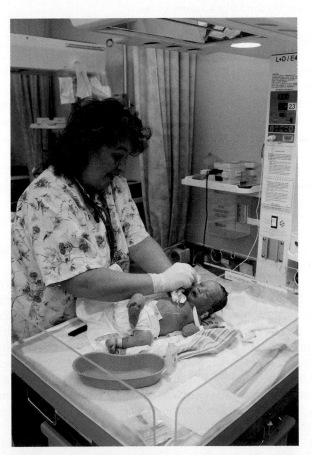

FIGURE **17.3** Bathing a newborn under a radiant warmer to prevent heat loss.

iron storage, carbohydrate metabolism, blood coagulation, and conjugation of bilirubin.

Iron Storage

As red blood cells are destroyed after birth, the iron is released and is stored by the liver until new red cells need to be produced. Newborn iron stores are determined by total body hemoglobin content and length of gestation. At birth, the term newborn has iron stores sufficient to last approximately 4 to 6 months (Garfunkel, Kaczorowski, & Christy, 2007).

Carbohydrate Metabolism

When the placenta is lost at birth, the maternal glucose supply is cut off. Initially, the newborn's serum glucose levels decline. Usually, a term newborn's blood glucose level is 70% to 80% of the maternal blood glucose level (Kenner & Lott, 2007).

Glucose is the main source of energy for the first several hours after birth. With the newborn's increased energy needs after birth, the liver releases glucose from glycogen stores for the first 24 hours. Initiating feedings helps to stabilize the newborn's blood glucose levels. Typically a newborn's blood glucose levels are assessed using a heel stick sample of blood on admission to the nursery and again at approximately 4 hours of age.

Bilirubin Conjugation

The liver is also responsible for the conjugation of bilirubin—a yellow to orange bile pigment produced by the breakdown of red blood cells. In utero, elimination of bilirubin in the blood is handled by the placenta and the mother's liver. However, once the cord is cut, the newborn must now assume this function.

Bilirubin normally circulates in plasma, is taken up by liver cells, and is changed to a water-soluble pigment that is excreted in the bile. This conjugated form of bilirubin is excreted from liver cells as a constituent of bile.

The principal source of bilirubin in the newborn is the hemolysis of erythrocytes. This is a normal occurrence after birth, when fewer red blood cells are needed to maintain extrauterine life.

When red blood cells die after approximately 80 days of life, the heme in their hemoglobin is converted to bilirubin. Bilirubin is released in an unconjugated form called indirect bilirubin, which is fat-soluble. Enzymes, proteins, and different cells in the reticuloendothelial system and liver process the unconjugated bilirubin into conjugated bilirubin or direct bilirubin. This form is water-soluble and now enters the gastrointestinal system via the bile and is eventually excreted through feces. The kidneys also excrete a small amount.

Newborns produce bilirubin at a rate of approximately 6 to 8 mg/kg/day. This is more than twice the production rate in adults, primarily because of relative polycythemia and increased red blood cell turnover. Bilirubin produc-

tion typically declines to the adult level within 10 to 14 days after birth (Maisels, 2006). In addition, the metabolic pathways of the liver are relatively immature and thus cannot conjugate bilirubin as quickly as needed.

Failure of the liver cells to break down and excrete bilirubin can cause an increased amount of bilirubin in the bloodstream, leading to jaundice (Stokowski, 2006). Bilirubin is toxic to the body and must be excreted. Blood tests ordered to determine bilirubin levels measure bilirubin in the serum. Total bilirubin is a combination of indirect (unconjugated) and direct (conjugated) bilirubin.

When unconjugated bilirubin pigment is deposited in the skin and mucous membranes, jaundice typically results. **Jaundice**, also known as icterus, refers to the yellowing of the skin, sclera, and mucous membranes that results from increased bilirubin blood levels. Visible jaundice as a result of increased blood bilirubin levels occurs in more than half of all healthy newborns. Even in healthy term newborns, extremely elevated blood levels of bilirubin during the first week of life can cause kernicterus, a permanent and devastating form of brain damage (W. R. Hansen, 2007).

Common risk factors for the development of jaundice include fetal–maternal blood group incompatibility, prematurity, breastfeeding, drugs (such as diazepam [Valium], oxytocin [Pitocin], sulfisoxazole/erythromycin [Pediazole], and chloramphenicol [Chloromycetin]), maternal gestational diabetes, infrequent feedings, male gender, trauma during birth resulting in cephalhematoma, cutaneous bruising, polycythemia, previous sibling with hyperbilirubinemia, infections such as TORCH (toxoplasmosis, other viruses, rubella, cytomegalovirus, herpes simplex viruses), and ethnicity such as Asian or Native American (W. R. Hansen, 2007).

The causes of newborn jaundice can be classified into three groups based on the mechanism of accumulation:

1. Bilirubin overproduction, such as from blood incompatibility (Rh or ABO), drugs, trauma at birth, polycythemia, delayed cord clamping, and breast milk jaundice
2. Decreased bilirubin conjugation, as seen in physiologic jaundice, hypothyroidism, and breastfeeding
3. Impaired bilirubin excretion, as seen in biliary obstruction (biliary atresia, gallstones, neoplasm), sepsis, chromosomal abnormality (Turner syndrome, trisomy 18 and 21), and drugs (aspirin, acetaminophen, sulfa, alcohol, steroids, antibiotics) (Stokowski, 2006)

Jaundice in the newborn is discussed in more detail in Chapter 24.

Gastrointestinal System Adaptations

The full-term newborn has the capacity to swallow, digest, metabolize, and absorb food taken in soon after birth. At birth, the pH of the stomach contents is mildly acidic, reflecting the pH of the amniotic fluid. The once-sterile gut changes rapidly, depending on what feeding is received.

Mucosal Barrier Protection

An important adaptation of the gastrointestinal system is the development of a mucosal barrier to prevent the penetration of harmful substances (bacteria, toxins, and antigens) present within the intestinal lumen. At birth, the newborn must be prepared to deal with bacterial colonization of the gut. Colonization is dependent on oral intake. It usually occurs within 24 hours of age and is required for the production of vitamin K (Kenner & Lott, 2007). If harmful substances are allowed to penetrate the mucosal epithelial barrier under pathologic conditions, they can cause inflammatory and allergic reactions (Blackburn, 2007).

▶ **Take** NOTE!

Human breast milk provides a passive mechanism to protect the newborn against the dangers of a deficient intestinal defense system. It contains antibodies, viable leukocytes, and many other substances that can interfere with bacterial colonization and prevent harmful penetration.

Stomach and Digestion

The stomach of the newborn has a capacity ranging from 30 to 90 mL, with a variable emptying time of 2 to 4 hours. The cardiac sphincter and nervous control of the stomach is immature, which may lead to uncoordinated peristaltic activity and frequent regurgitation. Immaturity of the pharyngoesophageal sphincter and absence of lower esophageal peristaltic waves also contribute to the reflux of gastric contents. Avoiding overfeeding and stimulating frequent burping may minimize regurgitation. Most digestive enzymes are available at birth, allowing newborns to digest simple carbohydrates and protein. However, they have limited ability to digest complex carbohydrates and fats, because amylase and lipase levels are low at birth. As a result, newborns excrete a fair amount of lipids, resulting in fatty stools.

Adequate digestion and absorption are essential for newborn growth and development. Normally, term newborns lose 5% to 10% of their birthweight as a result of insufficient caloric intake within the first week after birth, shifting of intracellular water to extracellular space, and insensible water loss. To gain weight, the term newborn requires an intake of 108 kcal/kg/day from birth to 6 months of age (Begany & Mascarenhas, 2007).

Bowel Elimination

The frequency, consistency, and type of stool passed by newborns vary widely. The evolution of a stool pattern begins with a newborn's first stool, which is meconium. **Meconium** is composed of amniotic fluid, shed mucosal cells, intestinal secretions, and blood. It is greenish black, has a tarry consistency, and is usually passed within 12 to 24 hours of birth. The first meconium stool passed is sterile, but this changes rapidly with ingestion of bacteria through feedings. After feedings are initiated, a transitional stool develops, which is greenish brown to yellowish brown, thinner in consistency, and seedy in appearance.

▶ **Take** NOTE!

Newborns who are fed early pass stools sooner, which helps to reduce bilirubin buildup.

The last development in the stool pattern is the milk stool. The characteristics differ in breast-fed and formula-fed newborns. The stools of the breast-fed newborn are yellow-gold, loose and stringy to pasty in consistency, and typically sour-smelling. The stools of the formula-fed newborn vary depending on the type of formula ingested. They may be yellow, yellow-green, or greenish and loose, pasty, or formed in consistency, and they have an unpleasant odor.

Renal System Changes

The majority of term newborns void immediately after birth, indicating adequate renal function. Although the newborn's kidneys can produce urine, they are limited in their ability to concentrate it until about 3 months of age, when the kidneys mature. Until that time, a newborn voids frequently and the urine has a low specific gravity (1.001 to 1.020). About six to eight voidings daily is average for most newborns; this indicates adequate fluid intake (Arenson & Drake, 2007).

The renal cortex is relatively underdeveloped at birth and does not reach maturity until 12 to 18 months of age. At birth, the glomerular filtration rate (GFR) is approximately 30% of normal adult values, reaching approximately 50% of normal adult values by the 10th day of life and full adult values by the first year of life (Blackburn, 2007). The low GFR and the limited excretion and conservation capability of the kidney affect the newborn's ability to excrete salt, water loads, and drugs.

▶ **Take** NOTE!

The possibility of fluid overload is increased in newborns; keep this in mind when administering intravenous therapy to a newborn.

Immune System Adaptations

Essential to the newborn's survival is the ability to respond effectively to hostile environmental forces. The newborn's immune system begins working early in gestation, but many of the responses do not function adequately during the early neonatal period. The intrauterine environment usually protects the fetus from harmful microorganisms and the need for defensive immunologic responses. With exposure to a wide variety of microorganisms at birth, the newborn must develop a balance between its host defenses and the hostile environmental organisms to ensure a safe transition to the outside world.

Responses of the immune system serve three purposes: defense (protection from invading organisms), homeostasis (elimination of worn-out host cells), and surveillance (recognition and removal of enemy cells). The newborn's immune system response involves recognition of the pathogen or other foreign material, followed by activation of mechanisms to react against and eliminate it. All immune responses primarily involve leukocytes (white blood cells).

The immune system's responses can be divided into two categories: natural and acquired immunity. These mechanisms are interrelated and interdependent; both are required for immunocompetency.

Natural Immunity

Natural immunity includes responses or mechanisms that do not require previous exposure to the microorganism or antigen to operate efficiently. Physical barriers (such as intact skin and mucous membranes), chemical barriers (such as gastric acids and digestive enzymes), and resident nonpathologic organisms make up the newborn's natural immune system. Natural immunity involves the most basic host defense responses: ingestion and killing of microorganisms by phagocytic cells.

Acquired Immunity

Acquired immunity involves two primary processes: (1) the development of circulating antibodies or immunoglobulins capable of targeting specific invading agents (antigens) for destruction and (2) formation of activated lymphocytes designed to destroy foreign invaders. Acquired immunity is absent until after the first invasion by a foreign organism or toxin.

Immunoglobulins are subdivided into five classes: IgA, IgD, IgE, IgG, and IgM. The newborn depends largely on three immunoglobulins for defense mechanisms: IgG, IgA, and IgM.

IgG is the major immunoglobulin and the most abundant, making up about 80% of all circulating antibodies (Blackburn, 2007). It is found in serum and interstitial fluid. It is the only class able to cross the placenta, with active placental transfer beginning at approximately 20 to 22 weeks' gestation. IgG produces antibodies against bacteria, bacterial toxins, and viral agents.

IgA is the second most abundant immunoglobulin in the serum. IgA does not cross the placenta, and maximum levels are reached during childhood. This immunoglobulin is believed to protect mucous membranes from viruses and bacteria. IgA is predominantly found in the gastrointestinal and respiratory tracts, tears, saliva, colostrum, and breast milk.

> ▶ *Take* NOTE!
>
> *A major source of IgA is human breast milk, so breastfeeding is believed to have significant immunologic advantages over formula feeding (Blackburn, 2007).*

IgM is found in blood and lymph fluid and is the first immunoglobulin to respond to infection. It does not cross the placenta, and levels are generally low at birth unless there is a congenital intrauterine infection. IgM offers a major source of protection from blood-borne infections. The predominant antibodies formed during neonatal or intrauterine infection are of this class.

Integumentary System Adaptations

The most important function of the skin is to provide a protective barrier between the body and the environment. It limits the loss of water, prevents absorption of harmful agents, protects thermoregulation and fat storage, and protects against physical trauma. The epidermal barrier begins to develop during mid-gestation and is fully formed by about 32 weeks' gestation. Although the neonatal epidermis is similar to the adult epidermis in thickness and lipid composition, skin development is not complete at birth (Hale, 2007). Although the basic structure is the same as that of an adult, the less mature the newborn, the less mature the skin functions. Fewer fibrils connect the dermis and epidermis in the newborn compared with the adult. Also in a newborn, the risk of injury producing a break in the skin from tape, monitors, and handling is greater than for an adult. In addition, sweat glands are present at birth, but full adult functioning is not present until the second or third year of life (Blackburn, 2007). Exposure to air after birth accelerates epidermal development in all newborns (Hale, 2007).

Newborns vary greatly in appearance. Many of the variations are temporary and reflect the physiologic adaptations that the newborn is experiencing. Skin coloring varies, depending on the newborn's age, race or ethnic group, temperature, and whether he or she is crying. Skin color changes with both the environment and health status. At birth, the newborn's skin is dark red to purple. As the newborn begins to breathe air, the skin color changes to red. This redness normally begins to fade the first day.

Neurologic System Adaptations

The nervous system consists of the brain, spinal cord, 12 cranial nerves, and a variety of spinal nerves that come from the spinal cord. Neurologic development follows cephalocaudal (head to toe) and proximal–distal (center to outside) patterns. Myelin develops early on in sensory impulse transmitters. Thus, the newborn has an acute sense of hearing, smell, and taste. The newborn's sensory capabilities include:

- Hearing—well developed at birth, responds to noise by turning to sound
- Taste—ability to distinguish between sweet and sour by 72 hours old
- Smell—ability to distinguish between mother's breast milk and breast milk from others
- Touch—sensitivity to pain, responds to tactile stimuli
- Vision—ability to focus on objects only in close proximity (7–12 inches away); tracks objects in midline or beyond (90 inches); this is the least mature sense at birth (McLenan, 2007)

*R*emember Maria, the new mother who is worried that her daughter can't see? What might the new mother notice about her daughter's behavior? What might be the new mother's expectations?

Successful adaptations demonstrated by the respiratory, circulatory, thermoregulatory, and musculoskeletal systems indirectly indicate the central nervous system's successful transition from fetal to extrauterine life, because it plays a major role in all these adaptations. In the newborn, congenital reflexes are the hallmarks of maturity of the central nervous system, viability, and adaptation to extrauterine life.

The presence and strength of a reflex is an important indication of neurologic development and function. A **reflex** is an involuntary muscular response to a sensory stimulus. It is built into the nervous system and does not need the intervention of conscious thought to take effect (Arenson & Drake, 2007). Many neonatal reflexes disappear with maturation, although some remain throughout adulthood.

The arcs of these reflexes end at different levels of the spine and brain stem, reflecting the function of the cranial nerves and motor systems. The way newborns blink, move their limbs, focus on a caretaker's face, turn toward sound, suck, swallow, and respond to the environment are all indications of their neurologic abilities. Congenital defects within the central nervous system are frequently not overt but may be revealed in abnormalities in tone, posture, or behavior (Kenner & Lott, 2007). Damage to the nervous system (birth trauma, perinatal hypoxia) during the birthing process can cause delays in the normal growth, development, and functioning of the newborn. Early identification may help to identify the cause and to start early intervention to decrease long-term complications or permanent sequelae.

Newborn reflexes are assessed to evaluate neurologic function and development. Absent or abnormal reflexes in a newborn, persistence of a reflex past the age when it is normally lost, or redevelopment of an infantile reflex in an older child or adult may indicate neurologic pathology. (See Chapter 18 for a description of newborn reflex assessment.)

*T*he Healthy Start nurse explained to Maria that all newborns are born with some degree of myopia (can't see distances) and that 20/20 vision isn't generally achieved until 2 years of age. What developmental information should the nurse discuss with Maria?

Behavioral Adaptations

In addition to adapting physiologically, the newborn also adapts behaviorally. All newborns progress through a specific pattern of events after birth, regardless of their gestational age or the type of birth they experienced.

Behavioral Patterns

The newborn usually demonstrates a predictable pattern of behavior during the first several hours after birth, characterized by two periods of reactivity separated by a sleep phase. Behavioral adaptation is a defined progression of events triggered by stimuli from the extrauterine environment after birth.

First Period of Reactivity

The first period of reactivity begins at birth and lasts for 30 minutes. The newborn is alert and moving and may appear hungry. This period is characterized by myoclonic movements of the eyes, spontaneous Moro reflexes, sucking motions, chewing, rooting, and fine tremors of the extremities (Dabrowski, 2007). Respiration and heart rate are elevated but gradually begin to slow as the next period begins.

This period of alertness allows parents to interact with their newborn and to enjoy close contact with their new baby (Fig. 17.4). The appearance of sucking and rooting behaviors provides a good opportunity for initiating breastfeeding. Many newborns latch on the nipple and suck well at this first experience.

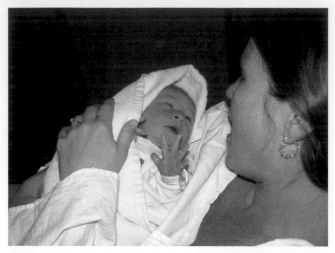

FIGURE 17.4 The first period of reactivity is an optimal time for interaction.

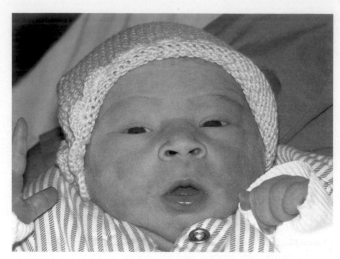

FIGURE 17.5 Newborn during the second period of reactivity. Note the newborn's wide-eyed interest.

Period of Deceased Responsiveness

At 30 to 120 minutes of age, the newborn enters the second stage of transition—that of sleep or a decrease in activity. This phase is referred to as a period of decreased responsiveness. Movements are less jerky and less frequent. Heart and respiratory rates decline as the newborn enters the sleep phase. The muscles become relaxed, and responsiveness to outside stimuli diminishes. During this phase, it is difficult to arouse or interact with the newborn. No interest in sucking is shown. This quiet time can be used for both mother and newborn to remain close and rest together after labor and the birthing experience.

Second Period of Reactivity

The second period of reactivity begins as the newborn awakens and shows an interest in environmental stimuli. This period lasts 2 to 8 hours in the normal newborn (Vandenberg, 2007). Heart and respiratory rates increase. Peristalsis also increases. Thus, it is not uncommon for the newborn to pass meconium during this period. In addition, motor activity and muscle tone increase in conjunction with an increase in muscular coordination (Fig. 17.5).

Interaction between the mother and the newborn during this second period of reactivity is encouraged if the mother has rested and desires it. This period also provides a good opportunity for the parents to examine their newborn and ask questions.

▶ **Take** NOTE!

Teaching about feeding, positioning for feeding, and diaper-changing techniques can be reinforced during this time.

Newborn Behavioral Responses

Newborns demonstrate several predictable responses when interacting with their environment. How they react to the world around them is termed a **neurobehavioral response**. It comprises predictable periods that are probably triggered by external stimuli.

Expected newborn behaviors include orientation, habituation, motor maturity, self-quieting ability, and social behaviors. Any deviation in behavioral responses requires further assessment, because it may indicate a complex neurobehavioral problem.

Orientation

The response of newborns to stimuli is called orientation. They become more alert when they sense a new stimulus in their environment. Orientation reflects newborns' response to auditory and visual stimuli, demonstrated by their movement of head and eyes to focus on that stimulus. Newborns prefer the human face and bright shiny objects. As the face or object comes into their line of vision, newborns respond by staring at the object intently. Newborns use this sensory capacity to become familiar with people and objects in their surroundings.

Remember Maria, who was concerned about her newborn daughter's vision? She told the nurse that her daughter didn't show any interest in her pastel-colored homemade mobile she had hung across the room from her crib. What suggestions can the nurse make to Maria regarding the placement of the mobile and the types and colors of objects used to promote orientation in her newborn daughter?

Habituation

Habituation is the newborn's ability to process and respond to visual and auditory stimuli—that is, how well and appropriately he or she responds to the environment. Habituation is the ability to block out external stimuli after the newborn has become accustomed to the activity. During the first 24 hours after birth, newborns should increase their ability to habituate to environmental stimuli and sleep. Habituation provides a useful indicator of their neurobehavioral intactness.

Motor Maturity

Motor maturity depends on gestational age and involves evaluation of posture, tone, coordination, and movements. These activities enable newborns to control and coordinate movement. When stimulated, newborns with good motor organization demonstrate movements that are rhythmic and spontaneous. Bringing the hand up to the mouth is an example of good motor organization. As newborns adapt to their new environment, smoother movements should be observed. Such motor behavior is a good indicator of the newborn's ability to respond and adapt accordingly—that is, process stimuli appropriately by the central nervous system.

Self-Quieting Ability

Self-quieting ability refers to newborns' ability to quiet and comfort themselves. Newborns vary in their ability to console themselves or to be consoled. "Consolability" is how newborns are able to change from the crying state to an active alert, quiet alert, drowsy, or sleep state. They console themselves by hand-to-mouth movements and sucking, alerting to external stimuli and motor activity (Arenson & Drake, 2007). Assisting parents to identify consoling behaviors to quiet their newborn if the newborn is not able to self-quiet is important. These behaviors include rocking, holding, gently patting, and softly singing to them.

Social Behaviors

Social behaviors include cuddling and snuggling into the arms of the parent when the newborn is held. Usually newborns are very sensitive to being touched, cuddled, and held. Cuddliness is very important to parents, because they frequently gauge their ability to care for their newborn by the newborn's acceptance or positive response to their actions. This can be assessed by the degree to which the newborn nestles into the contours of the holder's arms. Most newborns cuddle, but some will resist. Assisting parents to assume comforting behaviors (e.g., by cooing while holding their newborn) and praising them for their efforts can help foster cuddling behaviors.

■■■ Key Concepts

■ The neonatal period is defined as the first 28 days of life. As the newborn adapts to life after birth, numerous physiologic changes occur.

■ At birth, the cardiopulmonary system must switch from fetal to neonatal circulation and from placental to pulmonary gas exchange.

■ One of the most crucial adaptations that the newborn makes at birth is the adjustment of a fluid medium exchange from the placenta to the lungs and that of a gaseous environment.

■ Neonatal RBCs have a life span of 80 to 100 days in comparison with the adult RBC life span of 120 days, which causes several adjustment problems.

■ Thermoregulation is the maintenance of balance between heat loss and heat production. It is a critical physiologic function that is closely related to the transition and survival of the newborn.

■ The newborn's primary method of heat production is through nonshivering thermogenesis, a process in which brown fat (adipose tissue) is oxidized in response to cold exposure. Brown fat is a special kind of highly vascular fat found only in newborns.

■ Heat loss in the newborn is the result of four mechanisms: conduction, convection, evaporation, and radiation.

■ Responses of the immune system serve three purposes: defense (protection from invading organisms), homeostasis (elimination of worn-out host cells), and surveillance (recognition and removal of enemy cells).

■ In the newborn, congenital reflexes are the hallmarks of maturity of the central nervous system, viability, and adaptation to extrauterine life.

■ The newborn usually demonstrates a predictable pattern of behavior during the first several hours after birth, characterized by two periods of reactivity separated by a sleep phase.

REFERENCES

Arenson, J., & Drake, P. (2007). *Maternal and newborn health.* Sudbury, MA: Jones and Bartlett Publishers.

Begany, M., & Mascarenhas, M. (2007). Normal infant feeding. In R. E. Rakel & E. T. Bope (Eds.), *Conn's current therapy 2007* (Section 16, pp. 1210–1214). Philadelphia: Saunders Elsevier.

Blackburn, S. T. (2007). *Maternal fetal and neonatal physiology: A clinical perspective.* (3rd ed.). Philadelphia: Saunders Elsevier.

Cinar, N. D., & Filiz, T. M. (2006). Neonatal thermoregulation. *Journal of Neonatal Nursing, 12*(2), 69–74.

Dabrowski, G. A. (2007). Skin-to-skin contact: Giving birth back to mothers and babies. *AWHONN Lifelines, 11*(1), 64–71.

Garfunkel, L. C., Kaczorowski, J., & Christy, C. (2007). *Pediatric clinical advisor: Instant diagnosis and treatment* (2nd ed.). St. Louis, MO: Mosby Elsevier Health Sciences.

Hale, R. (2007). Protecting neonates' delicate skin. *British Journal of Midwifery, 15*(4), 231–235.

Hansen, T. W. (2007). Patency of the ductus arteriosus in the newborn—now you want it, now you don't. *Pediatric Critical Care Medicine, 8*(3), 302–303.

Hansen, W. R. (2007). Neonatal jaundice. *eMedicine.* Available at: http://www.emedicine.com/ped/topic1061.htm.

Kenner, C., & Lott, J. W. (2007). *Comprehensive neonatal care: An interdisciplinary approach* (4th ed.). St. Louis, MO: Saunders Elsevier.

Levy, T., & Blickstein, I. (2006). Timing of cord clamping revisited. *Journal of Perinatal Medicine, 34*(4), 293–297.

Maisels, M. J. (2006). Neonatal jaundice. *Pediatrics in Review, 27*(12), 443–454.

McLenan, D. (2007). Care of the high-risk neonate. In R. E. Rakel & E. T. Bope (Eds.), *Conn's current therapy 2007* (Section 16, pp. 1200–1210). Philadelphia: Saunders Elsevier.

Mercer, J. S., Erickson-Owens, D. A., Graves, B., & Haley, M. M. (2007). Evidence-based practices for the fetal to newborn transition. *Journal of Midwifery & Women's Health, 52*(3), 262–272.

Stokowski, L. A. (2006). Foundations in newborn care: Fundamentals of phototherapy for neonatal jaundice. *Advances in Neonatal Care, 6*(6), 303–312.

Vandenberg, K. A. (2007). State systems development in high-risk newborns in the neonatal intensive care unit: Identification and management of sleep, alertness, and crying. *Journal of Perinatal & Neonatal Nursing, 21*(2), 130–139.

Wheeler, D. S., & McCaffrey, M. J. (2007). Resuscitation of the newborn. In R. E. Rakel & E. T. Bope (Eds.), *Conn's current therapy 2007* (Section 16, pp. 1193–1200). Philadelphia: Saunders Elsevier.

WEBSITES

Academy of Neonatal Nursing: www.academyonline.org
American Academy of Pediatrics: www.aap.org
National Association of Neonatal Nurses: www.nann.org
Neonatal Network: www.neonatalnetwork.com

CHAPTER WORKSHEET

MULTIPLE CHOICE QUESTIONS

1. When assessing the term newborn, the following are observed: newborn is alert, heart and respiratory rates have stabilized, and meconium has been passed. The nurse determines that the newborn is exhibiting behaviors indicating:

   a. Initial period of reactivity

   b. Second period of reactivity

   c. Decreased responsiveness period

   d. Period of sleep

2. When caring for a newborn, the nurse ensures that the doors of the nursery are closed and minimizes opening of the isolette portholes to prevent heat loss via which mechanism?

   a. Conduction

   b. Evaporation

   c. Convection

   d. Radiation

3. After teaching a group of nursing students about thermoregulation and appropriate measures to prevent heat loss by evaporation, which of the following student behaviors would indicate successful teaching?

   a. Transporting the newborn in an isolette

   b. Maintaining a warm room temperature

   c. Placing the newborn on a warmed surface

   d. Drying the newborn immediately after birth

4. After birth, the nurse would expect which fetal structure to close as a result of increases in the pressure gradients on the left side of the heart?

   a. Foramen ovale

   b. Ductus arteriosus

   c. Ductus venosus

   d. Umbilical vein

5. Which of the following newborns could be described as breathing normally?

   a. Newborn A is breathing deeply, with a regular rhythm, at a rate of 20 bpm

   b. Newborn B is breathing diaphragmatically with sternal retractions, at a rate of 70 bpm

   c. Newborn C is breathing shallowly, with 40-second periods of apnea and cyanosis

   d. Newborn D is breathing shallowly, at a rate of 36 bpm, with short periods of apnea

6. When assessing a term newborn (6 hours old), the nurse auscultates bowel sounds and documents recent passing of meconium. These findings would indicate:

   a. Abnormal gastrointestinal newborn transition and need to be reported

   b. An intestinal anomaly that needs immediate surgery

   c. A patent anus with no bowel obstruction and normal peristalsis

   d. A malabsorption syndrome resulting in fatty stools

CRITICAL THINKING EXERCISES

1. As the nurse manager, you have been orienting a new nurse in the nursery for the past few weeks. Although she has been demonstrating adequacy with most procedures, today you observe her bathing several newborns without covering them, weighing them on the scale without a cover, leaving the storage door open with the transporter nearby, and leaving the newborns' head covers and blankets off after showing them to family members through the nursery observation window.

   a. What is your impression of this behavior?

   b. What principles concerning thermoregulation need to be reinforced?

   c. How will you evaluate whether your instructions have been effective?

2. The most important adaptations for the newborn to make after birth are to establish respirations, make cardiovascular adjustments, and establish thermoregulation. Nursing care focuses on monitoring and supporting adjustments to extrauterine adaptation. Write appropriate nursing intervention to help achieve the following newborn adaptations:

   a. Respiratory adaptation

   b. Safety, including prevention of infection

   c. Thermoregulation

STUDY ACTIVITIES

1. While in the nursery clinical setting, identify the period of behavioral reactivity (first, inactivity, or second period) for two newborns born at different times. Share your findings in post-conference that clinical day.

2. Obtain a set of vital signs (temperature, pulse, respiration) of a newborn on admission to the nursery. Repeat this procedure and compare changes in the values several hours later. Discuss what changes in the vital signs you would expect during this transitional period.

3. Find two websites about transition to extrauterine life that can be shared with other nursing students as well as nursery nurses. Critique the information presented in terms of how accurate and current it is.

4. The most common mechanism of heat loss in the newborn is _____.

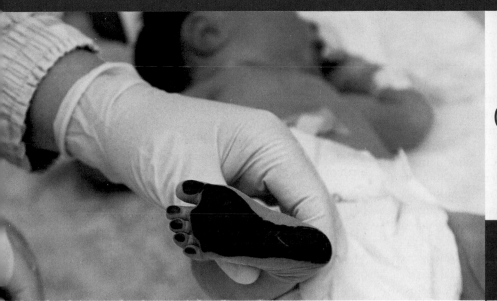

CHAPTER 18

NURSING MANAGEMENT OF THE NEWBORN

KEY TERMS

acrocyanosis
Apgar score
caput succedaneum
cephalhematoma
circumcision
Epstein's pearls
erythema toxicum

gestational age
harlequin sign
infant abduction
immunizations
milia
molding
Mongolian spots

nevus flammeus
nevus vasculosus
ophthalmia neonatorum
phototherapy
pseudomenstruation
stork bites
vernix caseosa

LEARNING OBJECTIVES

Upon completion of the chapter, the learner will be able to:

1. Define the key terms.
2. Discuss the assessments performed during the immediate newborn period.
3. Select interventions that meet the immediate needs of the term newborn.
4. List the components of a typical physical examination of a newborn.
5. Identify common variations that can be noted during a newborn's physical examination.
6. List common concerns in the newborn and appropriate interventions.
7. Compare the importance of the newborn screening tests.
8. Explain common interventions that are appropriate during the early newborn period.
9. Discuss the nurse's role in meeting the newborn's nutritional needs.
10. Outline discharge planning content and education needed for the family with a newborn.

Kelly, a 16-year-old first-time mother, calls the hospital maternity unit 3 days after being discharged home. She tells the nurse that her newborn son "looks like a canary" and "isn't nursing well." She wonders what is wrong.

Wow

You can send a more powerful message with your actions and behavior than with words alone.

Immediately after the birth of a newborn, all parents are faced with the task of learning and understanding as much as possible about caring for this new family member, even if the parents already have other children. In their new or expanded role as parents, they will face many demands and challenges. For most, this is a wonderful, exciting time filled with many discoveries and much information.

Parents learn as they watch the nurse interacting with their newborn. Nurses play a major role in teaching parents about normal newborn characteristics and about ways to foster optimal growth and development. This role is even more important today because of limited hospital stays.

The newborn has come from a dark, small, enclosed space in the mother's uterus into the bright, cold extrauterine environment. Nurses can easily forget that they are caring for a small human being who is experiencing his or her first taste of human interaction outside the uterus. The newborn period is an extremely important one, and two National Health Goals have been developed to address this critical period.

It is also easy to overlook the intensity with which parents and visitors observe the actions of nurses as they care for the new family member. Nurses need to serve as a model for giving nurturing care to newborns.

This chapter provides information about assessment and interventions in the period immediately following the birth of a newborn and during the early newborn period.

Nursing Management During the Immediate Newborn Period

The period of transition from intrauterine to extrauterine life occurs during the first several hours after birth. During this time, the newborn is undergoing numerous adaptations, many of which are occurring simultaneously (see Chap. 17 for more information on the newborn's adaptation). The neonate's temperature, respiration, and cardiovascular dynamics stabilize during this period. Close observation of the newborn's status is essential. Careful examination of the newborn at birth can detect anomalies, birth injuries, and disorders that can compromise adaptation to extrauterine life. Problems that occur during this critical time can have a lifelong impact.

Assessment

The initial newborn assessment is completed in the birthing area to determine whether the newborn is stable enough to stay with the parents or whether resuscitation or immediate interventions are necessary. A second assessment is done within the first 2 to 4 hours, when the newborn is admitted to the nursery. A third assessment is completed before discharge. The purpose of these assessments is to determine whether the baby is normal, to provide information to the parents, and to identify apparent physical abnormalities (Arenson & Drake, 2007).

During the initial newborn assessment, look for signs that might indicate a problem, including:

- Nasal flaring
- Chest retractions
- Grunting on exhalation
- Labored breathing
- Generalized cyanosis
- Abnormal breath sounds: rhonchi, crackles (rales), wheezing, stridor
- Abnormal respiratory rates (tachypnea, more than 60 breaths/minute; bradypnea, less than 25 breaths/minute)
- Flaccid body posture
- Abnormal heart rates (tachycardia, more than 160 bpm; bradycardia, less than 100 bpm)
- Abnormal newborn size: small or large for gestational age

If any of these findings are noted, medical intervention may be necessary.

HEALTHY PEOPLE 2010

Objective	Significance
Increase the proportion of mothers who breast-feed their babies during the early postpartum period from a baseline of 64% to 75%.	• Will emphasize the importance of breast milk as the most complete form of nutrition for infants
Increase the proportion of mothers who breast-feed at 6 months from a baseline of 29% to 50%.	• Will help to promote infant health, growth, immunity, and development throughout the newborn and infant periods
Increase the proportion of mothers who breast-feed at 1 year from a baseline of 16% to 25%.	• Will help to foster early detection and prompt treatment for conditions, thereby lessening the incidence of illness, disability, and death associated with these conditions and their overall effects on the newborn, infant, and family
Ensure appropriate newborn bloodspot screening, newborn hearing screening, follow-up testing, and referral services.	
Ensure that all newborns are screened at birth for conditions mandated by their state-sponsored newborn screening programs.	
Ensure that follow-up diagnostic testing for screening positives is performed within an appropriate time period.	

Source: U.S. DHHS, 2000.

Apgar Scoring

The **Apgar score**, introduced in 1952 by Dr. Virginia Apgar, is used to evaluate newborns at 1 minute and 5 minutes after birth. An additional Apgar assessment is done at 10 minutes if the 5-minute score is less than 7 points (Keenan, 2006). Assessment of the newborn at 1 minute provides data about the newborn's initial adaptation to extrauterine life. Assessment at 5 minutes provides a clearer indication of the newborn's overall central nervous system status.

Five parameters are assessed with Apgar scoring. A quick way to remember the parameters of Apgar scoring is as follows:

- A = appearance (color)
- P = pulse (heart rate)
- G = grimace (reflex irritability)
- A = activity (muscle tone)
- R = respiratory (respiratory effort)

Each parameter is assigned a score ranging from 0 to 2 points. A score of 0 points indicates an absent or poor response; a score of 2 points indicates a normal response (Table 18.1). A normal newborn's score should be 8 to 10 points. The higher the score, the better the condition of the newborn. If the Apgar score is 8 points or higher, no intervention is needed other than supporting normal respiratory efforts and maintaining thermoregulation. Scores of 4 to 7 points signify moderate difficulty and scores of 0 to 3 points represent severe distress in adjusting to extrauterine life. The Apgar score is influenced by the presence of infection, congenital anomalies, physiologic immaturity, maternal sedation via medications, and neuromuscular disorders (Keenan, 2006).

When the newborn experiences physiologic depression, the Apgar score characteristics disappear in a predictable manner: first the pink coloration is lost, next the respiratory effort, and then the tone, followed by reflex irritability and finally heart rate (Kenner & Lott, 2007).

> ▶ *Take* NOTE!
>
> *Although Apgar scoring is done at 1 and 5 minutes, it also can be used as a guide during the immediate newborn period to evaluate the newborn's status for any changes because it focuses on critical parameters that must be assessed throughout the early transition period.*

Length and Weight

Parents are eager to know their newborn's length and weight. These measurements are taken soon after birth. A disposable tape measure or a built-in measurement board located on the side of the scale can be used. Length is measured from the head of the newborn to the heel with the newborn unclothed (Fig. 18.1). Because of the flexed position of the newborn after birth, place the newborn in a supine position and extend the leg completely when measuring the length. The expected length of a full-term newborn is usually 48 to 53 cm (19 to 21 inches). Molding can affect measurement (Dillon, 2007).

TABLE 18.1 APGAR SCORING FOR NEWBORNS

Parameter (Assessment Technique)	0 Point	1 Point	2 Points
Heart rate (auscultation of apical heart rate for 1 full minute)	Absent	Slow (<100 bpm)	>100 bpm
Respiratory effort (observation of the volume and vigor of the newborn's cry; auscultation of depth and rate of respirations)	Apneic	Slow, irregular, shallow	Regular respirations (usually 30–60 breaths/minute), strong, good cry
Muscle tone (observation of extent of flexion in the newborn's extremities and newborn's resistance when the extremities are pulled away from the body)	Limp, flaccid	Some flexion, limited resistance to extension	Tight flexion, good resistance to extension with quick return to flexed position after extension
Reflex irritability (flicking of the soles of the feet or suctioning of the nose with a bulb syringe)	No response	Grimace or frown when irritated	Sneeze, cough, or vigorous cry
Skin color (inspection of trunk and extremities with the appropriate color for ethnicity appearing within minutes after birth)	Cyanotic or pale	Appropriate body color; blue extremities (acrocyanosis)	Completely appropriate color (pink on both trunk and extremities)

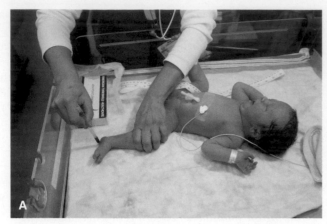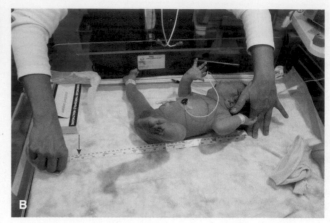

FIGURE 18.1 Measuring a newborn's length. (**A**) The nurse extends the newborn's leg and marks the pad at the heel. (**B**) The nurse measures from the newborn's head to the heel mark.

Most often, newborns are weighed using a digital scale that reads the weight in grams. Typically, the term newborn weighs 2,700 to 4,000 g (6 to 9 lb; Fig. 18.2). Birthweights less than 10% or more than 90% on a growth chart are outside the normal range and need further investigation. Weights taken at later times are compared with previous weights and are documented with regard to gain or loss on a nursing flow sheet. Newborns typically lose approximately 10% of their initial birth weight by 3 to 4 days of age secondary to loss of meconium, extracellular fluid, and limited food intake. This weight loss is usually regained by the 10th day of life (Kliegman et al., 2007).

Newborns can be classified by their birthweight regardless of their gestational age (AAP, 2007a) as follows:

- Low birthweight: <2,500 g (<5.5 lb)
- Very low birthweight: <1,500 g (<3.5 lb)
- Extremely low birthweight: <1,000 g (<2.5 lb)

Vital Signs

Heart rate and respiratory rate are assessed immediately after birth with Apgar scoring. Heart rate, obtained by taking an apical pulse for 1 full minute, typically is 120 to 160 bpm. Newborns' respirations are assessed when they are quiet or sleeping. Place a stethoscope on the right side of the chest and count the breaths for 1 full minute to identify any irregularities. The newborn respiratory rate is 30 to 60 breaths/minute with symmetric chest movement. Heart and respiratory rates are assessed every 30 minutes until stable for 2 hours after birth. Once stable, the heart rate and respiratory rates are checked every 8 hours (Kenner & Lott, 2007).

Axillary temperature is typically assessed not immediately after birth but on admission to the nursery or when the initial newborn assessment is carried out (e.g., the LDR room). The normal axillary temperature for a term newborn is 36.5° to 37.5°C (97.9° to 99.7°F). Rectal temperatures are no longer taken because of the risk of perforation (Blackburn, 2007). The thermometer or temperature probe is held in the midaxillary space according to manufacturer's directions and hospital protocol. Temperature is reassessed every 30 minutes until it has been stable for 2 hours, then every 8 hours until discharge (Kliegman et al., 2007).

Blood pressure is not usually assessed as part of a normal newborn examination unless there is a clinical indication or low Apgar scores. If assessed, an oscillometer (Dinamap) is used. The typical range is 50 to 75 mmHg

FIGURE 18.2 Weighing a newborn. Note how the nurse guards the newborn from above to prevent injury.

TABLE 18.2 NEWBORN VITAL SIGNS

Newborn Vital Signs	Ranges of values
Temperature	36.5° to 37.5°C (97.9° to 99.7°F)
Heart rate (pulse) to 180 during crying	120 to 160 bpm; can increase
Respirations	30 to 60 breaths/minute at rest; will increase with crying
Blood pressure	50 to 75 mmHg systolic, 30 to 45 mmHg diastolic

(systolic) and 30 to 45 mmHg (diastolic). Crying, moving, and late clamping of the umbilical cord will increase systolic pressure (Dillon, 2007).

Typical values for newborn vital signs are provided in Table 18.2.

Gestational Age Assessment

To determine a newborn's **gestational age** (the stage of maturity), physical signs and neurologic characteristics are assessed. Typically, gestational age is determined by using a tool such as the Dubowitz/Ballard or New Ballard Score system (Fig. 18.3). This scoring system provides an objective estimate of gestational age by scoring the specific parameters of physical and neuromuscular maturity. Points are given for each assessment parameter, with a low score of −1 point or −2 points for extreme immaturity to 4 or 5 points for postmaturity. The scores from each section are added together to correspond to a specific gestational age in weeks.

The physical maturity section of the examination is done during the first 2 hours after birth. The physical maturity assessment section of the Ballard examination evaluates physical characteristics that appear different at different stages depending on a newborn's gestational maturity. Newborns who are physically mature have higher scores than those who are not. The areas assessed on the physical maturity examination include:

- Skin texture—typically ranges from sticky and transparent to smooth, with varying degrees of peeling and cracking, to parchment-like or leathery with significant cracking and wrinkling
- Lanugo—soft downy hair on the newborn's body, which is absent in preterm newborns, appears with maturity, and then disappears again with postmaturity
- Plantar creases—creases on the soles of the feet, which range from absent to covering the entire foot, depending on maturity (the greater the number of creases, the greater the newborn's maturity)
- Breast tissue—the thickness and size of breast tissue and areola (the darkened ring around each nipple), which range from being imperceptible to full and budding

- Eyes and ears—eyelids can be fused or open and ear cartilage and stiffness determine the degree of maturity (the greater the amount of ear cartilage with stiffness, the greater the newborn's maturity)
- Genitals—in males, evidence of testicular descent and appearance of scrotum (which can range from smooth to covered with rugae) determine maturity; in females, appearance and size of clitoris and labia determine maturity (a prominent clitoris with flat labia suggests prematurity, whereas a clitoris covered by labia suggests greater maturity)

The neuromuscular maturity section typically is completed within 24 hours after birth. Six activities or maneuvers that the newborn performs with various body parts are evaluated to determine the newborn's degree of maturity:

1. Posture—How does the newborn hold his or her extremities in relation to the trunk? The greater the degree of flexion, the greater the maturity. For example, extension of arms and legs is scored as 0 point and full flexion of arms and legs is scored as 4 points.
2. Square window—How far can the newborn's hands be flexed toward the wrist? The angle is measured and scored from more than 90 degrees to 0 degrees to determine the maturity rating. As the angle decreases, the newborn's maturity increases. For example, an angle of more than 90 degrees is scored as −1 point and an angle of 0 degrees is scored as 4 points.
3. Arm recoil—How far do the newborn's arms "spring back" to a flexed position? This measure evaluates the degree of arm flexion and the strength of recoil. The reaction of the arm is then scored from 0 to 4 points based on the degree of flexion as the arms are returned to their normal flexed position. The higher the points assigned, the greater the neuromuscular maturity (for example, recoil less than a 90-degree angle is scored as 4 points).
4. Popliteal angle—How far will the newborn's knees extend? The angle created when the knee is extended is measured. An angle less than 90 degrees indicates greater maturity. For example, an angle of 180 degrees is scored as −1 point and an angle of less than 90 degrees is scored as 5 points.
5. Scarf sign—How far can the elbows be moved across the newborn's chest? An elbow that does not reach midline indicates greater maturity. For example, if the elbow reaches or nears the level of the opposite shoulder, this is scored as −1 point; if the elbow does not cross the proximate axillary line, it is scored as 4 points.
6. Heel to ear—How close can the newborn's feet be moved to the ears? This maneuver assesses hip flexibility: the lesser the flexibility, the greater the newborn's maturity. The heel-to-ear assessment is scored in the same manner as the scarf sign.

NEUROMUSCULAR MATURITY

NEUROMUSCULAR MATURITY SIGN	SCORE							RECORD SCORE HERE
	-1	0	1	2	3	4	5	
POSTURE								
SQUARE WINDOW (Wrist)	>90°	90°	60°	45°	30°	0°		
ARM RECOIL		180°	140°–180°	110°–140°	90°–110°	<90°		
POPLITEAL ANGLE	180°	160°	140°	120°	100°	90°	<90°	
SCARF SIGN								
HEEL TO EAR								
						TOTAL NEUROMUSCULAR MATURITY SCORE		

SCORE
Neuromuscular ____
Physical ____
Total ____

MATURITY RATING

Score	Weeks
-10	20
-5	22
0	24
5	26
10	28
15	30
20	32
25	34
30	36
35	38
40	40
45	42
50	44

PHYSICAL MATURITY

PHYSICAL MATURITY SIGN	SCORE							RECORD SCORE HERE
	-1	0	1	2	3	4	5	
SKIN	sticky, friable, transparent	gelatinous, red, translucent	smooth, pink, visible veins	superficial peeling and/or rash, few veins	cracking pale areas, rare veins	parchment, deep cracking, no vessels	leathery, cracked, wrinkled	
LANUGO	none	sparse	abundant	thinning	bald areas	mostly bald		
PLANTAR SURFACE	heel-toe 40–50 mm:-1 <40 mm:-2	>50 mm no crease	faint red marks	anterior transverse crease only	creases ant. 2/3	creases over entire sole		
BREAST	imperceptible	barely perceptible	flat areola no bud	stippled areola 1–2 mm bud	raised areola 3–4 mm bud	full areola 5–10 mm bud		
EYE-EAR	lids fused loosely: -1 tightly: -2	lids open pinna flat stays folded	sl. curved pinna; soft; slow recoil	well-curved pinna; soft but ready recoil	formed and firm instant recoil	thick cartilage, ear stiff		
GENITALS (Male)	scrotum flat, smooth	scrotum empty, faint rugae	testes in upper canal, rare rugae	testes descending, few rugae	testes down, good rugae	testes pendulous, deep rugae		
GENITALS (Female)	clitoris prominent and labia flat	prominent clitoris and small labia minora	prominent clitoris and enlarging minora	majora and minora equally prominent	majora large, minora small	majora cover clitoris and minora		
						TOTAL PHYSICAL MATURITY SCORE		

FIGURE **18.3** Gestational age assessment tool. (Ballard, J. L., Khoury, J. C., Wedig, K., et al. [1991]. New Ballard Score, expanded to include extremely premature infants. *Journal of Pediatrics, 119*[3], 417–423.)

After the scoring is completed, the 12 scores are totaled and then compared with standardized values to determine the appropriate gestational age in weeks. Scores range from very low in preterm newborns to very high for mature and postmature newborns.

Typically newborns are also classified according to gestational age as:

- Preterm or premature—born before 37 weeks' gestation, regardless of birthweight
- Term—born between 38 and 42 weeks' gestation
- Postterm or postdates—born after completion of week 42 of gestation
- Postmature—born after 42 weeks and demonstrating signs of placental aging

Using the information about gestational age and then considering birthweight, newborns can also be classified as follows:

- Small for gestational age (SGA)—weight less than the 10th percentile on standard growth charts (usually <5.5 lb)
- Appropriate for gestational age (AGA)—weight between 10th and 90th percentiles
- Large for gestational age (LGA)—weight more than the 90th percentile on standard growth charts (usually >9 lb)

Chapter 23 describes these variations in birthweight and gestational age in greater detail.

> ▶ **Take** NOTE!
>
> *Gestational age assessment is important because it allows the nurse to plot growth parameters and to anticipate problems related to prematurity, postmaturity, and growth abnormalities.*

Nursing Interventions

During the immediate newborn period, care focuses on helping the newborn to make the transition to extrauterine life. The nursing interventions include maintaining airway patency, ensuring proper identification, administering prescribed medications, and maintaining thermoregulation.

Maintaining Airway Patency

Immediately after birth, a newborn is suctioned to remove fluids and mucus from the mouth and nose. Typically, the newborn's mouth is suctioned first with a bulb syringe to remove debris and then the nose is suctioned. Suctioning in this manner helps to prevent aspiration of fluid into the lungs by an unexpected gasp.

When suctioning a newborn with a bulb syringe, compress the bulb before placing it into the oral or nasal cavity. Release bulb compression slowly, making sure the tip is placed away from the mucous membranes to draw up the excess secretions. Remove the bulb syringe from the mouth or nose, and then, while holding the bulb syringe tip over an emesis basin lined with paper towel or tissue, compress the bulb to expel the secretions. Repeat the procedure several times until all secretions are removed.

> ▶ **Take** NOTE!
>
> *Always keep a bulb syringe near the newborn in case he or she develops sudden choking or a blockage in the nose.*

Ensuring Proper Identification

Before the newborn and family leave the birthing area, be sure that agency policy about identification is followed. Typically, the mother and newborn, and possibly the father, receive matching identification bracelets. The newborn commonly receives two ID bracelets, one on a wrist and one on an ankle. The mother receives a matching one, usually on her wrist. The ID bands usually state name, gender, date and time of birth, and identification number. The same identification number is on the bracelets of all the family members.

These ID bracelets provide for the safety of the newborn and must be secured before the mother and newborn leave the birthing area. The ID bracelets are checked by all nurses to validate that the correct newborn is brought to the right mother if they are separated for any period of time (Fig. 18.4). They also serve as the official newborn identification and are checked before initiating any procedure on that newborn and on discharge from the unit (AAP, 2007). Taking the newborn's picture within 2 hours after birth with a color camera or color video/digital image also helps prevent mix-ups and abduction. Some facilities use electronic devices that sound an alarm if the newborn is removed from the area.

Newborns' footprints may also be taken, using a form that includes the mother's fingerprint, name, and date and time of the birth. Some states require footprints of the newborn, although many studies point out that birthing room staff members do not take consistently legible footprints suitable for identification purposes (Kenner & Lott, 2007). Many states have stopped requiring newborn footprints, and thus other means of identification are needed, such as collecting cord blood at the time of birth for DNA testing and live scans to capture digital forensic-quality prints that are suitable for identification purposes (Cohen, 2007).

Administering Prescribed Medications

During the immediate newborn period, two medications are commonly ordered: vitamin K and eye prophylaxis with

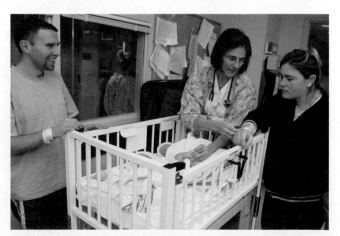

FIGURE **18.4** The nurse checks the newborn's identification band against the mother's.

either erythromycin or tetracycline ophthalmic ointment (Drug Guide 18.1).

Vitamin K

Vitamin K, a fat-soluble vitamin, promotes blood clotting by increasing the synthesis of prothrombin by the liver. A deficiency of this vitamin would delay clotting and might lead to hemorrhage.

Generally, the bacteria of the intestine produce vitamin K in adequate quantities. However, the newborn's bowel is sterile, so vitamin K is not produced in the intestine until after microorganisms are introduced, such as with the first feeding. Usually it takes about a week for the newborn to produce enough vitamin K to prevent vitamin K deficiency bleeding (Wasee, 2006).

The efficacy of vitamin K in preventing early vitamin K deficiency bleeding is firmly established and has been the standard of care since the AAP recommended it in the early 1960s. They recommend that vitamin K be administered to all newborns soon after birth in a single intramuscular dose of 0.5 to 1 mg (AAP, 2007) (Fig. 18.5). They suggest that additional research is needed to validate the efficacy and safety of oral forms of vitamin K, which have been used in many parts of the world but currently are not recommended in the United States.

Eye Prophylaxis

All newborns in the United States, whether delivered vaginally or by cesarean birth, must receive an instillation of a prophylactic agent in their eyes within an hour or two of birth. This is mandated in all 50 states to pre-

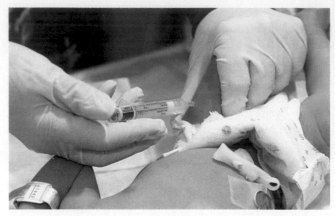

FIGURE **18.5** The nurse administers vitamin K IM to the newborn.

vent **ophthalmia neonatorum**, which can cause neonatal blindness (CDC, 2007). Ophthalmia neonatorum is a hyperacute purulent conjunctivitis occurring during the first 10 days of life. It is usually contracted during birth when the baby comes in contact with infected vaginal discharge of the mother (CDC, 2007). Most often both eyelids become swollen and red with purulent discharge.

Prophylactic agents that are currently recommended include erythromycin 0.5% ophthalmic ointment or tetracycline 1% ophthalmic ointment in a single application. Silver nitrate solution was formerly used but has little efficacy in preventing chlamydial eye disease (CDC, 2007).

Regardless of which agent is used, instillation should be done as soon as possible after birth (Fig. 18.6). If

---

DRUG GUIDE 18.1 DRUGS FOR THE NEWBORN

Drug	Action/Indication	Nursing Implications
Phytonadione (vitamin K [Aqua-MEPHYTON, Konakion, Mephyton])	Provides the newborn with vitamin K (necessary for production of adequate clotting factors II, VII, IX, and X by the liver) during the first week of birth until newborn can manufacture it Prevents vitamin K deficiency bleeding (VKDB) of the newborn	• Administer within 1 to 2 hours after birth. • Give as an IM injection at a 90-degree angle into the middle third of the vastus lateralis muscle. • Use a 25-gauge, 5/8-in needle for injection. • Hold the leg firmly and inject medication slowly after aspirating. • Adhere to standard precautions. • Assess for bleeding at injection site after administration.
Erythromycin ophthalmic ointment 0.5% or tetracycline ophthalmic ointment 1%	Provides bactericidal and bacteriostatic actions to prevent *Neisseria gonorrhoeae* and *Chlamydia trachomatis* conjunctivitis Prevents ophthalmia neonatorum	• Be alert for chemical conjunctivitis for 1–2 days. • Wear gloves, and open eyes by placing thumb and finger above and below the eye. • Gently squeeze the tube or ampoule to apply medication into the conjunctival sac from the inner canthus to the outer canthus of each eye. • Do not touch the tip to the eye. • Close the eye to make sure the medication permeates. • Wipe off excess ointment after 1 minute.

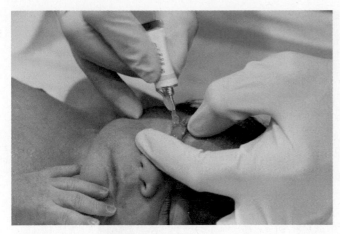

FIGURE 18.6 The nurse administers eye prophylaxis.

instillation is delayed to allow visualization and bonding, the nursery staff should make sure the agent is administered when the newborn reaches the nursery for observation and assessment.

Inform all parents about the eye treatment, including why it is recommended, what problems may arise if the treatment is not given, and possible adverse effects of the treatment.

> ▶ **Take** NOTE!
>
> *Parents have the right to refuse this treatment, but if they received adequate teaching about the treatment and understand its importance, they usually will consent to it.*

Maintaining Thermoregulation

Newborns have trouble regulating their temperature, especially during the first few hours after birth (see Chap. 17 for a complete discussion). Therefore, maintaining body temperature is crucial.

Assess body temperature frequently during the immediate newborn period. The baby's temperature should be taken every 30 minutes for the first 2 hours or until the temperature has stabilized, and then every 8 hours until discharge (AAP, 2007).

Commonly a thermistor probe (automatic sensor) is attached to the newborn to record body temperature on a monitoring device. The probe is taped to the newborn's abdomen, usually in the right upper quadrant, which allows for position changes without having to readjust the probe. The other end of the thermistor probe is inserted into the radiant heat control panel. Temperature parameters are set on an alarm system connected to the heat panel that will sound if the newborn's temperature falls out of the set range. Check the probe connection period-

ically to make sure that it remains secure. Remember the potential for heat loss in newborns, and perform all nursing interventions in a way that minimizes heat loss and prevents hypothermia.

Axillary temperatures can also be used to assess the newborn's body temperature. At one time, rectal thermometers were routinely used to monitor body temperature, but their use is no longer recommended because of the risk of traumatizing the rectal lining (Blackburn, 2007). A newborn's temperature typically is maintained at 36.5° to 37.5°C (97.7° to 99.7°F) (Kenner & Lott, 2007).

Nursing interventions to help maintain body temperature include:

• Dry the newborn immediately after birth to prevent heat loss through evaporation.
• Wrap the baby in warmed blankets to reduce heat loss via convection.
• Use a warmed cover on the scale to weigh the unclothed newborn.
• Warm stethoscopes and hands before examining the baby or providing care.
• Avoid placing newborns in drafts or near air vents to prevent heat loss through convection.
• Delay the initial bath until the baby's temperature has stabilized to prevent heat loss through evaporation.
• Avoid placing cribs near cold outer walls to prevent heat loss through radiation.
• Put a cap on the newborn's head after it is thoroughly dried after birth.
• Place the newborn under a temperature-controlled radiant warmer (Fig. 18.7).

Nursing Management During the Early Newborn Period

The early newborn period is a time of great adjustment for both the mother and the newborn, both of whom are adapting to many physiologic and psychological changes. In the past, mothers and newborns remained in the health care facility while these dramatic changes were taking place, with nurses and doctors readily available. However, today shorter hospital stays are the norm, and new mothers can easily be overwhelmed by having to go through all of these changes in such a short time: the woman gives birth, experiences marked physiologic and psychological changes, and must adapt to her newborn and learn the skills needed to care for herself and the baby, all within 24 to 48 hours.

The nurse's role is to assist the mother and her newborn through this dramatic transition period. The newborn needs continued health assessment, and the mother needs to be taught to care for the new baby. At discharge, the new mother may panic and feel insecure about her role as primary caretaker. Nurses play a major role in promoting the newborn's transition by providing ongoing assessment and

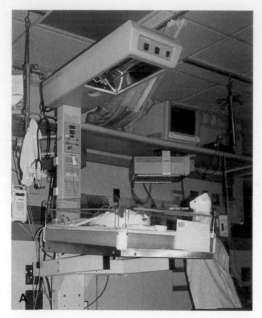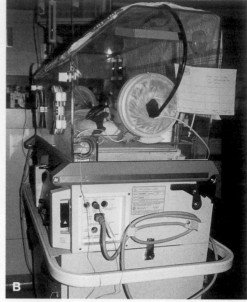

FIGURE 18.7 Maintaining thermoregulation. (**A**) Radiant warmer. (**B**) Isolette.

care and in promoting the woman's confidence by serving as a role model and teaching about proper newborn care.

Assessment

The newborn requires ongoing assessment after leaving the birthing area to ensure that his or her transition to extrauterine life is progressing without problems. The nurse uses the data gathered during the initial assessment as a baseline for comparison.

Perinatal History

Pertinent maternal and fetal data are vital to formulate a plan of care for the mother and her newborn. Historical information is obtained from the medical record and from interviewing the mother. Review the maternal history because it provides pertinent information, such as the presence of certain risk factors that could affect the newborn. Keep in mind that a comprehensive maternal history may not be available, especially if the mother has had limited or no prenatal care.

Historical information usually includes the following:

- Mother's name, medical record number, blood type, serology result, rubella and hepatitis status, and history of substance abuse
- Other maternal tests that are relevant to the newborn and care, such as HIV and group B streptococcus status
- Intrapartum maternal antibiotic therapy (type, dose, and duration)
- Maternal illness that can affect the pregnancy, evidence of chorioamnionitis, maternal use of medications such as steroids
- Prenatal care, including timing of first visit and subsequent visits

- Risk for blood group incompatibility, including Rh status and blood type
- Fetal distress or any nonreassuring fetal heart rate patterns during labor
- Known inherited conditions such as sickle cell anemia and phenylketonuria (PKU)
- Birthweights of previous live-born children, along with identification of any newborn problems
- Social history, including tobacco, alcohol, and recreational drug use
- History of depression or domestic violence
- Cultural factors, including primary language and educational level
- Pregnancy complications associated with abnormal fetal growth, fetal anomalies, or abnormal results from tests of fetal well-being
- Information on the progress of labor, birth, labor complications, duration of ruptured membranes, and presence of meconium in the amniotic fluid
- Medications given during labor, at birth, and immediately after birth
- Time and method of delivery, including presentation and the use of forceps or a vacuum extractor
- Status of the newborn at birth, including Apgar scores at 1 and 5 minutes, the need for suctioning, weight, gestational age, vital signs, and umbilical cord status
- Medications administered to the newborn
- Postbirth maternal information, including placental findings, positive cultures, and presence of fever

Newborn Physical Examination

The initial newborn physical examination, which may demonstrate subtle differences related to the newborn's age, is carried out within the first 24 hours after birth. For example, a newborn who is 30 minutes old has not yet completed the normal transition from intrauterine to extrauterine life, and thus variability may exist in vital signs and in respiratory, neurologic, gastrointestinal, skin, and cardiovascular systems. Therefore, a comprehensive examination should be delayed until after the newborn has completed the transition.

In a quiet newborn, begin the examination with the least invasive and noxious elements of the examination (auscultation of heart and lungs). Then examine the areas most likely to irritate the newborn (e.g., examining the hips and eliciting the Moro reflex). A general visual assessment provides an enormous amount of information about the well-being of a newborn. Initial observation gives an impression of a healthy (stable) versus an ill newborn and a term versus a preterm newborn.

A typical physical examination of a newborn includes a general survey of skin color, posture, state of alertness, head size, overall behavioral state, respiratory status, gender, and any obvious congenital anomalies. Check the overall appearance for anything unusual. Then complete the examination in a systematic fashion.

Remember Kelly, who called the home health nurse and said her newborn son "looks like a canary"? What additional information is needed about the baby? What might be causing his yellow color?

Anthropometric Measurements

Shortly after birth, after the gender of the child is revealed, most parents want to know the "vital statistics" of their newborn—length and weight—to report to their family and friends. Additional measurements, including head and chest circumference, are also taken and recorded. Abdominal measurements are not routinely obtained unless there is a suspicion of pathology that causes abdominal distention. The newborn's progress from that point on will be validated based on these early measurements. These measurements will be compared with future serial measurements to determine growth patterns, which are plotted on growth charts to evaluate normalcy. Therefore, accuracy is key.

Length

The average length of most newborns is 50 cm (20 in), but it can range from 45 to 55 cm (18 to 22 in). Measure length with the unclothed newborn lying on a warmed blanket placed on a flat surface with the knees held in an extended position. Then run a tape measure down the length of the newborn—from the head to the soles of the feet—and record this measurement in the newborn's record (see Fig. 18.1).

Weight

At birth the average newborn weighs 3,400 g (7.5 lb), but normal birthweights can range from 2,500 to 4,000 g (5 lb, 8 oz to 8 lb, 14 oz). Newborns are weighed immediately after birth and then daily. Newborns usually lose up to 10% of their birthweight within the first few days of life, but regain it in approximately 10 days. Newborns are weighed on admission to the nursery or are taken to a digital scale to be weighed and returned to the mother's room.

First, balance the scale if it is not balanced. Place a warmed protective cloth or paper as a barrier on the scale to prevent heat loss by conduction; recalibrate the scale to zero after applying the barrier. Next, place the unclothed newborn in the center of the scale. Keep a hand above the newborn for safety (see Fig. 18.2).

Weight is affected by racial origin, maternal age, size of the parents, maternal nutrition, and placental perfusion (Lawrence, 2006). Weight should be correlated with gestational age. A newborn who weighs more than normal might be LGA or an infant of a diabetic mother (IDM); a newborn who weighs less than normal might be SGA or preterm or might have a genetic syndrome. It is important to identify the cause for the deviation in size and to monitor the newborn for complications common to that etiology.

Head Circumference

The average newborn head circumference is 32 to 38 cm (13 to 15 in). Measure the circumference at the head's widest diameter (the occipitofrontal circumference). Wrap a flexible or paper measuring tape snugly around the newborn's head and record the measurement (Fig. 18.8A).

▶ **Take** NOTE!

Head circumference may need to be remeasured at a later time if the shape of the head is altered from birth.

The head circumference should be approximately one fourth of the newborn's length (Lawrence, 2006). A small head might indicate microcephaly caused by rubella, toxoplasmosis, or SGA status; an enlarged head might indicate hydrocephalus or increased intracranial pressure. Both need to be documented and reported for further investigation.

Chest Circumference

The average chest circumference is 30 to 36 cm (12 to 14 in). It is generally equal to or about 2 to 3 cm less than the head circumference (Burns et al., 2009). Place a flexible or paper tape measure around the unclothed newborn's chest at the nipple line without pulling it taut (see Fig. 18.8B).

▶ **Take** NOTE!

The head and chest circumferences are usually equal by about 1 year of age.

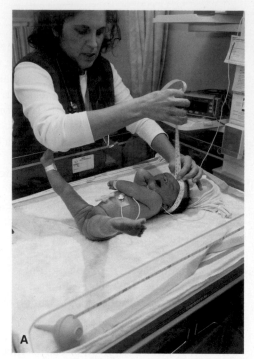 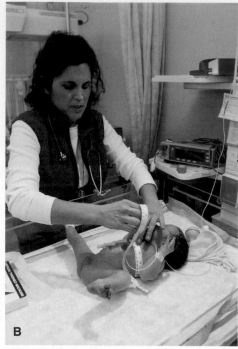

FIGURE 18.8 (**A**) Measuring head circumference. (**B**) Measuring chest circumference.

Vital Signs

In the newborn, temperature, pulse, and respirations are monitored frequently and compared with baseline data obtained immediately after birth. Generally, vital signs (excluding blood pressure) are taken:

- On admission to the nursery or in the LDR room after the parents are allowed to hold and bond with the newborn
- Once every 30 minutes until the newborn has been stable for 2 hours
- Then once every 4 to 8 hours until discharge (AAP, 2007)

Blood pressure is not routinely assessed in a normal newborn unless the baby's clinical condition warrants it. This schedule can change depending on the baby's health status.

Obtain a newborn's temperature by placing an electronic temperature probe in the midaxillary area or by monitoring the electronic thermistor probe that has been taped to the abdominal skin (applied when the newborn was placed under a radiant heat source).

Monitor the newborn's temperature hourly for changes until it stabilizes. On average, a newborn's temperature is 36.5° to 37.5°C (97.9° to 99.7°F). If the temperature is higher, adjust the environment, such as removing some clothing or blankets. If the temperature is lower, check the radiant warmer setting or add a warmed blanket. Report any abnormalities to the primary health care provider if simple adjustments to the environment do not change the baby's temperature.

Obtain an apical pulse by placing the stethoscope over the fourth intercostal space on the chest. Listen for a full minute, noting rate, rhythm, and abnormal sounds such as murmurs. In the typical newborn, the heart rate is 120 to 160 bpm, with wide fluctuations with activity and sleep. Sinus arrhythmia is a normal finding. Murmurs detected during the newborn period do not necessarily indicate congenital heart disease, but they need to be assessed frequently over the next several months to see if they persist.

Also palpate the apical, femoral, and brachial pulses for presence and equality (Fig. 18.9). Report any abnormalities to the primary health care provider for evaluation.

Assess respirations by observing the rise and fall of the chest for 1 full minute. Respirations should be symmetric, slightly irregular, shallow, and unlabored at a rate of 30 to 60 breaths/minute. The newborn's respirations are predominantly diaphragmatic, but they are synchronous with abdominal movements. Also auscultate breath sounds. Note any abnormalities, such as tachypnea, bradypnea, grunting, gasping, periods of apnea lasting longer than 20 seconds, asymmetry or decreased chest expansion, abnormal breath sounds (rhonchi, crackles), or sternal retractions. Some variations might exist early after birth, but if the abnormal pattern persists, notify the primary health care provider.

Skin

Observe the overall appearance of the skin, including color, texture, turgor, and integrity. The newborn's skin should be smooth and flexible, and the color should be consistent with genetic background.

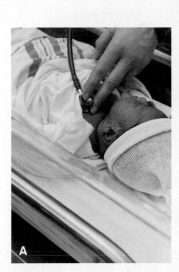 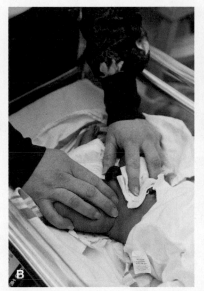 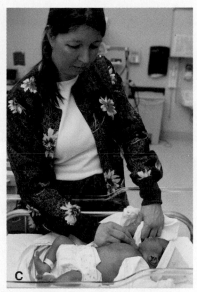

FIGURE 18.9 Assessing the newborn's vital signs. (**A**) Assessing the apical pulse. (**B**) Palpating the femoral pulse. (**C**) Palpating the brachial pulse.

Skin Condition and Color

Check skin turgor by pinching a small area of skin over the chest or abdomen and note how quickly it returns to its original position. In a well-hydrated newborn, the skin should return to its normal position immediately. Skin that remains "tented" after being pinched indicates dehydration. A small amount of lanugo (fine downy hair) may be observed over the shoulders and on the sides of the face and upper back. There may be some cracking and peeling of the skin. The skin should be warm to the touch and intact.

The newborn's skin often appears blotchy or mottled, especially in the extremities. Persistent cyanosis of fingers, hands, toes, and feet with mottled blue or red discoloration and coldness is called **acrocyanosis**. It may be seen in newborns during the first few weeks of life in response to exposure to cold. Acrocyanosis is normal and intermittent.

Newborn Skin Variations

While assessing the skin, note any rashes, ecchymoses or petechiae, nevi, or dark pigmentation. Skin lesions can be congenital or transient; they may be a result of infection or may result from the mode of birth. If any are present, observe the anatomic location, arrangement, type, and color. Bruising may result from the use of devices such as a vacuum extractor during delivery. Petechiae may be the result of pressure on the skin during the birth process. Forceps marks may be observed over the cheeks and ears. A small puncture mark may be seen if internal fetal scalp electrode monitoring was used during labor.

Common skin variations include vernix caseosa, stork bites or salmon patches, milia, Mongolian spots, erythema toxicum, harlequin sign, nevus flammeus, and nevus vasculosus (Fig. 18.10).

Vernix caseosa is a thick white substance that protects the skin of the fetus. It is formed by secretions from the fetus's oil glands and is found during the first 2 or 3 days after birth in body creases and the hair. It does not need to be removed because it will be absorbed into the skin.

Stork bites or salmon patches are superficial vascular areas found on the nape of the neck, on the eyelids, and between the eyes and upper lip (see Fig. 18.10A). The name comes from the marks on the back of the neck where, as myth goes, a stork may have picked up the baby. They are caused by a concentration of immature blood vessels and are most visible when the newborn is crying. They are considered a normal variant, and most fade and disappear completely within the first year.

Milia are unopened sebaceous glands frequently found on a newborn's nose. They may also appear on the chin and forehead (see Fig. 18.10B). They form from oil glands and disappear on their own within 2 to 4 weeks. When they occur in a newborn's mouth and gums, they are termed **Epstein's pearls**. They occur in approximately 60% of newborns (AAP, 2007b).

Mongolian spots are blue or purple splotches that appear on the lower back and buttocks of newborns (see Fig. 18.10C). They tend to occur in African-American, Asian, and Indian newborns but can occur in dark-skinned newborns of all races. The spots are caused by a concentration of pigmented cells and usually disappear within the first 4 years of life (Kliegman et al., 2007).

Erythema toxicum (newborn rash) is a benign, idiopathic, generalized, transient rash that occurs in up to 70% of all newborns during the first week of life. It consists of small papules or pustules on the skin resembling flea bites. The rash is common on the face, chest, and back (see Fig. 18.10D). One of the chief characteristics

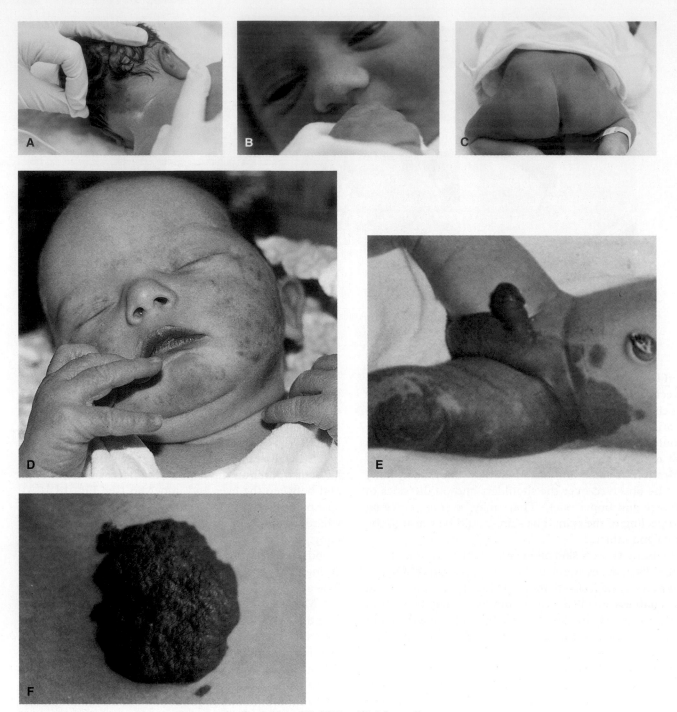

FIGURE 18.10 Common skin variations. (**A**) Stork bite. (**B**) Milia. (**C**) Mongolian spots.
(**D**) Erythema toxicum. (**E**) Nevus flammeus (port-wine stain). (**F**) Strawberry hemangioma.

of this rash is its lack of pattern. It is caused by the newborn's eosinophils reacting to the environment as the immune system matures (AAP, 2007b). It does not require
any treatment and disappears in a few days.

Harlequin sign refers to the dilation of blood vessels on only one side of the body, giving the newborn the
appearance of wearing a clown suit. It gives a distinct
midline demarcation, which is described as pale on the
nondependent side and red on the opposite, dependent

side. It results from immature autoregulation of blood
flow and is commonly seen in low-birthweight newborns
when there is a positional change (Dillon, 2007). It is transient, lasting as long as 20 minutes, and no intervention
is needed.

Nevus flammeus, also called a port wine stain, commonly appears on the newborn's face or other body areas
(see Fig. 18.10E). It is a capillary angioma located directly below the dermis. It is flat with sharp demarcations

and is purple–red. This skin lesion is made up of mature capillaries that are congested and dilated. It ranges in size from a few millimeters to large, occasionally involving as much as half the body surface. Although it does not grow in area or size, it is permanent and will not fade. Port wine stains may be associated with structural malformations, bony or muscular overgrowth, and certain cancers. Recent studies have noted an association between port wine birthmarks and childhood cancer, so newborns with these lesions should be monitored with periodic eye examinations, neurologic imaging, and extremity measurements (Johnson et al., 2007). Pulsed dye laser surgery has been used to remove larger lesions with some success (AAP, 2007b).

Nevus vasculosus, also called a strawberry mark or strawberry hemangioma, is a benign capillary hemangioma in the dermal and subdermal layers. It is raised, rough, dark red, and sharply demarcated (see Fig. 18.10F). It is commonly found in the head region within a few weeks after birth and can increase in size or number. Commonly seen in premature infants weighing less than 1,500 g (Kenner & Lott, 2007), these hemangiomas tend to resolve by age 3 without any treatment.

Head

Head size varies with age, gender, and ethnicity and has a general correlation with body size. Inspect a newborn's head from all angles. The head should appear symmetric and round. As many as 90% of the congenital malformations present at birth are visible on the head and neck, so careful assessment is very important (AAP, 2007a).

The newborn has two fontanels at the juncture of the cranial bones. The anterior fontanel is diamond-shaped and closes by 18 to 24 months. Typically it measures 4 to 6 cm at the largest diameter (bone to bone). The posterior one is triangular, smaller than the anterior fontanel (usually fingertip size or 0.5 to 1 cm), and closes by 6 to 12 weeks. Palpate both fontanels, which should be soft, flat, and open. Then palpate the skull. It should feel smooth and fused, except at the area of the fontanels. Also assess the size of the head and the anterior and posterior fontanels, and compare them with appropriate standards.

Variations in Head Size and Appearance

During inspection and palpation, be alert for common variations that may cause asymmetry. These include caput succedaneum, cephalhematoma, and molding.

Molding is the elongated shaping of the fetal head to accommodate passage through the birth canal (Fig. 18.11). It occurs with a vaginal birth from a vertex position in which elongation of the fetal head occurs with prominence of the occiput and overriding sagittal suture line. It typically resolves within a week after birth without intervention.

Caput succedaneum describes localized edema on the scalp that occurs from the pressure of the birth process. It is commonly observed after prolonged labor. Clinically,

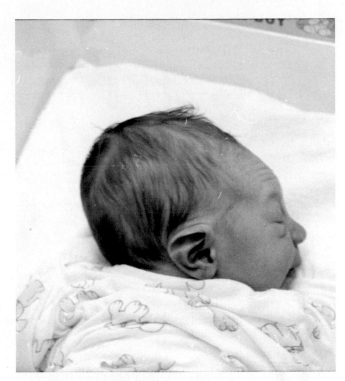

FIGURE **18.11** Molding in a newborn's head.

it appears as a poorly demarcated soft tissue swelling that crosses suture lines. Pitting edema and overlying petechiae and ecchymosis are noted (Fig. 18.12A). The swelling will gradually dissipate in about 3 days without any treatment. Newborns who were delivered via vacuum extraction usually have a caput in the area where the cup was used.

Cephalhematoma is a localized effusion of blood beneath the periosteum of the skull. This condition is due to disruption of the vessels during birth. It occurs after prolonged labor and use of obstetric interventions such as low forceps or vacuum extraction. The clinical features include a well-demarcated, often fluctuant swelling with no overlying skin discoloration. The swelling does not cross suture lines and is firmer to the touch than an edematous area (see Fig. 18.12B). Cephalhematoma usually appears on the second or third day after birth and disappears within weeks or months (Simonson et al., 2007).

Common Abnormalities in Head or Fontanel Size

Common abnormalities in head or fontanel size that may indicate a problem include:

- Microcephaly—a head circumference more than 2 standard deviations below average or less than 10% of normal parameters for gestational age, caused by failure of brain development (Cohen, 2007). It can be familial, with autosomal dominant or recessive inheritance, and it may be associated with infections (cytomegalovirus) and syndromes such as trisomy 13 and 18, and fetal alcohol syndrome (Kenner & Lott, 2007).

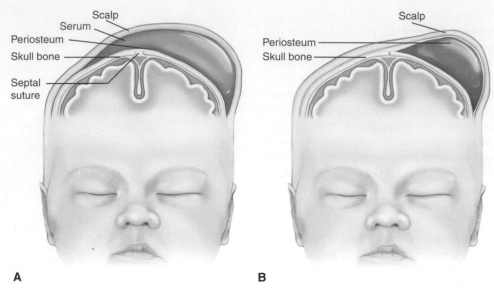

FIGURE 18.12 (**A**) Caput succedaneum involves the collection of serous fluid and often crosses the suture line. (**B**) Cephalhematoma involves the collection of blood and does not cross the suture line.

- Macrocephaly—a head circumference more than 90% of normal, typically related to hydrocephalus (Dillon, 2007). It is often familial (with autosomal dominant inheritance) and can be either an isolated anomaly or a manifestation of other anomalies, including hydrocephalus and skeletal disorders (achondroplasia).
- Large fontanels—more than 6 cm in the anterior diameter bone to bone or more than a 1-cm diameter in the posterior fontanel; possibly associated with malnutrition, hydrocephaly, congenital hypothyroidism, trisomies 13, 18, and 21, and various bone disorders such as osteogenesis imperfecta
- Small or closed fontanels—smaller-than-normal anterior and posterior diameters or fontanels that are closed at birth; associated with microcephaly or premature synostosis (union of two bones by osseous material) (Blackburn, 2007)

Face

Observe the newborn's face for fullness and symmetry. The face should have full cheeks and should be symmetric when the baby is resting and crying. If forceps were used during birth, the newborn may have bruising and reddened areas over both cheeks and parietal bones secondary to the pressure of the forceps blades. Reassure the parents that this resolves without treatment, and point out improvement each day.

Problems with the face can also involve facial nerve paralysis caused by trauma from the use of forceps. Paralysis is usually apparent on the first or second day of life. Typically, the newborn will demonstrate asymmetry of the face with the inability to close the eye and move the lips on the affected side. Newborns with facial nerve paralysis have difficulty making a seal around the nipple, and con-

sequently milk or formula drools from the paralyzed side of the mouth. Most facial nerve palsies resolve spontaneously within days, although full recovery may require weeks to months. Attempt to determine the cause from the newborn's history.

Nose

Inspect the nose for size, symmetry, position, and lesions. The newborn's nose is small and narrow. The nose should have a midline placement, patent nares, and an intact septum. The nostrils should be of equal size and should be patent. A slight mucus discharge may be present, but there should be no actual drainage. The newborn is a preferential nose breather and will use sneezing to clear the nose if needed. The newborn can smell after the nasal passages are cleared of amniotic fluid and mucus (AAP, 2007a).

Mouth

Inspect the newborn's mouth, lips, and interior structures. The lips should be intact with symmetric movement and positioned in the midline; there should not be any lesions. Inspect the lips for pink color, moisture, and cracking. The lips should encircle the examiner's finger to form a vacuum. Variations involving the lip might include cleft upper lip (separation extending up to the nose) or thin upper lip associated with fetal alcohol syndrome.

Assess the inside of the mouth for alignment of the mandible, intact soft and hard palate, sucking pads inside the cheeks, a midline uvula, a free-moving tongue, and working gag, swallow, and sucking reflexes. The mucous membranes lining the oral cavity should be pink and moist, with minimal saliva present.

Normal variations might include Epstein's pearls (small, white epidermal cysts on the gums and hard palate that disappear in weeks), erupted precocious teeth that may need to be removed to prevent aspiration, and thrush (white plaque inside the mouth caused by exposure to *Candida albicans* during birth), which cannot be wiped away with a cotton-tipped applicator.

Eyes

Inspect the external eye structures, including the eyelids, lashes, conjunctiva, sclera, iris, and pupils, for position, color, size, and movement. There may be marked edema of the eyelids and subconjunctival hemorrhages due to pressure during birth. The eyes should be clear and symmetrically placed. Test the blink reflex by bringing an object close to the eye; the newborn should respond quickly by blinking. Also test the newborn's pupillary reflex: pupils should be equal, round, and reactive to light bilaterally. Assess the newborn's gaze: he or she should be able to track objects to the midline. Movement may be uncoordinated during the first few weeks of life. Many newborns have transient strabismus (deviation or wandering of eyes independently) and searching nystagmus (involuntary repetitive eye movement), which is caused by immature muscular control. These are normal for the first 3 to 6 months of age.

Examine the internal eye structures. A red reflex (luminous red appearance seen on the retina) should be seen bilaterally on retinoscopy. The red reflex normally shows no dullness or irregularities.

Chemical conjunctivitis commonly occurs within 24 hours of instillation of eye prophylaxis after birth. There is lid edema with sterile discharge from both eyes. Usually it resolves within 48 hours without treatment.

Ears

Inspect the ears for size, shape, skin condition, placement, amount of cartilage, and patency of the auditory canal. The ears should be soft and pliable and should recoil quickly and easily when folded and released. Ears should be aligned with the outer canthi of the eyes. Low-set ears are characteristic of many syndromes and genetic abnormalities, such as trisomy 13 and 18, and internal organ abnormalities involving the renal system.

An otoscopic examination is not typically done because the newborn's ear canals are filled with amniotic fluid and vernix caseosa, which would make visualization of the tympanic membrane difficult.

Newborn hearing screening is required by law in most states (discussed later in the chapter). Hearing loss is the most common birth defect in the United States: One in 1,000 newborns is profoundly deaf and 2 to 3 in 1,000 have partial hearing loss (Wrightson, 2007). Delays in identification and intervention may affect the child's cognitive, verbal, behavioral, and emotional development. Screening at birth has reduced the age at which newborns with hearing loss are identified and has improved early intervention rates dramatically (AAP, 2007b). Prior to universal newborn screening, children were usually older than 2 years before significant congenital hearing loss was detected; by this time it had already affected their speech and language skills (USPSTF, 2006).

Causes of hearing loss can be conductive, sensorineural, or central. Risk factors for congenital hearing loss include cytomegalovirus infection and preterm birth necessitating a stay in the neonatal intensive care unit.

To assess for hearing ability generally, observe the newborn's response to noises and conversations. The newborn typically turns toward these noises and startles with loud ones.

Neck

Inspect the newborn's neck for movement and ability to support the head. The newborn's neck will appear almost nonexistent because it is so short. Creases are usually noted. The neck should move freely in all directions and should be capable of holding the head in a midline position. The newborn should have enough head control to be able to hold it up briefly without support. Report any deviations such as restricted neck movement or absence of head control.

Also inspect the clavicles, which should be straight and intact. The clavicles are the bones mostly commonly broken in infants, especially large ones. In most cases, the fractured clavicle is asymptomatic, but decreased or absent movement and pain or tenderness on movement of the arm on the affected side may be noted (Kenner & Lott, 2007). Treatment involves immobilization and minimizing pain.

Chest

Inspect the newborn's chest for size, shape, and symmetry. The newborn's chest should be round, symmetric, and 2 to 3 cm smaller than the head circumference. The xiphoid process may be prominent at birth, but it usually becomes less apparent when adipose tissue accumulates. Nipples may be engorged and may secrete a white discharge. This discharge, which occurs in both boys and girls, is a result of exposure to high levels of maternal estrogen while in utero. This enlargement and milky discharge usually dissipates within a few weeks. Some newborns may have extra nipples, called supernumerary nipples. They are typically small, raised, pigmented areas vertical to the main nipple line, 5 to 6 cm below the normal nipple (AAP, 2007a). They tend to be familial and do not contain glandular tissue. Reassure parents that these extra small nipples are harmless.

The newborn chest is usually barrel-shaped with equal anteroposterior and lateral diameters, and symmetric. Auscultate the lungs bilaterally for equal breath sounds. Normal breath sounds should be heard, with little difference between inspiration and expiration. Fine crackles can be heard on inspiration soon after birth as a result of clearing amniotic fluid from the lungs. Diminished breath sounds might indicate atelectasis, effusion, or poor respiratory effort (Dillon, 2007).

Listen to the heart when the newborn is quiet or sleeping. S1 and S2 heart sounds are accentuated at birth. The point of maximal impulse (PMI) is a lateral to midclavicular line located at the fourth intercostal space. A displaced PMI may indicate tension pneumothorax or cardiomegaly. Murmurs are often heard and are usually benign, but if present after the first 12 hours of life should be evaluated to rule out a cardiac disorder (Kliegman et al., 2007).

Abdomen

Inspect the abdomen for shape and movement. Typically the newborn's abdomen is protuberant but not distended. This contour is a result of the immaturity of the abdominal muscles. Abdominal movements are synchronous with respirations because newborns are, at times, abdominal breathers.

Auscultate bowel sounds in all four quadrants and then palpate the abdomen for consistency, masses, and tenderness. Perform auscultation and palpation systematically in a clockwise fashion until all four quadrants have been assessed. Palpate gently to feel the liver, the kidneys, and any masses. The liver is normally palpable 1 to 3 cm below the costal margin in the midclavicular line. The kidneys are 1 to 2 cm above and to both sides of the umbilicus. Normal findings would include bowel sounds in all four quadrants and no masses or tenderness on palpation. Absent or hyperactive bowel sounds might indicate an intestinal obstruction. Abdominal distention might indicate ascites, obstruction, infection, masses, or an enlarged abdominal organ (Cohen, 2007).

Inspect the umbilical cord area for the correct amount of blood vessels (two arteries and one vein). The umbilical vein is larger than the two umbilical arteries. Evidence of only a single umbilical artery is associated with renal and gastrointestinal anomalies. Also inspect the umbilical area for signs of bleeding, infection, granuloma, or abnormal communication with the intra-abdominal organs (Walsh, 2007).

Genitalia

Inspect the penis and scrotum in the male. In the circumcised male newborn, the glans should be smooth, with the meatus centered at the tip of the penis. It will appear reddened until it heals. For the uncircumcised male, the foreskin should cover the glans. Check the position of the urinary meatus: it should be in the midline at the glans tip. If it is on the ventral surface of the penis, hypospadias is present; if it is on the dorsal surface of the penis, it is termed epispadias. In either case, circumcision should be avoided until further evaluation.

Inspect the scrotum for size, symmetry, color, presence of rugae, and location of testes. The scrotum usually appears relatively large and should be pink in white neonates and dark brown in neonates of color. Rugae should be well formed and should cover the scrotal sac. There should not be bulging, edema, or discoloration (Fig. 18.13A).

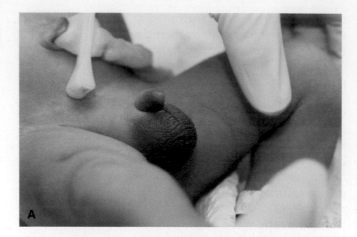

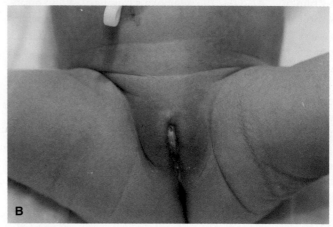

FIGURE **18.13** Newborn genitalia. (**A**) Male genitalia. Note the darkened color of the scrotum. (**B**) Female genitalia.

Palpate the scrotum for evidence of the testes, which should be in the scrotal sac. The testes should feel firm and smooth and should be of equal size on both sides of the scrotal sac in the term newborn. Undescended testes (cryptorchidism) might be palpated in the inguinal canal in preterm infants; they can be unilateral or bilateral. If the testes are not palpable within the scrotal sac, further investigation is needed.

In the female newborn, inspect the external genitalia. The urethral meatus is located below the clitoris in the midline (Dillon, 2007). In contrast to the male genitalia, the female genitalia will be engorged: the labia majora and minora may both be edematous. The labia majora is large and covers the labia minora. The clitoris is large and the hymen is thick. These findings are due to the maternal hormones estrogen and progesterone (see Fig. 18.13B). A vaginal discharge composed of mucus mixed with blood may also be present during the first few weeks of life. This discharge, called **pseudomenstruation**, requires no treatment. Explain this phenomenon to the parents.

Variations in female newborns may include a labial bulge, which might indicate an inguinal hernia; ambiguous genitalia; a rectovaginal fistula with feces present in the vagina; and an imperforate hymen.

Inspect the anus in both male and female newborns for position and patency. Passage of meconium indicates patency. If meconium is not passed, a lubricated rectal thermometer can be inserted or a digital examination can be performed to determine patency. Abnormal findings would include anal fissures or fistulas and no meconium passed within 24 hours after birth.

Extremities and Back

Inspect the newborn's upper extremities for appearance and movement. Inspect the hands for shape, number, and position of fingers and presence of palmar creases. The newborn's arms and hands should be symmetric and should move through range of motion without hesitation. Observe for spontaneous movement of the extremities. Each hand should have five digits. Note any extra digits (polydactyly) or fusing of two or more digits (syndactyly). Most newborns have three palmar creases on the hand. A single palmar crease, called a simian line, is frequently associated with Down syndrome.

A brachial plexus injury can occur during a difficult birth involving shoulder dystocia. Erb's palsy is an injury resulting from damage to the upper plexus during labor and birth. The affected arm hangs limp alongside the body, and the affected shoulder and arm are adducted, extended, and internally rotated with a pronated wrist. The Moro reflex is absent on the affected side in brachial palsy. Complete recovery may take 3 to 6 months (Adegbehingbe et al., 2007).

Assess the lower extremities in the same manner. They should of equal length, with symmetric skin folds. Inspect the feet for clubfoot (a turning-inward position), which is secondary to intrauterine positioning. This may be positional or structural. Perform the Ortolani and Barlow maneuvers to identify congenital hip dislocation, commonly termed developmental dysplasia of the hip (DDH). Nursing Procedure 18.1 highlights the steps for performing these maneuvers.

Inspect the back. The spine should appear straight and flat and should be easily flexed when the baby is held in a prone position. Observe for the presence of a tuft of

---

Nursing Procedure 18.1

PERFORMING ORTOLANI AND BARLOW MANEUVERS

Purpose: To Detect Congenital Developmental Dysplasia of the Hip

Ortolani Maneuver
1. Place the newborn in the supine position and flex the hips and knees to 90 degrees at the hip.
2. Grasp the inner aspect of the thighs and abduct the hips (usually to approximately 180 degrees) while applying upward pressure.

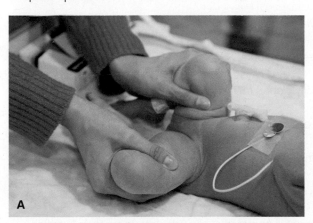

A

3. Listen for any sounds during the maneuver. There should be no "cluck" or "click" heard when the legs are abducted. Such a sound indicates the femoral head hitting the acetabulum as the head re-enters the area. This suggests developmental hip dysplasia.

Barlow Maneuver
1. With the newborn still lying supine and grasping the inner aspect of the thighs (as just mentioned), adduct the thighs while applying outward and downward pressure to the thighs.

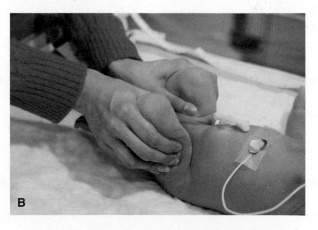

B

2. Feel for the femoral head slipping out of the acetabulum; also listen for a click (Dillon, 2007).

hair, a pilonidal dimple in the midline, a cyst, or a mass along the spine. These abnormal findings should be documented and reported to the primary health care provider.

Table 18.3 summarizes the newborn assessment.

Neurologic Status

Assess the newborn's state of alertness, posture, muscle tone, and reflexes.

Newborn Alertness, Posture, and Muscle Tone

The newborn should be alert and not persistently lethargic. The normal posture is hips abducted and partially flexed, with knees flexed. Arms are adducted and flexed at the elbow. Fists are often clenched, with fingers covering the thumb.

To assess for muscle tone, support the newborn with one hand under the chest. Observe how the neck muscles hold the head. The neck extensors should be able to hold the head in line briefly. There should be only slight head lag when pulling the newborn from a supine position to a sitting one.

Newborn Reflexes

Assess the newborn's reflexes to evaluate neurologic function and development. Absent or abnormal reflexes in a newborn, persistence of a reflex past the age when the reflex is normally lost, or return of an infantile reflex in an older child or adult may indicate neurologic pathology (Table 18.4). Reflexes commonly assessed in the newborn include sucking, Moro, stepping, tonic neck, root-

TABLE 18.3 NEWBORN ASSESSMENT SUMMARY

Assessment	Usual Findings	Variations and Common Problems
Anthropometric measurements	Head circumference: 33–37 cm (13–14 in) Chest circumference: 30–33 cm (12–13 in) Weight: 2,500–4,000 g (5.5–8.5 lb) Length: 45–55 cm (19–21 in)	SGA, LGA, preterm, postterm
Vital signs	Temperature: 36.5°–37.5°C (97°–99°F) Apical pulse: 120–160 bpm Respirations: 30–60 breaths/minute	
Skin	Normal: smooth, flexible, good skin turgor, warm	Jaundice, acrocyanosis, milia, Mongolian spots, stork bites
Head	Normal: varies with age, gender, ethnicity	Microcephaly, macrocephaly, enlarged fontanels
Face	Normal: full cheeks, facial features symmetric	Facial nerve paralysis, nevus flammeus, nevus vasculosus
Nose	Normal: small, placement in the midline and narrow, ability to smell	Malformation or blockage
Mouth	Normal: aligned in midline, symmetric, intact soft and hard palate	Epstein's pearls, erupted precocious teeth, thrush
Neck	Normal: short, creased, moves freely, baby holds head in midline	Restricted movement, clavicular fractures
Eyes	Normal: clear and symmetrically placed on face	Chemical conjunctivitis, subconjunctival hemorrhages
Ears	Normal: soft and pliable with quick recoil when folded and released	Low-set ears, hearing loss
Chest	Normal: round, symmetric, smaller than head	Nipple engorgement, whitish discharge
Abdomen	Normal: protuberant contour, soft, three vessels in umbilical cord	Distended, only two vessels in umbilical cord
Genitals	Normal male: smooth glans, meatus centered at tip of penis Normal female: swollen female genitals as a result of maternal estrogen	Edematous scrotum in males, vaginal discharge in females
Extremities and spine	Normal: extremities symmetric with free movement	Congenital hip dislocation; tuft or dimple on spine

TABLE 18.4 **NEWBORN REFLEXES: APPEARANCE AND DISAPPEARANCE**

Reflex	Appearance	Disappearance
Blinking	Newborn	Persists into adulthood
Moro	Newborn	3–6 mo
Grasp	Newborn	3–4 mo
Stepping	Birth	1–2 mo
Tonic neck	Newborn	3–4 mo
Sneeze	Newborn	Persists into adulthood
Rooting	Birth	4–6 mo
Gag reflex	Newborn	Persists into adulthood
Cough reflex	Newborn	Persists into adulthood
Babinski sign	Newborn	12 mo

ing, Babinski, and palmar grasp reflex. Spinal reflexes tested include truncal incurvation (Galant reflex) and anocutaneous reflex (anal wink).

The sucking reflex is elicited by gently stimulating the newborn's lips by touching them. The newborn will typically open the mouth and begin a sucking motion. Placing a gloved finger in the newborn's mouth will also elicit a sucking motion (Fig. 18.14A).

The Moro reflex, also called the embrace reflex, occurs when the neonate is startled. To elicit this reflex, place the newborn on his or her back. Support the upper body weight of the supine newborn by the arms, using a lifting motion, without lifting the newborn off the surface. Then release the arms suddenly. The newborn will throw the arms outward and flex the knees; the arms then return to the chest. The fingers also spread to form a C. The newborn initially appears startled and then relaxes to a normal resting position (see Fig. 18.14B).

Assess the stepping reflex by holding the newborn upright and inclined forward with the soles of the feet touching a flat surface. The baby should make a stepping motion or walking, alternating flexion and extension with the soles of the feet (see Fig. 18.14C).

The tonic neck reflex resembles the stance of a fencer and is often called the fencing reflex. Test this reflex by having the newborn lie on the back. Turn the baby's head to one side. The arm toward which the baby is facing should extend straight away from the body with the hand partially open, whereas the arm on the side away from the face is flexed and the fist is clenched tightly. Reversing the direction to which the face is turned reverses the position (see Fig. 18.14D).

Elicit the rooting reflex by stroking the newborn's cheek. The newborn should turn toward the side that was stroked and should begin to make sucking movements (see Fig. 18.14E).

The Babinski reflex should be present at birth and disappears at approximately 1 year of age. It is elicited by stroking the lateral sole of the newborn's foot from the heel toward and across the ball of the foot. The toes should fan out. A diminished response indicates a neurologic problem and needs follow-up (see Fig. 18.14F).

The newborn exhibits two grasp reflexes: palmar grasp and plantar grasp. Elicit the palmar grasp reflex by placing a finger on the newborn's open palm. The baby's hand will close around the finger. Attempting to remove the finger causes the grip to tighten. Newborns have strong

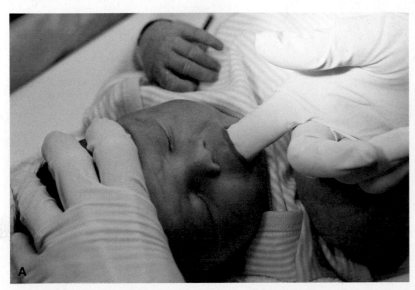
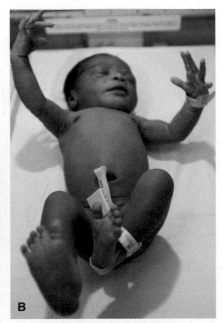

FIGURE **18.14** Newborn reflexes. (**A**) Sucking reflex. (**B**) Moro reflex. *(continued)*

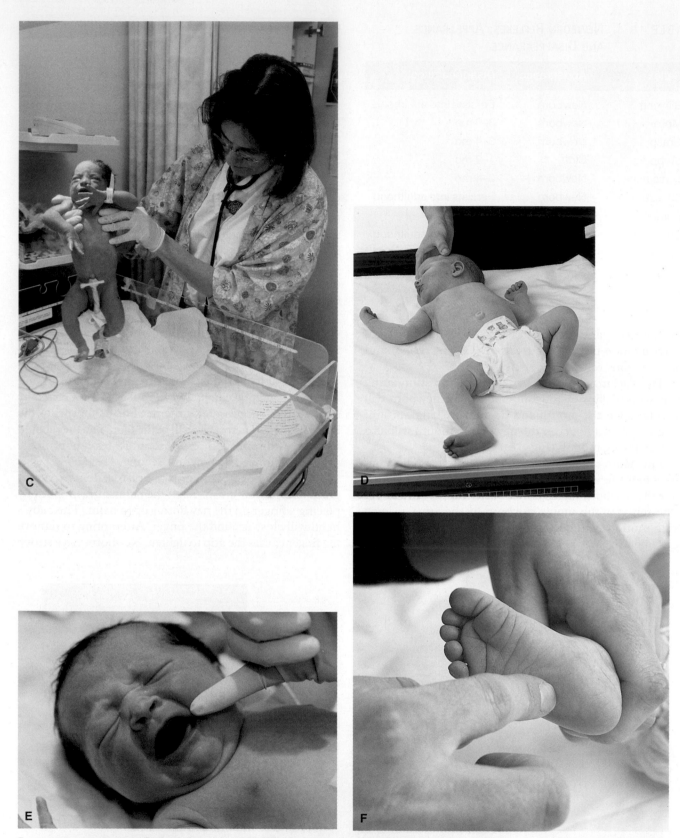

FIGURE **18.14** **(continued)** (**C**) Stepping reflex. (**D**) Tonic neck reflex. (**E**) Rooting reflex. (**F**) Babinski reflex. *(continued)*

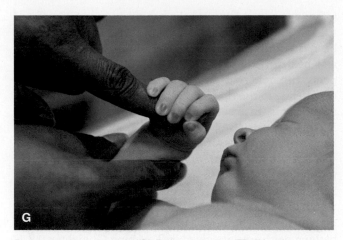

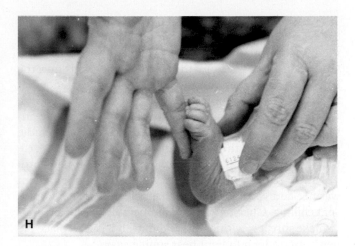

FIGURE 18.14   (continued) (**G**) Palmar grasp. (**H**) Plantar grasp.

grasps and can almost be lifted from a flat surface if both hands are used. The grasp should be equal bilaterally (see Fig. 18.14G).

The plantar grasp is similar to the palmar grasp. Place a finger just below the newborn's toes. The toes typically curl over the finger (see Fig. 18.14H).

Blinking, sneezing, gagging, and coughing are all protective reflexes and are elicited when an object or light is brought close to the eye (blinking), something irritating is swallowed or a bulb syringe is used for suctioning (gagging and coughing), or an irritant is brought close to the nose (sneezing).

The truncal incurvation reflex (Galant reflex) is present at birth and disappears in a few days to 4 weeks. With the newborn in a prone position or held in ventral suspension, apply firm pressure and run a finger down either side of the spine. This stroking will cause the pelvis to flex toward the stimulated side. This indicates T2–S1 innervation. Lack of response indicates a neurologic or spinal cord problem.

The anocutaneous reflex (anal wink) is elicited by stimulating the perianal skin close to the anus. The external sphincter will constrict (wink) immediately with stimulation. This indicates S4–5 innervation (Kenner & Lott, 2007).

Nursing Interventions

Developing confidence to care for their newborn is challenging for most couples. It takes time and patience and a great deal of instruction provided by the nurse. "Showing and telling" parents about their newborn and all the procedures (e.g., feeding, bathing, changing, handling) involved in daily care are key nursing interventions.

Providing General Newborn Care

Generally, newborn care involves bathing and hygiene, diaper care, cord care, circumcision care, use of appropriate clothing, environmental safety measures, and pre-

vention of infection. Nurses should teach these skills to parents and should serve as role models for appropriate and consistent interaction with newborns. Demonstrating respect for the newborn and family helps foster a positive atmosphere to promote the newborn's growth and development.

Bathing and Hygiene

Immediately after birth, drying the newborn and removing blood may minimize the risk of infection caused by hepatitis B, herpesvirus, and HIV, but the specific benefits of this practice remain unclear. Until the newborn has been thoroughly bathed, standard precautions should be used when handling the newborn.

Newborns are bathed primarily for aesthetic reasons, and bathing is postponed until thermal and cardiorespiratory stability is ensured. Traditional reasons why nurses bathe the newborn are so they can conduct a physical assessment, reduce the effect of hypothermia, and allow the mother to rest (Cohen, 2007). However, recent research suggests that nurses do not need to give the newborn an initial bath to reduce heat loss; rather, the parents could be given this opportunity, supported by nurses. A study found that the amount of heat loss was similar in newborns bathed by parents versus newborns who were bathed by nurses (Walsh, 2007).

Wear gloves, because of potential exposure to maternal blood on the newborn, and perform the bath quickly, drying the baby thoroughly to prevent heat loss by evaporation. Move from the "cleanest" area (the eyes) to the most soiled area (the diaper area) to prevent cross-contamination.

Use plain warm water on the face and eyes, adding a mild soap (e.g., Dove) to cleanse the remainder of the body. Instruct the parents to wash the face and neck gently after each feeding to prevent rashes and to prevent the odor that can develop when milk accumulates in the neck creases.

Wash the hair using running water so that the scalp can be thoroughly rinsed. A mild shampoo or soap can be used. Wash both fontanel areas. Frequently parents avoid these "soft spots" because they fear that they will "hurt the baby's brain" if they rub too hard. Reassure parents that there is a strong membrane providing protection. Urge the parents to clean and rinse these areas well. If the anterior fontanel is not rinsed well after shampooing, cradle cap (dry flakes on the scalp) can develop. In Figure 18.15, the nurse is showing the father how to bathe his newborn.

After bathing, place the newborn under the radiant warmer and wrap him or her securely in blankets to prevent chilling. Check the baby's temperature within an hour to make sure it is within normal limits. If it is low, place the newborn under a radiant heat source again.

The literature suggests that tub bathing for the first bath, as opposed to sponge bathing, can be done without significantly lowering the newborn's temperature or increasing rates of cord infection in healthy term newborns (AAP, 2007c).

After the initial bath, the newborn may not receive another full one during the stay in the birthing unit. The diaper area will be cleansed at each diaper change, and any milk spilled will be cleaned. Clear water and a mild soap are appropriate to cleanse the diaper area. The use of lotions, baby oil, and powders is not encouraged because oils and lotions can lead to skin irritation and can cause rashes. Powders should not be used because they can be inhaled, causing respiratory distress. If the parents want to use oils and lotions, have them apply a small amount onto their hand first, away from the newborn; this warms the lotion. Then the parents should apply the lotion or oil sparingly.

Instruct parents that a bath two or three times weekly is sufficient for the first year; more frequent bathing may dry the skin. Parents should not fully immerse the newborn into water until the umbilical cord area is healed—up to 2 weeks after birth. Encourage parents to give the infant a sponge bath until the umbilical cord falls off and the navel area is healed completely. If the newborn has been circumcised, advise parents to wait until that area has also healed (usually 1 to 2 weeks). Until then, clean the penis with mild soap and water and apply a small amount of Vaseline to the tip to prevent the diaper from adhering to the penis. Instruct parents to apply the diaper loosely and place the newly circumcised male infant on his side or back to prevent pressure and irritation on the penis.

Encourage the parents to gather all items needed before starting the bath: a soft, clean washcloth; two cotton balls to clean the eyes; mild, unscented soap and shampoo; towels or blankets; a tub or basin with warm water; a clean diaper; and a change of clothes. Other guidelines for bathing newborns are given in Teaching Guidelines 18.1.

Elimination and Diaper Area Care

Newborn elimination patterns are highly individualized. Usually the urine is light amber in color. Soaking 6 to 12 diapers a day indicates adequate hydration. Stools can

TEACHING GUIDELINES 18.1

Bathing a Newborn

- Select a warm room with a flat surface at a comfortable working height.
- Before the bath, gather all supplies needed so they will be within reach.
- Never leave the newborn alone or unattended at any time during the bath.
- Undress the newborn down to shirt and diaper.
- Always support the newborn's head and neck when moving or positioning him or her.
- Place a blanket or towel underneath the newborn for warmth and comfort.
- In this order, progressing from the cleanest to the dirtiest areas:
  - Wipe eyes with plain water, using either cotton balls or a washcloth. Wipe from the inner corner of the eyes to the outer with separate wipes.
  - Wash the rest of the face, including ears, with plain water.
  - Using baby shampoo, gently wash the hair and rinse with water.
  - Pay special attention to body creases, and dry thoroughly.
  - Wash extremities, trunk, and back. Wash, rinse, dry, cover.
  - Wash diaper area last, using soap and water, and dry; observe for rash.
- Put on a clean diaper and clean clothes after the bath.

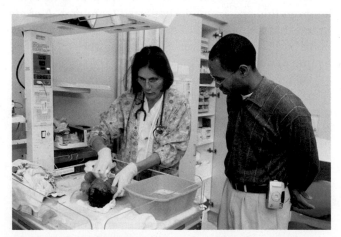

FIGURE **18.15** The nurse demonstrates bathing a newborn while the father watches.

change in color, texture, and frequency without signaling a problem. Meconium is passed for the first 48 hours after birth; the stools appear thick, tarry, sticky, and dark green. Transitional stools (thin, brown to green, less sticky than meconium) typically appear by day 3 after initiation of feeding. The stool characteristics after transitional stool depend on whether the newborn is breast-fed or bottle-fed. Breast-fed newborns typically pass mustard-colored, soft stool with a seedy consistency; formula-fed newborns pass yellow to brown, formed stool with a pasty consistency. As long as the newborn seems content, is eating normally, and shows no signs of illness, minor changes in bowel movements should not be a concern.

The newborn needs to be checked frequently to see whether a diaper change is needed, especially after feeding. Adhere to standard precautions when providing diaper area care. Instruct parents to keep the top edge of the diaper below the umbilical cord area to prevent irritation and to allow air to help dry the cord.

Meconium can be difficult to remove from the skin. Use plain water or special cleansing wipes if necessary to clean the area. Teach parents how to clean the diaper area properly and how to prevent skin irritation. Encourage them to avoid products such as powder and fragranced items, which could be irritating.

Discuss the pros and cons of using cloth diapers versus disposable diapers so that the parents can make informed decisions. Regardless of the type of diapers used, up to 10 diapers a day, or about 70 a week, will be needed.

Additional information about diapering might include:

- Before diapering, make sure all supplies are within reach, including clean diaper, cleaning agent or wipes, and ointment.
- Lay the newborn on a changing table and remove the dirty diaper.
- Use water and mild soap or wipes to gently wipe the genital area clean; wipe from front to back for girls to avoid urinary tract infections.
- Wash your hands thoroughly before and after changing diapers.

While performing diaper area care, parents should observe the area closely for irritation or rash. Tips for preventing or healing a diaper rash include:

- Change diapers frequently, especially after bowel movements.
- Apply a "barrier" cream, such as A & D ointment, after cleaning with mild soap and water.
- Use dye- and fragrance-free detergents to wash cloth diapers.
- Avoid the use of plastic pants, because they tend to hold in moisture.
- Expose the newborn's bottom to air several times a day.
- Place the newborn's buttocks in warm water after he or she had a diaper on all night.

▶ **Take** NOTE!

Advise parents that a rash that persists for more than 3 days may be fungal in origin and may require additional treatment. Encourage the parents to notify the health care provider.

Cord Care

The umbilical cord begins drying within hours after birth and is shriveled and blackened by the second or third day. Within 7 to 10 days, it sloughs off and the umbilicus heals. During this transition, frequent assessments of the area are necessary to detect any bleeding or signs of infection. Cord bleeding is abnormal and may occur if the cord clamp is loosened. Any cord drainage is also abnormal and is generally caused by infection, which requires immediate treatment.

To protect the cord area during each diaper change, apply the appropriate agent (e.g., triple dye, alcohol, or an antimicrobial agent), according to facility policy, to the cord stump to prevent any ascending infections. Single-use agents for cleaning are recommended to prevent cross-contamination with other newborns. Expect to remove the cord clamp approximately 24 hours after birth by using a cord-cutting clamp. However, if the cord is still moist, keep the clamp in place and ensure a referral to home health care so that the home care nurse can remove it after discharge. Always adhere to agency policies regarding cord care; changes in policy may be necessary based on new research findings.

Many parents avoid contact with the cord site to make sure they don't "bother" it. Teach them how to care for the cord site when they go home to prevent complications (Teaching Guidelines 18.2).

Circumcision Care

Circumcision is the surgical removal of all or part of the foreskin (prepuce) of the penis (AAP, 2007c). This has been traditionally done for hygiene and medical reasons and is the oldest known religious rite. In the Jewish faith, circumcision is a ritual that is performed by a *mohel* (ordained circumciser) on the eighth day after birth if possible. The circumcision is followed by a religious ceremony during which the newborn is named.

There are three commonly used methods of circumcision: the Gomco clamp, the Plastibell device, and the Mogen clamp. During the circumcision procedure, part of the foreskin is removed by clamping and cutting with a scalpel (Gomco or Mogen clamp) or by using a Plastibell. The Plastibell is fitted over the glans, and the excess foreskin is pulled over the plastic ring. A suture is tied around the rim to apply pressure to the blood vessels, creating hemostasis. The excess foreskin is cut away. The plastic rim remains in place until healing occurs.

Umbilical Cord Care

- Observe for bleeding, redness, drainage, or foul odor from the cord stump and report it to your newborn's primary care provider immediately.
- Avoid tub baths until the cord has fallen off and the area has healed.
- Expose the cord stump to the air as much as possible throughout the day.
- Fold diapers below the level of the cord to prevent contamination of the site and to promote air-drying of the cord.
- Observe the cord stump, which will change color from yellow to brown to black. This is normal.
- Never pull the cord or attempt to loosen it; it will fall off naturally.

The plastic ring typically loosens and falls off in approximately 1 week (Kenner & Lott, 2007) (Fig. 18.16).

The debate over routine newborn circumcision continues in the United States. For many years, the purported benefits and harms of circumcision have been debated in the medical literature and society at large, with no clear consensus to date. Despite the controversy, circumcision is the most common surgical procedure performed on newborns, and almost two thirds of American male newborns are circumcised (Cunningham et al., 2005).

A policy statement by the AAP indicates that newborn circumcision has potential disadvantages and risks as well as medical benefits and advantages. Risks to the newborn include infection, hemorrhage, skin dehiscence, adhesions, urethral fistula, and pain. Benefits to the newborn include the following:

- Urinary tract infections are slightly less common in circumcised boys; however, rates are low in both circumcised and uncircumcised boys and are easily treated without long-term sequelae.
- Sexually transmitted infections are less common in circumcised males, but the risk is believed to be related more to behavioral factors than to circumcision status. However, circumcised males have a 50% lower risk of acquiring HIV infection (Ridings & Amaya, 2007).
- There appears to be a slightly lower rate of penile cancer in circumcised males; however, penile cancer is rare and risk factors such as genital warts, infection with human papillomavirus (HPV), multiple sex partners, and cigarette smoking seem to play a much larger role in causing penile cancer than circumcision status (Kliegman et al., 2007).

The new AAP recommendations state that if parents decide to circumcise their newborn, pain relief must be provided. Research has found that newborns circumcised without analgesia experience pain and stress, indicated by changes in heart rate, blood pressure, oxygen saturation, and cortisol levels (Ridings & Amaya, 2007). Analgesic methods may include EMLA cream (a topical mixture of local anesthetics), a dorsal penile nerve block with buffered lidocaine, acetaminophen, a sucrose pacifier, and swaddling (Cunningham et al., 2005).

The AAP recommends that parents be given accurate and unbiased information about the risks and benefits of circumcision. As with other newborn procedures, research continues. Nurses must keep informed about current medical research to allow parents to make informed decisions. The absence of compelling medical evidence in favor of or against newborn circumcision makes informed consent of parents of paramount importance. The circumcision discussion involves cultural, religious, medical, and emotional considerations. Nurses may have difficulty remaining unbiased and unemotional as they present the facts to parents. Circumcision is a very personal decision for parents, and the nurse's major responsibility is to inform the parents of the risks and benefits of the pro-

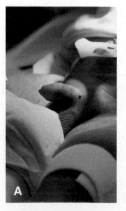
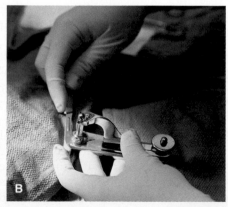
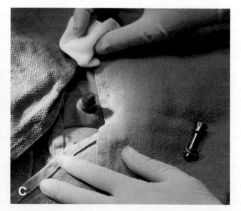

FIGURE **18.16** Circumcision. (**A**) Before the procedure. (**B**) Clamp applied and foreskin removed. (**C**) Appearance after circumcision.

cedure and to address concerns so that the parents can reach a fully informed decision.

▶ *Take* NOTE!

The decision to circumcise the male newborn is often a social one, with the strongest factor being whether the newborn's father is himself circumcised (AAP, 2007).

Immediately after circumcision, the tip of the penis is usually covered with petroleum jelly-coated gauze to keep the wound from sticking to the diaper. Continued care of this site includes:

- Assess for bleeding every 30 minutes for at least 2 hours.
- Document the first voiding to evaluate for urinary obstruction or edema.
- Squeeze soapy water over the area daily and then rinse with warm water. Pat dry.
- Apply a small amount of petroleum jelly with every diaper change if the Plastibell was used; clean with mild soap and water if other techniques were used.
- Fasten the diaper loosely over the penis and avoiding placing the newborn on his abdomen to prevent friction.

If a Plastibell has been used, it will fall off by itself in about a week. Inform parents of this and advise them not to pull it off sooner. Also instruct the parents to check daily for any foul-smelling drainage, bleeding, or unusual swelling.

If the newborn is uncircumcised, wash the penis with mild soap and water after each diaper change and do not force the foreskin back; it will retract normally over time.

Safety

Newborns are completely dependent on those around them to ensure their safety. Their safety must be ensured while in the health care facility and after they are discharged. Parental education is key, especially as the newborn grows and develops and begins to respond to and explore his or her surroundings (Teaching Guidelines 18.3).

Environmental Safety

People who enter a health care facility for treatment expect to be safe there until they return home, but ensuring a safe environment can be a daunting challenge to a health care facility.

Consider this scenario: A woman dressed in nurse's clothing entered the hospital room of a new mother soon after she had given birth. This "nurse" told the mother she needed to take her newborn to the nursery to have him weighed. Sometime later, a staff nurse making her routine rounds realized something was wrong when she

---

TEACHING GUIDELINES 18.3

General Newborn Safety

- Have emergency telephone numbers readily available, such as those for emergency medical assistance and the poison control center.
- Keep small or sharp objects out of reach to prevent them from being aspirated.
- Put safety plugs in wall sockets within the child's reach to prevent electrocution.
- Do not leave the infant alone in any room without a portable intercom on.
- Always supervise the newborn in the tub: a newborn can drown in 2 inches of water.
- Make sure the crib or changing table is sturdy, without any loose hardware, and is painted with lead-free paint.
- Avoid placing the crib or changing table near blinds or curtain cords.
- Provide a smoke-free environment for all infants.
- Place all infants on their backs to sleep to prevent sudden infant death syndrome.
- To prevent falls, do not leave the newborn alone on any elevated surface.
- Use sun shields on strollers and hats to avoid overexposing the newborn to the sun.
- To prevent infection, thoroughly wash your hands before preparing formula.
- Thoroughly investigate any infant care facility before using it.

Source: AAP, 2007b.

---

saw that the newborn's bassinet in the mother's room was empty and the mother was sound asleep in her bed. The staff nurse called security immediately because she suspected that a newborn abduction had taken place.

This is a typical abduction scenario that is repeated many times throughout the United States each year. In **infant abduction**, someone who is not a family member takes a child less than 1 year old (Cohen, 2007). Infant abductions are traumatic for the parents, the community, and the health care facility. The facility may also face huge financial liability if a lawsuit is filed by the parents.

Abductions typically occur during the day and are usually carried out by women who are not criminally sophisticated. Many of these women experienced a pregnancy loss in the past; they are often emotionally immature and compulsive, with low self-esteem. Most female abductors can play the role of a hospital employee convincingly (Healthcare Risk Management, 2007).

Health care agencies are challenged to prevent infant abduction by instituting sound security practices and systems (AWHONN Lifelines, 2007). Such measures include the following:

- All newborns must be transported in cribs and not carried.
- Nurses must respond immediately to any security alarm that sounds on the unit.
- Newborns must never be unattended at any time, especially in hallways.
- All staff must wear appropriate identification at all times.
- Scrubs should not be worn by nursing staff on the postpartum unit.
- Personnel should be wary of visitors who do not seem to be visiting a specific mother.
- The electronic security system should be checked to make sure it works.
- Proper functioning and placement of any electronic sensors used on newborns should be ensured.
- Parents should be taught what infant abduction is; why infant security is important; the schedule of nursery, feeding, and visiting hours; rules about visitor access; the facility's security policies and procedures; what parents can do to protect their infant in the hospital; which staff members are allowed to handle the newborn; and what a proper ID looks like.

Providing a safe and secure environment is a shared responsibility of the facility, staff, and parents. Preventing abductions requires everyone to learn and follow the rules and policies.

Car Safety

Every state requires the use of car seats for infants and children, because motor vehicle accidents are still the leading cause of unintentional injury and death in children under age 5 (AAP, 2007d). In more than half of these deaths, the child was unrestrained.

Despite evidence that the use of car seats can reduce the morbidity and mortality of motor vehicle crashes, parents who lack knowledge about them may underuse or misuse them (AAP, 2007d). Make sure that both parents understand the importance of safely transporting their newborn in a federally approved safety car seat every time the infant rides in a car. Do not release any newborn unless the parents have a car seat in place for their newborn's ride home (Fig. 18.17). If they cannot afford one, many community organizations will provide one for them. According to the AAP, no one car seat is considered to be the "safest" or the "best," but rather consistent and proper use is the key to preventing injuries and deaths. Instruct parents in the following:

- Select a car seat that is appropriate for the child's size and weight.
- Use the car seat correctly, every time the child is in the car.
- Use rear-facing car seats for infants until they are at least 1 year old and weigh 20 lb.

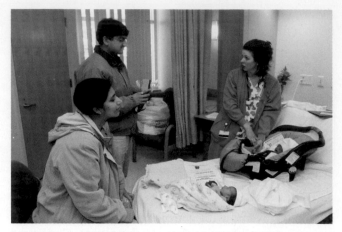

FIGURE **18.17** Newborn in a properly secured car seat.

- Make sure the harness (most seats have a three- to five-point harness) is in the slots at or below the shoulders.

Infection Prevention

The nurse plays a major role in preventing infection in the newborn environment. Ways to control infection are as follows:

- Minimize exposure of newborns to organisms.
- Wash your hands before and after providing care, and insist that all personnel wash their hands before handling any newborn.
- Do not allow ill staff or visitors to visit or handle newborns.
- Monitoring the umbilical cord stump and circumcision site for signs of infection.
- Providing eye prophylaxis by instilling prescribed medication soon after birth.
- Educate parents about appropriate home measures that will prevent infections, such as practicing good hand washing before and after diaper changes, keeping the newborn well hydrated, avoiding bringing the infant into crowds (which may expose him or her to colds and flu viruses), observing for early signs of infection (fever, vomiting, loss of appetite, lethargy, labored breathing, green watery stools, drainage from umbilical cord site or eyes), and keeping pediatrician appointments for routine immunizations.

Promoting Sleep

Although many parents feel their newborns need them every minute of the day, babies actually need to sleep much of the day initially. Usually newborns sleep up to 15 hours daily. They sleep for 2 to 4 hours at a time but do not sleep through the night because their stomach capacity is too small to go long periods without nourishment.

▶ *Take NOTE!*

All newborns develop their own sleep patterns and cycles, but it may take several months before the newborn sleeps through the night.

Parents should place the newborn on his or her back to sleep. To prevent suffocation, all fluffy bedding, quilts, sheepskins, stuffed animals, and pillows should be removed from the crib.

Parents should be informed that the practice of "co-sleeping" (sharing a bed) is not safe: for example, infants who sleep in adult beds are up to 40 times more likely to suffocate than those who sleep in cribs (Buswell & Spatz 2007). Suffocation can occur when the infant gets entangled in bedding or caught under pillows, or slips between the bed and the wall or the headboard and mattress. The parent may accidentally roll against or on top of the baby. The safest place for a newborn to sleep is in a crib, without any movable objects close by.

Teach parents to avoid other unsafe conditions, such as placing the newborn in the prone position, using a crib that does not meet federal safety guidelines, allowing window cords to hang loose and in close proximity to the crib, or setting the room temperature too high (can cause overheating) (Adler, Hyderi, & Hamilton, 2006).

Enhancing Bonding

Encourage and enhance parent–newborn interaction by involving both parents with the baby and demonstrating appropriate nurturing behaviors:

• Say "hello" and introduce yourself to the newborn.
• Ask the parents permission to care for and hold their newborn. This helps parents to realize that they are responsible for their child and reminds nurses of their role.
• Show parents the power of a soothing voice to calm the newborn.
• Provide care to the newborn in the least stressful way.
• Demonstrate ways to wake the newborn up gently to feed better.
• Tell parents what you are doing, why you are doing it, and how they can duplicate what you are doing at home.
• Offer the opportunity for parents to perform care while you observe them. Support their efforts to soothe the newborn throughout the care process.
• Help parents to interpret the communication cues the newborn uses.
• Point out the efforts the newborn is making to connect with the parents (e.g., alerting to the familiar voice, following the parents while they are speaking, quieting when held securely).

One of the most pleasurable aspects of newborn care is being close to them. Bonding begins soon after birth when parents cradle their newborn and gently stroke him or her with their fingers. Provide parents with opportunities for "skin-to-skin" contact with the newborn, holding the baby against their own skin when feeding or cradling. Many newborns respond very positively to gentle massage. If necessary, recommend books and videos that cover the subject.

For newborns, crying is their only way to communicate that something is wrong. Try to find out the reason why: Is the diaper wet? Is the room too hot or too cold? Is the baby uncomfortable (e.g., diaper rash or tight clothing)? Suggest the following ways in which parents can soothe an upset newborn:

• Try feeding or burping to relieve air or stomach gas.
• Lightly rub the newborn's back and speak softly to him or her.
• Gently sway side to side, or rock back and forth in a rocking chair.
• Talk with the newborn while making eye contact.
• Take the newborn for a walk in a stroller or carriage to get fresh air.
• Change the baby's position from back to side or vice versa.
• Try singing, reciting poetry and nursery rhymes, or reading to the baby.
• Turn on a musical mobile above the newborn's head.
• Give more physical contact by walking, rocking, or patting the newborn.
• Swaddle the newborn to provide a sense of security and comfort. To do this:
  • Spread out a receiving blanket, with one corner folded slightly.
  • Lay the newborn face up with head at the folded corner.
  • Wrap the left corner over the baby's body and tuck it beneath the baby.
  • Bring the bottom corner over the baby's feet.
  • Wrap the right corner around the baby, leaving only the head exposed.

Assisting With Screening Tests

Screening newborns for problems is important because some potentially life-threatening metabolic diseases may not be obvious at birth. Newborn screening tests that are required in most states before discharge are used to check for certain genetic and inborn errors of metabolism and hearing. Early identification and initiation of treatment can prevent significant complications and can minimize the negative effects of untreated disease.

Genetic and Inborn Errors of Metabolism Screening

Although each state mandates which conditions must be tested, the most common screening tests are for PKU, hypothyroidism, galactosemia, and sickle cell disease (Table 18.5).

TABLE 18.5 SELECTED CONDITIONS SCREENED FOR IN THE NEWBORN

Condition	Description	Clinical Picture/ Effect If Not Treated	Treatment	Timing of Screening
PKU	Autosomal recessive inherited deficiency in one of the enzymes necessary for the metabolism of phenylalanine to tyrosine—essential amino acids found in most foods	Irritability, vomiting of protein feedings, and a musty odor to the skin or body secretions of the newborn; if not treated, mental and motor retardation, seizures, microcephaly, and poor growth and development	Lifetime diet of foods low in phenylalanine (low protein) and monitoring of blood levels (Lawson, 2007); special newborn formulas available: Phenex and Lofenalac	Universally screened for in the United States; testing is done 24–48 hours after protein feeding (PKU)
Congenital hypothyroidism	Deficiency of thyroid hormone necessary for normal brain growth, calorie metabolism, and development; may result from maternal hypothyroidism	Increased risk in newborns with birthweight <2,000 g or >4,500 g, and those of Hispanic and Asian ethnic groups; feeding problems, growth and breathing problems; if not treated, irreversible brain damage and mental retardation	Lifelong thyroid replacement therapy (Dudek, 2006)	Testing (measures thyroxin [T4] and TSH) is done between days 4 and 6 of life.
Galactosemia	Absence of the enzyme needed for the conversion of the milk sugar galactose to glucose	Poor weight gain, vomiting, jaundice, mood changes, loss of eyesight, seizures, and mental retardation; if untreated, galactose buildup causing permanent damage to the brain, eyes, and liver, and eventually death	Eliminate milk from diet; substitute soy milk	First test done on discharge from the hospital with a follow-up test within 1 month
Sickle cell anemia	Recessively inherited abnormality in hemoglobin structure, most commonly found in African-American newborns	Anemia developing shortly after birth; increased risk for infection, growth restriction, vaso-occlusive crisis	Maintenance of hydration and hemodilution, rest, electrolyte replacement, pain management, blood replacement, and antibiotics	Bloodspot obtained at same time of other newborn screening tests or prior to 3 months of age

The trend toward early discharge of newborns can affect the timing of screening and the accuracy of some test results. For example, the newborn needs to ingest enough breast milk or formula to elevate phenylalanine levels for the screening test to identify PKU accurately, so newborn screening for PKU testing should not be performed before 24 hours of age.

Screening tests for genetic and inborn errors of metabolism require a few drops of blood taken from the newborn's heel (Fig. 18.18). These tests are usually per-

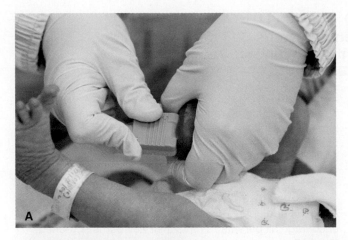

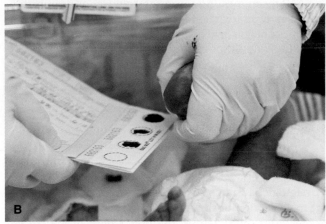

FIGURE 18.18 Screening for PKU. (A) Performing a heel stick. (B) Applying the blood specimen to the card for screening.

formed shortly before discharge. Newborns who are discharged before 24 hours of age need to have repeat tests done within a week in an outpatient facility.

Be aware of which conditions your state regularly screens for at birth to ensure that the parents are taught about the tests and the importance of early treatment. Also be familiar with the optimal time frame for screening and conditions that could affect the results. Ensure that a satisfactory specimen has been obtained at the appropriate time and that circumstances that could cause false results have been minimized. Send out specimens and completed forms within 24 hours of collection to the appropriate laboratory (Kenner & Lott, 2007).

Hearing Screening

Hearing loss is the most common birth disorder in the United States: approximately three to five newborns out of every 1,000 have some degree of hearing loss. Unlike a physical deformity, hearing loss is not clinically detectable at birth and thus remains difficult to assess (Wrightson, 2007). Factors associated with an increased risk of hearing loss include:

- Family history of childhood sensory hearing loss
- Congenital infections such as cytomegalovirus, rubella, toxoplasmosis, herpes

- Craniofacial anomalies involving the pinna or ear canal
- Low birthweight (less than 1,500 g)
- Postnatal infections such as bacterial meningitis
- Head trauma
- Hyperbilirubinemia requiring an exchange transfusion
- Exposure to ototoxic drugs, especially aminoglycosides
- Perinatal asphyxia (USPSTF, 2006)

Delays in identification and intervention may affect the child's language development, academic performance, and cognitive development. Detection before 3 months greatly improves outcomes. Because of this, auditory screening programs for all newborns are recommended by the AAP and are mandated by law in over 30 states. Screening only infants with risk factors is not enough, because as many as 50% of infants born with hearing loss have no known risk factors (AAP, 2007b). Early identification and intervention can prevent severe psychosocial, educational, and language development delays.

The current goals of *Healthy People 2010* (see the Healthy People 2010 display earlier in this chapter) are to screen all infants by 1 month of age, confirm hearing loss with an audiologic examination by 3 months of age, and treat with comprehensive early intervention services before 6 months of age (USDHHS, Volume II, Objective 16-20).

All newborns should be screened prior to discharge to ensure that any newborn with a hearing loss is not missed. Those with suspected hearing loss should be referred for follow-up assessment (Box 18.1 discusses screening methods). In addition, nurses should ensure that testing is accurate to facilitate early diagnosis and intervention services and to optimize the newborn's developmental potential.

BOX 18.1 Newborn Hearing Screening Methods

A newborn's hearing can be screened in one of two ways: otoacoustic emission (OAE) or automated auditory brain stem response (ABR). In OAE, an earphone is placed in the infant's ear canal and the sounds produced by the newborn's inner ear are measured in response to certain tones or clicks presented through the earphone. Preset parameters in the equipment decide whether the OAEs are sufficient for the newborn to pass or whether a referral is necessary for further evaluation.

In ABR, an earphone is placed in the ear canal or an earmuff is placed over the newborn's ear, and a soft, rapid tapping noise is presented. Electrodes placed around the newborn's head, neck, and shoulders record neural activity from the infant's brain stem in response to the tapping noises. The ABR tests how well the ear and the nerves leading to the brain work. Like OAEs, automated ABR screening is sensitive to more than mild degrees of hearing loss, but a "pass" does not guarantee normal hearing.

Source: AAP, 2007a.

EVIDENCE-BASED PRACTICE 18.1
Universal Neonatal Hearing Screening Versus Selective Screening as Part of the Management of Childhood Deafness

● Study

The principal factors that determine how deafness affects a child's development are the degree of hearing impairment and the age at which it is diagnosed. A number of factors are thought to increase the risk of hearing impairment, such as low birthweight, prematurity, and perinatal hypoxia and jaundice. The high incidence of deafness in children without risk factors and the introduction of simple new screening tests with high sensitivity and specificity have led many prestigious bodies to recommend universal early detection programs for deafness rather than screening that targets high-risk groups. A study was performed to compare the long-term effectiveness of a universal neonatal screening and early treatment program for hearing impairment versus screening and treatment of high-risk neonates only.

▲ Findings

This review found no randomized trials that compared the long-term results of these screening programs. Controlled trials and before-and-after studies are needed to address this issue.

■ Nursing Implications

Although additional research is needed, nurses should encourage all parents to have their newborns screened. The AAP recommends hearing screening for all newborns so that early interventions can be provided to prevent speech, language, and cognitive development impairments. This information should be stressed during discharge planning activities and follow-up tests if warranted.

Puig, T., Municio, A., & Medà, C. (2006). Universal neonatal hearing screening versus selective screening as part of the management of childhood deafness. *Cochrane Database of Systematic Reviews* 2006, Issue 2. Art. No.: CD003731. DOI: 10.1002/14651858.CD003731.pub2

Dealing With Common Concerns

During the newborn period of transition, certain conditions can develop that require intervention. These conditions, although not typically life-threatening, can be a source of anxiety for the parents. Common concerns include transient tachypnea of the newborn, physiologic jaundice, and hypoglycemia.

Transient Tachypnea of the Newborn

Transient tachypnea of the newborn appears soon after birth. It is accompanied by retractions, expiratory grunting, or cyanosis and is relieved by low-dose oxygen therapy. Mild or moderate respiratory distress typically is present at birth or within 6 hours of birth. This condition usually resolves within 3 days.

Transient tachypnea of the newborn occurs when the fetal liquid in the lungs is removed slowly or incompletely. This can be due to the lack of thoracic squeezing that occurs during a cesarean birth, or diminished respiratory effort if the mother received central nervous system depressant medication. Prolonged labor, macrosomia of the fetus, and maternal asthma also have been associated with this condition (Asenjo, 2007).

Nursing interventions include providing supportive care (giving oxygen, ensuring warmth, observing respiratory status frequently, and allowing time for the pulmonary capillaries and the lymphatics to remove the remaining fluid). The clinical course is relatively benign, but any newborn respiratory issue can be very frightening to the parents. Provide a thorough explanation and reassure them that the condition will resolve over time.

Physiologic Jaundice

Physiologic jaundice is very common in newborns, with the majority demonstrating yellowish skin, mucous membranes, and sclera within the first 3 days of life. In any given year, approximately 60% of the newborns in the United States will experience clinical jaundice (Deshpande & Ramer, 2007). Jaundice is the visible manifestation of hyperbilirubinemia. It typically results from the deposition of unconjugated bilirubin pigment in the skin and mucous membranes.

Factors that contribute to the development of physiologic jaundice in the newborn include an increased bilirubin load because of relative polycythemia, a shortened erythrocyte life span (80 days compared with the adult 120 days), and immature hepatic uptake and conjugation processes (Deshpande & Ramer, 2007). Normally the liver removes bilirubin from the blood and changes it to a form in which it can be excreted. As the red blood cell breakdown continues at a fast pace, the newborn's liver cannot keep up with bilirubin removal. Thus, bilirubin accumulates in the blood, causing a yellowish discoloration on the skin.

The AAP has recently released guidelines for the prevention and management of hyperbilirubinemia in newborns. These include:

• Promotion and support of successful breast-feeding practices to make sure the newborn is well hydrated and stooling frequently to promote elimination of bilirubin
• Completion of a systematic assessment before discharge for the risk of severe hyperbilirubinemia

- Early and focused follow-up based on the risk assessment
- When indicated, treatment of newborns with phototherapy or exchange transfusion to prevent kernicterus (AAP, 2006b)

Assess for jaundice in all newborns by pressing gently with a fingertip on the bridge of the nose, sternum, or forehead. If jaundice is present, the blanched area will appear yellow before the capillary refill (Kenner & Lott, 2007).

Measures that parents can take to reduce the risk of jaundice include exposing the newborn to natural sunlight for short periods of time throughout the day to help oxidize the bilirubin deposits on the skin, provide breastfeeding on demand to promote elimination of bilirubin through urine and stooling, and avoiding glucose water supplementation, which hinders elimination.

If or when the levels of unconjugated serum bilirubin increase and do not return to normal levels with increased hydration, phototherapy is used. The serum level of bilirubin at which phototherapy is initiated is a matter of clinical judgment by the physician, but it is often begun when bilirubin levels reach 12 to 15 mg/dL in the first 48 hours of life in a term newborn (Arenson & Drake, 2007). **Phototherapy** involves exposing the newborn to ultraviolet light, which converts unconjugated bilirubin into products that can be excreted through feces and urine.

> ▶ **Take** NOTE!
>
> *Exposure of newborns to sunlight represents the first documented use of phototherapy in the medical literature. Sister J. Ward, a charge nurse in Essex, England, in 1956 recognized that when jaundiced newborns were exposed to the sun they became less yellow. This observation changed the entire treatment of jaundice in newborns (Maisels, 2006).*

Phototherapy reduces bilirubin levels in the blood by breaking down unconjugated bilirubin into colorless compounds. These compounds can then be excreted in the bile. Phototherapy aims to curtail the increase in bilirubin blood levels, thereby preventing kernicterus, a condition in which unconjugated bilirubin enters the brain. If not treated, kernicterus can lead to brain damage and death.

During the past several decades, phototherapy has generally been administered with either banks of fluorescent lights or spotlights. Factors that determine the dose of phototherapy include spectrum of light emitted, irradiance of light source, design of light unit, surface area of newborn exposed to the light, and distance of the newborn from the light source (Cohen, 2006). For phototherapy to be effective, the rays must penetrate as much of the skin as possible. Thus, the newborn must be naked and turned frequently to ensure maximum exposure of the skin. Several side effects of standard phototherapy have been identified: frequent loose stools, increased insensible water loss, transient rash, and potential retinal damage if the newborn's eyes are not covered sufficiently.

Recently, fiberoptic pads (Biliblanket or Bilivest) have been developed that can be wrapped around the newborn or on which the newborn can lie. The light is delivered from a tungsten–halogen bulb through a fiberoptic cable and is emitted from the sides and ends of the fibers inside a plastic pad (Cohen, 2006). These products work on the premise that phototherapy can be improved by delivering higher-intensity therapeutic light to decrease bilirubin levels. The pads do not produce appreciable heat like the banks of lights or spotlights do, so insensible water loss is not increased. Eye patches also are not needed; thus, parents can feed and hold their newborns continuously to promote bonding.

When caring for newborns receiving phototherapy for jaundice, nurses must do the following:

- Closely monitor body temperature and fluid and electrolyte balance.
- Observe skin integrity (as a result of exposure to diarrhea and phototherapy lights).
- Provide eye protection to prevent corneal injury related to phototherapy exposure.
- Encourage parents to participate in their newborn's care to prevent parent–infant separation.

See Chapter 24 for a more detailed discussion of hyperbilirubinemia.

The home health nurse made a postpartum visit to Kelly to assess the situation. Kelly's son was slightly jaundiced when the home health nurse pressed gently over his sternum, but Kelly said he was nursing better compared with the previous 2 days. What home suggestions can the nurse make to Kelly to reduce the jaundice? What specific education about physiologic jaundice is needed?

Hypoglycemia

Hypoglycemia affects as many as 40% of all full-term newborns (Kenner & Lott, 2007). It is defined as a blood glucose level of less than 35 mg/dL or a plasma concentration of less than 40 mg/dL (Kenner & Lott, 2007). In newborns, blood glucose levels fall to a low point during the first few hours of life because the source of maternal glucose is removed when the placenta is expelled. This period of transition is usually smooth, but certain newborns are at greater risk for hypoglycemia: infants of diabetic mothers, preterm newborns, and newborns with IUGR, inadequate caloric intake, sepsis, asphyxia, hypothermia, polycythemia, glycogen storage disorders, and endocrine deficiencies (Kliegman et al., 2007).

Most newborns experience transient hypoglycemia and are asymptomatic. The symptoms, when present, are nonspecific and include jitteriness, lethargy, cyanosis, apnea, seizures, high-pitched or weak cry, and poor feeding. If hypoglycemia is prolonged or is left untreated, serious, long-term adverse neurologic sequelae such as learning disabilities and mental retardation can occur (Cohen, 2007). Subsequently, early diagnosis and appropriate intervention are essential for all newborns.

Nursing care of the hypoglycemic newborn includes monitoring for signs of hypoglycemia or identifying high-risk newborns prone to this disorder based on their perinatal history, physical examination, body measurements, and gestational age. Check the blood glucose level of all newborns within the first few hours after birth and every 4 hours thereafter. More frequent monitoring and early feeding may be necessary for newborns considered to be high risk. Prevent hypoglycemia in newborns at risk by initiating early feedings with breast milk or formula. If hypoglycemia persists despite feeding, notify the primary health care provider for orders such as intravenous therapy with dextrose solutions. Anticipate hypoglycemia in certain high-risk newborns and begin assessments immediately on nursery admission.

Promoting Nutrition

Several physiologic changes dictate the type and method of feeding throughout the newborn's first year. Some of these changes include the following:

- Stomach capacity is limited to about 90 mL at birth. The emptying time is short (2 to 3 hours) and peristalsis is rapid. Therefore, small, frequent feedings are needed at first, with amounts progressively increasing with maturity.
- The immune system is immature at birth, so the baby is at a high risk for food allergies during the first 4 to 6 months of life. Introducing solid foods prior to this time increases the risk of developing food allergies.
- Pancreatic enzymes and bile to assist in digestion of fat and starch are in limited supply until about 3 to 6 months of age. Infants cannot digest cereal prior to this time.
- The kidneys are immature and unable to concentrate urine until about 4 to 6 weeks of age. Excess protein and mineral intake can place a strain on kidney function and can lead to dehydration. Infants need to consume more water per unit of body weight than adults do as a result of their high body weight from water.
- Immature muscular control at birth changes over time to assist in the feeding process by improving head and neck control, hand–eye coordination, swallowing, and ability to sit, grasp, and chew. At about 4 to 6 months, inborn reflexes disappear, head control develops, and the infant can sit to be fed, making spoon-feeding possible (Dudek, 2006).

Newborn Nutritional Needs

As newborns grow, their energy and nutrient requirements change to meet their body's changing needs. During infancy, energy, protein, vitamin, and mineral requirements per pound of body weight are higher than at any other time of life. These high levels are needed to fuel the rapid growth and development during this stage of life. Generally, an infant's birthweight doubles in the first 4 to 6 months of life and triples within the first year (Dillon, 2007).

A newborn's caloric needs range from 80 to 120 cal/kg body weight. For the first 3 months, the infant needs 110 cal/kg/day; this decreases to 100 cal/kg/day from 3 to 6 months (Begany & Mascarenhas, 2007). Breast milk and formulas contain approximately 20 cal/oz, so the caloric needs of young infants can be met if several feedings are given throughout the day.

Fluid requirements for the newborn and infant range from 100 to 150 mL/kg daily. This requirement can be met through breast or bottle feedings. Additional water supplementation is not necessary. Adequate carbohydrates, fats, protein, and vitamins are achieved through consumption of breast milk or formula. The AAP recommends that bottle-fed infants be given iron supplementation, because iron levels are low in all types of formula milk. This can be achieved by giving iron-fortified formula from birth. The breast-fed infant draws on iron reserves for the first 6 months and then needs iron-rich foods or supplementation added at 6 months of age. The AAP (2007c) also has recommended that all infants (breast- and bottle-fed) receive a daily supplement of vitamin D starting within the first 2 months of life to prevent rickets and vitamin D deficiency. It is also recommended that fluoride supplementation be given to infants not receiving fluoridated water after the age of 6 months (AAP, 2007c).

Supporting the Choice of Feeding Method

Parents typically decide about the method of feeding well before the infant is born. Prenatal and childbirth classes present information about breast-feeding versus bottle feeding and allow the parents to make up their minds about which method is best for them. Various factors can influence their decision, including socioeconomic status, culture, employment, social support available, level of education, range of care interventions provided during pregnancy, childbirth, and the early postpartum period, and especially partner support (Pryor & Huggins, 2007). Nurses can provide evidence-based information to assist the couple in making their decision. Regardless of which method is chosen, the nurse needs to respect and support the couple.

Feeding the Newborn

The newborn can be fed at any time during the transition period if assessments are normal and a desire is demonstrated. Before the newborn can be fed, determine his or her ability to suck and swallow. Clear any mucus in the nares or mouth with a bulb syringe before initiating feeding. Auscultate bowel sounds, check for abdominal distention, and inspect the anus for patency. If these parameters are within normal limits, newborn feeding may be started. Most newborns are on demand feeding schedules and are allowed to feed when they awaken. When they go home, mothers are encouraged to feed their newborns every 2 to 4 hours during the day and only when the newborn awakens during the night for the first few days after birth.

Parents often have many questions about feeding. Generally, newborns should be fed on demand whenever they seem hungry. Most newborns will give clues about their hunger status by crying, placing their fingers or fist in their mouth, rooting around, and sucking.

Newborns differ in their feeding needs and preferences, but most breast-fed ones need to be fed every 2 to 3 hours, nursing for 10 to 20 minutes on each breast. The length of feedings is up to the mother and newborn. Encourage the mother to respond to cues from her infant and not feed according to a standard or preset schedule.

Formula-fed newborns usually feed every 3 to 4 hours, finishing a bottle in 30 minutes or less. Bottle-fed infants consume about 2 to 4 fluid ounces at first and double their intake within a few weeks of age (Begany & Mascarenhas, 2007). If the newborn seems satisfied, wets 6 to 10 diapers daily, produces several stools a day, sleeps well, and is gaining weight regularly, then he or she is probably receiving sufficient breast milk or formula.

Newborns swallow air during feedings, which causes discomfort and fussiness. Parents can prevent this by burping them frequently throughout the feeding. Tips about burping include:

- Hold the newborn upright with his or her head on the parent's shoulder (Fig. 18.19A).
- Support the head and neck while the parent gently pats or rubs the newborn's back (Fig.18.19B).
- Have the newborn sit on the parent's lap, while supporting the baby's chest and head. Gently rub the newborn's back with the other hand.
- Lay the newborn on the parent's lap with the baby's back facing up.
- Support the newborn's head in the crook of the parent's arm and gently pat or rub the back.

▶ *Take* NOTE!

It is the upright position, not the strength of the patting or rubbing, that allows the newborn to release air accumulated in the stomach.

Stress to parents that feeding time is more than an opportunity to get nutrients into their newborn; it is also a time for closeness and sharing. Feedings are as much

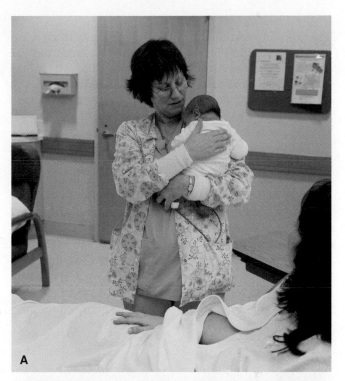

A

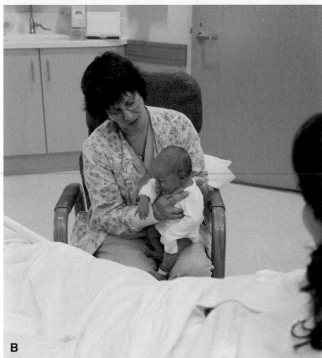

B

FIGURE **18.19** The nurse demonstrates holding the newborn upright over the shoulder (**A**) and sitting the newborn upright, supporting the neck and chin (**B**).

for the baby's emotional pleasure as his or her physical well-being. Encourage parents to maintain eye contact with the newborn during the feeding, hold him or her comfortably close to them, and talk softly during the feeding to promote closeness and security.

Breast-Feeding

There is consensus in the medical community that breast-feeding is optimal for all newborns. The AAP and the American Dietetic Association recommend breast-feeding exclusively for the first 6 months of life, continuing it in conjunction with other food at least until the newborn's first birthday (AAP, 2007c). Box 18.2 highlights the advantages of breast-feeding for the mother and newborn.

Mothers should continue to breast-feed during mild illnesses such as colds or the flu. However, in the United States mothers with HIV are advised not to breast-feed.

The composition of breast milk changes over time from colostrum, to transitional milk, and finally to mature milk. Colostrum is a thick, yellowish substance secreted during the first few days after birth. It is high in protein, minerals, and fat-soluble vitamins. It is rich in immunoglobulins (IgA), which help protect the newborn's gastrointestinal tract against infections. It is a natural laxative that helps rid the intestinal tract of meconium quickly (Pryor & Huggins, 2007).

BOX 18.2　Advantages of Breast-Feeding

Advantages for the Newborn
- Contributes to the development of a strong immune system
- Stimulates growth of positive bacteria in digestive tract
- Reduces incidence of stomach upset, diarrhea, and colic
- Begins the immunization process at birth by providing passive immunity
- Promotes optimal mother–infant bonding
- Reduces risk of newborn constipation
- Promotes greater developmental gains in preterm infants (AAP, 2006a, 2006b)
- Provides easily tolerated and digestible formula that is sterile, at proper temperature, and readily available with no artificial colorings, flavorings, or preservatives
- Is less likely to result in overfeeding, leading to obesity (AAP, 2006a, 2006b)
- Promotes better tooth and jaw development as a result of sucking hard
- Provides protection against food allergies
- Is associated with avoidance of type 1 diabetes and heart disease

Advantages for the Mother
- Can facilitate postpartum weight loss
- Stimulates uterine contractions to control bleeding
- Promotes uterine involution as a result of release of oxytocin
- Lowers risk of breast cancer and osteoporosis
- Affords some protection against conception, although it is not a reliable contraceptive method (Pryor & Huggins, 2007)

Transitional milk occurs between colostrum and mature milk and contains all the nutrients in colostrum, but it is thinner and less yellow than colostrum. This transitional milk is replaced by true or mature milk around day 10 after birth. Mature milk appears bluish and is not as thick as colostrum. It provides 20 cal/oz and contains:

- Protein—Although the content is lower than formula, it is ideal to support growth and development for the newborn. The majority of protein is whey, which is easy to digest.
- Fat—Approximately 58% of total calories are fat, but they are easy to digest. Essential fatty acid content is high, as is the level of cholesterol, which helps develop enzyme systems capable of handling cholesterol later in life.
- Carbohydrate—Approximately 35% to 40% of total calories are in the form of lactose, which stimulates the growth of natural defense bacteria in the gastrointestinal system and promotes calcium absorption.
- Water—Water, the major nutrient in breast milk, makes up 85% to 95% of the total volume. Total milk volume varies with the age of the infant and demand.
- Minerals—Breast milk contains calcium, phosphorus, chlorine, potassium, and sodium, with trace amounts of iron, copper, and manganese. Iron absorption is about 50%, compared with about 4% for iron-fortified formulas.
- Vitamins—All vitamins are present in breast milk; vitamin D is the lowest in amount. Debate about the need for vitamin D supplementation is ongoing.
- Enzymes—Lipase and amylase are found in breast milk to assist with digestion (Dudek, 2006).

Breast-Feeding Assistance

Breast-feeding can be initiated immediately after birth. If the newborn is healthy and stable, wipe the newborn from head to toe with a dry cloth and place him or her skin-to-skin on the mother's abdomen. Then cover the newborn and mother with another warmed blanket to hold in the warmth. Immediate mother–newborn contact takes advantage of the newborn's natural alertness after a vaginal birth and fosters bonding. This immediate contact also reduces maternal bleeding and stabilizes the newborn's temperature, blood glucose level, and respiratory rate (AAP, 2007c).

Left alone on the mother's abdomen, a healthy newborn scoots upward, pushing with the feet, pulling with the arms, and bobbing the head until finding and latching on to the mother's nipple. A newborn's sense of smell is highly developed, which also helps in finding the nipple. As the newborn moves to the nipple, the mother produces high levels of oxytocin, which contracts the uterus, thereby minimizing bleeding. Oxytocin also causes the breasts to release colostrum when the newborn sucks on the nipple. Colostrum is rich in antibodies and thus provides the newborn with her "first immunization" against infection.

Keys to successful breast-feeding include:

- Initiating breast-feeding within the first hour of life if the newborn is stable
- Following the newborn's feeding schedule—8 to 12 times in 24 hours
- Providing unrestricted periods of breast-feeding
- Offering no supplement unless medically indicated
- Having a lactation consultant observe a feeding session
- Avoiding artificial nipples and pacifiers except during a painful procedure
- Feeding from both breasts over each 24-hour period
- Watching for indicators of sufficient intake from infant:
  - Six to ten wet diapers daily
  - Waking up hungry 8 to 12 times in 24 hours
  - Acting content and falling asleep after feeding
- Keeping the newborn with the mother throughout the hospital stay

Help position the newborn so that latching-on is effective and is not painful for the mother. Placing pillows or a folded blanket under the mother's head may help, or rolling her to one side and tucking the newborn next to her. Assess both the mother and newborn during this initial session to determine needs for assistance and education. One tool used frequently in this assessment is the LATCH scoring tool (Table 18.6). The higher the score, the less nursing intervention is needed by the mother and baby.

Breast-Feeding Positioning

The mother and infant must be in comfortable positions to ensure breast-feeding success. The four most common positions for breast-feeding are the football, cradle, across-the-lap, and side-lying holds. Each mother, on experimentation, can decide which positions feel most comfortable for her (Fig. 18.20).

In the football hold, the mother holds the infant's back and shoulders in her palm and tucks the infant under her arm. Remind the mother to keep the infant's ear, shoulder, and hip in a straight line. The mother supports the breast with her hand and brings it to the infant's lips to latch on. She continues to support the breast until the infant begins to nurse. This position allows the mother to see the infant's mouth as she guides her infant to the nipple. This is a good choice for mothers who have had a cesarean birth because it avoids pressure on the incision.

The cradling position is the one most commonly used. The mother holds the baby in the crook of her arm, with the infant facing the mother. The mother supports the breast with her opposite hand.

In the across-the-lap position, the mother places a pillow across her lap, with the infant facing the mother. The mother supports the infant's back and shoulders with her palm and supports her breast from underneath. After the infant is in position, the infant is pulled forward to latch on.

In the side-lying position, the mother lies on her side with a pillow supporting her back and another pillow supporting the newborn in the front. To start, the mother props herself up on an elbow and supports the newborn with that arm, while holding her breast with the opposite hand. Once nursing is started, the mother lies down in a comfortable position.

To promote latching-on, instruct the mother to make a C or a V with her fingers. In the C hold, the mother places her thumb well above the areola and the other four fingers

TABLE 18.6 THE LATCH SCORING TOOL

Parameters	0 Point	1 Point	2 Points
L: Latch	Sleepy infant, no sustained latch achieved	Must hold nipple in infant's mouth to sustain latch and suck; must stimulate infant to continue to suck	Grasps nipple; tongue down; rhythmic sucking
A: Audible swallowing	None	A few observed with stimulation	Spontaneous and intermittent both <24 hours old and afterward
T: type of nipple	Inverted (drawn inward into breast tissue)	Flat (not protruding)	Everted or protruding out after stimulation
C: comfort of nipple	Engorged, cracked bleeding; severe discomfort	Filling; reddened, small blisters or bruises; mild to moderate discomfort	Soft, nontender
H: hold (positioning)	Nurse must hold infant to breast	Minimal assistance; help with positioning, then mother takes over	No assistance needed by nurse

Sources: AAP (2006a, 2006b, 2007); Pryor & Huggins (2007).

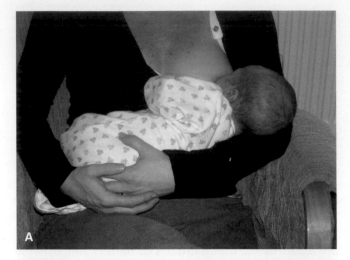

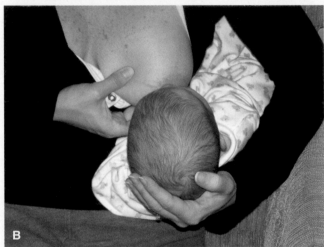

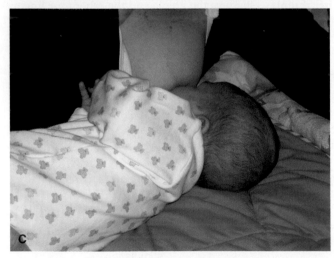

FIGURE 18.20 Breast-feeding positions.

below the areola and under the breast. In the V hold, the mother places her index finger above the areola and her other three fingers below the areola and under the breast. Either method can be used as long as the mother's hand is well away from the nipple so the infant can latch on.

Breast-Feeding Education

Breast-feeding is not an innate skill in human mothers. Almost all women have the potential to breast-feed successfully, but many fail because of inadequate knowledge. Nursing Care Plan 18.1 gives typical nursing diagnoses, outcomes, and interventions. For many mothers and newborns, breast-feeding goes smoothly from the start, but for others it is a struggle. Nurses can help throughout the experience by demonstrating techniques and offering encouragement and praise for success. Nurse should emphasize that the key to successful breast-feeding is correct positioning and latching-on.

Teaching by nurses has been shown to have a significant effect on both the ability to breast-feed successfully and the duration of lactation (Dudek, 2006). During the first few breast-feeding sessions, mothers want to know how often they should be nursing, whether breast-feeding is going well, if the newborn is getting enough nourishment, and what problems may ensue and how to cope with them. Education for the breast-feeding mother is highlighted in Teaching Guidelines 18.4.

*R*emember Kelly, who was concerned about jaundice in her newborn son? At her son's 2-week well-baby checkup at the clinic, his bilirubin level came back within normal limits. Kelly still felt he was not getting enough to eat and stated that she might switch to formula-feeding her son. What information can the nurse present to promote and reinforce breast-feeding? Should the nurse make a referral to the lactation consultant?

Breast Milk Storage and Expression

If the breast-feeding mother becomes separated from the newborn for any reason (e.g., work, travel, illness), she needs instruction on how to express and store milk safely. Expressing milk can be done manually (hand compression of breast) or by using a breast pump. Manual or hand pumps are inexpensive and can be used by mothers who occasionally need an extra bottle if they are going out. Electric breast pumps are used for mothers who experience a lengthy separation from their infants and need to pump their breasts regularly (Fig. 18.21).

To ensure the safety of expressed breast milk, instruct the mother in the following:

• Wash your hands before expressing milk or handling breast milk.
• Use clean containers to store expressed milk.
• Use sealed and chilled milk within 24 hours.
• Discard any milk that has been refrigerated more than 72 hours.
• Use any frozen expressed milk within 3 months.
• Do not use microwave ovens to warm chilled milk.
• Discard any used milk; never refreeze it.
• Store milk in quantities to be used for each feeding (2 to 4 oz).
• Thaw milk in warm water before using (AAP, 2007b).

Nursing Care Plan 18.1

OVERVIEW OF THE MOTHER AND NEWBORN HAVING DIFFICULTY WITH BREAST-FEEDING

Baby boy James, weight 7 lb, 4 oz, was born a few hours ago. His mother, Jane, is a 19-year-old gravida 1, para 1. His Apgar scores were 9 points at both 1 and 5 minutes. Labor and birth were unremarkable, and James was admitted to the nursery for assessment. After stabilization, James was brought to his mother, who had said she wished to breast-feed. The postpartum nurse assisted Jane with positioning and latching-on and left the room for a few minutes. On returning, Jane was upset, James was crying, and Jane stated she wanted a bottle of formula to feed him since she didn't have milk and her nipples hurt.

Assessment reveals a young, inexperienced mother placed in an uncomfortable situation with limited knowledge of breast-feeding. Anxiety from the mother transferred to James, resulting in crying. The mother, apprehensive about breast-feeding, needs additional help.

NURSING DIAGNOSIS: Knowledge deficit related to breast-feeding skills

Outcome Identification and Evaluation

Mother will demonstrate understanding of breast-feeding skills as evidenced by use of correct positioning and technique, and verbalization of appropriate information related to breast-feeding.

Interventions: Providing Education

- Instruct mother on proper positioning for breast-feeding; suggest use of football hold, side-lying position, modified cradle, and across-the-lap position to ensure comfort and *to promote ease in breast-feeding.*
- Review breast anatomy and milk letdown reflex *to enhance mother's understanding of lactation.*
- Observe newborn's ability to suck and latch on to the nipple *to assess whether newborn has adequate ability.*
- Monitor sucking and newborn swallowing for several minutes *to ensure adequate latching on and to assess intake.*
- Reinforce nipple care with water and exposure to air *to maintain nipple integrity.*

NURSING DIAGNOSIS: Anxiety related to breast-feeding ability and irritable, crying newborn

Outcome Identification and Evaluation

Mother will verbalize increased comfort with breast-feeding as evidenced by positive statements related to breast-feeding and verbalization of desire to continue to breast-feed newborn.

Interventions: Reducing Anxiety

- Ensure that the environment is calm and soothing without distractions *to promote maternal and newborn relaxation.*
- Show mother correct latching-on technique *to promote breast-feeding.*
- Assist in calming newborn by holding and talking *to ensure that the newborn is relaxed prior to latching on.*
- Reassure mother she can be successful at breast-feeding *to enhance her self-esteem and confidence.*
- Encourage frequent trials and attempts *to enhance confidence.*
- Encourage the mother to verbalize her anxiety/fears *to reduce anxiety.*

NURSING DIAGNOSIS: Pain related to breast-feeding and incorrect latching-on technique

Outcome Identification and Evaluation

Mother will experience a decrease in pain during breast-feeding as evidenced by statements of less nipple pain.

Interventions: Reducing Pain

- Suggest several alternate positions for breast-feeding *to increase comfort.*
- Demonstrate how to break suction before removing infant from breast *to minimize trauma to nipple.*
- Inspect nipple area *to promote early identification of trauma.*
- Reinforce correct latching-on technique *to prevent nipple trauma.*
- Administer pain medication if indicated *to relieve pain.*
- Instruct about nipple care between feedings *to maintain nipple integrity.*

TEACHING GUIDELINES 18.4

Breast-Feeding

- Set aside a quiet place where you can be relaxed and won't be disturbed. Relaxation promotes milk letdown.
- Sit in a comfortable chair or rocking chair or lie on a bed. Try to make each feeding calm, quiet, and leisurely. Avoid distractions.
- Listen to soothing music and sip a nutritious drink during feedings.
- Initially, nurse the newborn every few hours to stimulate milk production. Remember that the supply of milk is equal to the demand—the more sucking, the more milk.
- Watch for signals from the infant to indicate that he or she is hungry, such as:
  - Nuzzling against the mother's breasts
  - Demonstrating the rooting reflex by making sucking motions
  - Placing fist or hands in mouth to suck on
  - Crying and squirming
  - Smacking of the lips
- Stimulate the rooting reflex by touching the newborn's cheek to initiate sucking.
- Look for signs indicating that the newborn has latched on correctly: wide-open mouth with the nipple and much of the areola in the mouth, lips rolled outward, and tongue over lower gum, visible jaw movement drawing milk out, rhythmic sucking with an audible swallowing (soft "ka" or "ah" sound indicates the infant is swallowing milk).
- Hold the newborn closely, facing the breast, with the newborn's ear, shoulder, and hip in direct alignment.

- Nurse the infant on demand, not on a rigid schedule. Feed every 2 to 3 hours within a 24-hour period for a total of 8 to 12 feedings.
- Alternate the breast you offer first; identify with a safety pin on bra.
- Vary your position for each feeding to empty breasts and reduce soreness.
- Look for signs that the newborn is getting enough milk:
  - At least six wet diapers and two to five loose yellow stools daily
  - Steady weight gain after the first week of age
  - Pale-yellow urine, not deep yellow or orange
  - Sleeping well, yet looks alert and healthy when awake (AAP, 2007a)
- Wake up the newborn if he or she has nursed less than 5 minutes by unwrapping him or her.
- Before removing the baby from the breast, break the infant's suction by inserting a finger.
- Burp the infant to release air when changing breasts and at the end of the breast-feeding session.
- Avoid supplemental formula feedings to prevent "nipple confusion" (Pryor & Huggins, 2007)
- Do not take drugs or medications unless approved by the health care provider.
- Avoid drinking alcohol or caffeinated drinks because they pass through milk.
- Do not smoke while breast-feeding; it increases the risk of sudden infant death syndrome.
- Always wash your hands before expressing or handling milk to store.
- Wear nursing bras and clothes that are easy to undo.

Common Breast-Feeding Concerns

Breast-feeding women may experience problems such as cracked nipples, engorgement, or mastitis. Breast-feeding should not be painful for the mother. If she has sore, cracked nipples, the first step is to find the cause. Incorrect positioning or latching-on, removing the infant from the breast without first breaking the suction, or wearing a bra that is too tight can cause cracked or sore nipples. Cracked nipples can increase the risk of mastitis because a break in the skin may allow *Staphylococcus aureus* or other organisms to enter the body.

Sore nipples usually are caused by improper infant attachment, which traumatizes the tissue. The nurse should review techniques for proper positioning and latching-on. Recommend the following to the mother:

- Use only water, not soap, to clean the nipples to prevent dryness.

- Express some milk before feeding to stimulate the milk ejection reflex.
- Avoid using breast pads with plastic liners, and change pads when they are wet.
- Wear a comfortable bra that is not too tight.
- Apply a few drops of breast milk to the nipples after feeding.
- Rotate positions when feeding the infant to promote complete breast emptying.
- Leave the nursing bra flaps down after feeding to allow nipples to air-dry.
- Inspect the nipples daily for redness or cracks (Arenson & Drake, 2007).

To ease nipple pain and trauma, reinforce appropriate latching-on and remind the woman about the need to break the suction at the breast before removing the newborn from the breast. Additional measures may include

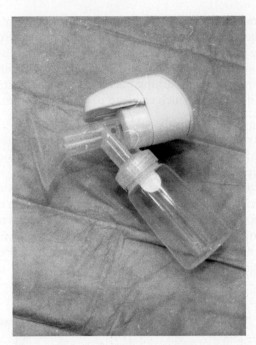

FIGURE **18.21** Hand-held breast pump.

applying cold compresses over the area and massaging breast milk onto the nipple after feeding.

Engorgement may occur as the milk comes in around day 3 or 4 after birth of the newborn. Explain to the mother that engorgement, though uncomfortable, is self-limited and will resolve as the newborn continues to nurse. The mother should continue to nurse during engorgement to avoid a plugged milk duct, which could lead to mastitis. Provide the following tips for relieving engorgement:

• Take warm to hot showers to encourage milk release.
• Express some milk manually before breast-feeding.
• Wear a supportive nursing bra 24 hours a day to provide support.
• Feed the newborn in a variety of positions—sitting up and then lying down.
• Massage the breasts from under the axillary area down toward the nipple.
• Increase the frequency of feedings.
• Apply warm compresses to the breasts prior to nursing.
• Stay relaxed while breast-feeding.
• Use a breast pump if nursing or manual expression is not effective.
• Remember that this condition is temporary and resolves quickly.

Mastitis, or inflammation of the breast, causes flu-like symptoms, chills, fever, and malaise. These symptoms may occur before the development of soreness, aching, swelling, and redness in the breast (usually the upper outer quadrant). This condition usually occurs in just one breast when a milk duct becomes blocked, causing inflammation, or through a cracked or damaged nipple, allowing bacteria to infect a portion of the breast. Treatment con-

sists of rest, warm compresses, antibiotics, breast support, and continued breast-feeding (the infection will not pass into the breast milk). Explain to the mother that it is important to keep the milk flowing in the infected breast, whether it is through nursing or manual expression or with a breast pump.

Formula Feeding

Despite the general acknowledgment that breast-feeding is the most desirable means of feeding infants, about 40% of mothers choose formula feeding and need education about this procedure. Formula-fed infants grow more rapidly than breast-fed infants not only in weight but also in length (Begany & Mascarenhas, 2007).

Formula feeding requires more than just opening, pouring, and feeding. Parents need information about the types of formula available, preparation and storage of formula, equipment, feeding positions, and the amount to feed their newborn. The mother also needs to know how to prevent lactation (see Chap. 16 for more information).

Commercially prepared formulas are regulated by the Food and Drug Administration (FDA) and are manufactured by Meade Johnson (Enfamil) or Ross Laboratories (Similac) in the United States. Normal full-term infants usually receive conventional cow's milk-based formula, but this decision is made by the health care provider. If the infant shows signs of a reaction or lactose intolerance, a switch to another formula type is recommended. The general recommendation is for all infants to receive iron-fortified formula until the age of 1 year. The latest generation of infant formulas includes some fortification with docosahexaenoic acid (DHA) and arachidonic acid (ARA), two natural components of breast milk. Researchers have found that formulas with DHA and ARA can enhance visual and cognitive development in children (Lawson, 2007).

Commercial formulas come in three forms: powder, concentrate, and easy to feed or ready to use. All are similar in terms of nutritional content but differ in expense. Powdered formula is the least expensive, with concentrated formula the next most expensive. Both must be mixed with water before using. Ready-to-feed formula is the most expensive; it can be opened and poured into a bottle and fed directly to the infant.

Parents need information about the equipment needed for formula feeding. Basic supplies are 4 to 6 4-oz bottles, 8 to 10 8-oz bottles, 8 to 10 nipple units, a bottle brush, and a nipple brush. A key area of instruction is assessing for flow of formula through the nipple and checking for any nipple damage. When the bottle is filled and turned upside down, the flow from the nipple should be approximately one drop per second. If the parents are using bottles with disposable bags, instruct them to make sure they have a tight-fitting nipple to prevent leaks. Frequent observation of the flow rate from the nipple and the condition of the nipple will prevent choking and aspiration associated with too fast a rate of delivery. Ask the parents to fill a bottle with formula and then turn it upside down and observe the rate at which the formula drips from the bottle. If it is too fast (more than one drop/second), then the nipple should be replaced.

Correct formula preparation is critical to the newborn's health and development. Mistakes in dilution may result if the parents do not understand how to prepare the formula or make measurement errors. The safety of the water supply should be considered. If well water is used, parents should sterilize the water by boiling it or should use bottled water. Many health care providers still recommend that all water used in formula preparation be brought to a rolling boil for 1 to 2 minutes and should be cooled to room temperature before use.

Opened cans of ready-made or concentrated formula should be covered and refrigerated after being prepared for the day (24 hours). Instruct parents to discard any unused portions after 48 hours.

> ▶ *Take* NOTE!
>
> *Any formula left in the bottle after feeding should also be discarded, because the infant's saliva has been mixed with it.*

To warm refrigerated formula, advise the parents to place the bottle in a pan of hot water and test the temperature by letting a few drops fall on the inside of the wrist. If it is comfortably warm to the mother, it is the correct temperature.

Formula-Feeding Assistance

The process of feeding a newborn formula from a bottle should mirror breast-feeding as closely as possible. Although nutrition is important, so are the emotional and interactive components of feeding. Encourage parents to cuddle their newborn closely and position him or her so that the head is in a comfortable position, not too far back or turned, which makes swallowing difficult. Also urge parents to communicate with their newborn during the feedings by talking and singing to him or her.

Although it may seem that bottle feeding is not a difficult task, many new parents find it awkward. At first glance, holding an infant and a bottle appears simple enough, but both the position of the baby and the angle of the bottle must be correct.

Formula-Feeding Positions

Advise mothers to feed their newborns in a relaxed and quiet setting to create a sense of calm for themselves and the baby. Make sure that comfort is a priority for both mother and newborn. The mother can sit in a comfortable chair, using a pillow to support the arm in which she is holding the baby. The mother can cradle the newborn in a semi-upright position, supporting the newborn's head in the crook of her arm. Holding the newborn close during feeding provides stimulation and helps prevent choking. Holding the newborn's head raised slightly will help prevent formula from washing backward into the eustachian tubes in the ears, which can lead to an ear infection.

Formula-Feeding Education

Parents require teaching about the correct preparation and storage of formula as well as the techniques for feeding. See Teaching Guidelines 18.5.

Proper positioning makes bottle feeding easier and more enjoyable for both mother and newborn. As in breast-feeding, frequent burping is key. Advise the parents to hold the bottle so that formula fills the nipple, thus allowing less air to enter. Infants get fussy when they swallow air during feedings and need to be relieved of it every 2 to 3 oz.

TEACHING GUIDELINES 18.5

Formula-Feeding

- Wash your hands with soap and water before preparing formula.
- Mix the formula and water amounts exactly as the label specifies.
- Always hold the newborn and bottle during feedings; never prop the bottle.
- Never freeze formula or warm it in the microwave.
- Place refrigerated formula in a pan of hot water for a few minutes to warm.
- Test the temperature of the formula by shaking a few drops on the wrist.
- Hold the bottle like a pencil, keeping it tipped to prevent air from entering. Position the bottle so that the nipple remains filled with milk.
- Burp the infant after every few ounces to allow air swallowed to escape.
- Move the nipple around in the infant's mouth to stimulate sucking.
- Always keep a bulb syringe close by to use if choking occurs.
- Avoid putting the infant to bed with a bottle to prevent "baby bottle tooth decay."
- Feed the newborn approximately every 3 to 4 hours.
- Use an iron-fortified formula for the first year.
- Prepare enough formula for the next 24 hours.
- Check nipples regularly and discard any that are sticky, cracked, or leaking.
- Store unmixed, open liquid formula in the refrigerator for up to 48 hours.
- Throw away any formula left in the bottle after each feeding.

Emphasize to parents that an electrolyte imbalance can occur in infants who are fed formula that has been incorrectly mixed. Hypernatremia can result from formula that is mixed too thickly; the high concentration of sodium is too much for the baby's immature kidneys to handle. As a result, sodium is excreted along with water, leading to dehydration. Mixing the formula with too much water in an effort to save money can lead to failure to thrive and lack of weight gain (AAP, 2007b).

Weaning and Introduction of Solid Foods

Eventually, breast-feeding or formula feeding ends. Weaning involves the transition from breast to bottle, from breast or bottle to cup, or from liquids to solids. Weaning from breast-feeding to cup has several advantages over weaning to a bottle because it eliminates the step of weaning first to a bottle and then to a cup. Another advantage is that the bottle does not become a security object for the infant.

Weaning can be done because the mother is returning to work and cannot keep breast-feeding, or because the infant is losing interest in breast-feeding and showing signs of independence. There is no "right" time to wean; it depends on the desires of the mother and infant. Weaning represents a significant change in the way the mother and infant interact, and each mother must decide for herself when she and her infant are ready to take that step. Either one can start the weaning process, but usually it occurs between 6 months and 1 year of age.

To begin weaning from the breast, instruct mothers to substitute breast-feeding with a cup or bottle. Often the midday feeding is the easiest feeding to replace. A trainer cup with two handles and a snap-on lid with a spout is appropriate and minimizes spilling. Because weaning is a gradual process, it may take months. Instruct parents to proceed slowly and let the infant's willingness and interest guide them.

Weaning from the bottle to the cup also needs to be timed appropriately for mother and infant. Typically, the night bottle is the last to be given up, with cup drinking substituted throughout the day. Slowly diluting the formula with water over a week can help in this process; the final result is an all-water bottle. To prevent the baby from sucking on the bottle during the night, remove it from the crib after the infant falls asleep.

When infants double their birthweight and weigh at least 13 lb, it is time to consider introducing solid foods. Readiness cues include:

- Consumption of 32 oz of formula or breast milk daily (estimated)
- Ability to sit up with minimal support and turn head away to indicate fullness
- Reduction of protrusion reflex so cereal can be propelled to back of throat
- Demonstration of interest in food others around them are eating
- Ability to open mouth automatically when food approaches it

When introducing solid foods, certain principles apply:

- Only one new single-ingredient food (e.g., rice cereal or carrots) should be introduced at a time to watch for allergies.
- Infants should be allowed to set the pace regarding how much they wish to eat.
- New foods should not be introduced more frequently than every 3 to 5 days.
- Fruits are added after cereals; then vegetables and meats are introduced; eggs are introduced last.
- A relaxed, unhurried, calm atmosphere for meals is important.
- A variety of foods are provided to ensure a balanced diet.
- Infants should never be force-fed (Lawson, 2007).

Nurses can promote good feeding practices by actively listening to new mothers, helping them clarify their feelings and discussing solutions. A warm, sincere manner and tone of voice will put an anxious mother at ease. Giving accurate information, making suggestions, and presenting options will enable the mother to decide what is best for her and her infant. Nurses should be sensitive to the individual, family, and economic and cultural differences among mothers before offering suggestions for feeding practices that may not be appropriate.

Preparing for Discharge

Preparing the parents for discharge is an essential task for the nurse. Because of today's shorter hospital stays, the nurse must identify the major teaching topics that need to be covered. Nurses should assess the parents' baseline knowledge and learning needs and plan how to meet them. Using the following principles fosters a learner-centered approach:

- Make the environment conducive to learning. Encourage the parents to feel comfortable during this intense time by using support and praise.
- Allow the parents to provide input about the content and the process of learning. What do they want and need to learn?
- Build the parents' self-esteem by confirming that their responses to the entire birthing process and aftercare are legitimate, and others have felt the same way.
- Ensure that what the parents learn is relevant to their day-to-day home situation.
- Encourage responsibility by reinforcing that their emotional and physical responses are within the normal range.
- Respect cultural beliefs and practices that are important to the family by taking into account their heritage and health beliefs regarding newborn care. Examples include placing a bellyband over the newborn's navel

(Hispanics and African-Americans), delaying naming the newborn (Asian-Americans and Haitians), and delaying breast-feeding (Native Americans; they regard colostrum as "bad") (Bowers, 2007).

While in the hospital, women have ready access to support and hands-on instruction regarding feeding and newborn care. When the new mother is discharged, this close supervision and support by nurses should not end abruptly. Providing the new parents with the phone number of the mother–baby unit will help them through this stressful transitional period. Giving the new family information and offering backup support via the telephone will increase parenting success.

▶ *Consider* THIS!

I have always prided myself on being very organized and in control in most situations, but survival at home after childbirth wasn't one of them. I left the hospital 24 hours after giving birth to my son because my doctor said I could. The postpartum nurse encouraged me to stay longer, but wanting to be in control and sleeping in my own bed again won out. I thought my baby would be sleeping while I sent out birth announcements to my friends and family—wrong! What happened instead was my son didn't sleep as I imagined and my nipples became sore after breast-feeding every few hours. I was weary and tired and wanted to sleep, but I couldn't. Somehow I thought I would be getting a full night's sleep because I was up throughout the day, but that was a fantasy too. At 2 o'clock in the morning when you are up feeding your baby, you feel you are the only one in the world up at that time and feel very much alone. My feelings of being organized and in control all the time have changed dramatically since I left the hospital. I have learned to yield to the important needs of my son and derive satisfaction from being able to bring comfort to him and to let go of my control.

Thoughts: It is interesting to see how a newborn changed this woman's need to organize and control her environment. What "tips of survival" could the nurse offer this woman to help in her transition to home with her newborn? How can friends and family help when women arrive home from the hospital with their newborns?

Ensuring Follow-Up Care

Most newborns are scheduled for their first health follow-up appointment within 2 to 4 days after discharge so they can have additional laboratory work done as part of the newborn screening series, especially if they were discharged within 48 hours. After this first visit, the typical schedule of health care visits is as follows: 2 to 4 weeks of age; 2, 4, and 6 months of age for checkups and vaccines; 9 months of age for a checkup; 12 months for a checkup and tuberculosis testing; 15 and 18 months for checkups and vaccines; and 2 years of age for a checkup. These appointments provide an opportunity for parents to ask questions and receive anticipatory guidance as their newborn grows and develops.

In addition to encouraging parents to keep follow-up appointments, advise parents to call their health care provider if they notice signs of illness in their newborn. They should know which over-the-counter medicines should be kept on hand. Review the following warning signs of illness with parents:

• Temperature of 38.3°C (101°F) or higher
• Forceful, persistent vomiting, not just spitting up
• Refusal to take feedings
• Two or more green, watery diarrheal stools
• Infrequent wet diapers and change in bowel movements from normal pattern
• Lethargy or excessive sleepiness
• Inconsolable crying and extreme fussiness
• Abdominal distention
• Difficult or labored breathing

Providing Immunization Information

Parents also need instructions about immunizations for their newborn. **Immunization** is the process of rendering an individual immune or of becoming immune to certain communicable diseases (AAP, 2007). The purpose of the immune system is to identify unknown (non-self) substances in the body and develop a defense against these invaders. Disease prevention by immunization is a public health priority and is one of the leading health indicators as part of *Healthy People 2010*. Despite many advances in vaccine delivery, the goal of universal immunization has not been reached (AAP, 2007). Nurses can help to meet this national goal by educating new parents about the importance of disease prevention through immunizations.

Immunity can be provided either passively or actively. Passive immunity is protection transferred via already formed antibodies from one person to another. Passive immunity includes transplacental passage of antibodies from a mother to her newborn, immunity passed through breast milk, and immunity from immunoglobulins. Passive immunity provides limited protection and decreases over a period of weeks or months (Blackburn, 2007). Active immunity is protection produced by an individual's own immune system. It can be obtained by having the actual disease or by receiving a vaccine that produces an immunologic response by that person's body. Active immunity may be lifelong either way.

Young infants and children are susceptible to various illnesses because their immune systems are not yet mature. Many of these illnesses can be prevented by following the recommended schedule of childhood immunizations; Figure 18.22 shows the 2008 Childhood Immunization

Recommended Immunization Schedule for Persons Aged 0–6 Years—UNITED STATES • 2008
For those who fall behind or start late, see the catch-up schedule

Vaccine ▼ Age ►	Birth	1 month	2 months	4 months	6 months	12 months	15 months	18 months	19–23 months	2–3 years	4–6 years
Hepatitis B[1]	HepB	HepB		see footnote 1		HepB					
Rotavirus[2]			Rota	Rota	Rota						
Diphtheria, Tetanus, Pertussis[3]			DTaP	DTaP	DTaP	see footnote 3	DTaP				DTaP
Haemophilus influenzae type b[4]			Hib	Hib	Hib[4]	Hib					
Pneumococcal[5]			PCV	PCV	PCV	PCV				PPV	
Inactivated Poliovirus			IPV	IPV		IPV					IPV
Influenza[6]						Influenza (Yearly)					
Measles, Mumps, Rubella[7]						MMR					MMR
Varicella[8]						Varicella					Varicella
Hepatitis A[9]						HepA (2 doses)				HepA Series	
Meningococcal[10]										MCV4	

Range of recommended ages

Certain high-risk groups

This schedule indicates the recommended ages for routine administration of currently licensed childhood vaccines, as of December 1, 2007, for children aged 0 through 6 years. Additional information is available at www.cdc.gov/vaccines/recs/schedules. Any dose not administered at the recommended age should be administered at any subsequent visit, when indicated and feasible. Additional vaccines may be licensed and recommended during the year. Licensed combination vaccines may be used whenever any components of the combination are indicated and other components of the vaccine are not contraindicated and if approved by the Food and Drug Administration for that dose of the series. Providers should consult the respective Advisory Committee on Immunization Practices statement for detailed recommendations, including for **high-risk conditions**: http://www.cdc.gov/vaccines/pubs/ACIP-list.htm. Clinically significant adverse events that follow immunization should be reported to the Vaccine Adverse Event Reporting System (VAERS). Guidance about how to obtain and complete a VAERS form is available at www.vaers.hhs.gov or by telephone, **800-822-7967**.

1. Hepatitis B vaccine (HepB). *(Minimum age: birth)*
  At birth:
  • Administer monovalent HepB to all newborns prior to hospital discharge.
  • If mother is hepatitis B surface antigen (HBsAg) positive, administer HepB and 0.5 mL of hepatitis B immune globulin (HBIG) within 12 hours of birth.
  • If mother's HBsAg status is unknown, administer HepB within 12 hours of birth. Determine the HBsAg status as soon as possible and if HBsAg positive, administer HBIG (no later than age 1 week).
  • If mother is HBsAg negative, the birth dose can be delayed, in rare cases, with a provider's order and a copy of the mother's negative HBsAg laboratory report in the infant's medical record.
  After the birth dose:
  • The HepB series should be completed with either monovalent HepB or a combination vaccine containing HepB. The second dose should be administered at age 1–2 months. The final dose should be administered no earlier than age 24 weeks. Infants born to HBsAg-positive mothers should be tested for HBsAg and antibody to HBsAg after completion of at least 3 doses of a licensed HepB series, at age 9–18 months (generally at the next well-child visit).
  4-month dose:
  • It is permissible to administer 4 doses of HepB when combination vaccines are administered after the birth dose. If monovalent HepB is used for doses after the birth dose, a dose at age 4 months is not needed.

2. Rotavirus vaccine (Rota). *(Minimum age: 6 weeks)*
  • Administer the first dose at age 6–12 weeks.
  • Do not start the series later than age 12 weeks.
  • Administer the final dose in the series by age 32 weeks. Do not administer any dose later than age 32 weeks.
  • Data on safety and efficacy outside of these age ranges are insufficient.

3. Diphtheria and tetanus toxoids and acellular pertussis vaccine (DTaP). *(Minimum age: 6 weeks)*
  • The fourth dose of DTaP may be administered as early as age 12 months, provided 6 months have elapsed since the third dose.
  • Administer the final dose in the series at age 4–6 years.

4. Haemophilus influenzae type b conjugate vaccine (Hib). *(Minimum age: 6 weeks)*
  • If PRP-OMP (PedvaxHIB® or ComVax® [Merck]) is administered at ages 2 and 4 months, a dose at age 6 months is not required.
  • TriHIBit® (DTaP/Hib) combination products should not be used for primary immunization but can be used as boosters following any Hib vaccine in children age 12 months or older.

5. Pneumococcal vaccine. *(Minimum age: 6 weeks for pneumococcal conjugate vaccine [PCV]; 2 years for pneumococcal polysaccharide vaccine [PPV])*
  • Administer one dose of PCV to all healthy children aged 24–59 months having any incomplete schedule.
  • Administer PPV to children aged 2 years and older with underlying medical conditions.

6. Influenza vaccine. *(Minimum age: 6 months for trivalent inactivated influenza vaccine [TIV]; 2 years for live, attenuated influenza vaccine [LAIV])*
  • Administer annually to children aged 6–59 months and to all eligible close contacts of children aged 0–59 months.
  • Administer annually to children 5 years of age and older with certain risk factors, to other persons (including household members) in close contact with persons in groups at higher risk, and to any child whose parents request vaccination.
  • For healthy persons (those who do not have underlying medical conditions that predispose them to influenza complications) ages 2–49 years, either LAIV or TIV may be used.
  • Children receiving TIV should receive 0.25 mL if age 6–35 months or 0.5 mL if age 3 years or older.
  • Administer 2 doses (separated by 4 weeks or longer) to children younger than 9 years who are receiving influenza vaccine for the first time or who were vaccinated for the first time last season but only received one dose.

7. Measles, mumps, and rubella vaccine (MMR). *(Minimum age: 12 months)*
  • Administer the second dose of MMR at age 4–6 years. MMR may be administered before age 4–6 years, provided 4 weeks or more have elapsed since the first dose.

8. Varicella vaccine. *(Minimum age: 12 months)*
  • Administer second dose at age 4–6 years; may be administered 3 months or more after first dose.
  • Do not repeat second dose if administered 28 days or more after first dose.

9. Hepatitis A vaccine (HepA). *(Minimum age: 12 months)*
  • Administer to all children aged 1 year (i.e., aged 12–23 months). Administer the 2 doses in the series at least 6 months apart.
  • Children not fully vaccinated by age 2 years can be vaccinated at subsequent visits.
  • HepA is recommended for certain other groups of children, including in areas where vaccination programs target older children.

10. Meningococcal vaccine. *(Minimum age: 2 years for meningococcal conjugate vaccine (MCV4) and for meningococcal polysaccharide vaccine (MPSV4))*
  • Administer MCV4 to children aged 2–10 years with terminal complement deficiencies or anatomic or functional asplenia and certain other high-risk groups. MPSV4 is also acceptable.
  • Administer MCV4 to persons who received MPSV4 3 or more years previously and remain at increased risk for meningococcal disease.

FIGURE **18.22** Recommended childhood immunization schedule.

Schedule. Readers can view the latest CDC immunization schedule by visiting www.cdc.gov/nip. The schedule for immunizations should be reviewed with parents, stressing the importance of continued follow-up health care to preserve their infant's health.

The newborn's first immunization (hepatitis B) is received in the hospital soon after birth. The first dose can also be given by age 2 months if the mother is HbsAg negative. If the mother is HbsAg positive, then the newborn should receive hepatitis B vaccine and hepatitis B immunoglobulin within 12 hours of birth (Cunningham et al., 2005).

Education for the parents should include the risks and benefits for each vaccine and possible adverse effects. Federal law requires a consent form to be signed before administering a vaccine. Parents have the right to refuse immunizations based on their religious beliefs and can sign a waiver noting their decision. The nurse administering the vaccine must document the date and time it was given, name and manufacturer, lot number and expiration date of the vaccine given, site and route of administration, and the name and title of the nurse who administered the vaccine.

■■■ Key Concepts

- The period of transition from intrauterine to extrauterine life occurs during the first several hours after birth. It is a time of stabilization for the newborn's temperature, respiration, and cardiovascular dynamics.
- The newborn's bowel is sterile at birth. It usually takes about a week for the newborn to produce vitamin K in sufficient quantities to prevent VKDB.
- It is recommended that all newborns in the United States receive an instillation of a prophylactic agent (erythromycin or tetracycline ophthalmic ointment) in their eyes within an hour or two of being born.
- Nursing measures to maintain newborns' body temperature include drying them immediately after birth to prevent heat loss through evaporation, wrapping them in prewarmed blankets, putting a hat on their head, and placing them under a temperature-controlled radiant warmer.
- The specific components of a typical newborn examination include a general survey of skin color, posture, state of alertness, head size, overall behavioral state, respiratory status, gender, and any obvious congenital anomalies.
- Gestational age assessment is pertinent because it allows the nurse to plot growth parameters and to anticipate potential problems related to prematurity/postmaturity and growth abnormalities such as SGA/LGA.
- After the newborn has passed the transitional period and stabilized, the nurse needs to complete ongoing assessments, vital signs, weight and measurements, cord care, hygiene measures, newborn screening tests, and various other tasks until the newborn is discharged home from the birthing unit.
- Important topics about which to educate parents include environmental safety, newborn characteristics, feeding and bathing, circumcision and cord care, sleep and elimination patterns of newborns, safe infant car seats, holding/positioning, and follow-up care.
- Newborn screening tests consist of hearing and certain genetic and inborn errors of metabolism tests required in most states for newborns before discharge from the birth facility.
- The AAP and the American Dietetic Association recommend breast-feeding exclusively for the first 6 months of life and that it continue along with other food at least until the first birthday.
- Parents who choose not to breast-feed need to know what types of formula are available, preparation and storage of formula, equipment, feeding positions, and how much to feed their infant.
- Common problems associated with the newborn include transient tachypnea, physiologic jaundice, and hypoglycemia.
- Transient tachypnea of the newborn appears soon after birth; is accompanied by retractions, expiratory grunting, or cyanosis; and is relieved by low-dose oxygen.
- Physiologic jaundice is a very common condition in newborns, with the majority demonstrating yellowish skin, mucous membranes, and sclera within the first 3 days of life. Newborns undergoing phototherapy in the treatment of jaundice require close monitoring of their body temperature, fluid, and electrolyte balance; observation of skin integrity; eye protection; and parental participation in their care.
- The newborn with hypoglycemia requires close monitoring for signs and symptoms of hypoglycemia if present. In addition, newborns at high risk need to be identified based on their perinatal history, physical examination, body measurements, and gestational age. Blood glucose levels of all newborns are checked within the first few hours after birth and every 4 hours thereafter.
- The schedule for immunizations should be reviewed with parents, stressing the importance of continual follow-up health care to preserve their infant's health.

REFERENCES

Adegbehingbe, O., Owa, J. A., Kuti, O., & Oginni, L. M. (2007). Orthopedic birth trauma: A reflection of current perinatal care. *Internet Journal of Gynecology and Obstetrics, 6*(2), 8–20.

Adler, M. R., Hyderi, A., & Hamilton, A. (2006). What are the safe sleeping arrangements for infants? *Journal of Family Practice, 55*(12), 1083–1087.

American Academy of Pediatrics (AAP). (2006a). *A woman's guide to breast-feeding.* Available at www.aap.org/family/brstguid.htm.

American Academy of Pediatrics (AAP). (2006b). Breast-feeding and the use of human milk. AAP policy statement. *Pediatrics, 115,* 496–506.

American Academy of Pediatrics (AAP). (2007a). *Bright futures guidelines for health supervision of infants, children, and adolescents.* Washington, DC: AAP.

American Academy of Pediatrics (AAP). (2007b). *Heading home with your newborn: From birth to reality.* Washington, DC: AAP.

American Academy of Pediatrics (AAP). (2007c). *Pediatric clinical practice guidelines and policies: A compendium of evidence-based research for pediatric practice* (7th ed.). Washington, DC: AAP.

American Academy of Pediatrics (AAP). (2007d). *Car safety seats: A guide for families 2007.* Available at www.aap.org/family/carseatguide.htm.

Arenson, J., & Drake, P. (2007). *Maternal and newborn health.* Sudbury, MA: Jones and Bartlett Publishers.

Asenjo, M. (2007). Transient tachypnea of the newborn. *eMedicine.* Available at www.emedicine.com/radio/topic710.htm.

AWHONN Lifelines. (2007). Preventing infant abduction: A parent's guide. *AWHONN Lifelines, 10*(6), 521–522.

Begany, M., & Mascarenhas, M. (2007). Normal infant feeding. In R. E. Rakel & E. T. Bope (Eds.), *Conn's current therapy 2007* (Section 16, pp. 1210–1214). Philadelphia: Saunders Elsevier.

Blackburn, S. T. (2007). *Maternal, fetal, and neonatal physiology: A clinical perspective* (3rd ed.). St. Louis: Saunders Elsevier.

Bowers, P. (2007). Cultural aspects of childbearing. *Nursing Spectrum.* Available at http://www.nurse.com/ce/syllabus.html?CCID=3245.

Burns, C. E., Dunn, A. M., Brady, M. A., Starr, N. B., & Blosser, C. G. (2009). *Pediatric primary care* (4th ed.). St. Louis: Saunders Elsevier.

Buswell, S. D., & Spatz, D. L. (2007). Parent-infant co-sleeping and its relationship to breastfeeding. *Journal of Pediatric Health Care, 21*(1), 22–28.

Centers for Disease Control and Prevention (CDC). (2007). *Sexually transmitted diseases treatment guidelines.* Available at www.cdc.gov/STD/treatment.

Cohen, S. (2007). *Critical thinking in the pediatric unit: Skills to assess, analyze and act.* Marblehead, MA: HCPro, Inc.

Cohen, S. M. (2006). Jaundice in the full-term newborn. *Pediatric Nursing, 32*(3), 202–208.

Cunningham, F. G., Leveno, K. J., Bloom, S. L., Hauth, J. C., Gilstrap, L. C., & Wenstrom, K. D. (2005). *Williams obstetrics* (22nd ed.). New York: McGraw-Hill Medical Publishing Division.

Deshpande, P. G., & Ramer, T. (2007). Breast milk jaundice. *eMedicine.* Available at http://www.emedicine.com/ped/topic282.htm.

Dillon, P. M. (2007). *Nursing health assessment: A critical thinking, case studies approach.* Philadelphia: F. A. Davis.

Dudek, S. G. (2006). *Nutrition essentials for nursing practice* (5th ed.). Philadelphia: Lippincott Williams & Wilkins.

Healthcare Risk Management. (2007). Infant abduction raises questions about health care security and vigilance. *Healthcare Risk Management, 29*(5), 49–60.

Johnson, K. J., Spector, L. G., Klebanoff, M. A., & Ross, J. A. (2007). Childhood cancer and birthmarks in the collaborative perinatal project. *Pediatrics, 119*(5), 1088–1093.

Keenan, W. (2006). Apgar score—How consistent is it? *Pediatric Alert, 31*(19), 113–114.

Kenner, C., & Lott, J. W. (2007). *Comprehensive neonatal care: An interdisciplinary approach* (4th ed.). St. Louis: Saunders Elsevier.

Kliegman, R. M., Behrman, R. E., Jenson, H. B., & Stanton, B. F. (2007). *Nelson's textbook of pediatrics* (18th ed.). St. Louis: Saunders Elsevier.

Lawrence, E. J. (2006). Focus on the physical. Part 1: A matter of size. *Advances in Neonatal Care, 6*(6), 313–322.

Lawson, M. (2007). Contemporary aspects of infant feeding. *Pediatric Nursing, 19*(2), 39–45.

Maisels, M. J. (2006). What's in a name? Physiologic and pathologic jaundice: The conundrum of defining normal bilirubin levels in the newborn. *Pediatrics, 118*(2), 805–807.

Mukherjee, S. (2007). Hyperbilirubinemia, unconjugated. *eMedicine.* Available at: http://www.emedicine.com/med/topic1066.htm.

Pryor, G., & Huggins, K. (2007). *Nursing mother, working mother: The essential guide to breastfeeding your baby before and after you return to work* (2nd ed.). Harvard, MA: The Harvard Common Press.

Ridings, H., & Amaya, M. (2007). Male neonatal circumcision: An evidence-based review. *Journal of the American Academy of Physician Assistants, 20*(2), 32–36.

Simonson, C., Barlow, P., Dehennin, N., Sphel, M., Toppet, V., Murillo, D., & Rozenberg, S. (2007). Neonatal complications of vacuum-assisted delivery. *Obstetrics and Gynecology, 109*(3), 626–633.

U.S. Department of Health and Human Services (USDHHS). (2000). *Healthy people 2010: Understanding and improving health* (2nd ed.). DHHS publication 017-001-00550-9. Washington, DC: Author.

U.S. Prevention Services Task Force (USPSTF). (2006). *The guide to clinical prevention services.* Agency for Healthcare Research and Quality. Washington, DC: AHRQ Pub.No. 06-0588.

Walsh, D. (2007). *Evidence-based care for normal labor and birth: A guide for midwives.* London: Taylor and Francis, Inc.

Wasee, M. (2006). Vitamin K and hemorrhagic disease of newborns. *Southern Medical Journal, 99*(11), 1199–1200.

Wrightson, A. S. (2007) Universal newborn hearing screening. *American Family Physician, 75*(9), 1349–1352.

WEBSITES

American Academy of Pediatrics, Newborn Screening Facts Sheets: www.aap.org/policy/01565.html

American Academy of Pediatrics, Breast-feeding and use of human milk: www.aap.org/policy/re9729.html

American Social Health Association: www.vaccines.ashastd.org

Baby Trend: www.babytrend.com

Breast-feeding information: www.breastfeeding.com

Bright Future Lactation Resource Center: www.bflrc.com

CDC's National Immunization Program: www.cdc.gov/nip

Graco/Century: www.gracobaby.com

Immunization Action Coalition: www.immunize.org

La Leche League International: www.lalecheleague.org

March of Dimes, newborn screening tests: www.marchofdimes.com/professionals/681–1200.asp

National Center for Missing and Exploited Children: www.missingkids.com

National Healthy Mothers, Healthy Babies Coalition: www.hmhb.org

National Institute of Child Health and Human Development: www.nih.gov

National Newborn Screening and Genetics Resource Center: http://genes-r-us.uthscsa.edu/resources/newborn/screestatus.htm

Neonatal Network: www.neonatalnetwork.com

Safeline Corporation: www.safelinekids.com

Vaccine Education Center: www.vaccine.chop.edu

CHAPTER WORKSHEET

MULTIPLE CHOICE QUESTIONS

1. At birth, a newborn's assessment reveals the following: heart rate of 140 bpm, loud crying, some flexion of extremities, crying when bulb syringe is introduced into the nares, and a pink body with blue extremities. The nurse would document the newborn's Apgar score as:

   a. 5 points

   b. 6 points

   c. 7 points

   d. 8 points

2. The nurse is explaining phototherapy to the parents of a newborn. The nurse would include which of the following as the purpose?

   a. Increase surfactant levels

   b. Stabilize the newborn's temperature

   c. Destroy Rh-negative antibodies

   d. Oxidize bilirubin on the skin

3. The nurse administers a single dose of vitamin K intramuscularly to a newborn after birth to promote:

   a. Conjugation of bilirubin

   b. Blood clotting

   c. Foreman ovale closure

   d. Digestion of complex proteins

4. A prophylactic agent is instilled in both eyes of all newborns to prevent which of the following conditions?

   a. Gonorrhea and chlamydia

   b. Thrush and Enterobacter

   c. *Staphylococcus* and syphilis

   d. Hepatitis B and herpes

5. The AAP recommends that all newborns be placed on their backs to sleep to reduce the risk of:

   a. Respiratory distress syndrome

   b. Bottle mouth syndrome

   c. Sudden infant death syndrome

   d. GI regurgitation syndrome

6. Which of the following immunizations is received by newborns before hospital discharge?

   a. Pneumococcus

   b. Varicella

   c. Hepatitis A

   d. Hepatitis B

7. Which condition would be missed if newborns are screened before they have tolerated protein feedings for at least 48 hours?

   a. Hypothyroidism

   b. Cystic fibrosis

   c. Phenylketonuria

   d. Sickle cell disease

CRITICAL THINKING EXERCISES

1. Linda Scott, an African-American mother who delivered her first baby and is on the mother–baby unit, calls the nursery nurse into her room and expresses concern about how her daughter looks. Ms. Scott tells the nurse that her baby's head looks like a "banana" and is mushy to the touch, and she has "white spots" all over her nose. In addition, there appear to be "big bluish bruises" all over her baby's buttocks. She wants to know what is wrong with her baby and whether these problems will go away.

   a. How should the nurse respond to Ms. Scott's questions?

   b. What additional newborn instruction might be appropriate at this time?

   c. What reassurance can be given to Ms. Scott regarding her daughter's appearance?

2. At approximately 12:30 a.m. on a Friday, a woman enters a hospital through a busy emergency room. She is wearing a white uniform and a lab coat with a stethoscope around her neck. She identifies herself as a new nurse coming back to check on something she had left on the unit on an earlier shift. She enters a postpartum client's room containing the mother's newborn, pushes the open crib down a hallway, and escapes through an exit. The security cameras aren't working. The infant isn't discovered missing until the 2 a.m. check by the nurse.

a. What impact does an infant abduction have on the family and the hospital?

b. What security measure was the weak link in the chain of security?

c. What can hospitals do to prevent infant abduction?

STUDY ACTIVITIES

1. Interview a new mother on the postpartum unit on her second day about the changes she has noticed in her newborn's appearance and behavior within the past 24 hours. Discuss your interview findings at post conference.

2. Demonstrate a newborn bath to a new mother in her room, using the principle of bathing from the cleanest to the dirtiest body part. Discuss the questions asked by the mother and her reaction to the demonstration in post conference.

3. Go to the La Leche League website (www.lalecheleague.org). Review the information it provides on breast-feeding. How helpful would it be to a new mother?

4. Debate the risks and benefits of neonatal circumcision within your nursing group at post conference. Did either side present a stronger position? What is your opinion, and why?

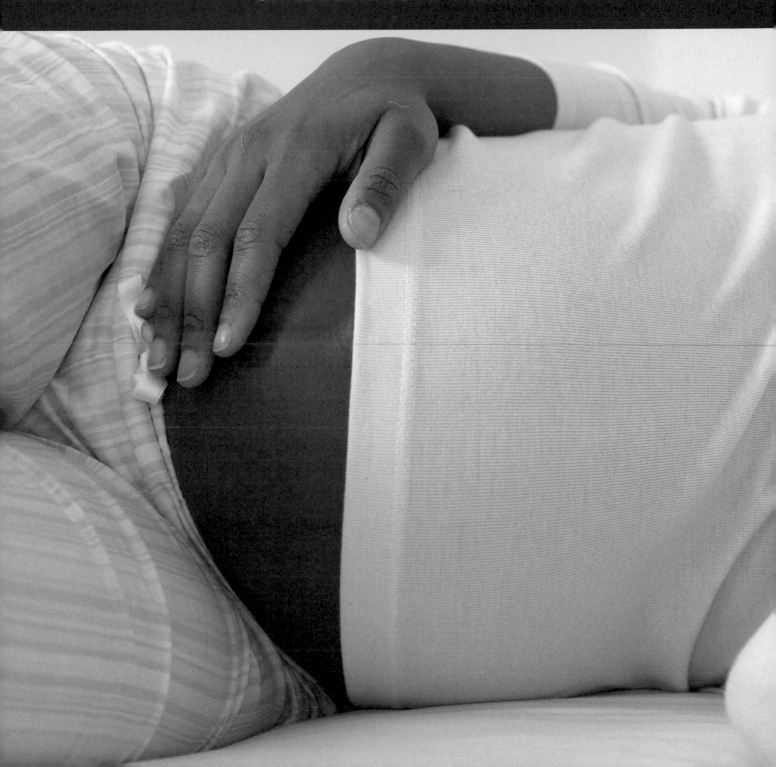

UNIT SEVEN

CHILDBEARING AT RISK

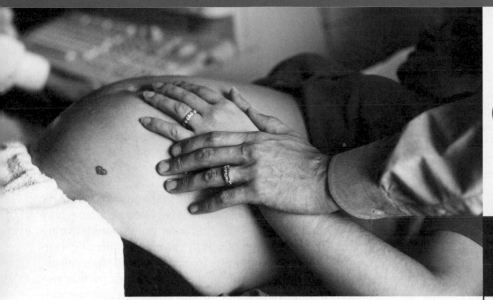

CHAPTER 19

NURSING MANAGEMENT OF PREGNANCY AT RISK: PREGNANCY-RELATED COMPLICATIONS

KEY TERMS

abortion
abruptio placentae
ectopic pregnancy
gestational hypertension
gestational trophoblastic
    disease (GTD)

high-risk pregnancy
hyperemesis gravidarum
multiple gestation
oligohydramnios
polyhydramnios
placenta previa

premature rupture of
    membranes (PROM)
preterm premature
    rupture of membranes
    (PPROM)

LEARNING OBJECTIVES

Upon completion of the chapter, the learner will be able to:

1. Define the term "high-risk pregnancy."
2. Explain common factors that might place a pregnancy at high risk.
3. Identify the causes of vaginal bleeding during early and late pregnancy.
4. Outline nursing assessment and management for the pregnant woman experiencing vaginal bleeding.
5. Develop a plan of care for the woman experiencing preeclampsia, eclampsia, and HELLP syndrome.
6. Explain the pathophysiology of polyhydramnios and subsequent management.
7. Select factors in a woman's prenatal history that place her at risk for premature rupture of membranes (PROM).
8. Formulate a teaching plan for maintaining the health of pregnant women experiencing a high-risk pregnancy.

*H*elen, a 35-year-old G5 P4, presented to the labor and birth suite with severe abdominal pain. She reports that the pain began suddenly about an hour ago while she was resting. She has had two prior cesarean births and thus far has had an uneventful past 32 weeks. Helen appears distressed and is moaning. What additional assessments do you need to care for Helen? What might be your immediate nursing action?

Wow

Detours and bumps along the road of life can be managed, but many cannot be entirely cured.

Most people view pregnancy as a natural process with a positive outcome—the birth of a healthy newborn. Unfortunately, conditions can occur that may result in negative outcomes for the fetus, mother, or both. A **high-risk pregnancy** is one in which a condition exists that jeopardizes the health of the mother, her fetus, or both. The condition may result from the pregnancy, or it may be a condition that was present before the woman became pregnant.

Approximately one in four pregnant women is considered to be at high risk or diagnosed with complications (Jung & Erogul, 2007). Women who are considered to be at high risk have a higher morbidity and mortality compared with mothers in the general population. The risk status of a woman and her fetus can change during the pregnancy, with a number of problems occurring during labor, birth, or afterward, even in women without any known previous antepartal risk. Examples of high-risk conditions include gestational diabetes and ectopic pregnancy. These conditions are specifically addressed in *Healthy People 2010*. Early identification of the woman at risk is essential to ensure that appropriate interventions are instituted promptly, increasing the opportunity to change the course of events and provide a positive outcome.

The term "risk" may mean different things to different groups. For example, health care professionals may focus on the disease processes and treatments to prevent complications. Nurses may focus on nursing care and on the psychosocial impact on the woman and her family. Insurance companies may concentrate on the economic issues related to the high-risk status. The woman's attention may be focused on her own needs and those of her family. Together, working as a collaborative team, the ultimate goal of care is to ensure the best possible outcome for the woman, her fetus, and her family.

Risk assessment begins at the first antepartal visit and continues with each subsequent visit because factors may be identified in later visits that were not apparent during earlier visits. For example, as the nurse and client develop a trusting relationship, previously unidentified or unsuspected factors (such as drug abuse or intimate partner violence) may be revealed. Through education and support, the nurse can encourage the client to inform her health care provider of these concerns, and necessary interventions or referrals can be made.

Various factors must be considered when determining a woman's risk for adverse pregnancy outcomes (Britt, Eden, & Evans, 2006), and a comprehensive approach to high-risk pregnancy is needed. For example, prenatal stress and distress have been shown to have significant consequences for the mother, child, and family (Price et al., 2007). Risks are grouped into broad categories based on threats to health and pregnancy outcome. Current categories of risk are biophysical, psychosocial, sociodemographic, and environmental (Gilbert, 2007) (Box 19.1).

This chapter describes the major conditions directly related to the pregnancy that can complicate a pregnancy, possibly affecting maternal and fetal outcomes. These include bleeding during pregnancy (spontaneous abortion, ectopic pregnancy, gestational trophoblastic disease, cervical insufficiency, placenta previa, and abruptio placentae), hyperemesis gravidarum, gestational hypertension, HELLP syndrome, gestational diabetes, blood incompatibility, amniotic fluid imbalances (hydramnios and oligohydramnios), multiple gestation, and premature rupture of membranes. Chapter 20 addresses preexisting conditions that can complicate a woman's pregnancy as well as populations that are considered to be at high risk.

Bleeding During Pregnancy

Bleeding at any time during pregnancy is potentially life-threatening. Bleeding can occur early or late in the pregnancy and may result from numerous conditions. Conditions commonly associated with early bleeding (first half of pregnancy) include spontaneous abortion, ectopic pregnancy, gestational trophoblastic disease, and conditions associated with midtrimester bleeding, such as cervical insufficiency. Conditions associated with late bleeding include placenta previa and abruptio placentae, which usually occur after the 20th week of gestation.

HEALTHY PEOPLE 2010

Objective	Significance
Decrease the proportion of pregnant women with gestational diabetes	• Will help to promote proper prepregnant and pregnancy glycemic control; foster careful perinatal obstetric monitoring, thereby helping to reduce perinatal death and congenital abnormalities • Will help to reinforce the importance of good nutrition during pregnancy as paramount in increasing better pregnancy outcomes
Reduce ectopic pregnancies	• Will help to focus attention on the need for initiating prenatal care early and for continued monitoring throughout pregnancy, thus helping to decrease maternal mortality related to ectopic pregnancies through early detection

Source: U.S. DHHS, 2000.

BOX 19.1 Factors Placing a Woman at Risk During Pregnancy

Biophysical Factors
- Genetic conditions
- Chromosomal abnormalities
- Multiple pregnancy
- Defective genes
- Inherited disorders
- ABO incompatibility
- Large fetal size
- Medical and obstetric conditions
- Preterm labor and birth
- Cardiovascular disease
- Chronic hypertension
- Incompetent cervix
- Placental abnormalities
- Infection
- Diabetes
- Maternal collagen diseases
- Pregnancy-induced hypertension
- Asthma
- Postterm pregnancy
- Hemoglobinopathies
- Nutritional status
- Inadequate dietary intake
- Food fads
- Excessive food intake
- Under- or overweight status
- Hematocrit value less than 33%
- Eating disorder

Psychosocial Factors
- Smoking
- Caffeine
- Alcohol
- Drugs
- Inadequate support system
- Situational crisis
- History of violence
- Emotional distress
- Unsafe cultural practices

Sociodemographic Factors
- Poverty status
- Lack of prenatal care
- Age younger than 15 years or older than 35 years
- Parity—all first pregnancies and more than five pregnancies
- Marital status—increased risk for unmarried
- Accessibility to health care
- Ethnicity—increased risk in nonwhite women

Environmental Factors
- Infections
- Radiation
- Pesticides
- Illicit drugs
- Industrial pollutants
- Second-hand cigarette smoke
- Personal stress (Gilbert, 2007; Blackburn, 2007)

Source: Blackburn, 2007; Gilbert, 2007.

▶ SPONTANEOUS ABORTION

An **abortion** is the loss of an early pregnancy, usually before week 20 of gestation. Abortion can be spontaneous or induced. A spontaneous abortion refers to the loss of a fetus resulting from natural causes—that is, not elective or therapeutically induced by a procedure. The term *miscarriage* is often used by nonmedical people to denote an abortion that has occurred spontaneously. A miscarriage can occur during early pregnancy, and many women who miscarry may not even be aware that they are pregnant. About 80% of spontaneous abortions occur within the first trimester.

The overall rate for spontaneous abortion in the United States is reported to be 15% to 20% of recognized pregnancies in the United States. However, with the development of highly sensitive assays for human chorionic gonadotropin (hCG) levels that detect pregnancies prior to the expected next menses, the incidence of pregnancy loss increases significantly—to about 60% to 70% (Puscheck & Pradhan, 2007).

Pathophysiology

The causes of spontaneous abortion are varied and often unknown. The most common cause for first-trimester abortions is fetal genetic abnormalities, usually unrelated to the mother. Those occurring during the second trimester are more likely related to maternal conditions, such as incompetent cervix, congenital or acquired anomaly of the uterine cavity, hypothyroidism, diabetes mellitus, chronic nephritis, use of crack cocaine, inherited and acquired thrombophilias, lupus, and acute infection such as rubella virus, cytomegalovirus, herpes simplex virus, bacterial vaginosis, and toxoplasmosis (Simpson, 2007).

Nursing Assessment

When a pregnant woman calls and reports vaginal bleeding, she must be seen as soon as possible by a health care professional to ascertain the etiology. Varying degrees of vaginal bleeding, low back pain, abdominal cramping, and passage of products of conception tissue may be reported.

Ask the woman about the color of the vaginal bleeding (bright red is significant) and the amount—for example, question her about the frequency with which she is changing her peripads (saturation of one peripad hourly is significant) and the passage of any clots or tissue. Instruct her to save any tissue or clots passed and bring them with her to the health care facility. Also, obtain a description of any other signs and symptoms the woman may be experiencing, along with a description of their severity and duration. It is important to remain calm and listen to the woman's description.

When the woman arrives at the health care facility, assess her vital signs and observe the amount, color, and characteristics of the bleeding. Ask her to rate her current pain level, using an appropriate pain assessment tool. Also, evaluate the amount and intensity of the woman's abdominal cramping or contractions, and assess the woman's level of understanding about what is happening to her. A thorough assessment helps in determining the type of spontaneous abortion, such as threatened abortion, inevitable abortion, incomplete abortion, complete abortion, missed abortion, and habitual abortion, that the woman may be experiencing (Table 19.1).

Nursing Management

Nursing management of the woman with a spontaneous abortion focuses on providing continued monitoring and psychological support, for the family is experiencing acute loss and grief. An important component of this support is reassuring the woman that spontaneous abortions usually result from an abnormality and that her actions did not cause the abortion.

Providing Continued Monitoring

Continued monitoring and ongoing assessments are essential for the woman experiencing a spontaneous abortion. Monitor the amount of vaginal bleeding through pad counts and observe for passage of products of conception tissue. Assess the woman's pain and provide appropriate pain management to address the cramping discomfort.

Assist in preparing the woman for procedures and treatments such as surgery to evacuate the uterus or medications such as misoprostol or PGE2. If the woman is Rh negative and not sensitized, expect to administer RhoGAM within 72 hours after the abortion is complete. Drug Guide 19.1 gives more information about these medications.

Providing Support

A woman's emotional reaction may vary depending on her desire for this pregnancy and her available support network. Provide both physical and emotional support. In addition, prepare the woman and her family for the assessment process, and answer their questions about what is happening.

Explaining some of the causes of spontaneous abortions can help the woman to understand what is happening and may allay her fears and guilt that she did something to cause this pregnancy loss. Most women experience an acute sense of loss and go through a grieving process with a spontaneous abortion. Providing sensitive listening, counseling, and anticipatory guidance to the woman and her family will allow them to verbalize their feelings and ask questions about future pregnancies.

The grieving period may last as long as 2 years after a pregnancy loss, with each person grieving in his or her own way. Encourage friends and family to be supportive but give the couple space and time to work through their loss. Referral to a community support group for parents who have experienced a miscarriage can be very helpful during this grief process.

► ECTOPIC PREGNANCY

An **ectopic pregnancy** is any pregnancy in which the fertilized ovum implants outside the uterine cavity. Ectopic pregnancies occur in from 1 in every 40 to 1 in every 100 pregnancies in the United States (March of Dimes, 2007). Their incidence has increased dramatically in the past few decades as a result of improved diagnostic techniques, such as more sensitive beta-hCG assays and the availability of transvaginal ultrasound (Silver, 2007).

With an ectopic pregnancy, rupture and hemorrhage may occur due to the growth of the embryo. A ruptured ectopic pregnancy is a medical emergency. It is a potentially life-threatening condition and involves pregnancy loss. It is the leading cause of maternal mortality in the first trimester and accounts for 10% to 15% of all pregnancy-related deaths (Lipscomb, 2007).

Pathophysiology

Normally, the fertilized ovum implants in the uterus. With an ectopic pregnancy, the ovum implants outside the uterus. The most common site for implantation is the fallopian tubes, but some ova may implant in the cornua of the uterus, the ovary, the cervix, or the abdominal cavity (Fig. 19.1) (Sepilian & Wood, 2007). None of these anatomic sites can accommodate placental attachment or a growing embryo.

Ectopic pregnancies usually result from conditions that obstruct or slow the passage of the fertilized ovum through the fallopian tube to the uterus. This may be a physical blockage in the tube, or failure of the tubal epithelium to move the zygote (the cell formed after the egg is fertilized) down the tube into the uterus. In the general population, most cases are the result of tubal scarring secondary to pelvic inflammatory disease. Organisms such

TABLE 19.1   **CATEGORIES OF ABORTION**

Category	Assessment Findings	Diagnosis	Therapeutic Management
Threatened abortion	Vaginal bleeding (often slight) early in a pregnancy No cervical dilation or change in cervical consistency Mild abdominal cramping Closed cervical os No passage of fetal tissue	Vaginal ultrasound to confirm if sac is empty Declining maternal serum hCG and progesterone levels to provide additional information about viability of pregnancy	Conservative supportive treatment Possible reduction in activity in conjunction with nutritious diet and adequate hydration
Inevitable abortion	Vaginal bleeding (greater than that associated with threatened abortion) Rupture of membranes Cervical dilation Strong abdominal cramping Possible passage of products of conception	Ultrasound and hCG levels to indicate pregnancy loss	Vacuum curettage if products of conception are not passed, to reduce risk of excessive bleeding and infection Prostaglandin analogs such as misoprostol to empty uterus of retained tissue (only used if fragments are not completely passed)
Incomplete abortion (passage of some of the products of conception)	Intense abdominal cramping Heavy vaginal bleeding Cervical dilation	Ultrasound confirmation that products of conception still in uterus	Client stabilization Evacuation of uterus via dilation and curettage (D&C) or prostaglandin analog
Complete abortion (passage of all products of conception)	History of vaginal bleeding and abdominal pain Passage of tissue with subsequent decrease in pain and significant decrease in vaginal bleeding	Ultrasound demonstrating an empty uterus	No medical or surgical intervention necessary Follow-up appointment to discuss family planning
Missed abortion (nonviable embryo retained in utero for at least 6 weeks)	Absent uterine contractions Irregular spotting Possible progression to inevitable abortion	Ultrasound to identify products of conception in uterus	Evacuation of uterus (if inevitable abortion does not occur): suction curettage during first trimester, dilation and evacuation during second trimester Induction of labor with intravaginal PGE2 suppository to empty uterus without surgical intervention
Habitual abortion	History of three or more consecutive spontaneous abortions Not carrying the pregnancy to viability or term	Validation via client's history	Identification and treatment of underlying cause (possible causes such as genetic or chromosomal abnormalities, reproductive tract abnormalities, chronic diseases or immunologic problems) Cervical cerclage in second trimester if incompetent cervix is the cause

DRUG GUIDE 19.1 MEDICATIONS USED WITH SPONTANEOUS ABORTIONS

Medication	Action/Indications	Nursing Implications
Misoprostol (Cytotec)	Stimulates uterine contractions to terminate a pregnancy; to evacuate the uterus after abortion to ensure passage of all the products of conception	• Monitor for side effects such as diarrhea, abdominal pain, nausea, vomiting, dyspepsia. • Assess vaginal bleeding and report any increased bleeding, pain, or fever. • Monitor for signs and symptoms of shock, such as tachycardia, hypotension, and anxiety.
Mifepristone (RU-486)	Acts as progesterone antagonist, allowing prostaglandins to stimulate uterine contractions; causes the endometrium to slough; may be followed by administration of misoprostol within 48 hours	• Monitor for headache, vomiting, diarrhea, and heavy bleeding. • Anticipate administration of antiemetic prior to use to reduce nausea and vomiting. • Encourage client to use acetaminophen to reduce discomfort from cramping.
PGE2, dinoprostone (Cervidil, Prepidil Gel, Prostin E2)	Stimulates uterine contractions, causing expulsion of uterine contents; to expel uterine contents in fetal death or missed abortion during second trimester, or to efface and dilate the cervix in pregnancy at term	• Bring gel to room temperature before administering. • Avoid contact with skin. • Use sterile technique to administer. • Keep client supine 30 minutes after administering. • Document time of insertion and dosing intervals. • Remove insert with retrieval system after 12 hours or at the onset of labor. • Explain purpose and expected response to client.
Rh(D) immunoglobulin (Gamulin, HydroRho-D, RhoGAM)	Suppresses immune response of nonsensitized Rh-negative patients who are exposed to Rh-positive blood; to prevent isoimmunization in Rh-negative women exposed to Rh-positive blood after abortions, miscarriages, and pregnancies	• Administer intramuscularly in deltoid area. • Give only MICRhoGAM for abortions and miscarriages <12 weeks unless fetus or father is Rh negative (unless patient is Rh positive, Rh antibodies are present). • Educate woman that she will need this after subsequent deliveries if newborns are Rh positive; also check lab study results prior to administering the drug.

as *Neisseria gonorrhoeae* and *Chlamydia trachomatis* preferentially attack the fallopian tubes, producing silent infections. A recent study reported a twofold increased risk for ectopic pregnancy in women with a history of a chlamydia infection (Bakken, Skjeldestad, & Nordbo, 2007). Even with early treatment, tubal damage can occur.

Therapeutic Management

The therapeutic management of ectopic pregnancy depends on whether the tube is intact or has ruptured. Historically, the treatment of ectopic pregnancy was limited to surgery, but medical therapy is currently available.

If the fallopian tube is still intact, medical management becomes an option. To be eligible for medical therapy, the client must be hemodynamically stable, with no signs of active bleeding in the peritoneal cavity, and the mass (which must measure less than 4 cm as determined by ultrasound) must be unruptured (Lipscomb, 2007). The potential advantages include avoidance of surgery, the preservation of tubal patency and function, and a lower cost. Methotrexate, prostaglandins, misoprostol, and actinomycin have all been used in the medical (nonsurgical) management of ectopic pregnancy, with a reported success rate of approximately 90% (Lipscomb, 2007).

Methotrexate, the agent most commonly used, is a folic acid antagonist that inhibits cell division in the developing embryo. It typically has been used as a chemotherapeutic agent in the treatment of leukemias, lymphomas, and carcinomas. It has been shown to produce results similar to that for surgical therapy in terms of high success rate, low complication rate, and good reproductive potential (Vitthala, Cheema, & Misra, 2007). Adverse effects associated with methotrexate include nausea, vomiting, stomatitis, diarrhea, gastric upset, increased abdominal pain, and dizziness. Prior to receiving the single-dose intramuscular injection to treat unruptured pregnancies, the woman needs to be counseled on the risks, benefits, adverse effects, and the possibility of failure of medical therapy, which would result in tubal rupture, necessitating surgery (Selway, 2006). The woman

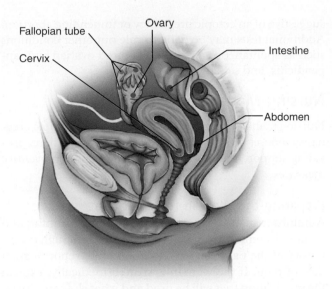

FIGURE 19.1 Possible sites for implantation with an ectopic pregnancy.

is then instructed to return weekly for follow-up laboratory studies for the next several weeks until beta-hCG titers decrease.

Surgical management for the unruptured fallopian tube might involve a linear salpingostomy to preserve the tube—an important consideration for the woman wanting to preserve her future fertility.

With a ruptured ectopic pregnancy, surgery is necessary as a result of possible uncontrolled hemorrhage. A laparotomy with a removal of the tube (salpingectomy) may be necessary. With earlier diagnosis and medical management, the focus has changed from preventing maternal death to facilitating rapid recovery and preserving fertility.

Regardless of the treatment approach (medical or surgical), the woman's beta-hCG level is monitored until it is undetectable to ensure that any residual trophoblastic tissue that forms the placenta is gone. Also, all Rh-negative unsensitized clients are given Rh immunoglobulin to prevent isoimmunization in future pregnancies.

Nursing Assessment

Nursing assessment focuses on determining the existence of an ectopic pregnancy and whether or not it has ruptured.

Health History and Physical Examination

Assess the client thoroughly for signs and symptoms that may suggest an ectopic pregnancy. The onset of signs and symptoms varies, but they usually begin at about the seventh or eighth week of gestation. A missed menstrual period, adnexal fullness, and tenderness may indicate an unruptured tubal pregnancy. As the tube stretches, the pain

---

EVIDENCE-BASED PRACTICE 19.1
Ectopic Pregnancy: Selecting the Best Intervention

● **Study**

The incidence of ectopic pregnancy, which involves implantation of the fertilized ovum outside the uterine cavity, has increased over the past several decades due to advances in diagnostic methods. The most common site for implantation is in the fallopian tube (thus the name tubal pregnancy). If left untreated, tubal rupture and hemorrhage can occur. At one time, surgery was the only available treatment option. However, treatment today may involve expectant care, medication therapy, or surgery (laparoscopic or open approach). Questions have arisen as to the effectiveness and safety of these treatments.

A study was conducted to evaluate the effectiveness of major types of treatment for ectopic pregnancy. Data were collected from 35 randomized controlled trials that compared the treatments for ectopic pregnancies.

▲ **Findings**

The open approach to surgery was significantly more effective in removing the ectopic pregnancy than the laparoscopic approach, but the laparoscopic approach was more cost-effective. Medication therapy involving fixed multiple doses of methotrexate was effective in women who had low pregnancy hormone levels without any evidence of bleeding. Expectant management was less successful than drug therapy, but the information on this treatment option was inadequate.

■ **Nursing Implications**

This study identified three important treatment options available to a woman with an ectopic pregnancy. Nurses can use this information in their practice as a basis for formulating a teaching plan about treatment options. Nurses can use the information from this study when reviewing the health care provider's recommendations for treatment. As a result, women can make a more informed decision. Nurses also can advocate for medication therapy for women who have low pregnancy hormone levels and no bleeding.

Hajenius, P. J., Mol, F., Mol, B. W. J., Bossuyt, P. M. M., Ankum, W. M., & van der Veen, F. (2007). Interventions for tubal ectopic pregnancy. *Cochrane Database of Systematic Reviews* 2007. Issue 1. Art. No.: CD000324.DOI: 10.1002/14651858.CD000324.pub2.

increases. Pain may be unilateral, bilateral, or diffuse over the abdomen.

> ▶ *Take* NOTE!
>
> *The hallmark of ectopic pregnancy is abdominal pain with spotting within 6 to 8 weeks after a missed menstrual period. Although this is the classic triad, all three of these signs and symptoms occur in only about 50% of cases. Many women have symptoms typical of early pregnancy, such as breast tenderness, nausea, fatigue, shoulder pain, and low back pain.*

In addition, review the client's history for possible contributing factors. These may include:

• Previous ectopic pregnancy
• History of sexually transmitted infections (STIs)
• Fallopian tube scarring from pelvic inflammatory disease
• In utero exposure to diethylstilbestrol
• Endometriosis
• Previous tubal or pelvic surgery
• Infertility and infertility treatments, including use of fertility drugs
• Uterine abnormalities such as fibroids
• Presence of intrauterine contraception
• Use of progestin-only mini-pill (slows ovum transport)
• Postpartum or post-abortion infection
• Increasing age (older than 35 years)
• Cigarette smoking (Brown-Guttovz, 2006)

If rupture or hemorrhage occurs before treatment begins, symptoms may worsen and include severe, sharp, and sudden pain in the lower abdomen as the tube tears open and the embryo is expelled into the pelvic cavity; feelings of faintness; referred pain to the shoulder area, indicating bleeding into the abdomen, caused by phrenic nerve irritation; hypotension; marked abdominal tenderness with distention; and hypovolemic shock.

Laboratory and Diagnostic Testing

The use of transvaginal ultrasound to visualize the misplaced pregnancy and low levels of serum beta-hCG assist in diagnosing an ectopic pregnancy. The ultrasound determines whether the pregnancy is intrauterine, assesses the size of the uterus, and provides evidence of fetal viability. The visualization of an adnexal mass and the absence of an intrauterine gestational sac are diagnostic of ectopic pregnancy (Condous, 2006). In a normal intrauterine pregnancy, beta-hCG levels typically double every 2 to 4 days until peak values are reached 60 to 90 days after conception. Concentrations of hCG decrease after 10 to 11 weeks and reach a plateau at low levels by 100 to 130 days (Blackburn, 2007). Therefore, low beta-hCG levels are suggestive of an ectopic pregnancy or impending abortion. Additional tests may be done to rule out other conditions such as spontaneous abortion, ruptured ovarian cyst, appendicitis, and salpingitis.

Nursing Management

Nursing management for the woman with an ectopic pregnancy focuses on preparing the woman for treatment, providing support, and providing education about preventive measures.

Preparing the Woman for Treatment

Administer analgesics as ordered to promote comfort and relieve discomfort from abdominal pain. Although the intensity of the pain can vary, women often report a great deal of pain. If the woman is treated medically, explain the medication that will be used and what she can expect. Also review signs and symptoms of possible adverse effects. If treatment will occur on an outpatient basis, outline the signs and symptoms of ectopic rupture (severe, sharp, stabbing, unilateral abdominal pain; vertigo/fainting; hypotension; and increased pulse) and advise the woman to seek medical help immediately if they occur.

If surgery is needed, close assessment and monitoring of the client's vital signs, bleeding (peritoneal or vaginal), and pain status are critical to identify hypovolemic shock, which may occur with tubal rupture. Prepare the client physiologically and psychologically for surgery or any procedure. Provide a clear explanation of the expected outcome. Astute vigilance and early referral will help reduce short- and long-term morbidity.

Providing Emotional Support

The woman with an ectopic pregnancy requires support throughout diagnosis, treatment, and aftercare. A woman's psychological reaction to an ectopic pregnancy is unpredictable. However, it is important to recognize she has experienced a pregnancy loss in addition to undergoing treatment for a potentially life-threatening condition. The woman may find it difficult to comprehend what has happened to her because events occur so quickly. In the woman's mind, she had just started a pregnancy and now it has ended abruptly. Help her to make this experience "more real" by encouraging her and her family to express their feelings and concerns openly, and validating that this is a loss of pregnancy and it is okay to grieve over the loss.

Provide emotional support, spiritual care, client education, and information about community support groups available (such as Resolve through Sharing) as the client grieves for the loss of her unborn child and comes to terms with the medical complications of the situation. Acknowledge the client's pregnancy and allow her to discuss her feelings about what the pregnancy means. Also, stress the need for follow-up blood testing for several weeks to monitor hCG titers until they return to zero, indicating resolution of the ectopic pregnancy. Ask about her feelings and concerns about her future fertility, and provide teaching about the need to use contraceptives for at least three menstrual cycles to allow her reproductive tract to heal and the tissue to be repaired. Include the woman's partner in this discussion to make sure both parties understand what has happened, what intervention is needed, and what the future holds regarding childbearing.

Educating the Client

Preventing ectopic pregnancies through screening and client education is essential. Many can be prevented by avoiding conditions that might cause scarring of the fallopian tubes. In addition, a contributing factor to the development of ectopic pregnancy is a previous ectopic pregnancy. Therefore, educating the woman is crucial.

Prevention education may include the following:

- Reduce risk factors such as sexual intercourse with multiple partners or intercourse without a condom.
- Avoid contracting STIs that lead to pelvic inflammatory disease (PID).
- Obtain early diagnosis and adequate treatment of STIs.
- Avoid the use of intrauterine contraceptive methods to reduce the risk of repeat ascending infections, which can be responsible for tubal scarring.
- Use condoms to decrease the risk of infections that cause tubal scarring.
- Seek prenatal care early to confirm the location of pregnancy.

▶ GESTATIONAL TROPHOBLASTIC DISEASE (GTD)

Gestational trophoblastic disease (GTD) comprises a spectrum of neoplastic disorders that originate in the placenta. Gestational tissue is present, but the pregnancy is not viable. The incidence is about 1 in 1,000 pregnancies in the United States; in Asian countries, the rate is as much as 15 times higher (Moore & Ware, 2007). The two most common types of GTD are hydatidiform mole (partial and complete) and choriocarcinoma.

Pathophysiology

Hydatidiform mole is a benign neoplasm of the chorion in which the chorionic villi degenerate and become transparent vesicles containing clear, viscid fluid. Hydatiform mole is classified as complete or partial, distinguished by differences in clinical presentation, pathology, genetics, and epidemiology (Garner et al., 2007). The complete mole contains no fetal tissue and develops from an "empty egg," which is fertilized by a normal sperm (the paternal chromosomes replicate, resulting in 46 all-paternal chromosomes). The embryo is not viable and dies. No circu-

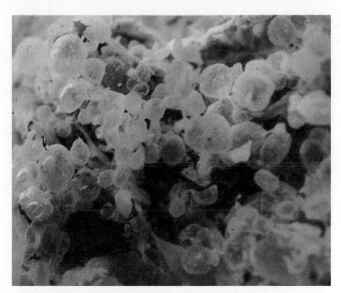

FIGURE 19.2 Complete hydatiform mole. The chorionic villi degenerate and become filled with a viscid fluid, forming transparent vesicles.

lation is established, and no embryonic tissue is found. The complete mole is associated with the development of choriocarcinoma. The partial mole has a triploid karyotype (69 chromosomes), because two sperm have provided a double contribution by fertilizing the ovum (Fig. 19.2).

▶ Consider THIS!

We had lived across the dorm hall from each other during nursing school but really didn't get to know each other except for a casual hello in passing. When we graduated, Rose went to work in the emergency room and I in OB. We saw each other occasionally in the employee cafeteria, but a quick hello was all that we usually exchanged. I heard she married one of the paramedics who worked in the ER and was soon pregnant. I finally got to say more than hello when she was admitted to the OB unit bleeding during her fourth month of pregnancy. What was discovered was gestational trophoblastic disease and not a normal pregnancy. I remember holding her in my arms as she wept. She was told she had a complete molar pregnancy after surgery, and she would need extensive follow-up for the next year. I lost track of her that summer as my life became busier. Around Thanksgiving time, I heard she had died from choriocarcinoma. I attended her funeral, finally, to get the time to say a final hello and good-bye, but this time with sadness and tears.

Thoughts: Rose was only 26 years old when she succumbed to this very virulent cancer. I think back

(continued)

▶ *Consider* THIS! *(continued)*

and realize I missed knowing this brave young woman and wished that I had taken the time to say more than hello. Could her outcome have been different? Why wasn't it recognized earlier? Did she not follow up after her diagnosis? I can only speculate regarding the whom, what, and where. She lived a short but purposeful life, and hopefully continued research will change other women's outcomes in the future.

The exact cause of molar pregnancy is unknown, but researchers are looking into a genetic basis. Studies have revealed some remarkable features about molar pregnancies, including:

- Ability to invade into the wall of the uterus
- Tendency to recur in subsequent pregnancies
- Possible development into choriocarcinoma, a virulent cancer with metastasis to other organs
- Influence of nutritional factors, such as protein deficiency
- Tendency to affect older women more often than younger women

Having a molar pregnancy (partial or complete) results in the loss of the pregnancy and the possibility of developing choriocarcinoma, a chorionic malignancy from the trophoblastic tissue. The most frequent sites of metastases are the lungs, lower genital tract, brain, liver, kidney and gastrointestinal tract (Hernandez, 2007).

Therapeutic Management

Treatment consists of immediate evacuation of the uterine contents as soon as the diagnosis is made and long-term follow-up of the client to detect any remaining trophoblastic tissue that might become malignant. Dilation and suction curettage (D&C) are used to empty the uterus. The tissue obtained is sent to the laboratory for analysis to evaluate for choriocarcinoma. Serial levels of hCG are used to detect residual trophoblastic tissue for 1 year. If any tissue remains, hCG levels will not regress. In 80% of women with a benign hydatidiform mole, serum hCG titers steadily drop to normal within 8 to 12 weeks after evacuation of the molar pregnancy. In the other 20% of women with a malignant hydatidiform mole, serum hCG levels begin to rise (Hernandez, 2007).

Due to the increased risk for cancer, the client is advised to receive extensive follow-up therapy for the next 12 months. The follow-up protocol may include:

- Baseline hCG level, chest radiograph, and pelvic ultrasound
- Weekly serum hCG level until it drops to zero and remains at that level for 3 consecutive weeks, then monthly for 6 months, then every 2 months for the remainder of the year
- Chest radiograph every 6 months to detect pulmonary metastasis
- Regular pelvic examinations to assess uterine and ovarian regression
- Systemic assessments for symptoms indicative of lung, brain, liver, or vaginal metastasis
- Strong recommendation to avoid pregnancy for 1 year because the pregnancy can interfere with the monitoring of hCG levels
- Use of a reliable contraceptive for at least 1 year (Gilbert, 2007)

Nursing Assessment

The nurse plays a crucial role in identifying and bringing this condition to the attention of the health care provider based on sound knowledge of the typical clinical manifestations and through astute antepartal assessments.

Clinical manifestations of GTD are very similar to those of spontaneous abortion at about 12 weeks of pregnancy. Assess the woman for potential clinical manifestations at each antepartal visit. Be alert for the following:

- Report of early signs of pregnancy, such as amenorrhea, breast tenderness, fatigue
- Brownish vaginal bleeding/spotting
- Anemia
- Severe morning sickness (due to high hCG levels)
- Fluid retention and swelling
- Uterine size larger than expected for pregnancy dates
- Extremely high hCG levels present; no single value considered diagnostic
- Early development of preeclampsia (usually not present until after 24 weeks)
- Absence of fetal heart rate or fetal activity
- Expulsion of grapelike vesicles (possible in some women)

The diagnosis is made by high hCG levels and the characteristic appearance of the vesicular molar pattern in the uterus via transvaginal ultrasound.

Nursing Management

Nursing management of the woman with GTD focuses on preparing her for a D&C, providing emotional support to deal with the loss and potential risks, and educating her about the risk that cancer may develop after a molar pregnancy and the strict adherence needed with the follow-up program. The woman must understand the need for the continued follow-up care regimen to improve her chances of future pregnancies and to ensure her continued quality of life.

Preparing the Client

Upon diagnosis, the client will need an immediate evacuation of the uterus. Perform preoperative care, preparing the client physically and psychologically for the procedure.

Providing Emotional Support

To aid the client and her family in coping with the loss of the pregnancy and the possibility of a cancer diagnosis, use the following interventions:

• Listen to their concerns and fears.
• Allow them time to grieve for the pregnancy loss.
• Acknowledge their loss and sad feelings (say you are sorry for their loss).
• Encourage them to express their grief; allow them to cry.
• Provide them with as much factual information as possible to help them make sense of what is happening.
• Enlist support from additional family and friends as appropriate and with the client's permission.

Educating the Client

After GTD is diagnosed, teach the client about the condition and appropriate interventions that may be necessary to save her life. Explain each phase of treatment accurately and provide support for the woman and her family as they go through the grieving process.

As with any facet of health care, be aware of the latest research and new therapies. Inform the client about her follow-up care, which will probably involve close clinical surveillance for approximately 1 year, and reinforce its importance in monitoring the client's condition. Tell the client that serial serum beta-hCG levels are used to detect residual trophoblastic tissue. Continued high or increasing hCG titers are abnormal and need further evaluation.

Inform the client about the possible use of chemotherapy, such as methotrexate, which may be started as prophylaxis. Strongly urge the client to use a reliable contraceptive to prevent pregnancy for 1 year, as a pregnancy would interfere with tracking the serial beta-hCG levels used to identify a potential malignancy. Stress the need for the client to cooperate and adhere to the plan of therapy throughout this year-long follow-up.

▶ CERVICAL INSUFFICIENCY

Cervical insufficiency, also called premature dilatation of the cervix, describes a weak, structurally defective cervix that spontaneously dilates in the absence of contractions in the second trimester, resulting in the loss of the pregnancy. The incidence of cervical insufficiency is less than 1%; estimates range from 1 in 500 to 1 in 2,000 pregnancies, accounting for approximately 20% to 25% of midtrimester losses (Fox & Chervenak, 2008).

Pathophysiology

The exact mechanism contributing to cervical insufficiency is not known. The incompetent cervix may have less elastin, less collagen, and greater amounts of smooth muscle than the normal cervix (Evans, 2007). Several theories have been proposed that focus on damage to the cervix as a key component.

Cervical insufficiency is likely to be the clinical endpoint of many pathologic processes, such as congenital cervical hypoplasia, in utero diethylstilbestrol (DES) exposure that caused cervical hypoplasia, trauma to the cervix (conization, amputation, obstetric laceration, or forced cervical dilatation [may occur during elective pregnancy termination]). Other conditions such as previous precipitous birth, a prolonged second stage of labor, or increased uterine volume (multiple gestation, hydramnios) are associated with cervical insufficiency (Vyas et al., 2006). However, the exact etiology of cervical insufficiency is not known.

Cervical length also has been associated with cervical insufficiency and subsequently preterm birth. Recent studies have examined the association between a short cervical length and the risk of preterm birth. Some have demonstrated a continuum of risk between a shorter cervix on ultrasound and a higher risk of preterm birth, leading to the hypothetical argument that women with a short cervix on ultrasound might benefit from cervical cerclage, but there have been conflicting results (Lotgering, 2007; Vidaeff & Ramin, 2007).

Therapeutic Management

Cervical insufficiency may be treated in a variety of ways: bed rest; pelvic rest; avoidance of heavy lifting; or surgically, via a procedure of a cervical cerclage in the second trimester. Cervical cerclage involves using a heavy pursestring suture to secure and reinforce the internal os of the cervix (Fig. 19.3).

According to the American College of Obstetricians & Gynecologists (ACOG) (2003), if a short cervix is identified at or after 20 weeks and no infection (chorioamnionitis) is present, the decision to proceed with cerclage should be made with caution. There have been limited numbers of well-designed randomized studies to support its efficacy. Suture displacement, rupture of membranes, and chorioamnionitis are the most common complications associated with cerclage placement, and their incidence varies widely in relation to the timing and indications for

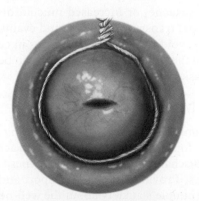

FIGURE **19.3** Cervical cerclage.

the cerclage (Ressel, 2004). The optimal timing for cerclage removal is unclear, according to ACOG (2003).

Nursing Assessment

Nursing assessment focuses on obtaining a thorough history to determine any risk factors that might have a bearing on this pregnancy—previous cervical trauma, preterm labor, fetal loss in the second trimester, or previous surgeries or procedures involving the cervix. History may reveal a previous loss of pregnancy around 20 weeks.

Also be alert for complaints of vaginal discharge or pelvic pressure. Commonly with cervical insufficiency the woman will report a pink-tinged vaginal discharge or an increase in pelvic pressure. Cervical dilation also occurs. If this continues, rupture of the membranes, release of amniotic fluid, and uterine contractions occur, subsequently resulting in delivery of the fetus, often before it is viable.

> ▶ *Take* NOTE!
>
> The diagnosis of cervical insufficiency remains difficult in many circumstances. The cornerstone of diagnosis is a history of midtrimester pregnancy loss associated with painless cervical dilatation without evidence of uterine activity.

Transvaginal ultrasound typically is done around 20 weeks' gestation to determine cervical length and evaluate for shortening. Cervical shortening occurs from the internal os outward and can be viewed on ultrasound as funneling. The amount of funneling can be determined by dividing funnel length by cervical length. The most common time at which a short cervix or funneling develops is 18 to 22 weeks, so ultrasound screening should be performed during this interval (Fox & Chervenak, 2008). A cervical length less than 25 mm is abnormal between 14 weeks and 24 weeks and may increase the risk of preterm labor.

Expect the woman (particularly a woman with pelvic pressure, backache, or increased mucoid discharge) to undergo serial transvaginal ultrasound evaluations every few days to avoid missing rapid changes in cervical dilation or until the trend in cervical length can be characterized (Bernasko et al., 2006).

Nursing Management

Nursing management focuses on monitoring the woman very closely for signs of preterm labor: backache, increase in vaginal discharge, rupture of membranes, and uterine contractions. Provide emotional support and education to allay the couple's anxiety about the well-being of their fetus. Provide preoperative care and teaching as indicated

if the woman will be undergoing cerclage. Teach the client and her family about the signs and symptoms of preterm labor and the need to report any changes immediately. Also reinforce the need for activity restrictions (if appropriate) and continued regular follow-up. Continuing surveillance throughout the pregnancy is important to promote a positive outcome for the family.

▶ PLACENTA PREVIA

Placenta previa is a bleeding condition that occurs during the last two trimesters of pregnancy. In placenta previa (literally, "afterbirth first"), the placenta implants over the cervical os. It may cause serious morbidity and mortality to the fetus and mother. It complicates approximately 5 of 1,000 births or 1 in every 200 pregnancies and is associated with potentially serious consequences from hemorrhage, abruption (separation) of the placenta, or emergency cesarean birth (Joy & Lyon, 2007).

Pathophysiology

The exact cause of placenta previa is unknown. It is initiated by implantation of the embryo in the lower uterus. With placental attachment and growth, the cervical os may become covered by the developing placenta. Placental vascularization is defective, allowing the placenta to attach directly to the myometrium (accreta), invade the myometrium (increta), or penetrate the myometrium (percreta).

Placenta previa is generally classified according to the degree of coverage or proximity to the internal os, as follows (Fig. 19.4):

• Total placenta previa: the internal cervical os is completely covered by the placenta
• Partial placenta previa: the internal os is partially covered by the placenta
• Marginal placenta previa: the placenta is at the margin or edge of the internal os
• Low-lying placenta previa: the placenta is implanted in the lower uterine segment and is near the internal os but does not reach it

Therapeutic Management

Therapeutic management depends on the extent of bleeding, the amount of placenta over the cervical os, whether the fetus is developed enough to survive outside the uterus, the position of the fetus, the mother's parity, and the presence or absence of labor (Zeltzer, 2007).

If the mother and fetus are both stable, therapeutic management may involve expectant ("wait-and-see") care. This care can be carried out at home or on an antepartal unit in the health care facility. If there is no active bleeding and the client has readily available access to reliable

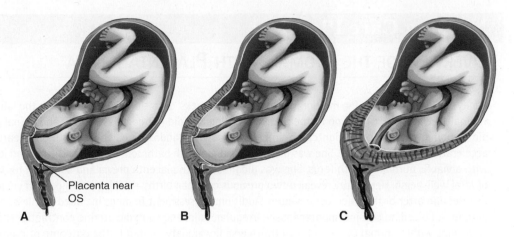

FIGURE 19.4 Classification of placenta previa. (**A**) Marginal. (**B**) Partial. (**C**) Complete.

Marginal   Partial   Complete

transportation, can maintain bed rest at home, and can comprehend instructions, expectant care at home is appropriate. However, if the client requires continuous care and monitoring and cannot meet the home care requirements, the antepartal unit is the best environment.

Nursing Assessment

Nursing assessment involves a thorough history, including possible risk factors, and physical examination. Evaluate the client closely for these risk factors:

- Advancing maternal age (more than 35 years)
- Previous cesarean birth
- Multiparity
- Uterine insult or injury
- Cocaine use
- Prior placenta previa
- Infertility treatment
- Asian ethnic background (incidence is increased in Asian cultural groups)
- Multiple gestations
- Previous induced surgical abortion
- Smoking
- Previous myomectomy to remove fibroids
- Smoking (Ko & Yoon, 2007)

Health History and Physical Examination

Ask the client if she has any problems associated with bleeding, now or in the recent past. The classical clinical presentation is painless, bright-red vaginal bleeding occurring during the second or third trimester. The initial bleeding usually is not profuse and it ceases spontaneously, only to recur again. The first episode of bleeding occurs (on average) at 27 to 32 weeks' gestation. The bleeding is thought to arise secondary to the thinning of the lower uterine segment in preparation for the onset of labor. When the bleeding occurs at the implantation site in the lower uterus, the uterus cannot contract adequately and stop the flow of blood from the open vessels. Typically with

normal placental implantation in the upper uterus, minor disruptive placental attachment is not a problem, because there is a larger volume of myometrial tissue able to contract and constrict bleeding vessels.

Assess the client for uterine contractions, which may or may not occur with the bleeding. Palpate the uterus; typically it is soft and nontender on examination. Auscultate the fetal heart rate; it commonly is within normal parameters. Fetal distress is usually absent but may occur when cord problems arise, such as umbilical cord prolapse or cord compression, or when the client has experienced blood loss to the extent that maternal shock or placental abruption has occurred (Oppenheimer, 2007).

Laboratory and Diagnostic Testing
To validate the position of the placenta, a transvaginal ultrasound is done. In addition, magnetic resonance imaging may be ordered when preparing for delivery because it allows identification of placenta accreta (placenta abnormally adherent to the myometrium), increta (placenta accreta with penetration of the myometrium), or percreta (placenta accreta with invasion of the myometrium to the peritoneal covering, causing rupture of the uterus) in addition to placenta previa. These placental abnormalities, although rare, carry a very high morbidity and mortality rate, possibly necessitating a hysterectomy at delivery.

Nursing Management

Whether the care setting is in the client's home or in the health care facility, the nurse focuses on monitoring the maternal–fetal status, including assessing for signs and symptoms of vaginal bleeding and fetal distress, and providing support and education to the client and her family, including what events and diagnostic studies are being performed. For the majority of women, a cesarean birth will be planned. Nursing Care Plan 19.1 discusses the nursing process for the woman with placenta previa.

Nursing Care Plan 19.1

OVERVIEW OF THE WOMAN WITH PLACENTA PREVIA

Sandy, a 39-year-old G5, P4, multigravida client at 32 weeks' gestation, was admitted to the labor and birth suite with sudden vaginal bleeding. Sandy had no further active bleeding and did not complain of any abdominal discomfort or tenderness. She did complain of occasional "tightening" in her stomach. Her abdomen palpated soft. Fetal heart rates were in the 140s with accelerations with movement. She was placed on bed rest with bathroom privileges. Ultrasound identified a low-lying placenta with a viable, normal-growth fetus. She was diagnosed with placenta previa and admitted for observation and surveillance of fetal well-being. Her history revealed two previous cesarean births, smoking half a pack of cigarettes per day, and endometritis infection after birth of her last newborn. Additional assessment findings included painless, bright-red vaginal bleeding with initial bleeding ceasing spontaneously; irregular, mild, and sporadic uterine contractions; fetal heart rate and maternal vital signs within normal range; fetus in transverse lie; anxiety related to the outcome of pregnancy; and expression of feelings of helplessness.

NURSING DIAGNOSIS: Ineffective tissue perfusion (fetal and maternal) related to blood loss

Outcome Identification and Evaluation
Client will maintain adequate tissue perfusion as evidenced by stable vital signs, decreased blood loss, few or no uterine contractions, normal fetal heart rate patterns and variability, and positive fetal movement

Interventions: Maintaining Adequate Tissue Perfusion
- Establish IV access *to allow for administration of fluids, blood, and medications as necessary.*
- Obtain type and cross-match for at least 2 U blood products *to ensure availability should bleeding continue.*
- Obtain specimens as ordered for blood studies, such as CBC and clotting studies *to establish a baseline and use for future comparison.*
- Monitor output *to evaluate adequacy of renal perfusion.*
- Administer IV fluid replacement therapy as ordered *to maintain blood pressure and blood volume.*
- Palpate for abdominal tenderness and rigidity *to determine bleeding and evidence of uterine contractions.*
- Institute bed rest *to reduce oxygen demands.*
- Assess for rupture of membranes *to evaluate for possible onset of labor.*
- Avoid vaginal examinations *to prevent further bleeding episodes.*
- Complete an Rh titer *to identify need for RhoGAM.*
- Avoid nipple stimulation *to prevent uterine contractions.*
- Continuously monitor for contractions or PROM *to allow for prompt intervention.*
- Administer tocolytic agents as ordered *to stall preterm labor.*
- Monitor vital signs frequently *to identify possible hypovolemia and infection.*
- Assess frequently for active vaginal bleeding *to minimize risk of hemorrhage.*
- Continuously monitor fetal heart rate with electronic fetal monitor *to evaluate fetal status.*
- Assist with fetal surveillance tests as ordered *to aid in determining fetal well-being.*
- Observe for abnormal fetal heart rate patterns, such as loss of variability, decelerations, tachycardia, *to identify fetal distress.*
- Position patient in side-lying position with wedge for support *to maximize placental perfusion.*
- Assess fetal movement *to evaluate for possible fetal hypoxia.*
- Teach woman to monitor fetal movement *to evaluate well-being.*
- Administer oxygen as ordered *to increase oxygenation to mother and fetus.*

Nursing Care Plan 19.1 (continued)

NURSING DIAGNOSIS: Anxiety related to threats to self and fetus

Outcome Identification and Evaluation
Client will experience a decrease in anxiety as evidenced by verbal reports of less anxiety, use of effective coping measures, and calm demeanor

Interventions: Minimizing Anxiety
- Provide factual information about diagnosis and treatment, and explain interventions and the rationale behind them *to provide client with understanding of her condition.*
- Answer questions about health status honestly *to establish a trusting relationship.*
- Speak calmly to patient and family members *to minimize environmental stress.*
- Encourage the use of past effective techniques for coping *to promote relaxation and feelings of control.*
- Acknowledge and facilitate the woman's spiritual needs *to promote effective coping.*
- Involve the woman and family in the decision-making process *to foster self-confidence and control over situation.*
- Maintain a presence during stressful periods *to allay anxiety.*
- Use the sense of touch if appropriate *to convey caring and concern.*
- Encourage talking as a means *to release tension.*

Monitoring Maternal–Fetal Status
Assess the degree of vaginal bleeding; inspect the perineal area for blood that may be pooled underneath the woman. Estimate and document the amount of bleeding. Perform a peripad count on an ongoing basis, making sure to report any changes in amount or frequency to the health care provider. If the woman is experiencing active bleeding, prepare for blood typing and cross-matching in the event a blood transfusion is needed.

> ▶ **Take** NOTE!
>
> *Avoid doing vaginal examinations in the woman with placenta previa. They may disrupt the placenta and cause hemorrhage.*

Monitor maternal vital signs and uterine contractility frequently for changes. Have the client rate her level of pain using an appropriate pain rating scale.

Assess fetal heart rates via Doppler or electronic monitoring to detect fetal distress. Monitor the woman's cardiopulmonary status, reporting any difficulties in respirations, changes in skin color, or complaints of difficulty breathing. Have oxygen equipment readily available should fetal or maternal distress develop. Encourage the client to lie on her side to enhance placental perfusion.

If the woman has an intravenous (IV) line inserted, inspect the IV site frequently. Alternately, anticipate the insertion of an intermittent IV access device such as a saline lock, which can be used if quick access is needed for fluid restoration and infusion of blood products. Obtain laboratory tests as ordered, including complete blood count (CBC), coagulation studies, and Rh status if appropriate.

Administer pharmacologic agents as necessary. Give Rh immunoglobulin if the client is Rh negative at 28 weeks' gestation. Monitor tocolytic medication if prevention of preterm labor is needed.

Providing Support and Education
Determine the woman's level of understanding about placenta previa and the associated procedures and treatment plan. Doing so is important to prevent confusion and gain her cooperation. Provide information about the condition and make sure that all information related is consistent with information from the primary care provider. Explain all assessments and treatment measures as needed. Act as a client advocate in obtaining information for the family.

Teach the woman how to perform and record daily fetal movement. This action serves two purposes. One, it provides valuable information about the fetus. Two, it is an activity that the client can participate in, thereby fostering some feeling of control over the situation.

If the woman will require prolonged hospitalization or home bed rest, assess the physical and emotional impact that this may have on her. Evaluate her coping mechanisms to help determine how well she will be able to adjust to and cooperate with the treatment plan. Allow the client to verbalize her feelings and fears and provide emotional support. Also, provide opportunities for distraction—educational videos, arts and crafts, computer games, reading books— and evaluate the client's response.

In addition to the emotional impact of prolonged bed rest, thoroughly assess the woman's skin to prevent skin breakdown and to help alleviate her discomfort secondary to limited physical activity. Instruct the woman in appropriate skin care measures. Encourage her to eat a balanced diet with adequate fluid intake to ensure adequate nutrition and hydration and prevent complications associated with urinary and bowel elimination secondary to bed rest.

Teach the client and family about any signs and symptoms that should be reported immediately. In addition, prepare the woman for the possibility of a cesarean birth. The woman must notify her health care provider about any bleeding episodes or backaches (may indicate preterm labor contractions) and must adhere to the prescribed bed rest regimen. To ensure compliance and a positive outcome, she needs to be aware of the purpose of all of the observations that need to be made.

▶ ABRUPTIO PLACENTAE

Abruptio placentae is the separation of a normally located placenta after the 20th week of gestation and prior to birth that leads to hemorrhage. It is a significant cause of third-trimester bleeding, with a high mortality rate. It occurs in about 1% of all pregnancies throughout the world (Gaufberg, 2007), or 1 in 120 pregnancies. The overall fetal mortality rate for placental abruption is 20% to 40%, depending on the extent of the abruption. Maternal mortality is approximately 6% in abruptio placentae and is related to cesarean birth and/or hemorrhage/coagulopathy (Deering & Satin, 2007).

Pathophysiology

The etiology of this condition is unknown; however, it has been proposed that abruption starts with degenerative changes in the small maternal arterioles, resulting in thrombosis, degeneration of the decidua, and possible rupture of a vessel. Bleeding from the vessel forms a retroplacental clot. The bleeding causes increased pressure behind the placenta and results in separation (Collins, 2007).

Fetal blood supply is compromised and fetal distress develops in proportion to the degree of placental separation. This is caused by the insult of the abruption itself and by issues related to prematurity when early birth is required to alleviate maternal or fetal distress.

Abruptio placentae is classified according to the extent of separation and the amount of blood loss from the maternal circulation. Classifications include:

- Mild (grade 1): minimal bleeding (less than 500 mL), marginal separation (10% to 20%), tender uterus, no coagulopathy, no signs of shock, no fetal distress
- Moderate (grade 2): moderate bleeding (1,000 to 1,500 mL), moderate separation (20% to 50%), continuous abdominal pain, mild shock
- Severe (grade 3): absent to moderate bleeding (more than 1,500 mL), severe separation (more than 50%), profound shock, agonizing abdominal pain, and development of disseminated intravascular coagulopathy (DIC) (Gilbert, 2007)

Abruptio placentae also may be classified as partial or complete, depending on the degree of separation. Al-ternately, it can be classified as concealed or apparent, by the type of bleeding (Fig. 19.5).

Remember Helen, the pregnant woman with severe abdominal pain? Electronic fetal monitoring revealed uterine hypertonicity with absent fetal heart sounds. Palpation of her abdomen revealed rigidity and extreme tenderness in all four quadrants. Her vital signs were as follows—temperature, afebrile; pulse 94; respirations 22; blood pressure 130/90 mm Hg. What might you suspect as the cause of Helen's abdominal pain? What course of action would you anticipate for Helen?

Therapeutic Management

Treatment of abruptio placentae is designed to assess, control, and restore the amount of blood lost; to provide a positive outcome for both mother and newborn; and to prevent coagulation disorders, such as DIC (Box 19.2). Emergency measures include starting two large-bore IV lines with normal saline or lactated Ringer's solution to combat hypovolemia, obtaining blood specimens for evaluating hemodynamic status values and for typing and cross-matching, and frequently monitoring fetal and maternal well-being. After the severity of abruption is determined and appropriate blood and fluid replacement is given, cesarean birth is done immediately if fetal distress is evident. If the fetus is not in distress, close monitoring continues, with delivery planned at the earliest signs of fetal distress. Because of the possibility of fetal blood loss through the placenta, a neonatal intensive care team should be available during the birth process to assess and treat the newborn immediately for shock, blood loss, and hypoxia.

If the woman develops DIC, treatment focuses on determining the underlying cause of DIC and correcting it. Replacement therapy of the coagulation factors is achieved by transfusion of fresh-frozen plasma along with cryoprecipitate to maintain the circulating volume and provide oxygen to the cells of the body. Anticoagulant therapy (low-molecular-weight heparin), packed red cells, platelet concentrates, antithrombin concentrates, and nonclotting protein-containing volume expanders, such as plasma protein fraction or albumin, are also used to combat this serious condition (Bick, 2007). Prompt identification and early intervention are essential for a woman with acute DIC associated with abruptio placentae to treat DIC and possibly save her life.

Nursing Assessment

Abruptio placentae is a medical emergency. The nurse plays a critical role in assessing the pregnant woman presenting with abdominal pain and/or experiencing vaginal bleeding, especially in a concealed hemorrhage, in which

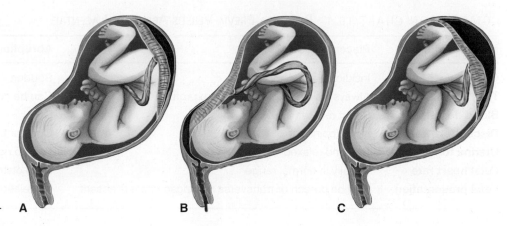

FIGURE **19.5** Classifications of abruptio placentae. (**A**) Partial abruption with concealed hemorrhage. (**B**) Partial abruption with apparent hemorrhage. (**C**) Complete abruption with concealed hemorrhage.

A Partial abruption, concealed hemorrhage

B Partial abruption, apparent hemorrhage

C Complete abruption, concealed hemorrhage

the extent of bleeding is not recognized. Rapid assessment is essential to ensure prompt, effective interventions to prevent maternal and fetal morbidity and mortality. Comparison Chart 19.1 compares placenta previa with abruptio placentae.

BOX 19.2 Disseminated Intravascular Coagulation (DIC)

DIC is a bleeding disorder characterized by an abnormal reduction in the elements involved in blood clotting resulting from their widespread intravascular clotting (Gilbert, 2007). This disorder can occur secondary to abruptio placentae.

Simply put, the clinical and pathologic manifestations of DIC can be described as a loss of balance between the clot-forming activity of thrombin and the clot-lysing activity of plasmin. Therefore, too much thrombin tips the balance toward the prothrombic state and the client develops clots. Alternately, too much clot lysis (fibrinolysis) results from plasmin formation and the client hemorrhages. Small clots form throughout the body, and eventually the blood-clotting factors are used up, rendering them unavailable to form clots at sites of tissue injury. Clot-dissolving mechanisms are also increased, which result in bleeding (possibly severe).

DIC can be stimulated by many factors, including sepsis, malignancy, and obstetric conditions such as placental abruption, missed abortion or retained dead fetus, amniotic fluid embolism, and eclampsia.

Laboratory studies that assist in the diagnosis include:
• Decreased fibrinogen and platelets
• Prolonged PT and aPTT
• Positive D-dimer tests and fibrin (split) degradation products (objective evidence of the simultaneous formation of thrombin and plasmin) (Furlong & Furlong, 2007)

Health History and Physical Examination

Begin the health history by assessing the woman for risk factors that may predispose her to abruptio placentae, such as maternal smoking, advanced maternal age (over 35 years old), poor nutrition, multiple gestation, excessive intrauterine pressure caused by hydramnios, hypertension, severe trauma (e.g., auto accident, intimate partner violence), cocaine use, alcohol ingestion, and multiparity (Norwitz & Schorge, 2006; Zeltzer, 2007). Ask the woman about her previous pregnancies to determine if she has experienced a prior abruption. In addition, be alert for other notable risk factors, such as male fetal gender, chorioamnionitis, prolonged premature ruptured membranes (more than 24 hours), oligohydramnios, preeclampsia, and low socioeconomic status (Deering & Satin, 2007).

Assess the woman for bleeding. As the placenta separates from the uterus, hemorrhage ensues. It can be apparent, appearing as vaginal bleeding, or it can be concealed. Vaginal bleeding is present in 80% of women diagnosed with abruptio placentae and may be significant enough to jeopardize both maternal and fetal health within a short time frame. The remaining 20% of abruptions are associated with a concealed hemorrhage and the absence of vaginal bleeding. Monitor the woman's level of consciousness, noting any signs or symptoms that may suggest shock.

▶ *Take* NOTE!

Vital signs can be within normal range, even with significant blood loss, because a pregnant woman can lose up to 40% of her total blood volume without showing signs of shock (Gilbert, 2007).

Assess the woman for complaints of pain, including the type, onset, and location. Ask if she has had any contractions. Palpate the abdomen, noting any contractions,

COMPARISON CHART 19.1 PLACENTA PREVIA VERSUS ABRUPTIO PLACENTAE

Manifestation	Placenta Previa	Abruptio Placentae
Onset	Insidious	Sudden
Type of bleeding	Always visible; slight, then more profuse	Can be concealed or visible
Blood description	Bright red	Dark
Discomfort/Pain	None (painless)	Constant; uterine tenderness on palpation
Uterine tone	Soft and relaxed	Firm to rigid
Fetal heart rate	Usually in normal range	Fetal distress or absent
Fetal presentation	May be breech or transverse lie; engagement is absent	No relationship

uterine tenderness, tenseness, or rigidity. Ask if she has noticed any changes in fetal movement and activity. Decreased fetal movement may be the presenting complaint, resulting from fetal jeopardy or fetal death (Oyelese & Ananth, 2006). Assess fetal heart rate and continue to monitor it electronically.

▶ **Take** NOTE!

Classic manifestations of abruptio placentae include painful, dark-red vaginal bleeding (port wine color) because the bleeding comes from the clot that was formed behind the placenta; "knife-like" abdominal pain; uterine tenderness; contractions; and decreased fetal movement. Rapid assessment is essential to ensure prompt, effective interventions to prevent maternal and fetal morbidity and mortality.

Laboratory and Diagnostic Testing

Laboratory and diagnostic tests may be helpful in diagnosing the condition and guiding management. These studies may include:

- CBC—determines the current hemodynamic status; however, it is not reliable for estimating acute blood loss
- Fibrinogen levels—typically are increased in pregnancy (hyperfibrinogenemia); thus, a moderate dip in fibrinogen levels might suggest coagulopathy (DIC) and, if profuse bleeding occurs, the clotting cascade might be compromised
- Prothrombin time (PT)/activated partial thromboplastin time (aPTT)—determines the client's coagulation status, especially if surgery is planned
- Type and cross-match—determines blood type if a transfusion is needed
- Kleihauer–Betke test—detects fetal red blood cells in the maternal circulation, determines the degree of fetal–maternal hemorrhage, and helps calculate the

appropriate dosage of RhoGAM to give to Rh-negative clients
- Nonstress test—demonstrates findings of fetal jeopardy manifested by late decelerations or bradycardia
- Biophysical profile—aids in evaluating clients with chronic abruption; a low score (less than 6 points) suggests possible fetal compromise (Collins, 2007)

Ultrasound is not useful for making a definitive diagnosis because the clot is sonographically visible in less than 50% of the cases (Zeltzer, 2007).

Nursing Management

Nursing management of the woman with abruptio placentae warrants immediate care to provide the best outcome for both mother and fetus.

Ensuring Adequate Tissue Perfusion

Upon arrival to the facility, place the woman on strict bed rest and in a left lateral position to prevent pressure on the vena cava. This position provides uninterrupted perfusion to the fetus. Expect to administer oxygen therapy via nasal cannula to ensure adequate tissue perfusion. Monitor oxygen saturation levels via pulse oximetry to evaluate the effectiveness of interventions.

Obtain maternal vital signs frequently, as often as every 15 minutes as indicated, depending on the woman's status and amount of blood loss. Observe for changes in vital signs suggesting hypovolemic shock and report them immediately. Also expect to insert an indwelling urinary (Foley) catheter to assess hourly urine output and initiate an IV infusion for fluid replacement using a large-bore catheter.

Assess fundal height for changes. An increase in size would indicate bleeding. Monitor the amount and characteristics of any vaginal bleeding as frequently as every 15 to 30 minutes. Be alert for signs and symptoms of DIC, such as bleeding gums, tachycardia, oozing from the IV insertion site, and petechiae, and administer blood products as ordered if DIC occurs.

Institute continuous electronic fetal monitoring. Assess uterine contractions and report any increased uterine tenseness or rigidity. Also observe the tracing for tetanic uterine contractions or changes in fetal heart rate patterns suggesting fetal compromise.

Providing Support and Education

A woman diagnosed with abruptio placentae may be filled with a sense of heightened anxiety and apprehension, for her own health as well as that of her fetus. Communicate empathy and understanding of the client's experience, and provide emotional support throughout this frightening time. Remain with the couple, acknowledge their emotions and fears, and address their spiritual and cultural needs. Answer their questions about the status of their fetus openly and honestly, being sure to explain indicators of fetal well-being. Provide information about the various diagnostic tests, treatments, and procedures that may be done, including the possible need for a cesarean birth.

Depending on the client's status, extent of bleeding, and length of gestation, the fetus may not survive. If the fetus does survive, he or she most likely will require neonatal intensive care. Assist the client and family to deal with the loss or with the birth of a newborn in the neonatal intensive care unit.

Although abruptio placentae is not a preventable condition, client education is important to help reduce the risk for a recurrence of this condition. Encourage the woman to avoid drinking, smoking, or using drugs during pregnancy. Urge her to seek early and continuous prenatal care and to receive prompt health care if any signs and symptoms occur in future pregnancies.

Think back to Helen, the pregnant woman described at the beginning of the chapter. She was diagnosed with abruptio placentae and was prepared for an emergency cesarean birth. On exploration, there was almost a 75% abruption, with approximately 800 mL of concealed blood between the uterus and the placenta. In addition, she lost an additional 500 mL during surgery. What in Helen's history may have placed her at increased risk for abruption? What assessments and interventions would be essential during her postpartum recovery secondary to her large blood loss? What psychosocial interventions would be necessary due to her fetal loss?

Hyperemesis Gravidarum

At least 80% of women experience nausea and vomiting during their pregnancy (Lane, 2007). The term *morning sickness* is often used to describe this condition when symptoms are relatively mild. Such symptoms usually disappear after the first trimester. This mild form mostly affects the quality of life of the woman and her family, whereas the severe form—hyperemesis gravidarum—results in dehydration, electrolyte imbalance, and the need for hospitalization (Wilcox & Edelman, 2007).

Unlike morning sickness, **hyperemesis gravidarum** is a complication of pregnancy characterized by persistent, uncontrollable nausea and vomiting that persists beyond the 20th week of pregnancy, causing weight loss of more than 5% of prepregnancy body weight, dehydration, metabolic acidosis from starvation, alkalosis from loss of hydrochloric acid, and hypokalemia (Lamondy, 2007).

Hyperemesis is estimated to occur in approximately 5 per 1,000 pregnancies. The prevalence increases in molar pregnancies and multiple gestations. Its peak incidence occurs between 8 and 12 weeks of pregnancy, and it usually resolves by week 16 (Ogunyemi, 2007).

> ▶ **Take** NOTE!
>
> *Every pregnant woman needs to be instructed to report any episodes of severe nausea and vomiting or episodes that extend beyond the first trimester.*

Pathophysiology

Although the exact cause of nausea and vomiting is unknown, its effects—decreased placental blood flow, decreased maternal blood flow, and acidosis—can threaten the health of the mother and fetus. Dehydration can also lead to preterm labor (Lane, 2007). Numerous theories abound, but few studies have produced scientific evidence to identify the etiology of this condition. It is likely that multiple factors contribute to it.

Elevated levels of hCG are present in all pregnant women during early pregnancy, usually declining after 12 weeks. This corresponds to the usual duration of morning sickness. In hyperemesis gravidarum, the hCG levels are often higher and extend beyond the first trimester. Symptoms exacerbate the disease. Decreased fluid intake and prolonged vomiting cause dehydration; dehydration increases the serum concentration of hCG, which in turn exacerbates the nausea and vomiting—a vicious cycle. A few other theories that have been proposed to explain its etiology include:

- Endocrine theory—high levels of hCG and estrogen during pregnancy
- Metabolic theory—vitamin B6 deficiency
- Psychological theory—psychological stress increases the symptoms

Therapeutic Management

Conservative management in the home is the first line of treatment for the woman with hyperemesis gravidarum. This usually focuses on dietary and lifestyle changes.

If conservative management fails to alleviate the client's symptoms and nausea and vomiting continue, hospitalization is necessary to reverse the effects of severe nausea and vomiting.

On admission to the hospital, blood tests are ordered to assess the severity of the client's dehydration, electrolyte imbalance, ketosis, and malnutrition. Parenteral fluids and drugs are ordered to rehydrate the woman and reduce the symptoms. The first choice for fluid replacement is generally 5% dextrose in lactated Ringer's solution with vitamins (pyridoxine [B6]) and electrolytes added. Oral food and fluids are withheld for the first 24 to 36 hours to allow the GI tract to rest. Antiemetics may be administered rectally or intravenously to control the nausea and vomiting initially because the woman is considered NPO. Once her condition stabilizes and she is allowed oral intake, medications may be administered orally.

If the client does not improve after several days of bed rest, "gut rest," IV fluids, and antiemetics, total parenteral nutrition or feeding through a percutaneous endoscopic gastrostomy tube is instituted to prevent malnutrition.

The FDA has not approved any drugs for the treatment of nausea and vomiting in pregnancy, but the risk of administration must be balanced against the sequelae of prolonged starvation and dehydration. Finding a drug that works for any given client is largely a matter of trial and error. If one drug is ineffective, another class of drugs with a different mechanism of action may help. Promethazine (Phenergan) and prochlorperazine (Compazine) are among the older preparations usually tried first. If they fail to relieve symptoms, newer drugs such as on-dansetron (Zofran) may be tried. Most drugs are given parenterally or rectally (Lane, 2007) (Drug Guide 19.2).

Few women receive complete relief of symptoms from any one therapy. Complementary and alternative medicine therapies appeal to many to help supplement traditional ones. Some popular therapies include acupressure, massage, therapeutic touch, ginger, and the wearing of Sea-bands to prevent nausea and vomiting. Recent research has reported a positive effect of using acupressure over the Neiguan point on the wrist by Sea-bands to control nausea and vomiting associated with pregnancy (Lane, 2007).

Nursing Assessment

Nursing assessment of the woman with hyperemesis gravidarum requires a thorough history and physical examination to identify signs and symptoms associated with this disorder. The client is extremely uncomfortable. She may experience many hours of lost work productivity and sleep, and hyperemesis may damage family relationships. If hyperemesis progresses untreated, it may cause neurologic disturbances, renal damage, retinal hemorrhage, or death (Lane, 2007). Laboratory and diagnostic tests aid in determining the severity of the disorder.

Health History and Physical Examination

Begin the history by asking the client about the onset, duration, and course of her nausea and vomiting. Ask her about any medications or treatments she used and how effective they were in relieving her nausea and vomiting. Obtain a diet history from the client, including a dietary

---

DRUG GUIDE 19.2 MEDICATIONS USED FOR HYPEREMESIS GRAVIDARUM

Medication	Action/Indications	Nursing Implications
Promethazine (Phenergan)	Diminishes vestibular stimulation and acts on the chemoreceptor trigger zone (CTZ). Symptomatic relief of nausea and vomiting, and motion sickness	Be alert for urinary retention, dizziness, hypotension, and involuntary movements. Institute safety measures to prevent injury secondary to sedative effects. Offer hard candy and frequent rinsing of mouth for dryness.
Prochlorperazine (Compazine)	Acts centrally to inhibit dopamine receptors in the CTZ and peripherally to block vagus nerve stimulation in the GI tract. Controls severe nausea and vomiting	Be alert for abnormal movements and for neuroleptic malignant syndrome such as seizures, hyper-/hypotension, tachycardia, and dyspnea. Assess mental status, intake/output. Caution patient not to drive as a result of drowsiness or dizziness. Advise to change position slowly to minimize effects of orthostatic hypotension.
Odansetron (Zofran)	Blocks serotonin peripherally, centrally, and in the small intestine. Prevents nausea and vomiting	Monitor for possible side effects such as diarrhea, constipation, abdominal pain, headache, dizziness, drowsiness, and fatigue. Monitor liver function studies as ordered.

Sources: Hodgson & Kizior, 2007; Lilley et al., 2007.

recall for the past week. Note the client's knowledge of nutrition and need for appropriate nutritional intake. Be alert for patterns that may contribute to or trigger her distress. Also ask about any complaints of ptyalism (excessive salivation), anorexia, indigestion, and abdominal pain or distention. Ask if she has noticed any blood or mucus in her stool.

Review the client's history for possible risk factors, such as young age, nausea and vomiting with previous pregnancy, history of intolerance of oral contraceptives, nulliparity, trophoblastic disease, multiple gestation, emotional or psychological stress, gastroesophageal reflux disease, primigravida status, obesity, hyperthyroidism, and *Helicobacter pylori* seropositivity (Ogunyemi, 2007). Weigh the client and compare this weight to her weight before she began experiencing symptoms and to her prepregnancy weight to estimate the degree of loss. With hyperemesis, weight loss usually exceeds 5% of body mass.

Inspect the mucous membranes for dryness and check skin turgor for evidence of fluid loss and dehydration. Assess blood pressure for changes, such as hypotension, that may suggest a fluid volume deficit. Also note any complaints of weakness, fatigue, activity intolerance, dizziness, or sleep disturbances.

Assess the client's perception of the situation. Note any evidence of depression, anxiety, irritability, mood changes, and decreased ability to concentrate, which can add to her emotional distress (Lamondy, 2007). Determine the woman's support systems that are available for help.

Laboratory and Diagnostic Testing

The results of laboratory and diagnostic tests may provide clues to the severity or etiology of the disorder: These may include:

- Liver enzymes—elevations of aspartate aminotransferase (AST) and alanine aminotransferase (ALT) are usually present
- CBC—elevated levels of red blood cells and hematocrit, indicating dehydration
- Urine ketones—positive when the body breaks down fat to provide energy in the absence of inadequate intake
- Blood urea nitrogen (BUN)—increased in the presence of salt and water depletion
- Urine specific gravity—greater than 1.025, possibly indicating concentrated urine linked to inadequate fluid intake or excessive fluid loss
- Serum electrolytes—decreased levels of potassium, sodium, and chloride resulting from excessive vomiting and loss of hydrochloric acid in stomach
- Ultrasound—evaluation for molar pregnancy or multiple gestation (Wilcox & Edelman, 2007)

Nursing Management

Nursing management for the client with hyperemesis gravidarum focuses on promoting comfort by controlling the client's nausea and vomiting and promoting adequate nutrition. In addition, the nurse plays a major role in supporting and educating the client and her family.

Promoting Comfort and Nutrition

During the initial period, expect to withhold all oral food and fluids, maintaining NPO status to allow the GI tract to rest. In addition, administer prescribed antiemetics to relieve the nausea and vomiting and IV fluids to replace fluid losses. Monitor the rate of infusion to prevent overload and assess the IV insertion site to prevent infiltration or infection. Also administer electrolyte replacement therapy as ordered to correct any imbalances, and periodically check serum electrolyte levels to evaluate the effectiveness of therapy.

Provide physical comfort measures such as hygiene measures and oral care. Pay special attention to the environment, making sure to keep the area free of pungent odors. As the client's nausea and vomiting subside, gradually introduce oral fluids and foods in small amounts. Monitor intake and output and assess the client's tolerance to the increase in intake.

Providing Support and Education

Women with hyperemesis gravidarum commonly are fatigued physically and emotionally. Many are exhausted, frustrated, and anxious. Offer reassurance that all interventions are directed toward promoting positive pregnancy outcomes for both the woman and her fetus. Providing information about the expected plan of care may help to alleviate the client's anxiety. Listen to her concerns and feelings, answering all questions honestly. Educate the woman and her family about the condition and its treatment options (Teaching Guidelines 19.1). Teach the client about therapeutic lifestyle changes, such as avoiding stressors and fatigue that may trigger nausea and vomiting. Offer ongoing support and encouragement and promote active participation in care decisions, thereby empowering the client and her family. Attempting to provide the client with a sense of control may help her overcome the feeling that she has lost control. If necessary, refer the client to a spiritual advisor or counseling. Also suggest possible local or national support groups that the client may contact for additional information.

Arrange for possible home care follow-up for the client and reinforce discharge instructions to promote understanding. Collaborate with community resources to ensure continuity of care.

Gestational Hypertension

Gestational hypertension is characterized by hypertension without proteinuria after 20 weeks of gestation and a return of the blood pressure to normal postpartum. Previously, gestational hypertension was known as pregnancy-induced hypertension or toxemia of pregnancy, but these terms are no longer used. Gestational hypertension is clin-

Teaching to Minimize Nausea and Vomiting

- Avoid noxious stimuli—such as strong flavors, perfumes, or strong odors such as frying bacon—that might trigger nausea and vomiting.
- Avoid tight waistbands to minimize pressure on abdomen.
- Eat small, frequent meals throughout the day—six small meals.
- Separate fluids from solids by consuming fluids in between meals.
- Avoid lying down or reclining for at least 2 hours after eating.
- Use high-protein supplement drinks.
- Avoid foods high in fat.
- Increase your intake of carbonated beverages.
- Increase your exposure to fresh air to improve symptoms.
- Eat when you are hungry, regardless of normal mealtimes.
- Drink herbal teas containing peppermint or ginger.
- Avoid fatigue and learn how to mange stress in life.
- Schedule daily rest periods to avoid becoming overtired.
- Eat foods that settle the stomach, such as dry crackers, toast, or soda.

ically characterized by a blood pressure of 140/90 mm Hg or more on two occasions at least 6 hours apart (Gibson & Carson, 2007). Gestational hypertension can be differentiated from chronic hypertension, which appears before the 20th week of gestation; or hypertension before the current pregnancy, which continues after the woman gives birth.

Gestational hypertension is the second leading cause of maternal death in the United States after thromboembolism, accounting for almost 15% of such deaths, and the most common complication reported during pregnancy. Hypertension complicates 12% to 20% of pregnancies and the rate has increased steadily, approximately 30% to 40% since 1990, for all ages, races, and ethnic groups. The highest rates are in women younger than 20 or older than 40 (Weismiller, 2007).

ACOG (2007a) and the National High Blood Pressure Education Program (2000) have identified a classification system for hypertensive disorders. Hypertension may be a preexisting condition (chronic hypertension) or it may present for the first time during pregnancy (gestational hypertension). Regardless of its onset, hypertension jeopardizes the well-being of the mother as well as the fetus.

The National High Blood Pressure Education Program Working Group on High Blood Pressure in Pregnancy has defined four categories of hypertension in pregnancy:

- Gestational hypertension: new onset, nonproteinuric hypertension after week 20 of gestation
- Chronic hypertension: maternal blood pressure of 140/90 or > on two occasions; week 20 of gestation, and persisting beyond week 12 of postpartum
- Preeclampsia: new-onset hypertension with proteinuria (>300 mg or 1+ on dipstick) after week 20 of gestation
- Preeclampsia superimposed on chronic hypertension: presence of new onset of proteinuria; hypertension and proteinuria before week 20 of gestation; sudden increase in blood pressure or proteinuria; or increase in liver enzymes or thrombocytopenia

Gestational hypertension can be classified as preeclampsia or eclampsia. Each is associated with specific criteria. Preeclampsia is further categorized as mild or severe. Comparison Chart 19.2 highlights these classifications.

Pathophysiology

Gestational hypertension remains an enigma. The condition can be devastating to both the mother and fetus, and yet the etiology still remains a mystery to medical science despite decades of research. Many theories exist, but none have truly explained the widespread pathologic changes that result in pulmonary edema, oliguria, seizures, thrombocytopenia, and abnormal liver enzymes (Podymow & August, 2007). Despite the results of several research studies, the use of aspirin or supplementation with calcium, magnesium, zinc, or antioxidant therapy (vitamin C and E), salt restriction, diuretic therapy, or fish oils has not proved to prevent this destructive condition.

The underlying mechanisms involved with this disorder are vasospasm and hypoperfusion. In addition, endothelial injury occurs, leading to platelet adherence, fibrin deposition, and the presence of schistocytes (fragment of an erythrocyte).

Generalized vasospasm results in elevation of blood pressure and reduced blood flow to the brain, liver, kidneys, placenta, and lungs. Decreased liver perfusion leads to impaired liver function and subcapsular hemorrhage. This is demonstrated by epigastric pain and elevated liver enzymes in the maternal serum. Decreased brain perfusion leads to small cerebral hemorrhages and symptoms of arterial vasospasm such as headaches, visual disturbances, blurred vision, and hyperactive deep tendon reflexes (DTRs). A thromboxane/prostacyclin imbalance leads to increased thromboxane (potent vasoconstrictor and stimulator of platelet aggregation) and decreased prostacyclin (potent vasodilator and inhibitor of platelet aggregation), which contribute to the hypertensive state. Decreased kidney perfusion reduces the glomerular filtra-

COMPARISON CHART 19.2 PREECLAMPSIA VERSUS ECLAMPSIA

	Mild Preeclampsia	Severe Preeclampsia	Eclampsia
Blood pressure	>140/90 mm Hg after 20 weeks' gestation	>160/110 mm Hg	Same as severe preeclampsia
Proteinuria	300 mg/24 h or greater than 1+ protein on a random dipstick urine sample	>500 mg/24 hours; greater than 3+ on random dipstick urine sample	Marked proteinuria
Seizures/coma	No	No	Yes
Hyperreflexia	No	Yes	Yes
Other signs and symptoms	Mild facial or hand edema Weight gain	Headache Oliguria Blurred vision, scotomata (blind spots) Pulmonary edema Thrombocytopenia (platelet count <100,000 platelets/mm^3) Cerebral disturbances Epigastric or RUQ pain HELLP	Severe headache Generalized edema RUQ or epigastric pain Visual disturbances Cerebral hemorrhage Renal failure HELLP

tion rate (GFR), resulting in decreased urine output and increased serum levels of sodium, BUN, uric acid, and creatinine, further increasing extracellular fluid and edema. Increased capillary permeability in the kidneys allows albumin to escape, which reduces plasma colloid osmotic pressure and moves more fluid into extracellular spaces; this leads to pulmonary edema and generalized edema. Poor placental perfusion resulting from prolonged vasoconstriction helps to contribute to intrauterine growth restriction, premature separation of the placenta (abruptio placentae), persistent fetal hypoxia, and acidosis. In addition, hemoconcentration (resulting from decreased intravascular volume) causes increased blood viscosity and elevated hematocrit (ACOG, 2007a).

Therapeutic Management

Management of the woman with gestational hypertension varies depending on the severity of her condition and its effects on the fetus. Typically the woman is managed conservatively if she is experiencing mild symptoms. However, if the condition progresses, management becomes more aggressive.

Management for Mild Preeclampsia

Conservative strategies for mild preeclampsia are used if the woman exhibits no signs of renal or hepatic dysfunction or coagulopathy. A woman with mild elevations in blood pressure may be placed on bed rest at home. She is encouraged to rest as much as possible in the lateral recumbent position to improve uteroplacental blood flow, reduce her blood pressure, and promote diuresis. In addition, antepartal visits and diagnostic testing—such as CBC, clotting studies, liver enzymes, and platelet levels—

increase in frequency. The woman will be asked to monitor her blood pressure daily (every 4 to 6 hours while awake) and report any increased readings; she will also measure the amount of protein found in urine using a dipstick and will weigh herself for any weight gain. Daily fetal movement counts also are implemented. If there is any decrease in movement, the woman needs to be evaluated by her health care provider that day. A balanced, nutritional diet with no sodium restriction is advised. In addition, she is encouraged to drink six to eight 8-oz glasses of water daily.

If home management fails to reduce the blood pressure, admission to the hospital is warranted and the treatment strategy is individualized based on the severity of the condition and the gestational age at the time of diagnosis. During the hospitalization, the woman with mild preeclampsia is monitored closely for signs and symptoms of severe preeclampsia or impending eclampsia (e.g., persistent headache, hyperreflexia). Blood pressure measurements are frequently recorded along with daily weights to detect excessive weight gain resulting from edema. Fetal surveillance is instituted in the form of daily fetal movement counts, nonstress testing, and serial ultrasounds to evaluate fetal growth and amniotic fluid volume to confirm fetal well-being. Expectant management usually continues until the pregnancy reaches term, fetal lung maturity is documented, or complications develop that warrant immediate birth (Mundy, 2006).

Prevention of disease progression is the focus of treatment during labor. Blood pressure is monitored frequently and a quiet environment is important to minimize the risk of stimulation and to promote rest. IV magnesium sulfate is infused to prevent any seizure activity, along with antihypertensives if blood pressure values begin to rise. Calcium gluconate is kept at the bedside in case the magnesium level becomes toxic. Continued close monitoring of neurologic status is warranted to detect any signs or symptoms of hypoxemia, impending seizure activity, or increased intracranial pressure. An indwelling urinary (Foley) catheter usually is inserted to allow for accurate measurement of urine output.

Management for Severe Preeclampsia

Severe preeclampsia may develop suddenly and bring with it high blood pressure of more than 160/110 mmHg, proteinuria of more than 5 g in 24 hours, oliguria of less than 400 mL in 24 hours, cerebral and visual symptoms, and rapid weight gain. This clinical picture signals severe preeclampsia, and immediate hospitalization is needed.

Treatment is highly individualized and based on disease severity and fetal age. Birth of the infant is the only cure, because preeclampsia depends on the presence of trophoblastic tissue. Therefore, the exact age of the fetus is assessed to determine viability.

Severe preeclampsia is treated aggressively because hypertension poses a serious threat to mother and fetus. The goal of care is to stabilize the mother–fetus dyad and prepare for birth. Therapy focuses on controlling hypertension, preventing seizures, preventing long-term morbidity, and preventing maternal, fetal, or newborn death (Weismiller, 2007). Intense maternal and fetal surveillance starts when the mother enters the hospital and continues throughout her stay.

The woman in labor with severe preeclampsia typically receives oxytocin to stimulate uterine contractions and magnesium sulfate to prevent seizure activity. Oxytocin and magnesium sulfate can be given simultaneously via infusion pumps to ensure both are administered at the prescribed rate. The client is evaluated closely for magnesium toxicity. If at all possible, a vaginal delivery is preferable to a cesarean birth. PGE2 gel may be used to ripen the cervix. A cesarean birth may be performed if the client is seriously ill. A pediatrician/neonatologist must be available in the birthing room to care for the newborn. A newborn whose mother received high doses of magnesium sulfate needs to be monitored for respiratory depression, hypocalcemia, and hypotonia (Blackburn, 2007).

Management of Eclampsia

In the woman who develops an eclamptic seizure, the convulsive activity begins with facial twitching, followed by generalized muscle rigidity. Respirations cease for the duration of the seizure, resulting from muscle spasms, thus compromising fetal oxygenation. Coma usually follows the seizure activity, with respiration resuming. Eclamptic seizures are life-threatening emergencies and require immediate treatment to decrease maternal morbidity and mortality.

As with any seizure, the initial management is to clear the airway and administer adequate oxygen. Positioning the woman on her left side and protecting her from injury during the seizure are key. Suction equipment must be readily available to remove secretions from her mouth after the seizure is over. IV fluids are administered after the seizure at a rate to replace urine output and additional insensible losses. Fetal heart rate is monitored closely. Magnesium sulfate is administered IV to prevent further seizures. Hypertension is controlled with antihypertensive medications. After the seizures are controlled, the woman's stability is assessed and birth via induction or cesarean birth is performed (Blincoe, 2007).

If the woman's condition remains stable, she will be transferred to the postpartum unit for care. If she becomes unstable after giving birth, she may be transferred to the critical care unit for closer observation.

Nursing Assessment

Preventing complications related to hypertension during pregnancy requires the use of assessment, advocacy, and counseling skills. Assessment begins with the accurate measurement of the client's blood pressure at each encounter. In addition, nurses need to assess for subjective complaints that may indicate progression of the disease—visual changes, severe headaches, unusual bleeding or bruising, or epigastric pain (Blincoe, 2007). The significant signs of gestational hypertension—proteinuria and hypertension—occur without the woman's awareness. Unfortunately, by the time symptoms are noticed, gestational hypertension can be severe.

> ▶ **Take** NOTE!
>
> *The absolute blood pressure (value that validates elevation) of 140/90 mmHg should be obtained on two occasions 6 hours apart to be diagnostic of gestational hypertension. Proteinuria is defined as 300 mg or more of urinary protein per 24 hours or more than 1+ protein by chemical reagent strip or dipstick of at least two random urine samples collected at least 6 hours apart with no evidence of UTI (ACOG, 2007a).*

Health History and Physical Examination

Take a thorough history during the first antepartal visit to identify whether the woman is at risk for preeclampsia. Risk factors include:

- Primigravida status
- Chromosomal abnormalities
- Structural congenital anomalies
- Multifetal pregnancy
- History of preeclampsia in a previous pregnancy
- Excessive placental tissue, as is seen in women with GTD

- Chronic stress
- Family history of preeclampsia (mother or sister)
- Lower socioeconomic group
- History of diabetes, hypertension, or renal disease
- Poor nutrition
- African-American ethnicity
- Age extremes (younger than 20 or older than 40)
- Obesity (Weismiller, 2007)

In addition, complete a nutritional assessment that includes the woman's usual intake of protein, calcium, daily calories, and fluids.

Women at risk for preeclampsia require more frequent prenatal visits throughout their pregnancy, and they require teaching about problems so that they can report them promptly.

Blood pressure must be measured carefully and consistently. Obtain all measurements with the woman in the same position (blood pressure is highest in the sitting position and lowest in the side-lying position) and by using the same technique (automated vs. manual). This standardization in position and technique will yield the most accurate readings (Weismiller, 2007).

Obtain the client's weight (noting gain since last visit), and assess for amount and location of edema. Asking questions such as, "Do your rings still fit on your fingers?" or "Is your face puffy when you get up in the morning?" will help to determine whether fluid retention is present or if the woman's status has changed since her last visit.

▶ **Take** *NOTE!*

Although edema is not a cardinal sign of preeclampsia, weight should be monitored frequently to identify sudden gains in a short time span. Current research relies less on the classic triad of symptoms (hypertension, proteinuria, and edema or weight gain) and more on decreased organ perfusion, endothelial dysfunction (capillary leaking and proteinuria), and elevated blood pressure as key indicators (Gibson & Carson, 2007).

If edema is present, assess the distribution, degree, and pitting. Document your findings and identify whether the edema is dependent or pitting. Dependent edema is present on the lower half of the body if the client is ambulatory, where hydrostatic pressure is greatest. It is usually observed in the feet and ankles or in the sacral area if the client is on bed rest.

Pitting edema is edema that leaves a small depression or pit after finger pressure is applied to a swollen area (Gibson & Carson, 2007). Record the depth of pitting demonstrated when pressure is applied. Although subjective, the following is used to record relative degrees:

- 1+ pitting edema = 2-mm depression into skin; disappears rapidly
- 2+ pitting edema = 4-mm skin depression; disappears in 10 to 15 seconds
- 3+ pitting edema = 6-mm depression into skin; lasts more than 1 minute
- 4+ pitting edema = 8-mm depression into skin; lasts 2 to 3 minutes

At every antepartal visit, assess the fetal heart rate with a Doppler device. Also check a clean-catch urine specimen for protein using a dipstick.

Laboratory and Diagnostic Testing

Various laboratory tests may be performed to evaluate the woman's status. Typically these include a CBC, serum electrolytes, BUN, creatinine, and hepatic enzyme levels. Urine specimens are checked for protein; if levels are 1-2+ or greater, a 24-hour urine collection is completed.

Nursing Management

Nursing management of the woman with gestational hypertension focuses on close monitoring of blood pressure and ongoing assessment for evidence of disease progression. Throughout the client's pregnancy, fetal surveillance is key.

Intervening With Preeclampsia

The woman with mild preeclampsia requires frequent monitoring to detect changes because preeclampsia can progress rapidly. Instruct all women in the signs and symptoms of preeclampsia and urge them to contact their health care professional for immediate evaluation should any occur.

Typically women with mild preeclampsia can be managed at home if they have a good understanding of the disease process, are stable, have no abnormal laboratory test results, and demonstrate good fetal movement (Teaching Guidelines 19.2). The home care nurse makes frequent visits and follow-up phone calls to assess the woman's condition, to assist with scheduling periodic evaluations of the fetus (such as nonstress tests), and to evaluate any changes that might suggest a worsening of the woman's condition.

Early detection and management of mild preeclampsia is associated with the greatest success in reducing progression of this condition. As long as the client carries out the guidelines of care as outlined by the health care provider and she remains stable, home care can continue to maintain the pregnancy until the fetus is mature. If disease progression occurs, hospitalization is required.

Intervening With Severe Preeclampsia

The woman with severe preeclampsia requires hospitalization. Maintain the client on complete bed rest in the left lateral lying position. Ensure that the room is dark

TEACHING GUIDELINES 19.2

Teaching for the Woman With Mild Preeclampsia

- Rest in a quiet environment to prevent cerebral disturbances.
- Drink 8 to 10 glasses of water daily.
- Consume a balanced, high-protein diet including high-fiber foods.
- Obtain intermittent bed rest to improve circulation to the heart and uterus.
- Limit your physical activity to promote urination and subsequent decrease in blood pressure.
- Enlist the aid of your family so that you can obtain appropriate rest time.
- Perform self-monitoring as instructed, including
  - Taking your own blood pressure twice daily
  - Checking and recording weight daily
  - Performing urine dipstick twice daily
  - Recording the number of fetal kicks daily
- Contact the home health nurse if any of the following occurs:
  - Increase in blood pressure
  - Protein present in urine
  - Gain of more than 1 lb in 1 week
  - Burning or frequency when urinating
  - Decrease in fetal activity or movement
  - Headache (forehead or posterior neck region)
  - Dizziness or visual disturbances
  - Increase in swelling in hands, feet, legs, and face
  - Stomach pain, excessive heartburn, or epigastric pain
  - Decreased or infrequent urination
  - Contractions or low back pain
  - Easy or excessive bruising
  - Sudden onset of abdominal pain
  - Nausea and vomiting

and quiet to reduce stimulation. Give sedatives as ordered to encourage quiet bed rest. The client is at risk for seizures if the condition progresses. Therefore, institute and maintain seizure precautions, such as padding the side rails and having oxygen, suction equipment, and call light readily available to protect the client from injury.

▶ *Take* NOTE!

Preeclampsia increases the risk of placental abruption, preterm birth, intrauterine growth restriction, and fetal distress during childbirth. Be prepared!

Closely monitor the client's blood pressure. Administer antihypertensives as ordered to reduce blood pressure (Drug Guide 19.3). Assess the client's vision and level of consciousness. Report any changes and any complaints of headache or visual disturbances. Offer a high-protein diet with 8 to 10 glasses of water daily. Monitor the client's intake and output every hour and administer fluid and electrolyte replacements as ordered. Assess the woman for signs and symptoms of pulmonary edema, such as crackles and wheezing heard on auscultation, dyspnea, decreased oxygen saturation levels, cough, neck vein distention, anxiety, and restlessness (Blincoe, 2007).

To achieve a safe outcome for the fetus, prepare the woman for possible testing to evaluate fetal status as preeclampsia progresses. These may include the nonstress test, serial ultrasounds to track fetal growth, amniocentesis to determine fetal lung maturity, Doppler velocimetry to screen for fetal compromise, and biophysical profile to evaluate ongoing fetal well-being (Jung & Erogul, 2007).

Other laboratory tests may be performed to monitor the disease process and to determine if it is progressing into HELLP syndrome. These include liver enzymes such as lactic dehydrogenase (LDH), ALT, and AST; chemistry panel, such as creatinine, BUN, uric acid, and glucose; CBC, including platelet count; coagulation studies, such as PT, PTT, fibrinogen, and bleeding time; and a 24-hour urine collection for protein and creatinine clearance.

Administer parenteral magnesium sulfate as ordered to prevent seizures. Assess deep tendon reflexes (DTRs) to evaluate the effectiveness of therapy. Clients with preeclampsia commonly present with hyperreflexia. Severe preeclampsia causes changes in the cortex, which disrupts the equilibrium of impulses between the cerebral cortex and the spinal cord. Brisk reflexes (hyperreflexia) are the result of an irritable cortex and indicate central nervous system involvement (Warden & Euerle, 2007).

Diminished or absent reflexes occur when the client develops magnesium toxicity. Because magnesium is a potent neuromuscular blockade, the afferent and efferent nerve pathways do not relay messages properly and hyporeflexia develops. Common sites used to assess DTRs are biceps reflex, triceps reflex, patellar reflex, Achilles reflex, and plantar reflex. Nursing Procedure 19.1 highlights the steps for assessing the patellar reflex.

The National Institute of Neurological Disorders and Stroke (NINDS), a division of the National Institutes of Health, published a scale in the early 1990s that, although subjective, is used widely today. It grades reflexes from 0 to 4+. Grades 2+ and 3+ are considered normal, whereas grades 0 and 4 may indicate pathology (Table 19.2). Because these are subjective assessments, to improve communication of reflex results, condensed descriptor categories such as absent, average, brisk, or clonus should be used rather than numeric codes (Gilbert, 2007).

Clonus is the presence of rhythmic involuntary contractions, most often at the foot or ankle. Sustained clonus

DRUG GUIDE 19.3   MEDICATIONS USED WITH PREECLAMPSIA AND ECLAMPSIA

Medication	Action/Indications	Nursing Implications
Magnesium sulfate	Blockage of neuromuscular transmission, vasodilation Prevention and treatment of eclamptic seizures.	Administer IV loading dose of 4–6 g over 30 minutes, continue maintenance infusion of 2–4 g/hour as ordered. Monitor serum magnesium levels closely. Assess DTRs and check for ankle clonus. Have calcium gluconate readily available in case of toxicity. Monitor for signs and symptoms of toxicity, such as flushing, sweating, hypotension, and cardiac and central nervous system depression.
Hydralazine hydrochloride (Apresoline)	Vascular smooth muscle relaxant, thus improving perfusion to renal, uterine, and cerebral areas Reduction in blood pressure	Administer 5–10 mg by slow IV bolus every 20 minutes. Use parenteral form immediately after opening ampule. Withdraw drug slowly to prevent possible rebound hypertension. Monitor for adverse effects such as palpitations, headache, tachycardia, anorexia, nausea, vomiting, and diarrhea.
Labetalol hydrochloride (Normodyne)	Alpha 1 and beta blocker Reduction in blood pressure	Be aware that drug lowers blood pressure without decreasing maternal heart rate or cardiac output. Administer IV bolus dose of 10–20 mg and then administer IV infusion of 2 mg/minute until desired blood pressure value achieved. Monitor for possible adverse effects such as gastric pain, flatulence, constipation, dizziness, vertigo, and fatigue.
Nifedipine (Procardia)	Calcium channel blocker/dilation of coronary arteries, arterioles, and peripheral arterioles Reduction in blood pressure, stoppage of preterm labor	Administer 10 mg orally for three doses and then every 4–8 hours. Monitor for possible adverse effects such as dizziness, peripheral edema, angina, diarrhea, nasal congestions, cough.
Sodium nitroprusside	Rapid vasodilation (arterial and venous) Severe hypertension requiring rapid reduction in blood pressure	Administer via continuous IV infusion with dose titrated according to blood pressure levels. Wrap IV infusion solution in foil or opaque material to protect from light. Monitor for possible adverse effects, such as apprehension, restlessness, retrosternal pressure, palpitations, diaphoresis, abdominal pain.
Furosemide (Lasix)	Diuretic action, inhibiting the reabsorption of sodium and chloride from the ascending loop of Henle Pulmonary edema (used only if condition is present)	Administer via slow IV bolus at a dose of 10–40 mg over 1–2 minutes. Monitor urine output hourly. Assess for possible adverse effects such as dizziness, vertigo, orthostatic hypotension, anorexia, vomiting, electrolyte imbalances, muscle cramps, and muscle spasms.

Sources: Hodgson & Kizior, 2007; Lilley et al., 2007.

Nursing Procedure 19.1

ASSESSING THE PATELLAR REFLEX

Purpose: To Evaluate for Nervous System Irritability Related to Preeclampsia

1. Place the woman in the supine position (or sitting upright with the legs dangling freely over the side of the bed or examination table).
2. If lying supine, have the woman flex her knee slightly.
3. Place a hand under the knee to support the leg and locate the patellar tendon. It should be midline just below the knee cap.
4. Using a reflex hammer or the side of your hand, strike the area of the patellar tendon firmly and quickly.
5. Note the movement of the leg and foot. A patellar reflex occurs when the leg and foot move (documented as 2+).
6. Repeat the procedure on the opposite leg.

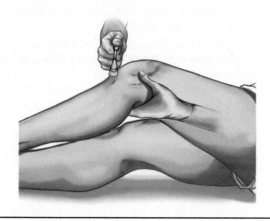

confirms central nervous system involvement. Nursing Procedure 19.2 highlights the steps when testing for ankle clonus.

With magnesium sulfate administration, the client is at risk for magnesium toxicity. Closely assess the client for signs of toxicity, which include a respiratory rate of

TABLE 19.2   GRADING DEEP TENDON REFLEXES

Description of Finding	Grade
Reflex absent, no response detected	0
Hypoactive response, diminished	1
Reflex in lower half of normal range	2
Reflex in upper half of normal range	3
Hyperactive, brisk, clonus present	4

Sources: Arenson & Drake, 2007; Weber, 2007.

Nursing Procedure 19.2

TESTING FOR ANKLE CLONUS

Purpose: To Evaluate for Nervous System Irritability Related to Preeclampsia

1. Place the woman in the supine position.
2. Have the client slightly bend her knee and place a hand under the knee to support it.
3. Dorsiflex the foot briskly and then quickly release it.
4. Watch for the foot to rebound smoothly against your hand. If the movement is smooth without any rapid contractions of the ankle or calf muscle, then clonus is not present; if the movement is jerky and rapid, clonus is present.
5. Repeat on the opposite side.

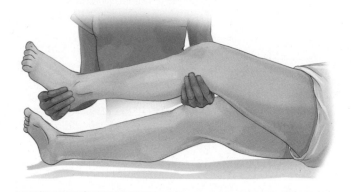

less than 12 breaths per minute, absence of deep tendon reflexes, and a decrease in urinary output, below 30 mL per hour. Also monitor serum magnesium levels. Although exact levels may vary among agencies, serum magnesium levels ranging from 4 to 7 mEq/L are considered therapeutic, whereas levels more than 8 mEq/dL are generally considered toxic. As levels increase, the woman is at risk for severe problems:

- 10 mEq/L: possible loss of DTRs
- 15 mEq/L: possible respiratory depression
- 25 mEq/L: possible cardiac arrest (Podymow & August, 2007)

If signs and symptoms of magnesium toxicity develop, expect to administer calcium gluconate as the antidote.

Throughout the client's stay, closely monitor her for signs and symptoms of labor. Perform continuous electronic fetal monitoring to assess fetal well-being. Note trends in baseline rate and presence or absence of accelerations or decelerations. Also observe for signs of fetal distress and report them immediately. Administer glucocorticoid treatment as ordered to enhance fetal lung maturity and prepare for labor induction if the mother's condition warrants.

Keep the client and family informed of the woman's condition and educate them about the course of treatment. Provide emotional support for the client and family. Severe preeclampsia is very frightening for the client and her family, and most expectant mothers are very anxious about their own health as well as that of the fetus. To allay anxiety, use light touch to comfort and reassure her that the necessary actions are being taken. Actively listening to her concerns and fears and communicating them to the health care provider is important in keeping lines of communication open. Offering praise for small accomplishments can provide positive reinforcement for behaviors that should be continued.

Intervening for Eclampsia

The onset of seizure activity identifies eclampsia. Typically, eclamptic seizures are generalized and start with facial twitching. The body then becomes rigid, in a state of tonic muscular contraction. The clonic phase of the seizure involves alternating contraction and relaxation of all body muscles. Respirations stop during seizure activity and resume shortly after it ends. Client safety is the primary concern during eclamptic seizures. If possible, turn the client to her side and remain with her. Make sure that the side rails are up and padded. Dim the lights and keep the room quiet.

Document the time and sequence of events as soon as possible. After the seizure activity has ceased, suction the nasopharynx as necessary and administer oxygen. Continue the magnesium sulfate infusion to prevent further seizures. Ensure continuous electronic fetal monitoring, evaluating fetal status for changes. Also assess the client for uterine contractions. After the client is stabilized, prepare her for the birthing process as soon as possible to reduce the risk of perinatal mortality.

Providing Follow-Up Care

After delivery of the newborn, continue to monitor the client for signs and symptoms of preeclampsia/eclampsia for at least 48 hours. Expect to continue to administer magnesium sulfate infusion for 24 hours to prevent seizure activity, and monitor serum magnesium levels for toxicity.

Assess vital signs at least every 4 hours, along with routine postpartum assessments—fundus, lochia, breasts, bladder, bowels, and emotional state attention when performing the fundal assessment and assessing lochia. Monitor urine output closely. Diuresis is a positive sign that, along with a decrease in proteinuria, signals resolution of the disease.

HELLP

HELLP is an acronym for hemolysis, elevated liver enzymes, and low platelets. HELLP syndrome occurs in about 20% of pregnant women diagnosed with severe preeclampsia. Although it has been reported as early as 17 weeks' gestation, most of the time it is diagnosed between 22 and 36 weeks' gestation (White, 2006). HELLP syndrome leads to an increased maternal risk for developing liver hematoma or rupture, stroke, cardiac arrest, seizure, pulmonary edema, DIC, subendocardial hemorrhage, adult respiratory distress syndrome, renal damage, sepsis, hypoxic encephalopathy, and maternal or fetal death (White, 2006).

Pathophysiology

The hemolysis that occurs is termed microangiopathic hemolytic anemia. It is thought to happen when red blood cells become fragmented as they pass through small, damaged blood vessels. Elevated liver enzymes are the result of reduced blood flow to the liver secondary to obstruction from fibrin deposits. Hyperbilirubinemia and jaundice result from liver impairment. Low platelets result from vascular damage, the result of vasospasm, and platelets aggregate at sites of damage, resulting in thrombocytopenia in multiple sites (Basama & Granger, 2007).

Therapeutic Management

The treatment for HELLP syndrome is based on the severity of the disease, the gestational age of the fetus, and the condition of the mother and fetus. The client should be admitted or transferred to a tertiary center with a neonatal intensive care unit. Additional treatments include magnesium sulfate, antihypertensives, and correction of the coagulopathies that accompany HELLP syndrome. After this syndrome is diagnosed and the woman's condition is stable, birth of the infant is indicated.

Magnesium sulfate is used prophylactically to prevent seizures. Antihypertensives such as hydralazine or labetalol are given to control blood pressure. Blood component therapy—such as fresh-frozen plasma, packed red cells, or platelets—is transfused to address the microangiopathic hemolytic anemia. Birth may be delayed up to 96 hours so that betamethasone or dexamethasone can be given to stimulate lung maturation in the preterm fetus.

Nursing Assessment

Nursing assessment of the woman with HELLP is similar to that for the woman with severe preeclampsia. Be alert for complaints of nausea (with or without vomiting), malaise, epigastric or right upper quadrant pain, and demonstrable edema. Perform systematic assessments frequently, as indicated by the woman's condition and response to therapy.

A diagnosis of HELLP syndrome is made based on laboratory test results, including:

- Low hematocrit that is not explained by any blood loss
- Elevated LDH (liver impairment)
- Elevated AST (liver impairment)
- Elevated ALT (liver impairment)

- Elevated BUN
- Elevated bilirubin level
- Elevated uric acid and creatinine levels (renal involvement)
- Low platelet count (less than 100,000 cells/mm³)

Nursing Management

Nursing management of the woman diagnosed with HELLP syndrome is the same as that for the woman with severe preeclampsia. Closely monitor the client for changes and provide ongoing support throughout this experience.

Gestational Diabetes

Gestational diabetes is a condition involving glucose intolerance that occurs during pregnancy. It is discussed in greater detail in Chapter 20.

Blood Incompatibility

Blood incompatibility most commonly involves blood type or the Rh factor. Blood type incompatibility, also known as ABO incompatibility, is not as severe a condition as Rh incompatibility. ABO incompatibility rarely causes significant hemolysis, and antepartum treatment is not warranted. Rh sensitization occurs in approximately 1 in 1,000 births to Rh-negative women (Salem, 2007).

According to the CDC (2007), Rh disease affected 16,000 newborns in the United States annually before RhoGAM administration was used to prevent it. Despite prevention measures, there still are approximately 4,000 infants annually affected with Rh disease.

Pathophysiology

Hemolysis associated with ABO incompatibility is limited to type O mothers with fetuses who have type A or B blood. In mothers with type A and B blood, naturally occurring antibodies are of IgM class, which do not cross the placenta, whereas in type O mothers, the antibodies are predominantly IgG in nature. Because A and B antigens are widely expressed in a variety of tissues besides red blood cells, only a small portion of antibodies crossing the placenta are available to bind to fetal red cells. In addition, fetal red cells appear to have less surface expression of A or B antigen, resulting in few reactive sites—hence the low incidence of significant hemolysis in affected neonates.

With ABO incompatibility, usually the mother is blood type O, with anti-A and anti-B antibodies in her serum; the infant is blood type A, B, or AB. The incompatibility arises as a result of the interaction of antibodies present in maternal serum and the antigen sites on the fetal red cells.

Rh incompatibility is a condition that develops when a woman with Rh-negative blood type is exposed to Rh-positive blood cells and subsequently develops circulating titers of Rh antibodies. Individuals with Rh-positive blood type have the D antigen present on their red cells, whereas individuals with an Rh-negative blood type do not. The presence or absence of the Rh antigen on the red blood cell membrane is genetically controlled.

In the United States, 15% of the population lack the Rh surface antigen on the erythrocyte and are considered Rh negative. The vast majority (85%) of individuals are considered Rh positive (Alan, 2007).

Rh incompatibility most commonly arises with exposure of an Rh-negative mother to Rh-positive fetal blood during pregnancy or birth, during which time erythrocytes from the fetal circulation leak into the maternal circulation. After a significant exposure, alloimmunization or sensitization occurs. As a result, maternal antibodies are produced against the foreign Rh antigen.

Theoretically, fetal and maternal blood does not mix during pregnancy. In reality, however, small placental accidents (transplacental bleeds secondary to minor separation), abortions, ectopic pregnancy, abdominal trauma, trophoblastic disease, amniocentesis, placenta previa, and abruptio placentae allow fetal blood to enter the maternal circulation and initiate the production of antibodies to destroy Rh-positive blood. The amount of fetal blood necessary to produce Rh incompatibility varies. In one study, less than 1 mL of Rh-positive blood was shown to result in sensitization of women who are Rh negative (Salem, 2007).

Once sensitized, it takes approximately a month for Rh antibodies in the maternal circulation to cross over into the fetal circulation. In 90% of cases, sensitization occurs during delivery (Blackburn, 2007). Thus, most firstborn infants with Rh-positive blood type are not affected because the short period from first exposure of Rh-positive fetal erythrocytes to the birth of the infant is insufficient to produce a significant maternal IgG antibody response.

The risk and severity of alloimmune response increase with each subsequent pregnancy involving a fetus with Rh-positive blood. A second pregnancy with an Rh-positive fetus often produces a mildly anemic infant, whereas succeeding pregnancies produce infants with more serious hemolytic anemia.

Nursing Assessment

At the first prenatal visit, determine the woman's blood type and Rh status. Also obtain a thorough health history, noting any reports of previous events involving hemorrhage to delineate the risk for prior sensitization. When the client's history reveals an Rh-negative mother who may be pregnant with an Rh-positive fetus, prepare the client for an antibody screen (indirect Coombs test) to determine whether she has developed isoimmunity to the Rh antigen. This test detects unexpected circulating antibodies in a woman's serum that could be harmful to the fetus (Gilbert, 2007).

Nursing Management

If the indirect Coombs test is negative (meaning no antibodies are present), then the woman is a candidate for RhoGAM. If the test is positive, RhoGAM is of no value because isoimmunization has occurred. In this case, the fetus is carefully monitored for hemolytic disease.

The incidence of isoimmunization has declined dramatically as a result of prenatal and postnatal RhoGAM administration after any event in which blood transfer may occur. The standard dose is 300 µg, which is effective for 30 mL of fetal blood. Rh immunoglobulin helps to destroy any fetal cells in the maternal circulation before sensitization occurs, thus inhibiting maternal antibody production. This provides temporary passive immunity, thereby preventing maternal sensitization.

The current recommendation is that every Rh-negative nonimmunized woman receives RhoGAM at 28 weeks' gestation and again within 72 hours after giving birth. Other indications for RhoGAM include:

- Ectopic pregnancy
- Chorionic villus sampling
- Amniocentesis
- Prenatal hemorrhage
- Molar pregnancy
- Maternal trauma
- Percutaneous umbilical sampling
- Therapeutic or spontaneous abortion
- Fetal death
- Fetal surgery (Blackburn, 2007)

Despite the availability of RhoGAM and laboratory tests to identify women and newborns at risk, isoimmunization remains a serious clinical reality that continues to contribute to perinatal and neonatal mortality. Nurses, as client advocates, are in a unique position to make sure test results are brought to the health care provider's attention so appropriate interventions can be initiated. In addition, nurses must stay abreast of current literature and research regarding isoimmunization and its management. Stress to all women that early prenatal care can help identify and prevent this condition. Since Rh incompatibility is preventable with the use of RhoGAM, prevention remains the best treatment. Nurses can make a tremendous impact to ensure positive outcomes for the greatest possible number of pregnancies through education.

Amniotic Fluid Imbalances

Amniotic fluid develops from several maternal and fetal structures, including the amnion, chorion, maternal blood, fetal lungs, GI tract, kidneys, and skin. Any alteration in one or more of the various sources will alter the amount of amniotic fluid. Polyhydramnios and oligohydramnios are two imbalances associated with amniotic fluid.

▶ POLYHYDRAMNIOS

Polyhydramnios, also called hydramnios, is a condition in which there is too much amniotic fluid (more than 2,000 mL) surrounding the fetus between 32 and 36 weeks. It occurs in approximately 3% of all pregnancies and is associated with fetal anomalies of development (Rajiah & Banerjee, 2007). It is associated with poor fetal outcomes because of the increased incidence of preterm births, fetal malpresentation, and cord prolapse.

There are several causes of polyhydramnios. Generally, too much fluid is being produced, there is a problem with the fluid being taken up, or both. It can be associated with maternal disease and fetal anomalies, but it can also be idiopathic in nature.

Therapeutic Management

Treatment may include close monitoring and frequent follow-up visits with the health care provider if the hydramnios is mild to moderate. In severe cases in which the woman is in pain and experiencing shortness of breath, an amniocentesis or artificial rupture of the membranes is done to reduce the fluid and the pressure. Removal of fluid by amniocentesis is only transiently effective. A noninvasive treatment may involve the use of a prostaglandin synthesis inhibitor (indomethacin) to decrease amniotic fluid volume by decreasing fetal urinary output, but this may cause premature closure of the fetal ductus arteriosus (Boyd & Carter, 2007).

Nursing Assessment

Begin the assessment with a thorough history, being alert to risk factors such as maternal diabetes or multiple gestation. Review the maternal history for information about possible fetal anomalies, including fetal esophageal or intestinal atresia, neural tube defects, chromosomal deviations, fetal hydrops, central nervous system or cardiovascular anomalies, and hydrocephaly.

Determine the gestational age of the fetus and measure the woman's fundal height. With hydramnios, there is a discrepancy between fundal height and gestational age, or a rapid growth of the uterus is noted. Assess the woman for complaints of discomfort in her abdomen, such as being severely stretched and tight. Also note any reports of uterine contractions, which may result from overstretching of the uterus. Assess for shortness of breath resulting from pressure on her diaphragm and inspect her lower extremities for edema, which results from increased pressure on the vena cava.

Palpate the abdomen and obtain fetal heart rate. Often the fetal parts and heart rate are difficult to obtain because of the excess fluid present.

Prepare the woman for possible diagnostic testing to evaluate for the presence of possible fetal anomalies. An ultrasound usually is done to measure the pockets of amniotic fluid to estimate the total volume. In some cases, ultrasound also is helpful in finding the etiology of polyhydramnios, such as multiple pregnancy or a fetal structural anomaly.

Nursing Management

Nursing management of the woman with polyhydramnios focuses on ongoing assessment and monitoring for symptoms of abdominal pain, dyspnea, uterine contractions, and edema of the lower extremities. Explain to the woman and her family that this condition can cause her uterus to become overdistended and may lead to preterm labor and preterm rupture of membranes. Outline the signs and symptoms of both conditions and instruct the woman to contact her health care provider if they do occur. If a therapeutic amniocentesis is performed, assist the health care provider and monitor maternal and fetal status throughout for any changes.

▶ OLIGOHYDRAMNIOS

Oligohydramnios is a decreased amount of amniotic fluid (less than 500 mL) between 32 weeks and 36 weeks' gestation. It occurs in 5% to 8% of all pregnancies. Oligohydramnios may result from any condition that prevents the fetus from making urine or blocks it from going into the amniotic sac.

This condition puts the fetus at an increased risk of perinatal morbidity and mortality (Blackburn, 2007). Reduction in amniotic fluid reduces the ability of the fetus to move freely without risk of cord compression, which increases the risk for fetal death and intrapartal hypoxia.

Therapeutic Management

The woman with oligohydramnios can be managed on an outpatient basis with serial ultrasounds and fetal surveillance through nonstress testing and biophysical profiles. As long as fetal well-being is demonstrated with frequent testing, no intervention is necessary. If fetal well-being is compromised, however, birth is planned along with amnioinfusion (the transvaginal infusion of crystalloid fluid to compensate for the lost amniotic fluid). The fluid is introduced into the uterus through an intrauterine pressure catheter. The infusion is administered in a controlled fashion to prevent overdistention of the uterus. Amnioinfusion is thought to improve abnormal fetal heart rate patterns, decrease cesarean births, and possibly minimize the risk of neonatal meconium aspiration syndrome (Norwitz & Schorge, 2006).

Nursing Assessment

Review the maternal history for factors associated with oligohydramnios, including:

- Uteroplacental insufficiency
- Premature rupture of membranes prior to labor onset
- Hypertension of pregnancy
- Maternal diabetes
- Intrauterine growth restriction
- Postterm pregnancy
- Fetal renal agenesis
- Polycystic kidneys
- Urinary tract obstructions

Assess the client for complaints of fluid leaking from the vagina. Leaking of amniotic fluid from the vagina occurs with rupture of the amniotic sac. Leaking in conjunction with a uterus that is small for expected dates of gestation also suggests oligohydramnios. Unfortunately, the woman may not present with any symptoms. Typically, the reduced volume of amniotic fluid is identified on ultrasound.

Nursing Management

Nursing management of the woman with oligohydramnios involves continuous monitoring of fetal well-being during nonstress testing or during labor and birth by identifying nonreassuring patterns on the fetal monitor. Variable decelerations indicating cord compression are common. Changing the woman's position might be therapeutic in altering this fetal heart rate pattern. After the birth, evaluate the newborn for signs of postmaturity, congenital anomalies, and respiratory difficulty.

Assist with amnioinfusion as indicated and continue to assess the woman's vital signs, contraction status, and fetal heart rate throughout the procedure. Provide comfort measures such as changing the bed linens and the woman's bed clothes frequently because of the constant leakage of fluid from the vagina. Also provide frequent perineal care during the infusion.

Multiple Gestation

Multiple gestation is defined as more than one fetus being born to a pregnant woman. This includes twins, triplets, and higher-order multiples such as quadruplets on up. In the past two decades, the number of multiple gestations in the United States has jumped dramatically because of the widespread use of fertility drugs, older women having babies, and assisted reproductive technologies to treat infertility. About one third of live births from assisted reproductive technology result in more than one infant, and twins represent 85% of those multiple-birth children (Grainger, Frazier, & Rowland, 2006). In the United States, the overall prevalence of twins is approximately 12 per 1,000, and two thirds are dizygotic (Zach & Pramanik, 2007). The increasing number of multiple gestations is a concern because women who are expecting more than one infant are at high risk for preterm labor, hydramnios, hyperemesis gravidarum, anemia, preeclampsia, and antepartum hemorrhage. Fetal/newborn risks or complications include prematurity, respiratory distress syndrome, birth asphyxia/perinatal depression, congenital anomalies (central nervous system, cardiovascular, and GI defects), twin-to-twin transfusion syndrome (transfusion of blood from one twin [i.e., donor] to the other twin [i.e., recipient]), intrauterine growth restriction, and becoming conjoined twins (Zach & Pramanik, 2007).

The two types of twins are monozygotic and dizygotic (Fig. 19.6). Monozygotic twins develop when a single, fertilized ovum splits during the first 2 weeks after conception. Monozygotic twins also are called identical twins. Two sperm fertilizing two ova produce dizygotic twins, which are called fraternal twins. Separate amnions, chorions, and placentas are formed in dizygotic twins. Triplets can be monozygotic, dizygotic, or trizygotic.

Therapeutic Management

When a multiple gestation is confirmed, the woman is followed with serial ultrasounds to assess fetal growth patterns and development. Biophysical profiles along with nonstress tests are ordered to determine fetal well-being. Many women are hospitalized in late pregnancy to prevent preterm labor and receive closer surveillance. During the intrapartum period the woman is closely monitored, with a perinatal team available to assist after birth. Operative delivery is frequently needed due to fetal malpresentation.

Nursing Assessment

Obtain a health history and physical examination. Be alert for complaints of fatigue and severe nausea and vomiting. Assess the woman's abdomen and fundal height. Typically with a multiple gestation the uterus is larger than expected based on the estimated date of birth. Laboratory test results may reveal anemia. Prepare the woman for ultrasound, which typically confirms the diagnosis of a multiple gestation.

Nursing Management

During the prenatal period, care focuses on providing education and support for the woman in areas of nutrition, increased rest periods, and close observation for pregnancy complications—anemia, excessive weight gain, proteinuria, edema, vaginal bleeding, and hypertension. Instruct the woman to be alert for and report immediately any signs and symptoms of preterm labor—contractions, uterine cramping, low back ache, increase in vaginal discharge, loss of mucus plug, pelvic pain, and pressure.

With the onset of labor, expect to monitor fetal heart rates continuously. Prepare the woman for an ultrasound to assess the presentation of each fetus to determine the best delivery approach. Ensure that extra nursing staff and the perinatal team are available for any birth or newborn complications.

After the babies are born, closely assess the woman for hemorrhage by frequently assessing uterine involution. Palpate the uterine fundus and monitor the amount and characteristics of lochia.

Throughout the entire pregnancy, birth, and hospital stay, inform and support the woman and her family. Encourage them to ask questions and verbalize any fears and concerns.

Premature Rupture of Membranes

Premature rupture of membranes (**PROM**) is the rupture of the bag of waters before the onset of true labor. There are a number of associated conditions and complications, such as infection, prolapsed cord, abruptio placentae, and preterm labor. This is the single most common diagnosis associated with preterm births (Gilbert, 2007).

PROM occurs in approximately 12% of all births (ACOG, 2007b). If prolonged (greater than 24 hours), the woman's risk for infection (chorioamnionitis, endometritis, sepsis, and neonatal infections) increases and

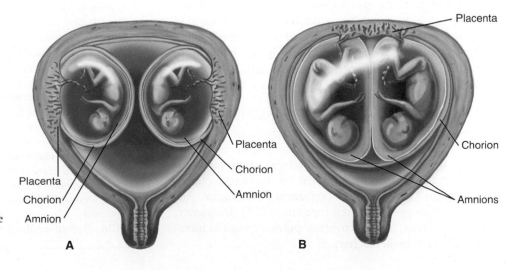

FIGURE **19.6** Multiple gestation with twins. (**A**) Dizygotic twins, where each fetus has its own placenta, amnion, and chorion. (**B**) Monozygotic twins, where the fetuses share one placenta, two amnions, and one chorion.

Placenta
Chorion
Amnion
Placenta
Chorion
Amnion
A

Placenta
Chorion
Amnions
B

this risk continues to increase as the duration of rupture time increases. The time interval from rupture of membranes to the onset of regular contractions is termed the latent period.

The terminology pertaining to PROM can be confusing. PROM is rupture of the membranes prior to the onset of labor and is used appropriately when referring to a woman who is beyond 37 weeks' gestation, has presented with spontaneous rupture of the membranes, and is not in labor. Related terms include **preterm premature rupture of membranes (PPROM)**, which is defined as rupture of membranes prior to the onset of labor in a woman who is *less* than 37 weeks of gestation. Perinatal risks associated with PPROM may stem from immaturity, including respiratory distress syndrome, intraventricular hemorrhage, patent ductus arteriosus, and necrotizing enterocolitis.

The exact cause of PROM is not known. In many cases, PROM occurs spontaneously.

Therapeutic Management

Treatment of PROM typically depends on the gestational age. Under no circumstances is an unsterile digital cervical examination done until the woman enters active labor, to minimize infection exposure. If the fetal lungs are mature, induction of labor is initiated. PROM is not a lone indicator for surgical birth. If the fetal lungs are immature, expectant management is carried out with adequate hydration, reduced physical activity, pelvic rest, and close observation for possible infection, such as with frequent monitoring of vital signs and laboratory test results (e.g., the white blood cell count). Corticosteroids may be given to enhance fetal lung maturity if lungs are immature, although this remains controversial. Recent studies have shown clear benefits of antibiotics to decrease neonatal morbidity associated with PPROM (ACOG, 2007b).

Nursing Assessment

Nursing assessment focuses on obtaining a complete health history and performing a physical examination to determine maternal and fetal status. An accurate assessment of the gestational age and knowledge of the maternal, fetal, and neonatal risks are essential to appropriate evaluation, counseling, and management of women with PROM and PPROM.

Health History and Physical Examination

Review the maternal history for risk factors such as infection, increased uterine size (hydramnios, macrosomia, multifetal gestation), uterine and fetal anomalies, lower socioeconomic status, STIs, cervical insufficiency, vaginal bleeding, and cigarette smoking during pregnancy. Ask about any history or current symptoms of UTI (frequency, urgency, dysuria, or flank pain) or pelvic or vaginal infection (pain or vaginal discharge).

Assess for signs and symptoms of labor, such as cramping, pelvic pressure, or back pain. Also assess her vital signs, noting any signs indicative of infection such as fever and elevated white blood cell count (more than 18,000 cells/mm^3) (Jazayeri & Galan, 2007).

Institute continuous electronic fetal heart rate monitoring to evaluate fetal well-being. Conduct a vaginal examination to ascertain the cervical status in PROM. If PPROM exists, a sterile speculum examination (where the examiner inspects the cervix but does not palpate it) is done rather than a digital cervical examination because it may diminish latency (period of time from rupture of membranes to birth) and increase newborn morbidity (Cunningham et al., 2005).

Observe the characteristics of the amniotic fluid. Note any evidence of meconium, or a foul odor. When meconium is present in the amniotic fluid, it typically indicates fetal distress related to hypoxia. Meconium stains the fluid yellow to greenish brown, depending on the amount present. A foul odor of amniotic fluid indicates infection. Also observe the amount of fluid. A decreased amount of amniotic fluid reduces the cushioning effect, thereby making cord compression a possibility. Key assessments are summarized in Box 19.3.

Laboratory and Diagnostic Testing

To diagnose PROM or PPROM, several procedures may be used: the Nitrazine test, fern test, or ultrasound. After the insertion of a sterile speculum, a sample of the fluid

---

BOX 19.3 Key Assessments With Premature Rupture of Membranes

For the woman with PROM, the following assessments are essential:

- Determining the date, time, and duration of membrane rupture by client interview
- Ascertaining gestational age of the fetus based on date of mother's LMP, fundal height, and ultrasound dating
- Questioning the woman about possible history of or recent UTI or vaginal infection that might have contributed to PROM
- Assessing for any associated labor symptoms, such as back pain or pelvic pressure
- Assisting with or performing diagnostic tests to validate leakage of fluid, such as Nitrazine test, "ferning" on slide, and ultrasound
- Continually assessing for signs of infection including
  - Elevation of maternal temperature and pulse rate
  - Abdominal/uterine tenderness
  - Fetal tachycardia more than 160 bpm
  - Elevated white blood cell count and C-reactive protein
  - Cloudy, foul-smelling amniotic fluid

in the vaginal area is obtained. With a Nitrazine test, pH of the fluid is tested; amniotic fluid is more basic (7.0) than normal vaginal secretions (4.5). Nitrazine paper turns blue in the presence of amniotic fluid. However, false-positive results can occur if blood, urine, semen, or antiseptic chemicals are also present; all will increase the pH.

For the fern test, a sample of vaginal fluid is place on a slide to be viewed directly under a microscope. Amniotic fluid will develop a fern-like pattern when it dries because of sodium chloride crystallization. If both of these tests are inconclusive, a transvaginal ultrasound can also be used to determine whether membranes have ruptured by demonstrating a decreased amount of amniotic fluid (oligohydramnios) in the uterus (Jazayeri & Galan, 2007).

Other laboratory and diagnostic tests that may be used include:

- Urinalysis and urine culture for UTI or asymptomatic bacteriuria
- Cervical test or culture for chlamydia or gonorrhea
- Vaginal culture for bacterial vaginosis and trichomoniasis
- Vaginal introital/rectal culture for group B streptococcus

Nursing Management

Nursing management for the woman with PROM or PPROM focuses on preventing infection and identifying uterine contractions. The risk for infection is great because of the break in the amniotic fluid membrane and its close proximity to vaginal bacteria. Therefore, monitor maternal vital signs closely. Be alert for a temperature elevation or an increase in pulse, which could indicate infection. Also monitor the fetal heart rate continuously, reporting any fetal tachycardia (which could indicate a maternal infection) or variable decelerations (suggesting cord compression). If variable decelerations are present, anticipate amnioinfusion based on agency policy. Evaluate the results of laboratory tests such as a CBC. An elevation in white blood cells would suggest infection. Administer antibiotics if ordered.

Encourage the woman and her partner to verbalize their feelings and concerns. Educate them about the purpose of the protective membranes and the implications of early rupture. Keep them informed about planned interventions, including potential complications and required therapy. As appropriate, prepare the woman for induction or augmentation of labor as appropriate if she is near term.

If labor doesn't start within 48 hours, the woman with PPROM may be discharged home on expectant management, which may include:

- Antibiotics if cervicovaginal cultures are positive
- Activity restrictions
- Education about signs and symptoms of infection and when to call with problems or concerns (Teaching Guidelines 19.3)

TEACHING GUIDELINES 19.3

Teaching for the Woman With PPROM

- Monitor your baby's activity by performing fetal kick counts daily.
- Check your temperature daily and report any temperature increases to your health care provider.
- Watch for signs related to the beginning of labor. Report any tightening of the abdomen or contractions.
- Avoid any touching or manipulating of your breasts, which could stimulate labor.
- Do not insert anything into your vagina or vaginal area.
- Maintain any specific activity restrictions as recommended.
- Wash your hands thoroughly after using the bathroom and make sure to wipe from front to back each time.
- Keep your perineal area clean and dry.
- Take your antibiotics as directed if your health care provider has prescribed them.
- Call your health care provider with changes in your condition, including fever, uterine tenderness, feeling like your heart is racing, and foul-smelling vaginal discharge.

- Frequent fetal testing for well-being
- Ultrasound every 3 to 4 weeks to assess amniotic fluid levels
- Possible corticosteroid treatment depending on gestational age
- Daily kick counts to assess fetal well-being

▪▪▪ Key Concepts

▪ Identifying risk factors early on and ongoing throughout the pregnancy is important to ensure the best outcome for every pregnancy. Risk assessment should start with the first prenatal visit and continue with subsequent visits.

▪ The three most common causes of hemorrhage early in pregnancy (first half of pregnancy) are spontaneous abortion, ectopic pregnancy, and GTD.

▪ Ectopic pregnancies occur in about 1 in 50 pregnancies and have increased dramatically during the past few decades.

▪ Having a molar pregnancy results in the loss of the pregnancy and the possibility of developing choriocarcinoma, a chronic malignancy from the trophoblastic tissue.

▪ The classic clinical picture presentation for placenta previa is painless, bright-red vaginal bleeding occurring during the third trimester.

- Treatment of abruptio placentae is designed to assess, control, and restore the amount of blood lost; to provide a positive outcome for both mother and infant; and to prevent coagulation disorders.

- DIC can be described in simplest terms as a loss of balance between the clot-forming activity of thrombin and the clot-lysing activity of plasmin.

- Hyperemesis gravidarum is a complication of pregnancy characterized by persistent, uncontrollable nausea and vomiting before the 20th week of gestation.

- Gestational hypertension is the leading cause of maternal death in the United States and the most common complication reported during pregnancy.

- HELLP is an acronym for hemolysis, elevated liver enzymes, and low platelets.

- Rh incompatibility is a condition that develops when a woman of Rh-negative blood type is exposed to Rh-positive fetal blood cells and subsequently develops circulating titers of Rh antibodies.

- Hydramnios occurs in approximately 3 to 4% of all pregnancies and is associated with fetal anomalies of development.

- Nursing care related to the woman with oligohydramnios involves continuous monitoring of fetal well-being during nonstress testing or during labor and birth by identifying nonreassuring patterns on the fetal monitor.

- The increasing number of multiple gestations is a concern because women who are expecting more than one infant are at high risk for preterm labor, hydramnios, hyperemesis gravidarum, anemia, preeclampsia, and antepartum hemorrhage.

- Nursing care related to PROM centers on infection prevention and identification of preterm labor contractions.

- Early identification of preterm labor would allow for appropriate interventions that may prolong the pregnancy, such as transferring the woman to a facility with a neonatal intensive care unit for prenatal care, administering glucocorticoids to the mother to promote fetal lung maturity, and giving appropriate antibiotics to treat infections to arrest the labor process.

- It is essential that nurses teach all pregnant women how to detect the early symptoms of preterm labor and what to do if they experience contractions or cramping that does not go away.

REFERENCES

Alan, R. (2007). *Rh incompatibility and isoimmunization.* March of Dimes. Available at: http://healthlibrary.epnet.com/Get Content.aspx?token=8482e079-8512-47c2-960c-a403c77a5e4c&chunkiid=11595.

American Academy of Pediatrics, American College of Obstetricians and Gynecologists. (2003). *Guidelines for perinatal care* (5th ed.). Washington, DC: Author.

American College of Obstetricians and Gynecologists (ACOG). (2003). ACOG practice bulletin: Cervical insufficiency. *Obstetrics and Gynecology, 102,* 1091–1099.

American College of Obstetricians and Gynecologists (ACOG). (2007a). *ACOG practice bulletin: Diagnosis and management of preeclampsia and eclampsia updated.* Number 33. Washington, DC: Author.

American College of Obstetricians and Gynecologists (ACOG). (2007b). ACOG Practice Bulletin No. 80: Premature rupture of membranes. *Obstetrics and Gynecology, 109*(4), 1007–1020.

Arenson, J., & Drake, P. (2007). *Maternal and newborn health.* Sudbury, MA: Jones and Bartlett Publishers.

Bakken, I. J., Skjeldestad, F. E., & Nordbo, S. A. (2007). *Chlamydia trachomatis* infections increase the risk for ectopic pregnancy: A population-based, nested case-control study. *Sexually Transmitted Diseases, 34*(3), 166–169.

Basama, F. M., & Granger, K. (2007). Case report: Postpartum class 1 HELLP syndrome. *Archives of Gynecology & Obstetrics, 275*(3), 187–189.

Bernasko, J., Lee, R., Pagano, M., & Kohn, N. (2006). Is routine prophylactic cervical cerclage associated with significant prolongation of triplet gestation? *Journal of Maternal-Fetal & Neonatal Medicine, 19*(9), 575–578.

Bick, R. L. (2007). Disseminated intravascular coagulation. In R. E. Rakel & E. T. Bope (Eds.), *Conn's current therapy 2007* (Section 6, pp. 502–505). Philadelphia: Saunders Elsevier.

Blackburn, S. (2007). *Maternal, fetal, and neonatal physiology: A clinical perspective* (3rd ed.). St. Louis: W. B. Saunders.

Blincoe, A. J. (2007). Hypertension in pregnancy: The importance of monitoring. *British Journal of Midwifery, 15*(1), 47–50.

Boyd, R. L., & Carter, B. S. (2007). Polyhydramnios and oligohydramnios. *eMedicine.* Available at: http://www.emedicine.com/ped/topic1854.htm.

Britt, D. W., Eden, R. D., & Evans, M. I. (2006). Matching risk and resources in high-risk pregnancies. *Journal of Maternal-Fetal and Neonatal Medicine, 19*(10), 645–650.

Brown-Guttovz, H. (2006). Myths and facts about ectopic pregnancy. *Nursing, 36*(8), 70.

Centers for Disease Control and Prevention (CDC). (2007). *Rh disease fact sheet.* Available at: http://www.marchofdimes.com/professionals/14332_1220.asp

Collins, N. J. (2007). Abruptio placentae. *Wild Iris Medical Education.* Available at: http://www.nursingceu.com/courses/81/index_nceu.html.

Condous, G. (2006). Ectopic pregnancy: Risk factors and diagnosis. *Australian Family Physician, 35*(11), 854–857.

Cunningham, F. G., Gant, N. F., Leveno, K. J., Gilstrap, L. C., Hauth, J. C., & Wenstrom, K. D. (2005). *Williams' obstetrics* (22nd ed.). New York: McGraw-Hill.

Deering, S. H., & Satin, A. (2007). Abruptio placentae. *eMedicine.* Available at www.emedicine.com/med/topic6.htm.

Evans, A. T. (2007). *Manual of Obstetrics* (7th ed.). Philadelphia: Lippincott Williams & Wilkins.

Fox, N. S., & Chervenak, F. A. (2008). Cervical cerclage: A review of the evidence. *Obstetrical & Gynecological Survey, 63*(1), 58–65.

Furlong, M. A., & Furlong, B. R. (2007). Disseminated intravascular coagulation. *eMedicine.* Available at: http://www.emedicine.com/emerg/topic150.htm.

Garner, E. I., Goldstein, D. P., Feltmate, C. M., & Berkowitz, R. S. (2007). Gestational trophoblastic disease. *Clinical Obstetrics & Gynecology, 50*(1), 112–122.

Gaufberg, S. V. (2007). Abruptio placentae. *eMedicine.* Available at www.emedicine.com/emerg/topic12.htm.

Gibson, P., & Carson, M. (2007). Hypertension and pregnancy. *eMedicine.* Available at: http://www.emedicine.com/med/topic3250.htm.

Gilbert, E. (2007). *Manual of high-risk pregnancy and delivery* (4th ed.). St. Louis: Mosby, Inc.

Grainger, D. A., Frazier, L. M., & Rowland, C. A. (2006). Preconception care and treatment with assisted reproductive technologies. *Maternal & Child Health Journal, 10*(5), Supplement: S161–164.

Hajenius, P. J., Mol, F., Mol, B. W. J., Bossuyt, P. M. M., Ankum, W. M., & van der Veen, F. (2007). Interventions for tubal ectopic pregnancy. *Cochrane Database of Systematic Reviews* 2007. Issue 1. Art. No.: CD000324.DOI: 10.1002/14651858.CD000324.pub2.

Hernandez, E. (2007). Gestational trophoblastic neoplasia. *eMedicine.* Available at: http://www.emedicine.com/med/topic866.htm.

Hodgson, B. B., & Kizior, R. J. (2007). *Saunders nursing drug handbook.* Philadelphia: Elsevier Health Sciences.

Jazayeri, A., & Galan, H. (2007). Premature rupture of membranes. *eMedicine*. Available at: http://www.emedicine.com/med/topic3256.htm.

Joy, S., & Lyon, D. (2007). Placenta previa. *eMedicine*. Available at: www.emedicine.com/med/topics3271/htm.

Jung, D. C., & Erogul, M. (2007). Pregnancy, preeclampsia. *eMedicine*. Available at: http://www.emedicine.com/emerg/topic480.htm.

Ko, P., & Yoon, Y. (2007). Placenta previa. *eMedicine*. Available at: www.emedicine.com/emerg/topic427.htm.

Lamondy, A. M. (2007). Managing hyperemesis gravidarum. *Nursing, 37*(2), 66–68.

Lane, C. A. (2007). Nausea and vomiting of pregnancy: A tailored approach treatment. *Clinical Obstetrics & Gynecology, 50*(1), 100–111.

Lilley, L. L., Harrington, S., & Snyder, J. S. (2007). *Pharmacology and the nursing process* (5th ed.). Philadelphia: Elsevier Health Sciences.

Lipscomb, G. H. (2007). Ectopic pregnancy. In R. E. Rakel & E. T. Bope (Eds.), *Conn's current therapy 2007* (Section 16, pp. 1175–1178). Philadelphia: Saunders Elsevier.

Lotgering, F. K. (2007). Clinical aspects of cervical insufficiency. *BMC Pregnancy and Childbirth, 7*(1), 17–20.

March of Dimes (2007). *Ectopic pregnancy*. Available at: http://www.marchofdimes.com/pnhec/188_851.asp.

Moore, L. E., & Ware, L. E. (2007). Hydatidiform mole. *eMedicine*. Available at: http://www.emedicine.com/med/topic1047.htm.

Mundy, D. C. (2006). *Diagnosis and management of preeclampsia/eclampsia*. Available at: www.acog.org/acog_sections/download/MOPreeclampsia20061016.ppt- 2007-03-14.

National High Blood Pressure Education Program. (2000). Working Group in High Blood Pressure in Pregnancy report. *American Journal of Obstetrics and Gynecology, 183*, S1–S22.

Norwitz, E. R., & Schorge, J. O. (2006). *Obstetrics and gynecology at a glance* (2nd ed.). Malden, MA: Blackwell Publishing Ltd.

O'Brien, J. M. (2006). Management of cervical insufficiency and bulging fetal membranes. *Obstetrics & Gynecology, 107*(6), 1421–1422.

Ogunyemi, D. A. (2007). Hyperemesis gravidarum. *eMedicine*. Available at: http://www.emedicine.com/med/topic1075.htm.

Oppenheimer, L. (2007). Diagnosis and management of placenta previa. *Journal of Obstetrics & Gynecology Canada, 29*(3), 261–266.

Oyelese, Y., & Ananth, C. V. (2006). Placental abruption. *Obstetrics and Gynecology, 108*(4), 1005–1016.

Podymow, T., & August, P. (2007). Hypertension in pregnancy. *Advances in Chronic Kidney Disease, 14*(2), 178–190.

Price, S., Lake, M., Breen, G., Carson, G., Quinn, C., & O'Connor, T. (2007). The spiritual experience of high risk pregnancy. *JOGNN, 36*(1), 63–70.

Puscheck, E., & Pradhan, A. (2007). First-trimester pregnancy loss. *eMedicine*. Available at: http://www.emedicine.com/med/topic3310.htm.

Rajiah, P., & Banerjee, B. (2007). Polyhydramnios. *eMedicine*. Available at: http://www.emedicine.com/radio/topic566.htm.

Ressel, G. W. (2004). Practice guidelines: ACOG releases bulletin on managing cervical insufficiency. *American Family Physician*. Available at www.aafp.org/afp/20040115/practice.html.

Salem, L. (2007). Rh incompatibility. *eMedicine*. Available at www.emedicine.com/emerg/topic507.htm.

Selway, J. (2006). The challenge of ectopic pregnancy. *Journal for Nurse Practitioners, 2*(9), 583–592.

Sepilian, V., & Wood, E. (2007). Ectopic pregnancy. *eMedicine*. Available at www.emedicine.com/med/topic3212.htm.

Silver, R. M. (2007). Fetal death. *Obstetrics & Gynecology, 109*(1), 153–167.

Simpson, J. L. (2007). Causes of fetal wastage. *Clinical Obstetrics & Gynecology, 50*(1), 10–30.

U.S. Department of Health and Human Services. (2000). *Healthy people 2010* (conference edition, in two volumes). Washington, DC: Author.

Vidaeff, A. C., & Ramin, S. M. (2007). From concept to practice: The recent history of preterm delivery prevention: cervical competence. *American Journal of Perinatology, 23*(1), 3–13.

Vitthala, S., Cheema, M. K., & Misra, P. K. (2007). Medical management of ectopic pregnancy using methotrexate. *Internet Journal of Gynecology & Obstetrics, 6*(2), 4–10.

Vyas, N. A., Vink, J. S., Ghidini, A., Pezzullo, J. C., Korker, V., Landy, H. J., & Poggi, S. H. (2006). Risk factors for cervical insufficiency after term delivery. *American Journal of Obstetrics & Gynecology, 195*(3), 787–791.

Warden, M., & Euerle, B. (2007). Preeclampsia. *eMedicine*. Available at: http://www.emedicine.com/med/topic1905.htm.

Weber, J. R. (2007). *Nurses' handbook of health assessment* (6th ed.). Philadelphia: Lippincott Williams & Wilkins.

Weismiller, D. G. (2007). Hypertension disorders of pregnancy. In R. E. Rakel & E. T. Bope (Eds.), *Conn's current therapy 2007* (Section 16, pp. 1180–1189). Philadelphia: Saunders Elsevier.

White, A. (2006). Emergency care for patients with HELLP syndrome. *Advanced Emergency Nursing Journal, 28*(4), 338–345.

Wilcox, S. R., & Edelman, A. (2007). Pregnancy, hyperemesis gravidarum. *eMedicine*. Available at www.emedicine.com/emerg/topic479.htm.

Zach, T., & Pramanik, A. (2007). Multiple births. *eMedicine*. Available at www.emedicine.com/ped/topic2599.htm.

Zeltzer, J. S. (2007). Vaginal bleeding in late pregnancy. In R. E. Rakel & E. T. Bope (Eds.), *Conn's current therapy 2007* (Section 16, pp. 1178–1180). Philadelphia: Saunders Elsevier.

WEBSITES

American Academy of Pediatrics: www.aap.org

American College of Obstetricians and Gynecologists: www.acog.org

Association of Women's Health, Obstetric & Neonatal Nurses: www.awhonn.org

March of Dimes: www.modimes.org

Resolve through Sharing: www.ectopicpregnancy.com

Sidelines High-Risk Pregnancy Support Office: www.sidelines.org

CHAPTER WORKSHEET

MULTIPLE CHOICE QUESTIONS

1. A woman diagnosed with preeclampsia is to receive magnesium sulfate. The rationale for this drug is to:

    a. Reduce CNS irritability to prevent seizures

    b. Provide supplementation of an important mineral she needs

    c. Prevent constipation during and after the birthing process

    d. Decrease musculoskeletal tone to augment labor

2. A woman is suspected of having abruptio placentae. Which of the following would the nurse expect to assess as a classic symptom?

    a. Painless, bright-red bleeding

    b. "Knife-like" abdominal pain

    c. Excessive nausea and vomiting

    d. Hypertension and headache

3. RhoGAM is given to Rh-negative women to prevent maternal sensitization. In addition to pregnancy, Rh-negative women would also receive this medication after which of the following?

    a. Therapeutic or spontaneous abortion

    b. Head injury from a car accident

    c. Blood transfusion after a hemorrhage

    d. Unsuccessful artificial insemination procedure

4. After teaching a woman about hyperemesis gravidarum and how it differs from the typical nausea and vomiting of pregnancy, which statement by the woman indicates that the teaching was successful?

    a. "I can expect the nausea to last through my second trimester."

    b. "I should drink fluids with my meals instead of in between them."

    c. "I need to avoid strong odors, perfumes, or flavors."

    d. "I should lie down after I eat for about 2 hours."

5. A pregnant woman, approximately 12 weeks' gestation, comes to the emergency department after calling her health care provider's office and reporting moderate vaginal bleeding. Assessment reveals cervical dilation and moderately strong abdominal cramps. She reports that she has passed some tissue with the bleeding. The nurse interprets these findings to suggest which of the following?

    a. Threatened abortion

    b. Inevitable abortion

    c. Incomplete abortion

    d. Missed abortion

CRITICAL THINKING EXERCISES

1. Suzanne, a 16-year-old primigravida, presents to the maternity clinic complaining of continual nausea and vomiting for the past 3 days. She states she is approximately 15 weeks pregnant and has been unable to hold anything down or take any fluids in without throwing up for the past 3 days. She reports she is dizzy and weak. On examination, Suzanne appears pale and anxious. Her mucous membranes are dry, skin turgor is poor, and her lips are dry and cracked.

    a. What is your impression of this condition?

    b. What risk factors does Suzanne have?

    c. What intervention is appropriate for this woman?

2. Gloria is an obese 39-year-old primigravida of African-American descent who is diagnosed with gestational hypertension. Her history reveals that her sister developed preeclampsia during her pregnancy. When describing her diet to the nurse, Gloria mentions that she tends to eat a lot of fast food.

    a. What risk factors does Gloria have that increase her risk for gestational hypertension?

    b. When assessing Gloria, what assessment findings would lead the nurse to suspect that Gloria has developed severe preeclampsia?

STUDY ACTIVITIES

1. Ask a community health maternity nurse how the signs and symptoms of gestational hypertension (including preeclampsia and eclampsia) are taught, and how effective efforts have been to reduce the incidence in the area.

2. Find a website designed to help parents who have suffered a pregnancy loss secondary to a spontaneous abortion. What is its audience level? Is the information up to date?

3. A pregnancy in which the blastocyst implants outside the uterus is an _____ pregnancy.

4. The most serious complication of hydatidiform mole is the development of _____ afterward.

5. Discuss various activities a woman with a multiple gestation could engage in to help pass the time when ordered to be on bed rest at home for 2 months.

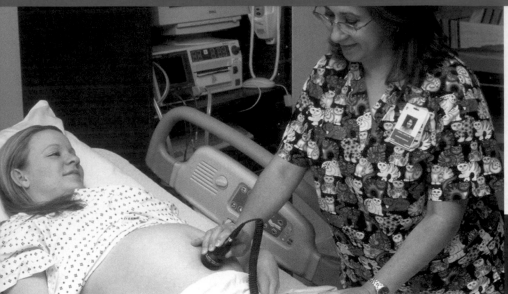

NURSING MANAGEMENT OF THE PREGNANCY AT RISK: SELECTED HEALTH CONDITIONS AND VULNERABLE POPULATIONS

KEY TERMS

acquired immunodeficiency
  syndrome (AIDS)
adolescence
anemia
fetal alcohol spectrum
  disorder (FASD)
gestational diabetes
  mellitus

glycosylated hemoglobin
  (HbA1C) level
human immunodeficiency
  virus (HIV)
impaired fasting glucose
impaired glucose tolerance
neonatal abstinence
  syndrome

perinatal drug abuse
pica
pregestational diabetes
teratogen
type 1 diabetes
type 2 diabetes

LEARNING OBJECTIVES

Upon completion of the chapter, the learner will be able to:

1. Identify at least two conditions present before pregnancy that can have a negative effect on a pregnancy.
2. Explain how a condition present before pregnancy can affect the woman physiologically and psychologically when she becomes pregnant.
3. Differentiate the nursing assessment and management for a pregnant woman with diabetes from that of a pregnant woman without diabetes.
4. Explore how congenital and acquired heart conditions can affect a woman's pregnancy.
5. Describe the nursing assessment and management of a pregnant woman with cardiovascular disorders and respiratory conditions.
6. Differentiate among the types of anemia affecting pregnant women in terms of prevention and management.
7. Describe the most common infections that can jeopardize a pregnancy, and propose possible preventive strategies.
8. Explain the nurse's role in the prevention and management of adolescent pregnancy.

Rose, a thin 16-year-old appearing very pregnant, came into the clinic wheezing and having difficulty catching her breath. She had missed several previous prenatal visits but arrived at the clinic today in distress. Rose has a history of asthma since she was 5 years old. How might Rose's current condition affect her pregnancy? Is this picture typical of the pregnant asthmatic?

Wow

As the sun sets each day, nurses should make sure they have done something for others, and should try to be understanding even under the most difficult of conditions.

LEARNING OBJECTIVES (continued)

9. Identify the impact of pregnancy on a woman over the age of 35.
10. Develop a plan of care for the pregnant woman who is HIV positive.
11. Examine the effects of substance abuse during pregnancy.

Pregnancy and childbirth are exciting yet complex facets within the continuum of women's health. Ideally the pregnant woman is free of any conditions that can affect a pregnancy, but in reality many women enter pregnancy with a multitude of health-related or psychosocial issues that can have a negative impact on the outcome.

Many pregnant women express the wish, "I hope my baby is born healthy." Nurses can play a major role in helping this become a reality by educating women before they become pregnant. Conditions such as diabetes, cardiac and respiratory disorders, anemias, and specific infections frequently can be controlled through close prenatal management so that their impact on pregnancy is minimized. Nurses can provide pregnancy-prevention strategies when counseling teenagers. Meeting the developmental needs of pregnant adolescents is a challenge. Finally, lifestyle choices can place many women at risk during pregnancy, and nurses need to remain non-judgmental in working with these special populations. Lifestyle choices such as use of alcohol, nicotine, and illicit substances during pregnancy are addressed in a National Health goal.

Chapter 19 described pregnancy-related conditions that place the woman at risk. This chapter addresses common conditions that can have a negative impact on the pregnancy and special populations at risk, outlining appropriate nursing assessment and management for each condition or situation. The unique skills of nurses, in conjunction with the other members of the health care team, can increase the potential for a positive outcome in many high-risk pregnancies.

Diabetes Mellitus

Diabetes mellitus is a chronic disease characterized by a relative lack of insulin or absence of the hormone, which is necessary for glucose metabolism. The chronic hyperglycemia of diabetes is associated with long-term damage, dysfunction, and failure of the eyes, kidneys, nerves, heart, and blood vessels. The prevalence of diabetes in the United States is increasing at an alarming rate, already reaching epidemic proportions. A contributing factor to these increasing rates is the incidence of obesity. Diabetes is a common endocrine disorder, affecting up to 14% of all pregnancies (American Diabetes Association [ADA], 2007a).

Diabetes commonly is classified based on disease etiology (ADA, 2007a). These groups include:

- **Type 1 diabetes**: absolute insulin deficiency (due to an autoimmune process); usually appears before the age of 30 years; approximately 10% of those diagnosed have type 1 diabetes
- **Type 2 diabetes**: insulin resistance or deficiency (related to obesity, sedentary lifestyle); diagnosed primarily in adults older than 30 years of age but is now being seen in children; accounts for 90% of all diagnosed cases.
- **Impaired fasting glucose** and **impaired glucose tolerance**: characterized by hyperglycemia at a level lower than what qualifies as a diagnosis of diabetes (fasting blood glucose level between 100 and 125 mg/dL; blood glucose level between 140 and 199 mg/dL after a 2-hour glucose tolerance test, respectively); symptoms of diabetes are absent; newborns are at risk for being large for gestational age (LGA)
- **Gestational diabetes mellitus**: glucose intolerance with its onset during pregnancy or first detected in pregnancy

During pregnancy, diabetes typically is categorized into two groups: **pregestational diabetes** (alteration in carbohydrate metabolism identified before conception), which includes women with type 1 or type 2 disease; and gestational diabetes, which develops during pregnancy.

HEALTHY PEOPLE 2010	
Objective	Significance
Increase abstinence from alcohol, cigarettes, and illicit drugs among pregnant women Increase in reported abstinence in the past month from substances by pregnant women Alcohol from a baseline of 86% to 94% Binge drinking from a baseline of 99% to 100% Cigarette smoking from abaseline of 87% to 99% Illicit drugs from a baseline of 98% to 100%	Will help to focus attention on measures for reducing substance exposure and use, thereby minimizing the effects of these substances on the fetus and newborn

USDHHS, 2000.

Pregestational diabetes complicates 0.2% to 0.3% of all pregnancies and affects more than 15,000 women annually. Gestational diabetes occurs in approximately 8% of all pregnant women, and those rates are higher among women of color. It is associated with either neonatal complications such as macrosomia, hypoglycemia, and birth trauma or maternal complications such as preeclampsia and cesarean birth. Gestational diabetes complicates more than 200,000 pregnancies annually in the United States and accounts for 90% of diabetic pregnancies (ADA, 2007a).

Before the discovery of insulin in 1922, most women with diabetes were infertile or experienced spontaneous abortion (March of Dimes, 2007b). Over the past several decades, great strides have been made in improving the outcomes of pregnancy in women with diabetes, but this chronic metabolic disorder remains a high-risk condition during pregnancy. A favorable outcome requires commitment on the woman's part to comply with frequent prenatal visits, dietary restrictions, self-monitoring of blood glucose levels, frequent laboratory tests, intensive fetal surveillance, and perhaps hospitalization.

Pathophysiology

With diabetes, there is a deficiency of or resistance to insulin. This alteration interferes with the body's ability to obtain essential nutrients for fuel and storage. If a pregnant woman has pregestational diabetes or develops gestational diabetes, the profound metabolic alterations that occur during pregnancy and that are necessary to support the growth and development of fetus can be affected.

▶ *Consider* THIS!

Scott and I had been busy all day setting up the new crib and nursery, and we finally sat down to rest. I was due any day, and we had been putting this off until we had a long weekend to complete the task. I was excited to think about all the frilly pinks that decorated her room. I was sure that my new daughter would love it as much as I loved her already. A few days later I barely noticed any fetal movement, but I thought that she must be as tired as I was by this point.

That night I went into labor and kept looking at the worried faces of the nurses and the midwife in attendance. I had been diagnosed with gestational diabetes a few months ago and had tried to follow the instructions regarding diet and exercise, but old habits are hard to change when you are 38 years old. I was finally told after a short time in the labor unit that they couldn't pick up a fetal heartbeat and an ultrasound was to be done—still no heartbeat was detected. Scott and I were finally told that our daughter was a stillborn. All I could think about was that she would never get to see all the pink colors in the nursery. . .

Maternal metabolism is directed toward supplying adequate nutrition for the fetus. In pregnancy, placental hormones cause insulin resistance at a level that tends to parallel the growth of the fetoplacental unit. As the placenta grows, more placental hormones are secreted. Human placental lactogen (hPL) and growth hormone (somatotropin) increase in direct correlation with the growth of placental tissue, rising throughout the last 20 weeks of pregnancy and causing insulin resistance. Subsequently, insulin secretion increases to overcome the resistance of these two hormones. In the nondiabetic pregnant woman, the pancreas can respond to the demands for increased insulin production to maintain normal glucose levels throughout the pregnancy (Cypryk et al., 2007). However, the woman with glucose intolerance or diabetes during pregnancy cannot cope with changes in metabolism resulting from insufficient insulin to meet the needs during gestation.

Over the course of pregnancy, insulin resistance changes. It peaks in the last trimester to provide more nutrients to the fetus. The insulin resistance typically results in postprandial hyperglycemia, although some women also have an elevated fasting blood glucose level (Homko & Reece, 2006). With this increased demand on the pancreas in late pregnancy, women with diabetes or glucose intolerance cannot accommodate the increased insulin demand; glucose levels rise as a result of insulin deficiency, leading to hyperglycemia. Subsequently, the mother and her fetus can experience major problems (Table 20.1).

Therapeutic Management

Preconception counseling is key for the woman with pregestational diabetes (the alteration in carbohydrate metabolism is identified before conception) to ensure that her disease state is stable. The goals of preconception care are to:

• Integrate the woman into the management of her diabetes
• Achieve the lowest glycosylated hemoglobin A1C test results without excessive hypoglycemia
• Ensure effective contraception until stable glycemia is achieved
• Identify and evaluate long-term diabetic complications such as retinopathy, nephropathy, neuropathy, cardiovascular disease, and hypertension (ADA, 2007b)

Excellent control of blood glucose, as evidenced by normal fasting blood glucose levels and a **glycosylated hemoglobin (HbA1C) level** (a measurement of the average glucose levels over the past 100 to 120 days), is crucial to achieve the best pregnancy outcome. A glycosylated hemoglobin level of less than 7% indicates good control; a value of more than 8% indicates poor control and warrants intervention (ADA, 2007b).

Preconception counseling also is important in helping to reduce the risk of congenital malformation. The most common malformations associated with diabetes occur in the renal, cardiac, skeletal, and central nervous systems. Since these defects occur by the eighth week of gestation, preconception counseling is critical. The rate of congenital anomalies in women with pregestational

TABLE 20.1 DIABETES AND PREGNANCY: EFFECTS ON THE MOTHER AND FETUS

Effects on the Mother	Effects on the Fetus/Neonate
• Polyhydramnios due to fetal diuresis caused by hyperglycemia • Gestational hypertension of unknown etiology • Ketoacidosis due to uncontrolled hyperglycemia • Preterm labor secondary to premature membrane rupture • Stillbirth in pregnancies complicated by ketoacidosis and poor glucose control • Hypoglycemia as glucose is diverted to the fetus (occurring in first trimester) • Urinary tract infections resulting from excess glucose in the urine (glucosuria), which promotes bacterial growth • Chronic monilial vaginitis due to glucosuria, which promotes growth of yeast • Difficult labor, cesarean birth, postpartum hemorrhage secondary to an overdistended uterus to accommodate a macrosomic infant	• Cord prolapse secondary to polyhydramnios and abnormal fetal presentation • Congenital anomaly due to hyperglycemia in the first trimester (cardiac problems, neural tube defects, skeletal deformities, and genitourinary problems) • Macrosomia resulting from hyperinsulinemia stimulated by fetal hyperglycemia • Birth trauma due to increased size of fetus, which complicates the birthing process (shoulder dystocia) • Preterm birth secondary to hydramnios and an aging placenta, which places the fetus in jeopardy if the pregnancy continues • Fetal asphyxia secondary to fetal hyperglycemia and hyperinsulinemia • Intrauterine growth restriction (IUGR) secondary to maternal vascular impairment and decreased placental perfusion, which restricts growth • Perinatal death due to poor placental perfusion and hypoxia • Respiratory distress syndrome (RDS) resulting from poor surfactant production secondary to hyperinsulinemia inhibiting the production of phospholipids, which make up surfactant • Polycythemia due to excessive red blood cell (RBC) production in response to hypoxia • Hyperbilirubinemia due to excessive RBC breakdown from hypoxia and an immature liver unable to break down bilirubin • Neonatal hypoglycemia resulting from ongoing hyperinsulinemia after the placenta is removed • Subsequent childhood obesity and carbohydrate intolerance

Sources: March of Dimes, 2007b; Gilbert, 2007; Blackburn, 2007.

diabetes can be reduced if excellent glycemic control is achieved at the time of conception (Varughese et al., 2007). This information needs to be stressed with all diabetic women contemplating a pregnancy.

In addition, the woman with pregestational diabetes needs to be evaluated for complications of diabetes. This evaluation should be part of baseline screening and continuing assessment during pregnancy.

Therapeutic management for the woman with gestational diabetes mellitus (defined as glucose intolerance with its onset during pregnancy or first detected during pregnancy) focuses on tight glucose control. The ADA (2007b) recommends maintaining a fasting blood glucose level below 95 mg/dL, with postprandial levels below 140 mg/dL and 2-hour postprandial levels below 120 mg/dL. In comparison, for pregnant women without diabetes, near-normal glucose values include a fasting value between 60 to 90 mg/dL, a 1-hour postprandial value of 100 to 120 mg/dL, and a 2-hour postprandial value of 60 to 120 mg/dL. Such tight control has been advocated because it is associated with a reduction in macrosomia (Scollan-Koliopoulos, Guadagno, & Walker, 2006).

Women with diabetes need comprehensive prenatal care. The primary goals of care are to maintain glycemic control and minimize the risks of the disease on the fetus. Key aspects of treatment include nutritional management, insulin regimens, and close maternal and fetal surveillance.

Nutritional management focuses on maintaining balanced glucose levels and providing enough energy and nutrients for the pregnant woman, while avoiding ketosis, and minimizing the risk of hypoglycemia in women treated with insulin (Edelstein & Herbold, 2007). Women who receive dietary instruction and follow it have been shown to have a better pregnancy outcome than those who don't receive dietary advice (Henriksen, 2006). For the woman with gestational diabetes, nutritional management may be all that is necessary.

Insulin, which doesn't cross the placenta, historically has been the medication of choice for treating hyperglycemia in pregnancy. Recent studies have examined the use of oral hypoglycemic medications in pregnancy. Several studies have used glyburide (Diabeta) with promising results. However, oral hypoglycemic agents are not usually recommended to control blood glucose levels in pregnant women by the ADA or ACOG because of insufficient research data. Many health care providers are using glyburide and metformin as an alternative to insulin therapy. Much debate and controversy remains about oral hypoglycemic use during pregnancy because the long-term effects of these medications on the mother and infant are still unknown (Simpson & Creehan, 2008). When oral agents are prescribed, additional treatment with insulin may be necessary as the pregnancy advances (Scollan-Koliopoulos, Guadagno, & Walker, 2006).

More research is indicated to establish the drug's safety and efficacy in managing diabetes in pregnancy before it can be considered an evidence-based practice (Homko & Reece, 2006; Rochon et al., 2006).

The ADA recommends that women diagnosed with gestational diabetes by a 3-hour glucose tolerance test receive nutritional counseling from a registered dietitian. The ADA also recommends insulin therapy if diet is unsuccessful in achieving a fasting glucose level below 105 mg/dL, a 1-hour postprandial level below 155 mg/dL, or 2-hour postprandial level below 130 mg/dL (ADA, 2007b).

The American College of Obstetricians and Gynecologists (ACOG) recommends the use of diet or insulin to achieve a 1-hour postprandial blood glucose level of 130 mg/dL. Both ADA and ACOG believe that further studies are needed to establish the safety of oral antidiabetic agents. Glycemic control—regardless of whether it involves diet, insulin, or oral agents—leads to fewer cases of shoulder dystocia, hyperbilirubinemia requiring phototherapy, nerve palsy, bone fracture, large for gestational age status, and fetal macrosomia (ADA, 2008).

Insulin remains the medication of choice for glycemic control in pregnant and lactating women with any type of diabetes (Ekpebegh et al., 2007). Generally, insulin doses are reduced in the first trimester to prevent hypoglycemia resulting from increased insulin sensitivity as well as from nausea and vomiting. Newer short-acting insulins such as lispo (Humalog) and aspart (Novolog), which do not cross the placenta, may help reduce postprandial hyperglycemia, episodes of hypoglycemia between meals (Hackley, Kriebs, & Rousseau, 2007). Target fasting glucose values of 60 to 90 mg/dL and 1-hour postprandial values less than 120 mg/dL are necessary to provide good glycemic control and good pregnancy outcomes (Frieden & Chan, 2007). Changes in diet and activity level add to the need for changes in insulin dosages throughout pregnancy.

Insulin regimens vary, and controversy remains over the best strategy for insulin delivery in pregnancy. Many health care providers use a split-dose therapy ($\frac{2}{3}$ of the daily dose in the morning and the remaining $\frac{1}{3}$ in the evening). Others advocate the use of an insulin pump to

---

EVIDENCE-BASED PRACTICE 20.1
Selecting Methods of Insulin Administration for Pregnant Women With Diabetes

● Study

A woman who has diabetes and becomes pregnant is at risk for various problems, both for herself and her fetus. The goal during pregnancy is to maintain optimal glucose control. For these women, insulin is the mainstay of treatment. Unfortunately blood glucose levels are not static and insulin requirements change throughout pregnancy.

Insulin typically is administered subcutaneously, commonly in multiple doses throughout the day. However, it also may be administered via a continuous subcutaneous infusion. The question arises as to which method of insulin administration affords the best control of blood glucose levels. The belief is that the continuous infusions would provide better blood glucose control and thus reduce the risks of problems for the mother and fetus.

A study was conducted comparing the effects of continuous subcutaneous insulin infusions with multiple daily doses of insulin therapy. The study involved a search of randomized controlled trials comparing these two methods of administration and their effect on neonatal birthweight, perinatal mortality, fetal anomalies, and maternal hypo- and hyperglycemia. Two studies consisting of 60 women were reviewed and a meta-analysis was performed.

▲ Findings

Women receiving continuous insulin infusions experienced an increase in birthweight of their infants compared to mothers receiving multiple daily doses of insulin. However, the researchers did not identify this difference as clinically significant. The researchers found no significant differences in perinatal mortality, fetal anomalies, or maternal hypo- and hyperglycemia between the two groups. The researchers attributed this to the small number of trials reviewed and the limited sample size of participants in the study. They concluded that there was insufficient evidence to support one method being better than the other. The researchers recommended additional research using a more vigorous approach and larger samples of women.

■ Nursing Implications

This study, although inconclusive, does underscore the need for glucose control in women with pregestational diabetes. Nurses need to be aware of these findings so that they can integrate knowledge of adequate blood glucose control when teaching pregnant women with diabetes about its potential effects, regardless of the method for insulin administration. Nurses also need to be cognizant of the various methods for insulin administration so that they can incorporate the information from this study to provide individualized care to the pregnant woman with diabetes, thereby promoting the best possible outcomes for the mother and her fetus.

Farrar, D., Tuffnell, D. J., & West, J. Continuous subcutaneous insulin infusion versus multiple daily injections of insulin for pregnant women with diabetes. *Cochrane Database of Systematic Reviews* 2007. Issue 3. Art. No.: CD005542.DOI: 10.1002/14651858.CD005542.pub2.

deliver a continuous subcutaneous insulin infusion. Regardless of which protocol is used, frequent blood glucose measurements are necessary, and the insulin dosage is adjusted on the basis of daily glucose levels.

Close maternal and fetal surveillance is also essential. Frequent laboratory tests are done during pregnancy to monitor the woman's status and glucose control. Fetal surveillance via diagnostic testing aids in evaluating fetal well-being and assisting in determining the best time for birth.

For the laboring woman with diabetes, intravenous saline is given and blood glucose levels are monitored every 1 to 2 hours. Glucose levels are maintained below 110 mg/dL throughout labor to reduce the likelihood of neonatal hypoglycemia. If necessary, an infusion of regular insulin may be given to maintain this level (ADA, 2007b). If the woman was receiving insulin during her pregnancy, adjustments in dosage may be necessary after birth since glucose diversion across the placenta to supply the growing fetus is no longer present and insulin resistance is now removed. Frequently, the woman with gestational diabetes can remain controlled through diet and weight management; the woman with type 1 diabetes usually returns to prepregnant levels of insulin administration (Modder, 2008).

Nursing Assessment

Nursing assessment begins at the first prenatal visit. A thorough history and physical examination in conjunction with specific laboratory and diagnostic testing aids in developing an individualized plan of care for the woman with diabetes.

Health History and Physical Examination

For the woman with pregestational diabetes, obtain a thorough history of the preexisting diabetic condition. Ask about her duration of disease, management of glucose levels (insulin injections, insulin pump, or oral hypoglycemic agents), dietary adjustments, presence of vascular complications and current vascular status, current insulin regimen, and technique used for glucose testing. Review any information that she may have received as part of her preconception counseling and measures that were implemented during this time.

Be knowledgeable about the woman's nutritional requirements and assess the adequacy and pattern of her dietary intake. Assess her blood glucose self-monitoring in terms of technique, frequency, and her ability to adjust the insulin dose based on the changing patterns. Ask about the frequency of episodes of hypoglycemia or hyperglycemia to ascertain the woman's ability to recognize and treat them. Continue to assess her for signs and symptoms of hypo- and hyperglycemia.

During antepartum visits, assess the client's knowledge about her disease, including the signs and symptoms of hypoglycemia, hyperglycemia, and diabetic ketoacidosis, insulin administration techniques, and the impact of pregnancy on her chronic condition. If possible have the woman demonstrate her technique for blood glucose monitoring and insulin administration if appropriate. Although the client may have had diabetes for some time, do not assume that she has a firm knowledge base about her disease process or management of it (Fig. 20.1).

Assess the woman's risk for gestational diabetes at the first prenatal visit. The ADA (2007b) recommends assessing all women for risk factors and then determining the need for additional testing in the high-risk group only. Factors that place a woman at high risk include:

- Previous infant with congenital anomaly (skeletal, renal, central nervous system, cardiac)
- History of gestational diabetes or hydramnios in a previous pregnancy
- Family history of diabetes
- Age 35 or older
- Previous infant weighing more than 9 pounds (4,000 g)
- Previous unexplained fetal demise or neonatal death
- Maternal obesity (Body Mass Index [BMI] > 30)
- Hypertension
- Hispanic, Native American, or African-American ethnicity
- Recurrent monilia infections that don't respond to treatment
- Signs and symptoms of glucose intolerance (polyuria, polyphagia, polydipsia, fatigue)
- Presence of glycosuria or proteinuria (Hackley, Kriebs, & Rousseau, 2007)

Women with clinical characteristics consistent with a high risk for gestational diabetes should undergo glucose testing as soon as feasible.

Provide close ongoing assessment throughout the antepartal period. Women with gestational diabetes mellitus are at increased risk for preeclampsia and glucose control-related complications such as hypoglycemia, hyperglycemia, and ketoacidosis. Gestational diabetes of any severity increases the risk of fetal macrosomia. It is also associated with an increased frequency of maternal hypertensive disorders and operative births. This may be the result of fetal growth disorders (ADA, 2007b).

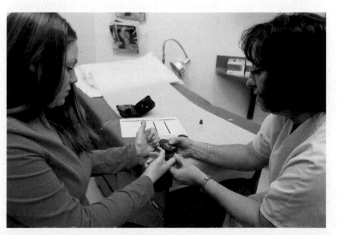

FIGURE 20.1 The nurse is demonstrating the technique for self-blood glucose monitoring with a pregnant client.

Even though gestational diabetes is diagnosed during pregnancy, the woman may have had glucose intolerance before the pregnancy. Therefore, monitor the woman closely for signs and symptoms of possible complications.

Also assess the woman's psychosocial adaptation to her condition. This assessment is critical to gain her co-operation for a change in regimen or the addition of a new regimen throughout pregnancy. Identify her support systems and note any financial constraints, as she will need more intense monitoring and frequent fetal surveillance.

Laboratory and Diagnostic Testing

The results of laboratory and diagnostic tests provide valuable information about maternal and fetal well-being. Women with pregestational diabetes and those discovered to have gestational diabetes require ongoing maternal and fetal surveillance to promote the best outcome.

Screening

ACOG and ADA currently recommend a risk analysis of all pregnant women at their first prenatal visit and additional screening of all high-risk pregnant women again at 24 to 28 weeks, or earlier if risk factors are present. If the initial screening risk assessment is low, additional screening may not be necessary. Pregnant women who fulfill all of the following criteria need not be screened:

- No history of glucose intolerance
- Less than 25 years old
- Normal body weight
- No family history (first-degree relative) of diabetes
- No history of poor obstetric outcome
- Not from an ethnic/racial group with a high prevalence of diabetes (ADA, 2007b)

If the initial risk assessment is high, rescreening should take place between 24 and 28 weeks. A woman with abnormal early results may have had diabetes before the pregnancy, and her fetus is a great risk for congenital anomalies. An elevated glycosylated hemoglobin supports the likelihood of gestational diabetes (D'Arrigo, 2007).

There is little consensus regarding the appropriate screening method. Typically, screening is based on a 50-g 1-hour glucose challenge test, usually performed between week 24 and 28 of gestation (ADA, 2007b). A 50-g oral glucose load is given, without regard to the timing or content of the last meal. Blood glucose is measured 1 hour later; a level above 140 mg/dL is abnormal. If the result is abnormal, a 3-hour glucose tolerance test is done. According to the ADA (2009), the normal plasma levels are:

- Fasting blood sugar level: less than 95 mg/dL
- At 1 hour: less than 180 mg/dL
- At 2 hours: less than 155 mg/dL
- At 3 hours: less than 140 mg/dL

A diagnosis of gestational diabetes can be made only after an abnormal result is obtained on the glucose toler-ance test. Two or more abnormal values confirm a diagnosis of gestational diabetes (ADA, 2007a).

Surveillance

Maternal surveillance may include the following:

- Urine check for protein (may indicate the need for further evaluation for preeclampsia) and for nitrates and leukocyte esterase (may indicate a urinary tract infection)
- Urine check for ketones (may indicate the need for evaluation of eating habits)
- Kidney function evaluation every trimester for creatinine clearance and protein levels
- Eye examination in the first trimester to evaluate the retina for vascular changes
- HbA1c every 4 to 6 weeks to monitor glucose trends (Hackley, Kriebs, & Rousseau, 2007)

Fetal surveillance may include ultrasound to provide information about fetal growth, activity, and amniotic fluid volume and to validate gestational age. Alpha-fetoprotein levels may be obtained to detect congenital anomalies such as an open neural tube or ventral wall defects of omphalocele or gastroschisis, and a fetal echocardiogram may be necessary to rule out cardiac anomalies. A biophysical profile helps to monitor fetal well-being and uteroplacental profusion, and nonstress tests commonly are performed weekly after 28 weeks' gestation to evaluate fetal well-being. As the pregnancy progresses, an amniocentesis may be done to determine the lecithin/sphingomyelin (L/S) ratio and the presence of phosphatidyl glycerol (PG) to evaluate whether the fetal lung is mature enough for birth (Frieden & Chan, 2007).

Nursing Management

The ideal outcome of every pregnancy is a healthy newborn and mother. Nurses can be pivotal in realizing this positive outcome for women with pregestational or gestational diabetes by implementing measures to minimize risks and complications. Since the woman with diabetes is considered to be at high risk, antepartal visits occur more frequently (every 2 weeks up to 28 weeks and then twice a week until birth), providing the nurse with numerous opportunities for ongoing assessment, education, and counseling (Nursing Care Plan 20.1).

Promoting Optimal Glucose Control

At each visit, review the mother's blood glucose levels, including any laboratory tests and self-monitoring results. Reinforce with the woman the need to perform blood glucose monitoring (usually four times a day, before meals and at bedtime) and to keep a record of the results. If appropriate, obtain a fingerstick blood glucose level to evaluate the accuracy of self-monitoring results. Also assess the woman's techniques for monitoring blood glucose levels and for administering insulin if ordered, and offer support and guidance. If the woman is receiving insulin

Nursing Care Plan 20.1

OVERVIEW OF THE PREGNANT WOMAN WITH TYPE 1 DIABETES

Donna, a 30-year-old woman with type 1 diabetes, presents to the maternity clinic for preconception care. She has been a diabetic for 8 years and takes insulin twice daily by injection. She does blood glucose self-monitoring four times daily. She reports that her disease is fairly well controlled, but "I'm worried about how my diabetes will affect a pregnancy and my baby. Will I need to make changes in my routine? Will my baby be normal?" She reports that she recently had a foot infection and needed to go to the emergency room because it led to an episode of ketoacidosis. She states that her last glycosylated hemoglobin A1c test results were abnormal.

NURSING DIAGNOSIS: Deficient knowledge related to type 1 diabetes, blood glucose control, and effects of condition on pregnancy as evidenced by questions about effect on pregnancy, possible changes in regimen, and pregnancy outcome

Outcome Identification and Evaluation

Client will demonstrate increased knowledge of type 1 diabetes and effects on pregnancy *as evidenced by proper techniques for blood glucose monitoring and insulin administration, ability to modify insulin doses and dietary intake to achieve control, and verbalization of need for glycemic control prior to pregnancy, with blood glucose levels remaining within normal range.*

Interventions: Providing Client Teaching

- Assess client's knowledge of diabetes and pregnancy *to establish a baseline from which to develop an individualized teaching plan.*
- Review the underlying problems associated with diabetes and how pregnancy affects glucose control *to provide client with a firm knowledge base for decision making.*
- Review signs and symptoms of hypoglycemia and hyperglycemia and prevention and management measures *to ensure client can deal with them should they occur.*
- Provide written materials describing diabetes and care needed for control *to provide opportunity for client's review and promote retention of learning.*
- Observe client administering insulin and self-glucose testing for technique and offer suggestions for improvement if needed *to ensure adequate self-care ability.*
- Discuss proper foot care *to prevent future infections.*
- Teach home treatment for symptomatic hypoglycemia *to minimize risk to client and fetus.*
- Outline acute and chronic diabetic complications *to reinforce the importance of glucose control.*
- Discuss use of contraceptives until blood glucose levels can be optimized before conception occurs *to promote best possible health status before conception.*
- Explain the rationale for good glucose control and the importance of achieving excellent glycemic control before pregnancy *to promote a positive pregnancy outcome.*
- Review self-care practices (blood glucose monitoring and frequency of testing; insulin administration; adjustment of insulin dosages based on blood glucose levels) *to foster independence in self-care and feelings of control over the situation.*
- Refer client for dietary counseling *to ensure optimal diet for glycemic control.*
- Outline obstetric management and fetal surveillance needed for pregnancy *to provide client with information on what to expect.*
- Discuss strategies for maintaining optimal glycemic control during pregnancy *to minimize risks to client and fetus.*

Nursing Care Plan 20.1 (continued)

NURSING DIAGNOSIS: Anxiety related to future pregnancy and its outcome secondary to underlying diabetes as evidenced by questions about her condition's effect on the baby and baby being normal

Outcome Identification and Evaluation
Client will openly express her feelings related to her diabetes and pregnancy *as evidenced by statements of feeling better about her pre-existing condition and pregnancy outlook, and statements of understanding related to future childbearing by linking good glucose control with positive outcomes for both herself and offspring.*

Interventions: Minimizing Anxiety
- Review the need for a physical examination *to evaluate for any effects of diabetes on the client's health status.*
- Explain the rationale for assessing client's blood pressure, vision, and peripheral pulses at each visit *to provide information related to possible effects of diabetes on health status.*
- Identify any alterations in present diabetic condition that need intervention *to aid in minimizing risks that may increase client's anxiety level.*
- Review potential effects of diabetes on pregnancy *to promote client understanding of risks and ways to control or minimize them.*
- Encourage active participation in decision making and planning pregnancy *to promote feelings of control over the situation and foster self-confidence.*
- Discuss feelings about future childbearing and managing pregnancy *to help reduce anxiety related to uncertainties.*
- Encourage client to ask questions or voice concerns *to help decrease anxiety related to the unknown.*
- Emphasize the use of frequent and continued surveillance of client and fetal status during pregnancy *to reduce the risk of complications and aid in alleviating anxieties related to the unknown.*
- Provide positive reinforcement for healthy behaviors and actions *to foster continued use and enhancement of self-esteem.*

---

therapy, assist with any changes needed if glucose levels are not controlled.

Obtain a urine specimen and check for glucose, protein, and ketones. Ask the woman if she has had any episodes of hypoglycemia and what she did to alleviate them.

Discuss dietary measures related to blood glucose control (Fig. 20.2). In addition, recommend the following:

- Avoid weight loss and dieting during pregnancy.
- Ensure that food intake is adequate to prevent ketone formation and promote weight gain.
- Eat three meals a day plus three snacks to promote glycemic control.
  –40% of calories from good-quality complex carbohydrates
  –35% of calories from protein sources
  –25% of calories from unsaturated fats (ADA, 2007b)

▶ *Take NOTE!*

Nutrient requirements and recommendations for weight gain for the pregnant woman with diabetes are the same as those for the pregnant nondiabetic woman.

If necessary, arrange for consultation with a dietitian or nutritionist to individualize the dietary plan. Also encourage the women to participate in an exercise program that includes at least three sessions lasting longer than 15 min-

utes per week. Exercise may lessen the need for insulin or dosage adjustments.

When caring for the laboring woman with pregestational or gestational diabetes, adjust the intravenous flow rate and the rate of supplemental regular insulin based on

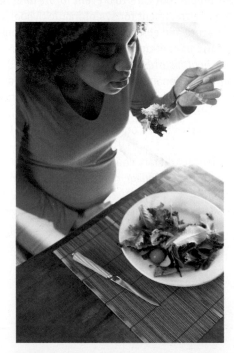

FIGURE 20.2 The pregnant client eating a nutritious meal to ensure adequate glucose control.

the blood glucose levels as ordered. Monitor blood glucose levels every 1 to 2 hours or more frequently if necessary. Keep a syringe with 50% dextrose solution available at the bedside to treat profound hypoglycemia. Monitor fetal heart rate patterns throughout labor to detect non-reassuring patterns. Assess maternal vital signs every hour, in addition to assessing the woman's urinary output with an indwelling catheter. If a cesarean birth is scheduled, monitor the woman's blood glucose levels hourly and administer short-acting insulin or glucose based on the blood glucose levels as ordered.

After birth, monitor blood glucose levels every 2 to 4 hours and continue intravenous fluid administration as ordered. Encourage breastfeeding to assist in maintaining good glucose control. For the woman with pregestational diabetes and type 1 or 2 diabetes, expect insulin needs to decrease rapidly after birth: they may be reduced by half of the antepartum dose as meals are started (Hackley, Kriebs, & Rousseau, 2007). Some women may return to their prepregnancy insulin dosage.

The therapy plan after childbirth is individualized for each woman. If recommended dietary modifications are carried out along with weight loss, the woman with gestational diabetes may return to her normal glucose levels. This is also true for the woman with pregestational diabetes, except that she will return to her prepregnancy insulin administration levels. This provides the nurse with a wonderful opportunity to reinforce healthy lifestyle interventions on the postpartum unit. Nurses can also become involved with community-based education to continue to offer their expertise.

Preventing Complications

Assess the woman closely for signs and symptoms of complications at each visit. Anticipate possible complications and plan appropriate interventions or referrals. Check the woman's blood pressure for changes and evaluate for proteinuria when obtaining a urine specimen. These might suggest the development of preeclampsia. Measure fundal height and review gestational age. Note any discrepancies between fundal height and gestational age or a sudden increase in uterine growth. These may suggest hydramnios.

Encourage the woman to perform daily fetal movement counts to monitor fetal well-being. Tell her specifically when she should notify her health care provider. Also prepare the woman for the need for frequent laboratory and diagnostic testing to evaluate fetal status. Assist with serial ultrasounds to monitor fetal growth and with nonstress tests and biophysical profiles to assess fetal well-being.

Providing Client Education and Counseling

The pregnant woman with diabetes requires counseling and education about the need for strict glucose monitoring, diet and exercise, and signs and symptoms of complications. Encourage the client and her family to make any lifestyle changes needed to optimize the pregnancy outcome. Providing dietary education and lifestyle advice that extends beyond pregnancy may lower the risk that the woman will have gestational diabetes in subsequent pregnancies as well as type 2 diabetes (Scollan-Koliopoulos, Guadagno, & Walker, 2006). At each visit stress the importance of performing blood glucose screening and documenting the results. With proper instruction, the client and her family will be able to cope with all the changes in her body during pregnancy (Teaching Guidelines 20.1).

Review discussions about the timing of birth and the rationale. Counsel the client about the possibility of cesarean birth for an LGA infant, or inform the woman who will be giving birth vaginally about the possible need for augmentation with oxytocin (Pitocin).

> ▶ **Take** NOTE!
>
> *In the woman with well-controlled diabetes, birth is typically not induced before term unless there are complications, such as preeclampsia or fetal compromise. An early delivery date might be set for the woman with poorly controlled diabetes who is having complications.*

Instruct the client about the benefits of breastfeeding related to blood glucose control. Breastfeeding helps to normalize blood glucose levels. Therefore, encourage the woman to breastfeed her newborn. Also teach the woman receiving insulin for her diabetes that her insulin needs after birth will drastically decrease. Inform her that she will need a repeat glucose challenge test at a postpartum visit (ADA, 2007b).

For the woman with gestational diabetes, the focus is on lifestyle education. Women with gestational diabetes have a greater than 50% increased risk of developing type 2 diabetes (ADA, 2007a). Inform the woman that screening most likely will be done at the postpartum follow-up appointment in 6 weeks. Women with normal results at that visit typically are screened every 3 years thereafter (ADA, 2007a). Teach her how to maintain an optimal weight to reduce her risk of developing diabetes. If necessary, refer the woman to a dietitian to help outline a balanced nutritious diet.

Cardiovascular Disorders

Every minute, an American woman dies of cardiovascular disease (American Heart Association [AHA], 2007). Cardiovascular disease is the leading cause of death for men and women in the United States. It kills nearly 500,000 women each year. Despite the prominent reduction in cardiovascular mortality among men, the rate has not declined for women. Cardiovascular disease has killed more women then men since 1984 (AHA, 2007). In addition to being the number-one killer of women, at

TEACHING GUIDELINES 20.1

Teaching for the Pregnant Woman With Diabetes

- Be sure to keep your appointments for frequent prenatal visits and tests for fetal well-being.
- Perform blood glucose self-monitoring as directed, usually before each meal and at bedtime. Keep a record of your results and call your healthcare provider with any levels outside the established range. Bring your results to each prenatal visit.
- Perform daily "fetal kick counts." Document them and report any decrease in activity.
- Drink 8 to 10 8-ounce glasses of water each day to prevent bladder infections and maintain hydration.
- Wear proper, well-fitted footwear when walking to prevent injury.
- Engage in a regular exercise program such as walking to aid in glucose control, but avoid exercising in temperature extremes.
- Consider breastfeeding your infant to lower your blood glucose levels.
- If you are taking insulin:
  - Administer the correct dose of insulin at the correct time every day.
  - Eat breakfast within 30 minutes after injecting regular insulin to prevent a reaction.
  - Plan meals at a fixed time and snacks to prevent extremes in glucose levels.
- Avoid simple sugars (cake, candy, cookies), which raise blood glucose levels.
- Know the signs and symptoms of hypoglycemia and treatment needed:
  - Sweating, tremors, cold, clammy skin, headache
  - Feeling hungry, blurred vision, disorientation, irritability
  - Treatment: Drink 8 ounces of milk and eat two crackers or glucose tablets
- Carry "glucose boosters" (such as Life Savers) to prevent hypoglycemia.
- Know the signs and symptoms of hyperglycemia and treatment needed:
  - Dry mouth, frequent urination, excessive thirst, rapid breathing
  - Feeling tired, flushed, hot skin, headache, drowsiness
  - Treatment: Notify health care provider, since hospitalization may be needed
- Wear a diabetic identification bracelet at all times.
- Wash your hands frequently to prevent infections.
- Report any signs and symptoms of illness, infection, and dehydration to your health care provider, because these can affect blood glucose control.

the time of diagnosis women have both a poorer overall prognosis and a higher risk of death than men diagnosed with heart disease (Peddicord, 2005). More women die of heart disease, stroke, and other cardiovascular diseases than men, yet many women do not realize they are at risk. These diseases kill more women each year than the next five causes of death combined (AHA, 2007).

Approximately 3% of pregnant women have cardiac disease, which is responsible for 10% to 25% of maternal deaths (Cunningham et al., 2005). The prevalence of cardiac disease is increasing as a result of lifestyle patterns, including cigarette smoking, diabetes, and stress. As women are delaying childbearing, the incidence of cardiac disease in pregnancy will continue to increase. Rheumatic heart disease used to represent the majority of cardiac conditions during pregnancy, but congenital heart disease now constitutes nearly half of all cases of heart disease encountered during pregnancy. Classic symptoms of heart disease mimic common symptoms of late pregnancy, such as palpitations, shortness of breath with exertion, and occasional chest pain. Few women with heart disease die during pregnancy, but they are at risk for other complications, such as heart failure, arrhythmias, and stroke. Their offspring are also at risk of complications, such as premature birth, low birthweight for gestational age, respiratory distress syndrome, intraventricular hemorrhage, and death (Abdin, 2006).

► CONGENITAL AND ACQUIRED HEART DISEASE

Congenital heart disease often involves structural defects that are present at birth but may not be discovered at that time (Table 20.2). Until recently women with congenital heart disease didn't live long enough to bear children. Today, due to new surgical techniques to correct these defects, many of these women can complete a successful pregnancy at relatively low risk when appropriate counseling and optimal care are provided. Increasing numbers of women with complex congenital heart disease are reaching childbearing age. Complications such as growth restriction and preterm and premature birth and fetal and neonatal mortality are more common among children of women with congenital heart disease. The risk of complications is determined by the severity of the cardiac lesion, the presence of cyanosis, the maternal functional class, and the use of anticoagulation (Karamermer & Roos-Hesselink, 2007).

Women with certain congenital conditions should avoid pregnancy. These include uncorrected tetralogy of Fallot or transposition of the great arteries, and Eisenmenger's syndrome, a defect with both cyanosis and pulmonary hypertension (Karamermer & Roos-Hesselink, 2007).

TABLE 20.2   **SELECTED HEART CONDITIONS AFFECTING PREGNANCY**

Condition	Description	Management
Tetralogy of Fallot	Congenital defect involving four structural anomalies: obstruction to pulmonary flow; ventricular septal defect (abnormal opening between the right and left ventricles); dextroposition of the aorta (aortic opening overriding the septum and receiving blood from both ventricles); and right ventricular hypertrophy (increase in volume of the myocardium of the right ventricle) (O'Toole, 2005)	Hospitalization and bed rest possible after the 20th week with hemodynamic monitoring via a pulmonary artery catheter to monitor volume status Oxygen therapy may be necessary during labor and birth.
Atrial septal defect (ASD)	Congenital heart defect involving a communication or opening between the atria with left-to-right shunting due to greater left-sided pressure Arrhythmias present in some women	Treatment with atrioventricular nodal blocking agents, and at times with electrical cardioversion (Gilbert & Harmon, 2006)
Ventricular septal defect (VSD)	Congenital heart defect involving an opening in the ventricular septum, permitting blood flow from the left to the right ventricle. Complications include arrhythmias, heart failure, and pulmonary hypertension (McMahon, 2007).	Rest with limited activity if symptomatic
Patent ductus arteriosus	Abnormal persistence of an open lumen in the ductus arteriosus between the aorta and the pulmonary artery after birth; results in increased pulmonary blood flow and redistribution of flow to other organs (Hermes-DeSantis & Clyman, 2006)	Surgical ligation of the open ductus during infancy; subsequent problems minimal after surgical correction
Mitral valve prolapse	Very common in the general population, occurring most often in younger women Leaflets of the mitral valve prolapse into the left atrium during ventricular contraction. The most common cause of mitral valve regurgitation if present during pregnancy (Wooley & Boudoulas, 2007) Usually improvement in mitral valve function due to increased blood volume and decreased systemic vascular resistance of pregnancy; most women are able to tolerate pregnancy well.	Most women are asymptomatic; diagnosis is made incidentally. Occasional palpations, chest pain, or arrhythmias in some women, possibly requiring beta-blockers Usually no special precautions are necessary during pregnancy.
Mitral valve stenosis	Most common chronic rheumatic valvular lesion in pregnancy Causes obstruction of blood flow from the atria to the ventricle, thereby decreasing ventricular filling and causing a fixed cardiac output Resultant pulmonary edema, pulmonary hypertension, and right ventricular failure (Barker et al., 2006) Most pregnant women with this condition can be managed medically.	General symptomatic improvement with medical management involving diuretics, beta-blockers, and anticoagulant therapy Activity restriction, reduction in sodium, and potentially bed rest if condition severe

(continued)

TABLE 20.2   SELECTED HEART CONDITIONS AFFECTING PREGNANCY (continued)

Condition	Description	Management
Aortic stenosis	Narrowing of the opening of the aortic valve, leading to an obstruction to left ventricular ejection (Balentine & Eisenhart, 2008). Women with mild disease can tolerate hypervolemia of pregnancy; with progressive narrowing of the opening, cardiac output becomes fixed. Diagnosis can be confirmed with echocardiography. Most women can be managed with medical therapy, bed rest, and close monitoring.	Diagnosis confirmed with echocardiography Pharmacologic treatment with beta-blockers and/or antiarrhythmic agents to reduce risk of heart failure and/or dysrhythmias Bed rest/limited activity and close monitoring
Peripartum cardiomyopathy	Rare congestive cardiomyopathy that may arise during pregnancy. Multiparity, age, multiple fetuses, hypertension, an infectious agent, autoimmune disease, or cocaine use may contribute to its presence (Mooney, 2007). Development of heart failure in the last month of pregnancy or within 5 months of giving birth without any preexisting heart disease or any identifiable cause	Preload reduction with diuretic therapy Afterload reduction with vasodilators Improvement in contractility with inotropic agents Nonpharmacologic approaches include salt restriction and daily exercise such as walking or biking. The question of whether another pregnancy should be attempted is controversial due to the high risk of repeat complications.
Myocardial infarction	Rare during pregnancy but incidence is expected to increase as older women are becoming pregnant and the risk factors for coronary artery disease become more prevalent Factors contributing to MI include family history, stress, smoking, age, obesity, multiple fetuses, hypercholesterolemia, and cocaine use (Gibson & Carson, 2007). Increased plasma volume and cardiac output during pregnancy increase the cardiac workload as well as the myocardial oxygen demands; imbalance in supply and demand may contribute to myocardial ischemia.	Usual treatment modalities for any acute MI along with consideration for the fetus Anticoagulant therapy, rest, and lifestyle changes to preserve the health of both parties

Sources: Balentine & Eisenhart, 2008; Gibson & Carson, 2007; McMahon, 2007; Mooney, 2007; O'Toole, 2005.

Acquired heart disease is typically rheumatic in origin (see Table 20.2). The incidence of rheumatic heart disease has declined dramatically in the past several decades because of prompt identification of streptococcal throat infections and treatment with antibiotics. When the heart is involved, valvular lesions such as mitral stenosis, prolapse, or aortic stenosis are common.

Many women are postponing childbearing until the fourth or fifth decade of life. With advancing maternal age, underlying medical conditions such as hypertension, diabetes, and hypercholesterolemia contributing to ischemic heart disease become more common and increase the incidence of acquired heart disease complicating pregnancy. Coronary artery disease and myocardial infarction may result.

A woman's ability to function during the pregnancy is often more important than the actual diagnosis of the cardiac condition. The following is a functional classification system developed by the Criteria Committee of the New York Heart Association (1994) based on past and present disability and physical signs:

- Class I: asymptomatic with no limitation of physical activity
- Class II: symptomatic (dyspnea, chest pain) with increased activity
- Class III: symptomatic (fatigue, palpitations) with normal activity
- Class IV: symptomatic at rest or with any physical activity

The classification may change as the pregnancy progresses and the woman's body must cope with the increasing stress on the cardiovascular system resulting from the numerous physiologic changes taking place. Typically, a woman with class I or II cardiac disease can go through a pregnancy without major complications. A woman with class III disease usually has to maintain bed rest during pregnancy. A woman with class IV disease should avoid pregnancy (McCann, 2007). Women with cardiac disease may benefit from preconception counseling so that they know the risks before deciding to become pregnant.

Maternal mortality varies directly with the functional class at pregnancy onset. ACOG has adopted a three-tiered classification according to the risk of death during pregnancy (Box 20.1).

BOX 20.1 Classification of Maternal Mortality Risk

Group I (minimal risk) has a mortality rate of 1% and comprises women with:
- Patent ductus arteriosus
- Tetralogy of Fallot, corrected
- Atrial septal defect
- Ventricular septal defect
- Mitral stenosis, class I and II

Group II (moderate risk) has a mortality rate of 5% to 15% and comprises women with:
- Tetralogy of Fallot, uncorrected
- Mitral stenosis with atrial fibrillation
- Aortic stenosis, class III and IV
- Aortic coarctation without valvular involvement
- Artificial valve replacement

Group III (major risk) has a 25% to 50% mortality rate and comprises women with:
- Pulmonary hypertension
- Complicated aortic coarctation
- Previous myocardial infarction

Sources: Gilbert & Harmon, 2006; Gilbert, 2007; Blackburn, 2007.

Pathophysiology

Numerous hemodynamic changes occur in all pregnant women. These normal physiologic changes can overstress the woman's cardiovascular system, increasing her risk for problems. Increased cardiac workload and greater myocardial oxygen demand during pregnancy place the woman's cardiovascular system at high risk for morbidity and mortality.

> ▶ **Take** NOTE!
>
> *Uterine blood flow increases by at least 1 liter per minute, requiring the body to produce more blood during pregnancy. This results in a 25% increase in red blood cells, a 50% expansion of plasma volume during pregnancy, and an overall hemodilution. In addition, the increase in total red blood cellular volume includes an increase in clotting factors and platelets, defining the hypercoagulable state of pregnancy (Dobbenga-Rhodes & Prive, 2006). These changes start as early as the second month of gestation.*

Similarly, cardiac output increases steadily during pregnancy by 30% to 50% over prepregnancy levels: stroke volume increases 20% to 30% from prepregnant levels, and the maternal heart rate increases by 10 to 20 beats per minute. The increase is due to both the expansion in blood volume and the augmentation of stroke volume and heart rate. Other hemodynamic changes associated with pregnancy include a decrease in both the systemic vascular resistance and pulmonary vascular resistance, thereby lowering the systolic and diastolic blood pressure. In addition, the hypercoagulability associated with pregnancy might increase the risk of arterial thrombosis and embolization. These normal physiologic changes are important for a successful adaptation to pregnancy but create unique physiologic challenges for the woman with cardiac disease (Comparison Chart 20.1).

Therapeutic Management

Ideally, a woman with a history of congenital or acquired heart disease should consult her health care provider before becoming pregnant and should undergo a risk assessment. This risk assessment must consider the woman's functional capacity, exercise tolerance, degree of cyanosis, medication needs, and history of arrhythmias. Data needed for risk assessment can be acquired from a thorough cardiovascular history and examination, a 12-lead electrocardiogram (ECG), and evaluation of oxygen saturation levels by pulse oximetry. The impact of heart disease on a woman's childbearing potential needs to be clearly explained, and information on how pregnancy may affect her and the fetus is important. This allows women to make an informed choice

COMPARISON CHART 20.1 CARDIOVASCULAR CHANGES: PREPREGNANCY VS PREGNANCY

Measurement	Prepregnancy	Pregnancy
Heart rate	72 (±10 bpm)	+10–20%
Cardiac output	4.3 (±0.9 L/min)	+30% to 50%
Blood volume	5 L	+20% to 50%
Stroke volume	73.3 (±9 mL)	+30%
Systemic vascular resistance	1,530 (±520 dyne/cm/sec)	–20%
Oxygen consumption	250 mL/minute	+20–30%

Sources: Blincoe, 2007; Blackburn, 2007; Harvey, 2007.

whether they wish to accept the risks associated with pregnancy. When possible, any surgical procedures, such as valve replacement, should be done before pregnancy to improve fetal and maternal outcomes (Uebing et al., 2006).

If the woman presents for care after she has become pregnant, prenatal counseling focuses on the impact of the hemodynamic changes of pregnancy, the signs and symptoms of cardiac compromise, and dietary and lifestyle changes needed. More frequent prenatal visits (every 2 weeks until the last month and then weekly) are usually needed to ensure the health and safety of the mother and fetus.

Nursing Assessment

Frequent and thorough assessments are crucial during the antepartum period to ensure early detection of and prompt intervention for problems. Assess the woman's vital signs, noting any changes. Auscultate the apical heart rate and heart sounds, being especially alert for abnormalities, including irregularities in rhythm or murmurs. Check the client's weight and compare to baseline and weights obtained on previous visits. Report any weight gain outside recommended parameters. Inspect the extremities for edema and note any pitting.

Question the woman about fetal activity, and ask if she has noticed any changes. Report any changes such as a decrease in fetal movements. Ask the woman about any symptoms of preterm labor, such as low back pain, uterine contractions, and increased pelvic pressure and vaginal discharge, and report them immediately. Assess the fetal heart rate and review serial ultrasound results to monitor fetal growth.

Assess the client's lifestyle and her ability to cope with the changes of pregnancy and its effect on her cardiac status and ability to function. Evaluate the client's understanding of her condition and what restrictions and lifestyle changes may be needed to provide the best outcome for her and her fetus. A healthy infant and mother at the end of pregnancy is the ultimate goal. As the client's pregnancy advances, expect her functional class to be revised based on her level of disability. Suggest realistic modifications.

The nurse plays a major role in recognizing the signs and symptoms of cardiac decompensation. Decompensation refers to the heart's inability to maintain adequate circulation. As a result, tissue perfusion in the mother and the fetus is impaired. The pregnant woman is most vulnerable for this complication from 28 to 32 weeks of gestation and in the first 48 hours postpartum (Witcher & Harvey, 2006). Assess the woman for the following signs and symptoms:

- Shortness of breath on exertion, dyspnea
- Cyanosis of lips and nail beds
- Swelling of face, hands, and feet
- Jugular vein engorgement
- Rapid respirations
- Abnormal heartbeats, reports of heart racing or palpitations
- Chest pain with effort or emotion
- Syncope with exertion
- Increasing fatigue
- Moist, frequent cough

▶ *Take* NOTE!

Assessing the pregnant woman with heart disease for cardiac decompensation is vital because the mother's hemodynamic status determines the health of the fetus.

Nursing Management

Nursing management of the pregnant woman with heart disease focuses on assisting with measures to stabilize the mother's hemodynamic status, because a decrease in maternal blood pressure or volume will cause blood to be shunted away from the uterus, thus reducing placental perfusion. Pregnant women with cardiac disease also need assistance in reducing risks that would lead to complications or further cardiac compromise. Therefore, education and counseling are critical. Collaboration between the cardiologist, obstetrician, perinatologist, and nurse is needed to promote the best possible outcome.

Encourage the woman to continue taking her cardiac medications as prescribed. Review the indications, actions, and potential side effects of the medications. Reinforce the importance of frequent antepartal visits and close medical supervision throughout the pregnancy.

Discuss the need to conserve energy. Help the client to prioritize household chores and childcare to allow rest periods. Encourage the client to rest in the side-lying position, which enhances placental perfusion.

Encourage the client to eat nutritious foods and consume a high-fiber diet to prevent straining and constipation. Discuss limiting sodium intake if indicated to reduce fluid retention. Contact a dietitian to assist the woman in planning nutritionally appropriate meals.

Assist the woman in preparing for diagnostic tests to evaluate fetal well-being. Describe the tests that may be done, such as ECG and echocardiogram, and explain the need for serial nonstress testing, usually beginning at approximately 32 weeks.

Instruct the woman in how to monitor fetal activity and movements. Urge her to do this daily and report any changes in activity immediately.

Although the morbidity and mortality rates of pregnant women with cardiac disease have decreased greatly, congestive heart failure, cardiac arrhythmia, thromboembolism, angina, hypoxemia, and infective endocarditis can occur (Witcher & Harvey, 2006). Explain the signs and symptoms of these complications and review the sign and symptoms of cardiac decompensation, encouraging the woman to notify her health care provider if any occur.

Provide support and encouragement throughout the antepartal period. Assess the support systems available to the client and her family, and encourage her to use them. If necessary, assist with referrals to community services for additional support.

During labor, anticipate the need for invasive hemodynamic monitoring, and make sure the woman has been prepared for this beforehand. Monitor her fluid volume carefully to prevent overload. Anticipate the use of epidural anesthesia if a vaginal birth is planned. After birth, assess the client for fluid overload as peripheral fluids mobilize. This fluid shift from the periphery to the central circulation taxes the heart, and signs of heart failure such as cough, progressive dyspnea, edema, palpitations, and crackles in the lung bases may ensue before postpartum diuresis begins. Because hemodynamics do not return to baseline for several days after childbirth, women at intermediate or high risk require monitoring for at least 48 hours postpartum (Barker et al., 2006).

▶ CHRONIC HYPERTENSION

Chronic hypertension exists when the woman has high blood pressure before pregnancy or before the 20th week of gestation, or when hypertension persists for more than 12 weeks postpartum. The Seventh Report of the Joint National Committee on Prevention, Detection, Evaluation, and Treatment of High Blood Pressure (JNC, 2003) has classified blood pressure as follows:

- Normal: systolic less than 120 mmHg, diastolic less than 80 mmHg
- Prehypertension: systolic 120 to 139 mmHg, diastolic 80 to 89 mmHg
- Mild hypertension: systolic 140 to 159 mmHg, diastolic 90 to 99 mmHg
- Severe hypertension: systolic 160 mm Hg or higher, diastolic 100 mm Hg or higher

Chronic hypertension occurs in up to 22% of women of childbearing age, with the prevalence varying according to age, race, and BMI. It complicates at least 5% of pregnancies, with 1 in 4 women developing preeclampsia during pregnancy (Blincoe, 2007). Chronic hypertension is typically seen in older, obese women with glucose intolerance. The most common complication is preeclampsia, which is seen in approximately 25% of women who enter the pregnancy with hypertension (Podymow & August, 2007; Tihtonen et al., 2007). (See Chapter 19 for more information about preeclampsia.)

Therapeutic Management

Preconception counseling is important in fostering positive outcomes. Typically, it involves lifestyle changes such as diet, exercise, weight loss, and smoking cessation.

Treatment for women with chronic hypertension focuses on maintaining normal blood pressure, preventing superimposed preeclampsia/eclampsia, and ensuring normal fetal development. Once the woman is pregnant, antihypertensive agents are typically reserved for severe hypertension (150 to 160 mmHg/100 to 110 mmHg). Methyldopa (Aldomet) is commonly prescribed because of its safety record during pregnancy. This slow-acting antihypertensive agent helps to improve uterine perfusion. Other antihypertensive agents that can be used include labetalol (Transdate), atenolol (Tenorium), and nifedipine (Procardia) (Gibson & Carson, 2007).

Lifestyle changes are needed and should continue throughout gestation. The woman with chronic hypertension will be seen more frequently (every 2 weeks until 28 weeks and then weekly until birth) to monitor her blood pressure and to assess for any signs of preeclampsia. At approximately 24 weeks' gestation, the woman will be instructed to document fetal movement. At this same time, serial ultrasounds will be ordered to monitor fetal growth and amniotic fluid volume. Additional tests will be included if the client's status changes.

Nursing Assessment

Nursing assessment of the woman with chronic hypertension involves a thorough history and physical examination. Review the woman's history closely for risk factors. The pathogenesis of hypertension is multifactorial and includes many modifiable risk factors such as smoking, obesity, caffeine intake, excessive alcohol intake, excessive salt intake, and use of nonsteroidal anti-inflammatory drugs. Also be alert for nonmodifiable risk factors such as increasing age and African-American race (Sharp, 2006). Ask if the woman has received any preconceptual counseling and what measures have been used to prevent or control hypertension.

Assess the woman's vital signs, in particular her blood pressure. Evaluate her blood pressure in all three positions (sitting, lying, and standing) and note any major differences in the readings. Assess her for orthostatic hypertension when she changes her position from sitting to standing. Document your findings.

Ask the woman if she monitors her blood pressure at home; if so, inquire about the typical readings. Ask the woman if she uses any medications for blood pressure control, including the drug, dosage, and frequency of administration, as well as any side effects. Ask the woman about lifestyle modifications that she has used to address any modifiable risk factors, and their effectiveness.

Hypertension during pregnancy decreases uteroplacental perfusion. Therefore, fetal well-being must be assessed and closely monitored. Anticipate serial ultrasounds to assess fetal growth and amniotic fluid volume. Question the woman about fetal movement and evaluate her report of daily "kick counts." Assess fetal heart rate at every visit.

Nursing Management

Preconception counseling is the ideal time to discuss lifestyle changes to prevent or control hypertension. One area to cover during this visit would be the Dietary Approaches to Stop Hypertension (DASH) diet, which contains an adequate intake of potassium, magnesium, and calcium. Sodium is usually limited to 2.4 g. Suggest aerobic exercise, although the woman should cease it once the pregnancy is confirmed. Encourage smoking cessation and avoidance of alcohol. If the woman is overweight, encourage her to lose weight before becoming pregnant, not during the pregnancy (Dudek, 2006). Stressing the positive benefits of a healthy lifestyle might help motivate the woman to make the modifications and change unhealthy habits.

Assist the woman in scheduling appointments for antepartum visits every 2 weeks until 28 weeks' gestation and then weekly. Prepare the woman for frequent fetal assessments. Explaining the rationale for the need to monitor fetal growth is important to gain the woman's cooperation. Carefully monitor the woman for signs and symptoms of abruptio placentae (abdominal pain, rigid abdomen, vaginal bleeding), as well as superimposed preeclampsia (elevation in blood pressure, weight gain, edema, proteinuria). Alerting the woman to these risks allows early identification and prompt intervention.

Stress the importance of daily periods of rest (1 hour) in the left lateral recumbent position to maximize placental perfusion. Encourage women with chronic hypertension to use home blood pressure monitoring devices. Urge the woman to report any elevations. As necessary, instruct the woman and her family how to take and record a daily blood pressure, and reinforce the need for her to take her medications as prescribed to control her blood pressure and to ensure the well-being of her unborn child. Praising her for her efforts at each prenatal visit may motivate her to continue the regimen throughout her pregnancy.

The close monitoring of the woman with chronic hypertension continues during labor and birth and during the postpartum period to prevent or identify the onset of preeclampsia. Accurate and frequent blood pressure readings and careful administration of antihypertensive medications, if prescribed, are essential components of care. Stressing the need for continued medical supervision after childbirth is vital to motivate the woman to maintain or initiate lifestyle changes and dietary habits and stay compliant with her medication regimen.

Respiratory Conditions

During pregnancy, the respiratory system is affected by hormonal changes, mechanical changes, and prior respiratory conditions. These changes can cause a woman with a history of compromised respiration to decompensate during pregnancy. While upper respiratory infections are typically self-limiting, chronic respiratory conditions, such as asthma or tuberculosis, can have a negative effect on the growing fetus when alterations in oxygenation occur in the mother. The outcome of pregnancy in a woman with a respiratory condition depends on the severity of the oxygen alteration as well as the degree and duration of hypoxia on the fetus.

▶ ASTHMA

Asthma affects approximately 1% to 4% of pregnancies. It affects 20 million Americans and is one of the most common and potentially serious medical conditions to complicate pregnancy (Arenson & Drake, 2007). Maternal asthma is associated with an increased risk of infant death, preeclampsia, intrauterine growth retardation (IUGR), preterm birth, and low birthweight. These risks are linked to the severity of asthma: more severe asthma increases the risk (National Asthma Education Prevention Program [NAEPP], 2007).

Remember Rose, the pregnant teenager with asthma in acute distress described at the beginning of the chapter? What therapies might be offered to control her symptoms? Should she be treated differently than someone who is not pregnant? Why or why not?

Pathophysiology

Asthma, an allergic-type inflammatory response of the respiratory tract to various stimuli, is also known as reactive airway disease because the bronchioles constrict in response to allergens, irritants, and infections. In addition to bronchoconstriction, inflammation of the airways produces thick mucus that further limits the movement of air and makes breathing difficult.

The normal physiologic changes of pregnancy affect the respiratory system. While the respiratory rate does not change, hyperventilation increases at term by 48% due to high progesterone levels. Diaphragmatic elevation and a decrease in functional lung residual capacity occur late in pregnancy, which may reduce the woman's ability to inspire deeply to take in more oxygen. Oxygen consumption and the metabolic rate both increase, placing additional stress on the woman's respiratory system (American Academy of Allergy, Asthma, and Immunology [AAAAI], 2007).

Both the woman and her fetus are at risk if asthma is not well managed during pregnancy. When a pregnant woman has trouble breathing, her fetus also has trouble getting the oxygen it needs for adequate growth and development. Severe persistent asthma has been linked to the development of maternal hypertension, preeclampsia, placenta previa, uterine hemorrhage, and oligohydramnios. Women whose asthma is poorly controlled during pregnancy are at increased risk of preterm birth, low birthweight, and stillbirth (Hackley, Kriebs, & Rousseau, 2007).

The severity of the condition improves in one third of pregnant women, remains unchanged in one third, and worsens in one third (Hackley, Kriebs, & Rousseau, 2007). However, the effect of pregnancy on asthma is unpredictable. The greatest increase in asthma attacks usually occurs between 24 and 36 weeks' gestation; flare-ups are rare during the last 4 weeks of pregnancy and during labor (AAAAI, 2007).

Therapeutic Management

Asthma should be treated as aggressively in pregnant women as in nonpregnant women because the benefits of averting an asthma attack outweigh the risks of medications. The goals of treatment are to prevent hospitalization, emergency room visits, work loss, and chronic disability. NAEPP recommends three specific drugs to be used during pregnancy to control asthma:

- Budesonide (inhaled-corticosteroid)
- Albuterol (short-acting beta2 agonist)
- Salmeterol (long-acting beta2 agonist)

Oral corticosteroids are not recommended for the treatment of asthma during pregnancy, but they can be used to treat severe asthma attacks during pregnancy (AAAAI, 2007).

Nursing Assessment

Obtain a thorough history of the disease, including the woman's usual therapy and control measures. Question the woman about asthma triggers and strategies used to reduce exposure to them (Box 20.2). Review the client's medication therapy regimen.

Auscultate the lungs and assess respiratory and heart rates. Include the rate, rhythm, and depth of respirations; skin color; blood pressure and pulse rate; and signs of fatigue. Patients with an acute asthma attack often present with wheezing, chest tightness, tachypnea, nonproductive coughing, shortness of breath, and dyspnea. Lung auscultation findings might include diffuse wheezes and rhonchi, bronchovesicular sounds, and a more prominent expiratory phase of respiration compared to the inspiratory phase (More, 2007). If the pregnancy is far enough along, the fetal heart rate is measured and routine prenatal assessments (weight, blood pressure, fundal height, urine for protein) are completed.

Laboratory studies usually include a complete blood count with differential (to assess the degree of nonspecific inflammation and identify anemia) and pulmonary function tests (to assess the severity of an attack and to provide a baseline to evaluate the client's response to treatment).

Nursing Management

Nursing management focuses on client education about the condition and the skills necessary to manage it: self-monitoring, correct use of inhalers, identifying and limiting exposure to asthma triggers, and following a long-term plan for managing asthma and for promptly handling signs and symptoms of worsening asthma. Client education fosters adherence to the treatment regimen, thereby promoting an optimal environment for fetal growth and development.

Ensure that the woman understands drug actions and interactions, the uses and potential abuses of asthma

---

BOX 20.2   Common Asthma Triggers

- Smoke and chemical irritants
- Air pollution
- Dust mites
- Animal dander
- Seasonal changes with pollen, molds, and spores
- Upper respiratory infections
- Esophageal reflux
- Medications, such as aspirin and nonsteroidal anti-inflammatory drugs (NSAIDs)
- Exercise
- Cold air
- Emotional stress

Sources: AAAAI, 2007; Little & Sinert, 2008; Gilbert, 2007.

medications, and the signs and symptoms that require medical evaluation. Reviewing potential perinatal complications with the woman is helpful in motivating her to adhere to the prescribed regimen. At each antepartum visit, reassess the efficacy of the treatment plan to determine whether adjustments are needed.

Taking control of asthma in pregnancy is the responsibility of the client along with her health care team. Providing the client with the knowledge and tools to monitor her condition, control triggers and her environment (Teaching Guidelines 20.2), and use medications to prevent acute exacerbations assist the client in taking control. Facilitating a partnership with the woman will improve perinatal outcomes.

When teaching the pregnant woman with asthma, cover the following topics:

- Signs and symptoms of asthma progression and exacerbation
- Importance and safety of medication to the fetus and to herself
- Warning signs that indicate the need to contact the health care provider
- Potential harm to the fetus and to herself by under-treatment or delay in seeking help
- Prevention and avoidance of known triggers
- Home use of metered-dose inhalers
- Adverse effects of medications

During labor, monitor the client's oxygenation saturation by pulse oximetry and provide pain management

---

TEACHING GUIDELINES 20.2

Teaching to Control Environmental Triggers

- Remove any carpeting in the house, especially the bedroom, to reduce dust mites.
- Use allergen-proof encasing on the mattress, box spring, and pillows.
- Wash all bedding in hot water.
- Remove dust collectors in house, such as stuffed animals, books, knick-knacks.
- Avoid pets in the house to reduce exposure to pet dander.
- Use a high-efficiency particulate air-filtering system in the bedroom.
- Do not smoke, and avoid places where you can be exposed to passive cigarette smoke from others.
- Stay indoors and use air conditioning when the pollen or mold count is high or air quality is poor.
- Wear a covering over your nose and mouth when going outside in the cold weather.
- Avoid exposure to persons with colds, flu, or viruses.

---

through epidural analgesia to reduce stress, which may trigger an acute attack. Continuously monitor the fetus for distress during labor and assess fetal heart rate patterns for hypoxia. Assess the newborn for signs and symptoms of hypoxia.

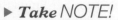

▶ *Take* NOTE!

Successful asthma management can reduce adverse perinatal outcomes: preeclampsia, preterm birth, and low birthweight.

Rose, the pregnant teenager described earlier, is concerned about passing her asthma on to her baby. What should the nurse discuss with her? What questions should the nurse ask to help in identifying triggers in Rose's environment to prevent future asthma attacks?

▶ TUBERCULOSIS

Tuberculosis (TB) is a disease that has been around for years but never seems to go away completely. Globally, TB is second only to HIV/AIDS as a cause of illness and death in adults, accounting for over 9 million cases of active disease and 2 million deaths each year. Someone in the world is newly infected with TB every second. Overall, one third of the world's population is currently infected with TB (World Health Organization [WHO], 2007). Although it is not prevalent in the United States, a resurgence was noted starting in the mid-1980s secondary to the AIDS epidemic and immigration. Left undiagnosed and untreated, each person with active TB will infect on average between 10 and 15 people each year (WHO, 2007). With the large numbers of immigrants coming to the United States, all nurses must be skilled in screening for and managing this condition.

A person becomes infected by inhaling the infectious organism, *Mycobacterium tuberculosis*, which is carried on a droplet nuclei and spread by airborne transmission. The lung is the major site of involvement, but the lymph glands, meninges, bones, joints, and kidneys can become infected. Women can remain asymptomatic for long periods of time as the organism may lie dormant. Pregnant women with untreated TB are more likely to have preeclampsia, miscarriage, preterm labor, an underweight infant, an infant with a low Apgar score, and perinatal death (Bothamley, 2006). The newborn is at risk of postnatally acquired TB if the mother still has active TB at the time of birth. Therefore, prenatal diagnosis and effective treatment of the mother are essential.

Therapeutic Management

Therapeutic management of TB during pregnancy is essentially the same as that for the general population. Medications are the cornerstone of treatment to prevent infection from progressing. The medical therapy for pregnant women is a combination of medications such as isoniazid, rifampin, and ethambutol, taken daily for up to 9 months. These anti-TB agents appear to have minimal teratogenic risks and may be started as soon as the diagnosis of TB is made. However, extensive research has not been done to determine the definitive safety of these drugs (Herchline & Amorosa, 2007).

Nursing Assessment

Review the woman's history for risk factors such as immunocompromised status, recent immigration status, homelessness or overcrowded living conditions, and injectable drug use. Women emigrating from developing countries such as Latin America, Asia, the Indian subcontinent, Eastern Europe, Russia, China, Mexico, Haiti, and Africa with high rates of TB also are at risk.

At antepartum visits, be alert for clinical manifestations of TB, including fatigue, fever or night sweats, nonproductive cough, slow weight loss, anemia, hemoptysis, and anorexia (Noyes & Popay, 2007). If TB is suspected or the woman is at risk for developing TB, anticipate screening with purified protein derivative (PPD) administered by intradermal injection. If the client has been exposed to TB, a reddened induration will appear within 72 hours. If the test is positive, anticipate a follow-up chest x-ray with lead shielding over the abdomen and sputum cultures to confirm the diagnosis.

Nursing Management

Compliance with the multidrug therapy is critical to protect the woman and her fetus from progression of TB. Provide education about the disease process, the mode of transmission, prevention, potential complications, and the importance of adhering to the treatment regimen.

Stressing the importance of health-promotion activities throughout the pregnancy is important. Some suggestions might include avoiding crowded living conditions, avoiding sick people, maintaining adequate hydration, eating a nutritious, well-balanced diet, keeping all prenatal appointments to evaluate fetal growth and well-being, and getting plenty of fresh air by going outside frequently. Determining the woman's understanding of her condition and treatment plan is important for compliance. A language interpreter may be needed to validate and reinforce her understanding if she does not speak English.

Breastfeeding is not contraindicated during the medication regimen and should in fact be encouraged. Management of the newborn of a mother with TB involves preventing transmission by teaching the parents not to cough, sneeze, or talk directly into the newborn's face. Nurses need to stay current about new therapies and screening techniques to treat this centuries-old disease.

Hematologic Conditions

Anemia, a reduction in red blood cell volume, is measured by hematocrit (Hct) or a decrease in the concentration of hemoglobin (Hgb) in the peripheral blood. This results in reduced capacity of the blood to carry oxygen to the vital organs of the mother and fetus. Anemia is a sign of an underlying problem but does not indicate its origin.

▶ IRON DEFICIENCY ANEMIA

Iron deficiency anemia affects one in four pregnancies and is usually related to an inadequate dietary intake of iron (McCann, 2007). It is a very common state in pregnant women. Anemia during the early part of pregnancy can increase the likelihood of preterm birth, low birthweight, and perinatal mortality (Blackburn, 2007). With significant maternal iron depletion, the fetus will attempt to store iron, but at the cost to the mother. Anemia at term increases the perinatal risk for both the mother and newborn. The risks of hemorrhage (impaired platelet function) and infection during and after birth also are increased.

Therapeutic Management

The goals of treatment for iron deficiency anemia in pregnancy are to eliminate symptoms, correct the deficiency, and replenish iron stores. The CDC recommends routine iron supplementation for all pregnant women at a low dose of 30 mg/day beginning at the first prenatal visit. Attempting to meet maternal iron requirements solely through diet in the face of diminished iron stores is difficult.

Nursing Assessment

Review the mother's history for factors that may contribute to the development of iron deficiency anemia, including poor nutrition, hemolysis, **pica** (consuming non-food substances), multiple gestation, limited intervals between pregnancies, and blood loss. Assess the woman's dietary intake as well as the quantity and timing of ingestion of substances that interfere with iron absorption, such as tea, coffee, chocolate, and high-fiber foods. Ask the woman if she has fatigue, weakness, malaise, anorexia, or increased susceptibility to infection, such as frequent colds. Inspect the skin and mucous membranes, noting any pallor. Obtain vital signs and report any tachycardia.

Prepare the woman for laboratory testing. Laboratory tests usually reveal low Hgb (<11 g/dL), low Hct (<35%), low serum iron (<30 ug/dL), microcytic and hypochromic cells, and low serum ferritin (<100 mg/dL).

> ▶ *Take NOTE!*

Hemoglobin and hematocrit decrease normally during pregnancy in response to an increase in blood plasma in comparison to red blood cells. This hemodilution can lead to physiologic anemia of pregnancy, which is expected in the second trimester of pregnancy. This hemodilution phenomenon should not be confused with an iron deficiency anemia, in which the Hgb would be below 11 g/100 mL and Hct below 35%.

Nursing Management

Nursing management of the woman with iron deficiency anemia focuses on encouraging compliance with drug therapy and providing dietary instruction about the intake of foods high in iron. Although iron constitutes a minimal percentage of the body's total weight, it has several major roles: it assists in the transport of oxygen and carbon dioxide throughout the body, it aids in the production of red blood cells, and it plays a role in the body's immune response.

Stress the importance of taking the prenatal vitamin and iron supplement consistently. Encourage the woman to take the iron supplement with vitamin C-containing fluids such as orange juice, which will promote absorption, rather than milk, which can inhibit iron absorption. Taking iron on an empty stomach improves its absorption, but many women cannot tolerate the gastrointestinal discomfort it causes. In such cases, advise the woman to take it with meals. Instruct the woman about adverse effects, which are predominantly gastrointestinal and include gastric discomfort, nausea, vomiting, anorexia, diarrhea, metallic taste, and constipation. Suggest that the woman take the iron supplement with meals and increase her intake of fiber and fluids to help overcome the most common side effects.

Provide dietary counseling. Recommend foods high in iron, such as dried fruits, whole grains, green leafy vegetables, meats, peanut butter, and iron-fortified cereals (Dudek, 2006). Anticipate the need for a referral to a dietitian. Teaching Guidelines 20.3 highlights instructions for the pregnant woman with iron deficiency anemia.

▶ THALASSEMIA

Thalassemia is a group of hereditary anemias in which synthesis of one or both chains of the hemoglobin molecule (alpha and beta) is defective. A low Hgb and a microcytic, hypochromic anemia result. The prevalence and severity of thalassemia depend on the woman's racial

TEACHING GUIDELINES 20.3

Teaching for the Woman With Iron Deficiency Anemia

- Take your prenatal vitamin daily; if you miss a dose, take it as soon as you remember.
- For best absorption, take iron supplement between meals.
- Avoid taking iron supplement with coffee, tea, chocolate, and high-fiber food.
- Eat foods rich in iron, such as:
  - Meats, green leafy vegetables, legumes, dried fruits, whole grains
  - Peanut butter, bean dip, whole-wheat fortified breads and cereals
- For best iron absorption from foods, consume the food along with a food high in vitamin C.
- Increase your exercise, fluids, and high-fiber foods to reduce constipation.
- Plan frequent rest periods during the day.

background: persons of Mediterranean, Asian, Italian, or Greek heritage and African-Americans are most frequently affected. Beta-thalassemia is the most common form found in the United States (Curran & Poggi, 2007).

Thalassemia occurs in two forms: alpha-thalassemia and beta-thalassemia. Alpha-thalassemia (minor), the heterozygous form, results from the inheritance of one abnormal gene from either parent, placing the offspring in a carrier trait state. These women have little or no hematologic disease and are clinically asymptomatic (silent carrier state). Beta-thalassemia (major) is the form involving inheritance of the gene from both parents. Beta-thalassemia major can be very severe. Genetic counseling might be necessary when decisions about childbearing are being made.

Thalassemia minor has little effect on the pregnancy, although the woman will have mild, persistent anemia. This anemia does not respond to iron therapy, and iron supplements should not be prescribed. Women with thalassemia major do not usually become pregnant because of lifelong severe hemolysis, anemia, and premature death (Hackley, Kriebs, & Rousseau, 2007).

Management of thalassemia during pregnancy depends on the severity of the disease. Identification and screening are important to plan care. The woman's ethnic background, medical history, and blood studies are analyzed. If the woman is determined to be a carrier, screening of the father of the child is indicated. Knowledge of the carrier state of each parent provides the genetic counselor with knowledge about the risk that the fetus will be a carrier or will have the disease (Curran & Poggi, 2007).

Mild anemia may be present, and instructions to rest and avoid infections are helpful. Nurses should provide supportive care and expectant management throughout the pregnancy.

SICKLE CELL ANEMIA

Sickle cell anemia is an autosomal recessive inherited condition that results from a defective hemoglobin molecule (hemoglobin S). It is found most commonly in African-Americans, Southeast Asians, and Middle Eastern populations. About 1 in 10 African-Americans are carriers of the trait, while approximately 3 in 800 are affected with the disease (McCann, 2007). People with only one gene for the trait (heterozygous) will have sickle cell trait without obvious symptoms of the disease and with little effect on the pregnancy.

Pathophysiology

In the human body, the hemoglobin molecule serves as the oxygen-carrying component of the red blood cells. Most people have several types of circulating hemoglobin (HbA and HbA2) that make up the majority of their circulatory system. In sickle cell disease, the abnormal hemoglobin S (HbS) replaces HbA and HbA2. This abnormal hemoglobin (HbS) becomes sickle-shaped as a result of any stress or trauma such as infection, fever, acidosis, dehydration, physical exertion, excessive cold exposure, or hypoxia. Significant anemia results. (See Chapter 46 for more information about sickle cell disease.)

Sickle cell anemia during pregnancy is associated with more severe anemia and frequent vaso-occlusive crises, with increased maternal and perinatal morbidity and mortality. In pregnant women with sickle cell anemia, complications can occur at any time during gestation, labor and birth, or postpartum. This is believed to be secondary to hormonal modifications, hypercoagulable state, and increased susceptibility to infection. Microvascular sickling in the placental circulation is associated with miscarriages, placental abruption, preeclampsia, preterm labor, intrauterine growth restriction, and low birthweight (El-sayegh & Shapiro, 2007).

Therapeutic Management

Ideally, women with hemoglobinopathies are screened before conception and are made aware of the risks of sickle cell anemia to themselves and to the fetus. A blood hemoglobin electrophoresis is done for all women from high-risk ancestry at their first prenatal visit to determine the types and percentages of hemoglobin present. This information should help them in making reproductive decisions.

Treatment depends on the health status of the woman. During pregnancy, only supportive therapy is used: blood transfusions for severe anemia, analgesics for pain, and antibiotics for infection.

Nursing Assessment

Assess the woman for signs and symptoms of sickle cell anemia. Ask the woman if she has anorexia, dyspnea, or malaise. Inspect the color of the skin and mucous membranes, noting any pallor. Be alert for indicators of sickle cell crisis, including severe abdominal pain, muscle spasms, leg pains, joint pain, fever, stiff neck, nausea and vomiting, and seizures (McCann, 2007).

Nursing Management

Clients require emotional support, education, and follow-up care to deal with this chronic condition, which can have a great impact on the woman and her family. Monitor vital signs, fetal heart rate, weight gain, and fetal growth. Assess hydration status at each visit and urge the client to drink 8 to 10 glasses of fluid daily to prevent dehydration. Teach the client about the need to avoid infections (including meticulous handwashing), cigarette smoking, alcohol consumption, and temperature extremes.

Assist the woman in scheduling frequent fetal well-being assessments, such as biophysical profiles, nonstress tests, and contraction stress tests, and monitor laboratory test results for changes. Throughout the antepartal period, be alert for early signs and symptoms of crisis.

During labor, encourage rest and provide pain management. Oxygen supplementation is typically used throughout labor, along with intravenous fluids to maintain hydration. The fetal heart rate is monitored closely. After giving birth, the woman is fitted with antiembolism stockings to prevent blood clot formation. Before discharge from the facility after birth of the newborn, discuss family planning options.

Infections

A wide variety of infections can affect the progression of pregnancy, possibly having a negative impact on the outcome. The effect of the infection depends on the timing and severity of the infection and the body systems involved. Common viral infections include cytomegalovirus (CMV), rubella, herpes simplex, hepatitis B, varicella, parvovirus B19, and several sexually transmitted infections (Table 20.3). Toxoplasmosis and group B streptococcus are common nonviral infections. Only the most common infections will be discussed here.

CYTOMEGALOVIRUS

Cytomegalovirus (CMV) is the most common congenital and perinatal viral infection in the world, possibly affecting up to 3% of all newborns (Ross, Jones, & Lynch,

TABLE 20.3   SEXUALLY TRANSMITTED INFECTIONS AFFECTING PREGNANCY

Infection/Organism	Effect on Pregnancy and Fetus/Newborn	Implications
Syphilis (*Treponema pallidum*)	Maternal infection increases risk of premature labor and birth. Newborn may be born with congenital syphilis—jaundice, rhinitis, anemia, IUGR, and CNS involvement.	All pregnant women should be screened for this STI and treated with benzathine penicillin G 2.4 million units IM to prevent placental transmission.
Gonorrhea (*Neisseria gonorrhoeae*)	Majority of women are asymptomatic. It causes ophthalmia neonatorum in the newborn from birth through infected birth canal.	All pregnant women should be screened at first prenatal visit, with repeat screening in the third trimester. All newborns receive mandatory eye prophylaxis with tetracycline or erythromycin within the first hour of life. Mother is treated with ceftriaxone (Rocephin) 125 mg IM in single dose before going home.
Chlamydia (*Chlamydia trachomatis*)	Majority of women are asymptomatic. Infection is associated with infertility and ectopic pregnancy, spontaneous abortions, preterm labor, premature rupture of membranes, low birthweight, stillbirth, and neonatal mortality. Infection is transmitted to newborn through vaginal birth. Neonate may develop conjunctivitis or pneumonia.	All pregnant women should be screened at first prenatal visit and treated with erythromycin.
Human papillomavirus (HPV)	Infection causes warts in the anogenital area, known as condylomata acuminata. These warts may grow large enough to block a vaginal birth. Fetal exposure to HPV during birth is associated with laryngeal papillomas.	Warts are treated with trichlorocetic acid, liquid nitrogen, or laser therapy under colposcopy. A quadrivalent HPV vaccine (Gardasil) against the viral types most likely to cause cervical cancer (types 16 and 18) and genital warts (types 6 and 11) has been licensed in the United States for girls and women 9 to 26 years old. The vaccine is 95% to 100% effective (Zimmerman, 2007). It is hoped that this vaccine will reduce the number of HPV-positive pregnant women in the future.
Trichomonas (*Trichomonas vaginalis*)	Infection produces itching and burning, dysuria, strawberry patches on cervix, and vaginal discharge. Infection is associated with premature rupture of membranes and preterm birth.	Treatment is with a single 2-g dose of metronidazole (Flagyl).

Sources: CDC STD Treatment Guidelines, 2006; Moore & Saybold, 2007.

2006). Pregnant women acquire active disease primarily from sexual contact, blood transfusions, kissing, and contact with children in daycare centers. The virus can be found in virtually all body fluids. Prevalence rates in women in the United States range from 50% to 85% (Hoerst & Samson, 2007). The incidence of primary CMV infection in pregnant women in the United States ranges from 1% to 3% (Hoerst & Samson, 2007). CMV infection during pregnancy may result in abortion, stillbirth, low birthweight, IUGR, microcephaly, deafness, blindness, mental retardation, jaundice, or congenital or neonatal infection. The first or primary infection, if it occurs during pregnancy, is the most dangerous to the fetus: the fetus has a 40% to 50% chance of being infected.

Most women are asymptomatic and don't know they have been exposed to CMV. Symptoms of CMV in the fetus and newborn, known as cytomegalovirus inclusion disease (CID), include hepatomegaly, thrombocytopenia, IUGR, jaundice, microcephaly, hearing loss, chorioretinitis, and mental retardation (Hoerst & Samson, 2007). Since there is no therapy that prevents or treats CMV infections, nurses are responsible for educating and supporting childbearing-age women at risk for CMV infection. Stressing the importance of good handwashing and use of sound hygiene practices can help to reduce transmission of the virus.

▶ RUBELLA

Rubella, commonly called German measles, is spread by droplets or through direct contact with a contaminated object. The risk of a pregnant woman transmitting this virus through the placenta to her fetus increases with earlier exposure to the virus. When infection occurs within the first month after conception, 50% of fetuses show signs of infection; in the second month following conception, 25% of fetuses will be infected; and in the third month, 10% of fetuses will be affected (Santis et al., 2006).

Education for primary prevention is key. Ideally, all women have been vaccinated and have adequate immunity against rubella. However, all women are still screened at their first prenatal visit to determine their status. A rubella antibody titer 1:8 or greater proves evidence of immunity. Women who are not immune should be vaccinated during the immediate postpartum period so they will be immune before becoming pregnant again (CDC, 2007c). Nurses need to check the rubella immune status of all new mothers and should make sure all mothers with a titer of less than 1:8 are immunized prior to discharge after birth of the newborn.

▶ HERPES SIMPLEX VIRUS

Approximately 50 million people are infected with genital herpes in the United States, and 500,000 new cases are diagnosed annually. Despite strategies designed to prevent perinatal transmission, the number of cases of newborn herpes simplex virus (HSV) infection continues to rise, mirroring the rising prevalence of genital herpes infection in women of childbearing age (Fischer, 2007).

HSV is a DNA virus with two subtypes: HSV-1 and HSV-2. HSV-1 infections were traditionally associated with oral lesions (fever blisters), whereas HSV-2 infections occurred in the genital region. Currently, either type can be found in either location (Fischer, 2007).

Infection occurs by direct contact of the skin or mucous membranes with an active lesion through such activities as kissing, sexual (vaginal, oral, anal) contact, or routine skin-to-skin contact. HSV is associated with infections of the genital tract that when acquired during pregnancy can result in severe systemic symptoms in the mother and significant morbidity and mortality in the newborn (Baker, 2007). Once the virus enters the body, it never leaves.

Infants born to mothers with a primary HSV infection have a 30% to 50% risk of acquiring the infection via perinatal transmission near or during birth. Recurrent genital herpes simplex infections carry a 1% to 3% risk of neonatal infection if the recurrence occurs around the time of vaginal birth (Xu et al., 2007).

The greatest risk of transmission is when the mother develops a primary infection near term and it is not recognized. Most neonatal infections are acquired at or around the time of birth through either ascending infection after ruptured membranes or contact with the virus at the time of birth. The method and timing of birth in a woman with genital herpes are controversial. The CDC recommends that in the absence of active lesions, a vaginal birth is acceptable, but if the woman has active herpetic lesions near or at term, a cesarean birth should be planned (CDC, 2008). All invasive procedures that might cause a break in the infant's skin should be avoided, such as artificial rupture of membranes, fetal scalp electrode, or forceps and vacuum extraction (Gilbert, 2007).

Management for the woman with genital herpes during pregnancy involves caring for her as well as reducing the risk of newborn herpes. Since the majority of newborn herpes cases result from perinatal transmission of the virus during vaginal birth, and because transmission can result in severe neurologic impairment or death, treatment of the mother with an antiviral agent such as acyclovir must be started as soon as the culture comes back positive. Universal screening for herpes is not economically sound, so nurses need to remain knowledgeable about current practice to provide accurate and sensitive care to all women.

▶ HEPATITIS B VIRUS

Hepatitis B virus (HBV) is one of the most prevalent chronic diseases in the world. HBV can be transmitted through contaminated blood, illicit drug use, and sexual contact. The virus is 100 times more infectious than HIV and, unlike HIV, it can live outside the body in dried blood for more than a week (Hoerst & Samson, 2007).

Sexual transmission accounts for most adult HBV infections in the United States. Acutely infected women develop hepatitis with anorexia, nausea, vomiting, fever, abdominal pain, and jaundice. In women with acute hepatitis B, vertical transmission occurs in approximately 10% of newborns when infection occurs in the first trimester and in 80% to 90% of newborns when acute infection occurs in the third trimester. Without intervention, 70% to 90% of infants born to women who are positive for hepatitis B will have chronic hepatitis B by 6 months of age (Kripke, 2007).

In addition, hepatitis B infection during pregnancy is associated with an increased risk of preterm birth, low birthweight, and neonatal death. Newborns infected with HBV are likely to become chronic carriers of the virus, becoming reservoirs for continued infection in the population (CDC, 2007e). The fetus is at particular risk during birth because of the possible contact with contaminated blood at this time.

Nursing Assessment

Review the woman's history for factors placing her at high risk:

- History of sexually transmitted infections
- Household contacts with HBV-infected persons
- Employment as a health care worker
- Abuse of intravenous drugs
- Sex worker (prostitute)
- Foreign born
- Multiple sexual partners
- Chinese, Southeast Asian, or African heritage
- Sexual partners who are HBV infected (CDC, 2007e)

At the first prenatal visit, all pregnant women should be screened for hepatitis B surface antigen (HbsAg) via blood studies. Expect to repeat this screening later in pregnancy for women in high-risk groups (Hoerst & Samson, 2007).

Nursing Management

If a woman tests positive for HBV, expect to administer HBV immune globulin (HBIG, Hep-B-Gammagee). The newborn receives HBV vaccine (Recombivax-HB, Engerix-B) within 12 hours of birth. The second and third doses of the vaccine are given at 1 month and 6 months of age (CDC, 2007e). The CDC recommends routine vaccination of all newborns.

Women who are HbsAg-negative may be vaccinated safely during pregnancy. No current research supports the use of surgical births to reduce vertical transmission of HBV. Breastfeeding by mothers with chronic HBV infection does not increase the risk of viral transmission to their newborns (Pyrsopoulos & Reddy, 2007).

Client education related to prevention of HBV is essential. Teach the woman about safer sex practices, good handwashing techniques, and the use of standard precautions (Teaching Guidelines 20.4). Protection can be afforded with the highly effective hepatitis B vaccine.

Permanent remission of the disease even with treatment rarely occurs. Therefore, therapy is directed at long-term suppression of viral replication and prevention of end-stage liver disease. Urge the woman to consume a

TEACHING GUIDELINES 20.4

Teaching to Prevent Hepatitis B Virus

- Abstain from alcohol.
- Avoid intravenous drug exposure or sharing of needles.
- Encourage all household contacts and sexual partners to be vaccinated.
- Receive immediate treatment for any sexually transmitted infection.
- Know that your newborn will receive the hepatitis B vaccine soon after birth.
- Use good handwashing techniques at all times.
- Avoid contact with blood or body fluids.
- Use barrier methods such as condoms during sexual intercourse.
- Avoid sharing any personal items, such as razors, toothbrushes, or eating utensils.

high-protein diet and avoid fatigue. A healthy lifestyle can help delay disease progression. Initiate an open discussion about the modes of transmission and use of condoms to prevent spread.

▶ VARICELLA ZOSTER VIRUS

Varicella zoster virus (VZV), a member of the herpesvirus family, is the virus that causes both varicella (chickenpox) and herpes zoster (shingles). Pregnant women are at risk for developing varicella when they come in close contact with children who have active infection. Maternal varicella can be transmitted to the fetus through the placenta, leading to congenital varicella syndrome, if the mother is infected during the first half of pregnancy, via an ascending infection during birth, or by direct contact with infectious lesions, leading to infection after birth. Varicella occurs in approximately 1 to 7 of 10,000 pregnancies (Anderson & Safdar, 2007).

Congenital varicella syndrome can occur in newborns of mothers infected during early pregnancy. It is characterized by low birthweight, skin lesions in a dermatomal distribution, spontaneous abortion, chorioretinitis, cataracts, cutaneous scarring, limb hypoplasia, microcephaly, ocular abnormalities, mental retardation, and early death (Laartz & Gompf, 2007).

Preconception counseling is important for preventing this condition. A major component of counseling involves determining the woman's varicella immunity. The vaccine is administered if needed. Provide education to women who work in occupations that increase the risk of exposure to the virus, such as daycare workers, teachers of young children, and staff caring for children in institutional settings.

Varicella during pregnancy can be associated with severe illnesses for both the mother and her newborn. If contracted in the first half of pregnancy, some pregnant women are at risk for developing varicella pneumonia, which may put them at risk of life-threatening ventilatory compromise and death (Sauerbrei & Wutzler, 2007). If the mother develops varicella rashes close to her due date, generalized neonatal varicella leading to death in about 20% of cases can be expected (Gardella & Brown, 2007). Maternal infection is preventable by preconception vaccination.

▶ PARVOVIRUS B19

Parvovirus B19 infection occurs worldwide. The incidence of acute B19 infection in pregnancy is about 3% (Malee, 2007). Parvovirus B19 is a common, self-limiting benign childhood virus that causes erythema infectiosum, also known as fifth disease (referring to its "fifth place" in a list of common childhood infections). Approximately 50% to 65% of women of reproductive age have developed immunity to parvovirus B19 (Broliden, Tolfvenstam, & Norbeck, 2006).

Pathophysiology

The infection is spread transplacentally, by the oropharyngeal route in casual contact, and through infected blood. Infection of the fetus occurs through transplacental passage of the virus. Acute infection in pregnancy can cause B19 infection in the fetus, leading to nonimmune fetal hydrops secondary to severe anemia or fetal loss, depending on the gestational age at the time of infection. The risk to the fetus is greatest when the woman is exposed and infected within the first 20 weeks of gestation. In addition to hydrops, other fetal effects of parvovirus include spontaneous abortion, congenital anomalies (central nervous system, craniofacial, and eye), and long-term effects such as hepatic insufficiency, myocarditis, and learning disabilities (Cunningham & Rennels, 2006).

Therapeutic Management

Generally, diagnosis of parvovirus is based on clinical symptoms and serologic antibody testing for parvovirus immunoglobulin G and parvovirus immunoglobulin M (IgM). Parvovirus B19 infection is followed by lifelong immunity, which is shown by positive serum B19 IgG. Pregnant women who have been exposed to or who develop symptoms of parvovirus B19 require assessment to determine whether they are susceptible to infection (nonimmune). If the woman is immune, she can be reassured

that she will not develop infection and that the virus will not adversely affect her pregnancy. If she is nonimmune, then referral to a perinatologist is recommended and counseling regarding the risks of fetal transmission, fetal loss, and hydrops is necessary. Knowledge of how best to manage it during pregnancy lags behind our understanding of the potential adverse consequences.

Intrauterine B19 infection is a cause of fetal anemia, hydrops, and demise, and perhaps also of congenital anomalies. The best strategy for surveillance of the infected pregnant woman is serial ultrasounds for detection of hydropic changes and fetal anemia, and treatment for severe fetal anemia. Serial ultrasounds are advocated because the rates of fetal death and complications peak 4 to 6 weeks after exposure, but they can occur as late as 3 months following onset of symptoms (Elbaz et al., 2007).

The infected newborn is assessed for any anomaly and followed for up to 6 years to identify any sequelae (Cunningham & Rennels, 2006).

Nursing Assessment

Review the mother's history for any risk factors. Schoolteachers, daycare workers, and women living with school-aged children are at highest risk for being seropositive for parvovirus B19, especially if a recent outbreak has occurred in those settings. Also assess the woman for specific signs and symptoms. The characteristic rash starts on the face with a "slapped-cheeks" appearance and is followed by a generalized maculopapular rash. Fever, arthralgia, and generalized malaise are usually present in the mother. Prepare the mother for antibody testing.

Nursing Management

Prevention is the best strategy. Stress the need for handwashing after handling children; cleaning toys and surfaces that children have been in contact with; and avoiding the sharing of food and drinks. Screening for parvovirus B19 during early pregnancy may help in early diagnosis, but the cost-effectiveness of a national screening program has not been accepted to date. The nurse can provide information regarding risk factors and potential complications if exposed and support the parent's decision.

▶ GROUP B STREPTOCOCCUS

Group B streptococcus (GBS) is a naturally occurring bacterium found in 10% to 35% of healthy adults. Women who test positive for the GBS bacteria are considered carriers. Carrier status is transient and doesn't indicate illness. Approximately 25% of pregnant women carry GBS in the rectum or vagina, thus introducing the risk of colonization of the fetus during birth. GBS affects about 1 in every 2,000 newborns in the United States

(March of Dimes, 2007d). Approximately 1 out of every 100 to 200 newborns born to mothers who carry GBS will develop signs and symptoms of GBS disease. Although GBS is rarely serious in adults, it can be life-threatening to newborns. GBS is the most common cause of sepsis and meningitis in newborns and is a frequent cause of newborn pneumonia (Moos, 2006). Newborns with early-onset (within a week after birth) GBS infections may have pneumonia or sepsis, whereas late-onset (after the first week) infections often manifest with meningitis (CDC, 2007b).

Genital tract colonization poses the most threat to the newborn because of exposure during birth and to the mother because of ascending infection after the membranes rupture. GBS colonization in the mother is thought to cause chorioamnionitis, endometritis, and postpartum wound infection.

Therapeutic Management

Antibiotic therapy usually is effective in treating women with GBS infections of the urinary tract or uterus, or chorioamnionitis without any sequelae. According to the 2002 CDC guidelines, all pregnant women should be screened for GBS at 35 to 37 weeks' gestation. Vaginal and rectal specimens are cultured for the presence of the bacterium. If positive, the woman should be treated with intravenous antibiotics during labor.

Penicillin G is the treatment of choice for GBS infection because of its narrow spectrum. Alternative antibiotics can be prescribed for clients with a penicillin allergy. The drug is usually administered intravenously at least 4 hours before birth so that it can reach adequate levels in the serum and amniotic fluid to reduce the risk of newborn colonization. Close monitoring is required during the administration of intravenous antibiotics because severe allergic reactions can occur rapidly.

Nursing Assessment

Review the woman's prenatal history, asking about any previous infection. Determine if the woman's membranes have ruptured and the time of rupture. Rupture of amniotic membranes greater than 18 hours increases the risk for infection. Monitor the mother's vital signs, reporting any maternal fever greater than 100.4°F. Assess the woman for other risk factors for perinatal transmission of GBS, including previous colonization with GBS, low socioeconomic status, African-American race, age less than 20 years, positive colonization at 35 to 37 weeks' gestation, GBS in urine sample, previous birth of GBS-positive newborn, preterm birth, and use of invasive obstetric procedures (March of Dimes, 2007d). Document this information to help prevent vertical transmission to the newborn.

Many women with GBS infection are asymptomatic, but they may have urinary tract infections, uterine infections, and chorioamnionitis.

Nursing Management

Nurses play major roles as educators and advocates for all women and newborns to reduce the incidence of GBS infections. Ensure that pregnant women between 35 and 37 weeks' gestation are screened for GBS infection during a prenatal visit. Record the results and notify the birth attendant if the woman has tested positive for GBS. During labor, be prepared to administer intravenous antibiotics to all women who are GBS positive.

▶ TOXOPLASMOSIS

Toxoplasmosis is a relatively widespread parasitic infection caused by a one-celled organism, *Toxoplasma gondii*. When a pregnant woman is exposed to this protozoan, the infection can pose serious risks to her fetus. Between 1 in 1,000 and 8,000 newborns are born infected with toxoplasmosis in the United States (Hokelek & Safdar, 2006). It is transferred by hand to mouth after touching cat feces while changing the cat litter box or through gardening in contaminated soil. Consuming undercooked meat, such as pork, lamb, or venison, can also transmit this organism.

A pregnant woman who contracts toxoplasmosis for the first time has approximately a 40% chance of passing the infection to her fetus (March of Dimes, 2007e). Although the woman typically remains asymptomatic, transmission to her fetus can occur throughout pregnancy. A fetus that contracts congenital toxoplasmosis typically has a low birthweight, enlarged liver and spleen, chorioretinitis, jaundice, neurologic damage, and anemia (Peyron et al., 2006).

Treatment of the woman during pregnancy to reduce the risk of congenital infection is a combination of pyrimethamine and sulfadiazine. Treatment with sulfonamides during pregnancy has been shown to reduce the risk of congenital infection.

Prevention is the key to managing this infection. Nurses play a key role in educating the woman about measures to prevent toxoplasmosis (Teaching Guidelines 20.5).

Vulnerable Populations

Every year there are an estimated 220 million pregnancies worldwide, with about 6 million of them in the United States (Alan Guttmacher Institute, 2007). Each pregnancy runs the risk of an adverse outcome for the mother and the baby, but risks are dramatically increased for certain vulnerable populations: adolescents, women over the age of 35, women who are HIV positive, and women who abuse substances. While risks cannot be totally eliminated once pregnancy has begun, they can be reduced through appropriate and timely interventions.

TEACHING GUIDELINES 20.5

Teaching to Prevent Toxoplasmosis

- Avoid eating raw or undercooked meat, especially lamb or pork. Cook all meat to an internal temperature of 160°F throughout.
- Clean cutting boards, work surfaces, and utensils with hot soapy water after contact with raw meat or unwashed fruits and vegetables.
- Peel or thoroughly wash all raw fruits and vegetables before eating them.
- Wash hands thoroughly with warm water and soap after handling raw meat.
- Avoid feeding the cat raw or undercooked meats.
- Avoid emptying or cleaning the cat's litter box. Have someone else do it daily.
- Keep the cat indoors to prevent it from hunting and eating birds or rodents.
- Avoid uncooked eggs and unpasteurized milk.
- Wear gardening gloves when in contact with outdoor soil.
- Avoid contact with children's sandboxes, because cats can use them as litter boxes.

Every woman's experience with pregnancy is unique and personal. The circumstances each one faces and what pregnancy means to her involve emotions and experiences that belong solely to her. Many women in these special population groups go through this experience in confusion and isolation, feeling desperately in need of help but not knowing where to go. Although all pregnant women experience these emotions to a certain extent, but they are heightened in women who have numerous psychosocial issues. Pregnancy is a stressful time. Pregnant women face wide-ranging changes in their lives, relationships, and bodies as they move toward parenthood. These changes can be challenging for a woman without any additional stresses but are even more so in the face of age extremes, illness, or substance abuse.

Skilled nursing interventions are essential to promote the best outcome for the client and her baby. Timely support and appropriate interventions during the perinatal period can have long-standing implications for the mother and her newborn, ultimately with the goal of stability and integration of the family as a unit.

▶ PREGNANT ADOLESCENT

Adolescence lasts from the onset of puberty to the cessation of physical growth, roughly from 11 to 19 years of age. Adolescents vacillate between being children and

being adults. They need to adjust to the physiologic changes their bodies are undergoing and establish a sexual identity during this time. They search for personal identity and desire freedom and independence of thought and action. However, they continue to have a strong dependence on their parents (O'Toole, 2005).

Each year in the United States, approximately 1 million adolescents, or 10% of girls between the ages of 15 to 19 years, become pregnant. These pregnancies, which account for 11% of all births, are typically unintended and occur outside of marriage (Alan Guttmacher Institute, 2006). In addition, about half of all teen pregnancies occur within 6 months of first having sexual intercourse. Of girls who become pregnant, one in six will have a repeat pregnancy within 1 year. Most of these girls are unmarried, and many are not ready for the emotional, psychological, and financial responsibilities of parenthood (March of Dimes, 2007a). Adolescent pregnancy is further complicated by the adolescent's lack of financial resources: the income of teen mothers is half that of women who have given birth in their 20s (March of Dimes, 2007a).

Although the incidence of teenage pregnancy has steadily declined since the early 1990s, it continues to be higher in the United States than in any other industrialized country (Alan Guttmacher Institute, 2006). Even this reduced incidence represents what is considered an unacceptably high level of pregnancy in an age group that is likely to suffer the social consequences of early pregnancy most. Subsequently, adolescent pregnancy is considered a major health problem and is addressed in Healthy People 2010.

Impact of Pregnancy in Adolescence

Adolescents are a unique group with special needs related to their stage of development. Adolescent pregnancy can be an emotionally charged situation, laden with ethical dilemmas and decisions. Topics such as abstinence, safer sex, abortion, and the decision to have a child are sensitive issues.

HEALTHY PEOPLE 2010

Objective	Significance
Reduce pregnancy among adolescent females from a baseline of 68 pregnancies per 1,000 adolescent girls to 43 pregnancies per 1,000 adolescent girls	Will help to foster a continued decline in adolescent pregnancy rates by focusing on interventions related to pregnancy prevention, including safe sex practices and teaching about the complications associated with adolescent pregnancy

USDHHS, 2000.

Adolescent pregnancy is an area when a nurse's moral convictions may influence the care that he or she provides to clients. Nurses need to examine their own beliefs about teen sexuality to identify personal assumptions. Putting aside one's moral convictions may be difficult, but it is necessary when working with pregnant adolescents. To be effective, health care providers must be able to communicate with adolescents in a manner they can understand and respect them as individuals.

Developmental Issues

An adolescent must accomplish certain developmental tasks to advance to the next stage of maturity. These developmental tasks include:

• Seeking economic and social stability
• Developing a personal value system
• Building meaningful relationships with others (Fig. 20.3)
• Becoming comfortable with their changing bodies
• Working to become independent from their parents
• Learning to verbalize conceptually (Zarrett & Eccles, 2006)

Adolescents have special needs when working to accomplish their developmental tasks and making a smooth transition to young adulthood. One of the biggest areas of need is sexual health. Adolescents commonly lack the information, skills, and services necessary to make informed choices related to their sexual and reproductive health. Developmentally, adolescents are trying to figure out who they are and how they fit into society. As adolescents mature, their parents become less influential and peers become more influential. Peer pressure can lead adolescents to participate in sexual activity, as can the typical adolescent's belief that "it won't happen to me" (Box 20.3).

As a result, unplanned pregnancies occur. Work on the developmental tasks of adolescence, especially identity, can be interrupted as the adolescent attempts to integrate the tasks of pregnancy, bonding, and preparing to

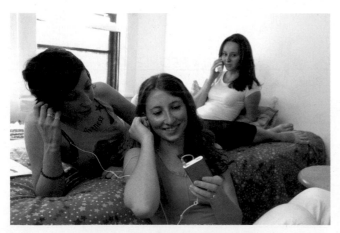

FIGURE 20.3 Adolescent girls sharing time together.

> ### BOX 20.3   Possible Factors Contributing to Adolescent Pregnancy
>
> • Early menarche
> • Peer pressure to become sexually active
> • Sexual or other abuse as a child
> • Lack of accurate contraceptive information
> • Fear of telling parents about sexual activity
> • Feelings of invulnerability
> • Poverty (85% of births occur in poor families)
> • Culture or ethnicity (high incidence in Hispanic and African-American girls)
> • Unprotected sex
> • Low self-esteem and inability to negotiate
> • Lack of appropriate role models
> • Strong need for someone to love
> • Drug use, truancy from school, or other behavioral problems
> • Wish to escape a bad home situation
> • Early dating without supervision

Sources: March of Dimes, 2008; Langille, 2007.

---

care for another with the tasks of developing self-identity and independence. A pregnant adolescent must try to meet her own needs along with those of her fetus. The process of learning how to separate from the parents while learning how to bond and attach to a newborn brings conflict and stress. A pregnancy can exacerbate an adolescent's feeling of loss of control (Secco et al., 2007).

Health and Social Issues

Adolescent pregnancy has a negative impact in terms of both health and social consequences. For example, seven out of ten adolescents will drop out of school. More than 75% will receive public assistance within 5 years of having their first child. In addition, children of adolescent mothers are at greater risk of preterm birth, low birthweight, child abuse, neglect, poverty, and death (As-Sanie, Gantt, & Rosenthal, 2004). The younger the adolescent is at the time of the first pregnancy, the more likely it is that she will have another pregnancy during her teens (Holub et al., 2007).

The psychosocial risks associated with early childbearing often have an even greater impact on mothers, families, and society than the obstetric or medical risks (Zeck et al., 2007). Pregnant adolescents experience higher rates of domestic violence and substance abuse. Those experiencing abuse are more likely to abuse substances, receive inadequate prenatal care, and have lower pregnancy weight compared with those who are not (Magill & Wilcox, 2007). Moreover, substance abuse (cigarettes, alcohol, or illicit drugs) can contribute to low birthweight, IUGR, preterm births, newborn addiction, and sepsis (March of Dimes, 2007a).

Although early childbearing (12 to 19 years of age) occurs in all socioeconomic groups, it is more prevalent among poor women and those from minority backgrounds, who face more obstetric and newborn risks than their more affluent counterparts (March of Dimes, 2007a). Poverty often contributes to delayed prenatal care and medical complications related to poor nutrition, such as anemia.

The financial burden of adolescent pregnancy is high and costs taxpayers an estimated $7 billion to $15 billion annually in the United States (Alan Guttmacher Institute, 2007). Much of the expense stems from Medicaid, food stamps, state health department maternity clinics, Aid to Families and Children, and direct payments to health care providers. However, this amount does not address the costs to society in terms of the loss of human resources and the far-reaching intergenerational effects of adolescent parenting.

For some adolescents, pregnancy may be seen as a hopeless situation: a grim story of poverty and lost dreams, of being trapped in a life that was never wanted. Health-related behaviors, such as smoking, diet, sexual behavior, and help-seeking behaviors, that are developed during adolescence often endure into later life (Goodman et al., 2007). The consequences associated with an adolescent's less-than-optimal health status at this age due to pregnancy can ultimately affect her long-term health and that of her children.

However, some adolescents can create a happy, stable life for themselves and their children by facing their challenges and working hard to beat the odds.

Recall Rose, the pregnant teenager with asthma. What issues would be important for the nurse to discuss with her related to her pregnancy, her asthma, and her age?

Nursing Assessment

Assessment of the pregnant adolescent is the same as that for any pregnant woman. However, when dealing with pregnant teens, the nurse also needs to ask:

• How does the girl see herself in the future?
• Are realistic role models available to her?
• How much does she know about child development?
• What financial resources are available to her?
• Does she work? Does she go to school?
• What emotional support is available to her?
• Can she resolve conflicts and manage anger?
• What does she know about health and nutrition for herself and her child?
• Will she need help dealing with the challenges of the new parenting role?
• Does she need information about community resources?

Having an honest regard for adolescents requires getting to know them and being able to appreciate the important aspects of their life. Doing so forms a basis for the nurse's clinical judgment and promotes care that takes into account the concerns and practical circumstances of the teen and her family. Skillful practice includes knowing how and when to advise a teen and when to listen and refrain from giving advice. Giving advice can be misinterpreted as "preaching," and the adolescent will probably ignore the information. The nurse must be perceptive, flexible, and sensitive and must work to establish a therapeutic relationship.

Nursing Management

For adolescents, as for all women, pregnancy can be a physically, emotionally, and socially stressful time. The pregnancy is often both the result of and cause of social problems and stressors that can be overwhelming to them. Nurses must support adolescents during the transition from childhood into adulthood, which is complicated by their emergence into motherhood. Assist the adolescent in identifying family and friends who want to be involved and provide support throughout the pregnancy.

Help the adolescent identify the options for this pregnancy, such as abortion, self-parenting of the child, temporary foster care for the baby or herself, or placement of the child for adoption. Explore with the adolescent why she became pregnant. Becoming aware of why she decided to have a child is necessary to help with the development of the adolescent and her ability to parent. Identify barriers to seeking prenatal care, such as lack of transportation, too many problems at home, financial concerns, the long wait for an appointment, and lack of sensitivity on the part of the health care system. Encourage the girl to set goals and work toward them. Assist her in returning to school and furthering her education. As appropriate, initiate a referral for career or job counseling.

Stress that the girl's physical well-being is important for both her and her developing fetus, which depends on her for its own health-related needs. Assist with arrangements for care, including stress management and self-care.

Having a healthy newborn eases the transition to motherhood somewhat, rather than having to deal with the added stress of caring for an unhealthy baby (Secco et al., 2007). Monitor weight gain, sleep and rest patterns, and nutritional status to promote positive outcomes for both. Stress the importance of attending prenatal education classes. Provide appropriate teaching based on the adolescent's developmental level and emphasize the importance of continued prenatal and follow-up care. Monitor maternal and fetal well-being throughout pregnancy and labor (Fig. 20.4).

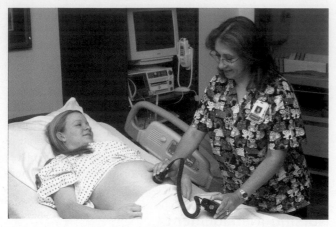

FIGURE 20.4 A pregnant adolescent receiving care during labor.

Nurses can also play a major role in preventing adolescent pregnancies, perhaps by volunteering to talk to teen groups. Box 20.4 highlights the key areas for teaching adolescents about pregnancy prevention.

Tackling the many issues surrounding adolescent pregnancy is difficult. Making connections with clients is crucial regardless of how complex their situation is. The future challenges nurses to find solutions to teenage pregnancies. Nurses must take proactive positions while working with adolescents, parents, schools, and communities to reduce the problems associated with early childbearing.

BOX 20.4 Topics for Teaching Adolescents to Prevent Pregnancy

- High-risk behaviors that lead to pregnancy
- Involvement in programs such as Free Teens, Teen Advisors, or Postponing Sexual Involvement
- Planning and goal setting to visualize their futures in terms of career, college, travel, and education
- Choice of abstinence or taking a step back to become a "second-time virgin"
- Discussions about sexuality with a wiser adult—someone they respect can help put things in perspective
- Protection against sexually transmitted infections and pregnancy if they choose to remain sexually active
- Critical observation and review of peers and friends to make sure they are creating the right atmosphere for friendship
- Empowerment to make choices that will shape their life for years to come, including getting control of their own lives now
- Appropriate use of recreational time, such as sports, drama, volunteer work, music, jobs, church activities, and school clubs

Sources: March of Dimes, 2007a; King-Jones, 2008; Lesesne et al., 2008.

▶ THE PREGNANT WOMAN OVER AGE 35

The term "elderly primip" is used to describe women ages 35 or older who are pregnant for the first time. A few decades ago, a woman having a baby after the age of 35 probably was giving birth to the last of several children, but today she may be having her first. With advances in technology and the tendency of women to seek career advancement prior to childbearing, the dramatic increase in women having first pregnancies after the age of 35 will likely continue.

Impact of Pregnancy on the Older Woman

Whether childbearing is delayed by choice or by chance, starting a family at age 35 is different and not without risks. Women in this age group may already have chronic health conditions that may put the pregnancy at risk. In addition, numerous studies have shown that increasing maternal age is a risk factor for infertility and spontaneous abortions, gestational diabetes, chronic hypertension, preeclampsia, preterm labor and birth, multiple pregnancy, genetic disorders and chromosomal abnormalities, placenta previa, IUGR, low Apgar scores, and surgical births (Hilton, 2006). However, even though increased age implies increased complications, most women today who become pregnant after age 35 have healthy pregnancies and healthy newborns (March of Dimes, 2007c).

Nursing Assessment

Nursing assessment of the pregnant woman over age 35 is the same as that for any pregnant woman. For a woman of this age, a preconception visit is important to identify chronic health problems that might affect the pregnancy and also to address lifestyle issues that may take time to modify. Encourage the older woman to plan for the pregnancy by seeing her health care provider before getting pregnant to discuss preexisting medical conditions, medications, and lifestyle choices. Assess the woman for risk factors such as cigarette smoking, poor nutrition, overweight or underweight, alcohol use, or illicit drug use.

A preconception visit also provides the opportunity to educate the woman about risk factors and provide information on how to modify her lifestyle habits to improve the pregnancy outcome. Assist the woman with lifestyle changes so that she can begin pregnancy in an optimal state of health. For example, if the woman is overweight, educate her about weight loss so that she can start the pregnancy at a healthy weight. If the woman smokes, encourage smoking cessation to reduce the effects of nicotine on herself and her fetus.

Prepare the woman for laboratory and diagnostic testing to establish a baseline for future comparisons. The risk of having a baby with Down syndrome increases with age, especially over age 35. Amniocentesis is routinely offered to all older women to allow the early detection of numerous chromosomal abnormalities, including Down syndrome. Additionally, a quadruple blood test screen (alpha fetoprotein [AFP], human chorionic gonadotropin [hCG], unconjugated estriol [UE], and inhibin A [placental hormone]) drawn between 15 and 20 weeks of pregnancy can be helpful in screening for Down syndrome and neural tube defects.

Nursing Management

During routine prenatal visits, the nurse can play a key role in promoting a healthy pregnancy. Consider social, genetic, and environmental factors that are unique to the older pregnant women and prepare to address these factors when providing care. Although research has shown increases in preterm labor and births, low-birthweight newborns, and operative interventions for older women, many carry their pregnancies to term without incident (Tough et al., 2007).

Assess the woman's knowledge about risk factors and measures to reduce them. Educate her about measures to promote a positive outcome. Encourage her to get early and regular prenatal care. Advise her to eat a variety of nutritious foods, especially fortified cereals, enriched grain products, and fresh fruits and vegetables, and drink at least six to eight glasses of water daily and to take the prescribed vitamin containing 400 micrograms of folic acid daily. Also stress the need for her to avoid alcohol intake during pregnancy, avoid exposure to second-hand smoke, and take no drugs unless they are prescribed. Provide continued surveillance of the mother and fetus throughout the pregnancy.

▶ WOMEN WHO ARE HIV POSITIVE

Human immunodeficiency virus (HIV) is a retrovirus that is transmitted by blood and body fluids. The number of people living with HIV infection in 2006 was estimated at nearly 40 million, including approximately 20 million women of childbearing age and 2.5 million children, most of whom acquired HIV from mother-to-child transmission (CDC, 2007a).

Despite the revolutionary strides that have been made in treatment and detection and recent clinical advances and cautious optimism associated with combination therapies and vaccines, the number of individuals who are HIV positive continues to climb worldwide. Intensive efforts notwithstanding, there still remains no real "cure" on the horizon (Lampe, 2006).

Historically, HIV/AIDS was associated with the male homosexual community and intravenous drug users, but currently the prevalence of HIV/AIDS is now increasing more rapidly among women than men. Women are the fastest-growing segment of persons becoming infected with HIV; transmission in women occurs most frequently from sexual contact (64%) and from intravenous drug use (33%) (CDC, 2007a). Most women, a large number of whom are mothers, have acquired the disease through heterosexual contact. The risk of acquiring HIV through heterosexual contact is greater for women due to exposure to the higher viral concentration in semen. In addition, sexual intercourse may cause breaks in the vaginal lining, increasing the chances that the virus will enter the woman's body. Fifty percent of all the HIV/AIDS cases worldwide occur in women. AIDS is the third leading cause of death among all U.S. women aged 25 to 44 years and the leading cause of death among African-American women in this age group (CDC, 2007a).

Pathophysiology

The three recognized modes of HIV transmission are unprotected sexual intercourse with an infected partner, contact with infected blood or blood products, and perinatal transmission.

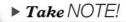

▶ **Take** NOTE!

HIV is not transmitted by doorknobs, faucets, toilets, dirty dishes, mosquitoes, wet towels, coughing or sneezing, shaking hands, or being hugged or by any other indirect method.

The virus attacks the T4 cells, decreases the CD4 cell count, and disables the immune system. The HIV condition can progress to a severe immunosuppressed state termed **acquired immunodeficiency syndrome (AIDS)**. AIDS is a progressive, debilitating disease that suppresses cellular immunity, predisposing the infected person to opportunistic infections and malignancies. The CDC defines AIDS as an HIV-infected person with a specific opportunistic infection or a CD4 count of less than 200. Eventually, death occurs. The time from infection with HIV to development of AIDS is a median of 11 years but varies depending on whether the patient is taking current antiretroviral therapy (Johnsen, 2007). Research indicates that pregnancy does not accelerate the progression of HIV to AIDS or death (Cressey & Lallemant, 2007).

Once infected with HIV, the woman develops antibodies that can be detected with the enzyme-linked immunosorbent assay (ELISA) and confirmed with the Western blot test. Antibodies develop within 6 to 12 weeks after exposure, although this latent period is much longer in some women. Table 20.4 highlights the four stages of HIV infection according to the CDC (2007a).

Impact of HIV on Pregnancy

When a woman who is infected with HIV becomes pregnant, the risks to herself, her fetus, and the newborn are great. The risks are compounded by problems such as drug abuse, lack of access to prenatal care, poverty, poor nutrition, and high-risk behaviors such as unsafe sex practices and multiple sex partners, which can predispose the woman to additional sexually transmitted infections such as herpes, syphilis, or human papillomavirus (HPV). Additional risk factors to assess for include women who exchange sex for money or drugs or have sex partners who do; women whose past or present sex partners were HIV infected; and women who had a blood transfusion between 1978 and 1985 (U.S. Preventive Services Task Force [USPSTF], 2006b). Subsequently, pregnant women who are HIV positive are at risk for preterm delivery, premature rupture of membranes, intrapartal or postpartum hemorrhage, postpartum infection, poor wound healing, and genitourinary tract infections (CDC, 2007a).

Perinatal transmission of HIV (from the mother to the fetus or child) also can occur. However, such cases have decreased in the past several years in the United States, primarily due to the use of zidovudine (ZDV) therapy in pregnant women infected with HIV. This has not been the case in poor countries without similar resources. The Joint United Nations programs on HIV/AIDS (UNAIDS) estimates that over 600,000 new infections due to mother-to-child transmission occur annually. This number is expected to increase rapidly as the prevalence rises in Southeast Asia (Johnsen, 2007). Perinatal transmission rates are as high as 35% when there is no intervention (antiretroviral therapy) and below 5% when antiretroviral treatment and appropriate care are available.

With perinatal transmission, approximately 25% to 50% of children manifest AIDS within the first year of life, and about 80% have clinical symptoms of the disease within 3 to 5 years (Johnsen, 2007). Breastfeeding is a major contributing factor for mother-to-child transmission, and the infected mother must be informed about this (Dao et al., 2007). The U.S. Public Health Service recommends that women who are HIV positive should avoid breastfeeding to prevent HIV transmission to the newborn. Given the devastating effects of HIV infection on children, preventing its transmission is critical (Lampe, 2006).

In addition to perinatal transmission, the fetus and newborn also are at risk for prematurity, IUGR, low birthweight, and infection. Prompt treatment with antiretroviral medications for the HIV-infected infant may slow the progression of the disease.

Therapeutic Management

Women who are seropositive for HIV require counseling about the risk of perinatal transmission and the potential for obstetric complications. The risk of perinatal transmission directly correlates with the viral load (Johnsen, 2007). A discussion of the options on continuing the pregnancy, medication therapy, risks, perinatal outcomes, and treatment is warranted. Women who elect to continue with the pregnancy should be treated with antiretroviral therapy regardless of their CD4 count or viral load.

Drug therapy is the mainstay of treatment for pregnant women infected with HIV. The standard treatment is

---

TABLE 20.4 **STAGES OF HIV INFECTION OUTLINED BY THE CDC**

Stages	Description	Clinical Picture
I	Acute infection	Early stage with pervasive viral production Flu-like symptoms 2–4 weeks after exposure Signs and symptoms: weight loss, low-grade fever, fatigue, sore throat, night sweats, and myalgia
II	Asymptomatic infection	Viral replication continues within lymphatics Usually free of symptoms; lymphadenopathy
III	Persistent generalized lymphadenopathy	Possibly remaining in this stage for years; AIDS develops in most within 7–10 years Opportunistic infections occur
IV	End-stage disease (AIDS)	Severe immune deficiency High viral load and low CD4 counts Signs and symptoms: bacterial, viral, or fungal opportunistic infections, fever, wasting syndrome, fatigue, neoplasms, and cognitive changes

oral antiretroviral drugs given twice daily from 14 weeks' gestation until giving birth, intravenous administration during labor, and oral syrup for the newborn in the first 6 weeks of life (Hackley, Kriebs, & Rousseau, 2007). The goal of therapy is to reduce the viral load as much as possible, which reduces the risk of transmission to the fetus.

Decisions about the birthing method to be used are made on an individual basis based on several factors involving the woman's health. Some reports suggest that cesarean birth may reduce the risk of HIV infection (Johnsen, 2007). Efforts to reduce instrumentation, such as avoiding the use of an episiotomy, fetal scalp electrodes, and fetal scalp sampling, will reduce the newborn's exposure to bodily fluids.

With appropriate therapies, the prognosis for pregnant women with HIV infection has improved significantly. In addition, the newborns of women with HIV infection who have received treatment usually do not become infected. Unfortunately, therapy is complicated and medications are expensive. Moreover, the medications are associated with numerous adverse effects and possible toxic reactions. These therapies offer a dual purpose: reduce the likelihood of mother-to-infant transmission and provide optimal suppression of the viral load in the mother. The core goal of all medical therapy is to bring the client's viral load to an undetectable level, thus minimizing the risk of transmission to the fetus and newborn.

Nursing Assessment

Nursing assessment begins with a thorough history and physical examination. In addition, the woman is offered screening for HIV antibodies.

Health History and Physical Examination

Review the woman's history for risk factors, such as unsafe sex practices, multiple sex partners, and injectable drug use. Also have the woman complete a risk assessment survey. In addition, question the woman about any flu-like symptoms such as a low-grade fever, fatigue, sore throat, night sweats, diarrhea, cough, skin lesions, or muscle pain.

Perform a complete physical examination. Obtain the woman's weight and determine if she has lost weight recently. Assess for signs and symptoms of sexually transmitted infections (STIs), such as vulvovaginal candidiasis, bacterial vaginosis, HSV, chancroid, CMV, or chlamydia because of the increased risk for STIs.

▶ **Take** NOTE!

Women who request an HIV test despite reporting no individual risk factors should be considered at risk, since many are not likely to disclose their high-risk behaviors.

Laboratory and Diagnostic Testing

The U.S. Public Health Service recommends that all pregnant women be offered HIV antibody testing, regardless of their risk of infection, and that testing be done during the initial prenatal evaluation (Lampe, 2006). Testing is essential because treatments are available that can reduce the likelihood of perinatal transmission and maintain the health of the woman.

▶ **Take** NOTE!

Screening only women who are identified as high risk based on their histories is inadequate due to the prolonged latency period that can exist after exposure. Also, research indicating that treatment with antiretroviral agents could reduce vertical transmission from the infected mother to the newborn has dramatically increased the importance of HIV antibody screening in pregnancy.

Offer all women who are pregnant or planning a pregnancy HIV testing using ELISA. Prepare the woman with a reactive screening test for an additional test, such as the Western blot or an immunofluorescence assay. The Western blot is the confirmatory diagnostic test. A positive antibody test confirmed by a supplemental test indicates that the woman has been infected with HIV and can pass it on to others. HIV antibodies are detectable in at least 95% of women within 3 months after infection (Cressey & Lallemant, 2007).

In addition to the usual screening tests done in normal pregnancy, additional testing for STIs may be necessary. Women infected with HIV have high rates of STIs, especially HPV, vulvovaginal candidiasis, bacterial vaginosis, syphilis, HSV, chancroid, CMV, gonorrhea, chlamydia, and hepatitis B (Hackley, Kriebs, & Rousseau, 2007).

Nursing Management

Women infected with HIV should have comprehensive prenatal care, which starts with pretest and posttest counseling. In pretest counseling, the client completes a risk assessment survey and the nurse explains the meaning of positive versus negative test results, obtains informed consent for HIV testing, and educates the woman on how to prevent HIV infection by changing lifestyle behaviors if needed. Posttest counseling includes informing the client of the test results, reviewing the meaning of the results again, and reinforcing safer sex guidelines. All pretest and posttest counseling should be documented in the client's chart.

Educating the Client

Pregnant clients are dealing with many issues at their first prenatal visit. The confirmation of pregnancy may be accompanied by feelings of joy, anxiety, depression, or other emotions. Simultaneously, the client is given many pamphlets and receives advice and counseling about many important health issues (e.g., nutrition, prenatal development, appointment schedules). This health teaching may be done while the woman feels excited, tired, and anxious. To expect women to understand detailed explanations of a complex disease entity (HIV/AIDS) too may be unrealistic. Determine the client's readiness for this discussion.

Identify the client's individual needs for teaching, emotional support, and physical care. Approach education and counseling of HIV-positive pregnant women in a caring, sensitive manner. Address the following information:

- Infection control issues at home
- Safer sex precautions
- Stages of the HIV disease process and treatment for each stage
- Symptoms of opportunistic infections
- Preventive drug therapies for her unborn infant
- Avoidance of breastfeeding
- Referrals to community support, counseling, and financial aid
- Client's support system and potential caretaker
- Importance of continual prenatal care
- Need for a well-balanced diet
- Measures to reduce exposure to infections

Be knowledgeable about HIV infection and how HIV is transmitted and share this knowledge with all women. Nurses also can work to influence legislators, public health officials, and the entire health establishment toward policies to address the HIV epidemic. Research toward treatment and cure is tremendously important, but the major key to prevention of the spread of the virus is education. Nurses play a major role in this education.

Supporting the Client

Be aware of the psychosocial sequelae of HIV/AIDS. A diagnosis of HIV can put a woman into an emotional tailspin, where she is worried about her own health and that of her unborn infant. She may experience grief, fear, or anxiety about the future of her children. Along with the medications that are so important to her health maintenance, address the woman's mental health needs, family dynamics, capacity to work, and social concerns and provide appropriate support and guidance.

Be aware of your personal beliefs and attitudes toward women who are HIV positive or have AIDS. Incorporate this awareness in your actions as you help the woman face the reality of the diagnosis and treatment options. Empathy, understanding, caring, and assistance are key to helping the client and her family.

Preparing for Labor, Birth, and Afterward

Current evidence suggests that cesarean birth performed before the onset of labor and before the rupture of membranes significantly reduces the rate of perinatal transmission. ACOG recommends that HIV-positive women be offered elective cesarean birth to reduce the rate of transmission beyond that which may be achieved through antiretroviral therapy. They further suggest that operative births be performed at 38 weeks' gestation and that amniocentesis be avoided to prevent contamination of the amniotic fluid with maternal blood. Decisions concerning the method of delivery should be based on the woman's viral load, the duration of ruptured membranes, the progress of labor, and other pertinent clinical factors (USPHSTF, 2006b).

Prepare the woman physically and emotionally for the possibility of cesarean birth and assist as necessary. Ensure that she understands the rationale for the surgical birth.

After the birth of the newborn, the motivation for taking antiretroviral medications may be lower, thus affecting the woman's compliance with therapy. Encourage the woman to continue therapy for her own sake as well as that of the newborn. Nurses can make a difference in helping women to adhere to their complex drug regimens.

Reinforce family planning methods during this time, incorporating a realistic view of her disease status. The use of oral contraceptives with concurrent use of condoms is recommended (Lampe, 2006). Advise the woman that breastfeeding is not recommended. Instruct the HIV-positive woman in self-care measures, including the proper method for disposing of perineal pads to reduce the risk of exposing others to infected body fluids. Finally, teach the HIV-positive woman the signs and symptoms of infection in newborns and infants, encouraging her to report any to the health care provider.

▶ *Take* NOTE!

*When providing direct care, **ALWAYS** follow standard precautions.*

◆ THE PREGNANT WOMAN WITH SUBSTANCE ABUSE

Perinatal drug abuse is the use of alcohol and other drugs by pregnant women. The incidence of substance abuse during pregnancy is highly variable because most pregnant women are reluctant to reveal the extent of their use. The National Institute on Drug Abuse estimates that 6% of the women in the United States have used illicit drugs while pregnant. These include cocaine, marijuana, heroin, and psychotherapeutic drugs that were not prescribed by a health care professional. More than 18% used alcohol and 21% smoked cigarettes during their pregnancy (National Institute on Drug Abuse [NIDA], 2007a).

Impact of Substance Abuse on Pregnancy

The use of drugs, legal or not, increases the risk of medical complications in the mother and poor birth outcomes in the newborn. The placenta acts as an active transport mechanism, not as a barrier, and substances pass from a mother to her fetus through the placenta. Thus, the fetus as well as the mother experiences substance use, abuse, and addiction. Additionally, fetal vulnerability to drugs is much greater because the fetus has not developed the enzymatic system needed to metabolize drugs (Hackley, Kriebs, & Rousseau, 2007).

A woman who claims to have taken no drugs while pregnant may be unaware that substances such as hair dye, diet cola, paint, or over-the-counter (OTC) medications for colds or headaches are still considered drugs. Thus, it is very difficult to get a true picture of the real use of drugs by pregnant women.

Many drugs are considered to have a teratogenic effect on growing fetuses. A **teratogen** is any environmental substance that can cause physical defects in the developing embryo and fetus. Pregnant women with substance abuse commonly present with polysubstance abuse, which is likely to be more damaging than the use of any single substance. Thus, it is inherently difficult to ascribe a specific perinatal effect to any one substance (Rassool & Villar-Luis, 2006).

Effects of Addiction

Addiction is a multifaceted process that is affected by environmental, psychological, family, and physical factors. Women who use drugs, alcohol, or tobacco come from all socioeconomic backgrounds, cultures, and lifestyles. Factors associated with substance abuse during a pregnancy may include low self-esteem, inadequate support systems, low self-expectations, high levels of anxiety, socioeconomic barriers, involvement in abusive relationships, chaotic familial and social systems, and a history of psychiatric illness or depression. Women often become substance abusers to relieve their anxieties, depression, and feelings of worthlessness (Jones, 2006).

Societal attitudes regarding women and substance abuse may prohibit them from admitting the problem and seeking treatment. Society sanctions women for failing to live up to expectations of how a pregnant woman "should" behave, thereby possibly driving them further away from the treatment they so desperately need. For many reasons, pregnant women who abuse substances feel unwelcome in prenatal clinics or medical settings. Often they seek prenatal care late or not at all. They may fear being shamed or reported to legal or child protection authorities. A nonjudgmental atmosphere and unbiased teaching to all pregnant women regardless of their lifestyle is crucial. A caring, concerned manner is critical to help these women feel safe and respond honestly to assessment questions.

Pregnancy can be a motivator for some who want to try treatment. The goal of therapy is to help the client deal with pregnancy by developing a trusting relationship. Providing a full spectrum of medical, social, and emotional care is needed.

Effects of Commonly Abused Substances

Substance abuse during pregnancy, particularly in the first trimester, has a negative effect on the health of the mother and the growth and development of the fetus. The fetus experiences the same systemic effects as the mother, but often more severely. The fetus cannot metabolize drugs as efficiently as the expectant mother and will experience the effects long after the drugs have left the women's system. Substance abuse during pregnancy is associated with preterm labor, abortion, IUGR, abruptio placentae, low birthweight, neurobehavioral abnormalities, and long-term childhood developmental consequences (Rassool & Villar-Luis, 2006). Table 20.5 summarizes the effects of selected drugs during pregnancy.

TABLE 20.5 EFFECTS OF SELECTED DRUGS ON PREGNANCY

Substance	Effect on Pregnancy
Alcohol	Spontaneous abortion, inadequate weight gain, IUGR, fetal alcohol spectrum disorder, the leading cause of mental retardation
Caffeine	Vasoconstriction and mild diuresis in mother; fetal stimulation, but teratogenic effects not documented via research
Nicotine	Vasoconstriction, reduced uteroplacental blood flow, decreased birthweight, abortion, prematurity, abruptio placentae, fetal demise
Cocaine	Vasoconstriction, gestational hypertension, abruptio placentae, abortion, "snow baby syndrome," CNS defects, IUGR
Marijuana	Anemia, inadequate weight gain, "amotivational syndrome," hyperactive startle reflex, newborn tremors, prematurity, IUGR
Narcotics	Maternal and fetal withdrawal, abruptio placentae, preterm labor, premature rupture of membranes, perinatal asphyxia, newborn sepsis and death, intellectual impairment, malnutrition
Sedatives	CNS depression, newborn withdrawal, maternal seizures in labor, newborn abstinence syndrome, delayed lung maturity

Sources: CDC, 2007d; Gilbert & Harmon, 2006; Jones, 2006.

Alcohol

Alcohol abuse is a major public health issue in the United States. Alcohol is a teratogen, a substance known to be toxic to human development. Approximately 10% of pregnant women report alcohol consumption (CDC, 2007d). Theoretically, no mother would give a glass of wine, beer, or hard liquor to her newborn, but when she drinks, her embryo or fetus is exposed to the same blood alcohol concentration as she is. The teratogenic effects of heavy maternal drinking have been recognized since 1973, when fetal alcohol syndrome was first described. Fetal alcohol syndrome is now a classification under the broader term of **fetal alcohol spectrum disorder (FASD)**; this disorder includes the full range of birth defects, such as structural anomalies and behavioral and neurocognitive disabilities caused by prenatal exposure to alcohol (Green, 2007). The incidence of FASD in the United States is estimated to be one or two cases per 1,000 live births (National Organization on Fetal Alcohol Syndrome [NoFAS], 2007). It is the leading cause of mental retardation (CDC, 2007d).

Not every woman who drinks during pregnancy will give birth to an affected child. Based on the best research available, the following is known about alcohol consumption during pregnancy:

- Intake increases the risk of alcohol-related birth defects, including growth deficiencies, facial abnormalities, central nervous system impairment, behavioral disorders, and intellectual development.
- No amount of alcohol consumption is considered safe during pregnancy.
- Damage to the fetus can occur at any stage of pregnancy, even before a woman knows she is pregnant.
- Cognitive defects and behavioral problems resulting from prenatal exposure are lifelong.
- Alcohol-related birth defects are completely preventable (U.S. Department of Health and Human Services [USDHHS], 2007).

Risk factors for giving birth to an alcohol-affected newborn include maternal age, socioeconomic status, ethnicity, genetic factors, poor nutrition, depression, family disorganization, unplanned pregnancy, and late prenatal care (Hackley, Kriebs, & Rousseau, 2007). Identification of risk factors strongly associated with alcohol-related birth outcomes could help identify high-risk pregnancies requiring intervention.

Characteristics of FASD include craniofacial dysmorphia (thin upper lip, small head circumference, and small eyes), IUGR, microcephaly, and congenital anomalies such as limb abnormalities and cardiac defects. Long-term sequelae include postnatal growth restriction, attention deficits, delayed reaction time, and poor scholastic performance (NoFAS, 2007). The complex neurobehavioral problems typically manifest themselves insidiously. Children with prenatal alcohol exposure struggle with cognitive, academic, social, emotional, and behavioral challenges.

> **BOX 20.5** **Common Cognitive and Behavioral Problems Associated With FASD**
>
> - Attention-deficit/hyperactivity disorder (ADHD)
> - Inability to foresee consequences
> - Inability to learn from previous experience
> - Lack of organization
> - Learning difficulties
> - Poor abstract thinking
> - Poor impulse control
> - Speech and language problems
> - Poor judgment

These challenges reduce the child's ability to learn and function successfully in many structured environments (Green, 2007). Common cognitive and behavioral problems are listed in Box 20.5, and Figure 20.5 illustrates the characteristic facial features. See Chapter 24 for a more detailed discussion of the newborn with FASD.

One of the biggest challenges in determining the true prevalence of FASD is how to recognize the syndrome, which depends in part on the age and physical features of the person being assessed. Difficulty in identifying alcohol abuse is due to the client's denial of alcohol use, unwillingness to report alcohol consumption, underreporting, and limited ability to recollect the frequency, quantity, and type of alcohol consumed. This makes it difficult to identify women who are drinking during pregnancy, institute preventive measures, or refer them for treatment.

Women who drink excessively while pregnant are at high risk for giving birth to children with birth defects. To prevent these defects, women should stop drinking during

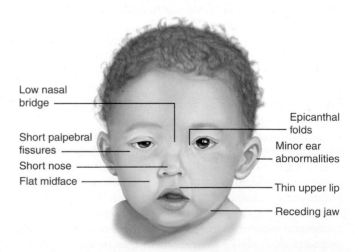

Low nasal bridge

Short palpebral fissures

Short nose

Flat midface

Epicanthal folds

Minor ear abnormalities

Thin upper lip

Receding jaw

FIGURE 20.5 Typical facial characteristics of a newborn with FASD.

all phases of a pregnancy. Unfortunately, many women continue to drink during their pregnancy despite warnings from professionals.

Currently, it is not known whether there is a minimal amount of alcohol safe to drink during pregnancy; an occasional glass of wine might be harmless or might not be. Therefore, eliminating alcohol consumption during pregnancy is the ultimate goal to prevent FASD. Most women know they shouldn't drink during pregnancy, but the "window of vulnerability"—the time lag between conception and the discovery of pregnancy—may put substantial numbers of children at risk. Additionally, traditional alcohol-screening questionnaires, such as the Michigan Alcoholism Screening Test (MAST) and the CAGE Questionnaire, are not sensitive enough to detect low levels of alcohol consumption among women.

Several challenges remain in preventing birth defects due to alcohol consumption:

- Ways to improve clinical recognition of high-risk women who drink alcohol
- Ways to intervene more effectively to modify drinking behaviors
- In utero approaches to prevent or minimize fetal injury
- Strategies to address the neurodevelopmental problems of children affected by maternal alcohol ingestion

Caffeine

Caffeine, a CNS stimulant, is present in varying amounts in such common products as coffee, tea, colas, and chocolate. It is also in cold remedies and analgesics. Birth defects have not been linked to caffeine consumption, but maternal coffee consumption decreases iron absorption and may increase the risk of anemia during pregnancy. The FDA recommends that pregnant women eliminate or limit their consumption of caffeine to less than 300 mg/day, or the equivalent of three cups of coffee or cola (Hoffman & Brown, 2006).

Nicotine

Nicotine, found in cigarettes, is another substance that is harmful to the pregnant women and her fetus. Nicotine, which causes vasoconstriction, transfers across the placenta and reduces blood flow to the fetus, contributing to fetal hypoxia. When compared with alcohol, marijuana, and other illicit drug use, tobacco use is less likely to decline as the pregnancy progresses (Wang, 2007). Smoking is associated with adverse pregnancy outcomes. However, these adverse outcomes can be avoided if the woman stops smoking before becoming pregnant.

Smoking increases the risk of spontaneous abortion, preterm labor and birth, maternal hypertension, placenta previa, and abruptio placentae. The perinatal death rate among infants of smoking mothers is 20% to 35% higher (Raatikainen, Huurinainen, & Heinonen, 2007).

Smoking has also been considered an important risk factor for low birthweight, sudden infant death syndrome (SIDS), and cognitive deficits, especially in language, reading, and vocabulary, as well as poorer performances on tests of reasoning and memory. Researchers have also reported behavior problems, such as increased activity, inattention, impulsivity, opposition, and aggression (Wang, 2007).

Women who smoke during the pregnancy also continue to smoke after giving birth, and thus the infant will be exposed to nicotine after birth. This environmental or passive exposure affects the child's development and increases the risk of childhood respiratory disorders.

Cocaine

Cocaine use is second only to marijuana in women who abuse drugs during pregnancy. The incidence of cocaine exposure in utero is 1 to 10 per 1,000 live births (Weekes & Lee, 2006).

Cocaine is a psychoactive drug derived from the leaves of the coca plant, which grows in the Andes Mountains of Peru, Ecuador, and Bolivia. The freebase form, called "crack" because of the cracking or popping noise made in its preparation, is less expensive, easily made, and smokable. Cocaine is a powerful vasoconstrictor. When sniffed into the mucous membranes of the nose, it produces an intense "rush" that some have compared to an orgasmic experience. Smoked crack is absorbed rapidly by the pulmonary vasculature and reaches the brain's circulation in 6 to 8 seconds (NIDA, 2007b).

Cocaine use produces vasoconstriction, tachycardia, and hypertension in both the mother and the fetus (Weekes & Lee, 2006). Uteroplacental insufficiency may result from reduced blood flow and placental perfusion. Chronic use can result in low birthweight, the most common effect of cocaine use in pregnancy (NIDA, 2007b).

Studies suggest that perinatal cocaine use increases the risk of preterm labor, abortion, abruptio placentae, IUGR, intrauterine fetal distress and demise, seizures, withdrawal, and cerebral infarcts. Cocaine may increase the risk of uterine rupture and congenital anomalies (NIDA, 2007b). Fetal anomalies associated with cocaine use in early pregnancy involve neurologic problems such as neural tube defects and microcephaly; cardiovascular anomalies such as congenital heart defects; genitourinary conditions such as prune belly syndrome, hydronephrosis, and ambiguous genitalia; and gastrointestinal system problems such as necrotizing enterocolitis (Jones, 2006). Some infants exposed to cocaine in utero show increased irritability and are difficult to calm and soothe to sleep.

Marijuana

Marijuana is the most commonly used illicit drug in America, with over 90 million people having tried it at least once. It is often called pot, reefer, herb, widow, hash, grass, weed, Mary Jane, or MJ (NIDA, 2007c). Marijuana is a preparation of the leaves and flowering tops of *Cannabis sativa,* the hemp plant, which contains a number of pharmacologically active agents. Tetrahydrocannabinol (THC) is the most active ingredient of marijuana. With heavy smoking, THC narrows the bronchi and bronchioles and produces inflammation of the mucous membranes. Smoking marijuana causes tachycardia and a reduction in blood pressure, resulting in orthostatic hypotension.

The effects of marijuana smoking on pregnancy are not yet fully understood because there are very few studies on its long-term effects on child development. One can speculate that the effects of marijuana on the immature nervous system may be subtle and not detected until more complex functions are required, usually in a formal educational setting. There is some evidence that marijuana increases the risk of spontaneous abortion and preterm delivery (Barros et al., 2006). Although marijuana is not considered teratogenic, many newborns display altered responses to visual stimuli, increased tremulousness, and a high-pitched cry, which might indicate CNS insults (Wang, 2007). A strong correlation exists between the use of marijuana and the use of alcohol and cigarettes.

Opiates and Narcotics

Opiates and narcotics include opium, heroin (known as horse, junk, smack, downtown), morphine, codeine, hydromorphone (Dilaudid; little D), oxycodone (Percodan, perkies), meperidine (Demerol, demise), and methadone (meth, dollies). These drugs are central nervous system depressants that soothe and lull. They may be used medically for pain, but all have a high potential for abuse. Most cause an intense addiction in both mother and newborn.

Narcotic dependence is particularly problematic in pregnant women. It leads to medical, nutritional, and social neglect by the woman due to the long-term risks of physical dependence, malnutrition, compromised immunity, hepatitis, and fatal overdose (Alexander et al., 2007). Taking opiates or narcotics during pregnancy places the woman at increased risk for preterm labor, IUGR, and preeclampsia (Wang, 2007).

Heroin is the most common illicitly used opioid. It is derived from the seeds of the poppy plant and can be sniffed, smoked, or injected. It crosses the placenta via simple diffusion within 1 hour of maternal consumption (Dodge, Brady, & Maguire, 2007). Use of heroin during pregnancy is believed to affect the developing brain of the fetus and may cause behavioral abnormalities in childhood (Alexander et al., 2007).

The most common harmful effect of heroin and other narcotics on newborns is withdrawal, or **neonatal abstinence syndrome** (see Chapter 24). This collection of symptoms may include irritability, hypertonicity, a high-pitched cry, vomiting, diarrhea, respiratory distress, disturbed sleeping, sneezing, diaphoresis, fever, poor sucking, tremors, and seizures (Ebner et al., 2007).

Withdrawal from opiates during pregnancy is extremely dangerous for the fetus, so a prescribed oral methadone maintenance program combined with psychotherapy is recommended for the pregnant woman. This closely supervised treatment program reduces withdrawal symptoms in the newborn, reduces drug cravings, and blocks the euphoric effects of narcotic drugs in order to reduce illicit drug use. Methadone maintenance provides a steady state of opiate levels, thus reducing the risk of withdrawal to the fetus and exposure to HIV and other STIs because the mother is no longer injecting drugs. However, methadone has the same withdrawal consequences for women and newborns as heroin does (Burns et al., 2007).

Sedatives

Sedatives relax the central nervous system and are used medically for inducing relaxation and sleep, relieving tension, and treating seizures. Sedatives easily cross the placenta and can cause birth defects and behavioral problems. Infants born to mothers who abuse sedatives during pregnancy may be physically dependent on the drugs themselves and are more prone to respiratory problems, feeding difficulties, disturbed sleep, sweating, irritability, and fever (Alexander et al., 2007).

Methamphetamines

Methamphetamine use among pregnant women has increased rapidly in the United States. This highly addictive stimulant is commonly known as speed, meth, or chalk. In its smoked form, it is often referred to as ice, crystal, crank, and glass. It is a white, odorless, bitter-tasting powder that was developed from its parent drug, amphetamine, and was used originally in nasal decongestants and bronchial inhalers. The maternal effects include increased energy and alertness, an intense rush, decreased appetite, tachycardia, and tachypnea. Chronic use can lead to psychosis, including paranoia, hallucinations, memory loss, and aggressive or violent behavior (Derlet & Albertson, 2006). Few studies have been done on the effects of methamphetamine abuse during pregnancy, but the few done indicate an increased risk for preterm births, placental abruption, fetal growth restriction, and congenital anomalies (NIDA, 2007d). These findings are hard to interpret, however, due to small sample size and polydrug use of the participants.

Nursing Assessment

Complete a thorough history and physical examination to evaluate a client for substance use and abuse. Substance abuse screening in pregnancy is done to detect the use of any substance known or suspected to exert a deleterious effect on the client or her fetus. Routinely ask about substance abuse with all women of childbearing age, inform them of the risks involved, and advise them against continuing. Screening questionnaires are helpful in identifying potential users, may reduce the stigma of asking clients about substance abuse, and result in a more accurate and consistent evaluation. The questions in Box 20.6 may be helpful in assessing a client who is at risk for substance abuse during pregnancy. Using "accepting" terminology may encourage the woman to give honest answers without fear of reproach.

A urine toxicology screen may also be helpful in determining drug use, although a urine screen identifies only recent or heavy use of drugs. The length of time a drug is present in urine is as follows:

- Cocaine: 24 to 48 hours in an adult, 72 to 96 hours in an infant
- Heroin: 24 hours in an adult, 24 to 48 hours in an infant
- Marijuana: 1 week to 1 month in an adult, up to a month or longer in an infant
- Methadone: up to 10 days in an infant (Wang, 2007)

Nursing Management

If the woman's drug screen is positive, use this as an opportunity to discuss prenatal exposure to substances that may be harmful. The discussion may lead the nurse to refer the client for a diagnostic assessment or identify an intervention such as counseling that may be helpful. Being nonjudgmental is a key to success; a client is more apt to

---

BOX 20.6 **Sample Questions for Assessing Substance Use**

- Have you ever used recreational drugs? If so, when and what?
- Have you ever taken a prescription drug other than as intended?
- What are your feelings about drug use during pregnancy?
- How often do you smoke cigarettes? How many per day?
- How often do you drink alcohol?

If the assessment reveals substance use, obtain additional information by using the RAFFT questions, which are a sensitive screening instrument for identifying substance abuse (Weekes & Lee, 2006):

R: Do you drink or take drugs to **R**elax, improve your self-image, or fit in?

A: Do you ever drink or take drugs while **A**lone?

F: Do you have any close **F**riends who drink or take drugs?

F: Does a close **F**amily member have a problem with alcohol or drugs?

T: Have you ever gotten in **T**rouble from drinking or taking drugs?

---

trust and reveal patterns of abuse if the nurse does not judge her and her lifestyle choices.

A positive drug screen in a newborn warrants an investigation by the state protection agency. In the interim, institute measures to reduce stress and stimuli to promote the newborn's comfort (see Chapter 24 for a more in-depth discussion).

Be proactive, supportive, and accepting when caring for the client. Assure women with substance abuse problems that sharing information of a confidential nature with health care providers will not render them liable to criminal prosecution. Provide counseling and education, emphasizing the following:

- Effects of substance exposure on the fetus
- Interventions to improve mother–child attachment and improve parenting
- Psychosocial support if treatment is needed to reduce substance abuse
- Referral to outreach programs to improve access to treatment facilities
- Hazardous legal substances to avoid during pregnancy
- Follow-up of children born to substance-dependent mothers
- Dietary counseling to improve the pregnancy outcome for both mother and child
- Drug screening to identify all drugs a client is using
- More frequent prenatal visits to monitor fetal well-being
- Maternal and fetal benefits of remaining drug-free
- Cultural sensitivity
- Coping skills, support systems, and vocational assistance

Substance abuse is a complex problem that requires sensitivity to each woman's unique situation and contributing factors. Be sure to address individual psychological and sociocultural factors to help the woman to regain control of her life. Treatment must combine different approaches and provide ongoing support for women learning to live drug-free. Developing personal strengths, such as communication skills and assertiveness, and self-confidence will help the woman in resisting the drug use. Encourage the use of appropriate coping skills. Enhancing self-esteem also helps provides a foundation to avoid drugs.

■■■ Key Concepts

- Preconception counseling for the woman with diabetes is helpful in promoting blood glucose control to prevent congenital anomalies.
- The classification system for diabetes commonly used is based on disease etiology and not pharmacology management; the classification includes type 1 diabetes, type 2 diabetes, gestational diabetes, and impaired fasting glucose and impaired glucose tolerance.
- A functional classification for heart disease during pregnancy is based on past and present disability: class I,

asymptomatic with no limitation of physical activity; class II, symptomatic (dyspnea, chest pain) with increased activity; class III, symptomatic (fatigue, palpitation) with normal activity; and class IV, symptomatic at rest or with any physical activity.

■ Chronic hypertension exists when the woman has a blood pressure of 140/90 mm Hg or higher before pregnancy or before the 20th week of gestation or when hypertension persists for more than 12 weeks postpartum.

■ Successful management of asthma in pregnancy involves elimination of environmental triggers, drug therapy, and client education.

■ Ideally, women with hematologic conditions are screened before conception and are made aware of the risks to themselves and to a pregnancy.

■ A wide variety of infections, such as rubella, herpes simplex, hepatitis B, varicella, parvovirus B19, and many sexually transmitted infections can affect the pregnancy, having a negative impact on its outcome.

■ The younger the adolescent is at the time of the first pregnancy, the more likely it is that she will have another pregnancy during her teens. About 1 million teenagers between the ages of 15 and 19 become pregnant each year; about half give birth and keep their infants.

■ The nurse's role in caring for the pregnant adolescent is to assist her in identifying the options for this pregnancy, including abortion, self-parenting of the child, temporary foster care for the baby or herself, or placement for adoption.

■ The prevalence of HIV/AIDS is increasing more rapidly among women then men: half of all the HIV/AIDS cases worldwide now occur in women. There are only three recognized modes of HIV transmission: unprotected sexual intercourse with an infected partner, contact with infected blood or blood products, and perinatal transmission. Breastfeeding is a major contributing factor in mother-to-child transmission of HIV.

■ Cases of perinatal AIDS have decreased in the past several years in the United States, primarily because of the use of zidovudine (ZDV) therapy in pregnant women with HIV. The U.S. Public Health Service recommends that all pregnant women should be offered HIV antibody testing regardless of their risk of infection, and that testing should be done during the initial prenatal evaluation.

■ Pregnant women with substance abuse problems commonly abuse several substance, making it difficult to ascribe a specific perinatal effect to any one substance. Societal attitudes regarding pregnant women and substance abuse may prohibit them from admitting the problem and seeking treatment.

■ Substance abuse during pregnancy is associated with preterm labor, abortion, low birthweight, CNS and fetal anomalies, and long-term childhood developmental consequences.

■ Fetal alcohol spectrum disorder is a lifelong yet completely preventable set of physical, mental, and neurobehavioral birth defects; it is the leading cause of mental retardation in the United States.

■ Nursing management for the woman with substance abuse focuses on screening and preventing substance abuse to reduce the high incidence of obstetric and medical complications as well as the morbidity and mortality among passively addicted newborns.

REFERENCES

Abdin, S. (2006). Care of pregnant women with heart disease: A multidisciplinary approach. *British Journal of Midwifery, 14*(10), 592–595.

Alan Guttmacher Institute. (2006). *U.S. teenager pregnancy statistics: National and state trends and trends by race and ethnicity.* New York: Author, 1–56.

Alan Guttmacher Institute. (2007). *In the know about pregnancy, contraception and abortion.* Available at: http://www.guttmacher.org/in-the-know/pregnancy.html.

Alexander, L. L., LaRosa, J. H., Bader, H., & Garfield, S. (2007). *New dimensions in women's health* (4th ed.). Sudbury: Jones & Bartlett Publishers.

American Academy of Allergy, Asthma & Immunology (AAAAI). (2007). *Managing asthma during pregnancy.* The National Asthma Education Prevention Program. Available at: http://www.aaaai.org/patients/topicofthemonth/0506/.

American Diabetes Association (ADA). (2008). Standards of medical care in diabetes in 2008. *Diabetes Care,* Supplement 1, S12–54.

American Diabetes Association (ADA). (2007a). Diagnosis and classification of diabetes mellitus. *Diabetes Care, 30*(Supplement 1), S42–47.

American Diabetes Association (ADA). (2007b). Standards of medical care in diabetes—2007. *Diabetes Care, 30*(Supplement 1), S4–S41.

American Heart Association (AHA). (2007). *Women and heart disease facts.* Available at: http://www.americanheart.org/presenter.jhtml?identifier=3039318.

Anderson, W. E., & Safdar, A. (2007). Varicella-zoster virus. *eMedicine.* Available at: http://emedicine.com/med/topic2361.htm.

Arenson, J., & Drake, P. (2007). *Maternal and newborn health.* Sudbury, MA: Jones and Bartlett Publishers.

As-Sanie, S., Gantt, A., & Rosenthal, M. S. (2004). Pregnancy prevention in adolescents. *American Family Physician, 70*(8), 1517–1524.

Baker, D. A. (2007). Consequences of herpes simplex virus in pregnancy and their prevention. *Current Opinion in Infectious Diseases, 20*(1), 73–76.

Balentine, J. & Eisenhart, A. (2008). Aortic stenosis. *eMedicine* [Online]. Available at: http://www.emedicine.com/EMERG/topic40.htm.

Barker, D., Lewis, N., Mason, G., & Tan, L. (2006). Maternal cardiovascular medicine: Toward better care for pregnant women with heart disease. *British Journal of Cardiology, 13*(6), 399–402.

Barros, M. C., Guinburg, R., Peres, C., Mitsuhiro, S., Chalem, E., & Laranjeira, R. R. (2006). Exposure to marijuana during pregnancy alters neurobehavior in the early neonatal period. *Journal of Pediatrics, 149,* 781–787.

Blackburn, S. T. (2007). *Maternal, fetal, & neonatal physiology: A clinical perspective* (3rd ed.). Philadelphia: Saunders.

Blincoe, A. J. (2007). Hypertension in pregnancy: The importance of monitoring. *British Journal of Midwifery, 15*(1), 50–53.

Bothamley, J. (2006). Tuberculosis in pregnancy: The role for midwives in diagnosis and treatment. *British Journal of Midwifery, 14*(4), 182–185.

Broliden, K., Tolfvenstam, T., & Norbeck, O. (2006). Clinical aspects of parvovirus B19 infection. *Journal of Internal Medicine, 260,* 285–304.

Burns, L., Mattick, R. P., Lim, K., & Wallace, C. (2007). Methadone in pregnancy: Treatment, retention and neonatal outcomes. *Addiction, 102*(2), 264–270.

CDC. (2006). *STD treatment guidelines.* Available at: http://www.cdc.gov/std/treatment/2006/toc.htm.

CDC. (2007a). *HIV/AIDS among women.* Available at: http://www.cdc.gov/hiv/topics/women/resources/factsheets/print/women.htm.

CDC. (2007b). *Prevention of perinatal group B streptococcal disease: revised guidelines from CDC.* Available at: http://www.cdc.gov/groupbstrep/hospitals/hospitals_guidelines_summary.htm.

CDC. (2007c). *Rubella.* Available at: www.cdc.gov/nip/publications/pink/rubella.pdf.

CDC (2007d). Fact sheet: Alcohol consumption among women who are pregnant. *Morbidity and Mortality Weekly Report, 54*(9), 229–230.

CDC. (2007e). *Fact sheet: Viral hepatitis B.* Available at: http://www.cdc.gov/ncidod/diseases/hepatitis/b/fact.htm.

CDC. (2008). *Genital herpes: CDC fact sheet* [Online]. Available at: http:www.cdc.gov/std/herpes/STDFact-herpes.htm.

Cressey, T. R., & Lallemant, M. (2007). Pharmacogenetics of antiretroviral drugs for the treatment of HIV-infected patients: An update. *Infection, Genetics & Evolution, 7*(2), 333–342.

Criteria Committee of the New York Heart Association. (1994). *Nomenclature and criteria for diagnosis of diseases of the heart and great vessels* (9th ed.). Dallas: American Heart Association.

Cunningham, D., & Rennels, M. B. (2006). Parvovirus B19 infection. *eMedicine.* Available at: http://www.emedicine.com/ped/topic192.htm.

Cunningham, F. G., Gant, N. F., Leveno, K. J., et al. (2005). *Williams' obstetrics* (22nd ed.). New York: McGraw-Hill.

Curran, D., & Poggi, S. H. (2007). Hematologic disease and pregnancy. *eMedicine.* Available at: http://www.emedicine.com/med/topic3254.htm.

Cypryk, K., Vilsboll, T., Nadel, I., Smyczynska, J., Holst J., & Lewinski, A. (2007). Normal secretion of the incretin hormones glucose-dependent insulinotropic polypeptide and glucagon-like peptide-1 during gestational diabetes mellitus. *Gynecologic Endocrinology, 23*(1), 58–62.

Dao, H., Mofenson, L. M., Ekpini, R., Gilks, C. F., Barnhart, M., Bolu, O., & Shaffer, N. (2007). International recommendations on antiretroviral drugs for treatment of HIV-infected women and prevention of mother-to-child HIV transmission in resource-limited settings. *American Journal of Obstetrics & Gynecology, 197*(3), S42–S55.

D'Arrigo, T. (2007). Pre-pregnant care cuts risks. *Diabetes Forecast, 60*(2), 16–17.

Derlet, R., & Albertson, T. (2006). Methamphetamine. *eMedicine.* Available at: http://www.emedicine.com/EMERG/topic859.htm.

Dobbenga-Rhodes, Y. A., & Prive, A. M. (2006). Assessment and evaluation of the woman with cardiac disease during pregnancy. *Journal of Perinatal & Neonatal Nursing, 20*(4), 295–233.

Dodge, P., Brady, M., & Maguire, B. (2007). Initiation of a nurse-developed interdisciplinary plan of care for opiate addiction in pregnant women and their infants. *International Journal of Childbirth Education, 21*(2), 21–24.

Dudek, S. G. (2006). *Nutrition essentials for nursing practice* (5th ed.). Philadelphia: Lippincott Williams & Wilkins.

Ebner, N., Rohrmeister, K., Winklbaur, B., Baewert, A., Jagsch, R., Peternell, A., Thau, K., & Fischer, G. (2007). Management of neonatal abstinence syndrome in neonates born to opioid maintained women. *Drug and Alcohol Dependence, 87*(2/3), 131–138.

Edelstein, S., & Herbold, N. (2007). *Nurse's pocket guide to nutrition.* Sudbury, MA: Jones and Bartlett Publishers.

Ekpebegh, C. O., Coetzee, E. J., van der Merwe, L., & Levitt, N. S. (2007). A 10-year retrospective analysis of pregnancy outcome in pregestational type 2 diabetes: Comparison of insulin and oral glucose-lowering agents. *Diabetic Medicine, 24*(3), 253–258.

Elbaz, W. F., Coyle, P., Hunter, A., & Farrag, S. (2007). Erythrovirus B19 as a potential cause of fetal hydrops: Assessing awareness. *British Journal of Midwifery, 15*(7), 440–444.

Elsayegh, D., & Shapiro, J. M. (2007). Sickle cell vasoocclusive crisis and acute chest syndrome at term pregnancy. *Southern Medical Journal, 100*(1), 77–79.

Farrar, D., Tuffnell, D. J., & West, J. Continuous subcutaneous insulin infusion versus multiple daily injections of insulin for pregnant women with diabetes. *Cochrane Database of Systematic*

Reviews 2007. Issue 3. Art. No.: CD005542.DOI: 10.1002/14651858.CD005542.pub2.

Fischer, R. (2007). Genital herpes in pregnancy. *eMedicine.* Available at: http://www.emedicine.com/med/topic3554.htm.

Frieden, F. J., & Chan, Y. (2007). Diabetes mellitus in pregnancy. In R. E. Rakel & E. T. Bope (Eds.), *Conn's current therapy 2007* (pp. 1169–1271). Philadelphia: Saunders Elsevier.

Gardella, C., & Brown, Z. A. (2007). Managing varicella zoster infection in pregnancy. *Cleveland Clinic Journal of Medicine, 74*(4), 290–296.

Gibson, P., & Carson, M. (2007). Hypertension and pregnancy. *eMedicine* Available at: http://emedicine.com/med/topic3250.htm.

Gilbert, E., & Harmon, J. (2006). *Manual of high-risk pregnancy and delivery* (4th ed.). St. Louis: Mosby.

Gilbert, E. S. (2007). *Manual of high risk pregnancy and delivery* (4th ed.). St. Louis: Mosby Elsevier.

Goodman, D., Klerman, L., Johnson, K., Chang, C., & Marth, N. (2007). Geographic access to family planning facilities and the risk of unintended and teenage pregnancy. *Maternal & Child Health Journal, 11*(2), 145–152.

Green, J. H. (2007). Fetal alcohol spectrum disorders: Understanding the effects of prenatal alcohol exposure and supporting students. *Journal of School Health, 77*(3), 103–108.

Hackley, B., Kriebs, J. M., & Rousseau, M. E. (2007). *Primary care of women: A guide for midwives and women's health providers.* Sudbury, MA: Jones and Bartlett Publishers.

Harner, H. M. (2004). Domestic violence and trauma care in teenage pregnancy: does paternal age make a difference? *JOGNN, 33*(3), 312–319.

Harvey, E. A. (2007). Hypertensive disorders or pregnancy. *Nursing Spectrum.* Available at: http://nsweb.nursingspectrum.com/ce/m23c-1.htm.

Henriksen, T. (2006). Nutrition and pregnancy outcome. *Nutrition Reviews, 64*(5), 19–23.

Herchline, T., & Amorosa, J. K. (2007). Tuberculosis. *Emedicine.* Available at: http://www.emedicine.com/MED/topic2324.htm.

Hermes-DeSantis, E. R., & Clyman, R. I. (2006). Patent ductus arteriosus: Pathophysiology and management. *Journal of Perinatology,* Supplement, 26, S14–S18.

Hilton, L. (2006). Pregnancy after 40: What's the risk? *Nursing Spectrum, 18A*(20), 19, 31.

Hoerst, B., & Samson, L. (2007). Perinatal infections. *Nursing Spectrum.* Available at: http://www.nurse.com/ce/course.html?CCID=2803.

Hoffman, D. J., & Brown, G. D. (2006). Neonatal abstinence syndrome secondary to in-utero caffeine exposure. *Neonatal Intensive Care, 19*(6), 24–25.

Hokelek, M., & Safdar, A. (2006). Toxoplasmosis. *eMedicine.* Available at: http://www.emedicine.com/med/topic2294.htm.

Holub, C., Kershaw, T., Ethier, K., Lewis, J., Milan, S., & Ickovics, J. (2007). Prenatal and parenting stress on adolescent maternal adjustment: Identifying a high-risk subgroup. *Maternal & Child Health Journal, 11*(2), 153–159.

Homko, C. J., & Reece, E. A. (2006). Insulins and oral hypoglycemic agents in pregnancy. *Journal of Maternal-Fetal and Neonatal Medicine, 19*(11), 679–686.

Johnsen, C. (2007). Preventing perinatal HIV transmission. *Nursing Spectrum.* Available at: http://www.nurse.com/ce/course.html?CCID=3239.

Joint National Committee (JNC). (2003). *Seventh Report of the Joint National Committee on Prevention, Detection, Evaluation, and Treatment of High Blood Pressure.* National Institutes of Health (NIH), National Heart, Lung, and Blood Institute. NIH Publication No. 035233. Washington, DC: NIH.

Jones, H. E. (2006). Drug addiction during pregnancy: Advances in maternal treatment and understanding child outcomes. *Current Directions in Psychological Science, 15*(3), 126–130.

Karamermer, Y., & Roos-Hesselink, J. W. (2007). Pregnancy and adult congenital heart disease. *Expert Review of Cardiovascular Therapy, 5*(5), 859–869.

King-Jones, T. C. (2008). Caring for pregnant adolescents: Perils and pearls of communication. *Nursing for Women's Health, 12*(2), 114–119.

Kripke, C. (2007). Hepatitis B vaccine for infants of HbsAg-positive mothers. *American Family Physician, 75*(1), 49–50.

Laartz, B., & Gompf, S. G. (2007). Viral infections and pregnancy. *EMedicine.* Available at: http://www.emedicine.com/med/topic3270.htm.

Lampe, M. A. (2006). Human immunodeficiency virus-1 and pre-conceptual care. *Maternal & Child Health Journal,* Supplement 10, 195–197.

Langille, D. B. (2007). Teenage pregnancy: Trends, contributing factors and the physicians' role. *Canadian Medical Association Journal, 176*(11), 1601–1602.

Lesesne, C. A., Lewis, K. M., White, C. P., Green, D. C., Duffy, J. L., & Wandersman, A. (2008). Promoting science-based approaches to teen pregnancy prevention: Proactively engaging the three systems of interactive systems framework. *American Journal of Community Psychology, 41*(3/4), 379–392.

Little, M. & Sinert, R. (2008). Pregnancy, asthma. *eMedicine* [Online]. Available at: http://www.emedicine.com/emerg/TOPIC476.HTM.

Magill, M. K., & Wilcox, R. (2007). Adolescent pregnancy and associated risks: Not just a result of maternal age. *American Family Physician, 75*(9), 1310–1311.

Malee, M. P. (2007). Parvovirus B19 infection. *Contemporary OB/GYN, 52*(5), 70–74.

March of Dimes. (2007a). *Teenage pregnancy.* Available at: http://www.marchofdimes.com/professionals/681_1159.asp.

March of Dimes. (2007b). *Diabetes in pregnancy.* Available at: http://marchofdimes.com/professionals/14332_1197.asp.

March of Dimes. (2007c). *Pregnancy after 35: Quick reference and fact sheet.* Available at: http://www.modimes.org/professionals/681_1155.asp.

March of Dimes. (2007d). *Group B strep infection.* Available at: http://www.marchofdimes.com/professionals/681_1205.asp.

March of Dimes. (2007e). *Toxoplasmosis.* Available at: http://www.marchofdimes.com/printableArticles/681_1228.asp?printable=true.

McCann, J. A. S. (2007). *Maternal-neonatal nursing made incredibly easy* (2nd ed.). Philadelphia: Lippincott Williams & Wilkins.

McMahon, W. S. (2007). Congenital heart disease. In R. E. Rakel & E. T. Bope (Eds.), *Conn's current therapy 2007* (Section 5, pp. 378–379). Philadelphia: Saunders Elsevier.

Menato, G., Bo, S., Signorile, A., Gallo, M., Cotrino, I., Poala, C., & Massobrio, M. (2008). Current management of gestational diabetes mellitus. *Expert Review of Obstetrics Gynecology, 3*(1), 73–91.

Modder, J. (2008). Diabetes in pregnancy: Can we make a difference? *International Journal of Obstetrics & Gynecology, 115*(4), 419–420.

Mooney, M. (2007). Managing cardiac disease in pregnancy. *British Journal of Midwifery, 15*(2), 76–78.

Moore, S. L., & Seybold, V. K. (2007). HPV vaccine. *Clinical Reviews, 17*(1), 36–41.

Moos, M. K. (2006) Group B strep: A prevention success story. *AWHONN Lifelines, 9*(6), 484–486.

More, D. (2007). Asthma in pregnancy. *About allergies.* Available at: http://allergies.about.com/od/allergiesandpregnancy/a/asthmapregnancy.htm.

National Asthma Education and Prevention Program (NAEPP). (2007). NAEPP Expert Panel Report: Managing asthma during pregnancy. *Journal of Allergy & Clinical Immunology, 115,* 36–46.

National Institute on Drug Abuse (NIDA). (2007a). *Drug use during pregnancy.* Available at: http://search2.google.cit.nih.gov/search?q=pregnancy&site=NIDA&client=NIDA_frontnd&proxystylesheet=NIDA_frontend&output=xml_no_dtd&filter=0&getfields=*&btnG.x=16&btnG.y=11.

National Institute on Drug Abuse (NIDA). (2007b). *Cocaine abuse and addiction.* Available at: http://www.nida.nih.gov/ResearchReports/Cocaine/cocaine4.html#maternal.

National Institute on Drug Abuse (NIDA). (2007c). *Marijuana.* Available at: http://www.drugabuse.gov/Infofacts/marijuana.html.

National Institute on Drug Abuse (NIDA). (2007d). *Methamphetamine abuse and addiction.* Available at: http://www.drugabuse.gov/ResearchReports/methamph/methamph5.html.

National Organization on Fetal Alcohol Syndrome (NoFAS). (2007). *What is fetal alcohol syndrome?* Available at: http://www.nofas.org/main/what_is_FAS.htm.

Noyes, J., & Popay, J. (2007). Directly observed therapy and tuberculosis: How can a systemic review of qualitative research contribute to improving services? A qualitative meta-synthesis. *Journal of Advanced Nursing, 57*(3), 227–243.

O'Toole, M. T. (2005). *Encyclopedia and dictionary of medicine, nursing, and allied health* (7th ed.). Philadelphia: Saunders.

Peddicord, K. (2005). Healthy hearts for women. *AWHONN Lifelines, 9*(1), 35–38.

Peyron, F., Wallon, M., Liou, C., & Garner, P. (2006). Treatments for toxoplasmosis in pregnancy. *Cochrane Library* (4), CD001684.

Podymow, T., & August, P. (2007). Hypertension in pregnancy. *Advances in Chronic Kidney Disease, 14*(2), 178–190.

Pyrsopoulos, N. T., & Reddy, K. R. (2007). Hepatitis B. *eMedicine.* Available at: http://www.emedicine.com/med/topic992.htm.

Raatikainen, K., Huurinainen, P., & Heinonen, S. (2007). Smoking in early gestation or through pregnancy: A decision crucial to pregnancy outcome. *Preventive Medicine, 44*(1), 59–63.

Rassool, G. H., & Villar-Luis, M. (2006). Reproductive risks of alcohol and illicit drugs: An overview. *Journal of Addictions Nursing, 17,* 211–213.

Rochon, M., Rand, L., Roth, L., & Gaddipati, S. (2006). Glyburide for the management of gestational diabetes: Risk factors predictive of failure associated pregnancy outcomes. *American Journal of Obstetrics and Gynecology, 195*(4), 1090–1094.

Ross, D. S., Jones, J. L., & Lynch, M. F. (2006). Toxoplasmosis, cytomegalovirus, listeriosis, and preconception care. *Maternal & Child Health Journal, 10*(5), Supplement: S187–S191.

Samson, L., Ferguson, H. W., & Scanlon, R. M. (2007). Chronic medical conditions and pregnancy, part I. *Nursing Spectrum.* Available at: http://nsweb.nursingspectrum.com/ce/m23ac.htm.

Santis, M., Cavaliere, A. F., Straface, G., & Caruso, A. (2006). Rubella infection in pregnancy. *Reproductive Toxicology, 21*(4), 390–398.

Sauerbrei, A., & Wutzler, P. (2007). Varicella-zoster virus infection during pregnancy: Current concepts of prevention, diagnosis and therapy. *Medical Microbiology & Immunology, 196*(2), 95–102.

Scollan-Koliopoulos, M., Guadagno, S., & Walker, E. A. (2006). Gestational diabetes management: Guidelines to a healthy pregnancy. *Nurse Practitioner, 31*(6), 14–25.

Secco, M. L., Profit, S., Kennedy, E., Walsh, A., Letourneau, N., & Stewart, M. (2007). Factors affecting postpartum depressive symptoms of adolescent mothers. *JOGNN, 36*(1), 47–54.

Sharp, K. (2006). Hypertension: Just the facts. *Clinical Journal of Oncology Nursing, 10*(6), 727–730.

Simpson, K. R., & Creehan, P. A. (2008). *AWHONN's perinatal nursing* (3rd ed.). Philadelphia: Lippincott Williams & Wilkins.

Tihtonen, K., Koobi, T., Huhtala, H., & Uotila, J. (2007). Hemodynamic adaptation during pregnancy in chronic hypertension. *Hypertension in Pregnancy, 26*(3), 315–328.

Tough, S., Benzies, K., Fraser-Lee, N., & Newburn-Cook, C. (2007). Factors influencing childbearing decisions and knowledge of perinatal risks among Canadian men and women. *Maternal & Child Health Journal, 11*(2), 189–198.

Uebing, A., Steer, P. J., Yentis, S. M., & Gatzoulis, M. A. (2006). Pregnancy and congenital heart disease. *British Medical Journal, 332,* 401–406.

U.S. Department of Health and Human Services (USDHHS). (2000). *Healthy people 2010* (Conference Edition, vol. 1). Washington, DC.

U.S. Department of Health and Human Services (USDHHS). (2007). *U.S. Surgeon General releases advisory on alcohol use in pregnancy.* HHS Office of the Surgeon General. Available at: http://hhs.gov/surgeongeneral/pressreleases/sg02222007.html.

U.S. Preventive Services Task Force (USPSTF). (2006a). *The guide to clinical preventive services 2006.* USDHHS: AHRQ Pub. No. 06-0588.

U.S. Preventive Services Task Force (USPSTF). (2006b). *Updated USPHSTF recommendations for the use of antiretroviral drugs in pregnant HIV-1-infected women for maternal health and interventions to reduce perinatal HIV-1 transmission in the United States.* Available at: http://aidsinfo.nih.gov.

Varughese, G. I., Chowdhury, S. R., Warner, D. P., & Barton, D. M. (2007). Preconception care of women attending adult general diabetes clinics—Are we doing enough? *Diabetes Research & Clinical Practice, 76*(1), 142–145.

Wang, M. (2007). Perinatal drug abuse and neonatal withdrawal. *eMedicine.* Available at: http://www.emedicine.com/ped/topic 2631.htm.

Weekes, A. J., & Lee, D. S. (2006). Substance abuse: Cocaine. *eMedicine.* Available at: http://www.emedicine.com/ped/topic2666.htm.

Witcher, P. M., & Harvey, C. J. (2006). Modifying labor routines for the woman with cardiac disease. *Journal of Perinatal & Neonatal Nursing, 20*(4), 303–311.

Wooley, C. F., & Boudoulas, H. (2007). Mitral valve prolapse: The floppy mitral valve, mitral valve prolapse, and mitral valvular regurgitation. In R. E. Rakel & E. T. Bope (Eds.), *Conn's current therapy 2007* (Section 5, pp. 386–390). Philadelphia: Saunders Elsevier.

World Health Organization (WHO). (2007). *Tuberculosis.* Available at: http://www.who.int/mediacentre/factsheets/fs104/en/.

Xu, F., Markowitz, L. E., Gottlieb, S. L., & Berman, S. M. (2007). Seroprevalence of herpes simplex virus types 1 and 2 in pregnant women in the United States. *American Journal of Obstetrics & Gynecology, 196*(1), 43–46.

Zarrett, N., & Eccles, J. (2006). The passage to adulthood: Challenges of late adolescence. *New Directions for Youth Development,* Fall (111), 13–28.

Zeck, W., Bjelic-Radisic, V., Haas, J., & Greimel, E. (2007). Impact of adolescent pregnancy on the future life of young mothers in terms of social, familial, and educational changes. *Journal of Adolescent Health, 41*(4), 380–388.

WEBSITES

Alan Guttmacher Institute: www.agi-usa.org
Alcoholics Anonymous: www.alcoholics-anonymous.org
American Academy of Pediatrics: www.aap.org
American College of Obstetricians and Gynecologists: www.acog.org
American Diabetes Association: www.diabetes.org
American Lung Association: www.lungusa.org
American Medical Association HIV/AIDS Resource Center:
    www.ama-assn.org/special/hiv
American Society of Addiction Medicine: www.asam.org
Association of Nurses in AIDS Care: www.anacnet.org
Association of Women's Health, Obstetric & Neonatal Nurses:
    www.awhonn.org
Asthma and Allergy Foundation of America: www.aafa.org
Allergy & Asthma Network of Mothers of Asthmatics:
    www.breatherville.org
CDC National Prevention Information Network: 1-800-458-5231,
    www.cdcnpin.org
HIV websites: www.hivinsite.ucsf.edu, www.hivatis.org
International Nurses Society on Addictions: www.intnsa.org
March of Dimes: www.modimes.org
Narcotics Anonymous: www.na.org
National Campaign to Prevent Teen Pregnancy:
    www.teenpregnancy.org
National Clearinghouse for Alcohol and Drug Abuse Information:
    www.health.org
National Heart, Lung and Blood Institute of NIH: www.nhlbi.nih.gov
National Institute on Drug Abuse: www.nida.nih.gov
National Organization for Fetal Alcohol Syndrome: www.nofas.org
Planned Parenthood: www.plannedparenthood.org
Sex Information and Education Council of United States:
    www.siecus.org
Sidelines High Risk Pregnancy Support Office: www.sidelines.org
Tobacco Information and Prevention Source (TIPS):
    www.cdc.gov/tobacco
Women for Sobriety Support Group: www.womenforsobriety.org

CHAPTER WORKSHEET

MULTIPLE CHOICE QUESTIONS

1. Which of the following would the nurse include when teaching a pregnant woman about the pathophysiologic mechanisms associated with gestational diabetes?

   a. Pregnancy fosters the development of carbohydrate cravings.

   b. There is progressive resistance to the effects of insulin.

   c. Hypoinsulinemia develops early in the first trimester.

   d. Glucose levels decrease to accommodate fetal growth.

2. When providing prenatal education to a pregnant woman with asthma, which of the following would be important for the nurse to do?

   a. Explain that she should avoid steroids during her pregnancy.

   b. Demonstrate how to assess her blood glucose levels.

   c. Teach correct administration of subcutaneous bronchodilators.

   d. Ensure she seeks treatment for any acute exacerbation.

3. Which of the following conditions would most likely cause a pregnant woman with type 1 diabetes the greatest difficulty during her pregnancy?

   a. Placenta previa

   b. Hyperemesis gravidarum

   c. Abruptio placentae

   d. Rh incompatibility

4. Women who drink alcohol during pregnancy:

   a. Often produce more alcohol dehydrogenase

   b. Usually become intoxicated faster than before

   c. Can give birth to an infant with fetal alcohol spectrum disorder

   d. Gain fewer pounds throughout the gestation

5. When explaining to a pregnant woman about HIV infection and transmission, which of the following would the nurse include?

   a. It primarily occurs when there is a large viral load in the blood.

   b. HIV is most commonly transmitted via sexual contact.

   c. It affects the majority of infants of mothers with HIV infection.

   d. Nurses are most frequently affected due to needle sticks.

CRITICAL THINKING EXERCISES

1. A client at 26 weeks' gestation came to the clinic to follow up on her previous 1-hour glucose screening. Her results had come back outside the accepted screening range, and a 3-hour glucose tolerance test (GTT) had been ordered. It resulted in three abnormal values, confirming a diagnosis of gestational diabetes. As the nurse in the prenatal clinic you are seeing her for the first time.

   a. What additional information will you need to provide care for her?

   b. What education will she need to address this new diagnosis?

   c. How will you evaluate the effectiveness of your interventions?

2. A 14-year-old girl comes to the public health clinic with her mother. The mother tells you that her daughter has been "out messing around and has gotten herself pregnant." The girl is crying quietly in the corner and avoids eye contact with you. The mother reports that her daughter "must be following in my footsteps" because she became pregnant when she was only 15 years old. The client's mother goes back out into the waiting room and leaves the client with you.

   a. What is your first approach with the client to gain her trust?

   b. List the client's educational needs during this pregnancy.

   c. What prevention strategies are needed to prevent a second pregnancy?

3. Linda, a 27-year-old G3P2, is admitted to the labor and birth suite because of preterm rupture of membranes at an estimated 35 weeks' gestation. She has received no prenatal care and reports this was an unplanned pregnancy. Linda appears distracted and very thin. She reports that her two previous children have been in foster care since birth because the child welfare authorities "didn't think I was an adequate mother." She denies any recent use of alcohol or

drugs, but you smell alcohol on her breath. She has a spontaneous vaginal birth a few hours later, producing a 4-lb baby boy with Apgar scores of 8 at 1 minute and 9 at 5 minutes.

a. What aspects of this woman's history may lead the nurse to suspect that this infant may be at risk for fetal alcohol spectrum disorder?

b. What additional screening or laboratory tests might validate your suspicion?

c. What physical and neurodevelopmental deficits might present later in life if the infant has fetal alcohol spectrum disorder?

STUDY ACTIVITIES

1. In the maternity clinic or hospital setting, interview a pregnant woman with a preexisting medical condition (e.g., diabetes, asthma, sickle cell anemia) and find out how this condition affects her life and this pregnancy, especially her lifestyle choices.

2. You have a close friend who has a problem with alcohol but denies it. She now admits to you that she thinks she is pregnant because she missed her period. What specific information and advice should you give her concerning alcohol use during pregnancy?

3. Should marijuana be legalized in the United States? What impact might your view (pro or con) have on pregnant women and their offspring?

4. Outline a discussion you might have with an HIV-positive pregnant woman who doesn't see the need to take antiretroviral agents to prevent perinatal transmission.

5. The nurse is preparing a teaching session about breastfeeding for a group of pregnant women who have various infections listed below. The nurse would include women with which of the following conditions? Select all that apply.

a. Hepatitis B

b. Parvovirus B19

c. Herpesvirus type 2

d. HIV-positive status

e. Cytomegalovirus

f. Varicella-zoster virus

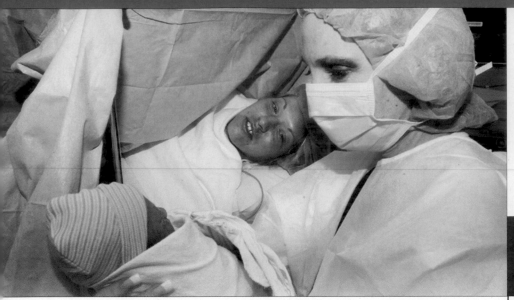

CHAPTER 21

NURSING MANAGEMENT OF LABOR AND BIRTH AT RISK

KEY TERMS

amnioinfusion
cesarean birth
dystocia
forceps
hypertonic uterine
   dysfunction
hypotonic uterine
   dysfunction

labor induction
macrosomia
postterm pregnancy
precipitous labor
preterm labor
shoulder dystocia

tocolytic
umbilical cord prolapse
vacuum extractor
vaginal birth after
   cesarean (VBAC)

LEARNING OBJECTIVES

Upon completion of the chapter, the learner will be able to:

1. Define dystocia.
2. Identify the four major abnormalities or problems associated with dysfunctional labor patterns, giving examples of each problem.
3. Describe the nursing management for the woman with dysfunctional labor experiencing a problem with the powers, passenger, passageway, and psyche.
4. Develop a plan of care for the woman experiencing preterm labor.
5. Discuss the nursing assessment and management of the woman experiencing a postterm pregnancy.
6. Explain four obstetric emergencies that can complicate labor and birth, including appropriate management for each.
7. Compare and contrast the nursing management for the woman undergoing labor induction or augmentation, forceps- and vacuum-assisted birth.
8. Summarize the plan of care for a woman who is to undergo a cesarean birth.
9. Discuss the key areas to be addressed when caring for a woman who is to undergo vaginal birth after cesarean (VBAC).

*J*ennifer, a 29 year-old G1P0, is at 41 weeks' gestation. Her health care provider has recommended that she come in for induction. She is very anxious about doing this since she has heard "horror stories" about the "hard painful contractions" that can result. What can the nurse do to calm her fears?

Wow

In face of a crisis or a potentially bad outcome, add a mixture of warmth and serenity to your technical abilities.

Most women describe pregnancy as an exciting time in their life, but the development of an unexpected problem can suddenly change this description dramatically. Consider the woman who has had a problem-free pregnancy and then suddenly develops a condition during labor, changing a routine situation into a possible crisis. Many complications occur with little or no warning and present challenges for the perinatal health care team as well as the family. The nurse plays a major role in identifying the problem quickly and coordinating immediate intervention, ultimately achieving a positive outcome.

National Health Goals address maternal and newborn outcomes involving complications of labor and birth and cesarean birth (USDHHS, 2000). These goals are highlighted in Healthy People 2010 21.1.

This chapter will address several conditions occurring during labor and birth that may increase the risk of an adverse outcome for the mother and fetus. It also describes birth-related procedures that may be necessary for the woman who develops a condition that increases her risk or that may be needed to reduce the woman's risk for developing a condition, thus promoting optimal maternal and fetal outcomes. Nursing management of the woman and her family focuses on professional support and compassionate care.

Dystocia

Dystocia, defined as abnormal or difficult labor, can be influenced by a vast number of maternal and fetal factors. Dystocia is said to exist when the progress of labor deviates from normal; it is characterized by a slow and abnormal progression of labor. It occurs in approximately 8% to 11% of all labors and is the leading indicator for primary cesarean birth in the United States (Joy & Lyon, 2007).

To characterize a labor as abnormal, a basic understanding of normal labor is essential. Normal labor starts with regular uterine contractions that are strong enough to result in cervical effacement and dilation. Early in labor, uterine contractions are irregular and cervical effacement and dilation occur gradually. When cervical dilation reaches 4 cm and uterine contractions become more powerful, the active phase of labor begins. It is usually during the active phase that dystocia becomes apparent. Because dystocia cannot be predicted or diagnosed with certainty, the term "failure to progress" is often used. This term includes lack of progressive cervical dilation, lack of descent of the fetal head, or both. An adequate trial of labor is needed to declare with confidence that dystocia or "failure to progress" exists.

Early identification of and prompt interventions for dystocia are essential to minimize risk to the woman and fetus. According to American College of Obstetrics and Gynecology (ACOG, 2003a), factors associated with an increased risk for dystocia include epidural analgesia, excessive analgesia, multiple gestation, hydramnios, maternal exhaustion, ineffective maternal pushing technique, occiput posterior position, longer first stage of labor, nulliparity, short maternal stature (less than 5 feet tall), fetal birth weight (more than 8.8 lb), shoulder dystocia, abnormal fetal presentation or position (breech), fetal anomalies (hydrocephalus), maternal age older than 35 years, gestational age more than 41 weeks, chorioamnionitis, ineffective uterine contractions, and high fetal station at complete cervical dilation.

Dystocia can result from problems or abnormalities involving the expulsive forces (known as the "powers"); presentation, position, and fetal development (the "passenger"); the maternal bony pelvis or birth canal (the "passageway"); and maternal stress (the "psyche"). Table 21.1 summarizes the diagnosis, therapeutic management, and nursing management of the common problems associated with dystocia.

HEALTHY PEOPLE 2010

Objective	Significance
Reduce maternal illness and complications due to pregnancy	• Will help to focus attention on the need for close antepartum surveillance and identification of risk factors for maternal illness and complications, particularly those most likely to be associated with maternal death
Reduce maternal complications during hospitalized labor and delivery from a baseline of 31.2/100 deliveries to a target of 24/100 deliveries	
Reduce cesarean births among low-risk (full term, singleton, vertex presentation) women	
Reduce the number of cesarean births in women giving birth for the first time from a baseline of 18% to 15%	• Will help to promote development of specific guidelines for trials of labor and labor management, continual labor support, and practice patterns, while helping to ensure positive maternal and newborn outcomes
Reduce the number of cesarean births in women with prior cesarean birth from 72% to 63%	

USDHHS, 2000.

▶ PROBLEMS WITH THE POWERS

When the expulsive forces of the uterus become dysfunctional, the uterus may either never fully relax (hypertonic contractions), placing the fetus in jeopardy, or relax too much (hypotonic contractions), causing ineffective contractions. Still another dysfunction can occur when the uterus contracts so frequently and with such intensity that a very rapid birth will take place (precipitous labor).

(text continues on page 619)

TABLE 21.1 DIAGNOSIS AND MANAGEMENT OF COMMON PROBLEMS ASSOCIATED WITH DYSTOCIA

	Description	Diagnosis	Therapeutic Management	Nursing Management
Problems with the powers				
Hypertonic uterine dysfunction	Occurring in the latent phase of the first stage of labor (cervical dilation of <4 cm); uncoordinated. Force of contraction typically in the midsection of uterus at the junction of the active upper and passive lower segments of the uterus rather than in the fundus. Loss of downward pressure to push the presenting part against the cervix (Gilbert & Harmon, 2007). Woman commonly becomes discouraged due to lack of progress; also has increased pain secondary to uterine anoxia.	Characteristic hypertonicity of the contractions and the lack of labor progress	Therapeutic rest with the use of sedatives to promote relaxation and stop the abnormal activity of the uterus. Identification and intervention of any contributing factors. Ruling out abruptio placentae (also associated with high resting tone and persistent pain). Onset of a normal labor pattern occurs in many women after a 4- to 6-hour rest period (Gilbert, 2007).	Institute bed rest and sedation to promote relaxation and reduce pain. Assist with measures to rule out fetopelvic disproportion and fetal malpresentation. Evaluate fetal tolerance to labor pattern, such as monitoring of FHR patterns. Assess for signs of maternal infection. Promote adequate hydration through IV therapy. Provide pain management via epidural or IV analgesics. Assist with amniotomy to augment labor. Explain to woman and family about dysfunctional pattern. Plan for operative birth if normal labor pattern is not achieved.
Hypotonic uterine dysfunction	Often termed secondary uterine inertia because the labor begins normally and then the frequency and intensity of contractions decrease (Joy & Lyon, 2007). Possible contributing factors: overdistended uterus with multifetal pregnancy or large single fetus, too much pain medicine given too early in labor, fetal malposition, and regional anesthesia (Bonilla & Forouzan, 2007).	Evaluation of the woman's labor to confirm that she is having hypotonic active labor rather than a long latent phase. Evaluation of maternal pelvis and fetal presentation and position to ensure that they are not contributing to the prolonged labor without noticeable progress.	Identification of possible cause of inefficient uterine action (a malpositioned fetus, a too small maternal pelvis, overdistention of the uterus with fluid or a macrosomic fetus). Rupture of amniotic sac (amniotomy) if all causes ruled out. Possible augmentation with oxytocin (Pitocin) to stimulate effective uterine contractions. Cesarean birth if amniotomy and augmentation ineffective.	Administer oxytocin as ordered once fetopelvic disproportion is ruled out. Assist with amniotomy if membranes are intact. Provide continuous electronic fetal monitoring. Monitor vital signs, contractions, and cervix continually. Assess for signs of maternal and fetal infection. Explain to woman and family about dysfunctional pattern. Plan for surgical birth if normal labor pattern is not achieved or fetal distress occurs.

Problem	Description	Identification	Expected Outcome	Nursing Interventions
Precipitous labor	Abrupt onset of higher-intensity contractions occurring in a shorter period of time instead of the more gradual increase in frequency, duration, and intensity that typifies most spontaneous labors	Identification based on the rapidity of progress through the stages of labor	Vaginal delivery if maternal pelvis is adequate	Closely monitor woman with previous history. Anticipate use of scheduled induction to control labor rate. Administer pharmacologic agents, such as tocolytics, to slow labor. Stay in constant attendance to monitor progress.
Problems with the passenger Persistent occiput posterior position	Engagement of fetal head in the left or right occipito-transverse position with the occiput rotating posteriorly rather than into the more favorable occiput anterior position (fetus born facing upward instead of the normal downward position) (Bonilla & Forouzan, 2007). Labor usually much longer and more uncomfortable (causing increased back pain during labor) if fetus remains in this position. Possible extensive caput succedaneum and molding from the sustained occiput posterior position.	Leopold maneuvers and vaginal examination to determine position of fetal head in conjunct on with the mother's complaints of severe back pain (back of fetal head pressing on mother's sacrum and coccyx).	Labor to proceed, preparing the woman for a long labor (spontaneous resolution possible). Comfort measures and maternal positioning to help promote fetal head rotation.	Assess for complaints of intense back pain in first stage of labor. Anticipate possible use of forceps to rotate to anterior position at birth or manual rotation to anterior position at end of second stage. Assess for prolonged second stage of labor with arrest of descent (common with this malposition). Encourage maternal position changes to promote fetal head rotation: hands and knees and rocking pelvis back and forth; side-lying position; side lunges during contractions; sitting; kneeling, or standing while leaning forward; squatting position to give birth and enlarge pelvic outlet. Prepare for possible cesarean birth if rotation is not achieved. Administer agents as ordered for pain relief (effective pain relief crucial to help the woman to tolerate the back discomfort). Apply low back counterpressure during contractions to ease the discomfort. Use other

(continued)

TABLE 21.1 DIAGNOSIS AND MANAGEMENT OF COMMON PROBLEMS ASSOCIATED WITH DYSTOCIA (continued)

	Description	Diagnosis	Therapeutic Management	Nursing Management
				helpful measures to attempt to rotate the fetal head, including lateral abdominal stroking in the direction that the fetal head should rotate; assisting the client into a hands-and-knees position (all fours); and squatting, pelvic rocking, stair climbing, assuming a side-lying position toward the side that the fetus should rotate, and side lunges (WHO, 2007). Provide measures to reduce anxiety. Continuously reinforce the woman's progress. Teach woman about measures to facilitate fetal head rotation.
Face and brow presentation	Face presentation with complete extension of the fetal head. Brow presentation: fetal head between full extension and full flexion so that the largest fetal skull diameter presents to the pelvis.	Diagnosis only once labor is well established via vaginal examination; palpation of facial features as the presenting part rather than the fetal head	Vaginal birth possible with face presentation with an adequate maternal pelvis and fetal head rotation; cesarean birth if head rotates backward. Cesarean birth for brow presentation unless head flexes.	Assist with evaluating for fetopelvic disproportion. Anticipate cesarean birth if vertex position is not achieved. Explain fetal malposition to the woman and her partner. Provide close observation for any signs of fetal hypoxia, as evidenced by late decelerations on the fetal monitor.
Breech presentation	Fetal buttocks, or breech, presenting first rather than the head. 1. Frank breech: buttock as the presenting part, with hips flexed and legs and knees extended upward 2. Complete breech (or full breech): buttock as presenting part, with hips flexed and knees flexed in a "cannonball" position	Vaginal examination to determine breech presentation. Ideally, ultrasound to confirm a clinically suspected presentation and to identify any fetal anomalies.	The optimal method of birth is controversial: cesarean birth by some providers unless the fetus is small and the mother has a large pelvis; vaginal birth by others with each occurrence treated individually and labor monitored very closely.	Assess for associated conditions such as placenta previa, hydramnios, fetal anomalies, and multiple gestation. Arrange for ultrasound to confirm fetal presentation. Assist with external cephalic version possible after 36 weeks and administer tocolytics to assist with external cephalic version.

3. Footling or incomplete breech: One or two feet as the presenting part, with one or both hips extended

Regardless of the birth method selected, the risk for trauma is high. Breech vaginal births are not recommended by ACOG and come with a higher risk to the mother and infant than a planned surgical birth (ACOG, 2001). Vaginal delivery: fetus allowed to spontaneously deliver up to the umbilicus; then maneuvers to assist in the delivery of the remainder of the body, arms, and head; fetal membranes left intact as long as possible to act as a dilating wedge and to prevent cord prolapse; anesthesiologist and pediatrician present.

Caesarean birth; Use of external cephalic version to reduce the chance of breech presentation at birth; attempted after the 36th week of gestation but before the start of labor (some fetuses spontaneously turn to a cephalic presentation on their own toward term, and some will return to the breech presentation if external cephalic version is attempted too early [Fischer, 2007]); variable success rates, with risk for fractured bones, ruptured viscera, abruptio placentae, fetomaternal hemorrhage, and umbilical cord

Anticipate trial labor for 4 to 6 hours to evaluate progress if version is unsuccessful. Plan for cesarean birth if no progress is seen or fetal distress occurs.
After external cephalic version, administer RhoGAM to the Rh-negative woman to prevent a sensitization reaction if trauma has occurred and the potential for mixing of blood exists (Gilbert, 2007).

(continued)

TABLE 21.1 **DIAGNOSIS AND MANAGEMENT OF COMMON PROBLEMS ASSOCIATED WITH DYSTOCIA** (continued)

	Description	Diagnosis	Therapeutic Management	Nursing Management
			entanglement (Fischer, 2007). Tocolytic drugs to relax the uterus, as well as other methods, to facilitate external cephalic version at term (Jenis, 2007). Individual evaluation of each woman for all factors before any interventions are initiated.	
Shoulder dystocia	Delivery of fetal head with neck not appearing; retraction of chin against the perineum; shoulders remaining wedged behind the mother's pubic bone, causing a difficult birth with potential for injury to both mother and baby. If shoulders still above the brim at this stage, no advancement. Newborn's chest trapped within the vaginal vault; chest unable to expand with respiration (although nose and mouth are outside). Risk of umbilical cord compression between the fetal body and the maternal pelvis.	Emergency, often unexpected complication. Diagnosis made when newborn's head delivers without delivery of neck and remaining body structures. Primary risk factors, including suspected infant macrosomia (weight >4,500 g), maternal diabetes mellitus, excessive maternal weight gain, abnormal maternal pelvic anatomy, maternal obesity, postdates pregnancy, short stature, a history of previous shoulder dystocia, and use of epidural analgesia (Gurewitsch et al., 2006).	If anticipated, preparatory tasks instituted: alerting of key personnel; education of woman and family regarding steps to be taken in the event of a difficult birth; emptying of woman's bladder to allow additional room for possible maneuvers needed for the birth. McRobert's maneuver. Suprapubic pressure (not fundal) (see Fig. 21.1). Combination of maneuvers effective in more than 50% of cases of shoulder dystocia (Abenhaim et al., 2007). Newborn resuscitation team readily available.	Intervene immediately due to cord compression. Perform McRobert's maneuver and application of suprapubic pressure. Assist with positioning the woman in squatting position, hands-and-knees position, or lateral recumbent position for birth to free shoulder. Anticipate cesarean birth if no success in dislodging shoulders. Clear room of unnecessary clutter to make room for additional personnel and equipment (Anderson, 2007). After the birth, assess newborn for crepitus, deformity, Erb's palsy, or bruising, which might suggest neurologic damage or a fracture (Arenson & Drake, 2007).
Multiple gestation	More than one fetus, leading to uterine overdistention and possibly resulting in hypotonic contractions and abnormal presentations of the fetuses. Fetal hypoxia during labor a significant threat due to placenta providing oxygen and nutrients to more than one fetus.	Nearly all multiples are now diagnosed early by ultrasound. Most women go into labor before 37 weeks.	Admission to facility with specialized care unit if woman goes into labor. Spontaneous progression of labor if woman has no complicating factors and first fetus is in longitudinal lie. Separate monitoring of each fetal heart rate during labor and birth.	Assess for hypotonic labor pattern due to overdistention. Evaluate for fetal presentation, maternal pelvic size, and gestational age to determine mode of delivery. Ensure presence of neonatal team for birth of multiples. Anticipate need for cesarean birth, which is common in multiple gestations.

(continued)

			After birth of first fetus, clamping of cord and lie of the second twin assessed. Possible external cephalic version necessary to assist in providing a longitudinal lie. Second and subsequent fetuses at greater risk for birth-related complications, such as umbilical cord prolapse, malpresentation, and abruptio placentae (Zach & Pramanik, 2007). Cesarean birth if risk factors high.	Assess for inability of fetus to descend. Anticipate need for vacuum and forceps-assisted births (common). Plan for cesarean birth if maternal parameters are inadequate to give birth to large fetus.
Excessive fetal size and abnormalities	Macrosomia leading to fetopelvic disproportion (fetus unable to fit through the maternal pelvis to be born vaginally). Reduced contraction strength due to overdistention by large fetus leading to a prolonged labor and the potential for birth injury and trauma. Fetal abnormalities possibly interfering with fetal descent, leading to prolonged labor and difficult birth.	A diagnosis of fetal macrosomia can be confirmed by measuring the birthweight after birth. Suspicion of macrosomia based on the findings of an ultrasound examination before onset of labor (if suspected due to conditions such as maternal diabetes or obesity, estimation of fetal weight via ultrasound). Leopold's maneuvers to estimate fetal weight and position on admission to labor and birth unit.	Scheduled cesarean birth if diagnosis is made before the onset of labor to reduce the risk of injury to both the newborn and the mother. If identified by Leopold's maneuvers, possible trial of labor to evaluate progress; however, providers usually opt to proceed with a cesarean birth in a primigravida with a macrosomic fetus (Catalano, 2007).	
Problems with the passageway	Contraction of one or more of the three planes of the pelvis. Poorer prognosis for vaginal birth in women with android and platypelloid types of pelvis. Contracted pelvis involving reduction in one or more of the pelvic diameters interfering with progress	Shortest A-P diameter <10 cm or greatest transverse diameter <12 cm. (Approximation of A-P diameter via measurement of diagonal conjugate, which in the contracted pelvis is <11.5 cm). X-ray pelvimetry to determine the smallest A-P diameter	Focus on allowing natural forces of labor contractions to push the largest diameter (biparietal) of the fetal head beyond the obstruction or narrow passage. Possible forceps and vacuum extraction to assist navigation through this passageway.	Assess for poor contractions, slow dilation, prolonged labor. Evaluate bowel and bladder status to reduce soft tissue obstruction and allow increased pelvic space. Anticipate trial of labor; if no labor progression after an adequate trial, plan for cesarean birth.

TABLE 21.1 DIAGNOSIS AND MANAGEMENT OF COMMON PROBLEMS ASSOCIATED WITH DYSTOCIA (continued)

Description	Diagnosis	Therapeutic Management	Nursing Management
of labor: inlet, midpelvis, and outlet contracture. Obstruction in the birth canal, such as placenta previa that partially or completely obstructs the internal os of the cervix, fibroids in the lower uterine segment, a full bladder or rectum, an edematous cervix caused by premature bearing-down efforts, and human papillomavirus (HPV) warts.	through which the fetal head must pass. Interischial tuberous diameter of <8 cm possibly compromising outlet contracture (outlet and midpelvic contractures frequently occur together).		
Problems with the psyche	Release of stress-related hormones (catecholamines, cortisol, epinephrine, beta-endorphin), which act on smooth muscle (uterus) and reduce uterine contractility. Excessive release of catecholamines and other stress-related hormones not therapeutic. Release also results in decreased uteroplacental perfusion and increased risk for poor newborn adjustment (Gilbert, 2007).	Ruling out of other possible causes of dystocia	Treatment dependent on woman's responses such as anxiety, fear, anger, frustration, or denial (highly variable due to woman's understanding of the condition itself, past experiences, previous coping mechanisms, and the amount of family and nursing support received). Appropriate medical or surgical interventions depending on the underlying condition.	Provide comfortable environment—dim lighting, music. Encourage partner to participate. Provide pain management to reduce anxiety and stress. Ensure continuous presence of staff to allay anxiety. Provide frequent updates concerning fetal status and progress. Provide ongoing encouragement to minimize the woman's stress and help her to cope with labor and to promote a positive, timely outcome. Assist in relaxation and comfort measures to help her body work more effectively with the forces of labor. Engage the woman in conversation about her emotional well-being; offer anticipatory guidance and reassurance to increase her self-esteem and ability to cope, decrease frustration, and encourage cooperation.

Hypertonic uterine dysfunction occurs when the uterus never fully relaxes between contractions. Subsequently, contractions are erratic and poorly coordinated because more than one uterine pacemaker is sending signals for contraction. Placental perfusion becomes compromised, thereby reducing oxygen to the fetus. These hypertonic contractions exhaust the mother, who is experiencing frequent, intense, and painful contractions with little progression. This dysfunctional pattern occurs in early labor and affects nulliparous women more than multiparous women (Cheng & Caughey, 2007).

Hypotonic uterine dysfunction occurs during active labor (dilation more than 4 cm) when contractions become poor in quality and lack sufficient intensity to dilate and efface the cervix. The major risk with this complication is hemorrhage after giving birth because the uterus cannot contract effectively to compress blood vessels.

Precipitous labor is one that is completed in less than 3 hours. Women experiencing precipitous labor typically have soft perineal tissues that stretch readily, permitting the fetus to pass through the pelvis quickly and easily. Maternal complications are rare if the maternal pelvis is adequate and the soft tissues yield to a fast fetal descent. Potential fetal complications may include head trauma, such as intracranial hemorrhage or nerve damage, and hypoxia due to the rapid progression of labor (Sharf et al., 2007).

▶ PROBLEMS WITH THE PASSENGER

Any presentation other than occiput anterior or a slight variation of the fetal position or size increases the probability of dystocia. These variations can affect the contractions or fetal descent through the maternal pelvis. Common problems involving the fetus include occiput posterior position, breech presentation, multifetal pregnancy, excessive size (macrosomia) as it relates to cephalopelvic disproportion (CPD), and structural anomalies.

Persistent occiput posterior is the most common malposition, occurring in about 15% of laboring women. The reasons for this malposition are often unclear. This position presents slightly larger diameters to the maternal pelvis, thus slowing fetal descent. A fetal head that is poorly flexed may be responsible. In addition, poor uterine contractions may not push the fetal head down into the pelvic floor to the extent that the fetal occiput sinks into it rather than being pushed to rotate in an anterior direction.

Face and brow presentations are rare and are associated with fetal abnormalities (anencephaly), pelvic contractures, high parity, placenta previa, hydramnios, low birthweight, or a large fetus (WHO, 2007).

Breech presentation, which occurs in 3% to 4% of labors, is frequently associated with multifetal pregnancies, grand multiparity (more than five births), advanced maternal age, placenta previa, hydramnios, preterm births, and fetal anomalies such as hydrocephaly (Lee, El-Sayed, & Gould, 2007). In a persistent breech presentation, an increased frequency of prolapsed cord, placenta previa, low birthweight from preterm birth, fetal or uterine anomalies, and perinatal morbidity and mortality from a difficult birth may occur (Cunningham et al., 2005). Perinatal mortality is increased two- to four-fold with a breech presentation, regardless of the mode of delivery (Lee, El-Sayed, & Gould, 2007).

Shoulder dystocia is defined as the obstruction of fetal descent and birth by the axis of the fetal shoulders after the fetal head has been delivered. The incidence of shoulder dystocia is increasing due to increasing birthweight, with reports of it in up to 2% of vaginal births. It is one of the most anxiety-provoking emergencies encountered in labor. Failure of the shoulders to deliver spontaneously places both the woman and the fetus at risk for injury. Postpartum hemorrhage, secondary to uterine atony or vaginal lacerations, is the major complication to the mother. Transient Erb's or Duchenne's brachial plexus palsies and clavicular or humeral fractures are the most common fetal injuries encountered with shoulder dystocia (WHO, 2007). Newborns experiencing shoulder dystocia typically have greater shoulder-to-head and chest-to-head disproportions compared with those delivered without dystocia (Cunningham et al., 2005). Prompt recognition and appropriate management, such as with McRobert's maneuver or suprapubic pressure, can reduce the severity of injuries to the mother and newborn (Fig. 21.1).

▶ **Take** NOTE!

Prompt recognition and appropriate management of shoulder dystocia can reduce the severity of injuries to the mother and infant. Immediately assess the infant for signs of trauma such as a fractured clavicle, Erb's palsy, or neonatal asphyxia. Assess the mother for excessive vaginal bleeding and blood in the urine from bladder trauma.

Multiple gestation refers to twins, triplets, or more infants within a single pregnancy (Box 21.1). The incidence is increasing, primarily as a result of infertility treatment (both ovarian stimulation and in vitro fertilization) and an increased number of women giving birth at older ages (March of Dimes, 2007b). The incidence of twins is approximately 1 in 30 conceptions, with about two thirds of them due to the fertilization of two ova (dizygotic or fraternal) and about one third occurring from the splitting of one fertilized ovum (monozygotic or identical twins). One in approximately 8,100 pregnancies results in triplets (March of Dimes, 2007b). The most

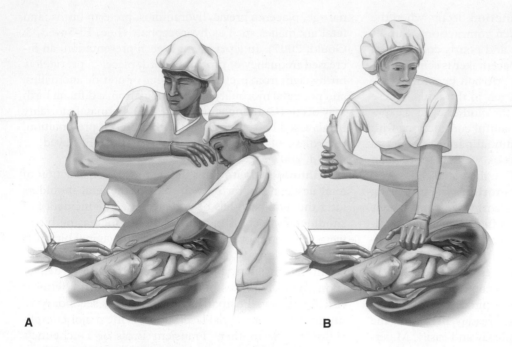

A   **B**

FIGURE 21.1 Maneuvers to relieve shoulder dystocia. (**A**) McRobert's maneuver. The mother's thighs are flexed and abducted as much as possible to straighten the pelvic curve. (**B**) Suprapubic pressure. Pressure is applied just above the pubic bone, pushing the fetal anterior shoulder downward to displace it from above the mother's symphysis pubis. The newborn's head is depressed toward the mother's anus while suprapubic pressure is applied.

BOX 21.1 Multiple Gestation

As the name implies, multiple gestation involves more than one fetus. These fetuses can result from fertilization of a single ovum or multiple ova. Twin pregnancies that are single-ovum conceptions (monozygotic twins) share one chorion (membrane closest to the uterus), and each twin has his or her own amnion (membrane surrounding the amniotic fluid). One fertilized ovum splits into two separate individuals who are said to be natural clones. They have separate amniotic sacs and placentas, are identical in appearance, and are always the same gender. Twin pregnancies that are multiple-ova conceptions (dizygotic twins) result from two ova fertilized by two sperm. Genetically, dizygotic twins are as alike (or unlike) as any other pair or siblings.

The fetuses of a twin gestation, whether monozygotic or dizygotic, are slightly "squashed" because two fetuses develop in a space usually occupied by one. This compression is reflected in the slowing of weight gain in both twins compared to that for singletons (Zach & Pramanik, 2007).

Multiple births other than twins can be of the identical type, the fraternal type, or combinations of the two. Triplets can occur from the division of one zygote into two, with one dividing again, producing identical triplets, or they can come from two zygotes, one dividing into a set of identical twins, and the second zygote developing as a single fraternal sibling, or from three separate zygotes. Triplets are said to occur once in 7,000 births and quadruplets once in 660,000 births (March of Dimes, 2007b). In recent years, fertility drugs used to induce ovulation have resulted in a greater frequency of quadruplets, quintuplets, sextuplets, and even octuplets.

---

common maternal complication is postpartum hemorrhage resulting from uterine atony.

Excessive fetal size and abnormalities can also contribute to labor and birth dysfunctions. **Macrosomia**, in which a newborn weighs 4,000 to 4,500 g (8.13 to 9.15 lb) or more at birth, complicates approximately 10% of all pregnancies (Jazayeri & Contreras, 2007). Fetal abnormalities may include hydrocephalus, ascites, or a large mass on the neck or head. Complications associated with dystocia related to excessive fetal size and anomalies include an increased risk for postpartum hemorrhage, dysfunctional labor, fetopelvic disproportion, soft tissue laceration during vaginal birth, fetal injuries or fractures, and asphyxia (Joy & Lyon, 2007).

▶ PROBLEMS WITH THE PASSAGEWAY

Problems with the passageway (pelvis and birth canal) are related to a contraction of one or more of the three planes of the maternal pelvis: inlet, midpelvis, and outlet. The female pelvis can be classified into four types based on the shape of the pelvic inlet, which is bounded anteriorly by the posterior border of the symphysis pubis, posteriorly by the sacral promontory, and laterally by the linea terminalis. The four basic types are gynecoid, anthropoid, android, and platypelloid (see Chapter 12 for additional information). Contraction of the midpelvis is more common than inlet contraction and typically causes an arrest of fetal descent. Obstructions in the maternal birth canal, such as swelling of the soft maternal tissue and cervix, termed soft tissue dystocia, also can hamper fetal descent and impede labor progression outside the maternal bony pelvis.

▶ PROBLEMS WITH THE PSYCHE

Many women experience an array of emotions during labor, which may include fear, anxiety, helplessness, being alone, and weariness. These emotions can lead to psychological stress, which indirectly can cause dystocia.

Nursing Assessment

Begin the assessment by reviewing the client's history to look for risk factors for dystocia. Include in the assessment the mother's frame of mind to identify fear, anxiety, stress, lack of support, and pain, which can interfere with uterine contractions and impede labor progress. Helping the woman to relax will promote normal labor progress.

Assess the woman's vital signs. Note any elevation in temperature (might suggest an infection) or changes in heart rate or blood pressure (might signal hypovolemia). Evaluate the uterine contractions for frequency and intensity. Question the woman about any changes in her contraction pattern, such as a decrease or increase in frequency or intensity, and report these. Assess fetal heart rate and pattern, reporting any abnormal patterns immediately.

Assess fetal position via Leopold's maneuvers to identify any deviations in presentation or position, and report any deviations. Assist with or perform a vaginal examination to determine cervical dilation, effacement, and engagement of the fetal presenting part. Evaluate for evidence of membrane rupture. Report any malodorous fluid.

Nursing Management

Nursing management of the woman with dystocia, regardless of the etiology, requires patience. The nurse should provide physical and emotional support to the client and her family. The final outcome of any labor depends on the size and shape of the maternal pelvis, the quality of the uterine contractions, and the size, presentation, and position of the fetus. Thus, dystocia is diagnosed not at the start of labor but rather after it has progressed for a time.

Promoting the Progress of Labor
The nurse plays a major role in determining the progress of labor. Continue to assess the woman, frequently monitoring cervical dilation and effacement, uterine contractions, and fetal descent, and document that all assessed parameters are progressing. Evaluate progress in active labor by using the simple rule of 1 cm/hour for cervical dilation. When the woman's membranes rupture, if they have not already ruptured, observe for visible cord prolapse.

> ▶ *Take NOTE!*
>
> *If a dysfunctional labor occurs, contractions will slow or fail to advance in frequency, duration, or intensity; the cervix will fail to respond to uterine contractions by dilating and effacing; and the fetus will fail to descend.*

Throughout labor, assess the woman's fluid balance status. Check skin turgor and mucous membranes. Monitor intake and output. Also monitor the client's bladder for distention at least every 2 hours and encourage her to empty her bladder often. In addition, monitor her bowel status. A full bladder or rectum can impede descent.

Continue to monitor fetal well-being. If the fetus is in the breech position, be especially observant for visible cord prolapse and note any variable decelerations in heart rate. If either occurs, report it immediately.

Be prepared to administer a labor stimulant such as oxytocin (Pitocin) if ordered to treat hypotonic labor contractions. Anticipate the need to assist with manipulations if shoulder dystocia is diagnosed. Prepare the woman and her family for the possibility of a cesarean birth if labor does not progress.

Providing Physical and Emotional Comfort
Employ physical comfort measures to promote relaxation and reduce stress. Offer blankets for warmth and a backrub, if the client wishes, to reduce muscle tension. Provide an environment conducive to rest so the woman can conserve her energy. Lower the lights and reduce external noise by closing the hallway door. Offer a warm shower to promote relaxation (if not contraindicated). Use pillows to support the woman in a comfortable position, changing her position every 30 minutes to reduce tension and to enhance uterine activity and efficiency. Offer her fluids/food as appropriate to moisten her mouth and replenish her energy (Fig. 21.2).

Assist with providing counterpressure along with backrubs if the fetus is in the occiput posterior position. Encourage the woman to assume different positions to promote fetal rotation. Upright positions are helpful in facilitating fetal rotation and descent. Also encourage the woman to visualize the descent and birth of the fetus.

Assess the woman's level of pain and degree of distress. Administer analgesics as ordered or according to the facility's protocol.

Evaluate the mother's level of fatigue throughout labor, such as verbal expressions of feeling exhausted, inability to cope in early labor, or inability to rest or calm down between contractions. Praise the woman and her partner for their efforts. Provide empathetic listening to increase the client's coping ability, and remain with the client to demonstrate caring.

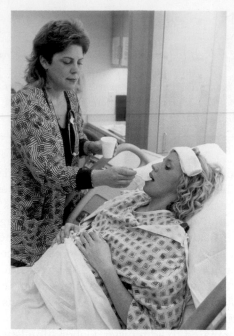

FIGURE 21.2 The nurse applies a cool, moist washcloth to the client's forehead and offers her ice chips to combat thirst and provide comfort for the woman experiencing dystocia.

Promoting Empowerment

Educate the client and family about dysfunctional labor and its causes and therapies. Explain therapeutic interventions that may be needed to assist with the labor process. Encourage the client and her partner to participate in decision making about interventions.

Assist the woman and partner in expressing their fears and anxieties. Provide encouragement to help them to maintain control. Support the client and her partner in their coping efforts. Keep the woman and her partner informed of progress and advocate for them.

Preterm Labor

Preterm labor is defined as the occurrence of regular uterine contractions accompanied by cervical effacement and dilation before the end of the 37th week of gestation. If not halted, it leads to preterm birth.

Preterm births remain one of the biggest contributors to perinatal morbidity and mortality in the world. According to the March of Dimes (2007c, 2007d, 2007e), about 12% of births (one in eight infants) in the United States are premature.

Preterm birth is one of the most common obstetric complications, and its sequelae have a profound effect on the survival and health of the newborn. The rate of preterm births in the United States has increased 35% in the past 20 years. Preterm births account for 75% of neurodevelopmental disorders and other serious morbidities,

as well as behavioral and social problems. They account for 85% of all perinatal morbidity and mortality. In addition, up to $30 billion is spent on maternal and infant care related to prematurity (March of Dimes, 2007c). Infants born prematurely also are at risk for serious sequelae such as respiratory distress syndrome, infections, congenital heart defects, thermoregulation problems that can lead to acidosis and weight loss, intraventricular hemorrhage, feeding difficulties resulting from diminished stomach capacity and an underdeveloped suck reflex, and neurologic disorders related to hypoxia and trauma at birth (Gray, 2006). Although great strides have been made in neonatal intensive care, prematurity remains the leading cause of death within the first month of life and is the second leading cause of all infant deaths (March of Dimes, 2007c).

The exact cause of preterm labor is not known. Currently, prevention is the goal.

Therapeutic Management

Predicting the risk of preterm labor is valuable only if there is an available intervention that is likely to improve the situation. According to ACOG, many factors must be considered before selecting an intervention. Many factors influence the decision to intervene when women present with symptoms of preterm labor, including the probability of progressive labor, gestational age, and the risks of treatment. ACOG (2003b) recommends the following as guidelines:

- There are no clear first-line **tocolytic** drugs (drugs that promote uterine relaxation by interfering with uterine contractions) to manage preterm labor. Clinical circumstances and the health care provider's preference should dictate treatment.
- Antibiotics do not appear to prolong gestation and should be reserved for group B streptococcal prophylaxis in women in whom birth is imminent.
- Tocolytic drugs may prolong pregnancy for 2 to 7 days; during this time, steroids can be given to improve fetal lung maturity and the woman can be transported to a tertiary care center.

Despite these recommendations, health care providers continue to prescribe pharmacologic treatment for preterm labor at home and in the hospital setting. This treatment often includes oral or intravenous tocolytics and varying degrees of activity restriction (Fig. 21.3). Antibiotics may also be prescribed to treat presumed or confirmed infections. Steroids may be given to enhance fetal lung maturity between 24 weeks and 34 weeks' gestation.

Tocolytic Therapy

The decision to stop preterm labor is individualized based on risk factors, extent of cervical dilation, membrane status, fetal gestational age, and presence or absence of infection. Tocolytic therapy is most likely ordered if preterm

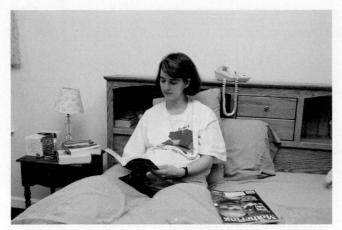

FIGURE 21.3 The mother with preterm labor resting in bed at home.

labor occurs before the 34th week of gestation in an attempt to delay birth and thereby to reduce the severity of respiratory distress syndrome and other complications associated with prematurity. Tocolytic therapy does not typically prevent preterm birth, but it may delay it. It is contraindicated for abruptio placentae, acute fetal distress or death, eclampsia or severe preeclampsia, active vaginal bleeding, dilation of more than 6 cm, chorioamnionitis, and maternal hemodynamic instability (Griffin, 2007).

Medications most commonly used for tocolysis include magnesium sulfate (which reduces the muscle's ability to contract), terbutaline (Brethine, a beta-adrenergic), indomethacin (Indocin, a prostaglandin synthetase inhibitor), and nifedipine (Procardia, a calcium channel blocker). These drugs are used "off label": this means they are effective for this purpose but have not been officially tested and developed for this purpose by the FDA (Tan et al., 2006). All these medications have serious side effects, and the woman needs close supervision when they are being administered (Drug Guide 21.1).

Corticosteroids

Corticosteroids given to the mother in preterm labor can help prevent or reduce the frequency and severity of respiratory distress syndrome in premature infants delivered between 24 weeks and 34 weeks' gestation. The beneficial effects of corticosteroids on fetal lung maturation have been reported within 48 hours of initial administration (Blackburn, 2007). These drugs require at least 24 hours to become effective, so timely administration is crucial.

Nursing Assessment

The preterm birth rate cannot be reduced until there are ways to predict the risk for preterm birth. Because the etiology is often multifactorial, an individualized approach is needed.

Health History and Physical Examination

The signs of preterm labor are subtle and may be overlooked by the client as well as the health care professional. Obtain a thorough health history and be alert for risk factors associated with preterm labor and birth (Box 21.2).

Frequently, women are unaware that uterine contractions, effacement, and dilation are occurring, thus making early intervention ineffective in arresting preterm labor and preventing the birth of a premature newborn. Ask the woman about any complaints, being alert for the subtle symptoms of preterm labor, which may include:

- Change or increase in vaginal discharge
- Pelvic pressure (pushing-down sensation)
- Low, dull backache
- Menstrual-like cramps
- Heaviness or aching in the thighs
- Uterine contractions, with or without pain
- Intestinal cramping, with or without diarrhea (Gilbert, 2007; Gray, 2006)

Assess the pattern of the contractions: the contractions must be persistent, such that four contractions occur every 20 minutes or eight contractions occur in 1 hour. Evaluate cervical dilation and effacement: cervical effacement is 80% or greater and cervical dilation is greater than 1 cm (AAP & ACOG, 2003). On examination, engagement of the fetal presenting part will be noted.

Laboratory and Diagnostic Testing

Commonly used diagnostic testing for preterm labor risk assessment includes a complete blood count to detect infection, which may be a contributing factor to preterm labor; urinalysis to detect bacteria and nitrites, which are indicative of a urinary tract infection; and an amniotic fluid analysis to determine fetal lung maturity and the presence of subclinical chorioamnionitis.

Four other tests may be used for preterm labor prediction: fetal fibronectin testing, cervical length evaluation by transvaginal ultrasound, salivary estriol, and home monitoring of uterine activity to recognize preterm contractions. Fetal fibronectin and cervical length examinations have a high negative predictive value and are thus better at predicting which pregnant women are unlikely to have a preterm birth as opposed to predicting those who will (Grimes-Dennis & Berghella, 2007).

Fetal Fibronectin

Fetal fibronectin, a glycoprotein produced by the chorion, is found at the junction of the chorion and decidua (fetal membranes and uterus). It is present in cervicovaginal fluid prior to delivery, regardless of gestational age. It is not found in vaginal secretions unless there has been a disruption between the chorion and decidua. The test is a useful marker for impending membrane rupture within 7 to 14 days if the level increases to greater than 0.05 ug/mL. Conversely, if fetal fibronectin is not present, there is a

DRUG GUIDE 21.1 MEDICATIONS USED WITH PRETERM LABOR

Drug	Action/Indication	Nursing Implications
Magnesium sulfate	Relaxes uterine muscles to stop irritability and contractions, to arrest uterine contractions for preterm labor (off-label use). Has been used in seizure prophylaxis and treatment of seizures in preeclamptic and eclamptic patients for almost 100 years (Lilley, Harrington, & Snyder, 2007).	Administer IV with a loading dose of 4–6 g over 15–30 minutes initially, and then maintain infusion at 1–4 g per hour. Assess vital signs and deep tendon reflexes (DTRs) hourly; report any hypotension or depressed or absent DTRs. Monitor level of consciousness; report any headache, blurred vision, dizziness, or altered level of consciousness. Perform continuous electronic fetal monitoring; report any decreased fetal heart rate variability, hypotonia, or respiratory depression. Monitor intake and output hourly; report any decrease in output (<30 mL/hour). Assess respiratory rate; report respiratory rate <12 breaths/minute; auscultate lung sounds for evidence of pulmonary edema. Monitor for common maternal side effects, including flushing, nausea and vomiting, dry mouth, lethargy, blurred vision, and headache. Assess for nausea, vomiting, transient hypotension, lethargy. Assess for signs and symptoms of magnesium toxicity, such as decreased level of consciousness, depressed respirations and DTRs, slurred speech, weakness, and respiratory and/or cardiac arrest. Have calcium gluconate readily available at the bedside to reverse magnesium toxicity.
Terbutaline sulfate (Brethine)	Relaxes smooth muscles to calm uterus, inhibits uterine activity to arrest preterm labor	This drug is usually effective in delaying birth for up to 48 hours (Tan et al., 2006). Monitor the mother for adverse effects such as tachycardia, hypotension, palpitations, tremors, chest pain, hypokalemia, water retention, nausea, vomiting, diarrhea, hyperglycemia, decreased urinary output, and nervousness. Monitor fetal well-being, noting any adverse effects such as tachycardia or heart failure. Adverse effects are dose-related and will increase as dose is increased. Perform cardiac assessment of woman to rule out preexisting cardiac disease and diabetes. Institute continuous fetal monitoring. Assess vital signs frequently for changes. Discontinue drug for the following: maternal tachycardia >120 bpm, hypotension <90/60 mmHg, fetal heart rate >180 bpm, signs of maternal pulmonary edema. Have propranolol (Inderal) available to reverse cardiac adverse effects.
Indomethacin (Indocin)	Inhibits prostaglandins, which stimulate contractions; inhibits uterine activity to arrest preterm labor	Continuously assess vital signs, uterine activity, and fetal heart rate. Administer oral form with food to reduce GI irritation.

Drug	Action/Indication	Nursing Implications
		Do not give to women with peptic ulcer disease. Schedule ultrasound to assess amniotic fluid volume and function of ductus arteriosus before initiating therapy; monitor for signs of maternal hemorrhage. Be alert for maternal adverse effects such as nausea, vomiting, heartburn, rash, prolonged bleeding time, oligohydramnios, and hypertension. Monitor for neonatal adverse effects, including constriction of ductus arteriosus, premature ductus closure, necrotizing enterocolitis, oligohydramnios, and pulmonary hypertension.
Nifedipine (Procardia)	Blocks calcium movement into muscle cells, inhibits uterine activity to arrest preterm labor	Use caution if giving this drug with magnesium sulfate because of increased risk for hypotension. Monitor blood pressure hourly if giving with magnesium sulfate; report a pulse rate >110 bpm. Monitor for fetal effects such as decreased uteroplacental blood flow manifested by fetal bradycardia, which can lead to fetal hypoxia. Monitor for adverse effects, such as flushing of the skin, headache, transient tachycardia, palpitations, postural hypertension, peripheral edema, and transient fetal tachycardia.
Betamethasone (Celestone)	Promotes fetal lung maturity by stimulating surfactant production, prevents or reduces risk of respiratory distress syndrome and intraventricular hemorrhage in the preterm neonate less than 34 weeks' gestation	Administer two doses intramuscularly 24 hours apart. Monitor for maternal infection or pulmonary edema. Educate parents about potential benefits of drug to preterm infant. Assess maternal lung sounds and monitor for signs of infection.

98% chance that the woman will not go into preterm labor (Incerti et al., 2007).

A sterile applicator is used to collect a cervicovaginal sample during a speculum examination. The result is either positive (fetal fibronectin is present) or negative (fetal fibronectin is not present). Interpretation of fetal fibronectin results must always be viewed in conjunction with the clinical findings; it is not used as a lone indicator for predicting preterm labor.

Transvaginal Ultrasound

Transvaginal ultrasound of the cervix has been used as a tool to predict preterm labor in high-risk pregnancies and to differentiate between true and false preterm labor. Three parameters are evaluated during the transvaginal ultrasound: cervical length and width, funnel width and length, and percentage of funneling. Measurement of the closed portion of the cervix visualized during the transvaginal ultrasound is the single most reliable parameter

for prediction of preterm delivery in high-risk women (Blackburn, 2007).

Cervical length varies during pregnancy and can be measured fairly reliably after 16 weeks' gestation using an ultrasound probe inserted in the vagina. A cervical length of 3 cm or more indicates that delivery within 14 days is unlikely. Women with a short cervical length of 2.5 cm during the mid-trimester have a substantially greater risk of preterm birth prior to 35 weeks' gestation. As with fetal fibronectin testing, negative results can be reassuring and prevent unnecessary interventions (Grimes-Dennis & Berghella, 2007).

Home Uterine Activity Monitoring

Home monitoring of uterine activity can identify women in preterm labor at an early stage to reduce the rate of preterm birth (Gilbert, 2007). Home uterine activity monitoring does not prevent preterm labor or birth; rather, it provides supplemental client education and

BOX 21.2 **Risk Factors Associated With Preterm Labor and Birth**

- African-American race (double the risk)
- Maternal age extremes less than 16 years and more than 40 years old
- Low socioeconomic status
- Alcohol or other drug use, especially cocaine
- Poor maternal nutrition
- Maternal periodontal disease
- Cigarette smoking
- Low level of education
- History of prior preterm birth (triples the risk)
- Uterine abnormalities, such as fibroids
- Low pregnancy weight for height
- Preexisting diabetes or hypertension
- Multiple gestation
- PROM
- Late or no prenatal care
- Short cervical length
- STIs: gonorrhea, *Chlamydia,* trichomoniasis
- Bacterial vaginosis (50% increased risk) (Pretorius et al., 2007)
- Chorioamnionitis
- Hydramnios
- Gestational hypertension
- Cervical insufficiency
- Short interpregnancy interval: less than 1 year between births
- Placental problems, such as placenta previa and abruption placenta
- Maternal anemia
- UTI
- Domestic violence
- Stress, acute and chronic (March of Dimes, 2007c)

clinical data for the health care provider in an effort to prolong gestation and maximize pregnancy outcomes through timely clinical interventions. It involves client education, daily client assessment, data collection, and data interpretation (Gray, 2007).

The woman is asked to wear an ambulatory tocodynamometer and transmit data to the nurse or health care provider daily via telephone lines. Uterine and fetal activity data are transmitted to perinatal nurses who are available around the clock for detection of uterine contractions, in addition to picking up the fetal heart rate. Women are also asked to record uterine activity (uterine pressure, back pain, or cramps) they experience for an hour twice a day and then speak to a perinatal nurse, who analyzes the results.

If the number of contractions exceeds a predetermined threshold, the woman drinks 8 to 12 oz of water, rests, empties her bladder, and then repeats uterine monitoring. The effectiveness of this type of screening remains controversial (Morrison & Chauhan, 2003).

Nursing Management

Nurses play a key role in reducing preterm labor and births to improve pregnancy outcomes for both mothers and their infants. Early detection of preterm labor is currently the best strategy to improve outcomes. Because of the numerous factors associated with preterm labor, it is challenging to identify and address all of them, especially when women experiencing contractions are frequently falsely reassured and not assessed thoroughly to determine the cause. This delay impedes initiation of interventions to reduce infant death and morbidity.

Preterm birth prevention programs for women at high risk have used self-monitoring of symptoms and patterns, weekly cervical examinations, telephone monitoring, home visiting, and home uterine activity monitoring, alone or in combination, with mixed results (Gray, 2006).

Nursing management of the woman with preterm labor involves administering tocolytic therapy if indicated, thoroughly educating the client, and providing psychological support during the process.

Administering Tocolytic Therapy

A firm diagnosis of preterm labor is necessary before treatment is considered. Diagnosis requires the presence of both uterine contractions and cervical change (or an initial cervical examination of more than 2 cm and/or more than 80% effacement in a nulliparous client). A cause for preterm labor should always be sought. Absolute contraindications to tocolytic agents include intrauterine infection, fetal distress, vaginal bleeding, prolonged premature rupture of the membranes, and intrauterine demise (Norwitz & Schorge, 2006). Bed rest and hydration are commonly recommended, but without proven efficacy.

Short-term pharmacologic therapy remains the cornerstone of management. However, there are no studies to suggest that any tocolytic agent can delay birth for longer than 48 hours (Stein, 2007). No single agent has a clear therapeutic advantage.

Magnesium sulfate may be ordered. This agent acts as a physiologic calcium antagonist and a general inhibitor of neurotransmission. Expect to administer it intravenously. Monitor the woman for nausea, vomiting, headache, weakness, hypotension, and cardiopulmonary arrest. Assess the fetus for decreased fetal heart rate variability, drowsiness, and hypotonia. Magnesium has a wide margin of safety and is commonly used as a first choice.

Although calcium channel blockers may be prescribed to manage preterm labor, available literature provides little evidence that they have better efficacy in treating preterm labor than magnesium sulfate (ACOG, 2003b). Administer calcium channel blockers (nifedipine) orally or sublingually every 4 to 8 hours as ordered. Monitor the woman for hypotension, reflex tachycardia, headache, nausea, and facial flushing.

If beta-adrenergic agonists (terbutaline) are ordered, expect to administer the agent intravenously during the initial period and then switch to the oral route for maintenance therapy. Closely assess the woman for side effects, including jitteriness, anxiety, restlessness, nausea, and tachycardia. Assess the fetus for tachycardia, hypotension, and hypoglycemia.

Supportive nursing care is needed for the woman in preterm labor whether the contractions are stopped with tocolytic therapy or not. Nursing tasks include monitoring vital signs, measuring intake and output, encouraging bed rest on the woman's left side to enhance placental perfusion, monitoring the fetal heart rate via an external monitor continuously, limiting vaginal examinations to prevent an ascending infection, and monitoring the mother and fetus closely for any adverse effects from the tocolytic agents. Offering the couple ongoing explanations will help prepare them for the birth.

Educating the Client

Ensure that every pregnant woman receives basic education about preterm labor, including information about harmful lifestyles, the signs of genitourinary infections and preterm labor, and the appropriate response to these symptoms. Teach the client how to palpate for and time uterine contractions. Provide written materials to support this education at a level and in a language appropriate for the client. Also educate clients about the importance of prenatal care, risk reduction, and recognizing the signs and symptoms of preterm labor. Teaching Guidelines 21.1 highlights important instructions related to preventing preterm labor.

Explaining to the couple what is happening in terms of labor progress, the treatment regimen, and the status of the fetus is important to reduce the anxiety associated with the risk of giving birth to a preterm infant. Educate them about the importance of promotion of fetal lung maturity with corticosteroids. Include supportive family members in all education. Allow time for the woman and her family to express their concerns about the possible outcome for the infant and the possible side effects of the tocolytic therapy. Encourage them to vent any feelings, fears, and anger they may experience. Provide the woman and her family with an honest appraisal of the situation and plan of treatment throughout her care.

Providing Psychological Support

Preterm labor and birth present multifactorial challenges for everyone involved. If the woman's activities are restricted, additional stresses may be placed on the family, contributing to the crisis. Assess the stress levels of the client and family, and make appropriate referrals. Emphasize the need for more frequent supervision and office visits, and encourage clients to talk to their health care provider for reassurance.

Every case of spontaneous preterm labor is unique. Care must take into account the clinical circumstances, and the full and informed consent of the woman and her

TEACHING GUIDELINES 21.1

Teaching to Prevent Preterm Labor

- Avoid traveling for long distances in cars, trains, planes, or buses.
- Avoid lifting heavy objects, such as laundry, groceries, or a young child.
- Avoid performing hard, physical work, such as yard work, moving of furniture, or construction.
- Visit a dentist in early pregnancy to evaluate and treat periodontal disease.
- Enroll in a smoking cessation program if you are unable to quit on your own.
- Curtail sexual activity until after 37 weeks if experiencing preterm labor symptoms.
- Consume a well-balanced nutritional diet to gain appropriate weight.
- Avoid the use of substances such as marijuana, cocaine, and heroin.
- Identify factors and areas of stress in your life, and use stress management techniques to reduce them.
- If you are experiencing intimate partner violence, seek resources to modify the situation.

Recognize the signs and symptoms of preterm labor and notify your birth attendant if any occur:

- Uterine contractions, cramping, or low back pain
- Feeling of pelvic pressure or fullness
- Increase in vaginal discharge
- Nausea, vomiting, and diarrhea
- Leaking of fluid from vagina

If you are experiencing any of these signs or symptoms, do the following:

- Stop what you are doing and rest for 1 hour.
- Empty your bladder.
- Lie down on your side.
- Drink two to three glasses of water.
- Feel your abdomen and make note of the hardness of the contraction. Call your health care provider and describe the contraction as
  - Mild if it feels like the tip of the nose
  - Moderate if it feels like the tip of the chin
  - Strong if it feels like your forehead (Simhan & Caritis, 2007)

partner is needed. Half of all women who ultimately give birth prematurely have no identifiable risk factors. Nurses should be sensitive to any complaint and should provide appropriate assessment, information, and follow-up. Sensitivity to the subtle differences between normal pregnancy sensations and the prodromal symptoms of preterm labor is a key factor in ensuring timely care. Offer clarification and validation of the woman's symptoms.

If tocolytic therapy isn't successful in stopping uterine contractions, support the couple through this stressful period to prepare them for the birth. Keep them informed of all progress and changes; for example, continuously monitor maternal and fetal vital signs, especially the maternal temperature to detect signs of early infection. Offer one-on-one contact and be available throughout this difficult and anxiety-producing period.

Postterm Labor

A term pregnancy usually lasts 38 to 42 weeks. A **postterm pregnancy** is one that continues past the end of the 42nd week of gestation, or 294 days from the first day of the last menstrual period. Postterm pregnancies account for about 3% to 12% of births (Butler & Wilkes, 2007). Incorrect dates account for the majority of these cases: many women have irregular menses and thus cannot identify the date of their last menstrual period accurately.

*R**ecall Jennifer described at the beginning of the chapter, who was at 41 weeks' gestation. What information would be most important to determine on admission to the facility? What interventions might the nurse anticipate when she arrives?*

The exact etiology of a postterm pregnancy is unknown because the mechanism for the initiation of labor is not completely understood. Theories suggest there may be a deficiency of estrogen and continued secretion of progesterone that prohibits the uterus from contracting, but no evidence has validated this. A woman who has one postterm pregnancy is at greater risk for another in subsequent pregnancies.

Postterm pregnancies may adversely affect both the mother and fetus or newborn. Maternal risk is related to the large size of the fetus at birth, which increases the chances that a cesarean birth will be needed. Other issues might include dystocia, birth trauma, postpartum hemorrhage, and infection. Mechanical or artificial interventions such as forceps or vacuum-assisted birth and labor induction with oxytocin may be necessary. In addition, maternal exhaustion and feelings of despair over this prolonged gestation can add to the woman's anxiety level and reduce her coping ability.

Fetal risks associated with a postterm pregnancy include macrosomia, shoulder dystocia, brachial plexus injuries, and cephalopelvic disproportion. All of these conditions predispose this fetus to birth trauma or a surgical birth. The perinatal mortality rate at more than 42 weeks of gestation is twice that at term and increases six-fold and higher at 43 weeks of gestation and beyond. Uteroplacental insufficiency, meconium aspiration, and intrauterine infection contribute to the increased rate of perinatal deaths (Heimstad et al., 2006). As the placenta ages, its

perfusion decreases and it becomes less efficient at delivering oxygen and nutrients to the fetus. Amniotic fluid volume also begins to decline by 40 weeks of gestation, possibly leading to oligohydramnios, subsequently resulting in fetal hypoxia and an increased risk of cord compression because the cushioning effect offered by adequate fluid is no longer present. Hypoxia and oligohydramnios predispose the fetus to aspiration of meconium, which is released by the fetus in response to a hypoxic insult (Gümezoglu, Crowther, & Middleton, 2006). All of these issues can compromise fetal well-being and lead to fetal distress.

Nursing Assessment

Obtain a thorough history to determine the estimated date of birth. Many women are unsure of the date of their last menstrual period, so the date given may be unreliable. Despite numerous methods used to date pregnancies, many are still misdated. Accurate gestational dating via ultrasound is essential.

Antepartum assessment for a postterm pregnancy typically includes daily fetal movement counts done by the woman, nonstress tests done twice weekly, amniotic fluid assessments as part of the biophysical profile, and weekly cervical examinations to evaluate for ripening. In addition, assess the following:

• Client's understanding of the various fetal well-being tests
• Client's stress and anxiety concerning her lateness
• Client's coping ability and support network

Nursing Management

Once the dates are established and postdate status is confirmed, monitoring fetal well-being becomes critical. When determining the plan of care for a woman with a postterm pregnancy, the first decision is whether to deliver the baby or wait. If the decision is to wait, then fetal surveillance is key. If the decision is to have the woman deliver, labor induction is initiated. Both decisions remain controversial, and there is no clear answer about which option is more appropriate. Therefore, the plan must be individualized.

*T**hink back to Jennifer, who is scheduled for labor induction. What ongoing nursing assessments would be important when providing care for her?*

Providing Support

The intense surveillance is time-consuming and intrusive, adding to the anxiety and worry already being experienced by the woman about her overdue status. Be alert to the woman's anxiety and allow her to discuss her feelings. Provide reassurance about the expected time range for birth

EVIDENCE-BASED PRACTICE 21.1
Labor Induction and Outcomes for Women Beyond Term

● **Study**

Postterm pregnancies may adversely affect both the mother and fetus or newborn. Placental perfusion decreases as the placenta ages and becomes less efficient at delivering oxygen and nutrients to the fetus. Amniotic fluid volume also begins to decline by 40 weeks of gestation, increasing the fetus's risk for oligohydramnios, meconium aspiration, and cord compression. However, questions arise: What is the best time for inducing labor in a postterm pregnancy? Does labor induction improve maternal and fetal outcomes, or would it be better to wait for spontaneous labor to begin? A study was conducted to compare the effects of inducing labor in women at or beyond term with those of waiting for spontaneous labor to begin. A search was conducted for randomized controlled trials that compared labor induction with waiting for spontaneous labor to begin in women who were at term or postterm. Two review authors collected the data and analyzed the trials. A total of 19 trials involving almost 8,000 women were evaluated.

▲ **Findings**

Based on the trials analyzed, fewer perinatal deaths occurred in women who underwent labor induction at 41 completed weeks of gestation or later. Fewer newborns experienced meconium aspiration syndrome with induction at 41 weeks or more. Women at 37 to 40 weeks' gestation who received expectant management were more likely to undergo a cesarean birth compared to those in the same gestational week range who received induction. Statistical analysis, however, showed that these differences were not significant.

■ **Nursing Implications**

Although the study did not reveal results that were statistically significant, nurses need to be aware of the potential benefits and limitations associated with labor induction so that they can provide women and their families with the most appropriate information about options for a postterm pregnancy. Nurses can integrate information from this study in their teaching about the risks associated with postterm pregnancy. They can also use this information to help answer the couple's questions about induction and its effectiveness as well as provide anticipatory guidance about the procedure. Doing so fosters empowerment of the woman and her family, promoting optimal informed decision making.

Gülmezoglu, A. M., Crowther, C. A., & Middleton, P. (2006). Induction of labour for improving birth outcomes for women at or beyond term. *Cochrane Database of Systematic Reviews* 2006. Issue 4. Art. No.: CD004945.DOI:10.1002/14651858.CD004945.pub2.

and the well-being of the fetus based on the assessment tests. Validating the woman's stressful state due to the prolonged pregnancy provides an opportunity for her to verbalize her feelings openly.

Educating the Woman and Her Partner

Teach the woman and her partner about the testing required and the reasons for each test. Also describe the methods that may be used for cervical ripening if indicated. Explain about the possibility of induction if the woman's labor isn't spontaneous or if a dysfunctional labor pattern occurs. Also prepare the woman for the possibility of a surgical delivery if fetal distress occurs.

Providing Care During the Intrapartum Period

During the intrapartum period, continuously assess and monitor fetal heart rate (FHR) to identify potential fetal distress early (e.g., late or variable decelerations) so that interventions can be initiated. Also monitor the woman's hydration status to ensure maximal placental perfusion. When the membranes rupture, assess amniotic fluid characteristics (color, amount, and odor) to identify previous fetal hypoxia and prepare for prevention of meconium aspiration. Report meconium-stained amniotic fluid imme-

diately when the membranes rupture. Anticipate the need for amnioinfusion to minimize the risk of meconium aspiration by diluting the meconium in the amniotic fluid expelled by the hypoxic fetus. In addition, monitor the woman's labor pattern closely because dysfunctional patterns are common (Gilbert, 2007).

Encourage the woman to verbalize her feelings and concerns, and answer all her questions. Provide support, presence, information, and encouragement throughout this time.

Women Requiring Labor Induction and Augmentation

Ideally, all pregnancies go to term, with labor beginning spontaneously. However, many women need help to initiate or sustain the labor process. **Labor induction** involves the stimulation of uterine contractions by medical or surgical means to produce delivery before the onset of spontaneous labor. The labor induction rate is at an all-time high in the United States. The widespread use of artificial induction of labor for convenience has contributed to the recent increase in the number of cesarean births.

Evidence is compelling that elective induction of labor significantly increases the risk of cesarean birth, instrumented delivery, use of epidural analgesia, and neonatal intensive care unit admission, especially for nulliparous women (Crane, 2006).

Labor induction is not an isolated event: it brings about a cascade of other interventions that may or may not produce a favorable outcome. Labor induction also involves intravenous therapy, bed rest, continuous electronic fetal monitoring, significant discomfort from stimulating uterine contractions, epidural analgesia/anesthesia, and a prolonged stay on the labor unit (Wing, 2006).

Labor augmentation enhances ineffective contractions after labor has begun. Continuous electronic FHR monitoring is necessary.

There are multiple medical and obstetric reasons for inducing labor, the most common being postterm gestation. Other indications for inductions include prolonged premature rupture of membranes, gestational hypertension, renal disease, chorioamnionitis, dystocia, intrauterine fetal demise, isoimmunization, and diabetes (Bueno et al., 2007). Contraindications to labor induction include complete placenta previa, abruptio placentae, transverse fetal lie, prolapsed umbilical cord, a prior classic uterine incision that entered the uterine cavity, pelvic structure abnormality, previous myomectomy, vaginal bleeding with unknown cause, invasive cervical cancer, active genital herpes infection, and abnormal FHR patterns (ACOG, 2004b). In general, labor induction is indicated when the benefits of birth outweigh the risks to the mother or fetus for continuing the pregnancy. However, the balance between risk and benefit remains controversial.

> ▶ *Take* NOTE!
>
> *Before labor induction is started, fetal maturity (dating, ultrasound, amniotic fluid studies) and cervical readiness (vaginal examination, Bishop scoring) must be assessed. Both need to be favorable for a successful induction.*

Therapeutic Management

The decision to induce labor is based on a thorough evaluation of maternal and fetal status. Typically, this includes an ultrasound to evaluate fetal size, position, and gestational age and to locate the placenta; pelvimetry to rule out fetopelvic disproportion; a nonstress test to evaluate fetal well-being; a phosphatidylglycerol (PG) level to assess fetal lung maturity; Nitrazine paper and/or fern test to confirm ruptured membranes; complete blood count and urinalysis to rule out infection; and a vaginal examination to evaluate the cervix for inducibility (ACOG, 2004). Accurate dating of the pregnancy also is essential before cervical ripening and induction are initiated to prevent a preterm birth.

Cervical Ripening

There has been increasing awareness that if the cervix is unfavorable or unripe, a successful vaginal birth is unlikely. Cervical ripeness is an important variable when labor induction is being considered. A ripe cervix is shortened, centered (anterior), softened, and partially dilated. An unripe cervix is long, closed, posterior, and firm. Cervical ripening usually begins prior to the onset of labor contractions and is necessary for cervical dilatation and the passage of the fetus.

Various scoring systems to assess cervical ripeness have been introduced, but the Bishop score is most commonly used today. The Bishop score helps identify women who would be most likely to achieve a successful induction (Table 21.2). The duration of labor is inversely correlated with the Bishop score: a score over 8 indicates a successful vaginal birth. Bishop scores of less than 6 usually indicate that a cervical ripening method should be used prior to induction (Rai & Schreiber, 2007).

Nonpharmacologic Methods
Nonpharmacologic methods for cervical ripening are less frequently used today, but nurses need to be aware of them and question clients about their use. Methods may include herbal agents such as evening primrose oil, black haw, black and blue cohosh, and red raspberry leaves. In

TABLE 21.2 **BISHOP SCORING SYSTEM**

Score	Dilation (cm)	Effacement (%)	Station	Cervical Consistency	Position of Cervix
0	Closed	0–30%	–3	Firm	Posterior
1	1–2 cm	40–50%	–2	Medium	Midposition
2	3–4 cm	60–70%	–1 or 0	Soft	Anterior
3	5–6 cm	80%	+1 or +2	Very soft	Anterior

Modified from Bishop, E. H. (1964). Pelvic scoring for elective induction. *Obstetrics & Gynecology, 24*(2), 267.

addition, castor oil, hot baths, and enemas are used for cervical ripening and labor induction. The risks and benefits of these agents are unknown.

Another nonpharmacologic method suggested for labor induction is sexual intercourse along with breast stimulation. This promotes the release of oxytocin, which stimulates uterine contractions. In addition, human semen is a biological source of prostaglandins used for cervical ripening. According to a Cochrane Review, sexual intercourse with breast stimulation would appear beneficial, but safety issues have not been fully evaluated, nor can this activity be standardized (Kavanagh, Kelly, & Thomas, 2007). Therefore, its use as a method for labor induction is not validated by research.

Mechanical Methods

Mechanical methods are used to open the cervix and stimulate the progression of labor. All share a similar mechanism of action—application of local pressure stimulates the release of prostaglandins to ripen the cervix. Potential advantages of mechanical methods, compared with pharmacologic methods, may include simplicity or preservation of the cervical tissue or structure, lower cost, and fewer side effects. The risks associated with these methods include infection, bleeding, membrane rupture, and placental disruption (Boulvain et al., 2007).

For example, an indwelling (Foley) catheter (e.g., 26 French) can be inserted into the endocervical canal to ripen and dilate the cervix. The catheter is placed in the uterus, and the balloon is filled. Direct pressure is then applied to the lower segment of the uterus and the cervix. This direct pressure causes stress in the lower uterine segment and probably the local production of prostaglandins (Rai & Schreiber, 2007).

Hygroscopic dilators absorb endocervical and local tissue fluids; as they enlarge, they expand the endocervix and provide controlled mechanical pressure. The products available include natural osmotic dilators (laminaria, a type of dried seaweed) and synthetic dilators containing magnesium sulfate (Lamicel, Dilapan). Hygroscopic dilators are advantageous because they can be inserted on an outpatient basis and no fetal monitoring is needed. As many dilators are inserted in the cervix as will fit, and they expand over 12 to 24 hours as they absorb water. Absorption of water leads to expansion of the dilators and opening of the cervix. They are a reliable alternative when prostaglandins are contraindicated or unavailable (Gelber, 2006).

Surgical Methods

Surgical methods used to ripen the cervix and induce labor include stripping of the membranes and performing an amniotomy. Stripping of the membranes is accomplished by inserting a finger through the internal cervical os and moving it in a circular direction. This motion causes the membranes to detach. Manual separation of the amniotic membranes from the cervix is thought to induce cervical ripening and the onset of labor (Rai & Schreiber, 2007).

An amniotomy involves inserting a cervical hook (Amniohook) through the cervical os to deliberately rupture the membranes. This promotes pressure of the presenting part on the cervix and stimulates an increase in the activity of prostaglandins locally. Risks associated with these procedures include umbilical cord prolapse or compression, maternal or neonatal infection, FHR deceleration, bleeding, and client discomfort (Shobeiri, Tehranian, & Nazari, 2007).

When either of these techniques is used, amniotic fluid characteristics (such as whether it is clear or bloody, or meconium is present) and the FHR pattern must be monitored closely.

Pharmacologic Agents

The use of pharmacologic agents has revolutionized cervical ripening. The use of prostaglandins to attain cervical ripening has been found to be highly effective in producing cervical changes independent of uterine contractions (Sifakis et al., 2007). In some cases, women will go into labor, requiring no additional stimulants for induction. Induction of labor with prostaglandins offers the advantage of promoting both cervical ripening and uterine contractility. A drawback of prostaglandins is their ability to induce excessive uterine contractions, which can increase maternal and perinatal morbidity (Hofmeyr & Gulmezoglu, 2007). Prostaglandin analogs commonly used for cervical ripening include dinoprostone gel (Prepidil), dinoprostone inserts (Cervidil), and misoprostol (Cytotec). Misoprostol (Cytotec), a synthetic PGE1 analog, is a gastric cytoprotective agent used in the treatment and prevention of peptic ulcers. It can be administered intravaginally or orally to ripen the cervix or induce labor. It is available in 100-mcg or 200-mcg tablets, but doses of 25 to 50 mcg are typically used. However, it is not approved by the FDA for cervical ripening since several reports found higher levels of uterine rupture associated with its use (USFDA, 2007) (Drug Guide 21.2). Furthermore, it is contraindicated for women with prior uterine scars and therefore should not be used for cervical ripening in women attempting a VBAC.

Oxytocin

Oxytocin is a potent endogenous uterotonic agent used for both artificial induction and augmentation of labor. It is produced naturally by the posterior pituitary gland and stimulates contractions of the uterus. For women with low Bishop scores, cervical ripening is typically initiated before oxytocin is used. Once the cervix is ripe, oxytocin is the most popular pharmacologic agent used for inducing or augmenting labor. Frequently a woman with an unfavorable cervix is admitted the evening before induc-

DRUG GUIDE 21.2 DRUGS USED FOR CERVICAL RIPENING AND LABOR INDUCTION

Drug	Action/Indication	Nursing Implications
Dinoprostone (Cervidil insert; Prepidil gel)	Directly softens and dilates the cervix/to ripen cervix and induce labor	Provide emotional support. Administer pain medications as needed. Frequently assess degree of effacement and dilation. Monitor uterine contractions for frequency, duration, and strength. Assess maternal vital signs and FHR pattern frequently. Monitor woman for possible adverse effects such as headache, nausea and vomiting, and diarrhea.
Misoprostol (Cytotec)	Ripens cervix/to induce labor	Instruct client about purpose and possible adverse effects of medication. Ensure informed consent is signed per hospital policy. Assess vital signs and FHR patterns frequently. Monitor client's reaction to drug. Initiate oxytocin for labor induction at least 4 hours after last dose was administered. Monitor for possible adverse effects such as nausea and vomiting, diarrhea, uterine hyperstimulation, and non-reassuring FHR pattern.
Oxytocin (Pitocin)	Acts on uterine myofibrils to contract/to initiate or reinforce labor	Administer as an IV infusion via pump, increasing dose based on protocol until adequate labor progress is achieved. Assess baseline vital signs and FHR and then frequently after initiating oxytocin infusion. Determine frequency, duration, and strength of contractions frequently. Notify health care provider of any uterine hypertonicity or abnormal FHR patterns. Maintain careful I & O, being alert for water intoxication. Keep client informed of labor progress. Monitor for possible adverse effects such as hyperstimulation of the uterus, impaired uterine blood flow leading to fetal hypoxia, rapid labor leading to cervical lacerations or uterine rupture, water intoxication (if oxytocin is given in electrolyte-free solution or at a rate exceeding 20 mU/min), and hypotension.

tion to ripen her cervix with one of the prostaglandin agents. Then induction begins with oxytocin the next morning if she has not already gone into labor. Doing so markedly enhances the success of induction.

Response to oxytocin varies widely: some women are very sensitive to even small amounts. The most common adverse effect of oxytocin is uterine hyperstimulation, leading to fetal compromise and impaired oxygenation (Smith & Merrill, 2006). The response of the uterus to the drug is closely monitored throughout labor so that the oxytocin infusion can be titrated appropriately. In addition, oxytocin has an antidiuretic effect, resulting in decreased urine flow that may lead to water intoxication. Symptoms to watch for include headache and vomiting.

Oxytocin is administered via an intravenous infusion pump piggybacked into the main intravenous line at the port most proximal to the insertion site. Usually 10 units of oxytocin is added to 1 L of isotonic solution to achieve an infusion rate of 1 mU/min = 6 mL/hr. The dose is titrated according to protocol to achieve stable contractions every 2 to 3 minutes lasting 40 to 60 seconds (Briggs & Wan, 2006). The uterus should relax between contractions. If the resting uterine tone remains above 20 mmHg, uteroplacental insufficiency and fetal hypoxia can result. This underscores the importance of continuous FHR monitoring.

Oxytocin has many advantages: it is potent and easy to titrate, it has a short half-life (1 to 5 minutes), and it is generally well tolerated. Induction using oxytocin has side effects (water intoxication, hypotension, and uterine hypertonicity), but because the drug does not cross the placental barrier, no direct fetal problems have been observed (Khan, Khan, & Ashraf, 2007) (Fig. 21.4).

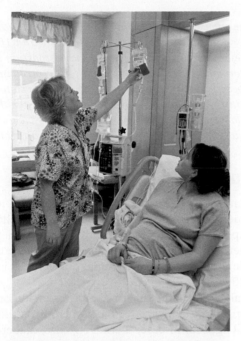

FIGURE **21.4** The nurse monitors an intravenous infusion of oxytocin being administered to a woman in labor.

*R*emember Jennifer, the young woman described at the beginning of the chapter? After her cervix is ripened, an oxytocin infusion is started and her progress is slow. What encouragement can the nurse offer? After a few hours, her contractions begin to increase in intensity and frequency. What typical pain management measures can the nurse implement, and how would the nurse evaluate the effectiveness of these measures?

Nursing Assessment

Nursing assessment of the woman who is undergoing labor induction or augmentation involves a thorough history and physical examination. Review the woman's history for relative indications for induction or augmentation, such as diabetes, hypertension, postterm status, dysfunctional labor pattern, prolonged ruptured membranes, and maternal or fetal infection, and for contraindications such as placenta previa, overdistended uterus, active genital herpes, fetopelvic disproportion, fetal malposition, or severe fetal distress.

Assist with determining the gestational age of the fetus to prevent a preterm birth. Assess fetal well-being to validate the client's and fetus's ability to withstand labor contractions. Evaluate the woman's cervical status, including cervical dilatation and effacement, and station via vaginal examination as appropriate before cervical ripening or induction is started. Determine the Bishop score to determine the probable success of induction.

▶ *Take* NOTE!

Nurses working with women in labor play an important role acting as the "eyes" and "ears" for the birth attendant because they remain at the client's bedside throughout the entire experience. Close, frequent assessment and follow-up interventions are essential to ensure the safety of the mother and her unborn child during cervical ripening and labor induction or augmentation.

Nursing Management

Explain to the woman and her partner about the induction or augmentation procedure clearly, using simple terms (Teaching Guidelines 21.2). Ensure that an informed consent has been signed after the client and her

TEACHING GUIDELINES 21.2

Teaching in Preparation for Labor Induction

- Your health care provider may recommend that you have your labor induced. This may be necessary for a variety of reasons, such as elevated blood pressure, a medical condition, prolonged pregnancy over 41 weeks, or problems with fetal heart rate patterns or fetal growth.
- Your health care provider may use one or more methods to induce labor, such as stripping the membranes, breaking the amniotic sac to release the fluid, administering medication close to or in the cervix to soften it, or administering a medication called oxytocin (Pitocin) to stimulate contractions.
- Labor induction is associated with some risks and disadvantages, such as overactivity of the uterus; nausea, vomiting, or diarrhea; and changes in fetal heart rate.
- Prior to inducing your labor, your health care provider may perform a procedure to ripen your cervix to help ensure a successful induction.
- Medication may be placed around cervix the day before you are scheduled to be induced.
- During the induction, your contractions may feel stronger than normal. However, the length of your labor may be reduced with induction.
- Medications for pain relief and comfort measures will be readily available.
- Health care staff will be present throughout labor.

partner have received complete information about the procedure, including its advantages, disadvantages, and potential risks. Ensure that the Bishop score has been determined before proceeding. Nursing Care Plan 21.1 presents an overview of the nursing care for a woman undergoing labor induction.

Administering Oxytocin

If not already done, prepare the oxytocin infusion by diluting 10 units of oxytocin in 1,000 mL of lactated Ringer's solution. Use an infusion pump on a secondary line connected to the primary infusion. Start the oxytocin infusion in mU/min or milliliters per hour as ordered. Typically, the initial dose is 0.5 to 1 mU/min; anticipate increasing the rate in increments of 1 to 2 mU/min every 30 to 60 minutes. Maintain the rate once the desired contraction frequency has been reached. To ensure adequate maternal and fetal surveillance during induction or augmentation, the nurse-to-client ratio should not exceed 1:2 (Briggs & Wan, 2006).

During induction or augmentation, monitoring of the maternal and fetal status is essential. Apply an external electronic fetal monitor or assist with placement of an internal device. Obtain the mother's vital signs and the FHR every 15 minutes during the first stage. Evaluate the contractions (frequency, duration, and intensity) and resting tone, and adjust the oxytocin infusion rate accordingly. Monitor the FHR, including baseline rate, baseline variability, and decelerations, to determine whether the oxytocin rate needs adjustment. Discontinue the oxytocin and notify the birth attendant if uterine hyperstimulation or a nonreassuring FHR pattern occurs. Perform or assist with periodic vaginal examinations to determine cervical dilation and fetal descent: cervical dilation of 1 cm/hour typically indicates satisfactory progress.

Continue to monitor the FHR continuously and document it every 15 minutes during the active phase of labor and every 5 minutes during the second stage. Assist with pushing efforts during the second stage.

Measure and record intake and output to prevent excess fluid volume. Encourage the client to empty her bladder every 2 hours to prevent soft tissue obstruction.

Providing Pain Relief and Support

Assess the woman's level of pain. Ask her frequently to rate her pain and provide pain management as needed. Offer position changes and other non-pharmacologic measures. Note her reaction to any medication given, and document its effect. Monitor her need for comfort measures as contractions increase.

Throughout induction and augmentation, frequently reassure the woman and her partner about the fetal status and labor progress. Provide them with frequent updates on the condition of the woman and the fetus. Assess the woman's ability to cope with stronger contractions (Kuczkowski, 2007). Provide support and encouragement as indicated.

After a very long day, Jennifer gives birth to a healthy baby boy with Apgar scores of 9 at 1 minute and 10 at 5 minutes. When transferring her to the postpartum unit, what information is essential to include for the accepting nurse? What specific nursing information should be given to the nursery nurse regarding the laboring experience? With such a lengthy labor, what assessments might the postpartum nurse be especially focused on for the first few hours after birth?

Intrauterine Fetal Demise

When an unborn life suddenly ends with fetal loss, the family members are profoundly affected. The sudden loss of an expected child is tragic and the family's grief can be very intense: it can last for years and can cause extreme psychological stress and emotional problems (Lindsey & Azad, 2007).

Fetal death can be due to numerous conditions, such as prolonged pregnancy, infection, hypertension, advanced maternal age, Rh disease, uterine rupture, diabetes, congenital anomalies, cord accident, abruption, premature rupture of membranes, or hemorrhage; it may go unexplained (Gilbert, 2007). Early pregnancy loss may be through a spontaneous abortion (miscarriage), an induced abortion (therapeutic abortion), or a ruptured ectopic pregnancy. A wide spectrum of feelings may be expressed, from relief to sadness and despair. A stillbirth can occur at any gestational age, and typically there is little or no warning other than reduced fetal movement.

The period following a fetal death is extremely difficult for the family. For many women, emotional healing takes much longer than physical healing. The feelings of loss can be intense. The grief response in some women may be so great that their relationships become strained, and healing can become hampered unless appropriate interventions and support are provided.

Fetal death also affects the health care staff. Despite the trauma that the loss of a fetus causes, some staff members avoid dealing with the bereaved family, never talking about or acknowledging their grief. This seems to imply that not discussing the problem will allow the grief to dissolve and vanish. As a result, the family's needs go unrecognized. Failing to keep the lines of communication open with a bereaved client and her family closes off some of the channels to recovery and healing that may be desperately needed. Subsequently, the bereaved family members may feel isolated.

Nursing Assessment

History and physical examination are of limited value in the diagnosis of fetal death, since the only history tends to be recent absence of fetal movement. An inability to obtain fetal heart sounds on examination suggests fetal demise, but an ultrasound is necessary to confirm the absence of fetal cardiac activity. Once fetal demise is confirmed, induction of labor is indicated.

Nursing Care Plan 21.1

OVERVIEW OF THE WOMAN UNDERGOING LABOR INDUCTION

Rose, a 29-year-old primipara, is admitted to the labor and birth suite at 40 weeks' gestation for induction of labor. Assessment reveals that her cervix is ripe and 80% effaced, and dilated to 2 cm. Rose says, "I'm a bit nervous about being induced. I've never been through labor before and I'm afraid that I'll have a lot of pain from the medicine used to start the contractions." She consents to being induced but wants reassurance that this procedure won't harm the baby. Upon examination, the fetus is engaged and in a cephalic presentation, with the vertex as the presenting part. Her partner is at her side. Induction is initiated with oxytocin. Rose reports that contractions have started and are beginning to get stronger.

NURSING DIAGNOSIS: Anxiety related to induction of labor and lack of experience with labor *as evidenced by statements about being nervous, not having gone through labor before and fear of pain*

Outcome Identification and Evaluation
Client will experience decrease in anxiety as evidenced by ability to verbalize understanding of procedures involved and use of positive coping skills to reduce anxious state.

Interventions: Minimizing Anxiety
- Provide a clear explanation of the labor induction process *to provide client and partner with a knowledge base.*
- Maintain continuous physical presence *to provide physical and emotional support and demonstrate concern for maternal and fetal well-being.*
- Explain each procedure before carrying it out and answer questions *to promote understanding of procedure and rationale for use and decrease fears of the unknown.*
- Review with client measures used in the past to deal with stressful situations *to determine effectiveness;* encourage use of past effective coping strategies *to aid in controlling anxiety.*
- Instruct client's partner in helpful measures to assist client in coping and encourage their use *to foster joint participation in the process and feelings of being in control and to provide support to the client.*
- Offer frequent reassurance of fetal status and labor progress *to help alleviate client's concerns and foster continued participation in the labor process.*

NURSING DIAGNOSIS: Risk for injury (maternal or fetal) related to induction procedure *as evidenced by client's concerns about fetal well-being and possible adverse effects of oxytocin administration*

Outcome Identification and Evaluation
Client will remain free of complications associated with induction *as evidenced by progression of labor as expected, delivery of healthy newborn, and absence of signs and symptoms of maternal and fetal adverse effects.*

Interventions: Promoting Maternal and Fetal Safety
- Follow agency's protocol for medication use and infusion rate *to ensure accurate, safe drug administration.*
- Set up oxytocin IV infusion to piggyback into the primary IV infusion line *to allow for prompt discontinuation should adverse effects occur.*
- Use an infusion pump *to deliver accurate dose as ordered.*
- Gradually increase oxytocin dose in increments of 1 to 2 mU/min every 30 to 60 minutes based on assessment findings and protocol *to promote effective uterine contractions.*
- Maintain oxytocin rate once desired frequency of contractions has been reached *to ensure continued progress in labor.*
- Accurately monitor contractions for frequency, duration, and intensity and resting tone *to prevent development of hypertonic contractions.*
- Maintain a nurse–client ratio of 1:2 *to ensure maternal and fetal safety.*
- Monitor FHR via electronic fetal monitoring during induction and continuously observe the FHR response to titrated medication rate *to ensure fetal well-being and identify adverse effects immediately.*
- Obtain maternal vital signs every 1 to 2 hours or as indicated by agency's protocol, reporting any deviations, *to promote maternal well-being and allow for prompt detection of problems.*
- Communicate with birth attendant frequently concerning progress *to ensure continuity of care.*

(continued)

Nursing Care Plan 21.1 (continued)

- Discontinue oxytocin infusion if tetanic contractions (>90 seconds), uterine hyperstimulation (<2 minutes apart), elevated uterine resting tone, or a nonreassuring FHR pattern occurs *to minimize risk of drug's adverse effects.*
- Provide client with frequent reassurance of maternal and fetal status *to minimize anxiety.*

NURSING DIAGNOSIS: Pain related to uterine contractions *as evidenced by client's statements about contractions increasing in intensity and expected effect of oxytocin administration*

Outcome Identification and Evaluation
Client will report a decrease in pain as evidenced by statements of increased comfort and pain rating of 3 or less on numeric pain rating scale.

Interventions: Promoting Comfort and Pain Relief
- Explain to the client that she will experience discomfort sooner than with naturally occurring labor *to promote client's awareness of events and prepare client for the experience.*
- Frequently assess client's pain using a pain rating scale *to quantify client's level of pain and evaluate effectiveness of pain-relief measures.*
- Provide comfort measures, such as hygiene, backrubs, music, and distraction, and encourage the use of breathing and relaxation techniques *to help promote relaxation.*
- Provide support for her partner *to aid in alleviating stress and concerns.*
- Employ nonpharmacologic methods, such as position changes, birthing ball, hydrotherapy, visual imagery, and effleurage, *to help in managing pain and foster feelings of control over situation.*
- Administer pharmacologic agents such as analgesia or anesthesia as appropriate and as ordered *to control pain.*
- Continuously reassess client's pain level *to evaluate effectiveness of pain management techniques used.*

Nursing Management

The nurse can play a major role in assisting the grieving family. With skillful intervention, the bereaved family may be better prepared to resolve their grief and move forward. To assist families in the grieving process, include the following measures:

- Provide accurate, understandable information to the family.
- Encourage discussion of the loss and venting of feelings of grief and guilt.
- Provide the family with baby mementos and pictures to validate the reality of death.
- Allow unlimited time with the stillborn infant after birth to validate the death; provide time for the family members to be together and grieve; offer the family the opportunity to see, touch, and hold the infant.
- Use appropriate touch, such as holding a hand or touching a shoulder.
- Inform the chaplain or the religious leader of the family's denomination about the death and request his or her presence.
- Assist the parents with the funeral arrangements or disposition of the body.
- Provide the parents with brochures offering advice about how to talk to other siblings about the loss.
- Refer the family to the support group SHARE Pregnancy and Infant Loss Support, Inc., which is designed for those who have lost an infant through abortion, miscarriage, fetal death, stillbirth, or other tragic circumstances.

- Make community referrals to promote a continuum of care after discharge.

Women Experiencing an Obstetric Emergency

Obstetric emergencies are challenging to all labor and birth personnel because of the increased risk of adverse outcomes for the mother and fetus. Quick clinical judgment and good critical decision making will increase the odds of a positive outcome for both mother and fetus. This chapter will discuss a few of these emergencies: umbilical cord prolapse, placental abruption, uterine rupture, and amniotic fluid embolism.

▶ UMBILICAL CORD PROLAPSE

An **umbilical cord prolapse** is the protrusion of the umbilical cord alongside (occult) or ahead of the presenting part of the fetus (Fig. 21.5). This condition occurs in 1 out of every 300 births and requires prompt recognition and intervention for a positive outcome (March of Dimes, 2007f). Cord prolapse occurs in 3% of deliveries when the fetus is in the vertex position and in 3.7% of deliveries when the fetus is in the breech position. The risk is increased further when the presenting part does not fill the lower uterine segment, as is the case with incomplete

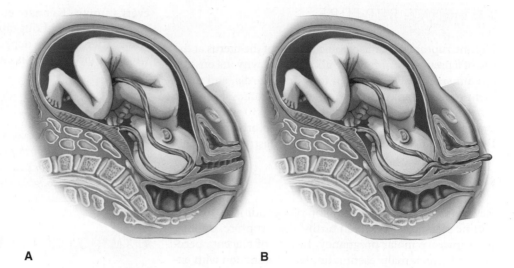

FIGURE 21.5 Prolapsed cord.
(**A**) Prolapse within the uterus.
(**B**) Prolapse with the cord visible
at the vulva.

A   **B**

breech presentations (5% to 10%), premature infants, and multiparous women (Morgan & Ross, 2007). With a 50% perinatal mortality rate, it is one of the most catastrophic events in the intrapartum period (Enakpene, Omigbodun, & Arowojolu, 2006).

Pathophysiology

Prolapse usually leads to total or partial occlusion of the cord. Since this is the fetus's only lifeline, fetal perfusion deteriorates rapidly. Complete occlusion renders the fetus helpless and oxygen-deprived. The fetus will die if the cord compression is not relieved.

Nursing Assessment

Prevention is the key to managing cord prolapse by identifying clients at risk for this condition. Carefully assess each client to help predict her risk status. Be aware that cord prolapse is more common in pregnancies involving malpresentation, growth restriction, prematurity, ruptured membranes with a fetus at a high station, hydramnios, grandmultiparity, and multifetal gestation (Dilbaz et al., 2006). Continuously assess the client and fetus to detect changes and to evaluate the effectiveness of any interventions performed.

▶ **Take** NOTE!

When the presenting part does not fully occupy the pelvic inlet, prolapse is more likely to occur.

Nursing Management

Prompt recognition of a prolapsed cord is essential to reduce the risk of fetal hypoxia resulting from prolonged cord compression. When membranes are artificially ruptured, assist with verifying that the presenting part is well applied to the cervix and engaged into the pelvis. If pressure or compression of the cord occurs, assist with measures to relieve the compression. Typically, the examiner places a sterile gloved hand into the vagina and holds the presenting part off the umbilical cord until delivery. Changing the woman's position to a modified Sims, Trendelenburg, or knee–chest position also helps relieve cord pressure. Monitor fetal heart rate, maintain bedrest, and administer oxygen if ordered. Provide emotional support and explanations as to what is going on to allay the woman's fears and anxiety. If the mother's cervix is not fully dilated, prepare the woman for an emergency cesarean birth to save the fetus's life.

▶ PLACENTAL ABRUPTION

Placental abruption refers to premature separation of a normally implanted placenta from the maternal myometrium. Abruptio placentae occurs in about 1% of all pregnancies throughout the world (March of Dimes, 2007a). Risk factors include preeclampsia, gestational hypertension, seizure activity, uterine rupture, trauma, smoking, cocaine use, coagulation defects, previous history of abruption, domestic violence, and placental pathology. These conditions may force blood into the underlayer of the placenta and cause it to detach (Deering & Satin, 2007).

Management of placental abruption depends on the gestational age, the extent of the hemorrhage, and maternal–fetal oxygenation perfusion/reserve status (see Chapter 19 for additional information on abruptio placentae). Treatment is based on the circumstances. Typically once the diagnosis is established, the focus is on maintaining the cardiovascular status of the mother and developing a plan to deliver the fetus quickly. A cesarean birth takes place if the fetus is still alive. A vaginal birth may take place if there is fetal demise.

UTERINE RUPTURE

Uterine rupture is a catastrophic tearing of the uterus at the site of a previous scar into the abdominal cavity. Its onset is often marked only by sudden fetal bradycardia, and treatment requires rapid surgery for good outcomes. From the time of diagnosis to delivery, only 10 to 30 minutes are available before clinically significant fetal morbidity occurs. Fetal morbidity occurs secondary to catastrophic hemorrhage, fetal anoxia, or both.

Nursing Assessment

Review the mother's history for risk conditions such as uterine scars, prior cesarean births, prior rupture, trauma, prior invasive molar pregnancy, history of placenta percreta or increta, malpresentation, labor induction with excessive uterine stimulation, and crack cocaine use (Nahum & Pham, 2007). Reviewing a client's history for risk factors might prove to be life-saving for both mother and fetus.

Generally, the first and most reliable symptom of uterine rupture is sudden fetal distress. Other signs may include acute and continuous abdominal pain with or without an epidural, vaginal bleeding, hematuria, irregular abdominal wall contour, loss of station in the fetal presenting part, and hypovolemic shock in the woman, fetus, or both (Nahum & Pham, 2007).

Timely management of uterine rupture depends on prompt detection. Because many women desire a trial of labor after a previous cesarean birth, the nurse must be familiar with the signs and symptoms of uterine rupture. It is difficult to prevent uterine rupture or to predict which women will experience rupture, so constant preparedness is necessary.

Screening all women with previous uterine surgical scars is important, and continuous electronic fetal monitoring should be used during labor because this may provide the only indication of an impending rupture.

Nursing Management

Because the presenting signs may be nonspecific, the initial management will be the same as that for any other cause of acute fetal distress. Urgent delivery by cesarean birth is usually indicated. Monitor maternal vital signs and observe for hypotension and tachycardia, which might indicate hypovolemic shock. Assist in preparing for an emergency cesarean birth by alerting the operating room staff, anesthesia provider, and neonatal team. Insert an indwelling urinary (Foley) catheter if one is not in place already. Inform the woman of the seriousness of this event and remind her that the health care staff will be working quickly to ensure her health and that of her fetus. Remain calm and provide reassurance that everything is being done to ensure a safe outcome for both.

The life-threatening nature of uterine rupture is underscored by the fact that the maternal circulatory system delivers approximately 500 mL of blood to the term uterus every minute (Kennare et al., 2007). Maternal death is a real possibility without rapid intervention. Newborn outcome after rupture depends largely on the speed with which surgical rescue is carried out.

> ▶ *Take* NOTE!
>
> *When excessive bleeding occurs during the childbirth process and it persists or signs such as bruising or petechiae appear, disseminated intravascular coagulation (DIC) should be suspected.*

AMNIOTIC FLUID EMBOLISM

Amniotic fluid embolism is a rare and often fatal event characterized by the sudden onset of hypotension, hypoxia, and coagulopathy. Amniotic fluid containing particles of debris (e.g., hair, skin, vernix, or meconium) enters the maternal circulation and obstructs the pulmonary vessels, causing respiratory distress and circulatory collapse (O'Shea & Eappen, 2007). The incidence is approximately 1 case per 8,000 to 80,000 pregnancies and carries a maternal mortality rate as high as 80% (Schoening, 2007).

Pathophysiology

Normally, amniotic fluid does not enter the maternal circulation because it is contained within the uterus, sealed off by the amniotic sac. An embolus occurs when the barrier between the maternal circulation and the amniotic fluid is broken and amniotic fluid enters the maternal venous system via the endocervical veins, the placental site (if the placenta is separated), or a site of uterine trauma. This condition has a high mortality rate: as many as 50% of women die within the first hour after the onset of symptoms, and about 85% of survivors have permanent hypoxia-induced neurologic damage (Moore, 2006).

Although medical science has supplied many answers to questions about this condition, health care providers remain largely unable to predict or prevent an amniotic fluid embolism or to decrease its mortality rate.

Nursing Assessment

No test can diagnose an amniotic fluid embolism. Therefore, the nurse's assessment skills are critical. Immediate recognition and diagnosis of this condition are essential to improve maternal and fetal outcomes. Until recently, the diagnosis could be made only after an autopsy of the mother revealed squamous cells, lanugo hair, or other fetal and amniotic material in the pulmonary arterial vasculature (Gilbert, 2007).

The clinical appearance is varied, but most women report difficulty breathing. Other symptoms include hypotension, cyanosis, seizures, tachycardia, coagulation failure, disseminated intravascular coagulation, pulmonary edema, uterine atony with subsequent hemorrhage, adult respiratory distress syndrome, and cardiac arrest (Moore & Ware, 2007).

▶ **Take** NOTE!

Amniotic fluid embolism should be suspected in any pregnant women with an acute onset of dyspnea, hypotension, and disseminated intravascular coagulation. By knowing how to intervene, the nurse can promote a better chance of survival for both the mother and her newborn.

Nursing Management

Upon recognizing the signs and symptoms, institute supportive measures: oxygenation (resuscitation and 100% oxygen), circulation (intravenous fluids, inotropic agents to maintain cardiac output and blood pressure), control of hemorrhage and coagulopathy (oxytocic agents to control uterine atony and bleeding), seizure precautions, and administration of steroids to control the inflammatory response (Schoening, 2007).

Care is largely supportive and aimed at maintaining oxygenation and hemodynamic function and correcting coagulopathy. There is no specific therapy that is lifesaving once this condition starts. Adequate oxygenation is necessary, with endotracheal intubation and mechanical ventilation for most women. Vasopressors are used to maintain hemodynamic stability. Management of disseminated intravascular coagulation may involve replacement with packed red blood cells or fresh-frozen plasma as necessary. Oxytocin infusions and prostaglandin analogs can be used to address uterine atony.

Explain to the client and family what is happening and what therapies are being instituted. The woman is usually transferred to a critical care unit for intensive observation and care. Assist the family to express their feelings and provide support as needed.

▶ WOMEN REQUIRING BIRTH-RELATED PROCEDURES

Most women can give birth without the need for operative obstetric interventions. Most will expect to have a "natural" birth experience and don't anticipate the need for medical intervention. However, in some situations interventions are necessary to safeguard the health of the mother and fetus. The most common birth-related procedures are amnioinfusion, episiotomy (see Chapter 14), forceps-assisted or vacuum-assisted birth, cesarean birth,

and vaginal birth following a previous cesarean birth. Nurses play a major role in helping the couple to cope with any unanticipated procedures by offering thorough explanations of the procedure, its anticipated benefits and risks, and any other options available.

▶ AMNIOINFUSION

Amnioinfusion is a technique in which a volume of warmed, sterile, normal saline or Ringer's lactate solution is introduced into the uterus through an intrauterine pressure catheter to increase the volume of fluid when oligohydramnios is present (Boyd & Carter, 2008). It is used to change the relationship of the uterus, placenta, cord, and fetus to improve placental and fetal oxygenation. Instilling an isotonic glucose-free solution into the uterus helps to cushion the umbilical cord or dilute thick meconium (Xu et al., 2007).

This procedure is commonly indicated for severe variable decelerations due to cord compression, oligohydramnios due to placental insufficiency, postmaturity or rupture of membranes, preterm labor with premature rupture of membranes, and thick meconium fluid. However, it does not prevent meconium aspiration syndrome (ACOG, 2006). Contraindications to amnioinfusion include vaginal bleeding of unknown origin, umbilical cord prolapse, amnionitis, uterine hypertonicity, and severe fetal distress (ACOG, 2006).

There is no standard protocol for amnioinfusion. After obtaining informed consent, a vaginal examination is performed to evaluate for cord prolapse, establish dilation, and confirm presentation. Next, 250 to 500 mL of warmed normal saline or lactated Ringer's solution is administered using an infusion pump over 20 to 30 minutes. Overdistention of the uterus is a risk, so the amount of fluid infused must be monitored closely (Boyd & Carter, 2008).

When caring for the woman who is receiving an amnioinfusion, include the following:

- Explain the need for the procedure, what it involves, and how it may solve the problem.
- Inform the mother that she will need to remain on bed rest during the procedure.
- Assess the mother's vital signs and associated discomfort level.
- Maintain intake and output records.
- Assess the duration and intensity of uterine contractions frequently to identify overdistention or increased uterine tone.
- Monitor the FHR pattern to determine whether the amnioinfusion is improving the fetal status.
- Prepare the mother for a possible cesarean birth if the FHR does not improve after the amnioinfusion.

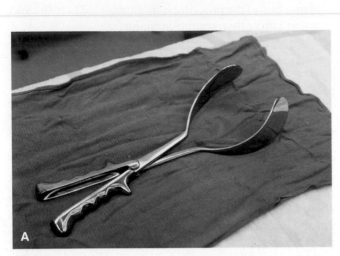

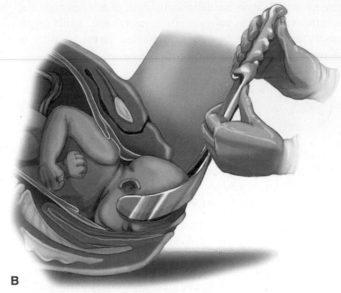

FIGURE 21.6 Forceps delivery. (**A**) Example of forceps. (**B**) Forceps being applied to the fetus.

FORCEPS- OR VACUUM-ASSISTED BIRTH

Forceps or a vacuum extractor may be used to apply traction to the fetal head or to provide a method of rotating the fetal head during birth. **Forceps** are stainless-steel instruments, similar to tongs, with rounded edges that fit around the fetus's head. Some forceps have open blades and some have solid blades. Outlet forceps are used when the fetal head is crowning and low forceps are used when the fetal head is at a +2 station or lower but not yet crowning. The forceps are applied to the sides of the fetal head. The type of forceps used is determined by the birth attendant. All forceps have a locking mechanism that prevents the blades from compressing the fetal skull (Fig. 21.6).

A **vacuum extractor** is a cup-shaped instrument attached to a suction pump used for extraction of the fetal head (Fig. 21.7). The suction cup is placed against the occiput of the fetal head. The pump is used to create negative pressure (suction) of approximately 50 to 60 mmHg. The birth attendant then applies traction until the fetal head emerges from the vagina.

The indications for the use of either method are similar and include a prolonged second stage of labor, a nonreassuring FHR pattern, failure of the presenting part to fully rotate and descend in the pelvis, limited sensation and inability to push effectively due to the effects of regional anesthesia, presumed fetal jeopardy or fetal distress, maternal heart disease, acute pulmonary edema, intrapartum infection, maternal fatigue, or infection (Pope & O'Grady, 2006).

The use of forceps or a vacuum extractor poses the risk of tissue trauma to the mother and the newborn. Maternal trauma may include lacerations of the cervix, vagina,

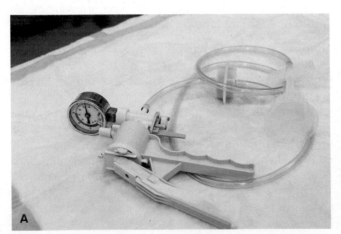

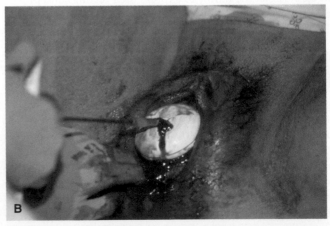

FIGURE 21.7 Vacuum extractor for delivery. (**A**) Example of a vacuum extractor. (**B**) Vacuum extractor applied to the fetal head to assist in delivery.

or perineum; hematoma; extension of the episiotomy incision into the anus; hemorrhage; and infection. Potential newborn trauma includes ecchymoses, facial and scalp lacerations, facial nerve injury, cephalhematoma, and caput succedaneum (Cunningham et al., 2005).

Prevention is key to reducing the use of these techniques. Preventive measures include frequently changing the client's position, encouraging ambulation if permitted, frequently reminding the client to empty her bladder to allow maximum space for birth, and providing adequate hydration throughout labor. Additional measures include assessing maternal vital signs, the contraction pattern, the fetal status, and the maternal response to the procedure. Provide a thorough explanation of the procedure and the rationale for its use. Reassure the mother that any marks or swelling on the newborn's head or face will disappear without treatment within 2 to 3 days. Alert the postpartum nursing staff about the use of the technique so that they can observe for any bleeding or infection related to genital lacerations.

▶ CESAREAN BIRTH

WATCH & LEARN

A **cesarean birth** is the delivery of the fetus through an incision in the abdomen and uterus. A classic (vertical) or low transverse incision may be used; today, the low transverse incision is more common (Fig. 21.8).

High cesarean birth rates are an international concern. The number of cesarean births has steadily risen in the United States: today approximately 29% or one in three births occur this way (ACOG, 2008). Although there has been some decline in rates since the 1980s, the

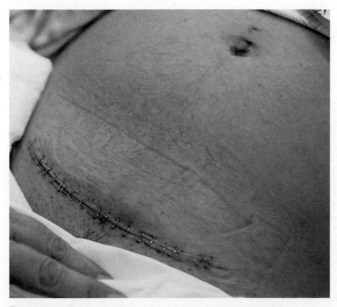

FIGURE 21.8 Low transverse incision for cesarean birth.

United States still has a way to go to reduce its surgical birth rates (USDHHS, 2000).

Several factors may explain this increased incidence of cesarean deliveries: the use of electronic fetal monitoring, which identifies fetal distress early; the reduced number of forceps-assisted births; older maternal age and reduced parity, with more nulliparous women having infants; convenience to the client and doctor; and a increase in malpractice suits (Katz, 2006).

Cesarean birth is a major surgical procedure with increased risks compared to a vaginal birth. The client is at risk for complications such as infection, hemorrhage, aspiration, pulmonary embolism, urinary tract trauma, thrombophlebitis, paralytic ileus, and atelectasis. Fetal injury and transient tachypnea of the newborn also may occur (Gagnon, Meir, & Waghorn, 2007).

Spinal, epidural, or general anesthesia is used for cesarean births. Epidural anesthesia is most commonly used today because it is associated with less risk and most women wish to be awake and aware of the birth experience.

Nursing Assessment

Review the woman's history for indications associated with cesarean birth and complete a physical examination. Any condition that prevents the safe passage of the fetus through the birth canal or that seriously compromises maternal or fetal well-being may be an indication for a cesarean birth. Examples include active genital herpes, fetal macrosomia, fetopelvic disproportion, prolapsed umbilical cord, placental abnormality (placenta previa or abruptio placentae), previous classic uterine incision or scar, gestational hypertension, diabetes, positive HIV status, and dystocia. Fetal indications include malpresentation (nonvertex presentation), congenital anomalies (fetal neural tube defects, hydrocephalus, abdominal wall defects), and fetal distress (Humenick, 2006).

Nursing Management

Once the decision has been made to proceed with a cesarean birth, assess the woman's knowledge of the procedure and necessary preparation. Assist with obtaining diagnostic tests as ordered. These tests are usually ordered to ensure the well-being of both parties and may include a complete blood count; urinalysis to rule out infection; blood type and cross-match so that blood is available for transfusion if needed; an ultrasound to determine fetal position and placental location; and an amniocentesis to determine fetal lung maturity if needed.

Although the nurse's role in a cesarean birth can be very technical and skill-oriented at times, the focus must remain on the woman, not the equipment surrounding the bed. Care should be centered on the family, not the surgery. Provide education and minimize separation of the mother, father, and newborn. Remember that the client is anxious and concerned about her welfare as well as that of her child. Use touch, eye contact, therapeutic communication, and genuine caring to provide couples with a positive birth experience, regardless of the type of delivery.

Providing Preoperative Care

Client preparation varies depending on whether the cesarean birth is planned or unplanned. The major difference is the time allotted for preparation and teaching. In an unplanned cesarean birth, institute measures quickly to ensure the best outcomes for the mother and fetus. Ensure that the woman has signed an informed consent, and allow for discussion of fears and expectations. Provide essential teaching and explanations to reduce the woman's fears and anxieties.

Ascertain the client's and family's understanding of the surgical procedure. Reinforce the reasons for surgery given by the surgeon. Outline the procedure and expectations of the surgical experience. Ensure that all diagnostic tests ordered have been completed, and evaluate the results. Explain to the woman and her family about what to expect postoperatively. Reassure the woman that pain management will be provided throughout the procedure and afterward. Encourage the woman to report any pain.

Ask the woman about the time she last had anything to eat or drink. Document the time and what was consumed. Throughout the preparations, assess maternal and fetal status frequently.

Provide preoperative teaching to reduce the risk of postoperative complications. Demonstrate the use of the incentive spirometer and deep-breathing and leg exercises. Instruct the woman on how to splint her incision.

Complete the preoperative procedures, which may include:

- Preparing the surgical site as ordered
- Starting an intravenous infusion for fluid replacement therapy as ordered
- Inserting an indwelling (Foley) catheter and informing the client about how long it will remain in place (usually 24 hours)
- Administering any preoperative medications as ordered; documenting the time administered and the client's reaction

Maintain a calm, confident manner in all interactions with the client and family. Help transport the client and her partner to the operative area.

Providing Postoperative Care

Postoperative care for the mother who has had a cesarean delivery is similar to that for one who has had a vaginal birth, with a few additional measures. Assess vital signs and lochia flow every 15 minutes for the first hour, then every 30 minutes for the next hour, and then every 4 hours if stable. Assist with perineal care and instruct the client in the same. Inspect the abdominal dressing and document

description, including any evidence of drainage. Assess uterine tone to determine fundal firmness. Check the patency of the intravenous line, making sure the infusion is flowing at the correct rate. Inspect the infusion site frequently for redness.

Assess the woman's level of consciousness if sedative drugs were administered. Institute safety precautions until the woman is fully alert and responsive. If a regional anesthetic was used, monitor for the return of sensation to the legs.

Assess for evidence of abdominal distention and auscultate bowel sounds. Assist with early ambulation to prevent respiratory and cardiovascular problems and to promote peristalsis. Monitor intake and output at least every 4 hours initially and then every 8 hours as indicated.

Encourage the woman to cough, perform deep-breathing exercises, and use the incentive spirometer every 2 hours. Administer analgesics as ordered and provide comfort measures, such as splinting the incision and pillows for positioning. Assist the client to move in bed and turn side to side to improve circulation. Also encourage the woman to ambulate to promote venous return from the extremities.

Encourage early touching and holding of the newborn to promote bonding. Assist with breastfeeding initiation and offer continued support. Suggest alternate positioning techniques to reduce incisional discomfort while breastfeeding.

Review with the couple their perception of the surgical birth experience. Allow them to verbalize their feelings and assist them in positive coping measures. Prior to discharge, teach the woman about the need for adequate rest, activity restrictions such as lifting, and signs and symptoms of infection.

▶ VAGINAL BIRTH AFTER CESAREAN

Vaginal birth after cesarean (VBAC) describes a woman who gives birth vaginally after having at least one previous cesarean birth. Despite evidence that some women who have had a cesarean birth are candidates for vaginal birth, most women who have had a cesarean birth once undergo another for subsequent pregnancies (Caughey, 2006).

The choice of a vaginal or a repeat cesarean birth can be offered to women who had a lower abdominal incision. However, controversy remains. The argument against VBAC focuses on the risk of uterine rupture and hemorrhage. Although the risk of uterine rupture is relatively low, the rate of fetal mortality in the event of a uterine rupture is extremely high.

Contraindications to VBAC include a prior classic uterine incision, prior transfundal uterine surgery (myomectomy), uterine scar other than low-transverse cesarean scar, contracted pelvis, and inadequate staff or facility if an emergency cesarean birth in the event of uterine rupture is required (Caughey, 2006). Most women go through a trial of labor to see how they progress, but this must be performed in an environment capable of handling the emergency of uterine rupture. The use of cervical ripening agents increases the risk of uterine rupture and thus is contraindicated in VBAC clients. The woman considering induction of labor after a previous cesarean birth needs to be informed of the increased risk of uterine rupture with an induction than with spontaneous labor (Meddings et al., 2007).

Women are the primary decision makers about the choice of birth method, but they need education about VBAC during their prenatal course. Management is similar for any women experiencing labor, but certain areas require special focus:

• Consent: Fully informed consent is essential for the woman who wants to have a trial of labor after cesarean birth. The client must be advised about the risks as well as the benefits. She must understand the ramifications of uterine rupture, even though the risk is small.
• Documentation: Recordkeeping is an important component of safe client care. If and when an emergency occurs, it is imperative to take care of the client, but also to keep track of the plan of care, interventions and their timing, and the client's response. Events and activities can be written right on the fetal monitoring tracing to correlate with the change in fetal status.
• Surveillance: A nonreassuring fetal monitor tracing in a woman undergoing a trial of labor after a cesarean birth should alert the nurse to the possibility of uterine rupture. Terminal bradycardia must be considered an emergency situation, and the nurse should prepare the team for an emergency delivery.
• Readiness for emergency: According to ACOG criteria for a safe trial of labor for a woman who has had a previous cesarean birth, the physician, anesthesia provider, and operating room team must be immediately available. Anything less would place the women and fetus at risk (ACOG, 2004a).

Nurses must act as advocates, giving input on the appropriate selection of women who wish to undergo VBAC. Nurses also need to become experts at reading fetal monitoring tracings to identify a nonreassuring pattern and set in motion an emergency delivery. Including all these nursing strategies will make VBAC safer for all.

■■■ Key Concepts

■ Risk factors for dystocia include epidural analgesia, occiput posterior position, longer first stage of labor, nulliparity, short maternal stature (<5 feet tall), high birth weight, maternal age older than 35 years, gestational age more than 41 weeks, chorioamnionitis, pelvic contractions, macrosomia, and high station at complete cervical dilation.
■ Dystocia may result from problems in the powers, passenger, passageway, or psyche.
■ Problems involving the powers that lead to dystocia include hypertonic uterine dysfunction, hypotonic uterine dysfunction, and precipitous labor.
■ Management of hypertonic labor pattern involves therapeutic rest with the use of sedatives to promote relaxation and stop the abnormal activity of the uterus.
■ Any presentation other than occiput or a slight variation of the fetal position or size increases the probability of dystocia.
■ Multiple gestation may result in dysfunctional labor due to uterine overdistention, which may lead to hypotonic dystocia, and abnormal presentations of the fetuses.
■ During labor, evaluation of fetal descent, cervical effacement and dilation, and characteristics of uterine contractions are paramount to determine progress or lack thereof.
■ Antepartum assessment for a postterm pregnancy typically includes daily fetal movement counts done by the woman, nonstress tests done twice weekly, amniotic fluid assessments as part of the biophysical profile, and weekly cervical examinations to check for ripening for induction.
■ Once the cervix is ripe, oxytocin is the most popular pharmacologic agent used for inducing or augmenting labor.
■ Generally, the first and most reliable symptom of uterine rupture is fetal distress.
■ Amniotic fluid embolism is a rare but often fatal event characterized by the sudden onset of hypotension, hypoxia, and coagulopathy.
■ Cesarean births have steadily risen in the United States; today, approximately one in five births occurs this way. Cesarean birth is a major surgical procedure and has increased risks over vaginal birth.

REFERENCES

Abenhaim, H., Kinch, R., Morin, L., Benjamin, A., & Usher, R. (2007). Effect of prepregnancy body mass index categories on obstetrical and neonatal outcomes. *Archives of Gynecology and Obstetrics, 275*(1), 39–43.
American Academy of Pediatrics (AAP) and American College of Obstetricians and Gynecologists (ACOG). (2003). *Guidelines for perinatal care* (5th ed.). Washington, DC: Author.
ACOG. (2001). ACOG committee opinion: Number 256. Mode of term single breech delivery. *International Journal of Gynecology and Obstetrics, 77*(1), 65–66.
ACOG. (2003a). *Dystocia and augmentation of labor. Clinical management guidelines for obstetricians-gynecologists.* ACOG Practice Bulletin No. 49. Washington, DC: Author.
ACOG. (2003b). ACOG practice bulletin: Management of preterm labor. *Obstetrics and Gynecology, 101,* 1039–1047.
ACOG. (2004a). Guidelines for VBAC. *American Family Physician, 70*(7), 1397–1399.

ACOG. (2004b). Management of postterm pregnancy (Practice Bulletin #55). *Obstetrics and Gynecology, 194,* 639–646.

ACOG. (2006). Amnioinfusion does not prevent meconium aspiration syndrome. ACOG Committee on Obstetric Practice, number 346. *Obstetrics & Gynecology, 108*(4), 1053–1055.

ACOG. (2008). Rising cesarean birth rates in U.S. tied to obesity, ACOG's 54th annual meeting. [online] Available at: http://www. medpagetoday.com/MeetingCoverage/ACOG/tb/3268.

Anderson, T. (2007). Cochrane made simple: Can midwives prevent shoulder dystocia? *Practicing Midwife, 10*(1), 36–37.

Arenson, J., & Drake, P. (2007). *Maternal and newborn health.* Sudbury, MA: Jones and Bartlett Publishers.

Blackburn, S. (2007). *Maternal, fetal, and neonatal physiology: A clinical perspective* (3rd ed.). St. Louis: W. B. Saunders.

Bonilla, M. M., & Forouzan, I. (2007). Dystocia. *eMedicine.* Available at: http://www.eMedicine.com/med/topic3280.htm.

Boulvain, M., Kelly, A., Lohse, C., Stan, C., & Irion, O. (2007). Mechanical methods for induction of labor. *Cochrane Database of Systematic Reviews 2007* Issue 1: DOI: 10.1002/14651858.CD001233.

Boyd, R. L., & Carter, B. S. (2008). Polyhydramnios and oligohydramnios. *eMedicine.* Available at: http://www.emedicine.com/ped/topic 1854.htm.

Briggs, G. G., & Wan, S. R. (2006). Drug therapy during labor and delivery. *American Journal of Health-System Pharmacists, 63*(12), 1131–1139.

Bueno, B., San-Frutos, L., Perez-Medina, T., Barbancho, C., & Bajo, J. (2007). The labor induction: Integrated clinical and sonographic variables that predict the outcome. *Journal of Perinatology, 27*(1), 4–8.

Butler, J. R., & Wilkes, P. T. (2007). Postterm pregnancy. *eMedicine.* Available at: http://www.emedicine.com/med/topic3248.htm.

Catalano, P. M. (2007). Management of obesity in pregnancy. *Obstetrics and Gynecology, 109*(2), 419–433.

Caughey, A. B. (2006). Vaginal birth after cesarean delivery. *eMedicine.* Available at: http://www.emedicine.com/med/topic3434.htm.

Cheng, Y. W., & Caughey, A. B. (2007). Normal labor and delivery. *eMedicine.* Available at: http://www.emedicine.com/med/topic 3239.htm.

Crane, J. M. (2006). Factors predicting labor induction success: A critical analysis. *Clinical Obstetrics & Gynecology, 49*(3), 573–584.

Cunningham, F. G., Leveno, K. J., Bloom, S. L., Hauth, J. C., Gilstrap, L., & Wenstrom, K. D. (2005). *Williams' obstetrics* (22nd ed.). New York: McGraw-Hill.

Deering, S. H., & Satin, A. (2007). Abruptio placentae. *eMedicine.* Available at: http://www.emedicine.com/med/topic6.htm.

Dilbaz, B., Ozturkoglu, E., Dilbaz, S., Ozturk, N., Sivaslioglu, A., & Haberal, A. (2006). Risk factors and perinatal outcomes associated with umbilical cord prolapse. *Archives of Gynecology & Obstetrics, 274*(2), 104–107.

Ecker, J., & Frigoletto, F. D. (2007). Cesarean delivery and the risk-benefit calculus. *New England Journal of Medicine, 356*(9), 885–888.

Enakpene, C. A., Omigbodun, A. O., & Arowojolu, A. O. (2006). Perinatal mortality following umbilical cord prolapse. *International Journal of Gynecology & Obstetrics, 95*(1), 44–45.

Fischer, R. (2007). Breech presentation. *eMedicine.* Available at: http://www.emedicine.com/med/topic3272.htm.

Gagnon, A. J., Meier, K. M., & Waghorn, K. (2007). Continuity of nursing care and its link to cesarean birth rate. *Birth: Issues in Perinatal Care, 34*(1), 26–31.

Gelber, S. (2006). Mechanical methods of cervical ripening and labor induction. *Clinical Obstetrics & Gynecology, 49*(3), 642–657.

Gilbert, E. (2007). *Manual of high-risk pregnancy and delivery* (4th ed.). St. Louis: Mosby.

Gray, B. A. (2006). How nurses can identify, treat and prevent preterm labor. *AWHONN Lifelines, 10*(5), 380–389.

Griffin, G. (2007). Are oral beta-mimetics effective maintenance therapies after threatened preterm labor? *American Family Physician, 75*(5), 648–649.

Grimes-Dennis, J., & Berghella, V. (2007). Cervical length and prediction of preterm delivery. *Current Opinion in Obstetrics & Gynecology, 19*(2), 191–195.

Gülmezoglu, A. M., Crowther, C. A., & Middleton, P. (2006). Induction of labour for improving birth outcomes for women at or beyond term. *Cochrane Database of Systematic Reviews 2006.* Issue 4. Art. No.: CD004945.DOI:10.1002/14651858.CD004945.pub2.

Gurewitsch, E. D., Johnson, E., Hamzehzadeh, S., & Allen, R. H. (2006). Risk factors for brachial plexus injury with and without shoulder dystocia. *American Journal of Obstetrics and Gynecology, 194,* 486–492.

Heimstad, R., Romundstad, P. R., Eik-Nes, S. H., & Salvesen, K. A. (2006). Outcomes of pregnancy beyond 37 weeks of gestation. *Obstetrics and Gynecology, 108*(3), 500–508.

Hofmeyr, G. J., & Gulmezoglu, A. M. (2007). Vaginal misoprostol for cervical ripening and induction of labor. *Cochrane Database of Systematic Reviews 2007* Issue 1. Art. No.: CD000941. DOI: 10.1002/14651858.CD000941.

Humenick, S. (2006). NIH weighs in on cesarean birth. *Journal of Perinatal Education, 15*(1), 3.

Incerti, M., Ghidini, A., Korker, V., & Pezzullo, J. (2007). Performance of cervicovaginal fetal fibronectin in a community hospital setting. *Archives of Gynecology & Obstetrics, 275*(5), 347–351.

Jazayeri, A., & Contreras, D. (2007). Macrosomia. *eMedicine.* Available at: http://emedicine.com/med/topic3279.htm.

Jenis, A. (2007). Pregnancy, breech delivery. *eMedicine.* Available at: http://www.emedicine.com/emerg/topic868.htm.

Joy, S., & Lyon, D. (2007). Diagnosis of abnormal labor. *eMedicine.* Available at: http://www.emedicine.com/med/topic3488.html.

Katz, V. L. (2006). Cesarean birth. *Obstetrics & Gynecology, 108*(1), 2–3.

Kavanagh, J., Kelly, A., & Thomas, J. (2007). Sexual intercourse for cervical ripening and induction of labor. *Cochrane Database of Systematic Reviews 2007* Issue 1: CD003093. DOI: 10.1002/14651858. CD003093.

Kennare, R., Tucker, G., Heard, A., & Chan, A. (2007). Risks of adverse outcomes in the next birth after a first cesarean delivery. *Obstetrics & Gynecology, 109*(2), 270–276.

Khan, R. A., Khan, Z. E., & Ashraf, O. (2007). Concurrent versus sequential methods for labor induction at term. *International Journal of Gynecology & Obstetrics, 96*(2), 94–97.

Kuczkowski, K. M. (2007). Labor pain and its management with the combined spinal-epidural analgesia: What does an obstetrician need to know? *Archives of Gynecology & Obstetrics, 275*(3), 183–185.

Lee, H. C., El-Sayed, Y. Y., & Gould, J. B. (2007). Delivery mode by race for breech presentation in the U.S. *Journal of Perinatology, 27*(3), 147–153.

Lilley, L. L., Harrington, S., & Snyder, J. S. (2007). *Pharmacology and the nursing process* (5th ed.). St. Louis: Elsevier Health Sciences.

Lindsey, J. L., & Azad, S. (2007). Evaluation of fetal death. *eMedicine.* Available at: http://www.emedicine.com/med/topic3235.htm.

March of Dimes. (2007a). *Placental abruption.* Available at: http://www.marchofdimes.com/pnhec/188_1135.asp.

March of Dimes. (2007b). *Multiples: Twins, triplets and beyond.* Available at: http://www.marchofdimes.com/professionals/681_4545.asp.

March of Dimes. (2007c). *Preterm labor and birth: A serious pregnancy complication.* Available at: http://www.marchofdimes.com/printable Articles/240_1080.asp?printable=true.

March of Dimes. (2007d). *Preterm birth.* Available at: http://www.marchofdimes.com/prematurity/5196_5799.asp.

March of Dimes. (2007e). *Preterm labor.* Available at: http://www.marchofdimes.com/pnhec/188_1080.asp.

March of Dimes. (2007f). *Umbilical cord abnormalities.* Available at: http://www.marchofdimes.com/professionals/681_4546.asp.

Meddings, F., Phipps, F. M., Haith-Cooper, M., & Haigh, J. (2007). Vaginal birth after cesarean section (VBAC): exploring women's perceptions. *Journal of Clinical Nursing, 16*(1), 160–167.

Moore, J. (2006). Amniotic fluid embolism: On the trail of an elusive diagnosis. *Lancet, 368*(9545), 1399–1401.

Moore, L. E., & Ware, D. (2007). Amniotic fluid embolism. *eMedicine.* Available at: http://emedicine.com/med/topic122.htm.

Morgan, B. L. G., & Ross, M. G. (2007). Umbilical cord complications. *eMedicine.* Available at: http://www.emedicine.com/med/topic3276.htm.

Morrison, J. C., & Chauhan, S. P. (2003). Current status of home uterine activity monitoring. *Clinics in Perinatology, 30*(4), 757–801.

Nahum, G. G., & Pham, K. Q. (2007). Uterine rupture in pregnancy. *eMedicine.* Available at: http://www.emedicine.com/med/topic3746.htm.

Norwitz, E. R., & Schorge, J. O. (2006). *Obstetrics and gynecology at a glance* (2nd ed.). Malden, MA: Blackwell Publishing, Ltd.

O'Shea, A., & Eappen, S. (2007). Amniotic fluid embolism. *International Anesthesiology Clinics, 45*(1), 17–28.

Pope, C. S., & O'Grady, J. P. (2006). Vacuum extraction. *eMedicine.* Available at: http://www.emedicine.com/med/topic3389.htm.

Pretorius, C., Jagatt, A., & Lamont, R. (2007). The relationship between periodontal disease, bacterial vaginosis, and preterm birth. *Journal of Perinatal Medicine, 35*(2), 93–99.

Rai, J., & Schreiber, J. R. (2007). Cervical ripening. *eMedicine.* Available at: http://www.emedicine.com/med/topic3282.htm.

Schoening, A. M. (2007). Amniotic fluid embolism: Recognizing trouble. *Nursing 2007, 37*(1), 64–67.

Sharf, Y., Farine, D., Batzalel, M., Megel, Y., Shenhav, M., Jaffa, A., & Barnea, O. (2007). Continuous monitoring of cervical dilatation and fetal head station during labor. *Medical Engineering & Physics, 29*(1), 61–71.

Shobeiri, F., Tehranian, N., & Nazari, M. (2007). Amniotomy in labor. *International Journal of Gynecology & Obstetrics, 96*(3), 197–198.

Sifakis, S., Angelakis, E., Avgoustinakis, E., Fragouli, Y., Mantas, N., Koukoura, O., Vardaki, E., & Koumantakis, E. (2007). A randomized comparison between intravaginal misoprostol and prostaglandin E2 for labor induction. *Archives of Gynecology and Obstetrics, 275*(4), 263–267.

Simhan, H., & Caritis, S. (2007). Prevention of preterm delivery. *New England Journal of Medicine, 357*(5), 477–487.

Smith, J. G., & Merrill, D. C. (2006). Oxytocin in induction of labor. *Clinical Obstetrics & Gynecology, 49*(3), 594–608.

Stein, A. M. (2007). *Maternity and women's health nursing.* Clifton Park, NY: Thomson Delmar Learning.

Tan, T. C., Devendra, K., Tan, L. K., & Tan, H. K. (2006). Tocolytic treatment for the management of preterm labor: A systematic review. *Singapore Medical Journal, 47*(5), 361–366.

U.S. Department of Health and Human Services (USDHHS), Public Health Service. (2000). *Healthy People 2010* (conference edition, in two volumes). U.S. Department of Health and Human Services. Washington, DC: U.S. Government Printing Office.

U.S. Food and Drug Administration (USFDA). (2007). *Misoprostol (marketed as Cytotec) information. FDA Alert—Risks of use in labor and delivery.* Available at: http://www.fda.gov/CDER/Drug/infopage/misoprostol/default.htm.

Wing, D. A. (2006). Symposium on cervical ripening and labor induction. *Clinical Obstetrics & Gynecology, 49*(3), 549–550.

World Health Organization (WHO). (2007). Malpositions and malpresentations: A guide for midwives and doctors. Available at: http://www.who.int/reproductive-health/impac/Symptoms/Malpositions__malpresetations_S69_S81.html.

Xu, H., Hofmeyr, J., Roy, C., & Fraser, W. D. (2007). Intrapartum amnioinfusion for meconium-stained amniotic fluid: A systematic review of randomized controlled trials. *International Journal of Obstetrics & Gynecology, 114*(4), 383–390.

Zach, T., & Pramanik, A. K. (2007). Multiple births. *eMedicine.* Available at: http://www.emedicine.com/ped/topic2599.htm.

WEBSITES

American Academy of Pediatrics: www.app.org
American College of Obstetricians and Gynecologists: www.acog.org
American Society of Reproductive Medicine: www.asrm.org
Association of Women's Health, Obstetric and Neonatal Nurses: www.awhonn.org
Birthrites: Healing after Cesarean, Inc.: www.birthrites.org
Department of Health and Human Services: www.4women.gov
International Cesarean Awareness Network: www.ican-online.org
March of Dimes: www.modimes.org
Mothers of Super Twins: www.mostonline.org
National Perinatal Association: www.nationalperinatal.org
SHARE Parents Support Group: www.nationalshareoffice.com/
Sidelines: High Risk Pregnancy Support Group: www.sidelines.org
Smoke-free Families: www.smokefreefamilies.org
VBAC: www.vbac.com

Chapter Worksheet

Multiple Choice Questions

1. When reviewing the medical record of a client, the nurse notes that the woman has a condition in which the fetus cannot physically pass through the maternal pelvis. The nurse interprets this as:

   a. Cervical insufficiency

   b. Contracted pelvis

   c. Maternal disproportion

   d. Fetopelvic disproportion

2. The nurse would anticipate a cesarean birth for a client who has which active infection present at the onset of labor?

   a. Hepatitis

   b. Herpes simplex virus

   c. Toxoplasmosis

   d. Human papillomavirus

3. After a vaginal examination, the nurse determines that the client's fetus is in an occiput posterior position. The nurse would anticipate that the client will have:

   a. Intense back pain

   b. Frequent leg cramps

   c. Nausea and vomiting

   d. A precipitous birth

4. When assessing the following women, which would the nurse identify as being at the greatest risk for preterm labor?

   a. Woman who had twins in a previous pregnancy

   b. Client living in a large city

   c. Woman working full-time as a computer programmer

   d. Client with a history of a previous preterm birth

5. The rationale for using a prostaglandin gel for a client prior to the induction of labor is to:

   a. Stimulate uterine contractions

   b. Numb cervical pain receptors

   c. Prevent cervical lacerations

   d. Soften and efface the cervix

6. A client who was in active labor and whose cervix had dilated to 4 cm experiences a weakening in the intensity and frequency of her contractions and exhibits no further progress in labor. The nurse interprets this as a sign of:

   a. Hypertonic labor

   b. Precipitous labor

   c. Hypotonic labor

   d. Dysfunctional labor

Critical Thinking Exercises

1. Marsha, a 26-year-old multipara, is admitted to the labor and birth suite in active labor. After a few hours, the nurse notices a change in her contraction pattern—poor contraction intensity and no progression of cervical dilatation beyond 5 cm. Marsha keeps asking about her labor progress and appears anxious about "how long this labor is taking."

   a. Based on the nurse's findings, what might you suspect is going on?

   b. How can the nurse address Marsha's anxiety?

   c. What are the appropriate interventions to change this labor pattern?

2. Marsha activates her call light and states, "I feel increased wetness down below."

   a. What might be occurring?

   b. How will the nurse confirm the suspicions?

   c. What interventions are appropriate for this finding?

Study Activities

1. Visit the SHARE Pregnancy and Infant Loss Support, Inc. website (http://www.nationalshareoffice.com/) and assess its helpfulness to parents.

2. Outline the fetal and maternal risks associated with a postterm pregnancy.

3. An abnormal or difficult labor describes _____.

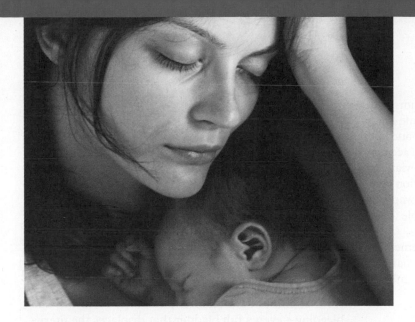

NURSING MANAGEMENT OF THE POSTPARTUM WOMAN AT RISK

KEY TERMS

mastitis
metritis
postpartum depression

postpartum hemorrhage
subinvolution
thrombophlebitis

uterine atony
uterine inversion

LEARNING OBJECTIVES

Upon completion of the chapter, the learner will be able to:

1. Define the major conditions that place the postpartum woman at risk.
2. Explain the risk factors, assessment, preventive measures, and nursing management of common postpartum complications.
3. Differentiate the causes of postpartum hemorrhage based on the underlying pathophysiologic mechanisms.
4. Outline the nurse's role in assessing and managing the care of a woman with a thromboembolic condition.
5. Discuss the nursing management of a woman who develops a postpartum infection.
6. Identify at least two affective disorders that can occur in women after birth, describing specific therapeutic management for each.

CHAPTER 22

Joan gave birth about an hour ago to her fifth baby boy, who weighed 10 pounds, and she is resting in bed when the nurse comes in to assess her. She tells the nurse that she feels like there is "something really wet" between her legs. She also feels a bit lightheaded. What would the nurse suspect is happening? What findings would support the nurse's suspicion? What should the nurse do first?

Wow

After holding their breath during the childbirth experience, nurses shouldn't let it out fully and relax until the woman and baby are discharged.

Typically, recovery from childbirth proceeds normally both physiologically and psychologically. It is a time filled with many changes and wide-ranging emotions, and the new mother commonly experiences a great sense of accomplishment. However, the woman can experience deviations from the norm, developing a postpartum condition that places her at risk. These high-risk conditions or complications can become life-threatening. Healthy People 2010 addresses these risks in two National Health Goals.

This chapter will address the nursing management of the most common conditions that place the postpartum woman at risk: hemorrhage, infection, thromboembolic disease, and postpartum affective disorders.

Postpartum Hemorrhage

Postpartum hemorrhage is a potentially life-threatening complication that can occur after both vaginal and cesarean births. It is the leading cause of maternal mortality worldwide: it is estimated that worldwide, 150,000 women die of postpartum hemorrhage annually—one every four minutes (American College of Obstetricians & Gynecologists [ACOG], 2006). More than half of all maternal deaths occur within 24 hours of giving birth, most commonly from excessive bleeding.

Postpartum hemorrhage is defined as a blood loss greater than 500 mL after vaginal birth or more than 1,000 mL after a cesarean birth. Blood loss that occurs within 24 hours of birth is termed *early postpartum hemorrhage;* blood loss that occurs 24 hours to 6 weeks after birth is termed *late postpartum hemorrhage.* However, this definition is arbitrary, because estimates of blood loss at birth are subjective and generally inaccurate. Studies have suggested that health care providers consistently underestimate actual blood loss (Smith & Brennan, 2007). A more objective definition of postpartum hemorrhage would be any amount of bleeding that places the mother in hemodynamic jeopardy.

Pathophysiology

Excessive bleeding can occur at any time between the separation of the placenta and its expulsion or removal. The most common cause of postpartum hemorrhage is **uterine atony**, failure of the uterus to contract and retract after birth. The uterus must remain contracted after birth to control bleeding from the placental site. Any factor that causes the uterus to relax after birth will cause bleeding—even a full bladder that displaces the uterus.

Over the course of a pregnancy, maternal blood volume increases by approximately 50% (from 4 to 6 L). The plasma volume increases twice as much in comparison to the total red blood cell volume. As a result, hemoglobin and hematocrit fall. The increase in blood volume meets the perfusion demands of the low-resistance uteroplacental unit and provides a reserve for the blood loss that occurs at delivery (Cunningham et al., 2005). Given this increase, the typical signs of hemorrhage (e.g., falling blood pressure, increasing pulse rate, and decreasing urinary output) do not appear until as much as 1,800 to 2,100 mL of blood has been lost (Gilbert and Harmon, 2007). In addition, accurate determination of actual blood loss is difficult because of blood pooling inside the uterus, on peripads, mattresses, and the floor. Since no universal clinical standard exists, nurses must remain vigilant, assessing for risk factors and checking clients carefully before the birth attendant leaves the birthing area.

Other causes of postpartum hemorrhage include lacerations of the genital tract, episiotomy, retained placental fragments, uterine inversion, coagulation disorders, and hematomas of the vulva, vagina, or subperitoneal areas (ACOG, 2006). A helpful way to remember the causes of postpartum hemorrhage is by using the "4 Ts": tone, tissue, trauma, and thrombosis (Anderson & Etches, 2007).

Tone

Altered uterine muscle tone most commonly results from overdistention of the uterus. Overdistention can be caused by multifetal gestation, fetal macrosomia, polyhydramnios, fetal abnormality, or placental fragments. Other causes might include prolonged or rapid, forceful labor, especially if stimulated; bacterial toxins (e.g., chorioamnionitis, endomyometritis, septicemia); use of anesthesia, especially halothane; and magnesium sulfate used in the treatment of preeclampsia (Nash, 2007). Overdistention of the uterus is a major risk factor for uterine atony, the most common cause of early postpartum hemorrhage, which can lead to hypovolemic shock.

HEALTHY PEOPLE *2010*	
Objective	Significance
Reduce maternal deaths from a baseline of 7.1 maternal deaths per 100,000 live births to 3.3 maternal deaths per 100,000 live births.	Will help foster the need for early identification of problems and prompt intervention to reduce the potential negative outcomes of pregnancy and birth
Reduce maternal illness and complications due to pregnancy	Will help to contribute to lower rates of rehospitalization, morbidity, and mortality by focusing on thorough assessments in the postpartum period
Related to postpartum complications, including postpartum depression	Will help to minimize the devastating effects of complications during the postpartum period and the woman's ability to care for her newborn

DHHS, 2000.

Tissue

Uterine contraction and retraction lead to detachment and expulsion of the placenta after birth. Classic signs of placental separation include a small gush of blood with lengthening of the umbilical cord and a slight rise of the uterus in the pelvis. Complete detachment and expulsion of the placenta permit continued contraction and optimal occlusion of blood vessels. Failure of complete placental separation and expulsion leads to retained fragments, which occupy space and prevent the uterus from contracting fully to clamp down on blood vessels; this can lead to hemorrhage. After the placenta is expelled, a thorough inspection is necessary to confirm its intactness; tears or fragments left inside may indicate an accessory lobe or placenta accreta (an uncommon condition in which the chorionic villi adhere to the myometrium, causing the placenta to adhere abnormally to the uterus and not separate and deliver spontaneously). Profuse hemorrhage results because the uterus cannot contract fully.

A prolapse of the uterine fundus to or through the cervix so that the uterus is turned inside out after birth is called **uterine inversion**. This condition is associated with grand multiparity, abnormal adherence of the placenta, excessive traction on the umbilical cord, vigorous fundal pressure, precipitous labor, or vigorous manual removal of the placenta. Acute postpartum uterine inversion is rare, with an estimated incidence of 1 in 2,000 births (Pope & O'Grady, 2006). Prompt recognition and rapid treatment to replace the inverted uterus will avoid morbidity and mortality for this serious complication (Smith & Brennan, 2006).

Subinvolution refers to incomplete involution of the uterus or failure to return to its normal size and condition after birth (Dorland, 2007). Complications of subinvolution include hemorrhage, pelvic peritonitis, salpingitis, and abscess formation (Weydert & Benda, 2006). Causes of subinvolution include retained placental fragments, distended bladder, uterine myoma, and infection. All of these conditions contribute to delayed postpartum bleeding. The clinical picture includes a postpartum fundal height that is higher than expected, with a boggy uterus; the lochia fails to change colors from red to serosa to alba within a few weeks. This condition is usually identified at the woman's postpartum examination 4 to 6 weeks after birth with a bimanual vaginal examination or ultrasound. Treatment is directed toward stimulating the uterus to expel fragments with a uterine stimulant, and antibiotics are given to prevent infection.

Trauma

Damage to the genital tract may occur spontaneously or through the manipulations used during birth. Lacerations and hematomas resulting from birth trauma can cause significant blood loss. Hematomas can present as pain or as a change in vital signs disproportionate to the amount of blood loss. Uterine inversion can occur secondary to pressure or pulling on the umbilical cord when the placenta is still firmly attached to the fundus after the infant has been born. Additionally, uterine rupture can cause damage to the genital tract and is more common in women with previous cesarean incisions or those who had undergone any procedure resulting in disruption of the uterine wall, including myomectomy, perforation of the uterus during a dilation and curettage (D&C), biopsy, or intrauterine device (IUD) insertion (Smith & Brennan, 2006).

Trauma can also occur after prolonged or vigorous labor, especially if the uterus has been stimulated with oxytocin or prostaglandins. Trauma can also occur after extrauterine or intrauterine manipulation of the fetus.

Cervical lacerations commonly occur during a forceps delivery or in mothers who have not been able to resist bearing down before the cervix is fully dilated. Vaginal sidewall lacerations are associated with operative vaginal births but may occur spontaneously, especially if the fetal hand presents with the head. Lacerations can arise during manipulations to resolve shoulder dystocia. Lacerations should always be suspected in the face of a contracted uterus with bright-red blood continuing to trickle out of the vagina.

Thrombosis

Thrombosis (blood clots) helps to prevent postpartum hemorrhage immediately after birth by providing hemostasis. Fibrin deposits and clots in supplying vessels play a significant role in the hours and days after birth. Disorders that interfere with the clot formation can lead to postpartum hemorrhage. Medication used to prevent hemorrhage by stimulating uterine contractions may delay the appearance of coagulation disorders. Coagulopathies should be suspected when postpartum bleeding persists without any identifiable cause (ACOG, 2006).

Ideally, the client's coagulation status is determined during pregnancy. However, if she received no prenatal care, coagulation studies should be ordered immediately to determine her status. Abnormal results typically include decreased platelet and fibrinogen levels, increased prothrombin time, partial thromboplastin time, and fibrin degradation products, and a prolonged bleeding time (Anderson & Etches, 2007). Conditions associated with coagulopathies in the postpartum client include idiopathic thrombocytopenic purpura, von Willebrand disease, and disseminated intravascular coagulation.

Idiopathic Thrombocytopenia Purpura

Idiopathic thrombocytopenia purpura (ITP) is a disorder of increased platelet destruction caused by the development of autoantibodies to platelet-membrane antigens. The incidence of ITP in adults is approximately 66 cases per 1 million per year (Silverman, 2007). Thrombocytopenia, capillary fragility, and increased bleeding time define the disorder, commonly manifested by easy bruising, bleeding from mucous membranes, menorrhagia, epistaxis, bleeding gums, hematomas, and severe hemorrhage after a cesarean birth or lacerations (Sood & Abrams, 2007). Glucocorticoids and immune globulin are the mainstays of medical therapy.

von Willebrand Disease

von Willebrand disease (vWD) is a congenital bleeding disorder, inherited as an autosomal dominant trait. It is characterized by a prolonged bleeding time, a deficiency of von Willebrand factor, and impairment of platelet adhesion (Dorland, 2007). In the United States, it is estimated to affect fewer than 3% of the population (Geil, 2007). Most cases remain undiagnosed due to lack of awareness, difficulty in diagnosis, a tendency to attribute bleeding to other causes, and variable symptoms (Kadir et al., 2007). The disorder is characterized by excessive bruising, prolonged nosebleeds, and prolonged oozing from wounds after surgery and after childbirth. The goal of therapy is to correct the defect in platelet adhesiveness by raising the level of von Willebrand factor with medications (Franchini & Lippi, 2007).

Disseminated Intravascular Coagulation

Disseminated intravascular coagulation (DIC) is a life-threatening, acquired pathologic process in which the clotting system is abnormally activated, resulting in widespread clot formation in the small vessels throughout the body (Levi & Schmaier, 2007). It can cause postpartum hemorrhage by altering the blood clotting mechanism. DIC is always a secondary diagnosis that occurs as a complication of abruptio placentae, amniotic fluid embolism, intrauterine fetal death with prolonged retention of the fetus, severe preeclampsia, septicemia, and hemorrhage. Clinical features include petechiae, ecchymoses, bleeding gums, fever, hypotension, acidosis, hematomas, tachycardia, proteinuria, uncontrolled bleeding during birth, and acute renal failure (Bick, 2007). Treatment goals are to maintain tissue perfusion through aggressive administration of fluid therapy, oxygen, heparin, and blood products.

Therapeutic Management

Therapeutic management focuses on the underlying cause of the hemorrhage. For example, uterine massage is used to treat uterine atony. If retained placental fragments are the cause, the fragments are usually manually separated and removed and a uterine stimulant is given to promote the uterus to expel fragments. Antibiotics are administered to prevent infection. Lacerations are sutured or repaired. Glucocorticoids and intravenous immunoglobulin, intravenous anti-RhoD, and platelet transfusions may be given. A splenectomy may be necessary if the bleeding tissues do not respond to medical management.

In vWD, there is a decrease in von Willebrand factor, which is necessary for platelet adhesion and aggregation. It binds to and stabilizes factor VIII of the coagulation cascade (Franchini & Lippi, 2007). Desmopressin, a syn-

thetic form of vasopressin (antidiuretic hormone), may be used to treat vWD. This drug stimulates the release of stored factor VIII and von Willebrand factor from the lining of blood vessels, which increases platelet adhesiveness and shortens bleeding time. Other treatments that may be ordered include clotting factor concentrates, replacement of von Willebrand factor and factor VIII (Alphanate, Humate-P); antifibrinolytics (Amicar); and nonsteroidal anti-inflammatory drugs (NSAIDs) that do not cause platelet dysfunction (Geil, 2007).

Nursing Assessment

Pregnancy and childbirth involve significant health risks, even for women with no preexisting health problems. There are an estimated 14 million cases of pregnancy-related hemorrhage every year, with some of these women bleeding to death. Most of these deaths occur within 4 hours of giving birth and are a result of problems during the third stage of labor (ACOG, 2006). The period after the birth and the first hours postpartum are crucial times for the prevention, assessment, and management of bleeding. Compared with other maternal risks such as infection, bleeding can rapidly become life-threatening, and nurses, along with other health care providers, need to identify this condition quickly and intervene appropriately.

Begin by reviewing the mother's history, including labor and birth history, for risk factors associated with postpartum hemorrhage (Box 22.1).

Since the most common cause of immediate severe postpartum hemorrhage is uterine atony (failure of the

---

BOX 22.1 **Factors Placing a Woman at Risk for Postpartum Hemorrhage**

- Prolonged first, second, or third stage of labor
- Previous history of postpartum hemorrhage
- Multiple gestation
- Fetal macrosomia
- Uterine infection
- Manual extraction of placenta
- Arrest of descent
- Maternal exhaustion, malnutrition, or anemia
- Mediolateral episiotomy
- Preeclampsia
- Precipitous birth
- Maternal hypotension
- Previous placenta previa
- Coagulation abnormalities
- Birth canal lacerations
- Operative birth (forceps or vacuum)
- Augmented labor with medication
- Coagulation abnormalities
- Grand multiparity
- Polyhydramnios (Anderson & Etches, 2007)

uterus to contract properly after birth), assess uterine tone after birth by palpating the fundus for firmness and location. A soft, boggy fundus indicates uterine atony.

> ▶ *Take* NOTE!
>
> *A soft, boggy uterus that deviates from the midline suggests that a full bladder is interfering with uterine involution. If the uterus is not in correct position (midline), it will not be able to contract to control bleeding.*

Assess the amount of bleeding. If bleeding continues even though there are no lacerations, suspect retained placental fragments. The uterus remains large with painless, dark-red bleeding mixed with clots. This cause of hemorrhage can be prevented by carefully inspecting the placenta for intactness.

If trauma is suspected, attempt to identify the source and document it. Typically, the uterus will be firm with a steady stream or trickle of unclotted bright-red blood noted in the perineum. Most deaths from postpartum hemorrhage are not due to gross bleeding, but rather to inadequate management of slow, steady blood loss (Anderson & Etches, 2007).

Assess for hematoma. The uterus would be firm, with bright-red bleeding. Observe for a localized bluish bulging area just under the skin surface in the perineal area (Fig. 22.1). Often the woman will report severe perineal or pelvic pain and will have difficulty voiding. In addition, she may exhibit hypotension, tachycardia, and anemia (Gilbert & Harmon, 2007).

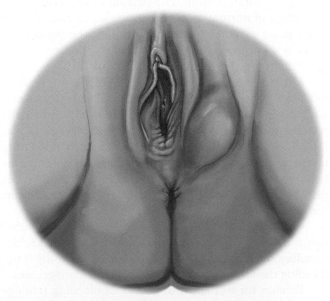

FIGURE 22.1 Perineal hematoma. Note the bulging swollen mass.

Inspect the skin and mucous membranes for gingival bleeding or petechiae and ecchymoses. Check venipuncture sites for oozing or prolonged bleeding. These findings might suggest a coagulopathy as a cause of postpartum hemorrhage. Also assess the amount of lochia, which would be much greater than usual. Urinary output would be diminished, with signs of acute renal failure. Vital signs would show an increased pulse rate and a decreased level of consciousness. However, signs of shock do not appear until hemorrhage is far advanced due to the increased fluid and blood volume of pregnancy.

Nursing Management

Massage the uterus if uterine atony is noted. The uterine muscles are sensitive to touch; massage stimulates the muscle fibers to contract. Massage the boggy uterus to stimulate contractions and expression of any accumulated blood clots while supporting the lower uterine segment. As blood pools in the vagina, stasis of blood causes clots to form; they need to be expelled as pressure is placed on the fundus. Overly forceful massage can tire the uterine muscles, resulting in further uterine atony and increased pain. See Nursing Procedure 22.1 for the steps in massaging the fundus.

If repeated fundal massage and expression of clots fail, medication is probably needed to cause the uterus to contract in order to control bleeding from the placental site. The injection of an uterotonic drug immediately after birth is an important intervention used to prevent postpartum hemorrhage. Oxytocin (Pitocin); methylergonovine maleate (Methergine); a synthetic analog of prostaglandin E1, misoprostol (Cytotec); and a derivative of prostaglandin (PGF2a), carboprost (Hemabate), are drugs used to manage postpartum hemorrhage (Drug Guide 22.1). However, misoprostol is not approved by the U.S. Food and Drug Association for this purpose. The choice of which uterotonic drug to use for management of bleeding depends on the judgment of the health care provider, the availability of drugs, and the risks and benefits of the drug.

*R*emember Joan, the woman described at the beginning of the chapter? The nurse assesses her and finds that her uterus is boggy. What would the nurse do next? What additional nursing measures might be used if Joan's fundus remains boggy? When should the health care provider be notified?

Maintain the primary IV infusion and be prepared to start a second infusion at another site if blood transfusions are necessary. Draw blood for type and cross-match and send it to the laboratory. Administer oxytocics as ordered, correlating and titrating the infusion rate to assessment findings of uterine firmness and lochia. Assess for visible vaginal bleeding, and count or weigh perineal pads.

Nursing Procedure 22.1

MASSAGING THE FUNDUS

Purpose: To Promote Uterine Contraction

1. After explaining the procedure to the woman, place one gloved hand (usually the dominant hand) on the fundus.
2. Place the other gloved hand on the area above the symphysis pubis (this helps to support the lower uterine segment).
3. With the hand on the fundus, gently massage the fundus in a circular manner. Be careful not to overmassage the fundus, which could lead to muscle fatigue and uterine relaxation.
4. Assess for uterine firmness (uterine tissue responds quickly to touch).
5. If firm, apply gentle yet firm pressure in a downward motion toward the vagina to express any clots that may have accumulated.
6. Do not attempt to express clots until the fundus is firm because the application of firm pressure on an uncontracted uterus could cause uterine inversion, leading to massive hemorrhage.
7. Assist the woman with perineal care and applying a new perineal pad.
8. Remove gloves and wash hands.

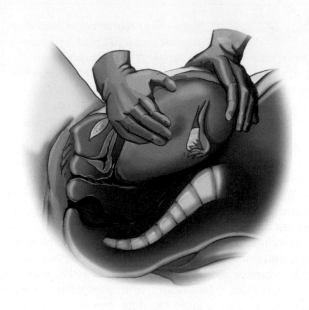

▶ *Take* NOTE!

When weighing perineal pads to determine blood loss, remember that 1 g of pad weight is equivalent to 1 mL of blood loss (Cohen, 2006).

Check vital signs every 15 to 30 minutes, depending on the acuity of the mother's health status. Monitor her complete blood count to identify any deficit or assess the adequacy of replacement. Assess the woman's level of consciousness to determine changes that may result from inadequate cerebral perfusion.

If a full bladder is present, assist the woman to empty her bladder to reduce displacement of the uterus. If the woman cannot void, anticipate the need to catheterize her to relieve bladder distention.

Prepare the woman for removal of retained placental fragments. These usually are manually separated and removed by the health care provider. Be sure that the health care provider remains long enough after birth to assess the bleeding status of the woman and determine the etiology. Assist the health care provider with suturing any lacerations immediately to control hemorrhage and repair the tissue.

Continually assess the woman for signs and symptoms of hemorrhagic shock, a condition in which inadequate perfusion of organs results in insufficient availability of oxygen to satisfy the metabolic needs of the tissues (Dorland, 2007). Subsequently a catabolic state develops, leading to inflammation, endothelial dysfunction, and disruption of normal metabolic processes in vital organs. Once these events become established, the process of shock is often irreversible, even if volume and red blood cell deficits are corrected (Cohen, 2006).

Monitor the woman's blood pressure, pulse, capillary refill, mental status, and urinary output. These assessments allow estimation of the severity of blood loss and help direct treatment. If the woman develops hemorrhagic shock, interventions focus on controlling the source of blood loss; restoring adequate oxygen-carrying capacity; and maintaining adequate tissue perfusion. Successful treatment depends on efficient collaboration among all health care team members to meet the woman's specific needs.

For the woman with ITP, expect to administer glucocorticoids, IV immunoglobulin, IV anti-RhoD, and platelet transfusions. Prepare the woman for a splenectomy if the bleeding tissues do not respond to medical management.

Be alert for women with abnormal bleeding tendencies, ensuring that they receive proper diagnosis and treatment. Teach them how to prevent severe hemorrhage by

DRUG GUIDE 22.1   DRUGS USED TO CONTROL POSTPARTUM HEMORRHAGE

Drug	Action/Indication	Nursing Implications
Oxytocin (Pitocin)	Stimulates the uterus to contract/ to contract the uterus to control bleeding from the placental site	Assess fundus for evidence of contraction and compare amount of bleeding every 15 minutes or according to orders. Monitor vital signs every 15 minutes. Monitor uterine tone to prevent hyperstimulation. Reassure client about the need for uterine contraction and administer analgesics for comfort. Offer explanation to client and family about what is happening and the purpose of the medication. Provide nonpharmacologic comfort measures to assist with pain management. Set up the IV infusion to be piggybacked into a primary IV line. This ensures that the medication can be discontinued readily if hyperstimulation or adverse effects occur while maintaining the IV site and primary infusion.
Methylergonovine maleate (Methergine)	Stimulates the uterus/to prevent and treat postpartum hemorrhage due to atony or subinvolution	Assess baseline bleeding, uterine tone, and vital signs every 15 minutes or according to protocol. Offer explanation to client and family about what is happening and the purpose of the medication. Monitor for possible adverse effects, such as hypertension, seizures, uterine cramping, nausea, vomiting, and palpitations. Report any complaints of chest pain promptly.
Prostaglandin (PGF-2α, Carboprost, Hemabate)	Stimulates uterine contractions/ to treat postpartum hemorrhage due to uterine atony when not controlled by other methods	Assess vital signs, uterine contractions, client's comfort level, and bleeding status as per protocol. Offer explanation to client and family about what is happening and the purpose of the medication. Monitor for possible adverse effects, such as fever, chills, headache, nausea, vomiting, diarrhea, flushing, and bronchospasm.

learning how to feel for and massage their fundus when boggy, assisting the nurse to keep track of the number of and amount of bleeding on perineal pads, and avoiding any medications with antiplatelet activity such as aspirin, antihistamines, or NSAIDs.

If the woman develops DIC, institute emergency measures to control bleeding and impending shock and prepare to transfer her to the intensive care unit. Identification of the underlying condition and elimination of the causative factor are essential to correct the coagulation problem. Be ready to replace fluid volume, administer blood component therapy, and optimize the mother's oxygenation and perfusion status to ensure adequate cardiac output and end-organ perfusion. Continually reassess the woman's coagulation status via laboratory studies.

Monitor vital signs closely, being alert for changes that signal an increase in bleeding or impending shock. Observe for signs of bleeding, including spontaneous bleeding from gums or nose, petechiae, excessive bleeding from the cesarean incision site, hematuria, and blood in the stool. These findings correlate with decreased blood volume, decreased organ and peripheral tissue perfusion, and clots in the microcirculation (Bick, 2007).

▶ **Take** NOTE!

Always remember the four causes of postpartum hemorrhage and the appropriate intervention for each: 1. Uterine atony—massage and oxytocics; 2. Retained placental tissue—evacuation and oxytocics; 3. Lacerations or hematoma—surgical repair; 4. Thrombosis (bleeding disorders)—blood products.

Institute measures to avoid tissue trauma or injury, such as giving injections and drawing blood. Also provide emotional support to the client and her family throughout this critical time by being readily available and providing explanations and reassurance.

An IV oxytocin infusion is started for Joan. What assessments will need to be done frequently to make sure Joan is not losing too much blood? What discharge instructions need to be reinforced with Joan?

Thromboembolic Conditions

A thrombosis (blood clot within a blood vessel) can cause an inflammation of the blood vessel lining (**thrombophlebitis**), which in turn can lead to a thromboembolism (obstruction of a blood vessel by a blood clot carried by the circulation from the site of origin). Thrombi can involve the superficial or deep veins in the legs or pelvis. Superficial venous thrombosis usually involves the saphenous venous system and is confined to the lower leg. Superficial thrombophlebitis may be caused by the use of the lithotomy position during birth. Deep venous thrombosis can involve deep veins from the foot to the calf, to the thighs, or pelvis. In both locations, thrombi can dislodge and migrate to the lungs, causing a pulmonary embolism.

The three most common thromboembolic conditions occurring during the postpartum period are superficial venous thrombosis, deep venous thrombosis, and pulmonary embolism. Although thromboembolic disorders occur in less than 1% of all postpartum women, pulmonary embolus can be fatal if a clot obstructs the lung circulation; thus, early identification and treatment are paramount.

Pathophysiology

Thrombus (blood clot) formation results typically results from venous stasis, injury to the innermost layer of the blood vessel, and hypercoagulation. Venous stasis and hypercoagulation are both common in the postpartum period.

If a clot dislodges and travels to the pulmonary circulation, pulmonary embolism can occur. Pulmonary embolism is a potentially fatal condition that occurs when the pulmonary artery is blocked by a blood clot that has traveled from another vein into the lungs, causing an obstruction and infarction. When the clot is large enough to block one or more of the pulmonary vessels that supply the lungs, it can result in sudden death. Pulmonary embolism is the leading cause of pregnancy-related death in the United States, occurring in 2 out of 100,000 live births (Shaughnessy, 2007).

Nursing Assessment

Assess the woman closely for risk factors and signs and symptoms of thrombophlebitis. Look for risk factors in the woman's history such as use of oral contraceptives before the pregnancy, smoking, employment that necessitates prolonged standing, history of thrombosis, thrombophlebitis, or endometritis, or evidence of current varicosities. Also look for other factors that can increase a woman's risk, such as prolonged bed rest, diabetes, obesity, cesarean birth, progesterone-induced distensibility of the veins of the lower legs during pregnancy, severe anemia, varicose veins, advanced maternal age (older than 35), and multiparity (Feied & Handler, 2007).

Ask the woman if she has pain or tenderness in the lower extremities. Suspect superficial venous thrombosis in a woman with varicose veins who reports tenderness and discomfort over the site of the thrombosis, most commonly in the calf area. The area appears reddened along the vein and is warm to the touch. The woman will report increased pain in the affected leg when she ambulates and bears weight.

Manifestations of deep venous thrombosis are often absent and diffuse. If they are present, they are caused by an inflammatory process and obstruction of venous return. Calf swelling, erythema, warmth, tenderness, and pedal edema may be noted. A positive Homans' sign (pain in the calf upon dorsiflexion) is not a definitive diagnostic sign and is no longer recommended as an indicator of deep vein thrombosis because calf pain can also be caused by a strained muscle or contusion (Feied & Handler, 2007).

Be alert for signs and symptoms of pulmonary embolism, including unexplained sudden onset of shortness of breath and severe chest pain. The woman may be apprehensive and diaphoretic. Additional manifestations may include tachypnea, tachycardia, hypotension, syncope, distention of the jugular vein, decreased oxygen saturation (shown by pulse oximetry), cardiac arrhythmias, hemoptysis, and a sudden change in mental status as a result of hypoxemia (Shaughnessy, 2007). Prepare the woman for a lung scan to confirm the diagnosis.

Nursing Management

Nursing management focuses on preventing thrombotic conditions, promoting adequate circulation if thrombosis occurs, and educating the client about preventive measures, anticoagulant therapy, and danger signs.

Preventing Thrombotic Conditions

Prevention of thrombotic conditions is an essential aspect of nursing management and can be achieved with the routine use of simple measures:

- Developing public awareness about risk factors, symptoms, and preventive measures
- Preventing venous stasis by encouraging activity that causes leg muscles to contract and promotes venous return (leg exercises and walking)
- Using intermittent sequential compression devices to produce passive leg muscle contractions until the woman is ambulatory
- Elevating the woman's legs above her heart level to promote venous return
- Stopping smoking to reduce or prevent vascular vasoconstriction
- Applying compression stockings and removing them daily for inspection of legs
- Performing passive range-of-motion exercises while in bed
- Using postoperative deep-breathing exercises to improve venous return by relieving the negative thoracic pressure on leg veins

- Reducing hypercoagulability with the use of warfarin, aspirin, and heparin
- Preventing venous pooling by avoiding pillows under knees, not crossing legs for long periods, and not leaving legs up in stirrups for long periods
- Padding stirrups to reduce pressure against the popliteal angle
- Avoiding sitting or standing in one position for prolonged periods
- Using a bed cradle to keep linens and blankets off extremities
- Avoiding trauma to legs to prevent injury to the vein wall
- Increasing fluid intake to prevent dehydration
- Avoiding the use of oral contraceptives

In women at risk, early ambulation is the easiest and most cost-effective method. Use of elastic compression stockings (TED hose or Jobst stockings) decrease distal calf vein thrombosis by decreasing venous stasis and augmenting venous return (Comerota & Chahwan, 2007). Women who are at a high risk for thromboembolic disease based on risk factors or a previous history of deep vein thrombosis or pulmonary embolism may be placed on prophylactic heparin therapy during pregnancy. Standard heparin or a low-molecular-weight heparin such as enoxaparin (Lovenox) can be given, since neither drug crosses the placenta. It is typically discontinued during labor and birth and then restarted during the postpartum period.

Promoting Adequate Circulation

For the woman with superficial venous thrombosis, administer NSAIDs for analgesia, provide for rest and elevation of the affected leg, apply warm compresses to the affected area to promote healing, and use antiembolism stockings to promote circulation to the extremities.

Implement bed rest and elevation of the affected extremity for the woman with deep vein thrombosis. These actions help to reduce interstitial swelling and promote venous return from that leg. Apply antiembolism stockings to both extremities as ordered. Fit the stockings correctly to avoid excess pressure and constriction and urge the woman to wear them at all times. Sequential compression devices can also be used for women with varicose veins, a history of thrombophlebitis, or a surgical birth.

Anticoagulant therapy using a continuous IV infusion of heparin usually is initiated to prolong the clotting time and prevent extension of the thrombosis. Monitor the woman's coagulation studies closely; these might include activated partial thromboplastin time (aPTT), whole blood partial thromboplastin time, and platelet levels. A therapeutic aPTT value typically ranges from 35 to 45 seconds, depending on which standard values are used (Pagana & Pagana, 2007). Also apply warm moist compresses to the affected leg and administer analgesics as ordered to decrease the discomfort.

After several days of IV heparin therapy, expect to begin oral anticoagulant therapy with warfarin (Coumadin) as ordered and monitor coagulation studies. In most cases, the woman will continue to take this medication for several months after discharge.

For the woman who develops a pulmonary embolism, institute emergency measures immediately. The objectives of treatment are to prevent growth or multiplication of thrombi in the lower extremities, prevent more thrombi from traveling to the pulmonary vascular system, and provide cardiopulmonary support if needed. Administer oxygen via mask or cannula as ordered and initiate IV heparin therapy titrated according to the results of the coagulation studies. Maintain the client on bed rest, and administer analgesics as ordered for pain relief. Be prepared to assist with administering thrombolytic agents, such as alteplase (tPA), which might be used to dissolve pulmonary emboli and the source of the thrombus in the pelvis or deep leg veins, thus reducing the potential for a recurrence.

Educating the Client

Provide teaching about the use of anticoagulant therapy and danger signs that should be reported (Teaching Guidelines 22.1). Provide anticipatory guidance, support, and education about associated signs of complications and risks. Focus teaching on the following issues:

- Elimination of modifiable risk factors for deep vein thrombosis (smoking, use of oral contraceptives, a sedentary lifestyle, and obesity)
- Importance of using compression stockings
- Avoidance of constrictive clothing and prolonged standing or sitting in a motionless, leg-dependent position
- Danger signs and symptoms (sudden onset of chest pain, dyspnea, and tachypnea) to report to the health care provider

Postpartum Infection

Infection during the postpartum period is a common cause of maternal morbidity and mortality. Overall, postpartum infection is estimated to occur in up to 8% of all births. There is a higher occurrence in cesarean births than in vaginal births (Gilbert & Harmon, 2007).

Postpartum infection is defined as a fever of 38°C or 100.4°F or higher after the first 24 hours after childbirth, occurring on at least 2 of the first 10 days after birth, exclusive of the first 24 hours (Dorland, 2007).

Infections can easily enter the female genital tract externally and ascend through the internal genital structures. In addition, the normal physiologic changes of childbirth increase the risk of infection by decreasing the vaginal acidity due to the presence of amniotic fluid, blood, and lochia, all of which are alkaline. An alkaline environment encourages the growth of bacteria.

Postpartum infections usually arise from organisms that constitute the normal vaginal flora, typically a mix of aerobic and anaerobic species. Generally, they are polymicrobial and involve the following microorganisms: *Staphylococcus aureus*, *Escherichia coli*, Klebsiella, *Gardnerella vaginalis,* gonococci, coliform bacteria, group A or B hemolytic streptococci, *Chlamydia trachomatis,* and the anaerobes that are common to bacterial vaginosis (Kennedy, 2007). Common postpartum infections include metritis, wound infections, urinary tract infections, and mastitis.

▶ METRITIS

Although usually referred to clinically as endometritis, postpartum uterine infections typically involve more than just the endometrial lining. **Metritis** is an infectious condition that involves the endometrium, decidua, and adjacent myometrium of the uterus. Extension of metritis can result in parametritis, which involves the broad ligament and possibly the ovaries and fallopian tubes, or septic pelvic thrombophlebitis, which results when the infection

spreads along venous routes into the pelvis (Simmons & Bammel, 2007).

The uterine cavity is sterile until rupture of the amniotic sac. As a consequence of labor, birth, and associated manipulations, anaerobic and aerobic bacteria can contaminate the uterus. In most cases, the bacteria responsible for pelvic infections are those that normally reside in the bowel, vagina, perineum, and cervix, such as *E. coli,* *Klebsiella pneumoniae,* or *G. vaginalis.*

The risk of metritis increases dramatically after a cesarean birth; it complicates from 10% to 20% of cesarean births. This is typically an extension of chorioamnionitis that was present before birth (indeed, that may have been why the cesarean birth was performed). In addition, trauma to the tissues and a break in the skin (incision) provide entrances for bacteria to enter the body and multiply (Kennedy, 2007).

▶ WOUND INFECTIONS

Any break in the skin or mucous membranes provides a portal for bacteria. In the postpartum woman, sites of wound infection include cesarean surgical incisions, the episiotomy site in the perineum, and genital tract lacerations (Fig. 22.2). Wound infections are usually not identified until the woman has been discharged from the hospital because symptoms may not show up until 24 to 48 hours after birth.

▶ URINARY TRACT INFECTIONS

Urinary tract infections are most commonly caused by bacteria often found in bowel flora, including *E. coli,* Klebsiella, Proteus, and Enterobacter species. Invasive manipulation of the urethra (e.g., urinary catheterization), frequent vaginal examinations, and genital trauma increase the likelihood of a urinary tract infection.

▶ MASTITIS

A common problem that may occur within the first 2 weeks postpartum is an inflammation of the breast, termed **mastitis**. It can result from any event that creates milk stasis: insufficient drainage of the breast, rapid weaning, oversupply of milk, pressure on the breast from a poorly fitting bra, a blocked duct, missed feedings, and breakdown of the nipple via fissures, cracks, or blisters (Betzold, 2007). The most common infecting organism is *S. aureus,* which comes from the breastfeeding infant's mouth or throat (Kennedy,

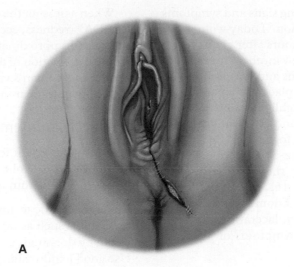
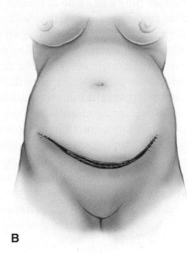

FIGURE 22.2 Postpartum wound infections. (**A**) Infected episiotomy site. (**B**) Infected cesarean birth incision.

A

B

2007). Infection can be transmitted from the lactiferous ducts to a secreting lobule, from a nipple fissure to periductal lymphatics, or by circulation (Gilbert & Harmon, 2007) (Fig. 22.3). A breast abscess may develop if mastitis is not treated adequately.

Therapeutic Management

When metritis occurs, broad-spectrum antibiotics are used to treat the infection. Management also includes measures to restore and promote fluid and electrolyte balance, provide analgesia, and provide emotional support. In most treated women, fever drops and symptoms cease within 48 to 72 hours after the start of antibiotic therapy.

Management for wound infections involves recognition of the infection, followed by opening of the wound to allow drainage. Aseptic wound management with sterile gloves and frequent dressing changes if applicable, good handwashing, frequent perineal pad changes, hydration, and ambulation to prevent venous stasis and improve circulation are initiated to prevent development of a more serious infection or spread of the infection to adjacent structures. Parenteral antibiotics are the mainstay of treatment. Analgesics are also important, because women often experience discomfort at the wound site.

If the woman develops a urinary tract infection, fluids are used to treat dehydration. Antibiotics may be ordered if appropriate.

Treatment of mastitis focuses on two areas: emptying the breasts and controlling the infection. The breast can be emptied either by the infant sucking or by manual expression. Increasing the frequency of nursing is advised. Lactation need not be suppressed. Control of infection is achieved with antibiotics. In addition, ice or warm packs and analgesics may be needed.

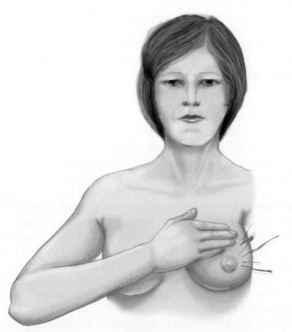

FIGURE 22.3 With mastitis, an area on one breast is tender, hot, red, and painful.

▶ *Take* NOTE!

Regardless of the etiology of mastitis, the focus is on reversing milk stasis, maintaining milk supply, and continuing breastfeeding, along with providing maternal comfort and preventing recurrence.

Nursing Assessment

Perinatal nurses are the primary caregivers for postpartum women and have a unique opportunity to identify subtle changes that place women at risk for infection.

Nurses play a key role in identifying signs and symptoms that suggest a postpartum infection. Today women are commonly discharged 24 to 48 hours after giving birth. Therefore, nurses must assess new mothers for risk factors and identify early, subtle signs and symptoms of an infectious process. Factors that place a woman at risk for a postpartum infection are highlighted in Box 22.2.

Review the client's history and physical examination and labor and birth record for factors that might increase her risk for developing an infection. Then complete the assessment (using the "BUBBLE-HE" parameters discussed in Chapter 16), paying particular attention to areas such as the abdomen and fundus, breasts, urinary tract, episiotomy, lacerations, or incisions, being alert for signs and symptoms of infection (Table 22.1).

▶ *Take* NOTE!

A postpartum infection is commonly associated with an elevated temperature, as mentioned previously. Other generalized signs and symptoms may include chills, foul-smelling vaginal discharge, headache, malaise, restlessness, anxiety, and tachycardia. In addition, the woman may have specific signs and symptoms based on the type and location of the infection.

When assessing the episiotomy site, use the acronym "REEDA" (redness, ecchymosis, edema, drainage or discharge, and approximation of wound edges) to ensure complete evaluation of the site (Arenson & Drake, 2007). Monitor the woman's vital signs, especially her temperature, for changes that may signal an infection.

Nursing Management

Nursing management focuses on preventing postpartum infections. Use the following guidelines to reduce the incidence of postpartum infections:

- Maintain aseptic technique when performing invasive procedures such as urinary catheterization, when changing dressings, and during all surgical procedures.
- Use good handwashing technique before and after each client care activity.
- Reinforce measures for maintaining good perineal hygiene.
- Use adequate lighting and turn the client to side to assess the episiotomy site.
- Screen all visitors for any signs of active infections to reduce the client's risk of exposure.
- Review the client's history for preexisting infections or chronic conditions.
- Monitor vital signs and laboratory results for any abnormal values.
- Monitor the frequency of vaginal examinations and length of labor.

BOX 22.2 **Factors Placing a Woman at Risk for Postpartum Infection**

- Prolonged (>18 to 24 hours) premature rupture of membranes (removes the barrier of amniotic fluid so bacteria can ascend)
- Cesarean birth (allows bacterial entry due to break in protective skin barrier)
- Urinary catheterization (could allow entry of bacteria into bladder due to break in aseptic technique)
- Regional anesthesia that decreases perception to void (causes urinary stasis and increases risk of urinary tract infection)
- Staff attending to woman are ill (promotes droplet infection from personnel)
- Compromised health status, such as anemia, obesity, smoking, drug abuse (reduces the body's immune system and decreases ability to fight infection)
- Preexisting colonization of lower genital tract with bacterial vaginosis, *Chlamydia trachomatis*, group B streptococci, *Staphylococcus aureus*, and *Escherichia coli* (allows microbes to ascend)
- Retained placental fragments (provides medium for bacterial growth)

- Manual removal of a retained placenta (causes trauma to the lining of the uterus and thus opens up sites for bacterial invasion)
- Insertion of fetal scalp electrode or intrauterine pressure catheters for internal fetal monitoring during labor (provides entry into uterine cavity)
- Instrument-assisted childbirth, such as forceps or vacuum extraction (increases risk of trauma to genital tract, which provides bacteria access to grow)
- Trauma to the genital tract, such as episiotomy or lacerations (provides a portal of entry for bacteria)
- Prolonged labor with frequent vaginal examinations to check progress (allows time for bacteria to multiply and increases potential exposure to microorganisms or trauma)
- Poor nutritional status (reduces body's ability to repair tissue)
- Gestational diabetes (decreases body's healing ability and provides higher glucose levels on skin and in urine, which encourages bacterial growth)
- Break in aseptic technique during surgery or birthing process (allows entry of bacteria)

TABLE 22.1 SIGNS AND SYMPTOMS OF POSTPARTUM INFECTIONS

Postpartum Infection	Signs and Symptoms
Metritis	Lower abdominal tenderness or pain on one or both sides
	Temperature elevation (>38°C)
	Foul-smelling lochia
	Anorexia
	Nausea
	Fatigue and lethargy
	Leukocytosis and elevated sedimentation rate
Wound infection	Weeping serosanguineous or purulent drainage
	Separation of or unapproximated wound edges
	Edema
	Erythema
	Tenderness
	Discomfort at the site
	Maternal fever
	Elevated white blood cell count
Urinary tract infection	Urgency
	Frequency
	Dysuria
	Flank pain
	Low-grade fever
	Urinary retention
	Hematuria
	Urine positive for nitrates
	Cloudy urine with strong odor
Mastitis	Flulike symptoms, including malaise, fever, and chills
	Tender, hot, red, painful area on one breast
	Inflammation of breast area
	Breast tenderness
	Cracking of skin or around nipple or areola
	Breast distention with milk

- Assess frequently for early signs of infection, especially fever and the appearance of lochia.
- Inspect wounds frequently for inflammation and drainage.
- Encourage rest, adequate hydration, and healthy eating habits.
- Reinforce preventive measures during any interaction with the client.

If the woman develops an infection, review treatment measures, such as antibiotic therapy if ordered, and any special care measures, such as dressing changes, that might be needed (Nursing Care Plan 22.1).

Client teaching is a priority due to today's short lengths of stay after delivery. Some infections may not manifest until after discharge. Review the signs and symptoms of infection, emphasizing the danger signs that need to be reported to the health care provider. Most importantly, stress proper handwashing, especially after perineal care and before and after breastfeeding. Also reinforce measures to promote breastfeeding, including proper breast care (see Chapter 16). Teaching Guidelines 22.2 highlights the major teaching points for a woman with a postpartum infection.

Postpartum Affective Disorders

The postpartum period involves extraordinary physiologic, psychological, and sociocultural changes in the life

Nursing Care Plan 22.1

OVERVIEW OF THE WOMAN WITH A POSTPARTUM COMPLICATION

Jennifer, a 16-year-old G1P1, gave birth to a boy 3 days ago. It was a cesarean birth due to cephalopelvic disproportion following 25 hours of labor with ruptured membranes. Her temperature is 102.6° F (39.2° C). She is complaining of chills and malaise and says, "My incision really hurts." Jennifer rates her pain as 7 to 8 out of 10. The incision site is red, swollen, and very warm to the touch. A 5-cm area of purulent drainage is noted on the dressing; a 3-cm area of the incision is slightly opened, with the wound edges separated. Jennifer's lochia is scant and dark red, with a strong odor. She asks the nurse to take her baby back to the nursery because she doesn't feel well enough to care for him.

NURSING DIAGNOSIS: Ineffective thermoregulation related to bacterial invasion *as evidenced by fever, complaints of chills and malaise, and statement of not feeling well*

Outcome Identification and Evaluation
Jennifer will exhibit a return to normothermia *as evidenced by a body temperature being maintained below 99° F, reports of a decrease in chills and malaise, and statements of feeling better.*

Interventions: Promoting Fever Reduction
- Assess vital signs every 2 to 4 hours and record results *to monitor progress of infection.*
- Administer antipyretics as ordered *to reduce temperature and help combat infection.*
- Encourage fluid intake *to promote fluid balance.*
- Document intake and output *to assess hydration status.*
- Offer cool bed bath or shower *to reduce temperature.*
- Place cool cloth on forehead and/or back of neck *for comfort.*
- Change bed linen and gown when damp from diaphoresis *to provide comfort and hygiene.*

NURSING DIAGNOSIS: Impaired skin integrity related to wound infection as *evidenced by purulent drainage, redness, swelling, and separation of wound edges*

Outcome Identification and Evaluation
Jennifer will experience a resolution of wound infection as *evidenced by a reduction in redness, swelling, and drainage from wound, absence of purulent drainage, and beginning signs and symptoms of wound healing.*

Interventions: Promoting Wound Healing
- Administer antibiotic therapy as ordered *to treat infection.*
- Perform frequent dressing changes and wound care as ordered *to promote wound healing;* monitor dressing for drainage, including amount, color, and characteristics, *to evaluate for resolution of infection.*
- Use aseptic technique *to prevent spread of infection.*
- Encourage fluid intake *to maintain fluid balance;* encourage adequate dietary intake, including protein, *to promote healing.*

NURSING DIAGNOSIS: Acute pain related to infectious process

Outcome Identification and Evaluation
Client reports a decrease in pain *as evidenced by pain rating of 0 or 1 on pain scale; verbalization of relief with pain management, and statements of feeling better and ability to rest comfortably.*

Interventions: Relieving Pain
- Place client in semi-Fowler's position *to facilitate drainage and relieve pressure.*
- Assess pain level on pain scale of 0 to 10 *to quantify pain level;* reassess pain level after intervening *to determine effectiveness of intervention.*
- Assess fundus gently *to ensure appropriate involution.*
- Administer analgesics as needed and on time as ordered *to maintain pain relief.*
- Provide for rest periods *to allow for healing.*
- Assist with positioning in bed with pillows *to promote comfort.*
- Offer nonpharmacologic pain measures such as a backrub *to ease aches and discomfort if desired and enhance effectiveness of analgesics.*

Nursing Care Plan 22.1 (continued)

NURSING DIAGNOSIS: Risk for impaired parent–infant attachment related to effects of postpartum infection *as evidenced by mother's request to take baby back to the nursery*

Outcome Identification and Evaluation

Jennifer begins to bond with newborn appropriately with each exposure *as evidenced by desire to spend time with newborn, expression of positive feelings toward newborn when holding him, increasing participation in care of newborn as client's condition improves, and statements about help and support at home to care for self and newborn.*

Interventions: Promoting Mother–Newborn Interaction

- Promote adequate rest and sleep *to ensure adequate energy for interaction and wound healing.*
- Bring newborn to mother after she is rested and had an analgesic *to allow mother to focus her energies on the child.*
- Progressively allow the client to care for her infant or comfort him as her energy level and pain level improve *to promote self-confidence in caring for the newborn.*
- Offer praise and positive reinforcement for caretaking tasks; stress positive attributes of newborn to mother while caring for him *to facilitate bonding and attachment.*
- Contact family members to participate in care of the newborn *to allow mother to rest and recover from infection.*
- Encourage mother to care for herself first and then the newborn *to ensure adequate energy for newborn's care.*
- Arrange for assistance and support after discharge from hospital *to provide necessary backup.*
- Refer to community health nurse for follow-up care of mother and newborn at home *to foster continued development of maternal–infant relationship.*

---

of a woman and her family. It is an exhilarating time for most women, but for others it may not be what they had expected. Women have varied reactions to their childbearing experiences, exhibiting a wide range of emotions. Typically, the delivery of a newborn is associated with positive feelings such as happiness, joy, and gratitude for the birth of a healthy infant. However, women may also feel weepy, overwhelmed, or unsure of what is happening to them. They may experience fear about loss of control; they may feel scared, alone, or guilty, or as if they have somehow failed.

Postpartum affective disorders have been documented for years, but only recently have they received medical attention. Plummeting levels of estrogen and progesterone immediately after birth can contribute to postpartum mood disorders. It is believed that the greater the change in these hormone levels between pregnancy and postpartum, the greater the chance for developing a mood disorder (Edler, Jones, & Venis, 2007).

Many types of affective disorders occur in the postpartum period. Although their description and classification may be controversial, the disorders are commonly classified on the basis of their severity as postpartum or baby blues, postpartum depression, and postpartum psychosis.

POSTPARTUM OR BABY BLUES

Many postpartum women (approximately 50% to 90%) experience the "baby blues" (ACOG, 2007). The woman exhibits mild depressive symptoms of anxiety, irritability, mood swings, tearfulness, increased sensitivity, feelings of being overwhelmed, and fatigue (Edler, Jones, & Venis, 2007). The "blues" typically peak on postpartum days 4 and 5 and usually resolve by postpartum day 10. Although the woman's symptoms may be distressing, they do not reflect psychopathology and usually do not affect the mother's ability to function and care for her infant.

Baby blues are usually self-limiting and require no formal treatment other than reassurance and validation of the woman's experience, as well as assistance in caring for herself and the newborn. However, follow-up of women with postpartum blues is important, because up to 20% go on to develop postpartum depression (Alexander et al., 2007).

POSTPARTUM DEPRESSION

Depression is more prevalent in women than in men, which may be related to biological, hormonal, and psychosocial factors. If the symptoms of postpartum blues last beyond 6 weeks and seem to get worse, the mother may be experiencing **postpartum depression**, a major depressive episode associated with childbirth (Edler, Jones, & Venis, 2007). As many as 20% of all mothers develop postpartum depression (ACOG, 2007). It affects approximately 500,000 mothers in the United States each year, and about half of these women receive no mental health evaluation or treatment (ACOG, 2007). Unlike the postpartum blues, women with postpartum depression feel

TEACHING GUIDELINES 22.2

Teaching for the Woman With a Postpartum Infection

- Continue your antibiotic therapy as prescribed.
  - Take the medication exactly as ordered and continue with the medication until it is finished.
  - Do not stop taking the medication even when you are feeling better.
- Check your temperature every day and call your health care provider if it is above 100.4°F (38°C).
- Watch for other signs and symptoms of infection, such as chills, increased abdominal pain, change in the color or odor of your lochia, or increased redness, warmth, swelling, or drainage from a wound site such as your cesarean incision or episiotomy. Report any of these to your health care provider immediately.
- Practice good infection prevention:
  - Always wash your hands thoroughly before and after eating, using the bathroom, touching your perineal area, or providing care for your newborn.
  - Wipe from front to back after using the bathroom.
  - Remove your perineal pad using a front-to-back motion. Fold the pad in half so that the inner sides of the pad that were touching your body are against each other. Wrap in toilet tissue or place in a plastic bag and discard.
  - Wash your hands before applying a new pad.
  - Apply a new perineal pad using a front-to-back motion. Handle the pad by the edges (top and bottom or sides) and avoid touching the inner aspect of the pad that will be against your body.
  - When performing perineal care with the peri-bottle, angle the spray of water to that it flows from front to back.
  - Drink plenty of fluids each day and eat a variety of foods that are high in vitamins, iron, and protein.
  - Be sure to get adequate rest at night and periodically throughout the day.

▶ *Consider* THIS!

As an assertive practicing attorney in her thirties, my first pregnancy was filled with nagging feelings of doubt about this upcoming event in my life. Throughout my pregnancy I was so busy with trial work that I never had time to really evaluate my feelings. I was always reading about the bodily changes that were taking place, and on one level I was feeling excited, but on another level I was emotionally drained. Shortly after the birth of my daughter, those suppressed nagging feelings of doubt surfaced big time and practically immobilized me. I felt exhausted all the time and was only too glad to have someone else care for my daughter. I didn't breastfeed because I thought it would tie me down too much. Although at the time I thought this "low mood" was normal for all new mothers, I have since found out it was postpartum depression. How could any woman be depressed about this wondrous event?

Thoughts: Now that postpartum depression has been "taken out of the closet" and recognized as a real emotional disorder, it can be treated. This woman showed tendencies during her pregnancy but was able to suppress the feelings and go forward. Her description of her depression is very typical of many women who suffer in silence, hoping to get over these feelings in time. What can nurses do to promote awareness of this disorder? Can it be prevented?

Practice 22.1). Prophylaxis starts with a prenatal risk assessment and education. Based on the woman's history of prior depression, prophylactic antidepressant therapy may be needed during the third trimester or immediately after giving birth. Management mirrors that of any major depression—a combination of antidepressant medication, antianxiety medication, and psychotherapy in an outpatient or inpatient setting (Jung et al., 2007). Marital counseling may be necessary if marital problems are contributing to the woman's depressive symptoms.

worse over time, and changes in mood and behavior do not go away on their own.

Postpartum depression affects not only the woman but also the entire family. Identifying depression early can substantially improve the client and family outcomes. Postpartum depression usually has a more gradual onset and becomes evident within the first 6 weeks postpartum.

Postpartum depression may lend itself to prophylactic intervention because its onset is predictable, the risk period for illness is well defined, and women at high risk potentially could be identified using a screening tool. This is not the case for all women, however (see Evidence-Based

▶ POSTPARTUM PSYCHOSIS

At the severe end of the continuum of postpartum emotional disorders is postpartum psychosis, which occurs in one or two women per 1,000 births (Edler, Jones, & Venis, 2007). It generally surfaces within 3 weeks of giving birth and is manifested by sleep disturbances, fatigue, depression, and hypomania. The mother will be tearful, confused, and preoccupied with feelings of guilt and worthlessness. Early symptoms resemble those of depression, but they may escalate to delirium, hallucinations, anger toward her-

EVIDENCE-BASED PRACTICE 22.1
Preventing Postpartum Depression Using Psychosocial Interventions

● Study

Postpartum depression can be a devastating condition for women and their families. There is a lack of knowledge about its cause, and women receive limited education about the possibility of depression after birth. Research has shown the effectiveness of treatment strategies that integrate psychosocial and psychological variables. The question then arises that if management addressing these variables is effective, would psychosocial interventions provided during pregnancy and the early postpartum period be effective in preventing postpartum depression?

Two reviewers searched multiple databases and contacted experts in the field. They also scanned secondary references and contacted several trial researchers for additional information. Both reviewers were involved in evaluating the methodology of the study and in extracting data. Information was gathered from all published and unpublished randomized controlled trials that compared psychosocial or psychological interventions with typical care during the antepartal, intrapartal, and postpartal periods. The researchers used relative risk for categorical data and weighted mean difference for continuous data. The study included 15 trials involving over 7,600 women.

▲ Findings

Women who received some type of psychosocial intervention had the same risk for developing postpartum depression as the women who received routine care; thus, the psychosocial intervention was not effective in preventing postpartum depression. However, statistical analysis found that intensive psychosocial support from public health nurses or midwives in the postpartum period was beneficial. The use of psychosocial interventions primarily during the postpartum period also was more effective than when these interventions were also used in the prenatal period. Interventions focusing on women at risk appear to be more effective than those geared to the overall maternal population. Individualized interventions were found to be more effective than those designed for groups. However, the risk for developing postpartum depression for either group did not differ significantly.

■ Nursing Implications

Although the study failed to identify effective measures for preventing postpartum depression, it did provide some useful information for nurses to incorporate when providing care to pregnant women throughout the perinatal period. Nurses need to remain alert for risk factors associated with postpartum depression so they can initiate appropriate interventions for these at-risk women. Nurses can implement psychosocial interventions during the prenatal period, keeping in mind that these interventions need to be continued throughout the postpartum period. They can also advocate for their clients upon discharge to ensure appropriate follow-up and support in the community.

Dennis, C.-L., & Creedy, D. (2004). Psychosocial and psychological interventions for preventing postpartum depression. *Cochrane Database of Systematic Reviews 2004,* Issue 4. Art. No.: CD001134. DOI:10.1002/14651858.CD001134.pub2.

---

self and her infant, bizarre behavior, manifestations of mania, and thoughts of hurting herself and the infant. The mother frequently loses touch with reality and experiences a severe regressive breakdown, associated with a high risk of suicide or infanticide (Johnson, 2007).

Most women with postpartum psychosis are hospitalized for up to several months. Psychotropic drugs are almost always part of treatment, along with individual psychotherapy and support group therapy.

> ▶ **Take** NOTE!
>
> *The greatest hazard of postpartum psychosis is suicide. Infanticide and child abuse are also risks if the woman is left alone with her infant. Early recognition and prompt treatment of this disorder are imperative.*

Nursing Assessment

Postpartum affective disorders are often overlooked and go unrecognized despite the large percentage of women who experience them. The postpartum period is a time of increased vulnerability, but few women receive education about the possibility of depression after birth. In addition, many women may feel ashamed of having negative emotions at a time when they "should" be happy; thus, they don't seek professional help. Nurses can play a major role in providing guidance about postpartum affective disorders, detecting manifestations, and assisting women to obtain appropriate care.

Begin the assessment by reviewing the history to identify general risk factors that could predispose a woman to depression:

- Poor coping skills
- Low self-esteem
- Numerous life stressors

- Mood swings and emotional stress
- Previous psychological problems or a family history of psychiatric disorders
- Substance abuse
- Limited or lack of social support network

Also review the history for specific pregnancy and birth factors that may increase the woman's risk for depression. These may include a history of postpartum depression, evidence of depression during the pregnancy, prenatal anxiety, a difficult or complicated pregnancy, traumatic birth experience, or birth of a high-risk or special-needs infant (Johnson, 2007).

Be alert for physical findings. Assess the woman's activity level, including her level of fatigue. Ask about her sleeping habits, noting any problems with insomnia. When interacting with the woman, observe for verbal and non-verbal indicators of anxiety as well as her ability to concentrate during the interaction. Difficulty concentrating and anxious behaviors suggest a problem. Also assess her nutritional intake: weight loss due to poor food intake may be seen. Assessment can identify women with a high-risk profile for depression, and the nurse can educate them and make referrals for individual or family counseling if needed. Some common assessment findings associated with postpartum depression are listed in Box 22.3.

Nursing Management

Nursing management focuses on assisting any postpartum woman to cope with the changes of this period. Encourage the client to verbalize what she is going through and emphasize the importance of keeping her expectations realistic. Assist the woman in structuring her day to regain a sense of control over the situation. Encourage her to seek help if necessary, using available support systems. Also reinforce the need for good nutrition and adequate exercise and sleep (Linter & Gray, 2006).

The nurse can play an important role in assisting women and their partners with postpartum adjustment. Providing facts about the enormous changes that occur during the postpartum period is critical. This information would include changes in the woman's body. Review the signs and symptoms of all three affective disorders. This information is typically included as part of prenatal visits and childbirth education classes. Know the risk factors associated with these disorders and review the history of clients and their families. Use specific, nonthreatening questions to aid in early detection, such as, "Have you felt down, depressed, or hopeless lately? Have you felt little interest or pleasure in doing things recently?"

Discuss factors that may increase a woman's vulnerability to stress during the postpartum period, such as sleep deprivation and unrealistic expectations, so couples can understand and respond to those problems if they occur. Stress that many women need help after childbirth and that help is available from many sources, including people they already know. Assisting women to learn how to ask for help is important so they can gain the support they need. Also provide educational materials about postpartum emotional disorders. Have available referral sources for psychotherapy and support groups appropriate for women experiencing postpartum adjustment difficulties.

■■■ Key Concepts

- Postpartum hemorrhage is a potentially life-threatening complication of both vaginal and cesarean births. It is the leading cause of maternal mortality in the United States.
- A good way to remember the causes of postpartum hemorrhage is the "4 Ts": tone, tissue, trauma, and thrombosis.
- Uterine atony is the most common cause of early postpartum hemorrhage, which can lead to hypovolemic shock.
- Oxytocin (Pitocin), methylergonovine maleate (Methergine), and prostaglandin PGF2a (Hemabate) are drugs used to manage postpartum hemorrhage.
- Failure of the placenta to separate completely and be expelled interferes with the ability of the uterus to contract fully, thereby leading to hemorrhage.
- Causes of subinvolution include retained placental fragments, distended bladder, uterine myoma, and infection.
- Lacerations should always be suspected when the uterus is contracted and bright-red blood continues to trickle out of the vagina.
- Conditions that cause coagulopathies may include idiopathic thrombocytopenic purpura (ITP), von Willebrand disease (vWD), and disseminated intravascular coagulation (DIC).

> ### BOX 22.3 Common Assessment Findings Associated With Postpartum Depression
>
> - Loss of pleasure or interest in life
> - Low mood, sadness, tearfulness
> - Exhaustion that is not relieved by sleep
> - Feelings of guilt
> - Irritability
> - Inability to concentrate
> - Anxiety
> - Despair
> - Compulsive thoughts
> - Loss of libido
> - Loss of confidence
> - Sleep difficulties (insomnia)
> - Loss of appetite
> - Feelings of failure as a mother (Litner & Gray, 2006)

■ Pulmonary embolism is a potentially fatal condition that occurs when the pulmonary artery is obstructed by a blood clot that has traveled from another vein into the lungs, causing obstruction and infarction.

■ The major causes of a thrombus formation (blood clot) are venous stasis and hypercoagulation, both common in the postpartum period.

■ Postpartum infection is defined as a fever of 38° C (100.4° F) or higher after the first 24 hours after childbirth, occurring on at least 2 of the first 10 days exclusive of the first 24 hours.

■ Common postpartum infections include metritis, wound infections, urinary tract infections, and mastitis.

■ Postpartum emotional disorders are commonly classified on the basis of their severity: "baby blues," postpartum depression, and postpartum psychosis.

■ Management of postpartum depression mirrors the treatment of any major depression—a combination of antidepressant medication, antianxiety medication, and psychotherapy in an outpatient or inpatient setting.

REFERENCES

Alexander, L. L., LaRosa, J. H., Bader, H., & Garfield, S. (2007). *New dimensions in women's health* (4th ed.). Sudbury, MA: Jones and Bartlett Publishers.

American College of Obstetricians and Gynecologists (ACOG). (2006). Clinical management guidelines: Postpartum hemorrhage. ACOG Practice Bulletin Number 76. *Obstetrics and Gynecology, 108*(4), 1039–1047.

American College of Obstetricians and Gynecologists (ACOG). (2007). *Spotlight on postpartum depression.* ACOG News Release. Available at: http://www.acog.org/from_home/publications/press_releases/nr02-30-07-2.cfm.

Anderson, J. M., & Etches, D. (2007). Prevention and management of postpartum hemorrhage. *American Family Physician, 75*(6), 875–882.

Arenson, J., & Drake, P. (2007). *Maternal and newborn health.* Sudbury, MA: Jones and Bartlett Publishers.

Betzold, C. M. (2007). An update on the recognition and management of lactational breast inflammation. *Journal of Midwifery & Women's Health, 52*(6), 595–605.

Bick, R. L. (2007). Disseminated intravascular coagulation. In R. E. Rakel & E. T. Bope (Eds.), *Conn's current therapy 2007* (Section 6, pp. 502–505). Philadelphia: Saunders Elsevier.

Cohen, W. R. (2006). Hemorrhagic shock in obstetrics. *Journal of Perinatal Medicine, 34*(4), 271–280.

Comerota, A. J., & Chahwan, S. (2007). Venous thrombosis. In R. E. Rakel & E. T. Bope (Eds.), *Conn's current therapy 2007* (Section 5, pp. 435–445). Philadelphia: Saunders Elsevier.

Cunningham, F. G., Gant, N. F., & Leveno, K. J. (2005). Conduct of normal labor and delivery. In: *Williams' obstetrics* (22nd ed., pp. 320–325). New York: McGraw-Hill.

Dennis, C. L., & Creedy, D. (2004). Psychosocial and psychological interventions for preventing postpartum depression. *Cochrane Database of Systematic Reviews 2004,* Issue 4. Art. No.: CD001134. DOI:10.1002/14651858.CD001134.pub2.

Dorland, W. A. N. (2007). *Dorland's illustrated medical dictionary* (30th ed.). St. Louis, MO: Saunders Elsevier.

Edler, C. R., Jones, H. W., & Venis, J. A. (2007). Beyond the baby blues: Postpartum depression. *Nursing Spectrum.* Available at: http://nsweb.nursingspectrum.com/ce/ce72d.htm.

Feied, C., & Handler, J. A. (2007). Thrombophlebitis. *eMedicine.* Available at: http://www.emedicine.com/emerg/topic582.htm.

Franchini, M., & Lippi, G. (2007). The role of von Willebrand factor in hemorrhagic and thrombotic disorders. *Critical Reviews in Clinical Laboratory Sciences, 44*(2), 115–149.

Geil, J. D. (2007). Von Willebrand disease. *eMedicine.* Available at: http://emedicine.com/ped/topic2419.htm.

Gilbert, E. S., & Harmon, J. S. (2007). *Manual of high-risk pregnancy and delivery* (4th ed.). St. Louis, MO: Mosby Elsevier.

Johnson, R. (2007). Mental illness in primary women's health care. In B. Hackley, J. M. Kriebs, & M. E. Rousseau (Eds.), *Primary care of women: A guide for midwives and women's health providers* (Chapter 9, pp. 249–312). Sudbury, MA: Jones and Bartlett Publishers.

Jung, V., Short, R., Letourneau, N., & Andrews, D. (2007). Interventions with depressed mothers and their infants: Modifying interactive behaviors. *Journal of Affective Disorders, 98*(3), 199–205.

Kadir, R. A., Kingman, C. E., Chi, C., Lee, C. A., & Economides, D. L. (2007). Is primary postpartum hemorrhage a good predictor of inherited bleeding disorders? *Hemophilia, 13*(2), 178–181.

Kennedy, E. (2007). Postpartum infections. *eMedicine.* Available at: http://www.emedicine.com/emerg/topic482.htm.

Levi, M., & Schmaier, A. H. (2007). Disseminated intravascular coagulation. *eMedicine.* Available at: http://www.emedicine.com/med/topic577.htm.

Lintner, N. C., & Gray, B. A. (2006). Childbearing and depression. *AWHONN Lifelines, 10*(1), 50–57.

MacMullen, N. J., Dulski, L. A., & Meagher, B. (2005). Red alert: Perinatal hemorrhage. *MCN, 30*(1), 46–51.

Nash, J. (2007). Postpartum care. In R. E. Rakel & E. T. Bope (Eds.), *Conn's current therapy 2007* (Section 16, pp. 1190–1193). Philadelphia: Saunders Elsevier.

Pagana, K. D., & Pagana, T. J. (2007). *Mosby's diagnostic and laboratory test reference* (8th ed.). St. Louis, MO: Mosby Elsevier.

Pope, C. S., & O'Grady, J. P. (2006). Malposition of the uterus. *eMedicine.* Available at: http://www.emedicine.com/med/topic3473.htm.

Shaughnessy, K. (2007). Massive pulmonary embolism. *Critical Care Nurse, 27*(1), 39–50.

Silverman, M. A. (2007). Idiopathic thrombocytopenic purpura. *eMedicine.* Available at: http://www.emedicine.com/emerg/topic282.htm.

Simmons, G. T., & Bammel, B. M. (2007). Endometritis. *eMedicine.* Available at: http://www.emedicine.com/MED/topic676.htm.

Smith, J. R., & Brennan, B. G. (2006). Management of the third stage of labor. *eMedicine.* Available at: http://www.emedicine.com/med/topic3569.htm.

Smith, J. R., & Brennan, B. G. (2007). Postpartum hemorrhage. *eMedicine.* Available at: http://emedicine.com/med/topic3568.htm.

Sood, S., & Abrams, C. S. (2007). Platelet-mediated bleeding disorders. In R. E. Rakel & E. T. Bope (Eds.), *Conn's current therapy 2007* (Section 6, pp. 499–501). Philadelphia: Saunders Elsevier.

U.S. Department of Health and Human Services (USDHHS), Public Health Service. (2000). *Healthy People 2010* (conference edition, in two volumes). U.S. Department of Health and Human Services. Washington, DC: U.S. Government Printing Office.

Weydert, J. A., & Benda, J. A. (2006). Subinvolution of the placental site as an anatomic cause of postpartum uterine bleeding. *Archives of Pathology & Laboratory Medicine, 130*(10), 1538–1542.

WEBSITES

A Place to Remember: www.aplacetoremember.com
Center for Postpartum Health: http://www.postpartumhealth.com
Depression: www.nimh.nih.gov/publicat/depwomenknows.cfm
Depression After Delivery, Inc. (D.A.D.): www.depressionafterdelivery.com
International Childbirth Educator's Association: www.icea.org
LaLeche League & Breastfeeding Resource Center: www.lalecheleague.org
Learning about von Willebrand Disease: www.allaboutbleeding.com
National Hemophilia Foundation: www.hemophilia.org
National Institute of Mental Health: www.nimh.nih.gov
National Women's Health Information Center: www.4women.gov
Parents Helping Parents: www.php.com
Postpartum Support International: www.postpartum.net
World Federation of Hemophilia: www.wfh.org

CHAPTER WORKSHEET

MULTIPLE CHOICE QUESTIONS

1. A postpartum mother appears very pale and states she is bleeding heavily. The nurse should first:

   a. Call the client's health care provider immediately.

   b. Immediately set up an intravenous infusion of magnesium sulfate.

   c. Assess the fundus and ask her about her voiding status.

   d. Reassure the mother that this is a normal finding after childbirth.

2. A postpartum woman reports hearing voices and says, "The voices are telling me to do bad things." The nurse interprets these findings as suggesting:

   a. Postpartum psychosis

   b. Postpartum anxiety disorder

   c. Postpartum depression

   d. Postpartum blues

3. When implementing the plan of care for a postpartum woman who gave birth just a few hours ago, the nurse vigilantly monitors the client for which complication?

   a. Deep vein thrombosis

   b. Postpartum psychosis

   c. Uterine infection

   d. Postpartum hemorrhage

4. Which of the following would the nurse expect to include in the plan of care for a woman with mastitis who is receiving antibiotic therapy?

   a. Stop breastfeeding and apply lanolin.

   b. Administer analgesics and bind both breasts.

   c. Apply warm or cold compresses and administer analgesics.

   d. Remove the nursing bra and expose the breast to fresh air.

5. While assessing a postpartum multiparous woman, the nurse detects a boggy uterus midline 2 cm above the umbilicus. Which intervention would be the priority?

   a. Assessing vital signs immediately

   b. Measuring her next urinary output

   c. Massaging her fundus

   d. Notifying the woman's obstetrician

6. Methergine has been ordered for a postpartum woman because of excessive bleeding. The nurse should question this order if which of the following is present?

   a. Minimal lochia flow

   b. Tender inflamed breasts

   c. Pulse rate of 68 beats per minute

   d. Blood pressure of 158/96 mm Hg

CRITICAL THINKING EXERCISES

1. Mrs. Griffin had a 22-hour labor before a cesarean birth. Her membranes ruptured 20 hours before she came to the hospital. Her fetus showed signs of fetal distress, so internal electronic fetal monitoring was used. Her most recent test results indicate she is anemic.

   a. What postpartum complication is this new mother at highest risk for? Why?

   b. What assessments need to be done to detect this complication?

   c. What nursing measures will the nurse use to prevent this complication?

2. Tammy, a 32-year-old G9P9, had a spontaneous vaginal birth 2 hours ago. Tammy has been having a baby each year for the past 9 years. Her lochia has been heavy, with some clots. She hasn't been up to void since she had epidural anesthesia and has decreased sensation to her legs.

   a. What factors place Tammy at risk for postpartum hemorrhage?

   b. What assessments are needed before planning interventions?

   c. What nursing actions are needed to prevent a postpartum hemorrhage?

3. Lucy, a 25-year-old G2P2, gave birth 2 days ago and is expected to be discharged today. She had severe postpartum depression 2 years ago with her first child. Lucy has not been out of bed for the past 24 hours, is not eating, and provides no care for herself or her newborn. Lucy states she already has a boy at home and not having a girl this time is disappointing.

   a. What factors/behaviors place Lucy at risk for an affective disorder?

   b. Which interventions might be appropriate at this time?

   c. What education does the family need prior to discharge?

STUDY ACTIVITIES

1. Compare and contrast postpartum blues, postpartum depression, and postpartum psychosis in terms of their features and medical management.

2. Select a website from the ones listed at the end of the chapter. Critique it regarding its helpfulness to parents, the correctness of the information, and when it was last updated.

3. Interview a woman who has given birth and ask if she had any complications and what was most helpful to her during the experience.

4. The number-one cause of postpartum hemorrhage is _____.

5. When giving report to the nurse who will be caring for a woman and her newborn in the postpartum period, what information should the labor nurse convey?

UNIT EIGHT

THE NEWBORN AT RISK

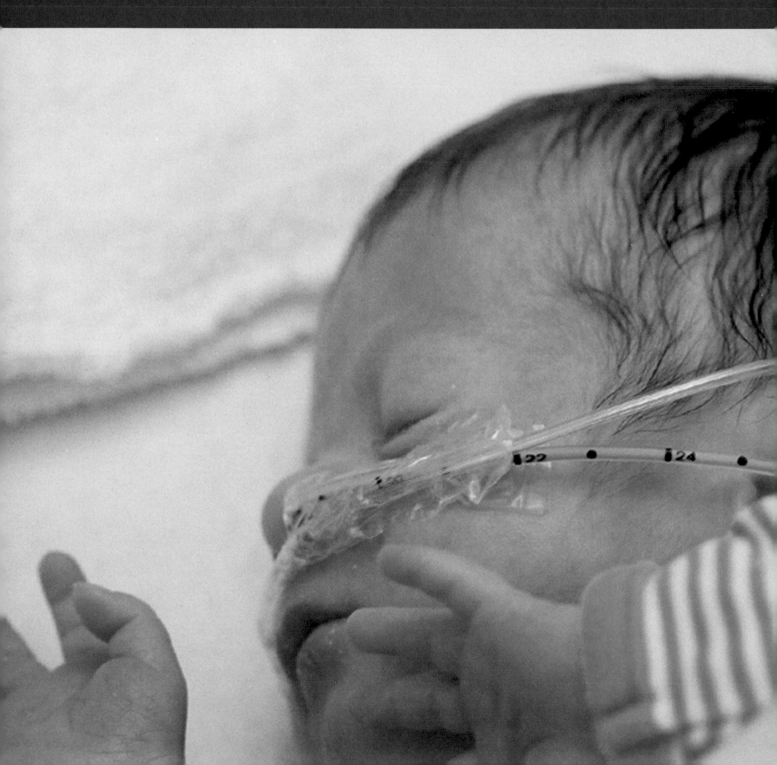

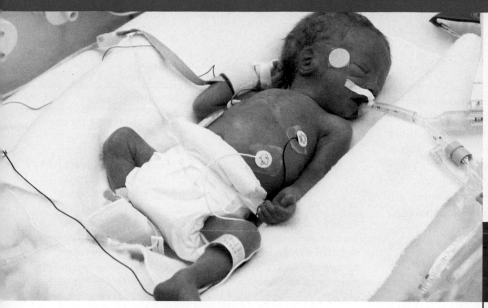

CHAPTER 23

NURSING CARE OF THE NEWBORN WITH SPECIAL NEEDS

KEY TERMS

appropriate for
   gestational age
asphyxia
extremely low birthweight
large for gestational age

late preterm newborn
low birthweight
postterm newborn
preterm newborn

retinopathy of prematurity
small for gestational age
term newborn
very low birthweight

LEARNING OBJECTIVES

Upon completion of the chapter, the learner will be able to:

1. Explain factors that assist in identifying a newborn at risk due to variations in birthweight and gestational age.
2. Select contributing factors and common complications associated with dysmature infants and their management.
3. Compare and contrast a small-for-gestational-age newborn and a large-for-gestational-age newborn; a postterm and preterm newborn.
4. Discuss associated conditions that affect the newborn with variations in birthweight and gestational age, including appropriate management.
5. Outline the nurse's role in helping parents experiencing perinatal grief or loss.
6. Integrate knowledge of the risks associated with late preterm births into nursing interventions, discharge planning, and parent education.

nna and her husband were stunned when she went into labor at 7 months' gestation. They couldn't understand what would cause her to give birth early, but it happened. When they approached the NICU, Anna took a deep breath and looked down at her tiny baby with tubes coming from everywhere. What feelings might they be experiencing at this moment? Do you think that guilt would be one of those feelings? If so, why?

Wow

Guiding a parent's hand to touch a frail or ill newborn demonstrates courage and compassion under very difficult circumstances and is a powerful tool in helping to deal with the newborn's special needs.

Most newborns are born between 38 and 40 weeks' gestation and weigh 6 to 8 lb, but variations in birthweight or gestational age can occur, and newborns with these variations have special needs. Gestational age at birth is inversely correlated with the risk that the infant will experience physical, neurologic, or developmental sequelae (March of Dimes, 2007b, 2007c). Some newborns are born very ill and need special advanced care to survive.

When a woman gives birth to a newborn with problems involving immaturity or birthweight, especially one who is considered high risk, she may go through a grieving process in which she mourns the loss of the healthy full-term newborn she had expected. Through this process she learns to come to terms with the experience she now faces.

The development of new technologies and regionalized care centers for the care of newborns with special needs has resulted in significant improvements. Nurses need to have a sound knowledge base to identify the newborn with special needs and to provide coordinated care.

The key to identifying a newborn with special needs related to birthweight or gestational age variation is an awareness of the factors that could place a newborn at risk. These factors are similar to those that would suggest a high-risk pregnancy and include:

- Maternal nutrition (malnutrition or overweight)
- Substandard living conditions
- Low socioeconomic status
- Maternal age of less than 20 or more than 35 years old
- Substance abuse
- Failure to seek prenatal care
- Smoking or exposure to passive smoke
- Periodontal disease
- Multiple gestation
- Extreme maternal stress
- Abuse and violence
- Placental complications (placenta previa or abruptio placentae)
- History of previous preterm birth
- Maternal disease (e.g., hypertension or diabetes)
- Maternal infection (e.g., urinary tract infection or chorioamnionitis)
- Exposure to occupational hazards (Gilbert, 2007)

Being able to anticipate the birth of a newborn at risk allows the birth to take place at a health care facility equipped with the resources to meet the mother's and newborn's needs. This is important in reducing mortality and morbidity.

Healthy People 2010 identifies preterm births and low birthweight as important national health goals (U.S. Department of Health and Human Services [USDHHS], 2000).

This chapter discusses the nursing management of newborns with special needs related to variations in birth-

HEALTHY PEOPLE 2010

Objective	Significance
Increase the proportion of very low birthweight (VLBW) infants born at level III hospitals or subspecialty perinatal centers	• Will help to promote the delivery of high-risk infants in settings that have the technological capacity to care for them, ultimately reducing the morbidity and mortality rates for these infants
Reduce low birthweight (LBW) from a baseline of 7.6% to a target of 5%; reduce very low birthweight (VLBW) from a baseline of 1.4% to 0.9%	• Will help to emphasize the issue of LBW as a risk factor associated with newborn death, helping to promote measures to reduce this risk factor and thus contributing to significant reductions in infant mortality
Reduce the total number of preterm births from a baseline of 11.6% to 7.6% Reduce the number of live births at 32 to 36 weeks' gestation from a baseline of 9.6% to 6.4% Reduce the number of live births at less than 32 weeks' gestation from a baseline of 2% to 1.1%	• Will help to emphasize the role of preterm birth as the leading cause of newborn deaths unrelated to birth defects • Will aid in promoting an overall reduction in infant illness, disability, and death

USDHHS, 2000.

weight and gestational age. It also describes selected associated conditions affecting these newborns. Due to the frailty of these newborns, the care of the family experiencing perinatal loss and the role of the nurse in helping the family cope also are addressed.

Birthweight Variations

Fetal growth is influenced by maternal nutrition, genetics, placental function, environment, and a multitude of other factors. Assigning size to a newborn is a way to measure and monitor the growth and development of the newborn at birth. Newborns can be classified according to their weight and weeks of gestation, and knowing the group into which a newborn fits is important.

Appropriate for gestational age (AGA) characterizes approximately 80% of newborns and describes a newborn with a normal height, weight, head circumference, and body mass index (BMI; Dorland, 2007). Being in the AGA group confers the lowest risk for any problems. These infants have lower morbidity and mortality than other groups.

Small-for-gestational-age (SGA) newborns typically weigh less than 2,500 g (5 lb 8 oz) at term due to less

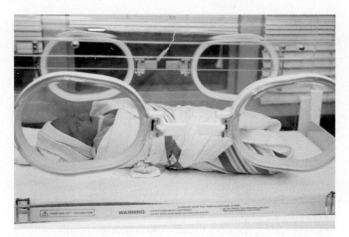

FIGURE 23.1 A low birthweight newborn in an isolette.

growth in utero than expected. A newborn is also classified as SGA if his or her birthweight is at or below the 10th percentile as correlated with the number of weeks of gestation on a growth chart.

Large-for-gestational-age (LGA) describes newborns whose birthweight is above the 90th percentile on a growth chart and who weigh more than 4,000 g (8 lb 13 oz) at term due to accelerated growth for length of gestation (Herranz et al., 2007).

The following terms describe other newborns with marginal weights at birth and of any gestational age:

• **Low birthweight**: less than 2,500 g (5.5 lb) (Fig. 23.1)
• **Very low birthweight**: less than 1,500 g (3 lb 5 oz)
• **Extremely low birthweight**: less than 1,000 g (2 lb 3 oz)

▶ SMALL-FOR-GESTATIONAL-AGE NEWBORNS

Newborns are considered SGA when they weigh less than two standard deviations for gestational age or fall below the 10th percentile on a growth chart for gestational age. These infants can be preterm, term, or postterm.

In some SGA newborns, the rate of growth does not meet the expected growth pattern. Termed intrauterine growth restriction (IUGR), these newborns also are considered at risk, with the perinatal morbidity and mortality rate increased substantially compared to that of the appropriate-for-age newborn (Cunningham et al., 2005). IUGR is the pathologic counterpart of SGA. However, an important distinction to make between SGA and IUGR newborns is that not all who are SGA have IUGR. The converse also is true: not all newborns who have IUGR are SGA. Some SGA newborns are constitutionally small: they are statistically small but otherwise healthy.

Conditions altering fetal growth produce insults that affect all organ systems and are known to produce two patterns of growth that depend on the timing of the insult to the developing embryo or fetus. An early insult (typically occurring before 28 weeks) results in overall growth restriction, with all organs being small. These SGA infants never catch up in size when compared with normal children. An insult later in gestation (after 28 weeks) results in intrauterine malnutrition, but optimal postnatal nutrition generally restores normal growth potential and carries a better prognosis than earlier insults (Kenner & Lott, 2007).

Historically, IUGR has been categorized as symmetric or asymmetric. Symmetric IUGR refers to fetuses with equally poor growth rates of the head, the abdomen, and the long bones. Asymmetric IUGR refers to infants whose head and long bones are spared compared to their abdomen and internal organs. The current belief is that in most cases IUGR is a continuum from symmetry (early stages) to asymmetry (late stages) (Harper & Lam, 2007).

Fetal growth is dependent on genetic, placental, and maternal factors. Cognitive and motor development during infancy forms the basis for children's subsequent development. Newborns who experience nutritional deficiencies in utero and are born SGA are at risk for cognitive deficits that can undermine their academic performance throughout their lives (Kristensen et al., 2007).

The fetus is thought to have an inherent growth potential that, under normal circumstances, yields a healthy newborn of appropriate size. The maternal–placental–fetal units act in harmony to meet the needs of the fetus during gestation. However, growth potential in the fetus can be limited, and this is analogous to failure to thrive in the infant. The causes of both can be intrinsic or environmental. Factors that can contribute to the birth of an SGA newborn are highlighted in Box 23.1.

Nursing Assessment

Assessment of the SGA infant begins by reviewing the maternal history to identify risk factors such as smoking, drug abuse, chronic maternal illness, hypertension, multiple gestation, or genetic disorders. This information allows the nurse to anticipate a possible problem and to be prepared to intervene quickly should one occur. At birth, perform a thorough physical examination, closely observing the newborn for typical characteristics, including:

• Head disproportionately large compared to rest of body
• Wasted appearance of extremities
• Reduced subcutaneous fat stores
• Decreased amount of breast tissue
• Scaphoid abdomen (sunken appearance)
• Wide skull sutures secondary to inadequate bone growth
• Poor muscle tone over buttocks and cheeks
• Loose and dry skin that appears oversized
• Thin umbilical cord

BOX 23.1 Factors Contributing to the Birth of SGA Newborns

- Maternal causes
  - Chronic hypertension
  - Diabetes mellitus with vascular disease
  - Autoimmune diseases
  - Living at a high altitude (hypoxia)
  - Smoking
  - Substance abuse (heroin, cocaine, methamphetamines)
  - Hemoglobinopathies (sickle cell anemia)
  - Preeclampsia
  - Chronic renal disease
  - Malnutrition
  - TORCH group infections
- Placental factors
  - Abnormal cord insertion

- Chronic abruption
- Decreased surface area, infarction
- Decreased placental weight
- Placenta previa
- Placental insufficiency
- Fetal factors
- Trisomy 13, 18, and 21
- Turner's syndrome
- Chronic fetal infection (cytomegalovirus [CMV], rubella, syphilis, toxoplasmosis)
- Congenital anomalies (heart, diaphragmatic hernia, tracheoesophageal fistula)
- Radiation exposure
- Multiple gestation

Sources: Harper & Lam, 2007; Kenner & Lott, 2007; and Neonatal Handbook, 2007e

---

Also assess the SGA newborn for any congenital malformations, neurologic insults, or indications of infection. SGA newborns commonly face problems after birth because of the decrease in placental function during gestation. Table 23.1 highlights some of the common problems associated with SGA newborns and others experiencing a variation in birthweight or gestational age. Anticipate the need for and provide resuscitation as indicated by the newborn's condition.

Nursing Management

Interventions for the SGA infant may include obtaining weight, length, and head circumference, comparing them to standards, and documenting the findings. Perform frequent serial blood glucose measurements as ordered and monitor vital signs, being particularly alert for changes in respiratory status that might indicate respiratory distress. Institute measures to maintain a neutral thermal environment to prevent cold stress and acidosis.

Initiate early and frequent oral feedings unless contraindicated. At birth the newborn's glucose level is 70% of the mother's serum glucose (Aylott, 2006a). Any newborn stressed at birth uses up available glucose stores with resulting hypoglycemia, a plasma glucose concentration at or below 40 mg/dL (Stanley, 2006). With the loss of the placenta at birth, the newborn now must assume control of glucose homeostasis through intermittent oral feedings. If oral feedings are not accepted, an intravenous infusion with 10% dextrose in water may be needed to maintain the glucose level above 40 mg/dL. Weigh the newborn daily and ensure that he or she has adequate rest periods to decrease metabolic requirements.

Observe for clinical signs of polycythemia and monitor blood results. Asymptomatic newborns with a hematocrit between 60% and 70% may simply be supported with fluids, close observation, and a repeat hematocrit

level in 4 to 6 hours (Kates & Kates, 2007). If the newborn is symptomatic, partial exchange transfusion may be used, but this treatment is considered controversial.

Provide anticipatory guidance to parents about any treatments and procedures that are being done. Emphasize the need for close follow-up and careful monitoring of the infant's growth in length, weight, and head circumference and feeding patterns throughout the first year of life to confirm any "catch-up" growth taking place.

▶ LARGE-FOR-GESTATIONAL-AGE NEWBORNS

A newborn whose weight is above the 90th percentile on growth charts or two standard deviations above the mean weight for gestational age is defined as LGA. The range of weight is 4,000 to 5,000 g, or more than 9 lb. LGA infants may be preterm, term, or postterm. Based on these definitions, up to 10% of all births involve an LGA newborn (March of Dimes, 2007a).

Because of the newborn's large size, vaginal birth may be difficult and occasionally results in birth injury. In addition, shoulder dystocia, clavicular fractures, and facial palsies are common. The incidence of cesarean births is very high with LGA newborns to avoid arrested labor and birth trauma.

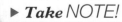 ▶ *Take* NOTE!

Diabetes is commonly associated with LGA newborns. However, due to poor placental perfusion, the newborn may experience IUGR and be SGA.

TABLE 23.1   COMMON PROBLEMS ASSOCIATED WITH NEWBORNS EXPERIENCING A VARIATION IN BIRTHWEIGHT OR GESTATIONAL AGE

Problem	Occurrence	Etiology/Pathophysiology	Assessment Findings	Nursing Implications
Perinatal asphyxia	SGA newborns (common)	Poor tolerance to stress of labor, frequently leading to acidosis and hypoxia Living in hypoxic environment prior to birth, leaving little to no oxygen reserves available to withstand stress of labor: —Uterine contractions increase hypoxic stress —Possible depletion of glycogen stores due to chronic hypoxic state, leading to fetal distress —Impaired uteroplacental circulation due to maternal and uterine conditions predisposing to perinatal depression Compromised newborn at birth experiencing difficulty adjusting to extrauterine environment	Fetal distress (bradycardia, decelerations) during labor Low Apgar scores (Deshpande, 2007)	Anticipate possible problem; assess for maternal risk factors. Initiate resuscitation measures immediately at birth.
	Postterm newborns	Placental deprivation or oligohydramnios, leading to cord compression and subsequent reduction in perfusion to fetus		
	Preterm newborns (common)	Surfactant deficiency Unstable chest wall Immaturity of respiratory control centers in the CNS Small respiratory passages, increasing risk for obstruction Inability to clear mucus from airways		
Difficulty with thermoregulation	SGA newborns (common)	Less muscle mass, less brown fat, less heat-preserving subcutaneous fat, and limited ability to control skin capillaries (Aylott, 2006b) Associated with depleted glycogen stores, poor subcutaneous fat stores, and disturbances in CNS thermoregulation due to hypoxia (Kenner & Lott, 2007)	Temperature <36.4° C; temperature instability; skin cool to touch; cyanosis of hands and feet Bradypnea (<25 bpm) and tachypnea (>60 breaths/min)	Maintain a neutral thermal environment to promote stabilization of newborn's temperature. Assess skin temperature and respiration characteristics. Monitor arterial blood gases and blood glucose levels.

(continued)

TABLE 23.1 COMMON PROBLEMS ASSOCIATED WITH NEWBORNS EXPERIENCING A VARIATION IN BIRTHWEIGHT OR GESTATIONAL AGE (continued)

Problem	Occurrence	Etiology/Pathophysiology	Assessment Findings	Nursing Implications
	Postterm newborns	Increased risk for acidosis and hypoglycemia secondary to metabolic stress (Neonatal Handbook, 2007j) Loss of subcutaneous fat second to placental insufficiency Use of stored nutrients for nutrition due to lost ability of placenta to nourish fetus Subsequent wasting of subcutaneous fat, muscle, or both (Aylott, 2006b) Loss of natural insulation (subcutaneous fat) important in temperature regulation	Tremors, irritability Wheezing, crackles, retractions Restlessness, lethargy Hypotonia Weak or high-pitched cry Seizures Poor feeding Grunting (Galligan, 2006) Acidosis	Eliminate sources of heat loss: —Dry newborn thoroughly. —Wrap in warmed blanket with stockinette cap on head. —Use radiant heat source.
	Preterm newborns (common) Late preterm infant (common)	Immaturity of CNS (temperature-regulating center) interferes with ability to regulate body temperature Inadequate amounts of subcutaneous fat Lack of muscle tone and flexion to conserve heat Inadequate brown fat to generate heat Limited muscle mass activity, reducing ability to produce own heat Inability to shiver to generate heat		
Hypoglycemia	SGA newborns (common) LGA newborns (common)	Increased metabolic rate and lack of adequate glycogen stores to meet newborn's metabolic needs Commonly associated with infants of diabetic mothers Abrupt cessation of high-glucose maternal blood supply with birth and continued insulin production by the newborn Limited ability to release glucagons and catecholamines, which normally stimulate glucagon breakdown and glucose release	Often subtle Lethargy, tachycardia Respiratory distress Jitteriness Drowsiness Poor feeding, feeble sucking Hypothermia, temperature instability Diaphoresis Weak cry Seizures Hypotonia	Monitor blood glucose levels, initially on arrival to nursery and hourly thereafter. Maintain fluid and electrolyte balance. Watch for subtle changes. Initiate early oral feedings if possible; if not, administer IV infusion with 10% dextrose in water.

Problem	Occurrence	Etiology/Pathophysiology	Assessment Findings	Nursing Implications
	Postterm newborns	Hypoxia secondary to depleted glycogen reserves Placental insufficiency secondary to placental aging contributing to chronic fetal nutritional deficiency further depleting glycogen stores	Blood glucose levels <40 mg/dL for term newborns, <20 mg/dL for preterm newborns (Kenner & Lott, 2007)	
	Preterm newborns Late preterm infants	Immature sucking and swallowing leading to insufficient intake Perinatal hypoxia Increased energy expenditure Decreased subcutaneous and brown fat with little to no glycogen stores		
Polycythemia	SGA newborns	Chronic mild hypoxia secondary to placental insufficiency Stimulation of erythropoietin release, leading to increased RBC production	Venous hematocrit >65% Plethora (ruddy appearance) Weak sucking reflex Tachypnea Jaundice Lethargy Jitteriness Hypotonia Irritability Feeding difficulties Difficulty in arousing Seizures	Ensure adequate hydration (orally or IV). Monitor hematocrit levels (goal is ~60%). Administer partial exchange transfusion, albumin or normal saline IV to reduce RBC volume and increase fluid volume (controversial).
	LGA newborns	Secondary to fetal hypoxia, trauma with bleeding, increased erythropoietin production, or delayed cord clamping (Lessaris, 2007)		
	Postterm newborns	Intrauterine hypoxia triggers increased RBC cell production to compensate for lower oxygen levels.		
Meconium aspiration	SGA newborns	Release of meconium into amniotic fluid prior to birth Inhalation of meconium-containing amniotic fluid by the newborn, leading to aspiration	Green amniotic fluid with rupture of membranes during labor Green staining of the umbilical cord or fingernails Difficulty initiating respirations	Initiate resuscitation measures as necessary. Suction airways and support ventilation (see Chapter 24 for more information).
	Postterm newborns	Commonly associated with chronic intrauterine hypoxia Struggling by fetus making respiratory efforts and bearing down with abdominal muscles, leading to expulsion of meconium into amniotic fluid Normal sucking and swallowing by fetus leads to meconium filling airways.		

(continued)

TABLE 23.1 COMMON PROBLEMS ASSOCIATED WITH NEWBORNS EXPERIENCING A VARIATION IN BIRTHWEIGHT OR GESTATIONAL AGE (continued)

Problem	Occurrence	Etiology/Pathophysiology	Assessment Findings	Nursing Implications
Hyperbilirubinemia	LGA newborns (common)	Associated with polycythemia and RBC breakdown Inability to tolerate feedings in the first few days of life, leading to increased enterohepatic circulation of bilirubin Excessive bruising secondary to birth trauma, leading to higher-than-normal bilirubin levels	Elevated serum bilirubin levels Jaundice Tea-colored urine Clay-colored stools	Ensure adequate hydration. Institute early feedings if possible. Administer phototherapy (see Chapter 24 for more information).
	Preterm newborns Late preterm infants	Increased breakdown of RBCs and immature liver function to handle excess load		
Birth trauma	LGA newborns	Large size requiring use of operative birth procedure	Obvious deformities Bruising Edema Asymmetrical movement	Perform complete physical and neurologic assessment of the newborn. Note symmetry of structure and function. Assist parents in understanding situation (see Chapter 24 for more information).

Nursing Assessment

Assessment of the LGA newborn begins with a review of the maternal history, which can provide clues as to whether the woman has an increased risk of giving birth to an LGA newborn. Maternal factors that increase the chance of bearing an LGA newborn include maternal diabetes mellitus or glucose intolerance, multiparity, prior history of a macrosomic infant, postdates gestation, maternal obesity, male fetus, and genetics (Jazayeri, 2007).

At birth, assess the newborn for common characteristics. The typical LGA newborn has a large body and appears plump and full-faced. The increase in body size is proportional. However, the head circumference and body length are in the upper limits of intrauterine growth. These newborns have poor motor skills and have difficulty in regulating behavioral states. LGA newborns are more difficult to arouse to a quiet alert state (Neonatal Handbook, 2007f).

Thoroughly assess the LGA newborn at birth to identify traumatic birth injuries such as fractured clavicles, brachial palsy, facial paralysis, phrenic nerve palsy,

skull fractures, or hematomas. Perform a neurologic examination to identify any nerve palsies, looking for abnormalities such as immobility of the upper arm. Observe and document any injuries discovered to allow for early intervention and improved outcomes.

Obtain frequent blood glucose levels as ordered to evaluate for hypoglycemia. The clinical signs are often subtle and include lethargy, apathy, drowsiness, irritability, tachypnea, weak cry, temperature instability, jitteriness, seizures, apnea, bradycardia, cyanosis or pallor, feeble suck and poor feeding, hypotonia, and coma. Other disorders, including septicemia, severe respiratory distress, and congenital heart disease, may present with similar findings. In addition, be alert for other common problems, such as polycythemia and hyperbilirubinemia (see Table 23.1 earlier in this chapter).

Nursing Management

Assist in stabilizing the LGA newborn. Monitor blood glucose levels within 30 minutes of birth and repeat the screening every hour. Recheck levels before feedings and also immediately in any infant suspected of having or showing clinical signs of hypoglycemia, regardless of age (Aylott, 2006a). To help prevent hypoglycemia, initiate feedings, which can be formula or breast milk, with intravenous glucose supplementation as needed.

If the newborn's blood glucose level is below 25 mg/dL, institute immediate treatment with intravenous glucose, regardless of clinical symptoms (Aylott, 2006a). Monitor and record intake and output and obtain daily weights to aid in evaluating nutritional intake.

Observe for signs of polycythemia and hyperbilirubinemia and report any immediately to the health care provider so that early interventions can be taken to prevent poor long-term neurologic development outcomes. Polycythemia and hyperviscosity are associated with fine and gross motor delays, speech delays, and neurologic sequelae (Neonatal Handbook, 2007g). Increasing fluid volume aids in decreasing blood viscosity. Partial exchange transfusion with plasma or normal saline may be used to lower hematocrit and decrease blood viscosity, but this treatment remains controversial. Hydration, early feedings, and phototherapy are used to treat hyperbilirubinemia (see Chapter 24 for more information about hyperbilirubinemia). Provide parental guidance about the treatments and procedures being done and about the need for follow-up care for any abnormalities identified.

Gestational Age Variations

The mean duration of pregnancy, calculated from the first day of the last normal menstrual period, is approximately 280 days, or 40 weeks. Gestational age is typically measured in weeks: a newborn born before completion of 37 weeks is classified as a **preterm newborn** and one born after completion of 42 weeks is classified as a **postterm newborn**. An infant born from the first day of 38th week through 42 weeks is classified as a **term newborn**. As of 2006, a new classification has been added, the **late preterm newborn**—one who is born between 34 weeks and 36 weeks, 6 days of gestation.

Precise knowledge of a newborn's gestational age is imperative for effective postnatal management. Determination of gestational age by the nurse assists in planning appropriate care for the newborn and provides important information regarding potential problems that need interventions. See Chapter 18 for more information on assessing gestational age.

▶ **Take** NOTE!

Although preterm and postterm newborns may appear to be at opposite ends of the gestational age spectrum and are very different in size and appearance, both are at high risk and need special care.

▶ POSTTERM NEWBORN

A pregnancy that extends beyond 42 weeks' gestation produces a posterm newborn. Other terms used to describe these late births include postmature, prolonged pregnancy, or postdates pregnancy. Postterm newborns may be LGA, SGA, or dysmature (newborn weighs less than established normal parameters for estimated gestational age [IUGR]), depending on placental function.

The reason why some pregnancies last longer than others is not completely understood. What is known is that women who experience one posterm pregnancy are at increased risk in subsequent pregnancies. The incidence of prolonged pregnancy is approximately 10% (Gilbert, 2007).

The ability of the placenta to provide adequate oxygen and nutrients to the fetus after 42 weeks' gestation is thought to be compromised, leading to perinatal mortality and morbidity. As the placenta loses its ability to nourish the fetus, the fetus uses stored nutrients to stay alive, and wasting occurs. This wasted appearance at birth is secondary to the loss of muscle mass and subcutaneous fat.

▶ **Consider** THIS!

I had been waiting for this baby my whole married life and now I was told to wait even longer. I was into my third week past my due date and was just told that if I didn't go into labor on my own, the doctor would induce me on Monday. As I waddled out of his office into the hot summer sun, I thought about all the comments that would await me at the office: "You're not still pregnant, are you?" "Weren't you due last month?" "You look as big as a house." "Are you sure you aren't expecting triplets?" I started to get into my car when I felt warm fluid slide down my legs. Although I was embarrassed at my wetness, I was thrilled I wouldn't have to go back to the office and drove myself to the hospital. Within hours my wait was finally over with the birth of my son, a posterm infant with peeling skin and a thick head of hair. He was certainly worth the wait!

Thoughts: Although most due dates are within plus or minus 2 weeks, we can't "go to the bank with it" because so many factors influence the start of labor. This woman was anxious about her overdue status, but nature prevailed. The old adage "when the fruit is ripe, it will fall" doesn't always bring a good outcome: many women need a little push to bring a healthy newborn forth. What happens when the fetus stays inside the uterus too long? What other features are typical of posterm infants?

Nursing Assessment

A thorough assessment of the postterm newborn upon admission to the nursery provides a baseline from which to identify changes in clinical status. Review the maternal history for any risk factors associated with postterm birth. Also be aware of the common physical characteristics and be able to identify any deviation from the expected. Postterm newborns typically exhibit the following characteristics:

- Dry, cracked, wrinkled skin
- Long, thin extremities
- Creases that cover the entire soles of the feet
- Wide-eyed, alert expression
- Abundant hair on scalp
- Thin umbilical cord
- Limited vernix and lanugo
- Meconium-stained skin
- Long nails (Kenner & Lott, 2007)

Assess the newborn's gestational age and complete a physical examination to identify any abnormalities. Review the medical record to determine the color of the amniotic fluid when membranes ruptured and observe for a meconium-stained umbilical cord and fingernails to assess for possible meconium aspiration. Careful suctioning at the time of birth and afterwards, if the condition dictates it, reduces the incidence of meconium aspiration. Also be alert for other typical complications associated with a postterm newborn, such as perinatal asphyxia, hypoglycemia, hypothermia, and polycythemia, and be prepared to initiate early interventions (see Table 23.1 earlier in the chapter).

Nursing Management

The birth of a postterm newborn creates a crisis for the mother and her family. In most situations, birth of a newborn requiring special care was not anticipated. Postterm newborns are susceptible to several birth challenges secondary to placental dysfunction that place them at risk for asphyxia, hypoglycemia, and respiratory distress. The nurse must be vigilant for complications when managing these newborns.

The postterm newborn is at high risk for perinatal asphyxia, which is usually attributed to placental deprivation or oligohydramnios that leads to cord compression, thereby reducing perfusion to the fetus. Anticipating the need for newborn resuscitation is a priority. The newborn resuscitation team needs to be available in the birthing suite for immediate backup. The newborn may require transport to the neonatal intensive care unit (NICU) for continuous assessment, monitoring, and treatment, depending on his or her status after resuscitation.

Monitor and maintain the postterm newborn's blood glucose levels once stabilized. Intravenous dextrose 10% and/or early initiation of feedings will help stabilize the blood glucose levels to prevent central nervous system sequelae.

Also monitor the postterm newborn's skin temperature, respiration characteristics, results of blood studies, such as arterial blood gases (ABGs) and serum bilirubin levels, and neurologic status. Institute measures to prevent or reduce the risk of hypothermia by eliminating sources of heat loss: thoroughly dry the newborn at birth, wrap him or her in a warmed blanket, and place a stockinet cap on the newborn's head. Providing environmental warmth via a radiant heat source will help stabilize the newborn's temperature.

Closely assess all postterm newborns for polycythemia. Providing adequate hydration helps to reduce the viscosity of the newborn's blood to prevent thrombosis. Be alert to the early, often subtle signs to promote early identification and prompt treatment to prevent any neurodevelopmental delays.

▶ PRETERM NEWBORN

A preterm newborn is one who is born before the completion of 37 weeks of gestation. Although the national birth rate has been declining since the 1990s, the preterm birth rate has been climbing rapidly. Approximately one in eight babies, or 12%, is born before the 37th week of gestation (March of Dimes, 2007c). Prematurity is now the leading cause of death within the first month of life and the second leading cause of all infant deaths.

The etiology of half of all preterm births is unknown (March of Dimes, 2007b, 2007c). Preterm births take an enormous financial toll, estimated to be in the billions of dollars. They also take an emotional toll on those involved.

Changes in perinatal care practices, including regional care, have reduced newborn mortality rates. Transporting high-risk pregnant women to a tertiary center for birth rather than transferring the neonate after birth is associated with a reduction in neonatal mortality and morbidity (Vargo & Trotter, 2007). Despite increasing survival rates, preterm infants continue to be at high risk for neurodevelopmental disorders such as cerebral palsy or mental retardation, intraventricular hemorrhage, congenital anomalies, neurosensory impairment, behavioral problems, and chronic lung disease (Kipiani, Tatishvili, & Sirbiladze, 2007). Making sure that all pregnant women receive quality prenatal care throughout pregnancy is a major method for preventing preterm births.

Effects of Prematurity on Body Systems

Since the preterm newborn did not remain in utero long enough, every body system may be immature, affecting the newborn's transition from intrauterine to extrauterine life and placing him or her at risk for complications.

Without full development, organ systems are not capable of functioning at the level needed to maintain extrauterine homeostasis (March of Dimes, 2007b, 2007c).

Recall Anna, who was described at the beginning of the chapter; she gave birth to a newborn at 7 months' gestation. What problems would you anticipate that her newborn might have?

Respiratory System

The respiratory system is one of the last body systems to mature. Therefore, the preterm newborn is at great risk for respiratory complications. A few of the problems that affect the preterm newborn's breathing ability and adjustment to extrauterine life include:

• Surfactant deficiency, leading to the development of respiratory distress syndrome
• Unstable chest wall, leading to atelectasis
• Immature respiratory control centers, leading to apnea
• Smaller respiratory passages, leading to an increased risk for obstruction
• Inability to clear fluid from passages, leading to transient tachypnea

Cardiovascular System

The preterm newborn has great difficulty in making the transition from intrauterine to extrauterine life in terms of changing from a fetal to a newborn circulation pattern. Higher oxygen levels in the circulation once air breathing begins spur this transition. If the oxygen levels remain low secondary to perinatal asphyxia, the fetal pattern of circulation may persist, causing blood flow to bypass the lungs. Another problem affecting the cardiovascular system is the increased incidence of congenital anomalies associated with continued fetal circulation—patent ductus arteriosus and an open foramen ovale. In addition, impaired regulation of blood pressure in preterm newborns may cause fluctuations throughout the circulatory system. One of special note is cerebral blood flow, which may predispose the fragile blood vessels in the brain to rupture, causing intracranial hemorrhage (Lissauer & Weindling, 2006).

Gastrointestinal System

Preterm newborns usually lack the neuromuscular coordination required to maintain the suck, swallow, and breathing regimen necessary for sufficient calorie and fluid intake to support growth. Perinatal hypoxia causes shunting of blood from the gut to more important organs such as the heart and brain. Subsequently, ischemia and damage to the intestinal wall can occur. This combination of shunting, ischemia, damage to the intestinal wall, and poor sucking ability places the preterm infant at risk for malnutrition and weight loss.

In addition, preterm newborns have a small stomach capacity, weak abdominal muscles, compromised metabolic function, limited ability to digest proteins and absorb nutrients, and weak or absent suck and gag reflexes. All of these limitations place the preterm newborn at risk for nutritional deficiency and subsequent growth and development delays (Neonatal Handbook, 2007h).

Currently, minimal enteral feeding is used to prepare the preterm newborn's gut to overcome the many feeding difficulties associated with gastrointestinal immaturity. It involves the introduction of small amounts, usually 0.5 to 1 mL/kg/h, of enteral feeding to induce surges in gut hormones that enhance maturation of the intestine. This minute amount of breast milk or formula given via gavage feeding prepares the gut to absorb future introduction of nutrients. It builds mucosal bulk, stimulates development of enzymes, enhances pancreatic function, stimulates maturation of gastrointestinal hormones, reduces gastrointestinal distention and malabsorption, and enhances transition to oral feedings (Blackburn, 2007).

Renal System

The renal system of the preterm newborn is immature, reducing the baby's ability to concentrate urine and slowing the glomerular filtration rate. As a result, the risk for fluid retention, with subsequent fluid and electrolyte disturbances, increases. In addition, preterm newborns have limited ability to clear drugs from their systems, thereby increasing the risk of drug toxicity. Close monitoring of the preterm newborn's acid–base and electrolyte balance is critical to identify metabolic inconsistencies. Prescribed medications require strict evaluation to prevent overwhelming the preterm baby's immature renal system.

Immune System

The preterm newborn's immune system is very immature, increasing his or her susceptibility to infections. A deficiency of IgG may occur because transplacental transfer does not occur until after 34 weeks' gestation. This protection is lacking if the baby was born before this time. In addition, preterm newborns have an impaired ability to manufacture antibodies to fight infection if they were exposed to pathogens during the birth process. Moreover, the preterm newborn's thin skin and fragile blood vessels provide a limited protective barrier, adding to the increased risk for infection. Thus, anticipating and preventing infections is the goal; preventing infections has a better outcome than treating them.

Central Nervous System

The preterm newborn is susceptible to injury and insult to the central nervous system (CNS), increasing the potential for long-term disability into adulthood. Like all newborns, preterm newborns have difficulty in temperature regulation and maintaining stability. However, their risk for heat loss is compounded by inadequate amounts of insulating subcutaneous fat; lack of muscle tone and flexion to conserve heat; inadequate brown fat to generate heat; limited muscle mass activity, reducing the possibility of producing their own heat; inability to shiver to generate heat; and an immature temperature-regulating center in the brain (Blackburn, 2007). Preventing cold stress, which would increase the newborn's metabolic and oxygen needs, is crucial. The goal is to create a neutral thermal environment in which oxygen consumption is minimal but body temperature is maintained (Kenner & Lott, 2007).

In addition, the preterm newborn is especially susceptible to hypoglycemia due to immature glucose control mechanisms, decreased glucose stores, and a reduced availability of alternative fuels such as ketone bodies.

> ▶ *Take* NOTE!
>
> *Glucose is needed by the brain and CNS to maintain and support numerous body system functions.*

Nursing Assessment

Preterm newborns are at high risk for numerous problems and require special care. When preterm labor develops and cannot be stopped by medical interventions, plans for appropriate management of the mother and the preterm newborn are necessary, such as transporting them to a regional center with facilities to care for preterm newborns or notifying the facility's NICU. Depending on the degree of prematurity, the preterm newborn may be kept in the NICU for months.

A thorough assessment of the preterm newborn upon admission to the nursery provides a baseline from which to identify changes in clinical status. Be aware of the common physical characteristics and be able to identify any deviation from the expected (Fig. 23.2). Common physical characteristics of preterm infants may include:

- Birthweight of less than 5.5 lb
- Scrawny appearance
- Head disproportionately larger than chest circumference
- Poor muscle tone
- Minimal subcutaneous fat
- Undescended testes
- Plentiful lanugo (soft, downy hair), especially over the face and back
- Poorly formed ear pinna, with soft, pliable cartilage
- Fused eyelids
- Soft and spongy skull bones, especially along suture lines
- Matted scalp hair, wooly in appearance
- Absent to a few creases in the soles and palms
- Minimal scrotal rugae in male infants; prominent labia and clitoris in female infants

- Thin, transparent skin with visible veins
- Breast and nipples not clearly delineated
- Abundant vernix caseosa (Kenner & Lott, 2007)

Be alert for evidence that might suggest that the preterm newborn is developing a complication (see Table 23.1 earlier in the chapter).

Review the maternal history to identify risk factors for preterm birth and check antepartum and intrapartum records for maternal infections to anticipate the need for treatment. Maternal risk factors associated with preterm birth include a previous preterm delivery, low socioeconomic status, preeclampsia, hypertension, poor maternal nutrition, smoking, multiple gestation, infection, advanced maternal age, and substance abuse.

Assess the newborn's gestational age and assess for IUGR if appropriate. Inspect the newborn's skin closely, especially skin color. Assess vital signs, including temperature via skin probe to identify hypothermia or fever, and heart rate for tachycardia or bradycardia. Evaluate the newborn's respiratory effort and respiratory rate. Observe for periods of apnea lasting longer than 20 seconds. Monitor oxygen saturation levels by pulse oximetry to validate perfusion status. Note and report any signs of respiratory distress. Auscultate lung and heart sounds, being especially alert for possible murmur, which would indicate the presence of patent ductus arteriosus in a preterm newborn.

Assess neurologic status by observing the newborn's behavior. Note any restlessness, hypotonia, or weak cry or sucking effort and report unusual findings.

Monitor laboratory studies such as hemoglobin and hematocrit for signs of polycythemia. Screen for hypoglycemia upon admission and then hourly, always observing for nonspecific signs of hypoglycemia such as lethargy, poor feeding, and seizures. Evaluate serum bilirubin concentrations.

Also assess the mother and family members. Identify family strengths and coping mechanisms to establish a basis for intervention.

Nursing Management

The birth of a preterm newborn creates a crisis for the mother and family. Multiple studies have found that hospitalization for preterm newborns is often followed by negative mental health/behavioral outcomes, anxiety and depressive disorders, and developmental problems (Melnyk, Feinstein, & Fairbanks, 2006). Preterm newborns present with immaturity of all organ systems, abundant physiologic challenges, and significant morbidity and mortality (Kenner & Lott, 2007). The nurse must be vigilant for complications when managing preterm newborns (Fig. 23.3 and Nursing Care Plan 23.1).

Promoting Oxygenation

Newborns normally start to breathe without assistance and often cry after birth, being stimulated by a change in pres-

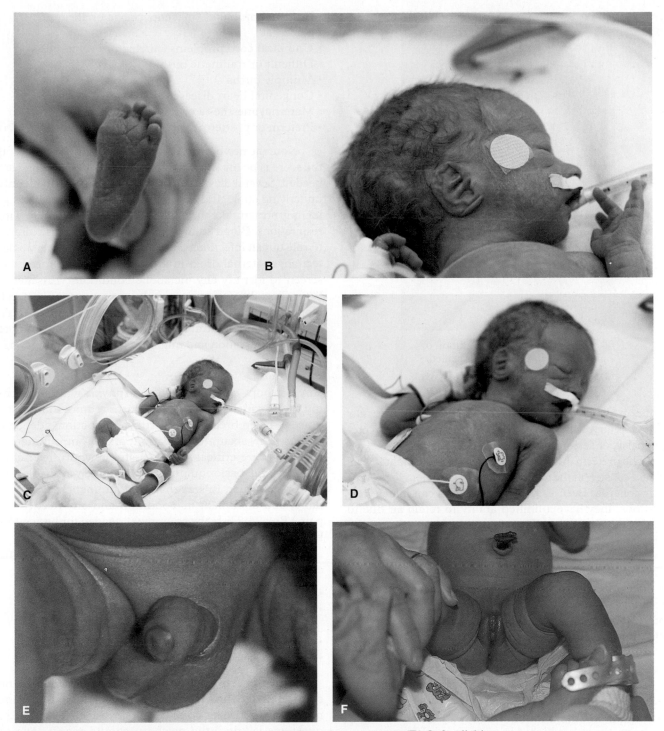

FIGURE 23.2 Characteristics of a preterm newborn. (**A**) Few plantar creases. (**B**) Soft, pliable ear cartilage, matted hair, and fused eyelids. (**C**) Lax posture with poor muscle tone. (**D**) Breast and nipple area barely visible. (**E**) Male genitalia with minimal rugae on scrotum. (**F**) Female genitalia with prominent labia and clitoris.

sure gradients and environmental temperature. The work of taking that first breath is primarily due to overcoming the surface tension of the walls of the terminal lung units at the gas–tissue interface. Subsequent breaths require less inspiratory pressure since there is an increase in functional capacity and air retained. By 1 minute of age, most new-

borns are breathing well. A newborn who fails to establish adequate, sustained respiration after birth is said to have **asphyxia**. On a physiologic level, it is defined as an impairment in gas exchange resulting in a decrease in oxygen in the blood (hypoxemia) and an excess of carbon dioxide or hypercapnia that leads to acidosis. Asphyxia is the most

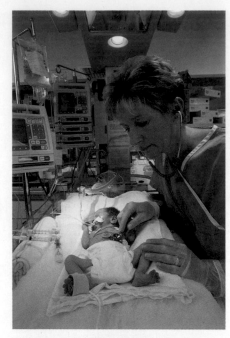

FIGURE 23.3 The physical condition of a preterm newborn demands skilled assessment and nursing care.

common clinical insult in the perinatal period that results in brain injury, which may lead to mental retardation, cerebral palsy, or seizures (Blackburn, 2007).

The preterm infant lacks surfactant. Surfactant lowers surface tension in the alveoli and stabilizes them to prevent their collapse. Even if preterm newborns can initiate respirations, they have a limited ability to retain air due to insufficient surfactant. Therefore, preterm newborns develop atelectasis quickly without alveoli stabilization. The inability to initiate and establish respirations leads to hypoxemia and ultimately hypoxia (decreased oxygen), acidosis (decreased pH), and hypercarbia (increased carbon dioxide). This change in the newborn's biochemical environment may inhibit the transition to extrauterine circulation, thus allowing fetal circulation patterns to persist.

Failure to initiate extrauterine breathing or failure to breathe well after birth leads to hypoxia (too little oxygen in the cells of the body). As a result, the heart rate falls, cyanosis develops, and the newborn becomes hypotonic and unresponsive. Although this can happen with any newborn, the risk is higher in preterm newborns.

Prevention and early identification of newborns at risk are key. Prenatal risk factors that can help identify the newborn who may need resuscitation at birth secondary to asphyxia include:

• History of substance abuse
• Gestational hypertension
• Fetal distress due to hypoxia before birth
• Chronic maternal diseases such as diabetes or a heart or renal condition
• Maternal or perinatal infection

• Placental problems (placenta previa or abruptio placentae)
• Umbilical cord problems (nuchal or prolapsed)
• Difficult or traumatic birth
• Multiple births
• Congenital heart disease
• Maternal anesthesia or recent analgesia
• Preterm or postterm birth (Neonatal Handbook, 2007i)

Note the newborn's Apgar score at 1 and 5 minutes. If the score is below 7 at either time, resuscitation efforts are needed. Several diagnostic studies may be done to identify underlying etiologies. For example, a chest x-ray helps to identify structural abnormalities that might interfere with respirations. Blood studies may be done, such as cultures to rule out an infectious process, a toxicology screen to detect any maternal drugs in the newborn, and a metabolic screen to identify any metabolic conditions (Lissauer & Weindling, 2007). Monitor vital signs continuously, check blood glucose levels for hypoglycemia secondary to stress, and maintain a neutral thermal environment to promote energy conservation and minimize oxygen consumption.

Resuscitating the Newborn

Any newborn can be born with asphyxia without warning. Approximately 10% of newborns require some assistance to begin breathing at birth. Anticipation, adequate preparation, accurate evaluation, and prompt initiation of support are critical for successful newborn resuscitation. Have all basic equipment immediately available and in working order. Ensure that the equipment is evaluated daily, and document its condition and any needed repairs. Box 23.2 lists the equipment needed for basic newborn resuscitation.

Determine the need for resuscitation by performing a rapid assessment using the following four questions:

• What is the gestational age of this newborn?
• Was the amniotic fluid clear of meconium or cloudy (infection present)?
• Is the newborn breathing or crying now?
• Does the newborn have good muscle tone?

If the answers are "yes" to all questions, then routine care is initiated: provide warmth, clear the airway, dry the newborn, and assess color. If the answer to any of these questions is "no," the newborn should receive one or more of the following actions, according to this sequence:

1. Stabilization—Dry the newborn thoroughly with a warm towel; provide warmth by placing him or her under a radiant heater to prevent rapid heat loss through evaporation; position the head in a neutral position to open the airway; clear the airway with a bulb syringe or suction catheter; stimulate breathing. At times, handling and rubbing the newborn with a dry towel may be all that is needed to stimulate respirations.

Nursing Care Plan 23.1

OVERVIEW OF THE CARE OF A PRETERM NEWBORN

Alice, an 18-year-old, felt she had done everything right during her first pregnancy and certainly didn't anticipate giving birth to a preterm newborn at 32 weeks' gestation. When Mary Kaye was born, she had respiratory distress and hypoglycemia and couldn't stabilize her temperature. Assessment revealed the following: newborn described as scrawny in appearance; skin thin and transparent with prominent veins over abdomen; hypotonia with lax, extended positioning; weak sucking reflex when nipple offered; respiratory distress with tachypnea (70 breaths/min), nasal flaring, and sternal retractions; low blood glucose level suggested by lethargy, tachycardia, jitteriness; axillary temperature of 36° C (96.8° F) despite warmed blanket; weight 2,146 g (4.73 lb); length 45 cm (17.72 inches).

NURSING DIAGNOSIS: Ineffective breathing pattern related to immature respiratory system and respiratory distress as evidenced by tachypnea, nasal flaring, and sternal retractions

Outcome Identification and Evaluation

Newborn's respiratory status returns to adequate level of functioning as evidenced by rate remaining within 30 to 60 breaths/min, maintenance of acceptable oxygen saturation levels, and minimal to absent signs of respiratory distress.

Interventions: Promoting Optimal Breathing Pattern

- Assess gestational age and risk factors for respiratory distress *to allow early detection.*
- Anticipate need for bag and mask setup and wall suction *to allow for prompt intervention should respiratory status continue to worsen.*
- Assess respiratory effort (rate, character, effort) *to identify changes.*
- Assess heart rate for tachycardia and auscultate heart sounds *to determine worsening of condition.*
- Observe for cues (grunting, shallow respirations, tachypnea, apnea, tachycardia, central cyanosis, hypotonia, increased effort) *to identify need for additional oxygen.*
- Maintain slight head elevation *to prevent upper airway obstruction.*
- Assess skin color *to evaluate tissue perfusion.*
- Monitor oxygen saturation level via pulse oximetry *to provide objective indication of perfusion status.*
- Provide supplemental oxygen as indicated and ordered *to ensure adequate tissue oxygenation.*
- Assist with any ordered diagnostic tests, such as chest x-ray and arterial blood gases, *to determine effectiveness of treatments.*
- Cluster nursing activities *to reduce oxygen consumption.*
- Maintain a neutral thermal environment *to reduce oxygen consumption.*
- Monitor hydration status *to prevent fluid volume deficit or overload.*
- Explain all events and procedures to the parents *to help alleviate anxiety and promote understanding of the newborn's condition.*

NURSING DIAGNOSIS: Ineffective thermoregulation related to lack of fat stores and hypotonia as evidenced by extended positioning, low axillary temperature despite warmed blanket, respiratory distress, and lethargy

Outcome Identification and Evaluation

Newborn will demonstrate ability to regulate temperature as evidenced by temperature remaining in normal range (36.5° to 37.5° C) and absent signs of cold stress.

Interventions: Promoting Thermoregulation

- Assess the axillary temperature every hour or use a thermistor probe *to monitor for changes.*
- Review maternal history *to identify risk factors contributing to problem.*
- Monitor vital signs, including heart rate and respiratory rate, every hour *to identify deviations.*
- Check radiant heat source or isolette *to ensure maintenance of appropriate temperature of the environment.*
- Assess environment for sources of heat loss or gain through evaporation, conduction, convection, or radiation *to minimize risk of heat loss.*
- Avoid bathing and exposing newborn *to prevent cold stress.*
- Warm all blankets and equipment that come in contact with newborn; place warmed cap on the newborn's head and keep it on *to minimize heat loss.*

(continued)

Nursing Care Plan 23.1 (continued)

- Encourage kangaroo care (mother or father holds preterm infant underneath clothing skin-to-skin and upright between breasts) *to provide warmth.*
- Educate parents on how to maintain a neutral thermal environment, including importance of keeping the newborn warm with a cap and double-wrapping with blankets and changing them frequently to keep dry *to promote newborn's adjustment.*
- Demonstrate ways to safeguard warmth and prevent heat loss.

NURSING DIAGNOSIS: Risk for imbalanced nutrition: less than body requirements related to poor sucking and lack of glycogen stores necessary to meet the newborn's increased metabolic demands as evidenced by weak sucking reflex, low birthweight, and signs and symptoms of hypoglycemia, including lethargy, tachycardia, and jitteriness

Outcome Identification and Evaluation
Newborn will demonstrate adequate nutritional intake, remaining free of signs of hypoglycemia as evidenced by blood glucose levels being maintained above 45 mg/dL, enhanced sucking ability, and appropriate weight gain.

Interventions: Promoting Optimal Nutrition
- Identify newborn at risk based on behavioral characteristics, body measurements, and gestational age *to establish a baseline and allow for early detection.*
- Assess blood glucose levels as ordered *to determine status and establish a baseline for interventions.*
- Obtain blood glucose measurements upon admission to nursery and every 1 to 2 hours as indicated *to evaluate for changes.*
- Observe behavior for signs of low blood glucose *to allow early identification.*
- Initiate early oral feedings or gavage feedings *to maintain blood glucose levels.*
- If oral or gavage feedings aren't tolerated, initiate an IV glucose infusion *to aid in stabilizing blood glucose levels.*
- Assess skin for pallor and sweating *to identify signs of hypoglycemia.*
- Assess neurologic status for tremors, seizures, jitteriness, and lethargy *to identify further drops in blood glucose levels.*
- Monitor weight daily for changes *to determine effectiveness of feedings.*
- Maintain temperature using warmed blankets, radiant warmer, or warmed isolette *to prevent heat loss and possible cold stress and reduce energy demands.*
- Monitor temperature *to prevent cold stress resulting in decreased blood glucose levels.*
- Offer opportunities for non-nutritive sucking on premature-size pacifier *to satisfy sucking needs.*
- Monitor for tolerance of oral feedings, including intake and output, *to determine effectiveness.*
- Administer IV dextrose if newborn is symptomatic *to raise blood glucose levels quickly.*
- Decrease energy requirements, including clustering care activities and providing rest periods, *to conserve glucose and glycogen stores.*
- Inform parents about procedures and treatments, including rationale for frequent blood glucose levels, *to help reduce their anxiety.*

---

2. Ventilation
3. Chest compressions
4. Administration of epinephrine and/or volume expansion (AHA/AAP, 2006).

The decision to progress from one set of actions to the next and the need for further resuscitative efforts is determined by the assessment of respirations, heart rate, and color (AHA/AAP, 2006).

When performing newborn resuscitation, use the mnemonic "ABCDs" (airway, breathing, circulation, and drugs) to remember the sequence of steps (Box 23.3).

Resuscitation measures are continued until the newborn has a pulse above 100 bpm, a good cry, or good breathing efforts and a pink tongue. This last sign indicates a good oxygen supply to the brain (AHA/AAP, 2006).

Throughout the resuscitation period, keep the parents informed of what is happening to their newborn and what is being done and why. Provide support through this initial crisis. Once the newborn is stabilized, encourage bonding by having them stroke, touch, and when appropriate hold the newborn.

Administering Oxygen
Oxygen administration is a common therapy in newborn nurseries. Although it has been used in newborns for over 75 years, there is no universal agreement on the most ap-

---

**BOX 23.2 Basic Equipment
for Newborn Resuscitation**

- A wall vacuum suction apparatus
- A wall source or tank source of 100% oxygen
  with a flow meter
- A neonatal self-inflating ventilation bag with
  correct-sized face masks
- A selection of endotracheal tubes (2.5, 3.0, or 3.5 mm)
  with introducers
- A laryngoscope with a small, straight blade and spare
  batteries and bulbs
- Ampules of naloxone (Narcan) with syringes and
  needles
- A wall clock to document timing of activities and events
- A supply of disposable gloves in a variety of sizes for
  staff to use

BOX 23.3 ABCDs of Newborn Resuscitation

- **A**irway
  - Place infant's head in "sniffing" position.
  - Suction mouth, then nose.
  - Suction trachea if meconium-stained and newborn is
    NOT vigorous (strong respiratory effort, good muscle
    tone, and heart rate > 100 bpm).
- **B**reathing
  - Use positive-pressure ventilation (PPV) for apnea,
    grasping, or pulse <100 bpm.
  - Ventilate at rate of 40 to 60 breaths/minute.
  - Listen for raising heart rate, audible breath sounds.
  - Look for slight chest movement with each breath.
  - Use carbon dioxide detector after intubation.
- **C**irculation
  - Start compressions if heart rate is <60 after 30 seconds
    of effective PPV.
  - Give 3 compressions: 1 breath every 2 seconds.
  - Compress one third of the anterior-posterior diameter
    of the chest.
- **D**rugs
  - Give epinephrine if heart rate is <60 after 30 seconds
    of compressions and ventilation.
  - *Caution:* Epinephrine dosage is different for
    endotracheal and IV routes!
    - Epinephrine: 1:10,000 concentration
      - 0.1 to 0.3 mL/kg IV
      - 0.3 to 1 ml/kg via endotracheal tube (AHA/AAP,
        2006)

---

propriate range at which oxygen levels should be maintained for newborns experiencing hypoxia, nor is there a standard time frame for oxygen to be administered (Neonatal Handbook, 2007d). While this uncertainty continues, nurses will experience a wide variation in practice in terms of modes of administration, monitoring, blood levels, and target ranges for both short- and long-term oxygen therapy.

A guiding principle, though, is that oxygen therapy should be targeted to levels appropriate to the condition, gestational age, and postnatal age of the newborn. Oxygen therapy must be used judiciously to prevent **retinopathy of prematurity (ROP)**, a major cause of blindness in preterm newborns in the past. ROP is a potentially blinding eye disorder that occurs when abnormal blood vessels grow and spread through the retina, eventually leading to retinal detachment. The incidence of ROP is inversely proportional to the preterm baby's birthweight. Approximately 400 to 600 children become blind because of ROP in the United States annually (Lyon & Warren, 2006).

Although the role of oxygen in the pathogenesis of ROP is unclear, current evidence suggests that it is linked to the duration of oxygen use rather than the concentration. Thus, the use of 100% oxygen to resuscitate a newborn should not pose a problem (National Eye Institute, 2007). However, an ophthalmology consult for follow-up after discharge is essential for preterm infants who have received extensive oxygen therapy. See Chapter 38 for a more in-depth discussion of this condition.

Respiratory distress in preterm infants is commonly caused by a deficiency of surfactant, retained fluid in the lungs (wet lung syndrome), meconium aspiration, pneumonia, hypothermia, or anemia. The principles of care are the same regardless of the cause of respiratory distress. First, keep the newborn warm, preferably in a warmed iso-

lette or with an overhead radiant warmer, to conserve the baby's energy and prevent cold stress. Handle the newborn as little as possible, because stimulation often increases the oxygen requirement. Provide energy through calories via intravenous dextrose or gavage or continuous tube feedings to prevent hypoglycemia. Treat cyanosis with an oxygen hood or blow-by oxygen placed near the newborn's face if respiratory distress is mild and short-term therapy is needed. Record the following important observations every hour or more frequently if indicated, and document any deterioration or changes in respiratory status:

- Respiratory rate, quality of respirations, and respiratory effort
- Airway patency, including removal of secretions per facility policy
- Skin color, including any changes to duskiness, blueness, or pallor
- Lung sounds on auscultation to differentiate breath sounds in upper and lower fields
- Equipment required for oxygen delivery, such as:
  - Blow-by oxygen delivered via mask or tube for short-term therapy

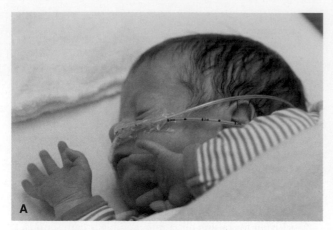 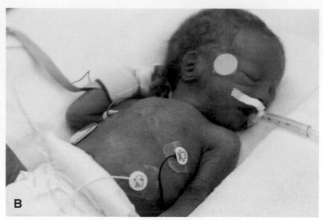

FIGURE 23.4 (**A**) A preterm newborn receiving oxygen therapy via a nasal cannula. The newborn also has an enteral feeding tube inserted for nutrition. (**B**) A preterm newborn receiving mechanical ventilation.

- Oxygen hood (oxygen is delivered via a plastic hood placed over the newborn's head)
- Nasal cannula (oxygen is delivered directly through the nares) (Fig. 23.4A)
- Continuous positive airway pressure (CPAP), which prevents collapse of unstable alveoli and delivers high levels of inspired oxygen into the lungs
- Mechanical ventilation, which delivers consistent assisted ventilation and oxygen therapy, reducing the work of breathing for the fatigued infant (see Fig. 23.4B)
- Correct placement of endotracheal tube (if present)
- Heart rate, including any changes
- Oxygen saturation levels via pulse oximetry to evaluate need for therapy modifications based on hemoglobin
- Maintenance of oxygen saturation level from 87% to 95% (Aylott, 2006b)
- Nutritional intake, including calories provided, to prevent hypoglycemia and method of feeding, such as gavage, intravenous, or continuous enteral feedings
- Hydration status, including any signs and symptoms of fluid overload
- Laboratory tests, including ABGs, to determine effectiveness of oxygen therapy
- Administration of medication, such as exogenous surfactant

If the newborn shows worsening cyanosis or if oxygen saturation levels fall below 87%, prepare to give additional oxygen as ordered. Throughout care, strict asepsis, including handwashing, is vital to reduce the risk of infection.

Maintaining Thermal Regulation

Immediately after birth, dry the newborn with a warmed towel and then place him or her in a second warm, dry towel before performing the assessment. This drying prevents rapid heat loss secondary to evaporation. Newborns who are active, breathing well, and crying are stable and can be placed on their mother's chest ("kangaroo care")

to promote warmth and prevent hypothermia. Preterm newborns who are not considered stable may be placed under a radiant warmer or in a warmed isolette after they are dried with a warmed towel.

Typically newborns use nonshivering thermogenesis for heat production by metabolizing their own brown adipose tissue. However, the preterm newborn has an inadequate supply of brown fat because he or she left the uterus before it was adequate. The preterm newborn also has decreased muscle tone and thus cannot assume the flexed fetal position, which reduces the amount of skin exposed to a cooler environment. In addition, preterm newborns have large body surface areas compared to weight. This allows an increased transfer of heat from their bodies to the environment.

Typically, a preterm newborn who is having problems with thermal regulation is cool to cold to the touch. The hands, feet, and tongue may appear cyanotic. Respirations are shallow or slow, or signs of respiratory distress are present. The newborn is lethargic and hypotonic, feeds poorly, and has a feeble cry. Blood glucose levels are probably low, leading to hypoglycemia, due to the energy expended to keep warm.

When promoting thermal regulation for the preterm newborn:

- Remember the four mechanisms for heat transfer and ways to prevent loss:
  - Convection: heat loss through air currents (avoid drafts near the newborn)
  - Conduction: heat loss through direct contact (warm everything the newborn comes in contact with, such as blankets, mattress, stethoscope)
  - Radiation: heat loss without direct contact (keep isolettes away from cold sources and provide insulation to prevent heat transfer)
  - Evaporation: heat loss by conversion of liquid into vapor (keep the newborn dry and delay the first bath until the baby's temperature is stable)

- Frequently assess the temperature of the isolette or radiant warmer, adjusting the temperature as necessary to prevent hypo- or hyperthermia.
- Assess the newborn's temperature every hour until stable.
- Observe for clinical signs of cold stress, such as respiratory distress, central cyanosis, hypoglycemia, lethargy, weak cry, abdominal distention, apnea, bradycardia, and acidosis.
- Remember the complications of hypothermia and frequently assess the newborn for signs:
  - Metabolic acidosis secondary to anaerobic metabolism used for heat production, which results in the production of lactic acid
  - Hypoglycemia due to depleted glycogen stores
  - Pulmonary hypertension secondary to pulmonary vasoconstriction
- Monitor the newborn for signs of hyperthermia such as tachycardia, tachypnea, apnea, warm to touch, flushed skin, lethargy, weak or absent cry, and CNS depression; adjust the environmental temperature appropriately.
- Explain to the parents the need to maintain the newborn's temperature, including the measures used; demonstrate ways to safeguard warmth and prevent heat loss.

Promoting Nutrition and Fluid Balance

Providing nutrition is challenging for preterm newborns because their needs are great but their ability to take in optimal amounts of energy/calories is reduced due to their compromised health status. Individual nutritional needs are highly variable.

Depending on their gestational age, preterm newborns receive nutrition orally, enterally, or parenterally via infusion. Several different methods can be used to provide nutrition: parenteral feedings administered through a percutaneous central venous catheter for long-term venous access with delivery of total parenteral nutrition (TPN), or enteral feedings, which can include oral feedings (formula or breast milk), continuous nasogastric tube feedings, or intermittent gavage tube feedings. Gavage feedings are commonly used for compromised newborns to allow them to rest during the feeding process. Many have a weak suck and become fatigued and thus cannot consume enough calories to meet their needs.

Most newborns born after 34 weeks' gestation without significant complications can feed orally. Those born before 34 weeks' gestation typically start with parenteral nutrition within the first 24 hours of life. Then enteral nutrition is introduced and advanced based on the degree of maturity and clinical condition. Ultimately, enteral nutrition methods replace parenteral nutrition.

To promote nutrition and fluid balance in the preterm newborn:

- Measure daily weight and plot it on a growth curve.
- Monitor intake; calculate fluid and caloric intake daily.

- Assess fluid status by monitoring weight; urinary output; urine specific gravity; laboratory test results such as serum electrolyte levels, blood urea nitrogen, creatinine, and hematocrit; skin turgor; and fontanels (Kenner & Lott, 2007). Be alert for signs of dehydration, such as a decrease in urinary output, sunken fontanels, temperature elevation, lethargy, and tachypnea.
- Continually assess for enteral feeding intolerance; measure abdominal girth, auscultate bowel sounds, and measure gastric residuals before the next tube feeding.
- Encourage and support breastfeeding by facilitating maternal breast pumping.
- Encourage nuzzling at the breast in conjunction with kangaroo care if the newborn is stable.

▶ **Take** NOTE!

When assessing the fluid status of a preterm newborn, palpate the fontanels. Sunken fontanels suggest dehydration; bulging fontanels suggest overhydration.

Preventing Infection

Prevention of infection is critical when caring for preterm newborns. Infections are the most common cause of morbidity and mortality in the NICU population (Kenner & Lott, 2007). Nursing assessment and early identification of problems are imperative to improve outcomes.

Preterm newborns are at risk for infection because their early birth deprived them of maternal antibodies needed for passive protection. Preterm newborns also are susceptible to infection because of their limited ability to produce antibodies, asphyxia at birth, and thin, friable skin that is easily traumatized, providing an entry portal for microorganisms.

Early detection is crucial. The clinical manifestations can be nonspecific and subtle: apnea, diminished activity, poor feeding, temperature instability, respiratory distress, seizures, tachycardia, hypotonia, irritability, pallor, jaundice, and hypoglycemia. Report any of these to the primary care provider immediately so that treatment can be instituted.

Include the following interventions when caring for a preterm or postterm newborn to prevent infection:

- Assess for risk factors in maternal history that place the newborn at increased risk.
- Monitor for changes in vital signs such as temperature instability, tachycardia, or tachypnea.
- Assess oxygen saturation levels and initiate oxygen therapy as ordered if oxygen saturation levels fall below acceptable parameters.
- Assess feeding tolerance, typically an early sign of infection.

- Monitor laboratory test results for changes.
- Avoid using tape on the newborn's skin to prevent tearing.
- Use equipment that can be thrown away after use.
- Adhere to standard precautions; use clean gloves to handle dirty diapers and dispose of them properly.
- Use sterile gloves when assisting with any invasive procedure; attempt to minimize the use of invasive procedures.
- Remove all jewelry on your hands prior to washing hands; wash hands upon entering the nursery and in between caring for newborns.
- Avoid coming to work when ill, and screen all visitors for contagious infections.

Preventing Complications

Preterm newborns face a myriad of possible complications as a result of their fragile health status or the procedures and treatments used. Some of the more common complications in preterm newborns include respiratory distress syndrome, periventricular-intraventricular hemorrhage, bronchopulmonary dysplasia, ROP, hyperbilirubinemia, anemia, necrotizing enterocolitis, hypoglycemia, infection or septicemia, delayed growth and development, and mental or motor delays (March of Dimes, 2007b). Several of these complications are described in Chapter 24.

Remember Anna, who was in a state of shock when she entered the NICU to see her preterm baby for the first time? How could the nurse have prepared her for this event? What information needs to be given at the isolette to reduce her anxiety and fear now?

Providing Appropriate Stimulation

Newborn stimulation involves a series of activities to encourage normal development. Research on developmental interventions shows that when preterm newborns, in particular, receive sensorimotor interventions such as rocking, skin-to-skin contact with parents, containment (swaddling and surrounded by blanket rolls), music, non-nutritive sucking, breastfeeding, massage, holding, or sleeping on waterbeds, they gain weight faster, progress in feeding abilities more quickly, and show improved interactive behavior compared to preterm newborns who were not stimulated (Field et al., 2006). Conversely, overstimulation may have negative effects by reducing oxygenation and causing stress. A newborn reacts to stress by flaying the hands or bringing an arm up to cover the face. When overstimulated, such as by noise, lights, excessive handling, alarms, and procedures, and stressed, heart and respiratory rates decrease and periods of apnea or bradycardia may follow (Blackburn, 2007).

Appropriate developmental stimulation that would not overtax the compromised newborn might include

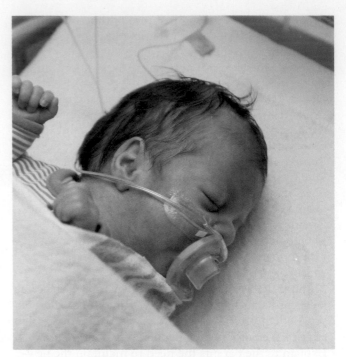

FIGURE 23.5 A preterm newborn receiving non-nutritive sucking.

kangaroo (skin-to-skin) holding, rocking, soft singing or music, cuddling, gentle stroking of the infant's skin, colorful mobiles, gentle massage, waterbed mattresses, and non-nutritive sucking opportunities (Fig. 23.5) or providing sucrose if tolerated.

The NICU environment can be altered to provide periods of calm and rest for the newborn by dimming the lights, lowering the volume and tone of conversations, closing doors gently, setting the telephone ringer to the lowest volume possible, clustering nursing activities, and covering the isolette with a blanket to act as a light shield to promote rest at night.

Encourage parents to hold and interact with their newborn. Doing so helps to acquaint the parents with their newborn, promotes self-confidence, and fosters parent–newborn attachment (Fig. 23.6).

Think back to Anna, the woman who gave birth to a preterm newborn at 7 months' gestation. Anna will be discharged but her newborn will be staying in the NICU for a while. What interventions would be appropriate to facilitate bonding despite their separation? What support can be provided specifically to her family?

Managing Pain

Pain is an unpleasant sensory and emotional experience felt by all humans. Newborns feel pain and require the same level of pain assessment and management as adults. Common indicators of pain in the newborn who is unable

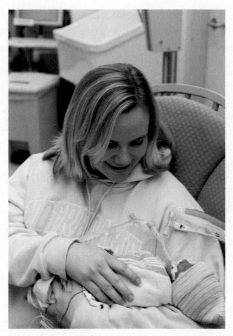

FIGURE **23.6** A mother bonding with her preterm newborn.

to vocalize include facial expressions, body movements, and physiologic changes (Kenner & Lott, 2007). Untreated pain in newborns may result in increased morbidity and length of stay in the NICU, exaggerated responses to pain in later life, and altered psychosocial development (Koeppel, 2007). Parents commonly expect that health care providers will use appropriate measure to prevent pain in their newborns, but there are gaps in knowledge about the most effective way to accomplish this.

Assessment of pain in the newborn remains a contentious and vexing problem. Newborns in the NICU are subjected to repeated procedures that cause them pain. Newborns, whether preterm, full term, or postterm, do experience pain, but the pain is difficult to validate with consistent behaviors. Considering that ill newborns undergo multiple noxious stimuli from invasive procedures, such as lumbar punctures, heel sticks, venipuncture, line insertions, chest tube placement, specimen collections, endotracheal intubation and suctioning, and mechanical ventilation, common sense would suggest that newborns experience pain from these many activities and interventions. However, pain management in infants was not addressed formally until various professional and accrediting organizations issued position statements and clinical recommendations in an effort to promote effective pain management (AAP, 2006a, 2006b). An international consortium established principles of newborn pain prevention and management that all nurses must be familiar with and apply (Box 23.4).

Several psychometric tools are available to assess pain in the newborn. Examples include the Pain Assessment Tool (PAT), which evaluates respirations, heart rate, oxy-

---

BOX 23.4 Newborn Pain Prevention and Management Guidelines

- Newborn pain frequently goes unrecognized and undertreated.
- Pain assessment is an essential activity prior to pain management.
- Newborns experience pain, and analgesics should be given.
- A procedure considered painful for an adult should also be considered painful for a newborn.
- Developmental maturity and health status must be considered when assessing for pain in newborns.
- Newborns may be more sensitive to pain than adults.
- Pain behavior is frequently mistaken for irritability and agitation.
- Newborns are more susceptible to the long-term effects of pain.
- Adequate pain management may reduce complications and mortality.
- Nonpharmacologic measures can prevent, reduce, or eliminate newborn pain.
- Sedation does not provide pain relief and may mask pain responses.
- A newborn's response to both pharmacologic and nonpharmacologic pain therapy should be assessed within 30 minutes of administration or intervention.
- Health care professionals are responsible for pain assessment and treatment.
- Written guidelines are needed on each newborn unit.

Source: Kenner & Lott, 2007.

---

gen saturation, and blood pressure; the Premature Infant Pain Profile (PIPP), which assesses heart rate and oxygen saturation; the CRIES tool (cry, requires oxygen, increased vital signs, expression and sleeplessness); and the Neonatal Infant Pain Scale (NIPS), which evaluates respiratory patterns. Most are based on facial expressions, crying patterns, change in vital signs, and body movements (AAP, 2006a).

Nurses play a key role in assessing a newborn's pain level. Assess the newborn frequently. Pain is considered the "fifth vital sign" and should be assessed as frequently as the other four vital signs. Differentiate pain from agitation by observing for changes in vital signs, behavior, facial expression, and body movement. Suspect pain if the newborn exhibits the following:

- Sudden high-pitched cry
- Facial grimace with furrowing of brow and quivering chin
- Increased muscle tone
- Oxygen desaturation

- Body posturing, such as squirming, kicking, arching
- Limb withdrawal and thrashing movements
- Increase in heart rate, blood pressure, pulse, and respirations
- Fussiness and irritability (Arenson & Drake, 2007)

The goals of pain management are to minimize the amount, duration, and severity of pain and to assist the newborn in coping. Effective pain management strategies for newborns include preventing, limiting, or avoiding noxious stimuli; using nonpharmacologic techniques to reduce pain; and administering pharmacologic agents when appropriate. Box 23.5 lists some of the more commonly used nonpharmacologic pain management techniques for the preterm newborn.

The number of analgesics available for use with preterm newborns is limited. Morphine and fentanyl, usually administered intravenously, are the most commonly used opioids for moderate to severe pain. Acetaminophen is effective for mild pain. Benzodiazepines are used as sedatives during painful procedures and can be combined with opioids for more effectiveness. Local or topical anesthetics (e.g., EMLA cream) also may be used before procedures such as venipuncture, lumbar puncture, and intravenous catheter insertion (AAP, 2006b).

Be vigilant in assessing for adverse effects (respiratory depression or hypotension) when administering pharmacologic agents for pain management, especially in preterm

newborns with neurologic impairment. These negative effects are usually dose- and route-related, so be knowledgeable about the pharmacokinetics and therapeutic dosing of any drug administered.

Promoting Growth and Development

In the late 1970s, researchers evaluated the NICU environment in terms of light and sound levels, caregiving activities, and handling of newborns. As a result of this research, many environmental modifications were made to reduce the stress and overstimulation of the NICU, and the concept of developmentally supportive care was introduced. Developmentally supportive care is defined as care of a newborn or infant to support positive growth and development. Developmental care focuses on what newborns or infants can do at that stage of development; it uses therapeutic interventions only to the point that they are beneficial; and it provides for the development of the newborn–family unit (Neonatal Handbook, 2007b).

Developmental care is a philosophy of care that requires rethinking the relationships between newborns, families, and health care providers. It includes a variety of activities designed to manage the environment and individualize the care of the preterm or high-risk ill newborn based on behavioral observations (see Evidence-Based Practice 23.1). The goal is to promote a stable, well-organized newborn who can conserve energy for growth and development (Hendricks-Munoz & Prendergast, 2007).

Developmental care includes these strategies:

- Clustering care to promote rest and conserve the infant's energy
- Flexed positioning to simulate in utero positioning
- Environmental management to reduce noise and visual stimulation
- Kangaroo care to promote skin-to-skin sensation
- Placement of twins in the same isolette or open crib to reduce stress
- Activities to promote self-regulation and state regulation:
  - Surrounding the newborn with nesting rolls/devices
  - Swaddling with a blanket to maintain the flexed position
  - Providing sheepskin or a waterbed to simulate the uterine environment
  - Providing non-nutritive sucking (calms the infant)
  - Providing objects to grasp (comforts the newborn)
- Promotion of parent–infant bonding by making parents feel welcome in the NICU
- Open, honest communication with parents and staff
- Collaboration with the parents in planning the infant's care (Davidson et al., 2007)

Developmental care can be fostered by clustering the lights in one area so that no lights are shining directly on newborns, installing visual alarm systems and limiting overhead pages to minimize noise, and monitoring continuous and peak noise levels. Nurses can play an active role

---

BOX 23.5 **Nonpharmacologic Techniques to Reduce Pain in the Preterm Newborn**

- Gentle handling, rocking, caressing, cuddling, and massaging
- Rest periods before and after painful procedures
- Kangaroo care (skin-to-skin contact) during procedure
- Breastfeeding, if able, to reduce pain from minor procedures
- Use of a facilitated tuck (holding arms and legs in a flexed position)
- Application of topical anesthetics prior to venipuncture or lumbar puncture
- Swaddling and positioning to establish physical boundaries
- Non-nutritive sucking (pacifier dipped in sucrose) prior to procedure
- Minimal use of tape, with gentle removal to avoid skin tears
- Warm blankets for wrapping to facilitate relaxation
- Reduction of environmental stimuli by removing or turning down noxious stimuli such as noise from alarms, beepers, loud conversations, and bright lights
- Distraction, such as with colored objects or mobiles (AAP, 2006a, 2006b)

EVIDENCE-BASED PRACTICE 23.1
Promoting Development and Preventing Morbidity in Preterm Infants

● Study

Preterm newborns are at risk due to their immature body systems. This is compounded by the newborn's increased risk for complications and illnesses and his or her exposure to numerous stimuli in the NICU environment. Together, these stressors can interfere with the newborn's growth and development. Developmental care is a philosophy that includes a wide range of activities to manage the environment and individualize care. The belief is that it can reduce the effects of these stressors. Activities typically associated with developmental care include controlling external stimuli, clustering care activities, and positioning and swaddling the preterm newborn.

A study was done to examine the effects of developmental care on preterm newborns. The study evaluated relevant outcomes such as neurodevelopment, weight gain, length of hospital stay, duration of mechanical ventilation, and physiologic stress. A computerized search of all articles, controlled trials, and conference and symposia proceedings was done. Two independent experts identified the data from all relevant randomized trials that compared the elements of developmental care to routine nursery care for newborns less than 37 weeks' gestation. The researchers identified 36 controlled trials.

▲ Findings

Assessing the benefits of developmental care was difficult because most of the studies reviewed included multiple interventions and many of the trials had small sample sizes. Therefore, the authors could not determine whether any one intervention was more effective than another. Overall, they reported that developmental care had limited benefits and no major harmful effects. It had a limited benefit on decreasing moderate to severe chronic lung disease, decreasing the incidence of necrotizing colitis, and improving family outcomes. Evidence was also limited related to the long-term positive effect on behavior and movement at 5 years corrected age. However, individualized developmental care activities showed some positive effects in improving neurodevelopmental outcomes.

■ Nursing Implications

Although the study found that developmental care for preterm newborns was of limited benefit, it emphasized that this type of care had no major harmful effects. Nurses can integrate these findings into their care for preterm newborns with the understanding that they are beneficial but that the effect may be limited. Nurses can advocate for individualizing the activities involved in developmental care based on the newborn's needs. They also can play a key role in fostering research to help determine which stressors seem to be the most troublesome and which specific activities are of the greatest benefit. In addition, nurses can assist in identifying appropriate short- and long-term outcome measures.

Symington, A., & Pinelli, J. (2006). Developmental care for promoting development and preventing morbidity in preterm infants. *Cochrane Database of Systematic Reviews* 2006. Issue 2. Art. No.: CD001814. DOI: 10.1002/14651858.CD001814.pub2.

---

by serving on committees that address these issues. In addition, nurses can provide direct developmentally supportive care. Doing so involves careful planning of nursing activities to provide the ideal environment for the newborn's development. For example:

- Dim the lights and cover isolettes at night to simulate nighttime.
- Support early extubation from mechanical ventilation.
- Encourage early and consistent feedings with breast milk.
- Administer prescribed antibiotics judiciously.
- Position the newborn as if he or she was still in utero (a nesting fetal position).
- Promote kangaroo care by encouraging parents to hold the newborn against the chest for extended periods each day.
- Coordinate care to respect sleep and awake states.

Throughout the newborn's stay, work with the parents, developing a collaborative partnership so they feel comfortable caring for their newborn. Be prepared to make referrals to community support groups to enhance coping (McGrath, 2006).

Promoting Parental Coping

Generally, pregnancy and the birth of a newborn are exciting times, but when the newborn has serious, perhaps life-threatening problems, the exciting experience suddenly changes to one of anxiety, fear, guilt, loss, and grief.

Parents are typically unprepared for the birth of a preterm newborn and commonly experience an array of emotions, including disappointment, fear for the survival of the newborn, and anxiety due to the separation from their newborn immediately after birth (Mok & Sui, 2006). Early interruptions in the bonding process and concern about the newborn's survival can create extreme anxiety and interfere with attachment (Mercer & Walker, 2006).

Nursing interventions aimed at reducing parental anxiety include:

- Reviewing with them the events that have occurred since birth
- Providing simple relaxation and calming techniques (visual imagery, breathing)
- Exploring their perception of the newborn's condition and offering explanations
- Validating their anxiety and behaviors as normal reactions to stress and trauma
- Providing a physical presence and support during emotional outbursts
- Exploring the coping strategies they used successfully in the past and encouraging their use now
- Encouraging frequent visits to the NICU
- Addressing their reactions to the NICU environment and explaining all equipment used
- Identifying family and community resources available to them (Franklin, 2006)

Preparing for Discharge

Discharge planning typically begins with evidence that recovery of the newborn is certain. However, the exact date of discharge may not be predictable. The goal of the discharge plan is to make a successful transition to home care. Essential elements for discharge are a physiologically stable infant, a family who can provide the necessary care with appropriate support services in place in the community, and a primary care physician available for ongoing care.

The care of each high-risk newborn after discharge requires careful coordination to provide ongoing multidisciplinary support for the family. The discharge planning team typically includes the parents, primary care physician, neonatologists, neonatal nurses, and a social worker. Other professionals, such as surgical specialists and pediatric subspecialists, occupational, physical, speech, and respiratory therapists, nutritionists, home health care nurses, and a case manager, may be included as needed. Critical components of discharge planning are summarized in Box 23.6.

Nurses involved in the discharge process are instrumental in bridging the gap between the hospital and home. Interventions typically include:

- Assessing the physical status of the mother and the newborn
- Discussing the early signs of complications and what to do if they occur
- Reinforcing instructions for infant care and safety
- Stressing the importance of proper car seat use
- Providing instructions for medication administration
- Reinforcing instructions for equipment operation, maintenance, and troubleshooting
- Teaching infant cardiopulmonary resuscitation and emergency care

---

BOX 23.6   Critical Components of Discharge Planning

- Parental education—involvement and support in newborn care during NICU stay will ensure their readiness to care for the infant at home
- Evaluation of unresolved medical problems—review of the active problem list and determination of what home care and follow-up is needed
- Implementation of primary care—completion of newborn screening tests, immunizations, examinations such as funduscopic exam for ROP, and hematologic status evaluation
- Development of home care plan, including assessment of:
  - Equipment and supplies needed for care
  - In-home caregiver's preparation and ability to care for infant
  - Adequacy of the physical facilities in the home
  - An emergency care and transport plan if needed
  - Financial resources for home care costs
  - Family needs and coping skills
  - Community resources, including how they can be accessed

- Demonstrating techniques for special care procedures such as dressings, ostomy care, artificial airway maintenance, chest physiotherapy, suctioning, and infant stimulation
- Providing breastfeeding support or instruction on gavage feedings
- Assisting with defining roles in the adjustment period at home
- Assessing the parents' emotional stability and coping status
- Providing support and reassurance to the family
- Reporting abnormal findings to the health care team for intervention
- Following up with parents to assure them that they have a "lifeline"

Dealing With Perinatal Loss

Perinatal loss is a profound experience for the family. It engenders a unique kind of mourning since the infant is so much a part of the parents' identity. Instead of celebrating a new life as they expected, parents are mourning the loss of dreams and hopes and the loss of an extension of themselves. NICU nurses face a difficult situation when caring for newborns who may not survive. Newborn death is incomprehensible to most parents. This makes the grieving process more difficult because what is happening "can't be real." Deciding whether to see, touch, or hold the dying newborn is extremely difficult for many parents. Nurses play a major role in assisting parents to make their dying newborn "real" to them by providing them with as many memories as possible and encouraging them to see, hold, touch, dress, and take care of the infant and take photographs. These actions help to validate the parents' sense of loss, relive the experience, and attach significance to the meaning of loss. A lock of hair, a name card, or an identification bracelet may serve as important mementoes that can ease the grieving process. The memories created by these interventions can be useful allies in the grieving process and in resolving grief (Callister, 2006).

Parent–newborn interaction is vital to the normal processes of attachment and bonding. The detachment process involved in a newborn's death is equally important for parents. Nurses can aid in this process by helping parents to see their newborn through the maze of equipment, explaining the various procedures and equipment, encouraging them to express their feelings about the newborn's status, and providing time for them to be with their dying newborn (Kavanaugh & Moro, 2006).

A common reaction by many people when learning that a newborn is not going to survive is one of avoidance. Nurses are no exception. It is difficult to initiate a conversation about such a sensitive issue without knowing how the parents are going to react and cope with the impending loss. One way to begin a conversation with the parents is to convey concern and acknowledge their loss. Active listening can give parents a safe place to begin the healing process. The relationship that the nurse establishes with the parents is a unique one, providing an opportunity for both the nurse and the parents to share their feelings.

Be aware of personal feelings about loss and how these feelings are part of one's own life and personal belief system. Actively listen to the parents when they are talking about their experiences. Communicate empathy (understanding and feeling what another person is feeling), respect their feelings, and respond to them in helpful and supportive ways (Kavanaugh & Moro, 2006). Table 23.2 highlights appropriate interventions for a family experiencing a perinatal loss before and after a newborn dies.

In a time of crisis or loss, individuals are often more sensitive to other people's reactions. For example, the parents may be extremely aware of the nurse's facial expressions, choice of words, and tone of voice. Talking quickly,

TABLE 23.2 ASSISTING PARENTS TO COPE WITH PERINATAL LOSS

Before the newborn's death	Respect variations in the family's spiritual needs and readiness.
	Assess cultural beliefs and practices that may bring comfort; respect culturally appropriate requests for truth telling and informed refusal.
	Initiate spiritual comfort by calling the hospital clergy if appropriate; offer to pray with the family if appropriate.
	Encourage the parents to take photographs, make memory boxes, and record their thoughts in a journal.
	Explore with family members how they dealt with previous losses.
	Discuss techniques to reduce stress, such as meditation and relaxation.
	Recommend that family members maintain a healthy diet and get adequate rest and exercise to preserve their health.
	Participate in early and repeated care conferencing to reduce family stress.
	Allow family to be present at both medical rounds and resuscitation; provide explanations of all procedures, treatments, and findings; answer questions honestly and as completely as possible.
	Provide opportunities for the family to hold the newborn if they choose to.
	Assess the family's support network.
	Provide suggestions as to how friends can be helpful to the family.
After the newborn's death	Help the family to accept the reality of death by using the word "died."
	Acknowledge their grief and the fact that their newborn has died.
	Help the family to work through their grief by validating and listening.
	Provide the family with realistic information about the causes of death.
	Offer condolences to the family in a sincere manner.
	Encourage the father to cry and grieve with his partner.
	Provide opportunities for the family to hold the newborn if they desire.
At the time of the release of the newborn's body	Reassure the family that their feelings and grieving responses are normal.
	Encourage the parents to have a funeral or memorial service to bring closure.
	Suggest that the parents plant a tree or flowers to remember the infant.
	Address attachment issues concerning subsequent pregnancies.
	Provide information about local support groups.
	Provide anticipatory guidance regarding the grieving process.
	Present information about any impact on future childbearing, and refer the parents to appropriate specialists or genetic resources.

Sources: Callister, 2006; Cote-Arsenault & Donato, 2007; Kobler, Limbo, & Kavanaugh, 2007.

in a businesslike fashion, or ignoring the loss may inhibit parents from discussing their pain or how they are coping with it. Parents may need to vent their frustrations and anger, and the nurse may become the target. Validate their feelings and attempt to reframe or refocus the anger toward the real issue of loss. An example would be to say, "I understand your frustration and anger about this situation. You have experienced a tremendous loss and it must be difficult not to have an explanation for it at this time." Doing so helps to defuse the anger while allowing them to express their feelings.

When assisting bereaved parents, start where the parents are in the grief process to avoid imposing your own agenda on them. You may feel uncomfortable at not being able to change the situation or take the pain away. The nurse's role is to provide immediate emotional support and facilitate the grieving process. Supporting and strengthening the family bond in the face of perinatal loss is essential.

▶ LATE PRETERM NEWBORN

A late preterm newborn is an infant born between 34 weeks and 36 weeks, 6 days of gestation. In recent years, the subject of late preterm birth has received much attention, since this population of preterm newborns represents more than 70% of all preterm births in the United States and has increased by 30% in the past 20 years (National Center for Health Statistics, 2006). With the sharp rise in the number of cesarean births performed, the incidence of late preterm newborns will also rise. Perinatal nurses need to understand the risks of late preterm births and the unique needs of this population to facilitate timely assessment and intervention to improve outcomes.

Some of the challenges facing the late preterm newborn include respiratory distress (secondary to cesarean births, maternal gestational diabetes, chorioamnionitis, premature rupture of membranes, and fetal distress); thermoregulation issues related to limited ability to flex the trunk and extremities to decrease exposed surface area; hypoglycemia related to the first two challenges (respiratory distress and cold stress); jaundice and hyperbilirubinemia related to a gestational age of 36 weeks or less; and feeding challenges related to immature suck and swallowing reflexes (Askin et al., 2007). These challenges are similar to those facing the preterm newborn and require similar management. Nurses and parents must be aware of the risks associated with late preterm births to optimize care and outcomes for this group of newborns.

■■■ Key Concepts

■ Variations in birthweight and gestational age can place a newborn at risk for problems that require special care.

■ Variations in birthweight include the following categories: small for gestational age, appropriate for gestational age, and large for gestational age. Newborns who are small or large for gestational age have special needs.

■ The small-for-gestational-age newborn faces problems related to a decrease in placental function in utero; these problems may include perinatal asphyxia, hypothermia, hypoglycemia, polycythemia, and meconium aspiration.

■ Risk factors for the birth of a large-for-gestational-age infant include maternal diabetes mellitus or glucose intolerance, multiparity, prior history of a macrosomic infant, postdates gestation, maternal obesity, male fetus, and genetics. Large-for-gestational-age newborns face problems such as birth trauma due to cephalopelvic disproportion, hypoglycemia, and jaundice secondary to hyperbilirubinemia.

■ Variations in gestational age include postterm and preterm newborns. Postterm newborns may be large or small for gestational age or dysmature, depending on placental function.

■ The postterm newborn may develop several complications after birth, including fetal hypoxia, hypoglycemia, hypothermia, polycythemia, and meconium aspiration.

■ Preterm birth is the leading cause of death within the first month of life and the second leading cause of all infant deaths.

■ The preterm newborn is at risk for complications because his or her organ systems are immature, thereby impeding the transition from intrauterine life to extrauterine life.

■ Newborns can experience pain, but their pain is difficult to validate with consistent behaviors.

■ Newborns with gestational age variations, primarily preterm newborns, benefit from developmental care, which includes a variety of activities designed to manage the environment and individualize the care based on behavioral observations.

■ Nurses play a key role in assisting the parents and family of a newborn with special needs to cope with this crisis situation, including dealing with the possibility that the newborn may not survive. Nurses working with parents experiencing a perinatal loss can help by actively listening, understanding the parents' experiences, and communicating empathy.

■ The goal of discharge planning is to make a successful transition to home care.

REFERENCES

American Academy of Pediatrics (AAP). (2006a). *Guidelines for neonatal resuscitation: Translating evidence-based guidelines for NRP.* Available at: http://www.aap.org/nrp/nrpmain.html.

American Academy of Pediatrics (AAP). (2006b). Prevention and management of pain in the neonate: An update. *Pediatrics, 118*(5), 2231–2241.

American Heart Association (AHA) and American Academy of Pediatrics (AAP). (2006). Neonatal resuscitation program (NRP). *Neonatal Network, 25*(2), 145–151.

Arenson, J., & Drake, P. (2007). *Maternal and newborn health.* Sudbury, MA: Jones and Bartlett Publishers.

Askin, D. F., Bakewell-Sachs, S., Medoff-Cooper, B., Rosenberg, S., & Santa-Donato, A. (2007). Late preterm infant assessment guide. *AWHONN,* Washington, DC.

Aylott, M. (2006a). The neonatal energy triangle. Part 1: Metabolic adaptation. *Pediatric Nursing, 18*(6), 38–42.

Aylott, M. (2006b). The neonatal energy triangle. Part 2: Thermo-regulation and respiratory adaptation. *Pediatric Nursing, 20*(7), 38–42.

Blackburn, S. (2007). *Maternal, fetal and neonatal physiology: A clinical perspective* (3rd ed.). Philadelphia: Saunders Elsevier.

Callister, L. C. (2006). Perinatal loss. *Journal of Perinatal & Neonatal Nursing, 20*(3), 227–234.

Clark, D. A., & Clark, M. B. (2007). Meconium aspiration syndrome. *eMedicine.* Available at: www.emedicine.com/ped/topic768.htm.

Côté-Arsenault, D., & Donato, K. (2007). Restrained expectations in late pregnancy following loss. *JOGNN: Journal of Obstetric, Gyne-cologic, & Neonatal Nursing, 36*(6), 550–557.

Cunningham, F. G., Leveno, K. J., Bloom, S. L., Hauth, J. C., Gilstrap, L. C., & Wenstrom, K. D. (2005). *Williams obstetrics* (22nd ed.). New York: McGraw-Hill.

Davidson, J. E., Powers, K., Hedayat, K. M., et al. (2007). Clinical practice guidelines for support of the family in the patient-centered intensive care unit: American College of Critical Care Medicine Task Force. *Critical Care Medicine, 35*(2), 605–622.

Deshpande, S. (2007). Early postnatal blood lactate predicts short-term outcome in infants with perinatal asphyxia. *Early Human Development, 83*(2), 128–129.

Dorland, W. A. N. (2007). *Dorland's illustrated medical dictionary* (30th ed.). St. Louis: Saunders Elsevier.

Field, T., Hernandez-Reif, M., Feijo, L., & Freedman, J. (2006). Pre-natal, perinatal and neonatal stimulation: A survey of neonatal nurseries. *Infant Behavior & Development, 29*(1), 24–31.

Franklin, C. (2006). The neonatal nurse's role in parental attachment in the NICU. *Critical Care Nursing Quarterly, 29*(1), 81–85.

Galligan, M. (2006). Proposed guidelines for skin-to-skin treatment of neonatal hypothermia. *MCN, 31*(5), 298–306.

Gilbert, E. S. (2007). *Manual of high-risk pregnancy and delivery* (4th ed.). St. Louis: Mosby.

Harper, T., & Lam, G. (2007). Fetal growth restriction. *eMedicine.* Available at: www.emedicine.com/med/topic3247.htm.

Hendricks-Munoz, K. D., & Prendergast, C. C. (2007). Barriers to provision of developmental care in the NICU: Neonatal nursing perceptions. *American Journal of Perinatology, 24*(2), 71–77.

Herranz, L., Pallardo, L., Hillman, N., et al. (2007). Maternal third trimester hyperglycemic excursions predict large-for-gestational-age infants in type 1 diabetic pregnancy. *Diabetes Research & Clinical Practice, 75*(1), 42–46.

Jazayeri, A. (2007). Macrosomia. *eMedicine.* Available at: http://www.emedicine.com/med/topic3279.htm.

Kates, E. H., & Kates, J. S. (2007). Anemia and polycythemia in the newborn. *Pediatrics in Review, 28*(1), 33–35.

Kavanaugh, K., & Morro, T. (2006). Supporting parents after still-birth or newborn death. *AJN, 106*(9), 74–79.

Kenner, C., & Lott, J. W. (2007). *Comprehensive neonatal care: An interdisciplinary approach* (4th ed.). St. Louis: Saunders.

Kipiani, T., Tatisvili, N., & Sirbiladze, T. (2007). Long-term neuro-logical developments of the preterm newborns. *Georgian Medical News, 142,* 42–45.

Kobler, K., Limbo, R., & Kavanaugh, K. (2007). Meaningful mo-ments: The use of ritual in perinatal and pediatric death. *MCN: The American Journal of Maternal Child Nursing, 32*(5), 288–297.

Koeppel, R. (2007). Assessment and management of acute pain in the newborn. *AWHONN.* Available at: http://www.awhonn.org.

Kristensen, S., Salihu, H., Keith, L., et al. (2007). SGA subtypes and mortality risk among singleton births. *Early Human Development, 83*(2), 99–105.

Laroia, N. (2006). Birth trauma. *eMedicine.* Available at: www.emedi-cine.com/ped/topic2836.htm.

Lessaris, K. J. (2007). Polycythemia of the newborn. *eMedicine.* Avail-able at: www.emedicine.com/ped/topic2479.htm.

Leu, M., & Diament, MJ. (2006). Meconium aspiration. *eMedicine.* Available at: www.emedicine.com/radio/topic426.htm.

Lissauer, T., & Weindling, A. (2006). *Neonatology at a glance.* Ames, IA: Blackwell Publishers.

Lyon, D. W., & Warren, D. F. (2006). A clinical guide to retinopathy of prematurity. *Review of Optometry, 143*(12), 53–61.

March of Dimes. (2007a). *Diabetes in pregnancy.* Available at: http://www.marchofdimes.com/professionals/14332_1197.asp.

March of Dimes. (2007b). *Complications of preterm birth.* Available at: www.marchofdimes.com/prematurity/5512.asp.

March of Dimes. (2007c). *Prematurity.* Available at: www.marchofdimes.com/prematurity/5408_5576.asp.

McGrath, J. M. (2006). Family-centered developmental care begins before birth. *Journal of Perinatal & Neonatal Nursing, 20*(3), 195–196.

Melnyk, B. M., Feinstein, N., & Fairbanks, E. (2006). Two decades of evidence to support implementation of the COPE program as standard practice with parents of young children unexpectedly hospitalized/critically ill children and premature infants. *Pediatric Nursing, 32*(5), 475–481.

Mercer, R. T., & Walker, L. O. (2006). A review of nursing interven-tions to foster becoming a mother. *JOGNN, 35*(5), 568–582.

Mok, E., & Sui, L. (2006). Nurses as providers of support for mothers of premature infants. *Journal of Clinical Nursing, 15*(6), 726–734.

National Center for Health Statistics (NCHS). (2006). Percent distri-bution of preterm births in the United States. *National Vital Statis-tics Reports, 55*(1), 22.

National Eye Institute. (2007). *Retinopathy of prematurity (ROP).* U.S. National Institutes of Health Resource Guide. Available at: http://nei.nih.gov/health/rop/index.asp.

Neonatal Handbook. (2007a). *Breastfeeding issues.* Available at: http://www.netsvic.org.au/nets/handbook/?doc_id=907.

Neonatal Handbook. (2007b). *Developmental care.* Available at: http://www.netsvic.org.au/nets/handbook/?doc_id=719.

Neonatal Handbook. (2007c). *Jaundice in the first two weeks of life.* Available at: http://www.netsvic.org.au/nets/handbook/?doc_id=458.

Neonatal Handbook. (2007d). *Respiratory distress syndrome.* Available at: http://www.rwh.org.au/nets/handbook/index.cfm?doc=603.

Neonatal Handbook. (2007e). *Small-for-gestational-age infants.* Avail-able at: http://www.netsvic.org.au/nets/handbook/?doc_id=821.

Neonatal Handbook. (2007f). *Infant of a diabetic mother.* Available at: http://www.netsvic.org.au/nets/handbook/?doc_id=889.

Neonatal Handbook. (2007g). *Polycythemia.* Available at: http://www.netsvic.org.au/nets/handbook/?doc_id=636.

Neonatal Handbook. (2007h). *Nutrition of the preterm infant.* Available at: http://www.rch.org.au/nets/handbook/index.cfm?doc_id=909.

Neonatal Handbook. (2007i). *Perinatal asphyxia.* Available at: http://www.rch.org.au/nets/handbook/index.cfm?doc_id=11236.

Neonatal Handbook. (2007j). *Metabolic diseases.* Available at: http://www.rch.org.au/nets/handbook/index.cfm?doc_id=895.

Stanley, C. A. (2006). Hypoglycemia in the neonate. *Pediatric Endo-crinology Reviews, 4*(1), 76–81.

U.S. Department of Health and Human Services (USDHHS), Public Health Service. (2000). *Healthy People 2010* (conference edition, in two volumes). Washington, DC.: U.S. Government Printing Office.

Vargo, L. E., & Trotter, C. W. (2007). The premature infant: Nurs-ing assessment and management. *March of Dimes Nursing Modules* (2nd ed.). #33-1995-05.

WEBSITES

March of Dimes: www.marchofdimes.com

National Association of Neonatal Nurses: www.nann.org

Neonatal Network: www.neonatalnetwork.com

Parental Guide for Developmentally Supportive Care: www.comeunity.com/premature/baby/supportive-care.html

Physical and Developmental Environment of the High-Risk Infant: www.med.usf.edu/tsinger

Premature Infant: www.premature-infant.com

CHAPTER WORKSHEET

MULTIPLE CHOICE QUESTIONS

1. The nurse documents that a newborn is postterm based on the understanding that he was born after:

   a. 38 weeks' gestation

   b. 40 weeks' gestation

   c. 42 weeks' gestation

   d. 44 weeks' gestation

2. SGA and LGA newborns have an excessive number of red blood cells because of:

   a. Hypoxia

   b. Hypoglycemia

   c. Hypocalcemia

   d. Hypothermia

3. Because subcutaneous and brown fat stores were used for survival in utero, the nurse would assess an SGA newborn for which of the following?

   a. Hyperbilirubinemia

   b. Hypothermia

   c. Polycythemia

   d. Hypoglycemia

4. In assessing a preterm newborn, which of the following findings would be of greatest concern?

   a. Milia over the bridge of the nose

   b. Thin transparent skin

   c. Poor muscle tone

   d. Heart murmur

5. In dealing with parents experiencing a perinatal loss, which of the following nursing interventions would be most appropriate?

   a. Sheltering the parents from the bad news

   b. Making all the decisions regarding care

   c. Encouraging them to participate in the newborn's care

   d. Leaving them by themselves to allow time to grieve

6. The nurse is providing care to several newborns with variations in gestational age and birthweight. When developing the plan of care for these newborns, the nurse focuses on energy conservation to promote growth and development. Which measures would the nurse include in the nursing plans of care? Select all that apply.

   a. Keeping the handling of the newborn to a minimum

   b. Maintaining a neutral thermal environment

   c. Decreasing environmental stimuli

   d. Initiating early oral feedings

   e. Using thermal warmers in all cribs

7. Which of the following concepts would the nurse incorporate into the plan of care when assessing pain in a newborn with special needs?

   a. Newborns experience pain primarily with surgical procedures.

   b. Preterm newborns in the NICU are at least risk for pain.

   c. Pain assessment needs to be comprehensive and frequent.

   d. A newborn's facial expression is the primary indicator of pain.

CRITICAL THINKING EXERCISES

1. After fetal distress was noted on the monitor, a postterm newborn was delivered via a difficult vacuum extraction. The newborn had low Apgar scores and had to be resuscitated before being transferred to the nursery. Once admitted, the nurse observed the following behaviors: jitteriness, tremors, hypotonia, lethargy, and rapid respirations.

   a. What might these behaviors indicate?

   b. For what other conditions might this newborn be at high risk?

   c. What intervention is needed to address this newborn's condition?

2. A preterm newborn was born at 35 weeks following an abruptio placentae due to a car accident. He was transported to the NICU at a nearby regional medical center. After being stabilized, he was placed in an isolette close to the door and placed on a cardiac monitor. A short time later, the nurse notices that he is cool to the touch and lethargic, has a weak cry, and has an axillary temperature of 36°C.

   a. What might have contributed to this newborn's hypothermic condition?

b. What transfer mechanism may have been a factor?

c. What intervention would be appropriate for the nurse to initiate?

3. A term SGA newborn weighing 4 lb was brought to the nursery for admission a short time after birth. The labor and birth nurse reports the mother was a heavy smoker and a cocaine addict and experienced physical abuse throughout her pregnancy. After stabilizing the newborn and correcting the hypoglycemia with oral feedings, the nurse observes the following: acrocyanosis, ruddy color, poor circulation to the extremities, tachypnea, and irritability.

a. What complication might this SGA newborn be manifesting?

b. What factors may have contributed to this complication?

c. What would be an appropriate intervention to manage this condition?

STUDY ACTIVITIES

1. At a community health department maternity clinic, secure permission to interview the parents of a special needs child. Ask about their feelings throughout the experience. How are they managing and coping now?

2. Visit the March of Dimes website and review this group's national campaign to reduce the incidence of prematurity. Are their strategies workable or not? Explain your reasoning.

3. A common metabolic disorder present in both SGA and LGA newborns after birth is

_____.

4. A 10-lb LGA newborn is brought to the nursery after a difficult vaginal birth. The nursery nurse should focus on detecting birth injuries such as

_____.

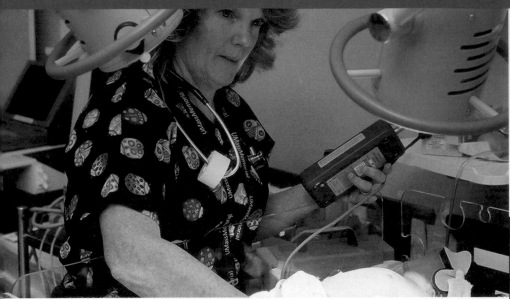

NURSING MANAGEMENT OF THE NEWBORN AT RISK: ACQUIRED AND CONGENITAL NEWBORN CONDITIONS

*K*elly, a 27-year-old G2P1, comes to the labor and birth area in active labor. She tells you she is overdue and relieved to finally be giving birth. Her membranes rupture on admission, revealing meconium-stained fluid. What additional nursing assessments need to be carried out now? What risk factors need to be considered when developing Kelly's plan of care?

KEY TERMS

alcohol–related birth
    defects
anencephaly
asphyxia
caput succedaneum
cephalhematoma
congenital diaphragmatic
    hernia
developmental dysplasia
    of the hip
epispadias

fetal alcohol spectrum
    disorder
fetal alcohol syndrome
gastrochisis
hydrocephalus
hyperbilirubinemia
hypospadias
infant of a diabetic mother
kernicterus
meconium aspiration
    syndrome

meningocele
microcephaly
myelomeningocele
neonatal abstinence
    syndrome
neonatal sepsis
neural tube defect (NTD)
omphalocele
respiratory distress
    syndrome
spina bifida

LEARNING OBJECTIVES

After completion of the chapter, the learner will be able to:

1. Identify the most common acquired conditions affecting the newborn.
2. Describe the nursing management of a newborn experiencing respiratory distress syndrome.
3. Outline the birthing room preparation and procedures necessary to prevent meconium aspiration syndrome in the newborn at birth.
4. Discuss parent education for the follow-up care needed by newborns with retinopathy of prematurity.
5. Discuss risk factors for the development of necrotizing enterocolitis.
6. Explain the impact of maternal diabetes on the newborn and the care needed.
7. Describe the assessment and interventions for a newborn experiencing substance withdrawal after birth.
8. Identify assessment and nursing management for newborns sustaining trauma and birth injuries.

Wow

Courage and faith in oneself project onto others, giving them the strength to persevere.

LEARNING OBJECTIVES (continued)

9. Outline the assessment, interventions, prevention, and management of hyperbilirubinemia in newborns.
10. Summarize the interventions appropriate for a newborn with neonatal sepsis.
11. Compare and contrast the four classifications of congenital heart disease.
12. Describe the major acquired congenital anomalies affecting the central nervous system, respiratory system, gastrointestinal system, genitourinary system, and musculoskeletal system that can occur in a newborn.
13. Discuss three inborn errors of metabolism.
14. Formulate a plan of care for a newborn with an acquired or congenital condition.
15. Discuss the importance of parental participation in care of the newborn with an acquired or congenital condition, including the nurse's role in facilitating parental involvement.

Advances in prenatal and neonatal medical and nursing care throughout the industrialized world have led to a marked increase in the number of newborns who have survived a high-risk pregnancy but experience acquired or congenital conditions. These newborns are considered at risk: that is, they are susceptible to morbidity and mortality because of the acquired or congenital disorder. Several National Health Goals address the issues of acquired and congenital conditions in newborns (Healthy People 2010).

Technological and pharmacologic advances, in conjunction with standardized policies and procedures, over the past several decades have significantly improved survival rates for at-risk newborns. However, morbidity remains an important sequela. For example, some of these newborns are at risk for continuing health problems that require long-term technological support. Other newborns remain at risk for physical and developmental problems into the school years and beyond. Providing the complex care needed to maintain the child's health and well-being will have a tremendous emotional and economic impact on the family. Nurses are challenged to provide support to mothers and their families when neonatal well-being is threatened.

Acquired disorders typically occur at or soon after birth. They may result from problems or conditions experienced by the woman during her pregnancy or at birth, such as diabetes, maternal infection, or substance abuse, or conditions associated with labor and birth, such as prolonged rupture of membranes or fetal distress. However, there may be no identifiable cause for the disorder.

Congenital disorders are disorders present at birth, usually due to some type of malformation that occurred during the antepartal period. Congenital disorders, which typically involve a problem with inheritance, include structural anomalies (commonly referred to as birth defects), chromosomal disorders, and inborn errors of metabolism. Most congenital disorders have a complex etiology, involving many interacting genes, gene products, and social and environmental factors during organogenesis. Some alterations can be prevented or compensated for with pharmacologic, nutritional, or other types of interventions, while others cannot be changed. Only through a better understanding of the complex interplay of genetic, environmental, social, and cultural factors can these devastating and life-changing outcomes be prevented (Arenson & Drake, 2007).

This chapter addresses selected acquired and congenital newborn conditions. In addition, it describes the nurse's role in assessment and management, emphasizing parental education and support. Nurses play a key role in helping the parents cope with the stress of having an ill newborn.

Acquired Disorders

▶ NEONATAL ASPHYXIA

As the newborn makes the transition to life outside the fluid-filled intrauterine environment, dramatic changes must occur to facilitate newborn respirations. Newborns normally start to breathe with routine warming, drying, airway suctioning, and mild stimulation. Most newborns make this transition such that by 1 minute of age, they are breathing well on their own. A newborn who fails to establish adequate, sustained respiration after birth is said to have **asphyxia**. Physiologically, asphyxia can be defined as impaired gas exchange resulting in a decrease in blood oxygen levels (hypoxemia) and an excess of carbon dioxide or hypercapnia that leads to acidosis.

HEALTHY PEOPLE 2010

Objective	Significance
1. Reduce fetal and infant deaths Decrease the number of all infant deaths (within 1 year) from a baseline of 7.2/1,000 live births to 4.5/1,000 live births. Decrease the number of neonatal deaths (within the first 28 days of life) from a baseline of 4.8 to 2.9 deaths/1,000 live births. Decrease the number of post-neonatal deaths from a baseline of 2.4 to 1.2 deaths/1,000 live births. Reduce the number of deaths related to all birth defects from a baseline of 1.6 to 1.1 deaths/1,000 live births.	• Will foster early and consistent prenatal care, including education to place infants on their backs for naps and sleeping to prevent SIDS and avoidance of exposing the newborn to cigarette smoke
2. Reduce the occurrence of developmental disabilities Reduce the number of children with mental retardation from a baseline of 131 to 124 children/10,000. Reduce the number of children with cerebral palsy from a baseline of 32.2 to 31.5 children/10,000. Reduce the number of children with autism spectrum disorder.	• Will promote measures for close antepartal and intrapartal monitoring of women at risk, subsequently reducing the incidence of disabilities, leading to a reduction in long-term effects and costs of care
3. Reduce the occurrence of spina bifida and other neural tube defects. Reduce the number of new cases of spina bifida or other neural tube defects from a baseline of 6 to 3 new cases/10,000 live births.	• Will help to increase awareness of the need for all women of childbearing age to take a multivitamin containing at least 400 mg of folic acid and consume foods high in folic acid.
4. Reduce the occurrence of fetal alcohol syndrome	• Will foster programs for at-risk groups, including adolescents, about the effects of substance abuse, especially alcohol, during pregnancy
5. Ensure appropriate newborn blood spot screening, follow-up testing, and referral to services. Ensure all newborns are screened at birth for conditions as mandated by their state-sponsored newborn screening programs. Ensure that follow-up diagnostic testing for screening positives is performed within an appropriate time period. Ensure that infants with diagnosed disorders are enrolled in appropriate service interventions within an appropriate time period.	• Will help in the development of protocols and procedures to ensure appropriate screening and follow-up for all newborns.

DHHS, 2000; available online at www.healthypeople.gov.

Asphyxia is the most common clinical insult in the perinatal period. As many as 10% of newborns require some degree of active resuscitation to stimulate breathing (Cunningham et al., 2005). According to the World Health Organization, 4 to 9 million cases of neonatal asphyxia occur annually worldwide, accounting for approximately 20% of all newborn deaths. More than a million newborns who survive asphyxia at birth develop long-term problems such as cerebral palsy, mental retardation, and speaking, hearing, visual, and learning disabilities (Maternal and Neonatal Health [MNH], 2007).

Pathophysiology

Asphyxia occurs when oxygen delivery is insufficient to meet metabolic demands, resulting in hypoxia, hypercarbia, and metabolic acidosis. Any condition that reduces oxygen delivery to the fetus can result in asphyxia. These conditions may include maternal hypoxia, such as from cardiac or respiratory disease, anemia, or postural hypotension; maternal vascular disease that leads to placental insufficiency, such as diabetes or hypertension; cord problems such as compression or prolapse; and postterm pregnancies, which may trigger meconium release into the amniotic fluid.

Initially, the newborn uses compensatory mechanisms including tachycardia and vasoconstriction to help bring oxygen to the vital organs for a time. However, without intervention, these mechanisms fail, leading to hypotension, bradycardia, and eventually cardiopulmonary arrest.

With failure to breathe well after birth, the newborn will develop hypoxia (too little oxygen in the cells of the body). As a result, the heart rate falls, cyanosis develops, and the newborn becomes hypotonic and unresponsive.

Think back to Kelly, described at the beginning of the chapter. She gives birth to a son weighing approximately 2,500 g; he appears postterm and small for gestational age. His skin is stained yellow-green and he is limp, cyanotic, and apneic at birth. The initial assessment once the newborn is under the radiant warmer indicates that resuscitation and tracheal suctioning are needed. What is the nurse's role during resuscitation? What assessments will be needed during this procedure?

Nursing Assessment

The key to successful treatment of newborn asphyxia is early identification and recognition of newborns who may be at risk. Review the perinatal history for risk factors, including:

- Trauma: injury to the central or peripheral nervous system secondary to a long or difficult labor, a precipitous birth, multiple gestation, abnormal presentation, cephalopelvic disproportion, shoulder dystocia, or extraction by forceps or vacuum
- Intrauterine asphyxia: for example, fetal hypoxia secondary to maternal hypoxia, diabetes, hypertension, anemia, cord compression, or meconium aspiration
- Sepsis: acquired bacterial or viral organisms from infected amniotic fluid, maternal infection, or direct contact while passing through the birth canal
- Malformation: congenital anomalies including facial or upper airway deformities, renal anomalies, pulmonary hypoplasia, neuromuscular disorders, esophageal atresia, or neural tube defects
- Hypovolemic shock: secondary to abruptio placentae, placenta previa, or cord rupture resulting in blood loss to the fetus
- Medication: drugs given to mother during labor that can affect the fetus by causing placental hypoperfusion and hypotension; use of hypnotics, analgesics, anesthetics, narcotics, oxytocin, and street drugs during pregnancy

At birth, assess the newborn immediately. Observe the infant's color, noting any pallor or cyanosis. Assess the work of breathing. Be alert for apnea, tachypnea, gasping respirations, grunting, nasal flaring, or retractions. Evaluate heart rate and note bradycardia. Assess the newborn's temperature, noting hypothermia. Determine the Apgar score at 1 and 5 minutes; an Apgar score below 7 at either time indicates that resuscitation is needed.

Anticipate diagnostic testing to identify etiologies for the newborn's asphyxia. For example, a chest x-ray may identify structural abnormalities that might interfere with respiration. A blood culture may identify an infectious process. A blood toxicology screen may detect any maternal drugs in the newborn (Kenner & Lott, 2007).

Nursing Management

Management of the newborn experiencing asphyxia includes immediate resuscitation. Ensure that the equipment needed for resuscitation is readily available and in working order. Essential equipment includes a wall suction apparatus, an oxygen source, a newborn ventilation bag, endotracheal tubes (2 to 3 mm), a laryngoscope, and ampules of naloxone (Narcan) with syringes and needles for administration (see Chapter 23 for a more detailed discussion of resuscitation).

Dry the newborn quickly with a warm towel and then place him or her under a radiant heater to prevent rapid heat loss through evaporation. Handling and rubbing the newborn with a dry towel may be all that is needed to stimulate breathing. If the newborn fails to respond to stimulation, then active resuscitation is needed.

The procedure for newborn resuscitation is easily remembered by the "ABCDs"—airway, breathing, circulation, and drugs (see Chapter 23, Box 23.3). Continue resuscitation until the newborn has a pulse above 100 bpm, a good cry, or good breathing efforts and a pink tongue. This last sign indicates a good oxygen supply to the brain (Brodsky & Ouellette, 2007).

> ▶ **Take** NOTE!
>
> *According to the American Heart Association and American Academy of Pediatrics Emergency Care Guidelines for Neonatal Resuscitation, resuscitation efforts may be stopped if the newborn exhibits no heart beat and no respiratory effort after 10 minutes of continuous and adequate resuscitation (AHA/AAP, 2005; Zaichkin, 2006).*

Provide continued observation and assessment of the newborn who has been successfully resuscitated. Monitor the newborn's vital signs and oxygen saturation levels closely for changes. Maintain a neutral thermal environment to prevent hypothermia, which would increase the newborn's metabolic and oxygen demands. Check the blood glucose level and observe for signs of hypoglycemia; if this develops, it can further stress the newborn.

The need for resuscitative measures can be extremely upsetting for the parents. Explain to them the initial resuscitation activities being performed and offer ongoing explanations about any procedures being done, equipment being used, or medications given. Provide physical and emotional support to the parents through the initial crisis and throughout the newborn's stay. When the newborn is stable, allow parents to spend time with their newborn to promote bonding (Fig. 24.1). Point out the newborn's positive attributes and give frequent updates on his or her status. Role-model techniques for holding,

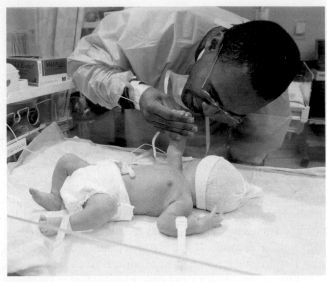

FIGURE 24.1 A father interacting with his newborn once the newborn's condition has stabilized.

interacting with, and caring for the newborn to decrease the parents' anxiety.

Remember Kelly, the young woman described at the beginning of the chapter? Her son is intubated and tracheal suctioning is performed. Positive-pressure ventilation is also started with a self-inflating bag and 50% oxygen. Ventilation is continued for 1 minute and then gradually discontinued. The heart rate is now 120 bpm, and spontaneous respirations are noted. When free-flow oxygen is administered, the newborn begins to cry and turn pink. What continued care is needed in the special care nursery? What explanation should be offered to Kelly regarding her son's treatment?

▶ TRANSIENT TACHYPNEA OF THE NEWBORN

Transient tachypnea of the newborn (TTN) is a condition involving a mild degree of respiratory distress. It is described as the retention of lung fluid or transient pulmonary edema (McLenan, 2007). It usually occurs within a few hours of birth and resolves by 72 hours of age. TTN occurs in approximately 11 per 1,000 live births (Asenjo, 2007).

Pathophysiology

Most newborns make the transition from fetal to newborn life without incident. During fetal life, the lungs are filled with a serous fluid because the placenta, not the lungs, is used for nutrient and gas exchange. During and after birth, this fluid must be removed and replaced with air. Passage through the birth canal during a vaginal birth compresses the thorax, which helps remove the majority of this fluid. Pulmonary circulation and the lymphatic drainage remove the remaining fluid shortly after birth. TTN occurs when the liquid in the lung is removed slowly or incompletely.

Nursing Assessment

Astutely observe the newborn with respiratory distress because TTN is a diagnosis of exclusion. Initially it might be difficult to distinguish this condition from respiratory distress syndrome or group B streptococcal pneumonia, since the clinical picture is similar. However, the symptoms of transient tachypnea rarely last more than 72 hours (McLenan, 2007).

Health History and Physical Examination

Review the perinatal history for contributing factors. TTN is commonly seen in newborns who are sedated or have been born via cesarean birth. Also check the history for evidence of a prolonged labor, fetal macrosomia, and maternal asthma and smoking. These factors are associated with a higher incidence of TTN.

Closely assess the newborn for signs of TTN. Within the first few hours of birth, observe for tachypnea, expiratory grunting, retractions, labored breathing, nasal flaring, and mild cyanosis (Asenjo, 2007). Mild to moderate respiratory distress is present by 6 hours of age, with respiratory rates as high as 100 to 140 breaths per minute (Kenner & Lott, 2007). Also inspect the newborn's chest for hyperextension or a barrel shape. Auscultate breath sounds, which may be slightly diminished secondary to reduced air entry.

Laboratory and Diagnostic Testing

To aid in the diagnosis, a chest x-ray may be done. It usually reveals mild symmetric lung overaeration and prominent perihilar interstitial markings and streaking. These findings correlate with lymphatic engorgement of retained fetal fluid (Asenjo, 2007).

Nursing Management

Nursing management focuses on providing adequate oxygenation and determining whether the newborn's respiratory manifestations appear to be resolving or persisting. Provide supportive care while the retained lung fluid is reabsorbed. Administer intravenous (IV) fluids and/or gavage feedings until the respiratory rate decreases enough to allow safe oral feeding. Provide supplemental oxygen via a nasal cannula or oxygen hood to maintain adequate oxygen saturation. Maintain a neutral thermal environment with minimal stimulation to minimize oxygen demand.

Provide ongoing assessment of the newborn's respiratory status. As TTN resolves, the newborn's respiratory rate declines to 60 breaths per minute or less, the oxygen requirement decreases, and the chest x-ray shows resolution of the perihilar streaking. Provide reassurance and progress reports to the parents to help them cope with this crisis.

▶ RESPIRATORY DISTRESS SYNDROME

Despite improved survival rates and advances in perinatal care, many high-risk newborns are at risk for respiratory problems, particularly **respiratory distress syndrome** (RDS), a breathing disorder resulting from lung immaturity and lack of alveolar surfactant. Since the link between RDS and surfactant deficiency was discovered more than 30 years ago, tremendous strides have been made in understanding the pathophysiology and treatment of this disorder. The introduction of prenatal steroids to accelerate lung maturity and the development of synthetic surfactant can be credited with the dramatic improvements in the outcome of newborns with RDS.

RDS affects an estimated 25,000 infants born alive in the United States annually. The incidence declines with degree of maturity at birth. It occurs in 60% of preterm newborns of less than 28 weeks' gestation, 30% of those born at 28 to 34 weeks, and less than 5% of those born after 34 weeks (American Lung Association [ALA], 2007). Intensive respiratory care, usually with mechanical ventilation, is necessary.

Pathophysiology

Lung immaturity and surfactant deficiency contribute to the development of RDS. Surfactant is a complex mixture of phospholipids and proteins that adheres to the alveolar surface of the lungs. Surfactant forms a coating over the inner surface of the alveoli, reducing the surface tension and preventing alveolar collapse at the end of expiration. In the affected newborn, surfactant is deficient or lacking, and this deficit results in stiff lungs and alveoli that tend to collapse, leading to diffuse atelectasis. The work of breathing is increased because increased pressure similar to that required to initiate the first breath is needed to inflate the lungs with each successive breath. Hypoxemia and acidemia result, leading to vasoconstriction of the pulmonary vasculature. Right-to-left shunting occurs and alveolar capillary circulation is limited, further inhibiting surfactant production. As the disease progresses, fluid and fibrin leak from the pulmonary capillaries, causing hyaline membranes to form in the bronchioles, alveolar ducts, and alveoli. These membranes further decrease gas exchange. A vicious circle is created, compounding the problem (Blackburn, 2007).

Nursing Assessment

Nursing assessment focuses on keen observation to identify the signs and symptoms of respiratory distress. In addition, assessment aids in differentiating RDS from other respiratory conditions, such as TTN or group B streptococcal pneumonia.

Health History and Physical Examination

Review the history for risk factors associated with RDS; these include perinatal asphyxia regardless of gestational age, cesarean birth in the absence of preceding labor (due to the lack of thoracic squeezing), male gender, and maternal diabetes. It is believed that each of these conditions has an impact on surfactant production, thus resulting in RDS in the term infant (Stoll & Kliegman, 2007).

> ▶ *Take NOTE!*
>
> *Prolonged rupture of membranes, intrauterine growth restriction (IUGR), gestational hypertension, maternal heroin addiction, and use of prenatal corticosteroids reduce the newborn's risk for RDS because of the physiologic stress imposed on the fetus. Chronic stress experienced by the fetus in utero accelerates the production of surfactant before the 35th week of gestation and thus reduces the incidence of RDS at birth.*

The newborn with RDS usually demonstrates signs at birth or within a few hours of birth. Observe the infant for expiratory grunting, nasal flaring, chest wall retractions, seesaw respirations, and generalized cyanosis. Auscultate the heart and lungs, noting tachycardia (rates above 150 to 180), fine inspiratory crackles, and tachypnea (rates above 60 breaths per minute). Use the Silverman-Anderson index assessment tool to determine the degree of respiratory distress. The index involves observation of five features, each of which is scored as 0, 1, or 2 (Fig. 24.2). The higher the score, the greater the respiratory distress. A score over 7 suggests severe respiratory distress.

Laboratory and Diagnostic Testing

The diagnosis of RDS is based on the clinical picture and x-ray findings. A chest x-ray reveals hypoaeration, underexpansion, and a "ground glass" pattern (Brodsky & Ouellete, 2007; Simpson & Creehan, 2008).

Nursing Management

If untreated, RDS will worsen. However, it appears to be a self-limiting disease, with respiratory symptoms declining after 72 hours. This decline parallels the production of surfactant in the alveoli (McLenan, 2007). The newborn needs supportive care until surfactant is produced. Effec-

Score

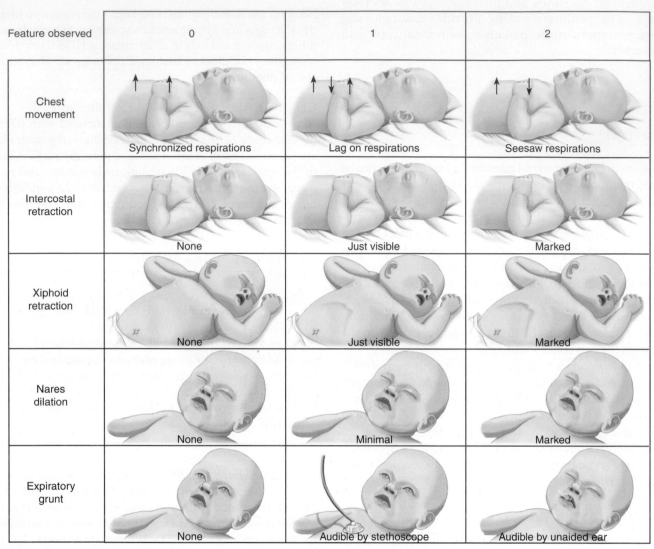

Feature observed	0	1	2
Chest movement	Synchronized respirations	Lag on respirations	Seesaw respirations
Intercostal retraction	None	Just visible	Marked
Xiphoid retraction	None	Just visible	Marked
Nares dilation	None	Minimal	Marked
Expiratory grunt	None	Audible by stethoscope	Audible by unaided ear

FIGURE 24.2 Assessing the degree of respiratory distress. (Used with permission from Silverman, W. A., & Anderson, D. H. [1956]. A controlled clinical trial of effects of water mist on obstructive respiratory signs, death rate, and necroscopy findings among premature infants. *Pediatrics, 17*[4], 1–9.)

tive therapies for established RDS include conventional mechanical ventilation, continuous positive airway pressure (CPAP), or positive end-expiratory pressure (PEEP) to prevent volume loss during expiration, and surfactant therapy. The use of exogenous surfactant replacement therapy to stabilize the newborn's lungs until postnatal surfactant synthesis matures has become a life-saver.

Care of the newborn with RDS is primarily supportive and requires a multidisciplinary approach to obtain the best outcomes. Therapy focuses on improving oxygenation and maintaining optimal lung volumes. Expect to transfer the newborn to the neonatal intensive care unit (NICU) soon after birth. Apply the basic principles of newborn care, such as thermoregulation, cardiovascular and nutritional support, normal glucose level maintenance, and infection

prevention, to achieve the therapeutic goals of reducing mortality and minimizing lung trauma.

Anticipate the administration of surfactant replacement therapy, prophylactically or as a rescue approach. With prophylactic administration, surfactant is given within minutes after birth, thus providing replacement surfactant before severe RDS develops. Rescue treatment is indicated for newborns with established RDS who require mechanical ventilation and supplemental oxygen. The earlier the surfactant is administered, the better the effect on gas exchange (Kenner & Lott, 2007).

Administer the prescribed oxygen concentration via nasal cannula. Anticipate the need for ventilator therapy, which has greatly improved in the past several years, with significant advances in conventional and high-frequency ventilation therapies (Fig. 24.3). Recent studies show no difference in outcomes for newborns who received early treatment with high-frequency oscillatory ventilation compared with those receiving conventional mechanical ventilation (Blackburn, 2007). Although mechanical ventilation has increased survival rates, it is also a contributing factor to bronchopulmonary dysplasia, pulmonary hypertension, and retinopathy of prematurity (Cunningham et al., 2005).

In addition, support the newborn with RDS using the following interventions:

- Continuously monitor the infant's cardiopulmonary status via invasive or noninvasive means (e.g., arterial lines or auscultation, respectively).
- Monitor oxygen saturation levels continuously; assess pulse oximeter values to determine oxygen saturation levels.
- Closely monitor vital signs, acid–base status, and arterial blood gases.
- Administer broad-spectrum antibiotics if blood cultures are positive.
- Administer sodium bicarbonate or acetate as ordered to correct metabolic acidosis.
- Provide fluids and vasopressor agents as needed to prevent or treat hypotension.
- Test blood glucose levels and administer dextrose as ordered for prevention or treatment of hypoglycemia.
- Cluster caretaking activities to avoid overtaxing and compromising the newborn.
- Place the newborn in the prone position to optimize respiratory status and reduce stress.
- Perform gentle suctioning to remove secretions and maintain a patent airway.
- Assess level of consciousness to identify intraventricular hemorrhage.
- Provide sufficient calories via gavage and IV feedings.
- Maintain adequate hydration and assess for signs of fluid overload.

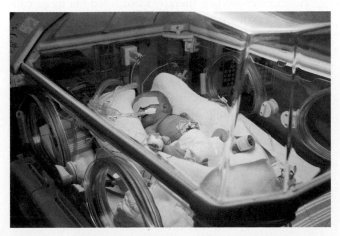

FIGURE 24.3 A newborn with RDS receiving mechanical ventilation.

- Provide information to the parents about treatment modalities; give thorough but simple explanations about the rationales for interventions and provide support.
- Encourage the parents to participate in care (Blackburn, 2007).

Provide ongoing assessment and be alert for complications. These may include air leak syndrome, bronchopulmonary dysplasia (chronic lung disease), patent ductus arteriosus, congestive heart failure, intraventricular hemorrhage, retinopathy of prematurity, necrotizing enterocolitis, complications resulting from intravenous catheter use (infection, thrombus formation), and developmental delay or disability (Stoll & Kliegman, 2007).

▶ MECONIUM ASPIRATION SYNDROME

Meconium is a viscous green substance composed primarily of water and other gastrointestinal secretions that can be noted in the fetal gastrointestinal tract as early as 10 to 16 weeks' gestation (Clark & Clark, 2007). It is expelled as the newborn's first stool after birth. **Meconium aspiration syndrome** occurs when the newborn inhales particulate meconium mixed with amniotic fluid into the lungs while still in utero or on taking the first breath after birth. It is a common cause of newborn respiratory distress and can lead to severe illness. Meconium staining of the amniotic fluid, with the possibility of aspiration, occurs in approximately 20% of pregnancies at term (Cunningham et al., 2005). Aspiration induces airway obstruction, surfactant dysfunction, hypoxia, and chemical pneumonitis with inflammation of pulmonary tissues. In severe cases, it progresses to persistent pulmonary hypertension and death (Cunningham et al., 2005). About 3% to 5% of infants with meconium aspiration syndrome die (Wiswell, Tin, & Ohler, 2007).

Pathophysiology

Meconium may be passed in utero secondary to hypoxic stress. Hypoxia induces the fetus to gasp or attempt to breathe. The fetus may bear down and pass meconium into the amniotic fluid or he or she may experience a vagal reflex that causes relaxation of the anal sphincter, allowing meconium to be passed into the amniotic fluid. The fetus then sucks or swallows this amniotic fluid in utero, or the infant may aspirate meconium with the first breath after birth as air rushes into the lungs.

Although the etiology is not well understood, the effects of meconium can be harmful to the fetus. Meconium alters the amniotic fluid by reducing antibacterial activity and subsequently increasing the risk of perinatal bacterial infection. Additionally, meconium is very irritating because it contains enzymes from the fetal pancreas.

When aspirated into the lungs, meconium blocks the bronchioles, causing an inflammatory reaction as well as a decrease in surfactant production. Gas exchange is impaired and atelectasis occurs. A ball–valve effect occurs when air is inspired into the alveoli but cannot be fully expired secondary to reduced airway diameter. Significant respiratory distress is followed by persistent pulmonary hypertension, right-to-left shunting of blood, and patent ductus arteriosus. Conventional mechanical ventilation, extracorporeal membrane oxygenation (ECMO), nitric oxide, high-frequency ventilation, or liquid ventilation may be necessary.

Nursing Assessment

Review prenatal and birth records to identify newborns who may be at high risk for meconium aspiration. Predisposing factors for meconium aspiration syndrome include postterm pregnancy; breech, forceps, or vacuum extraction births; prolonged or difficult labor associated with fetal distress in a term or postterm newborn; maternal hypertension or diabetes; oligohydramnios; IUGR; prolapsed cord; or acute or chronic placental insufficiency (Kenner & Lott, 2007).

Assess the amniotic fluid for meconium staining when the maternal membranes rupture. Green-stained amniotic fluid suggests the presence of meconium in the amniotic fluid and should be reported immediately. After birth, note any yellowish-green staining of the umbilical cord, nails, and skin. This staining indicates that meconium has been present for some time.

*C*onsider Kelly, the 27-year-old woman who gave birth to a son who required resuscitation. What findings would lead the nurse to suspect that her son aspirated meconium? What risk factors in Kelly's history would support the diagnosis of meconium aspiration syndrome?

▶ **Take** NOTE!

Standard prevention and treatment for meconium aspiration syndrome previously included suctioning the mouth and nares upon head delivery before body delivery. However, recent evidence suggests that aspiration occurs in utero, not at delivery; therefore, the infant's birth should not be impeded for suctioning. After full delivery, the infant should be handed to a neonatal team for evaluation and treatment. Although infants previously have been given intubation and airway suctioning, current evidence favors expectant management unless certain criteria (i.e., spontaneous respiration, heart rate greater than 100 beats per minute, and reasonable tone) are absent (Hermansen & Lorah, 2007).

Observe the newborn for a barrel-shaped chest with an increased anterior-posterior (AP) chest diameter (similar to that found in a patient with chronic obstructive pulmonary disease), prolonged tachypnea, progression from mild to severe respiratory distress, intercostal retractions, end-expiratory grunting, and cyanosis (Clark & Clark, 2007). Auscultate the lungs, noting coarse crackles and rhonchi.

Chest x-rays show patchy, fluffy infiltrates unevenly distributed throughout the lungs and marked hyperaeration mixed with areas of atelectasis. Arterial blood gas analysis will indicate metabolic acidosis with a low blood pH, decreased PaO_2, and increased $PaCO_2$ (Wiswell, Tin, & Ohler, 2007). Direct visualization of the vocal cords for meconium staining using a laryngoscope can confirm the presence of meconium below the larynx.

Nursing Management

Nursing management focuses on ensuring adequate tissue perfusion and minimizing oxygen demand and energy expenditure. Caring for the newborn with meconium aspiration begins in the birthing unit when the birth attendant identifies meconium-stained amniotic fluid with membrane rupture during labor. Upon delivery of the newborn's head, before the newborn takes the first breath, the nasal cavity and then the posterior pharynx are gently suctioned to decrease the potential for aspiration. If the newborn is significantly depressed at birth, secondary clearing of the lower airways by direct tracheal suctioning may be necessary. Repeated suctioning and stimulation are limited to prevent overstimulation and further depression (Clark & Clark, 2007). Usually the newborn is transferred to the NICU for close monitoring.

Maintain a neutral thermal environment, including placing the newborn under a radiant warmer or in a warmed isolette, to prevent hypothermia. In addition, minimize handling to reduce energy expenditure and oxygen consumption that could lead to further hypoxemia and acidosis.

Administer oxygen therapy as ordered via nasal cannula or with positive-pressure ventilation. Monitor oxygen saturation levels via pulse oximetry to evaluate the newborn's response to treatment and to detect changes. Increased pulmonary pressures associated with meconium aspiration may cause blood to be shunted away from the lungs. The newborn may exhibit uneven pulmonary ventilation, with hyperinflation in some areas and atelectasis in others. This leads to poor perfusion and subsequent hypoxemia, which in turn may increase pulmonary vasoconstriction, resulting in a worsening of hypoxemia and acidosis.

Expect to administer hyperoxygenation to dilate the pulmonary vasculature and close the ductus arteriosus or nitric oxide inhalation to decrease pulmonary vascular resistance, or to use high-frequency oscillatory ventilation to increase the chance of air trapping (Clark & Clark, 2007). In addition, administer vasopressors and pulmonary vasodilators as prescribed and administer surfactant as ordered to counteract inactivation by meconium. Monitor arterial blood gas results for changes and assist with measures to correct acid–base imbalances to facilitate perfusion of tissues and prevent pulmonary hypertension (Simpson & Creehan, 2008). If these measures are ineffective, be prepared to assist with the use of ECMO, a modified type of heart–lung machine.

In addition, perform the following interventions:

- Cluster newborn care to minimize oxygen demand.
- Administer broad-spectrum antibiotics to treat bacterial pneumonia.
- Administer sedation to reduce oxygen consumption and energy expenditure.
- Continuously monitor the newborn's condition.
- Provide continuous reassurance and support to the parents throughout the experience (McLenan, 2007).

▶ PERSISTENT PULMONARY HYPERTENSION OF THE NEWBORN

Persistent pulmonary hypertension of the newborn, previously referred to as persistent fetal circulation, is a cardiopulmonary disorder characterized by marked pulmonary hypertension that causes right-to-left extrapulmonary shunting of blood and hypoxemia. Persistent pulmonary hypertension can occur idiopathically or as a complication of perinatal asphyxia, meconium aspiration syndrome, pneumonia, congenital heart defects, metabolic disorders such as hypoglycemia, hypothermia, hypovolemia, hyperviscosity, acute hypoxia with delayed resuscitation, sepsis, and RDS. It occurs in 2 to 6 newborns per 1,000 live births of term, near-term, or postterm infants (Steinhorn, 2007).

Pathophysiology

Normally, pulmonary artery pressure decreases when the newborn takes the first breath. However, interference with this ability to breathe allows pulmonary pressures to remain increased. Hypoxemia and acidosis also occur, leading to vasoconstriction of the pulmonary artery. These events cause an elevation in pulmonary vascular resistance. Normally, the decrease in pulmonary artery pressure and pulmonary vascular resistance with breathing leads to the closure of the ductus arteriosus and foramen ovale. However, with persistent pulmonary hypertension, pulmonary vascular resistance is elevated to the point that venous blood is diverted to some degree through fetal structures, such as the ductus arteriosus or foramen ovale, causing them to remain open, leading to a right-to-left shunting of blood into the systemic circulation. This diversion of blood bypasses the lungs, resulting in systemic arterial hypoxemia.

Nursing Assessment

Assess the newborn's status closely. A newborn with persistent pulmonary hypertension demonstrates tachypnea within 12 hours after birth. Observe for marked cyanosis, grunting, and retractions. Auscultate the heart, noting a systolic ejection murmur, and measure blood pressure for hypotension resulting from both heart failure and persistent hypoxemia (Kenner & Lott, 2007). Measure oxygen saturation via pulse oximetry and report low values. Prepare the newborn for an echocardiogram, which will reveal right-to-left shunting of blood that confirms the diagnosis.

Nursing Management

When caring for the newborn with persistent pulmonary hypertension, pay meticulous attention to detail, with continuous monitoring of the newborn's oxygenation and perfusion status and blood pressure. The goals of therapy include improving alveolar oxygenation, inducing metabolic alkalosis by administering sodium bicarbonate, correcting hypovolemia and hypotension with the administration of volume replacement and vasopressors, and anticipating use of ECMO when support has failed to maintain acceptable oxygenation (Steinhorn, 2007).

Provide immediate resuscitation after birth and administer oxygen therapy as ordered. Early and effective resuscitation and correction of acidosis and hypoxia are helpful in preventing persistent pulmonary hypertension. Monitor arterial blood gases frequently to evaluate the effectiveness of oxygen therapy. Provide respiratory support, which frequently necessitates the use of mechanical ventilation. Administer prescribed medications, monitor cardiopulmonary status, cluster care to reduce stimulation, and provide ongoing support and education to the parents.

> ▶ **Take** NOTE!
>
> *Almost any procedure, such as suctioning, weighing, changing diapers, or positioning, can precipitate severe hypoxemia due to the instability of the pulmonary vasculature. Therefore, minimize the newborn's exposure to stimulation as much as possible.*

▶ BRONCHOPULMONARY DYSPLASIA

Bronchopulmonary dysplasia, currently referred to as chronic lung disease, commonly occurs in infants who have experienced a lung injury resulting in the need for continued use of oxygen after the initial neonatal period (28 days of life). Approximately 5,000 to 10,000 new cases of bronchopulmonary dysplasia occur each year.

White male infants seem to be at greatest risk for developing bronchopulmonary dysplasia (ALA, 2007). The overall costs of treating bronchopulmonary dysplasia in the United States are estimated to be $2.4 billion annually (ALA, 2007). Newborns with bronchopulmonary dysplasia need hospital care for several months after birth and home oxygen therapy after being discharged.

Pathophysiology

Bronchopulmonary dysplasia results from an underlying lung injury. However, the etiology of the lung injury is multifactorial: it is associated with surfactant deficiency, pulmonary edema, lung immaturity, barotrauma from mechanical ventilation, and fluid overload. Lung injury commonly occurs secondary to mechanical ventilation and oxygen toxicity, usually in infants who have had RDS. High inspired oxygen concentrations cause an inflammatory process in the lungs that leads to parenchymal damage (Driscoll & Davis, 2007). This damage includes epithelial stretching, invasion by macrophages and polymorphonuclear leukocytes, airway edema interfering with the growth and development of lung structures, loss of cilia, and a decrease in the number of alveoli.

Therapeutic Management

Bronchopulmonary dysplasia can be prevented by administering steroids to the mother in the antepartal period and exogenous surfactant to the newborn to help reduce the risk for RDS and its severity. In addition, using high-frequency ventilation and nitric oxide helps reduce the need for respiratory support with mechanical ventilation (Lowdermilk & Perry, 2007).

Supplemental oxygen, antibiotics, and fluid restriction and diuretics to decrease fluid accumulation in the lungs are used. Bronchodilators are used to open the airways. Intravenous feedings are given to meet the infant's nutrition needs, and physical therapy is used to improve muscle performance and to help the lungs expel mucus.

Nursing Assessment

Although bronchopulmonary dysplasia is most common in preterm newborns, it can also occur in full-term ones who had respiratory problems during their first days of life. Thus, it is essential to assess the newborn's history for risk factors, including male gender, preterm birth (<32 weeks), nutritional deficiencies, white race, excessive fluid intake during the first few days of life, presence of patent ductus arteriosus, severe RDS treated with mechanical ventilation for more than 1 week, and sepsis (Cutz & Chiasson, 2008). Also review the history for use of supplemental oxygen, the length of exposure to oxygen therapy, and the use of ventilatory support.

Assess the infant for signs and symptoms of bronchopulmonary dysplasia. These may include tachypnea, poor weight gain related to the increased metabolic work-load, tachycardia, sternal retractions, nasal flaring, and bronchospasm with abnormal breath sounds (crackles, rhonchi, and wheezes). Hypoxia, as evidenced by abnormal blood gas results, and acidosis and hypercapnia also are noted. Chest x-rays will show hyperinflation, infiltrates, and cardiomegaly.

Nursing Management

Nursing care includes providing continuous ventilatory and oxygen support and optimal nutrition to support growth, and administering bronchodilators, anti-inflammatory agents, and diuretics as ordered. Continuously monitor the newborn's respiratory status to determine the need for continued ventilatory assistance. When the newborn is clinically stable and ready, expect to wean him or her slowly so that he or she can compensate for the changes. Supplemental oxygen may be needed after discharge from the hospital. Provide a high caloric intake to promote growth and to compensate for the calories expended due to the increased work of breathing. Some infants may require high-calorie formulas to foster adequate growth.

Newborns with bronchopulmonary dysplasia may require continued care at home. When planning for discharge, educate the family caretaker about how to manage a chronically ill child who may be oxygen-dependent for an extended time. Provide ongoing support to parents as they learn to meet their infant's needs. Also instruct the family about the safe use of oxygen in the home, including the need to notify emergency medical services and utility companies that a technology-dependent child is living in their district. In addition, initiate a social service referral to help the family access community resources and obtain necessary support (Cutz & Chiasson, 2008).

▶ RETINOPATHY OF PREMATURITY

Retinopathy of prematurity (ROP) is a developmental abnormality that affects the immature blood vessels of the retina. The incidence of ROP in preterm newborns is inversely proportional to their birthweight. Of the approximately 4 million infants born in the United States annually, about 28,000 weigh 1,500 grams (2.75 lb) or less. About 14,000 to 16,000 of these infants are affected by some degree of ROP (National Eye Institute [NEI], 2008). ROP can lead to lifelong vision impairment and blindness (NEI, 2008). It can also lead to vitreous hemorrhage and retinal detachment (Greene, 2007).

Pathophysiology

The eye begins to develop early in gestation, at approximately 16 weeks. Blood vessels begin to form and grow to supply the retina, which transmits visual information to the brain, with oxygen and nutrients. These vessels continue to grow gradually until about the last 12 weeks of pregnancy (between 28 and 40 weeks' gestation), at which time the eye undergoes rapid development. Thus, an infant born at term has retinal vessels that are almost completely developed. However, when the infant is born preterm, normal blood vessel development may cease.

ROP typically develops in both eyes secondary to an injury such as hyperoxemia due to prolonged assistive ventilation and high oxygen exposure, acidosis, and shock. Exposure to high oxygen concentrations leads to severe retinal vasoconstriction with endothelial damage and vessel obliteration. Abnormal blood vessels develop in an attempt to nourish the retina. These vessels, which proliferate in the retina, are highly fragile and bleed easily, leading to the formation of scar tissue. They also can enlarge and twist, pulling the retina away from the wall of the eye and resulting in retinal detachment.

> ► **Take** NOTE!
>
> *Although the precise levels of hyperoxemia that can be sustained without causing retinopathy are not known, very immature newborns who develop respiratory distress often must be given high oxygen concentrations to maintain life (Cunningham et al., 2005).*

ROP is classified in five stages, ranging from mild (stage I) to severe (stage V). The degree of abnormal blood vessel growth and evidence of retinal detachment are used to stage this disorder.

Therapeutic Management

The key to treating ROP is prevention, by minimizing the risk of preterm birth through providing quality prenatal care and health counseling to all pregnant women. When ROP does develop, treatment depends on the stage and degree of retinal findings. Typically, stages I and II resolve on their own and require only periodic evaluation by the ophthalmologist. For more advanced stages, surgical intervention such as laser therapy or cryotherapy can be done. For later stages of ROP, scleral buckling surgery (stage IV or V) and/or vitrectomy (stage V) may be done.

Nursing Assessment

The newborn who develops ROP exhibits no signs or symptoms, so assessment involves identifying the newborn at risk. Review the maternal prenatal history for risk factors such as substance abuse, hypertension, preeclampsia, heavy cigarette smoking, or evidence of placental insufficiency. Also assess the newborn's gestational age and weight. Be especially alert for newborns weighing 1,500 grams or less or those born at 28 weeks' gestation or less. Evaluate the newborn's history for the duration of intubation and the use of oxygen therapy, intraventricular hemorrhage, and sepsis (Vision Channel, 2007). Prepare the infant for an ophthalmologic examination.

Nursing Management

Institute measures for prevention. Administer oxygen therapy cautiously and monitor oxygen saturation levels to ensure that the lowest oxygen concentration possible is used and for the shortest possible duration. Cover the isolette with a blanket and dim the surrounding lights to protect the newborn's eyes.

> ► **Take** NOTE!
>
> *Any newborn with a birthweight of less than 1,500 g or born at less than 28 weeks' gestation should be examined by a pediatric ophthalmologist within 4 to 6 weeks after birth.*

Assist with scheduling an ophthalmic examination for the newborn. Expect to administer a mydriatic eye agent to dilate the newborn's pupils approximately 1 hour prior to the examination as ordered. During this time, take extra care to protect the newborn's eyes from bright light. If necessary, provide assistance with the examination by holding the newborn's head. Assist with scheduling follow-up eye examinations, usually every 2 to 3 weeks depending on the severity of the clinical findings at the first examination (Clark & Mandal, 2008).

Provide support to the parents. This is an extremely difficult time for them: in addition to learning to meet the needs of their preterm newborn, they must also deal with the possibility that their baby may have a condition that could lead to blindness. Consider the family's needs and provide individualized support and guidance. Provide information about the newborn's condition and treatment options. Stress the need for follow-up vision screenings, because ROP is considered a life-long disease.

► PERIVENTRICULAR– INTRAVENTRICULAR HEMORRHAGE

Periventricular–intraventricular hemorrhage is defined as bleeding that usually originates in the subependymal germinal matrix region of the brain, with extension into the ventricular system (Brodsky & Ouellette, 2007). It is a common problem in preterm infants, especially in those born before 32 weeks. A significant number of these newborns will incur brain injury, leading to complications that may include hydrocephalus, seizure disorders, periventricular leukomalacia (an ischemic injury resulting from inadequate perfusion of the white matter adjacent to the ventricles), cerebral palsy, learning disabilities, vision or hearing deficits, and mental retardation. Identifying preventive strategies to reduce the incidence of these brain insults is a national public health priority (McLenan, 2007).

The incidence of ventricular hemorrhage depends on the gestational age at birth. Up to 50% of newborns weighing 1,500 g or less or born at 30 weeks' gestation or less will have evidence of hemorrhage, whereas only about 4% of term newborns show evidence of ventricular hemorrhage. Very-low-birthweight infants have the earliest onset of hemorrhage and the highest mortality rate (Brodsky & Ouellette, 2007).

Pathophysiology

The preterm newborn is at greatest risk for periventricular–intraventricular hemorrhage because cerebral vascular development is immature, making it more vulnerable to injury. The earlier the newborn is, the greater the likelihood for brain damage. While all areas of the brain can be injured, the periventricular area is the most vulnerable.

Each ventricular area contains a rich network of capillaries that are very thin and fragile and can rupture easily. The causes of rupture vary and include fluctuations in systemic and cerebral blood flow, increases in cerebral blood flow from hypertension, IV infusions, seizure activity, increases in cerebral venous pressure due to vaginal delivery, hypoxia, and respiratory distress. With a preterm birth, the fetus is suddenly transported from a well-controlled uterine environment into a highly stimulating one. This tremendous physiologic stress and shock may contribute to the rupture of periventricular capillaries and subsequent hemorrhage. Most hemorrhages occur in the first 72 hours after birth (Cunningham et al., 2005).

Periventricular–intraventricular hemorrhage is classified according to a grading system of I to V (least severe to most severe) (Blackburn, 2007). The prognosis is guarded, depending on the grade and severity of the hemorrhage. Generally, newborns with mild hemorrhage (grades I and II) have a much better developmental outcome than those with severe hemorrhage (grades III and IV).

Nursing Assessment

The signs of periventricular–intraventricular hemorrhage vary significantly; no clinical signs may be evident. Closely monitor newborns who are at an increased risk, such as those who are preterm or of low birthweight. Also assess for risk factors such as acidosis, asphyxia, unstable blood pressure, meningitis, seizures, acute blood loss, hypovolemia, respiratory distress with mechanical ventilation, intubation, apnea, hypoxia, suctioning, use of hyperosmo-

lar solutions, rapid volume expansion, and activities that involve handling.

Evaluate the newborn for an unexplained drop in hematocrit, pallor, and poor perfusion as evidenced by respiratory distress and oxygen desaturation. Note seizures, lethargy or other changes in level of consciousness, weak suck, high-pitched cry, or hypotonia. Palpate the anterior fontanel for tenseness. Assess vital signs, noting bradycardia and hypotension. Evaluate laboratory data for changes indicating metabolic acidosis or glucose instability (Annibale & Hill, 2007). Frequently a bleed can progress rapidly and result in shock and death. Prepare the newborn for cranial ultrasonography, the diagnostic tool of choice to detect hemorrhage.

Nursing Management

Prevention of preterm birth is essential in preventing periventricular–intraventricular hemorrhage. Promote community awareness of factors that may contribute to periventricular–intraventricular hemorrhage, such as a lack of prenatal care, maternal infection, alcohol consumption, and smoking (Kenner & Lott, 2007). Identify risk factors that can lead to hemorrhage, and focus care on interventions to decrease the risk of hemorrhage. For example, institute measures to prevent perinatal asphyxia and birth trauma and provide developmental care in the NICU. If a preterm birth is expected, having the mother deliver at a tertiary care facility with a NICU would be most appropriate.

Care of the newborn with periventricular–intraventricular hemorrhage is primarily supportive. Correct anemia, acidosis, and hypotension with fluids and medications. Administer fluids slowly to prevent fluctuations in blood pressure. Avoid rapid volume expansion to minimize changes in cerebral blood flow. Keep the newborn in a flexed, contained position with the head elevated to prevent or minimize fluctuations in intracranial pressure. Continuously monitor the newborn for signs of hemorrhage, such as changes in the level of consciousness, bulging fontanel, seizures, apnea, and reduced activity level. Also, measure head circumference daily.

Minimize handling of the newborn by clustering nursing care, and limit stimulation in the newborn's environment to reduce stress. Also reduce the newborn's exposure to noxious stimuli to avoid a fluctuation in blood pressure and energy expenditure. Provide adequate oxygenation to promote tissue perfusion but controlled ventilation to decrease the risk of pneumothorax.

Support for the parents to cope with the diagnosis and potential long-term sequelae is essential. The long-term neurodevelopmental outcome is determined by the severity of the bleed. Provide education and emotional support for the parents throughout the newborn's stay. Discuss expectations for short-term and long-term care needs with the parents and assist them in obtaining the necessary support from appropriate community resources.

♦ NECROTIZING ENTEROCOLITIS

Necrotizing enterocolitis (NEC) is a serious gastrointestinal disease occurring in newborns. It is the most common and most serious acquired gastrointestinal disorder among hospitalized preterm neonates and is associated with significant acute and chronic morbidity and mortality (Wiedmeier, 2008). NEC occurs in 1 to 3 cases per 1,000 live births, affecting 1% to 5% of all newborns in intensive care units (Stoll & Kliegman, 2007). Ways to improve gastrointestinal function and reduce the risk of NEC include enteral antibiotics, judicious administration of parenteral fluids, human milk feedings, antenatal corticosteroids, enteral probiotics (*Lactobacillus acidophilus*), and slow continuous drip feedings (Neu, 2007).

Pathophysiology

The pathophysiology of NEC is not clearly understood and is thought to be multifactorial in nature. Current research points to three major pathologic mechanisms that lead to NEC: bowel ischemia, bacterial flora, and the effect of feeding (Neu, 2007).

During perinatal or postnatal stress, oxygen is shunted away from the gut to more important organs such as the heart and brain. Ischemia and intestinal wall damage occur, allowing bacteria to invade. High-solute feedings allow bacteria to flourish. Mucosal or transmucosal necrosis of part of the intestine occurs (Wood, 2007). Although any region of the bowel can be affected, the distal ileum and proximal colon are the regions most commonly involved. NEC usually occurs between 3 and 12 days of life, but it can occur weeks later in some newborns.

Nursing Assessment

NEC can be devastating, and astute assessment is crucial. Assessing the newborn for the development of NEC includes the health history and physical examination as well as laboratory and diagnostic testing.

Health History and Physical Examination

Assess the newborn's history for risk factors associated with NEC. In addition to preterm birth, prenatal and postnatal predisposing risk factors are highlighted in Box 24.1.

Also observe the newborn for common signs and symptoms, which may include:

- Abdominal distention and tenderness
- Bloody stools
- Feeding intolerance, characterized by bilious vomiting
- Signs of sepsis
- Lethargy
- Apnea
- Shock

Always keep the possibility of NEC in mind when dealing with preterm newborns, especially when enteral

---

BOX 24.1 **Predisposing Factors for the Development of Necrotizing Enterocolitis**

Prenatal Factors
- Preterm labor
- Prolonged rupture of membranes
- Preeclampsia
- Maternal sepsis
- Amnionitis
- Uterine hypoxia

Postnatal Factors
- Respiratory distress syndrome
- Patent ductus arteriosus
- Congenital heart disease
- Exchange transfusion
- Low birthweight
- Low Apgar scores
- Umbilical catheterization
- Hypothermia
- Gastrointestinal infection
- Hypoglycemia
- Asphyxia

---

feedings are being administered. Note respiratory distress, cyanosis, lethargy, decreased activity level, temperature instability, feeding intolerance, diarrhea, bile-stained emesis, or grossly bloody stools. Assess blood pressure, noting hypotension. Evaluate the neonate's abdomen for distention, tenderness, and visible loops of bowel (Wiedmeier, 2008). Measure the abdominal circumference, noting an increase. Determine residual gastric volume prior to feeding; when it is elevated, be suspicious for NEC.

Laboratory and Diagnostic Testing

Common laboratory and diagnostic tests ordered for assessment of NEC include:

- Kidney, ureter, and bladder (KUB) x-ray: confirms the presence of pneumatosis intestinalis (air in the bowel wall) and persistently dilated loops of bowel (Srinivasan, Brandler, & D'Souza, 2008; Wood, 2007)
- Blood values: may demonstrate metabolic acidosis, increased white blood cells, thrombocytopenia, neutropenia, electrolyte imbalance, or disseminated intravascular coagulation (DIC)

Nursing Management

Nursing management of the newborn with NEC focuses on maintaining fluid and nutritional status, providing supportive care, and teaching the family about the condition and prognosis. Therapeutic management initially consists of bowel rest and antibiotic therapy. Serial KUB x-rays are used to assess the resolution or progression of NEC. If medical treatment fails to stabilize the newborn or if free air is present on a left lateral decubitus film, surgical intervention will be necessary to resect the portion of necrotic bowel. Surgery for NEC usually requires the placement of a proximal enterostomy until the anastomosis site is ready for reconnection.

Maintaining Fluid and Nutritional Status

If NEC is suspected, immediately stop enteral feedings until a diagnosis is made. Administer IV fluids initially to restore proper fluid balance. If ordered, administer total parenteral nutrition (TPN) to keep the newborn supported nutritionally. Give prescribed IV antibiotics to prevent sepsis from the necrotic bowel (if surgery is required, antibiotics may be needed for an extended period). Institute gastric decompression as ordered with an orogastric tube attached to low intermittent suction. Carefully monitor intake and output. Restart enteral feedings once the disease has resolved (normal abdominal examination and KUB negative for pneumatosis) or as determined postoperatively by the surgeon.

Providing Supportive Care

Manage pain by administering analgesics as ordered. Infection control is important, with an emphasis on careful handwashing. In addition, implement these interventions in an ongoing manner:

- Check stools for evidence of blood and report any positive findings.
- Measure the abdominal girth.
- Palpate the abdomen for tenderness and rigidity.
- Auscultate for normal bowel sounds.
- Observe the abdomen for redness or shininess, which indicates peritonitis.

Teaching the Family

The diagnosis of NEC may cause significant family anxiety. Listen to the family's worries and fears. Answer their questions honestly. Inform the family that medically treated NEC is usually limited to a short period and resolves within 48 hours of stopping oral feedings, but surgically treated NEC can be a much lengthier process. The amount of bowel that has necrosed, as determined during the bowel resection, significantly increases the likelihood of long-term medical problems. Short bowel syndrome may result from a large resection of the bowel. Reassure the family that although some infants have more involved cases of NEC, the improved parenteral nutrition formulations have improved the outcomes for these infants. Provide education about ostomy care if surgery is required. Promote interaction with the newborn.

▶ INFANTS OF DIABETIC MOTHERS

An **infant of a diabetic mother** is one born to a woman with pregestational or gestational diabetes (see Chapter 20 for additional information). The newborn of a diabetic woman is at high risk for numerous health-related complications, especially hypoglycemia. In light of the increasing incidence of type 2 diabetes among women of childbearing age, it is important to educate women about the potential impact of poor glycemic control on their offspring.

Impact of Diabetes on the Newborn

For more than a century, it has been known that diabetes during pregnancy can have severe adverse effects on fetal and newborn outcomes. Infants of diabetic mothers have increased morbidity and mortality in the perinatal period. The incidence of major congenital anomalies is much greater for these newborns than for other newborns. Poor glycemic control in the first trimester, during organogenesis, is thought to be a major reason for congenital malformations. The most common types of malformations in infants of diabetic mothers involve the cardiovascular, skeletal, central nervous, gastrointestinal, and genitourinary systems. Cardiac anomalies are the most common (Kwik et al., 2007).

Infants of diabetic mothers are longer and weigh more than newborns of similar gestational age. They also have increased organ weights (organomegaly) and excessive fat deposits on their shoulders and trunk, contributing to the increased overall body weight and predisposing them to shoulder dystocia. These newborns are macrosomic (an infant whose birthweight exceeds 4,500 g). These oversized newborns frequently require cesarean births for cephalopelvic disproportion and are often hypoglycemic in the first few hours after birth.

Despite their increased size and weight, they may be remarkably frail, showing behaviors similar to those of a preterm newborn. Thus, birthweight may not be a reliable criterion of maturity. Newborns of women with diabetes but without vascular complications often tend to be large for gestational age (LGA), whereas those of women with diabetes and vascular disease are usually small for gestational age (SGA).

Pathophysiology

The large size of the infant born to a diabetic mother occurs secondary to exposure to high levels of maternal glucose crossing the placenta into the fetal circulation. Maternal hyperglycemia acts as a fuel to stimulate increased production of fetal insulin, which in turn promotes somatic growth within the fetus. The fetus responds to these high levels by producing more insulin, which acts as a growth factor in the fetus (Blackburn, 2007). How the fetus will be affected and the problems that the newborn experiences depend on the severity, duration, and control of the diabetes in the mother. Table 24.1 summarizes the

TABLE 24.1   COMMON PROBLEMS OF INFANTS OF DIABETIC MOTHERS

Condition	Description	Effects
Macrosomia	Newborn with an excessive birthweight; arbitrarily defined as a birthweight >4,000 g (8 lb 13 oz) to 4,500 g (9 lb 15 oz) or >90% for gestational age Complication in 10% of all pregnancies in the United States	Increased risk for shoulder dystocia, traumatic birth injury, birth asphyxia Risks for newborn hypoglycemia and hypomagnesemia, polycythemia, and electrolyte disturbances Increased maternal risk for surgical birth, postpartum hemorrhage and infection, and birth canal lacerations Increased risk of developing type 2 diabetes later in life for both Higher weight and accumulation of fat in childhood and a higher rate of obesity in adults
Respiratory distress syndrome (RDS)	Cortisol-induced stimulation of lecithin/sphingomyelin (phospholipids) necessary for lung maturation is antagonized due to the high-insulin environment within the fetus due to mother's hyperglycemia. Less mature lung development than expected for gestational age Decrease in the phospholipid phosphatidylglycerol (PG), which stabilizes surfactant, compounding risk	Most commonly, baby is breathing normally at birth but develops labored, grunting respiration with cough and a hoarse complaining cry within a few hours, with chest retractions and varying degrees of cyanosis. Infants of diabetic mothers with vascular disease seldom develop RDS because the chronic stress of poor intrauterine perfusion leads to increased production of steroids, which accelerates lung maturation.
Hypoglycemia	Glucose is the major source of energy for organ function. Typical characteristics: – Poor feedings – Jitteriness – Lethargy – High-pitched or weak cry – Apnea – Cyanosis and seizures Some newborns are asymptomatic.	Low blood glucose levels are problematic during the early post-birth period due to abrupt cessation of high-glucose maternal blood supply and the continuation of insulin production by the newborn. Limited ability to release glucagon and catecholamines, which normally stimulate glucagon breakdown and glucose release Prolonged and untreated hypoglycemia leads to serious, long-term adverse neurologic sequelae such as learning disabilities and mental retardation.
Hypocalcemia and hypomagnesemia	Hypocalcemia (drop in calcium levels) is manifested by tremors, hypotonia, apnea, high-pitched cry, and seizures due to abrupt cessation of maternal transfer of calcium to the fetus, which occurs primarily in the third trimester and if the infant experiences birth asphyxia Associated hypomagnesemia is directly related to the maternal level before birth About half of infants of diabetic mothers are affected.	Newborn is at risk for a prolonged delay in parathyroid hormone production and cardiac dysrhythmias.
Polycythemia	Venous hematocrit of >65% in the newborn Increased oxygen consumption by neonate secondary to fetal hyperglycemia and hyperinsulinemia Increased fetal erythropoiesis secondary to intrauterine hypoxia due to placental insufficiency from maternal diabetes Hypoxic stimulation of increased red blood cell (RBC) production as compensatory mechanism	Increased viscosity, resulting in poor blood flow that predisposes newborn to decreased tissue oxygenation and development of microthrombi

(continued)

TABLE 24.1 COMMON PROBLEMS OF INFANTS OF DIABETIC MOTHERS (continued)

Condition	Description	Effects
Hyperbilirubinemia	Usually seen within the first few days after birth; manifested by a yellow appearance of the sclera and skin Excessive red cell hemolysis necessary to break down increased RBCs in circulation due to polycythemia Resultant elevated bilirubin levels Excessive bruising secondary to birth trauma of macrosomic infants, further adding to high bilirubin levels	If untreated, high levels of unconjugated bilirubin may lead to kernicterus (neurologic syndrome that results in irreversible damage) with long-term sequelae that include cerebral palsy, sensorineural hearing loss, and mental retardation.
Congenital anomalies	Occur in up to 10% of infants of diabetic mothers, accounting for 30% to 50% of perinatal deaths Incidence is greatest among small-for-gestational-age newborns. Overall, infants of diabetic mothers have ~3 times the usual incidence of congenital anomalies compared to newborns from the non-diabetic general population.	Most common anomalies: – Coarctation of the aorta – Atrial and ventricular septal defects – Transposition of the great vessels – Sacral agenesis – Hip and joint malformations – Anencephaly – Spina bifida – Caudal dysplasia – Hydrocephalus

Sources: Arenson & Drake, 2007; Blackburn, 2007; Kenner & Lott, 2007; McLenan, 2007.

common problems that may occur in infants of diabetic mothers.

Nursing Assessment

Assessment begins in the prenatal period by identifying women with diabetes and taking measures to control maternal glucose levels (see Chapter 20 for information on management of the pregnant woman with diabetes).

Physical Examination

At birth, inspect the newborn for these characteristic features:

- Full rosy cheeks with a ruddy skin color
- Short neck (some describe "no-neck" appearance)
- Buffalo hump over the nape of the neck
- Massive shoulders with a full intrascapular area
- Distended upper abdomen due to organ overgrowth
- Excessive subcutaneous fat tissue, producing fat extremities (Fig. 24.4)

Be alert for hypoglycemia, which may occur immediately or within an hour after birth. Assess blood glucose levels, which should remain above 40 mg/dL. Closely assess the newborn for signs of hypoglycemia, including listlessness, hypotonia, apathy, poor feeding, apneic episodes with a drop in oxygen saturation, cyanosis, temperature instability, pallor and sweating, tremors, irritability, and seizures.

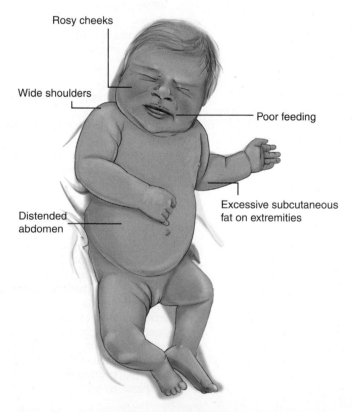

Rosy cheeks

Wide shoulders

Poor feeding

Distended abdomen

Excessive subcutaneous fat on extremities

FIGURE 24.4 Characteristics of an infant of a diabetic mother.

Assess the newborn for signs of birth trauma involving the head (tense, bulging fontanels, cephalhematoma, skull fractures, and facial nerve paralysis), shoulders and extremities (posturing, paralysis), and skin (bruising). Inspect the newborn for compromised oxygenation by examining the skin for cyanosis, pallor, mottling, and sluggish capillary refill. Take the newborn's temperature frequently and provide a neutral thermal environment to prevent cold stress, which would increase the glucose utilization and contribute to the hypoglycemic state.

Laboratory and Diagnostic Testing

Determine baseline serum calcium, magnesium, and bilirubin levels and monitor them frequently for changes (Table 24.2). Hypocalcemia is typically manifested in the first 2 to 3 days of life as a result of birth injury or a prolonged delay in parathyroid hormone production. Hypomagnesemia parallels calcium levels and is suspected only when hypocalcemia does not respond to calcium replacement therapy. Red blood cell breakdown leads to increased hematocrit and polycythemia. In addition, hyperbilirubinemia may be caused by slightly decreased extracellular fluid volume, hepatic immaturity, and birth trauma forming enclosed hemorrhages. It can appear within the first 24 hours of life (pathologic) or after 24 hours of life (physiologic).

Nursing Management

The focus of care for these infants is early detection and initiation of therapy to address potential problems (Nursing Care Plan 24.1). Perform a head-to-toe physical assessment to identify congenital anomalies. Institute measures to correct hypoglycemia, hypocalcemia, hypomagnesemia, dehydration, and jaundice. Provide oxygenation and ventilatory support as necessary.

Preventing Hypoglycemia

Prevent hypoglycemia by providing early oral feedings with formula or breast milk at frequent intervals (every 2 to 3 hours). Feedings help to control glucose levels, reduce hematocrit, and promote bilirubin excretion. Maintain a neutral thermal environment to avoid cold stress, which may stimulate the metabolic rate, thereby increasing the demand for glucose. Provide rest periods to decrease energy demand and expenditure.

Monitor blood glucose levels via heel stick every hour for the first 4 hours of life and then every 3 to 4 hours until stable. Document the results. Report unstable glucose values if oral feedings do not maintain and stabilize the newborn's blood glucose levels. If glucose levels are not stabilized, initiate IV glucose infusions as ordered and ensure that the infusions are flowing at the prescribed rate.

Maintaining Fluid and Electrolyte Balance

Monitor serum calcium levels for changes indicating the need for supplementation, such as with oral or IV calcium gluconate. Assess the newborn for signs of hypocalcemia, such as tremors, jitteriness, twitching, seizures, and high-pitched cry.

Also administer fluid therapy as ordered to maintain adequate hydration. Monitor serum bilirubin levels and institute phototherapy if the newborn is over 24 hours old.

Providing Parental Support

Assist the parents and family in understanding the newborn's condition and need for frequent monitoring. Offer support and information to the parents and family. They may erroneously interpret the newborn's large size as an indication that the newborn is free of problems. Encourage open communication and listen with empathy to the family's fears and concerns. Provide frequent opportunities for the parents to interact with their newborn. Make appropriate referrals to social services and community resources as necessary to help the family cope.

▶ BIRTH TRAUMA

Injuries to the newborn from the forces of labor and birth are categorized as birth trauma. In the past, numerous injuries were associated with difficult births requiring external or internal version or mid- or high forceps deliveries. Today, however, cesarean births have contributed to the decline in birth trauma.

Significant birth trauma accounts for fewer than 2% of neonatal deaths and stillbirths in the United States (Kenner & Lott, 2007). Improved prenatal diagnosis and monitoring during labor have helped to reduce the incidence of birth injuries today.

Pathophysiology

The process of birth is a blend of compression, contractions, torques, and traction. When fetal size, presentation, or neurologic immunity complicates this process, the forces of labor and birth may lead to tissue damage, edema, hemorrhage, or fracture in the newborn. For example, birth trauma may result from the pressure of birth, especially in

TABLE 24.2 **CRITICAL LABORATORY VALUES FOR INFANTS OF DIABETIC MOTHERS**

Hypoglycemia	<40 mg/dL
Hypocalcemia	<7 mg/dL
Hypomagnesemia	<1.5 mg/dL
Hyperbilirubinemia	>12 mg/dL (term infant)
Polycythemia	>65% (venous hematocrit)

Nursing Care Plan 24.1

OVERVIEW OF THE INFANT OF A DIABETIC MOTHER

Jamie, a 38-year-old Hispanic woman, gave birth to a term large-for-gestational-age newborn weighing 10 lb. She had a history of gestational diabetes but had not received any prenatal care. She arrived at the hospital in active labor. Despite macrosomia, the newborn's Apgar scores were 8 and 9 at 1 and 5 minutes respectively. No resuscitative measures were needed.

One hour after birth, assessment revealed a pale, irritable newborn with sweating and several episodes of apnea. A glucose level obtained at this time via a heel stick was 35 mg/dL. Two hours later, the newborn begins exhibiting signs of respiratory distress—grunting, nasal flaring, retractions, tachypnea (respiratory rate 72 breaths/minute), and tachycardia (heart rate 176 bpm).

NURSING DIAGNOSIS: Risk for unstable glucose level related to hypoglycemia secondary to intrauterine hyperinsulin state resulting from maternal gestational diabetes as evidenced by low blood glucose level, irritability, pallor, sweating, and apnea

Outcome Identification and Evaluation

The newborn will exhibit adequate glucose control *as evidenced by maintaining blood glucose levels above 40 mg/dL and an absence of clinical signs of hypoglycemia.*

Interventions: Promoting Glucose Control

- Monitor blood glucose levels hourly for the first 4 hours and then every 3 to 4 hours or as necessary *to detect hypoglycemia, which would be <40 mg/dL.*
- Continue to observe for manifestations of hypoglycemia, such as pallor, tremors, jitteriness, lethargy, and poor feeding, *to allow for early detection and prompt intervention, thereby minimizing the risk of complications associated with hypoglycemia.*
- Monitor temperature frequently and institute measures to maintain a neutral thermal environment *to prevent cold stress, which would increase metabolic demands and further deplete glycogen stores.*
- Initiate early feedings every 2 to 3 hours or as appropriate or administer glucose supplements as ordered *to prevent hypoglycemia caused by the newborn's hyperinsulin state.* Administer IV glucose infusions as ordered *to correct hypoglycemia if glucose levels do not stabilize with feeding.*
- Cluster infant care activities and provide for rest periods *to conserve the newborn's energy and reduce use of glucose and glycogen stores.*
- Reduce environmental stimuli by dimming lights and speaking softly *to reduce energy demands and further utilization of glucose.*
- Explain all events and procedures to the mother *to help alleviate anxiety and promote understanding of the newborn's condition.*

NURSING DIAGNOSIS: Impaired gas exchange related to respiratory distress secondary to delayed lung maturity resulting from inhibition of pulmonary surfactant production due to fetal hyperinsulinemia as evidenced by grunting, nasal flaring, retractions, tachypnea, and tachycardia

Outcome Identification and Evaluation

Newborn will demonstrate signs of adequate oxygenation without respiratory distress *as evidenced by respiratory rate and vital signs within acceptable parameters, absence of nasal flaring, retractions, and grunting, and oxygen saturation and arterial blood gas levels within acceptable parameters.*

Interventions: Promoting Oxygenation

- Monitor newborn's vital signs *to establish a baseline and evaluate for changes.*
- Assess airway patency and perform gentle suctioning as ordered *to ensure patency and allow for adequate oxygen intake.*
- Position the newborn prone *to optimize respiratory status and reduce stress.*
- Assess lung sounds for changes *to allow early detection of change in status.*
- Continuously monitor oxygen saturation levels via pulse oximetry *to determine adequacy of tissue perfusion.*
- Assess arterial blood gas results *to detect changes indicating acidosis, hypoxemia, or hypercarbia, which would suggest hypoxia.* Administer medications as ordered *to correct acidosis.*
- Administer oxygen as ordered *to promote adequate tissue perfusion.*
- Assess newborn's skin to identify cyanosis, pallor, and mottling *to detect changes indicating compromised oxygenation.*
- Administer surfactant replacement therapy as ordered *to aid in stabilizing the newborn's lungs until postnatal surfactant synthesis improves.*
- Institute measures to maintain normal blood glucose levels and a neutral thermal environment, cluster care activities, and reduce excessive stimuli *to reduce oxygen demand and consumption.*

a prolonged or abrupt labor, abnormal or difficult presentation, cephalopelvic disproportion, or mechanical forces, such as forceps or vacuum used during delivery. Table 24.3 summarizes the most common types of birth trauma.

Nursing Assessment

Recognition of trauma and birth injuries is imperative so that early treatment can be initiated. Review the labor and birth history for risk factors, such as a prolonged or abrupt labor, abnormal or difficult presentation, cephalopelvic disproportion, or mechanical forces, such as forceps or vacuum used during delivery. Also review the history for multiple fetus deliveries, large-for-date infants, extreme prematurity, large fetal head, or newborns with congenital anomalies.

Complete a careful physical and neurologic assessment of every newborn admitted to the nursery to establish whether injuries exist. Inspect the head for lumps, bumps, or bruises. Note if swelling or bruising crosses the suture line. Assess the eyes and face for facial paralysis, observing for asymmetry of the face with crying or appearance of the mouth being drawn to the unaffected side. Ensure that the newborn spontaneously moves all extremities. Note any absence of or decrease in deep tendon reflexes or abnormal positioning of extremities.

Assess and document symmetry of structure and function. Be prepared to assist with scheduling diagnostic studies to confirm trauma or injuries, which will be important in determining treatment modalities.

Nursing Management

Nursing management is primarily supportive and focuses on assessing for resolution of the trauma or any associated complications along with providing support and education to the parents. Provide the parents with explanations and reassurance that these injuries usually resolve with minimal or no treatment. Parents are alarmed when their newborn is unable to move an extremity or demonstrates asymmetric facial movements. Provide parents with a realistic picture of the situation to gain their understanding and trust. Be readily available to answer questions and teach them how to care for the newborn, including any modifications that might be necessary. Allow parents adequate time to understand the implications of the birth trauma or injury and what treatment modalities are needed, if any. Provide them with information about the length of time until the injury will resolve and when and if they need to seek further medical attention for the condition. Spending time with the parents and providing them with support, information, and teaching are important to allow them to make decisions and care for their newborn. Anticipate the need for community referral for ongoing follow-up and care, if necessary.

► NEWBORNS OF SUBSTANCE-ABUSING MOTHERS

It is generally assumed that all pregnant women want to provide a healthy environment for their unborn child and know how to avoid harm. However, for women who use substances such as drugs or alcohol, this may not be the case. Substance use during pregnancy exposes the fetus to the possibility of IUGR, prematurity, neurobehavioral and neurophysiologic dysfunction, birth defects, infections, and long-term developmental sequelae (Kenner & Lott, 2007).

It is difficult to establish the true prevalence of substance use in pregnant women; many women deny taking any nonprescribed substance because of the associated social stigma and legal implications. The National Institute on Drug Abuse (NIDA) suggests that approximately 1 in 10 newborns are exposed to one or more mood-altering drugs in utero (NIDA, 2007f). Drug exposure may go unrecognized in these newborns, and they may be discharged from the newborn nursery at risk for medical and social problems, including abuse and neglect.

Tobacco, alcohol, and marijuana are the substances most commonly abused during pregnancy. Other drugs may include opioids such as morphine, codeine, methadone, meperidine, and heroin; CNS stimulants such as amphetamines and cocaine; CNS depressants such as barbiturates, diazepam (Valium), and sedative–hypnotics; and hallucinogens, such as LSD, inhalants, glue, paint thinner, nail polish remover, and nitrous oxide (NIDA, 2007f). Table 24.4 highlights commonly used substances and their effects on the fetus and newborn.

► *Consider* THIS!

> I admit, I had led a reckless life since I was a teen. I rebelled against my mother's authority and started smoking and doing drugs just to "check out" of my painful world. It was one big blast after another with a high and then a low. I never considered the consequences of my behavior then and never thought it would hurt anyone until I learned I was about 4 months pregnant. I convinced myself that if I cut back, everything would be fine.
>
> Now, as I stand here in the NICU watching my tiny son struggle for air and tremble all over, I am not so convinced that I didn't hurt anyone except myself. As I witness my son fight against MY nicotine and drug addiction, my heart is heavy with guilt. I wonder how I could have thought that my troubles wouldn't become another's plight sooner or later. What must I have been thinking to isolate my addiction and not consider the impact that it would have on my mother and my son?

(text continues on page 725)

TABLE 24.3 COMMON TYPES OF BIRTH TRAUMA

Type	Description	Findings	Treatment
Fractures	Most often occur during breech births or shoulder dystocia in newborns with macrosomia Mid-clavicular fractures are the most common type of fracture, secondary to shoulder dystocia. Long bone fractures of humerus or femur, usually mid-shaft, also can occur.	Mid-clavicular fractures: The newborn is irritable and does not move the arm on the affected side either spontaneously or when the Moro reflex is elicited. Femoral or humeral long bone fractures: The newborn shows loss of spontaneous leg or arm motion respectively; usually swelling and pain accompany the limited movement. X-rays confirm the fracture.	Mid-clavicular fractures typically heal rapidly and uneventfully; arm motion may be limited by pinning the newborn's sleeve to the shirt. Femoral and humeral shaft fractures are treated with splinting. Healing and complete recovery are expected within 2 to 4 weeks without incident (Laroia, 2007). Explanation to the parents and reassurance are needed.
Brachial plexus injury	Primarily in large babies, babies with shoulder dystocia, or breech delivery Results from stretching, hemorrhage within a nerve, or tearing of the nerve or the roots associated with cervical cord injury Associated traumatic injuries include fracture of the clavicle or humerus or subluxations of the shoulder or cervical spine. Erb's palsy is an upper brachial plexus injury. Klumpke's palsy is an injury to the lower brachial plexus (lower brachial injuries are less common).	In Erb's palsy, the involved extremity usually presents adducted, prone, and internally rotated; shoulder movement is absent; Moro, bicep, and radial reflexes are absent, but the grasp reflex is usually present. Klumpke's palsy is manifested by weakness in the hand and wrist; grasp reflex is absent.	Erb's palsy usually involves immobilization of the upper arm across the upper abdomen/chest to protect the shoulder from excessive motion for the first week; then gentle passive range-of-motion exercises are performed daily to prevent contractures. There is usually no associated sensory loss, and this condition usually improves rapidly. Treatment for Klumpke's palsy involves placing the hand in a neutral position and using passive range-of-motion exercises. In some cases deficits may persist, requiring continuing observation.
Cranial nerve trauma	Most common is facial nerve palsy. Frequently attributed to pressure resulting from forceps May also result from pressure on the nerve in utero, related to fetal positioning such as the head lying against the shoulder	Physical findings include asymmetry of the face when crying; mouth may be drawn towards the unaffected side; wrinkles are deeper on the unaffected side. The paralyzed side may be smooth, with a swollen appearance. Eye is persistently open on the affected side.	Most infants begin to recover in the first week, but full resolution may take up to several months; parents need reassurance about this. In most cases, treatment is not necessary, only observation. If the eye is affected and unable to close, protection with patches and synthetic tears may be necessary. Parents need instruction about how to feed the newborn, since he or she cannot close the lips around the nipple without having milk seep out.

Type	Description	Findings	Treatment
Head trauma	Mild trauma can cause soft tissue injuries such as cephalhematoma and caput succedaneum; greater trauma can cause depressed skull fractures. **Cephalhematoma** (subperiosteal collection of blood secondary to the rupture of blood vessels between the skull and periosteum) occurs in 2.5% of all births and typically appears within hours after birth (Cunningham et al., 2005). **Caput succedaneum** (soft tissue swelling) is caused by edema of the head against the dilating cervix during the birth process. Subarachnoid hemorrhage (one of the most common types of intracranial trauma) may be due to hypoxia/ischemia, variations in blood pressure, and the pressure exerted on the head during labor. Bleeding is of venous origin, and underlying contusions also may occur (Laroia, 2007). Subdural hemorrhage (hematomas) occurs less often today because of improved obstetric techniques. Typically, tears of the major veins or venous sinuses overlying the cerebral hemispheres or cerebellum (most common in newborns of primaparas and large newborns, or after an instrumented birth) are the cause. Increased pressure on the blood vessels inside the skull leads to tears. Depressed skull fractures (rare) may result from the pressure of a forceps delivery; can also occur during spontaneous or cesarean births and may be associated with other head trauma causing subdural bleeding, subarachnoid hemorrhage, or brain trauma (Laroia, 2007).	In cephalhematoma, suture lines delineate its extent; usually located on one side, over the parietal bone. In caput succedaneum, swelling is not limited by suture lines: it extends across the midline and is associated with head molding. It does not usually cause complications other than a misshapen head. Swelling is maximal at birth and then rapidly decreases in size. In subarachnoid hemorrhage, some RBCs may appear in the CSF of full-term newborns. Newborns may present with apnea, seizures, lethargy, or abnormal findings on a neurologic examination (Barker, 2007). Subdural hemorrhage can be asymptomatic, or the neonate can exhibit seizures, enlarging head size, decreased level of consciousness, or abnormal findings on a neurologic examination, with hypotonia, a poor Moro reflex, or extensive retinal hemorrhages. Depressed skull fractures can be observed and palpated as depressions. Confirmation by x-ray is necessary.	Cephalhematoma resolves gradually over 2 to 3 weeks without treatment (see Chapter 18). Caput succedaneum usually resolves over the first few days without treatment (see Chapter 18). Subarachnoid hemorrhage requires minimal handling to reduce stress. Subdural hematoma requires aspiration; can be life-threatening if it is in an inaccessible location and cannot be aspirated (Laroia, 2007). Depressed skull fractures typically require a neurosurgical consultation.

TABLE 24.4   SUBSTANCES AND THEIR EFFECTS ON THE FETUS AND NEWBORN

Substance	Description	Effects on Fetus and Newborn	Nursing Implications
Alcohol	Consumption is pervasive and widely accepted, with use, abuse, and addiction affecting all levels of society. It is a common misconception that a substance sold to the public without restriction is safe.	Fetal alcohol syndrome (one of the most common known causes of mental retardation) Fetal alcohol spectrum disorders Alcohol-related birth defects	Provide education that decreasing or eliminating alcohol consumption during pregnancy is the only way to prevent fetal alcohol syndrome and fetal alcohol effects. Assist pregnant woman in finding a treatment program if possible. Inform all women who are pregnant or planning to become pregnant about the detrimental effects of alcohol during pregnancy. Educate women using a nonjudgmental, culturally connected approach. Warn women that there is no safe time to drink and that there is no safe amount of alcohol they can consume.
Tobacco/nicotine	Nicotine is an addictive substance. It causes epinephrine release from adrenal cortex, leading to initial stimulation followed by depression and fatigue, causing the user to seek more nicotine. Increased numbers of women are smoking (at least 11% smoke during pregnancy; March of Dimes, 2007c). Over 2,500 chemicals are found in cigarette smoke, including nicotine, tar, carbon monoxide, and cyanide. It is unknown which are harmful, but nicotine and carbon monoxide are believed to play a role in causing adverse pregnancy outcomes.	Impaired oxygenation of mother and fetus due to nicotine crossing placenta and carbon monoxide combining with hemoglobin Increased risk for low birthweight (risk almost doubled), small for gestational age, and preterm birth Increased risk for sudden infant death syndrome (SIDS) and chronic respiratory illness (MNH, 2007)	Provide teaching to women about healthy behaviors. Provide support for smoking cessation. Individualize counseling based on factors associated with the woman's smoking and challenges faced (why woman smokes, stressors in life, and social support network). Suggest options such as group smoking cessation programs, relaxation techniques, individual counseling, hypnosis, and partner-support counseling.

Substance	Description	Effects on Fetus and Newborn	Nursing Implications
Marijuana	Most widely used illicit psychoactive substance in Western world and most commonly used illicit drug in the United States (NIDA, 2007d) Derived from *Cannabis sativa* plant	Not shown to have teratogenic effects on fetus; no consistent types of malformations identified Intrauterine growth restriction (IUGR) is common due to delivery of carbon monoxide to fetus (NIDA, 2007d). Increased risk for small for gestational age Altered responses to visual stimuli, sleep-pattern abnormalities, photophobia, lack of motor control, hyperirritability, increased tremulousness, and high-pitched cry noted in infants of mothers who smoked marijuana Research on long-term effects is continuing (NIDA, 2007d).	Provide teaching to women about healthy behaviors. Provide support for cessation of marijuana use.
Methamphetamines	Addictive stimulant; use releases high levels of dopamine, which stimulates brain cells, enhancing mood and body movement High potential for abuse and addiction; can be inhaled, injected, smoked, or taken orally Many street names, such as speed, meth, ice, and chalk Primary effects include accelerated heart and respiratory rate, elevated blood pressure, papillary dilation; secondary effects include loss of appetite. Used medically as treatment for obesity and narcolepsy in adults and hyperactivity in children	Little research on use during pregnancy because its use is less common than cocaine or narcotics Fetal effects similar to cocaine (suggesting vasoconstriction as possible underlying mechanism) Possible maternal malnutrition, leading to problems with fetal growth and development Increased risk for preterm birth and low-birthweight newborns Infants may have withdrawal symptoms, including dysphoria, agitation, jitteriness, poor weight gain, abnormal sleep patterns, poor feeding, frantic fist sucking, high-pitched cry, respiratory distress soon after birth, frequent infections, and significant lassitude (Arenson & Drake, 2007). Long-term effects are not known.	Provide teaching to women about healthy behaviors. Provide support for cessation of methamphetamine use. Monitor the woman for weight changes; emphasize the need for adequate nutritional intake to support fetal growth and development.
Cocaine	Strong CNS stimulant that interferes with reabsorption of dopamine Physical effects: vasoconstriction; pupillary dilation; increased temperature, heart rate, and blood pressure Taken orally, sublingually, intranasally, intravenously, and via inhalation	Preterm birth and lower birthweight Unclear impact on later development Speculation that cocaine interferes with infant's cognitive development, leading to learning and memory difficulties later in life (Kenner & Lott, 2007)	Educate the woman about the effects of cocaine use on the fetus and newborn. Assess for use of other substances. Provide teaching to women about healthy behaviors.

(continued)

TABLE 24.4   SUBSTANCES AND THEIR EFFECTS ON THE FETUS AND NEWBORN (continued)

Substance	Description	Effects on Fetus and Newborn	Nursing Implications
	Estimated that 30% to 40% of cocaine addicts are female Maternal cocaine use during pregnancy is a significant health problem (March of Dimes, 2007b). Increased potential for use of multiple drugs if mother using cocaine	Associated congenital anomalies: GU, cardiac, and CNS defects, and prune belly syndrome Other typical newborn characteristics: smaller head circumference, piercing cry (indicative of neurologic dysfunction), limb defects, ambiguous genitalia, poor feeding, poor visual and auditory responses, poor sleep patterns, decreased impulse control, stiff, hyperextended positioning, irritability and hypersensitivity (hard to console when crying), inability to respond to caretaker (Blackburn, 2007)	Provide support and guidance for cessation of cocaine and other substance use.
Heroin	Illegal, highly addictive opiate derived from morphine that can be sniffed, smoked, or injected Possible consequences include HIV infection, tuberculosis, crime, violence, and family disruption. Severe physical addiction; CNS depressant producing mental dullness and drowsiness	Newborns of heroin-addicted mothers are born dependent on heroin. Increased risk for transmission of hepatitis B and C and HIV to newborns when mothers share needles Significantly increased rates of stillbirth, IUGR, preterm birth, and newborn mortality (3 to 7 times greater; NIDA, 2007b, 2007c) Small-for-gestational age newborns, meconium aspiration, high incidence of SIDS, and delayed effects from subacute withdrawal (restlessness, continual crying, agitation, sneezing, vomiting, fever, diarrhea, seizures, irritability, and poor socialization [possibly persisting for 4 to 6 months]; March of Dimes, 2007b) Intrauterine death or preterm birth is possible with abrupt cessation of heroin use.	Educate the woman about the effects of heroin use on the fetus and newborn. Assess for use of other substances. Provide teaching to women about healthy behaviors. Warn the woman not to abruptly stop heroin use. Encourage her to enroll in a methadone maintenance program.

Substance	Description	Effects on Fetus and Newborn	Nursing Implications
Methadone	Synthetic opiate narcotic used primarily as maintenance therapy for heroin addiction	Improvement in many of the detrimental fetal effects associated with heroin use Withdrawal symptoms are common in newborns. Possible low birthweight due to symmetric fetal growth restriction Increased severity and longer period of withdrawal (due to methadone's longer half-life) Seizures (commonly severe) do not usually occur until 2 to 3 weeks of age, when the newborn is at home. Increased rate of SIDS (3 to 4 times higher; Goff & O'Connor, 2007)	Methadone maintenance programs are the standard of care for women with narcotic addiction. Inform the woman about the benefits and risks of methadone use vs. heroin use. Advantages include improved fetal and newborn growth, reduced risk of fetal death, and reduced risk of HIV infections. Advise the woman that she will need to return consistently to receive the prescribed methadone dose. Reinforce the need for continued prenatal care. Inform the woman that she can breastfeed her newborn while receiving methadone. Teach mother and caregivers about signs and symptoms of methadone withdrawal.

▶ *Consider* THIS! *(continued)*

> *Thoughts: This woman honestly regrets what her addiction has done to her son as she stands watching him go through withdrawal. Her lifestyle choices do affect others, despite her previous denial. One problem with addiction is the difficulty in getting help after deciding to finally quit. There aren't enough rehab centers to deal with the large numbers needing their services and it can be difficult to get into one. What can be offered to pregnant women who abuse substances? How can nurses increase community awareness about the impact of this problem, especially during pregnancy?*

Substance abuse during pregnancy is the subject of much controversy. The timing of drug ingestion usually determines the type and severity of damage to the fetus. Frequently, the woman uses more than one substance, which compounds the problem. Nurses must be knowledgeable about the issues of substance abuse and must be alert for opportunities to identify, prevent, manage, and educate women and families about this key public health issue.

Fetal Alcohol Syndrome

The adverse effects of alcohol consumption have been recognized for centuries, but the associated pattern of fetal anomalies was not labeled until the early 1970s. The distinctive pattern identified three specific findings: growth restriction (prenatal and postnatal), craniofacial structural anomalies, and CNS dysfunction. These distinctive findings were called **fetal alcohol syndrome**, characterized by physical and mental disorders that appear at birth and remain problematic throughout the child's life. However, there are also circumstances in which the effects of prenatal alcohol exposure are apparent but the newborn does not meet all of the criteria. In an attempt to include those who do not meet the strict criteria, the terms "fetal alcohol effects," "alcohol-related birth defects," and "alcohol-related neurologic defects" are used to describe children with a variety of problems thought to be related to alcohol consumption during pregnancy. The Institutes of Medicine coined the term **fetal alcohol spectrum disorder** as a way of describing the broader effects of prenatal alcohol exposure. Children with fetal alcohol syndrome are at the severe end of the spectrum (Manning & Hoyme, 2007). Newborns with some but not all of the symptoms of fetal alcohol syndrome are described as having **alcohol-related birth defects**. Fetal alcohol effects may include such problems as low birthweight, developmental delays, and hyperactivity. Box 24.2 summarizes the manifestations of fetal alcohol syndrome.

Worldwide, the incidence of fetal alcohol syndrome is 1 to 3 cases per 1,000 live births, and that of fetal alcohol effects is 3 to 5 per 1,000 live births (March of Dimes, 2007a). Current estimates indicate that approximately 13% of women of childbearing age are either problem drinkers or alcoholics; therefore, the number of fetuses exposed to alcohol during utero increases dramatically (March of Dimes, 2007a).

Fetal alcohol syndrome is one of the most common known causes of mental retardation, and it is the only cause that is entirely preventable. The effects last a lifetime. Children with this syndrome have varying degrees of psychological and behavioral problems and often find it difficult to hold a job and live independently (CDC, 2007b).

Decreasing or eliminating alcohol consumption during pregnancy is the only way to prevent fetal alcohol syndrome and fetal alcohol effects. Unfortunately, few treatment programs address the needs of pregnant women, so many newborns are exposed to alcohol in utero.

Neonatal Abstinence Syndrome

Newborns of women who abuse tobacco, illicit substances, caffeine, and alcohol can exhibit withdrawal behavior. Withdrawal symptoms occur in 60% of all newborns exposed to drugs (Arenson & Drake, 2007). Drug dependency acquired in utero is manifested by a constellation of neurologic and physical behaviors and is known as **neonatal abstinence syndrome**. Although often treated as a single entity, neonatal abstinence syndrome is not a single pathologic condition. The manifestations of withdrawal are a function of the drug's half-life, the specific drug or combination of drugs used, dosage, route of administration, timing of drug exposure, and length of drug exposure (Kuschel, 2007). Typical newborn behaviors include CNS hypersensitivity, autonomic dysfunction, and gastrointestinal disturbances (Marcellus, 2007). Neonatal abstinence syndrome has both medical and developmental consequences for the newborn.

Nursing Assessment

Several assessment tools can be used to assess a drug-exposed newborn. Figure 24.5 shows an example. Regardless of the tool used for assessment, address these key areas:

- Maternal history to identify risk behaviors for substance abuse:
  - Previous unexplained fetal demise
  - Lack of prenatal care
  - History of missed prenatal appointments
  - Severe mood swings
  - Precipitous labor
  - Poor nutritional status
  - Abruptio placentae
  - Hypertensive episodes
  - History of drug abuse
- Laboratory test results (toxicology) to identify substances in mother and newborn
- Signs of neonatal abstinence syndrome (use the "WITHDRAWAL" acronym; see description below)
- Evidence of seizure activity and need for protective environment

The newborn's behavior often prompts the health care provider or nurse to suspect intrauterine drug exposure (Box 24.3). The newborn physical examination may

---

> ### BOX 24.2 Clinical Picture of Fetal Alcohol Syndrome
>
> - Microcephaly (head circumference <10th percentile)*
> - Small palpebral (eyelid) fissures*
> - Abnormally small eyes
> - Intrauterine growth restriction
> - Maxillary hypoplasia (flattened or absent)
> - Epicanthal folds (folds of skin of the upper eyelid over the eye)
> - Thin upper lip*
> - Missing vertical groove in median portion of upper lip*
> - Short upturned nose
> - Short birth length and low birthweight
> - Joint and limb defects
> - Altered palmar crease pattern
> - Prenatal or postnatal growth ≤10th percentile*
> - Congenital cardiac defects (septal defects)
> - Delayed fine and gross motor development
> - Poor eye–hand coordination
> - Clinically significant brain abnormalities*
> - Mental retardation
> - Narrow forehead
> - Performance substantially below expected level in cognitive or developmental functioning, executive or motor functioning, and attention or hyperactivity; social or language skills*
> - Inadequate sucking reflex and poor appetite
>
> ---
>
> *Diagnosis of fetal alcohol syndrome requires the presence of three findings:
> 1. Documentation of all three facial abnormalities
> 2. Documentation of growth deficits (height, weight or both below 10th percentile)
> 3. Documentation of CNS abnormalities (structural, neurologic, or functional)
>
> Source: National Center on Birth Defects and Developmental Disabilities (NCBDDD) (2007). Fetal alcohol syndrome: guidelines for referral and diagnosis (p. 20). Atlanta: Centers for Disease Control and Prevention (CDC), Department of Health and Human Services (DHHS).

CENTRAL NERVOUS SYSTEM DISTURBANCES													
SIGNS AND SYMPTOMS	**SCORE**	AM						PM					
Excessive high-pitched cry	2												
Continuous high-pitched cry	3												
Sleeps <1 hour after feeding	3												
Sleeps <2 hours after feeding	2												
Sleeps <3 hours after feeding	1												
Hyperactive Moro reflex	2												
Markedly hyperactive Moro reflex	3												
Mild tremors disturbed	1												
Moderate–severe tremors disturbed	2												
Mild tremors undisturbed	1												
Moderate–severe tremors undisturbed	4												
Increased muscle tone	2												
Excoloration (specify area)	1												
Myoclonic jerks	3												
Generalized convulsions	5												
METABOLIC / VASOMOTOR/RESPIRATORY DISTURBANCES													
Sweating													
Fever <101 (99–100.8°F/37.2–38.2°C)	1												
Fever >101 (38.2°C and higher)	2												
Frequent yawning (>3– 4 times/interval)	1												
Mottling	1												
Nasal stuffiness	1												
Sneezing (>3–4 times/interval)	1												
Nasal flaring	2												
Respiratory rate >60 / min	1												
Respiratory rate >60 / min, with retractions	2												
GASTROINTESTINAL DISTURBANCES													
Excessive sucking	1												
Poor feeding	2												
Regurgitation	2												
Projectile vomiting	3												
Loose stools	2												
Watery stools	3												
TOTAL SCORE													

FIGURE 24.5 Neonatal abstinence scoring system. (From Cloherty, J. P., & Stark, A. P. [1998]. *Manual of neonatal care* [4th ed., pp. 26–27]. Boston: Little, Brown.).

BOX 24.3 Manifestations of Neonatal Abstinence Syndrome

CNS Dysfunction
- Tremors
- Generalized seizures
- Hyperactive reflexes
- Restlessness
- Hypertonic muscle tone, constant movement
- Shrill, high-pitched cry
- Disturbed sleep patterns

Metabolic, Vasomotor, and Respiratory Disturbances
- Fever
- Frequent yawning
- Mottling of the skin
- Sweating
- Frequent sneezing
- Nasal flaring
- Tachypnea >60 bpm
- Apnea

Gastrointestinal Dysfunction
- Poor feeding
- Frantic sucking or rooting
- Loose or watery stools
- Regurgitation or projectile vomiting (Belik & Al-Hamad, 2007)

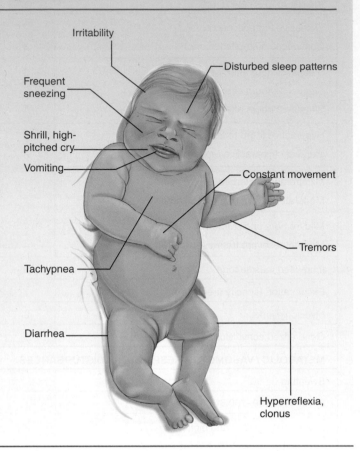

also reveal low birthweight for gestational age or drug- or alcohol-related birth defects and dysfunction.

▶ **Take** NOTE!

Cocaine-exposed newborns are typically fussy, irritable, and inconsolable at times. They demonstrate poor coordination of sucking and swallowing, making feeding time frustrating for the newborn and caregiver alike.

Assess the newborn for signs of neonatal abstinence syndrome. Use the acronym WITHDRAWAL to focus the assessment:

W = Wakefulness: sleep duration less than 1 to 3 hours after feeding
I = Irritability
T = Temperature variation, tachycardia, tremors
H = Hyperactivity, high-pitched persistent cry, hyperreflexia, hypertonus
D = Diarrhea, diaphoresis, disorganized suck
R = Respiratory distress, rub marks, rhinorrhea
A = Apneic attacks, autonomic dysfunction
W = Weight loss or failure to gain weight
A = Alkalosis (respiratory)
L = Lacrimation (Belik & Hawes, 2007)

Assist with obtaining diagnostic studies to identify the severity of withdrawal. In general, a urine screen signifies only recent newborn exposure to maternal use of drugs. It can detect marijuana use up to a month earlier, cocaine use up to 96 hours earlier, heroin use 24 to 48 hours earlier, and methadone use up to 10 days earlier (Belik & Hawes, 2007). Toxicology screening of the newborn's blood, urine, and meconium identifies the substances to which the newborn has been exposed.

Nursing Management

The needs of the substance-exposed newborn are multiple, complex, and costly, both to the health care system and to society. Substance abuse takes place among people of all colors, sizes, shapes, incomes, types, and conditions. Most pregnant women are unaware of the adverse impact their substance abuse can have on the newborn.

Nurses are in a unique position to help because they interact with high-risk mothers and newborns in many settings, including the community, health care facilities, and family agencies. It is the responsibility of all nurses to identify, educate, counsel, and refer pregnant women with substance-abusing problems. For example, nurses can be instrumental in increasing the number of pregnant women who make a serious attempt to quit smoking by using the "5 A's" approach:

- Ask: Ask all women if they smoke and would like to quit.
- Advise: Encourage the use of clinically proven treatment plans.
- Assess: Provide motivation by discussing the "5 R's":
  - Relevance of quitting to the woman
  - Risk of continued smoking to the fetus
  - Rewards of quitting for both
  - Roadblocks to quitting
  - Repeat at every visit
- Assist: Help the woman to protect her fetus and newborn from the negative effects of smoking.
- Arrange: Schedule follow-up visits to reinforce the woman's commitment to quit.

Although this approach is geared to smoking cessation, nurses can adapt it to focus on cessation for any substance use. Early, supportive, ongoing nursing care is critical to the well-being of the mother and her newborn.

Caring for a substance-exposed newborn remains a major challenge to health care professionals. The major goals include providing comfort to the newborn by relieving symptoms, improving feeding and weight gain, preventing seizures, promoting mother–newborn interactions, and reducing the incidence of newborn mortality and abnormal development (Belik & Hawes, 2007).

Promoting Comfort

Keep environmental stimuli to a minimum. For example, decrease stimuli by dimming the lights in the nursery, and swaddle the newborn tightly to decrease irritability behaviors. Other techniques such as gentle rocking, using a flexed position, and offering a pacifier can help manage CNS irritability. A pacifier also helps satisfy the newborn's need for nonnutritive sucking. Use a calm, gentle approach when handling the newborn and plan activities to avoid overstimulating the newborn, allowing time for rest periods.

Meeting Nutritional Needs

When feeding the newborn, use small amounts and position the newborn upright to prevent aspiration and to facilitate rhythmic sucking and swallowing. Breastfeeding is encouraged unless the mother is still using drugs. Monitor the newborn's weight daily to evaluate the success of food intake. Assess hydration; check skin turgor and fontanels. Assess the frequency and characteristics of bowel movements and monitor the newborn's fluid and electrolyte and acid–base status.

Preventing Complications

Pharmacologic treatment is warranted if conservative measures, such as swaddling and decreased environmental stimulation, are not adequate. The AAP recommends that for newborns with confirmed drug exposure, drug therapy is indicated if the newborn has seizures, diarrhea, and vomiting resulting in excessive weight loss and dehydration, poor feeding, inability to sleep, and fever unrelated to infection (AAP Committee on Substance Abuse, 2005). Common medications used in the management of newborn withdrawal include morphine, paregoric, phenobarbital, tincture of opium, methadone, clonidine, chlorpromazine, and diazepam (Marcellus, 2007). Administer the prescribed medications and document the newborn's behavioral responses.

The newborn is at risk for skin breakdown. Weight loss, diarrhea, dehydration, and irritability can contribute to this risk. Provide meticulous skin care and protect the newborn's elbows and knees against friction and abrasions.

Promoting Parent–Newborn Interaction

For a mother who abuses substances, the birth of a drug-exposed newborn is both a crisis and an opportunity. The mother may feel guilty about the newborn's condition. Many of these newborns are unresponsive and have disorganized sleeping and feeding patterns. When awake, they can be easily overstimulated and irritated. Such characteristics make parent–newborn interactions difficult and frustrating, leading to possible detachment and avoidance (Burd, 2007). In addition, the mother may be single and a victim of physical and sexual abuse and may have a limited support system. Many of these mothers may have had poor parenting themselves, lack information about characteristic infant behaviors, and have unrealistic expectations about the newborn's abilities (Goff & O'Connor, 2007). Instruct the mother or caretaker how to care for the newborn, including what to do after the newborn goes home (Teaching Guidelines 24.1).

On the other hand, the newborn may be a powerful motivator for the mother to undergo treatment and seek recovery. Refer the mother to community agencies to address her addiction and the infant's developmental needs (Gilbert, 2007). The nurse can play a pivotal role in assisting her to abstain from drug use and to promote effective parenting skills.

▶ HYPERBILIRUBINEMIA

Hyperbilirubinemia is a total serum bilirubin level above 5 mg/dL resulting from unconjugated bilirubin being deposited in the skin and mucous membranes

TEACHING GUIDELINES 24.1

Caring for Your Newborn at Home

- Position your newborn with the head elevated to prevent choking.
- To aid your newborn's sucking and swallowing during feeding, position the chin downward and support it with your hand.
- Place your newborn on his or her back to sleep or nap, never on the stomach.
- Keep a bulb syringe close by to suction your newborn's mouth in case of choking.
- Cluster newborn care (bathing, feeding, dressing) to prevent overstimulation.
- If your newborn is fussy or crying, try these measures to help calm him or her:
  - Wrap your newborn snugly in a blanket and gently rock in rocking chair.
  - Take the baby for a ride in the car (using a newborn car seat).
  - Play soothing music and "dance" with the newborn.
  - Use a wind-up swing with music.
- To help your newborn get to sleep, try these measures:
  - Schedule a bath with a gentle massage prior to bedtime.
  - Change diaper and clothes to make the baby comfortable.
  - Feed the baby just prior to bedtime.
  - If the newborn cries when put in crib and all needs are met, allow him or her to cry.
  - Use a rocking chair to feed and sing a soft lullaby.
- Call your primary care provider if you observe withdrawal behaviors such as:
  - Slight tremors (shaking) of hands and legs
  - Stiff posture when held in your arms
  - Irritability and frequent fussiness
  - High-pitched cry, excessive sucking motions
  - Erratic sleep pattern
  - Frequent yawning, nasal stuffiness, sweating
  - Prolonged time needed to feed
  - Frequent vomiting after feeding

(Blackburn, 2007). Hyperbilirubinemia is exhibited as jaundice (yellowing of the body tissues and fluids). Newborn jaundice is one of the most common reasons for hospital readmission. It occurs in 60% to 80% of term newborns in the first week of life and in virtually all preterm newborns (Fanaroff & Lissauer, 2008).

Pathophysiology

Newborn jaundice results from an imbalance in the rate of bilirubin production and bilirubin elimination. This imbalance determines the pattern and degree of newborn hyperbilirubinemia (Blackburn, 2007).

During the newborn period, a rapid transition from the intrauterine to the extrauterine pattern of bilirubin physiology occurs. Fetal unconjugated bilirubin is normally cleared by the placenta and the mother's liver in utero, so total bilirubin at birth is low. After the umbilical cord is cut, the newborn must conjugate bilirubin (convert a lipid-soluble pigment into a water-soluble pigment) in the liver on his or her own. The rate and amount of bilirubin conjugation depend on the rate of red blood cell breakdown, the bilirubin load, the maturity of the liver, and the number of albumin-binding sites (Kenner & Lott, 2007). Bilirubin production increases after birth mainly because of a shortened red blood cell lifespan (70 days in the newborn vs. 90 days in the adult) combined with an increased red blood cell mass. Therefore, the amount of bilirubin the newborn must deal with is large compared to that of an adult.

Bilirubin has two forms—unconjugated or indirect, which is fat-soluble and toxic to body tissues, and conjugated or direct, which is water-soluble and nontoxic. Elevated serum bilirubin levels are manifested as jaundice in the newborn. Typically the total serum bilirubin level rises over the first 3 to 5 days and then declines.

Physiologic Jaundice

Physiologic jaundice is the manifestation of the normal hyperbilirubinemia seen in newborns, appearing during the third to fourth days of life, due to the limitations and abnormalities of bilirubin metabolism. It occurs in 60% of term infants and up to 80% of preterm infants (Blackburn, 2007). Serum bilirubin levels reach up to 10 mg/dL and then decline rapidly over the first week after birth (Cunningham et al., 2005). Most newborns have been discharged by the time this jaundice peaks (at about 72 hours).

Physiologic jaundice may result from an increased bilirubin load because of relative polycythemia, a shortened red blood cell lifespan, immature hepatic uptake and conjugation process, and increased enterohepatic circulation (McLenan, 2007). Newborns with delayed passage of meconium are more likely to develop physiologic jaundice (Blackburn, 2007).

Physiologic jaundice differs between breastfed and bottle-fed newborns in relation to the onset of symptoms. Breastfed newborns typically have peak bilirubin levels on the fourth day of life; levels for bottle-fed newborns usually peak on the third day of life. The rate of bilirubin decline is less rapid in breastfed newborns compared to bottle-fed newborns because bottle-fed newborns tend to have more frequent bowel movements. Jaundice associated with breastfeeding presents in two distinct patterns: early-onset breastfeeding jaundice and late-onset breast milk jaundice.

Early-Onset Breastfeeding Jaundice

Early-onset breastfeeding jaundice is probably associated with ineffective breastfeeding practices because of relative caloric deprivation in the first few days of life. Decreased volume and frequency of feedings may result in mild dehydration and the delayed passage of meconium. This delayed defecation allows enterohepatic circulation reuptake of bilirubin and an increase in the serum level of unconjugated bilirubin. To prevent this, strategies to promote early effective breastfeeding are important. The AAP guidelines recommend early and frequent breastfeeding without supplemental water or dextrose-water unless medically indicated (AAP, 2005). Early frequent feedings can provide the newborn with adequate calories and fluid volume (via colostrum) to stimulate peristalsis and passage of meconium to eliminate bilirubin.

Late-Onset Breastfeeding Jaundice

Late-onset breastfeeding jaundice occurs later in the newborn period, with the bilirubin level usually peaking in the 6th to 14th day of life. Total serum bilirubin levels may be 12 to 20 mg/dL, but the levels are not considered pathologic (Simpson, 2007). The specific cause of late-onset breast milk jaundice is not entirely understood, but it may be related to a change in the milk composition resulting in enhanced enterohepatic circulation. Additional research is needed to determine the cause. Interrupting breastfeeding is not recommended unless bilirubin levels reach dangerous levels; if this occurs, breastfeeding is stopped for only 1 or 2 days. Substituting formula during this short break usually results in a prompt decline of bilirubin levels.

Pathologic Jaundice

Pathologic jaundice is manifested within the first 24 hours of life when total bilirubin levels increase by more than 5 mg/dL/day and the total serum bilirubin level is higher than 17 mg/dL in a full-term infant (Ozen & Mukherjee, 2007). Conditions that alter the production, transport, uptake, metabolism, excretion, or reabsorption of bilirubin can cause pathologic jaundice in the newborn. A few conditions that contribute to red blood cell breakdown and thus higher bilirubin levels include polycythemia, blood incompatibilities, and systemic acidosis. These altered conditions can lead to high levels of unconjugated bilirubin, possibly reaching toxic levels and resulting in a severe condition called kernicterus.

Kernicterus (yellow nucleus) or bilirubin encephalopathy is a preventable neurologic disorder characterized by encephalopathy, motor abnormalities, hearing and vision loss, and death (Maisels & Newman, 2007). Neurotoxicity develops because unconjugated bilirubin has a high affinity for brain tissue, and bilirubin not bound to albumin is free to cross the blood–brain barrier and damage cells of the CNS.

In the acute stage, the newborn becomes lethargic, irritable, and hypotonic and sucks poorly. If the hyperbilirubinemia is not treated, the newborn becomes hypertonic, with arching and seizures. A high-pitched cry may be noted. These changes can occur rapidly, so all newborns must be assessed for jaundice and tested if indicated so that treatment can be initiated.

The most common condition associated with pathologic jaundice is hemolytic disease of the newborn secondary to incompatibility of blood groups of the mother and the newborn. The most frequent conditions are Rh factor and ABO incompatibilities.

> ▶ **Take** NOTE!
>
> *Significant jaundice in a newborn less than 24 hours of age should be immediately reported to the physician, as it may indicate a pathologic process.*

Rh Isoimmunization

Rh incompatibility or isoimmunization develops when an Rh-negative woman who has experienced Rh isoimmunization subsequently becomes pregnant with an Rh-positive fetus. The maternal antibodies cross the placenta into the fetal circulation and begin to break down the red blood cells (Fig. 24.6). Destruction of the fetal red blood cells leads to

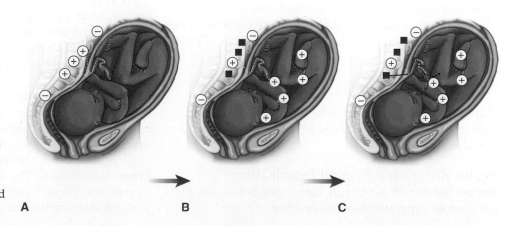

Subsequent Rh⊕fetus

FIGURE 24.6 Rh isoimmunization. (**A**) The Rh-negative mother is exposed to Rh-positive antigens. (**B**) Maternal antibodies form. (**C**) Rh antibodies are transferred to the fetus.

A   B   C

fetal anemia and hemolytic disease of the newborn. The severity of the fetal hemolytic process depends on the level and effectiveness of anti-D antibodies and the capacity of the fetal system to remove antibody-coated cells.

Intrauterine transfusions with Rh-negative, type O blood may be life-saving if done in time. The widespread administration of Rh immune globulin (RhoGAM), combined with aggressive fetal surveillance and transfusion, has reduced the incidence of hemolytic disease of the newborn.

Immune hydrops, also called hydrops fetalis, is a severe form of hemolytic disease of the newborn that occurs when pathologic changes develop in the organs of the fetus secondary to severe anemia. Hydrops fetalis results from fetal hypoxia, anemia, congestive heart failure, and hypoproteinemia secondary to hepatic dysfunction. ABO and Rh incompatibilities can both cause hydrops fetalis, but Rh disease is the more common cause. Typically, hydrops is not observed until the hemoglobin drops below approximately 4 g/dL (hematocrit <15%) (Huang et al., 2007). Fetuses with hydrops may die in utero from profound anemia and circulatory failure. The placenta is very enlarged and edematous. One sign of severe anemia and impending death is the sinusoidal fetal heart rate pattern (Cunningham et al., 2005).

ABO Incompatibility

ABO incompatibility is an immune reaction that occurs when the mother has type O blood and the fetus has type A, B, or AB blood. Although it occurs more frequently than Rh incompatibilities, it causes less severe problems and rarely results in hemolytic disease severe enough to be clinically diagnosed and treated. Enlargement of the spleen and liver may be found in newborns with ABO incompatibility, but hydrops fetalis is rare (Kenner & Lott, 2007). Because the antibodies resulting in ABO incompatibility occur naturally, it is impossible to eliminate this type of incompatibility.

Women with type O blood develop anti-A or anti-B antibodies throughout their life through foods they eat and exposure to infections. Most species of anti-A and anti-B antibodies are immunoglobin M (IgM), which cannot cross the placenta and thus cannot gain access to the fetal red blood cells. Some anti-A and anti-B antibodies from the mother may cross the placenta to the fetus during the first pregnancy and can cause hemolysis of fetal blood cells.

Nursing Assessment

Nurses play an important role in early detection and identification of jaundice in the newborn. Keen observation skills are essential.

Health History and Physical Examination

Review the history for factors that might predispose the newborn to hyperbilirubinemia, such as:

- Polycythemia
- Significant bruising or cephalhematoma, which increases bilirubin production
- Infections such as TORCH (toxoplasmosis, hepatitis B, rubella, cytomegalovirus, herpes simplex virus)
- Use of drugs during labor and birth such as diazepam (Valium) or oxytocin (Pitocin)
- Prematurity
- Gestational age of 34 to 36 weeks
- Hemolysis due to ABO incompatibility or Rh isoimmunization
- Macrosomic infant of a diabetic mother
- Delayed cord clamping, which increases the erythrocyte volume
- Decreased albumin binding sites to transport unconjugated bilirubin to the liver because of acidosis
- Delayed meconium passage, which increases the amount of bilirubin that returns to the unconjugated state and can be absorbed by the intestinal mucosa
- Siblings who had significant jaundice
- Inadequate breastfeeding leading to dehydration, decreased caloric intake, weight loss, and delayed passage of meconium
- Ethnicity, such as Asian-American, Mediterranean, or Native American
- Male gender (Kenner & Lott, 2007)

Perform a complete physical examination. Assess the skin, mucous membranes, sclerae, and bodily fluids (tears, urine) for a yellow color. Detect jaundice by observing the infant in a well-lit room and blanching the skin with digital pressure over a bony prominence. Typically, jaundice begins on the head and gradually progresses to the abdomen and extremities. Also inspect for pallor (anemia), excessive bruising (bleeding), and dehydration (sluggish circulation), which may contribute to the development of jaundice and the risk for kernicterus.

Assess the newborn for Rh incompatibility. Be alert for clinical manifestations such as ascites, congestive heart failure, edema, pallor, jaundice, hepatosplenomegaly, hydramnios, thick placenta, and dilation of the umbilical vein (Blackburn, 2007).

The hydropic newborn appears pale, edematous, and limp at birth and typically requires resuscitation. The newborn with immune hydrops exhibits severe generalized edema, organ hypertrophy and enlargement, and effusion of fluid into body cavities.

Laboratory and Diagnostic Testing

Determine maternal and fetal blood types, checking for incompatibilities (Comparison Chart 24.1). Assess laboratory values for bilirubin (both unconjugated and conjugated). Bilirubin levels establish the diagnosis of hyperbilirubinemia. The newborn with Rh incompatibility demonstrates a rapidly rising unconjugated bilirubin level at birth or in the first 24 hours. Also expect to obtain

COMPARISON CHART 24.1   RH VS. ABO INCOMPATIBILITY

Clinical Picture	Rh Incompatibility	ABO Incompatibility
First-born	Rare	Common
Later pregnancies	More severe	No increase in severity
Jaundice	Moderate to severe	Mild
Hydrops fetalis	Frequent	Rare
Anemia	Frequently severe	Rare
Ascites	Frequent	Rare
Hepatosplenomegaly	Frequent	Common

alkaline phosphatase, liver enzymes, and prothrombin time and partial thromboplastin time, as well as:

- Direct Coombs test—to identify hemolytic disease of the newborn; positive results indicate that the newborn's red blood cells have been coated with antibodies and thus are sensitized
- Hemoglobin concentration—for evidence of anemia
- Blood type—to determine Rh status and any incompatibility of the newborn
- Total serum protein—to detect reduced binding capacity of albumin
- Reticulocyte count—to identify an elevated level indicating increased hemolysis

Assist with obtaining blood specimens. Use cord blood for hemoglobin concentration measurements; use a heel stick for direct Coombs testing and bilirubin levels. Prepare the parents and newborn for radiologic evaluation if necessary to determine abnormalities that may be causing the jaundice.

Nursing Management

Nursing management of a newborn with hyperbilirubinemia requires a comprehensive approach. As members of the health care team, nurses share in the responsibility for early detection and identification, family education, management, and follow-up of the mother and newborn. Documentation of the timing of onset of jaundice is essential to differentiate between physiologic (>24 hours) and pathologic (<24 hours) jaundice. Nurses can improve care by offering their presence and support.

Reducing Bilirubin Levels

Encourage early initiation of feedings to prevent hypoglycemia and provide protein to maintain the albumin levels to transport bilirubin to the liver. Ensure newborn feedings (breast milk or formula) every 2 to 3 hours to promote prompt emptying of bilirubin from the bowel. Encourage the mother to breastfeed (8 to 12 feedings per day) to prevent inadequate intake and thus dehydration. Supplement breast milk with formula to supply protein if bilirubin levels continue to increase with breastfeeding

only. Monitor serum bilirubin levels frequently to reduce the risk of severe hyperbilirubinemia.

Phototherapy

For the newborn with jaundice, regardless of its etiology, phototherapy is used to convert unconjugated bilirubin to the less toxic water-soluble form that can be excreted. Phototherapy, via special lights placed above the newborn or a fiber-optic blanket placed under the newborn and wrapped around him or her, involves blue wavelengths of light to alter unconjugated bilirubin in the skin. For the newborn receiving phototherapy, place the newborn under the lights or on the fiberoptic blanket, exposing as much skin as possible. Cover the newborn's genitals and shield the eyes to protect them from becoming irritated or burned when using direct lights. Assess the intensity of the light source to prevent burns and excoriation (Fig. 24.7). Turn the newborn every 2 hours to maximize the area of exposure, removing the newborn from the lights only for feedings. Maintain a neutral thermal environment to decrease energy expenditure, and assess the newborn's neurologic status frequently.

Assess the newborn's temperature every 3 to 4 hours as indicated. Monitor fluid intake and output closely and assess daily weights for gains or losses. Check skin turgor for evidence of dehydration.

With feedings, remove the newborn from the lights and remove the eye shields to allow interaction with the newborn. Encourage breast or bottle feedings every 2 to 3 hours. Follow agency policy about removing the eye shields periodically to assess the eyes for discharge or corneal irritation secondary to eye shield pressure. Typically, the eyes are assessed and eye shields are removed once a shift.

Monitor stool for consistency and frequency. Unconjugated bilirubin excreted in the feces will produce a greenish appearance, and typically stools are loose. Lack of frequent green stools is a cause for concern.

Provide meticulous skin care. Assess skin surfaces frequently for dryness and irritation secondary to the dehydrating effects of phototherapy and irritation from highly acidic stool to prevent excoriation and skin breakdown (Simpson, 2007). Monitor the newborn's skin turgor.

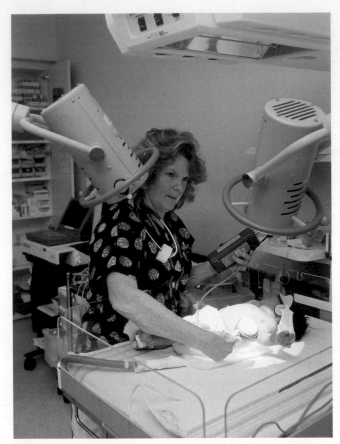

FIGURE 24.7 A newborn receiving phototherapy. Here the nurse is checking the intensity of the lights with a meter.

Exchange Transfusion

If the total serum bilirubin level remains elevated after intensive phototherapy, an exchange transfusion, the quickest method for lowering serum bilirubin levels, may be necessary (Springer & Annibale, 2007). In the presence of hemolytic disease, severe anemia, or a rapid rise in the total serum bilirubin level, an exchange transfusion is recommended. An exchange transfusion removes the newborn's blood and replaces it with nonhemolyzed red blood cells from a donor. During the transfusion, monitor the newborn's cardiovascular status continuously because serious complications can arise, such as acid–base imbalances, infection, hypovolemia, and fluid and electrolyte imbalances. Exchange transfusion is used only as a second-line therapy after phototherapy has failed to yield results. Intensive nursing care is needed.

Assist the physician with an exchange transfusion if necessary. Monitor the newborn's status closely for changes, especially in vital signs and heart rate and rhythm, before, during, and after the procedure.

Providing Parent Teaching and Support

Nurses can help the parents to understand the diagnostic tests and treatment modalities by offering individualized teaching. Explore with the family their understanding of jaundice and treatment modalities to reduce anxiety and gain their cooperation in monitoring the infant. Teach the parents about jaundice and its potential risk using written and verbal material. Also show the parents how to identify newborn behaviors that might indicate rising bilirubin levels. Emphasize the need to seek treatment from their pediatrician should any of the following occur:

• Lethargy, sleepiness, poor muscle tone, floppiness
• Poor sucking, lack of interest in feeding
• High-pitched cry

Teach the parents how to assess their newborn for signs of jaundice because physiologic jaundice may not occur until after the newborn is discharged. Reinforce the need for appropriate follow-up with the primary care provider within 48 to 72 hours after discharge to assess jaundice status (Keren & Bhutani, 2007).

The need for phototherapy can be anxiety-producing for the parents. Explain the rationale for the procedure and demonstrate techniques that the parents can use to interact with their newborn. Additional education about phototherapy may be necessary when home phototherapy is used (Teaching Guidelines 24.2).

▶ NEWBORN INFECTIONS

Newborns are susceptible to infections because their immune system is immature and slow to react. The antibodies that newborns received from the mother during pregnancy and from breast milk help protect them from invading organisms. However, these need time to reach optimal levels.

Bacterial infections of the newborn affect approximately 4 out of every 1,000 live births (McLenan, 2007). Making the diagnosis of sepsis in newborns is difficult due to its nonspecific symptoms. The mortality rate from newborn sepsis may be as high as 50% if untreated. Infection is a major cause of death during the first month of life, contributing to 13% to 15% of all neonatal deaths (Anderson-Berry & Bellig, 2007).

Pathophysiology

When a pathologic organism overcomes the newborn's defenses, infection and sepsis results. **Neonatal sepsis** is the presence of bacterial, fungal, or viral microorganisms or their toxins in blood or other tissues. Infections that have an onset within the first month of life are termed newborn infections. Exposure to a pathogenic organism, whether a virus, fungus, or bacteria, occurs, and it enters the newborn's body and begins to multiply.

Newborn infections are usually grouped into three classes according to their time of onset: congenital infection, acquired in utero (intrauterine infections) by vertical transmission with onset before birth; early-onset

TEACHING GUIDELINES 24.2

Caring for Your Newborn Receiving Home Phototherapy

- Inspect your newborn's skin, eyes, and mucous membranes for a yellow color.
- Remember that a home health nurse will come to visit and help you set up the light system.
- Keep the lights about 12 to 30 inches above your newborn.
- Cover your newborn's eyes with patches or cotton balls and gauze to protect them.
- Keep the newborn undressed except for the diaper area; fold the diaper down below the newborn's navel in the front and as far as possible in the back to expose as much skin as possible.
- Turn your newborn every 2 hours so that all areas of the body are exposed.
- Remove the newborn from the lights only for feeding.
- Remove the eye patches during feedings so that you can interact with your newborn.
- Record your newborn's temperature, weight, and fluid intake daily.
- Document the frequency, color, and consistency of all stools; the stools should be loose and green as the bilirubin is broken down.
- Keep the skin clean and dry to prevent irritation.
- Feed your newborn frequently, including supplemental glucose water if allowed to provide added fluid, protein, and calories.
- Rock, cuddle, or hold the newborn to promote bonding when out of the lights.
- Contact your pediatrician or home health care agency with any questions or changes, including refusing feedings, fewer than five wet diapers in one day, vomiting of complete amounts of feeding, or elevated temperature.
- Keep appointments for follow-up laboratory testing to monitor bilirubin levels.

infections, acquired by vertical transmission in the perinatal period, either shortly before or during birth; and late-onset infections, acquired by horizontal transmission in the nursery. As many as 80% to 90% of neonatal infections have their onset in the first 2 days of life (Rubarth, 2008). Comparison Chart 24.2 compares the three classes of newborn infections.

Nursing Assessment

Nursing assessment focuses on early identification of a newborn at risk for infection to allow for prompt treatment, thus reducing mortality and morbidity. Be aware of the myriad risk factors associated with newborn sepsis. Among the factors that contribute to the newborn's overall vulnerability to infection are poor skin integrity, invasive procedures, exposure to numerous caregivers, and an environment conducive to bacterial colonization (Kenner & Lott, 2007).

Few newborn infections are easy to recognize because manifestations usually are nonspecific. Early symptoms can be vague because of the newborn's inability to mount an inflammatory response. Often, the observation is that the newborn does not "look right." Assess the newborn for common nonspecific signs of infection, including:

- Hypothermia
- Pallor or duskiness
- Hypotonia
- Cyanosis
- Poor weight gain
- Irritability
- Seizures
- Jaundice
- Grunting
- Nasal flaring
- Apnea and bradycardia
- Lethargy
- Hypoglycemia
- Poor feeding (lack of interest in feeding)
- Abdominal distention (Anderson-Berry & Bellig, 2007)

Since infection can be confused with other newborn conditions, laboratory and radiographic tests are needed to confirm the presence of infection. Be prepared to coordinate the timing of the various tests and assist as necessary.

Evaluate the complete blood count with a differential to identify anemia, leukocytosis, or leukopenia. Elevated C-reactive protein levels may indicate inflammation. As ordered, obtain x-rays of the chest and abdomen, which may reveal infectious processes located there. Blood, cerebrospinal fluid, and urine cultures are indicated to identify the location and type of infection present. Positive cultures confirm that the newborn has an infection.

Nursing Management

To enhance the newborn's chance of survival, early recognition and diagnosis are key. Often the diagnosis of sepsis is based on a suspicious clinical picture. Antibiotic therapy is usually started before the laboratory results identify the infecting pathogen (see Evidence-Based Practice 24.1). Along with antibiotic therapy, circulatory, respiratory, nutritional, and developmental support is important. Antibiotic therapy is continued for 7 to 21 days if cultures are positive, or it is discontinued within 72 hours if cultures are negative. With the use of antibiotics along with early recognition and supportive care, mortality and morbidity rates have been reduced greatly.

COMPARISON CHART 24.2   INTRAUTERINE VS. EARLY-ONSET VS. LATE-ONSET NEWBORN INFECTIONS

	Intrauterine (Congenital)	Early-Onset Infections	Late-Onset Infections
Risk factors	– Immature immune system IgM, IgA, and T lymphocytes – Decreased gastric acid, which is needed to reduce organisms	– Prolonged rupture of membranes – Urinary tract infections – Preterm labor – Prolonged or difficult labor – Maternal fever – Colonization with group B streptococci – Maternal infections	– Low birthweight – Prematurity – Meconium staining – Need for resuscitation – Birth asphyxia – Improper handwashing
Common causative organisms	– Cytomegalovirus – Rubella – Toxoplasmosis – Syphilis	– *Escherichia coli* – Group B streptococci – *Klebsiella pneumoniae* – *Listeria monocytogenes* – Other enteric gram-negative bacilli	– *Candida albicans* – Coagulase-negative staphylococci – *Staphylococcus aureus* – *E. coli* – Enterobacter – Klebsiella – Serratia – Pseudomonas – Group B streptococci
Mechanism of infection	– Organism crossing placenta into fetal circulatory system; organism residing in amniotic fluid – Ascent of organism via the vagina, ultimately infecting membranes and causing rupture and leading to respiratory and gastrointestinal tract infections	Most occur during birthing process when newborn comes into contact with infected birth canal (newborn cannot defend against host organisms). – Newborn susceptibility to infection by exogenous organisms possibly due to inadequacy of physical barriers (thin, friable skin with little subcutaneous tissue) – Lack of gastric acidity, possibly resulting in easy colonization by environmental organisms – Aspiration of microorganisms during birth with development of pneumonia	More common in newborns undergoing invasive procedures such as endotracheal intubation or catheter insertion; break in skin or mucosal protection barrier

Sources: Blackburn, 2007; Brousseau & Sharieff, 2007; Kenner & Lott, 2007.

Nurses possess the education and assessment tools to decrease the incidence of and reduce the impact of infections on women (see Chapter 20 for additional information) and their newborns. Implement measures for prevention and early recognition, including:

• Formulating a sepsis prevention plan that includes education of all members of the health care team on identification and treatment of sepsis
• Screening all newborns daily for signs of sepsis
• Monitoring sepsis cases and outcomes to reinforce continued quality-improvement measures or to modify current practices
• Outlining and carrying out measures to prevent nosocomial infections, such as:

• Thorough handwashing hygiene for all staff
• Frequent oral care and inspections of mucous membranes
• Proper positioning and turning to prevent skin breakdown
• Use of strict aseptic technique for all wound care
• Frequent monitoring of invasive catheter sites for signs of infection
• Identifying newborns at risk for sepsis by reviewing risk factors
• Monitoring vital sign changes and observing for subtle signs of infection
• Monitoring for signs of organ system dysfunction:
  • Cardiovascular compromise—tachycardia and hypotension

EVIDENCE-BASED PRACTICE 24.1
Treating Neonatal Sepsis With Gentamicin Given as a Once-Daily Dose or as Multiple Doses per Day

Sepsis in a newborn can be fatal, and the signs and symptoms can be vague. Antibiotic therapy is usually initiated before the infection is confirmed by cultures. Gentamicin is an antibiotic commonly used to treat neonatal sepsis because it is effective against gram-negative pathogens. However, gentamicin, like other aminoglycosides, can have adverse effects on hearing and kidney function, leading to questions about the most effective dosing regimen. Studies have shown that once-a-day dosing is most effective in older children and adults, but these studies do not address the neonatal population.

● Study
A study involving neonates with confirmed or suspected sepsis was completed to evaluate the effectiveness and safety of two types of dosing regimens: once-a-day dosing and multiple-doses-per-day dosing. All randomized or quasi-randomized controlled trials involving a comparison of one daily dose with multiple doses per day of gentamicin to newborns less than 28 days of age were selected. Information about clinical effectiveness, pharmacokinetic effectiveness, ototoxicity, and nephrotoxicity was collected. Of the 24 studies initially selected, 11 were evaluated. Most of the studies used intravenous infusion of gentamicin as the method of administration. One study used a bolus dose of gentamicin administered over 1 minute; two other studies used intramuscular administration.

▲ Findings
Regardless of the dosing regimen, gentamicin was shown to be effective in treating the sepsis. The once-daily dosing regimen appeared to be more effective: appropriate peak and trough levels of the drug were obtained more frequently when compared to the multiple-dose regimen. The studies found no evidence of ototoxicity or nephrotoxicity with either regimen.

■ Nursing Implications
The study confirmed the effectiveness of gentamicin in the treatment of neonatal sepsis, but it did not determine whether a once-daily dose was more effective than multiple doses per day in treating sepsis. Nurses can integrate the findings of this study into their practice when caring for newborns who are at risk for or have developed sepsis. Regardless of the regimen ordered, nurses can be diligent in ensuring that peak and trough drug levels are monitored. Although the study showed no evidence of hearing and kidney adverse effects, nurses still need to monitor the newborns for this possibility.

Rao, S. C., Ahmed, M., & Hagan, R. (2006). One dose per day compared to multiple doses per day of gentamicin for treatment of suspected or proven sepsis in neonates. *Cochrane Database of Systematic Reviews* 2006. Issue 1. Art. No.: CD005091.

- Respiratory compromise—respiratory distress and tachypnea
- Renal compromise—oliguria or anuria
- Systemic compromise—abnormal blood values
- Providing comprehensive sepsis treatment:
- Circulatory support with fluids and vasopressors
- Supplemental oxygen and mechanical ventilation
- Obtaining culture samples as requested
- Antibiotic administration as ordered, observing for side effects
- Promoting newborn comfort
- Assessing the family's educational needs and providing instructions as necessary

Perinatal infections continue to be a public health problem, with severe consequences for those affected. By promoting a better understanding of newborn infections and appropriate use of therapies, nurses can lower the mortality rates associated with severe sepsis, especially with appropriate timing of interventions. The potential for nursing interventions to identify, prevent, and minimize the risk for sepsis is significant. Primary disease prevention must be a major focus for nurses. Family education plays a key role in the prevention of perinatal infections, in addition to following accepted practices in immunization.

Congenital Conditions

Congenital conditions can arise from many etiologies, including single-gene disorders, chromosome aberrations, exposure to teratogens, and many sporadic conditions of unknown cause. Congenital conditions may be inherited or sporadic, isolated or multiple, apparent or hidden, gross or microscopic. They cause nearly half of all deaths in term newborns and cause long-term sequelae for many. The incidence varies according to the type of defect. When a serious anomaly is identified prenatally, the parents can decide whether or not to continue the pregnancy. When an anomaly is identified at or after birth, parents need to be informed promptly and given a realistic appraisal of the severity of the condition, the prognosis, and treatment options so that they can participate in all decisions pertaining to their child.

Congenital conditions can affect virtually any body system. This chapter describes common congenital conditions identified at or after birth. Some of these conditions warrant immediate treatment soon after birth. Other conditions, although identified in the newborn period, are long-term with ongoing effects into childhood.

▶ CONGENITAL HEART DISEASE

Congenital heart disease is a structural defect involving the heart, the great vessels, or both that is present at birth (American Heart Association [AHA], 2008a, 2008b). It is a broad term that can describe a number of abnormalities affecting the heart. Approximately 8 newborns out of every 1,000 live births will have some form of congenital heart disease. Congenital heart disease causes more deaths during the first year of life than any other birth defect (AHA, 2008a). The defect may be very mild and the newborn appears healthy at birth, or it may be so severe that the newborn's life is in immediate jeopardy. Severe congenital cardiac defects usually present in the first few days or weeks of life, while the newborn's circulation is continuing to adapt to the demands of extrauterine life. Advances in diagnosis and medical and surgical interventions have led to dramatic increases in survival rates for newborns with serious heart defects.

Pathophysiology

In most cases, the exact cause of congenital heart disease is unknown. Most congenital heart defects develop during the first 8 weeks of gestation and are usually the result of genetic and environmental forces.

Typically, congenital heart disease is divided into four physiologic categories based on structural abnormalities and functional alterations (Table 24.5):

- Defects causing increased pulmonary blood flow, such as atrial septal defect and ventricular septal defect
- Defects causing obstructed blood flow out of the heart, such as pulmonary or aortic stenosis
- Defects causing decreased pulmonary blood flow, such as tetralogy of Fallot
- Defects involving mixing of saturated and desaturated blood, such as truncus arteriosus or transposition of the great arteries

These four categories are more descriptive than the system used previously, which classified the disorder only as cyanotic or acyanotic. This previous classification was imprecise because some newborns with "acyanotic" defects developed cyanosis and delayed symptoms that often became apparent during infancy and early childhood. With the hemodynamic classification, the clinical picture of each grouping is more uniform and predictable (Simpson & Creehan, 2008).

Therapeutic Management

If the defect is mild, typically no treatment is necessary. However, for most congenital defects corrective surgery is necessary.

Nursing Assessment

While most congenital heart defects cannot be prevented, several key areas need to be addressed to ensure the optimal health status for the woman and her fetus. A thorough health history of the woman and newborn and physical examination provide valuable information. Laboratory and diagnostic tests provide additional information about the defect and its severity.

Health History and Physical Examination

Ideally, nursing assessment begins prenatally by reviewing the maternal history for risk factors that might predispose the newborn to a congenital heart defect. Risk factors include:

- Maternal alcoholism
- Maternal diabetes mellitus
- Single-gene mutation or chromosomal disorders
- Maternal exposure to x-rays
- Maternal exposure to rubella infection
- Poor maternal nutrition during pregnancy
- Maternal age over 40
- Maternal use of amphetamines
- Genetic factors (family recurrence patterns)
- Maternal metabolic disorder of phenylketonuria
- Maternal use of anticonvulsants, estrogen, progesterone, lithium, warfarin (Coumadin), or isotretinoin (Accutane) (Simpson & Creehan, 2008)

After birth, carefully assess the newborn's cardiovascular and respiratory systems, looking for signs of respiratory distress, cyanosis, or congestive heart failure that might indicate a cardiac anomaly. Assess rate, rhythm, and heart sounds, reporting any abnormalities immediately. Note any signs of heart failure, including edema, diminished peripheral pulses, hepatomegaly, tachycardia, diaphoresis, respiratory distress with tachypnea, peripheral pallor, and irritability (Kenner & Lott, 2007).

Laboratory and Diagnostic Tests

Assist with diagnostic testing, such as:

- Arterial blood gases to determine oxygenation levels and to differentiate lung disease from heart disease as the cause of cyanosis
- Chest x-rays to identify cardiac size, shape, and position

TABLE 24.5 CLASSIFICATIONS OF CONGENITAL HEART DISEASE

Cardiac Defect	Examples	Pathophysiology	Clinical Picture
Increased pulmonary blood flow (left-to-right shunting)	Atrial septal defect (ASD) Ventricular septal defect (VSD) Patent ductus arteriosus (PDA)	Cardiac septum communication or abnormal connection between the great arteries permits blood to flow from higher pressure (left side of heart) to lower pressure (right side of heart).	Asymptomatic or murmur, fatigue with feedings, and symptoms of congestive heart failure (CHF): pallor, diminished peripheral blood flow, feeding difficulties, edema, diaphoresis, tachypnea, and tachycardia
Decreased pulmonary blood flow	Tetralogy of Fallot (TOF) Tricuspid atresia	Pulmonary blood flow obstruction accompanied by an anatomic defect such as ASD or VSD between the right and left sides of the heart, which allows desaturated blood to shunt right to left, causing desaturated blood to enter into the systemic circulation	Mild to severe oxygen desaturation, polycythemia, murmur, hypoxemia, dyspnea, increased cardiac workload, and marked exercise intolerance
Obstruction to blood flow out of the heart	Pulmonary stenosis Aortic stenosis Coarctation of the aorta	A narrowing or constriction of an opening causes pressure to rise in the area behind the obstruction and a decrease in blood available for systemic perfusion	CHF, decreased cardiac output, and pump failure
Mixed defects	Transposition of the great arteries Total anomalous pulmonary venous connection Truncus arteriosus Hypoplastic left heart syndrome	Fully saturated systemic blood flow mixes with desaturated pulmonary blood flow, causing desaturation of the systemic circulation. This leads to pulmonary congestion and a decrease in cardiac output. To support life, intervention must bring about a mixing of arterial and venous blood.	Decreased cardiac output, CHF, ruddiness, dusky or gray color, dyspnea

Sources: Bader, Huhta, & Hornberger, 2008; Kyle, 2008; Rudolph, 2007.

- Magnetic resonance imaging (MRI) to evaluate for cardiac malformations
- Electrocardiogram to detect atrial or ventricular hypertrophy and dysrhythmias
- Echocardiogram to evaluate heart anatomy and flow defects
- Blood studies to assess anemia, blood glucose, and electrolyte levels
- Catheterization to obtain data for definitive diagnosis or in preparation for cardiac surgery

Nursing Management

Like nursing assessment, nursing management ideally focuses on prevention with measures during the prenatal period. For example, ensure that all women are tested prior to pregnancy for immunity to rubella so that they can be immunized if necessary. Any chronic health problems, such as diabetes, hypertension, seizures, and phenylketonuria, should be controlled and any medication or dietary adjustments should be made before attempting conception.

Once pregnant, the woman should be encouraged to avoid alcohol, smoking, and the use of unprescribed drugs. Refer the woman and her partner for genetic counseling if cardiac defects are present in the family to provide the parents with a risk assessment for future offspring.

Some defects can be discovered on routine prenatal ultrasound. Therefore, stress the importance of receiving prenatal care throughout pregnancy so that appropriate interventions can be initiated early if the need arises.

After birth of the newborn, nursing management focuses on ensuring adequate cardiac functioning. Provide continuous monitoring of the newborn's cardiac and respiratory status. Administer medications as ordered. Provide comfort measures to the newborn who will be subjected to a variety of painful procedures. Be vigilant in ensuring the newborn's comfort, since he or she cannot report or describe pain. Assist in preventing pain as much as possible; interpret the newborn's cues suggesting pain and manage it appropriately.

Include the parents in the plan of care. Assess their ability to cope with the diagnosis, encouraging them to verbalize their feelings about the newborn's condition and treatment. Educate them about the specific cardiac defect; include written information and pictures to enhance understanding. Present an overview of the prognosis and possible interventions. Teach them about the medications prescribed, including side effects and doses, and how to observe for signs and symptoms indicating heart failure.

Assist them with making decisions about treatment, and support their decisions for the newborn's care. If surgical correction is planned, provide the parents with preoperative teaching and orient them to the NICU prior to surgery. Provide emotional support and guidance throughout the newborn's care.

The parents also need clear instructions about how to monitor the newborn at home, especially if the newborn will be discharged and then brought back later so the condition can be corrected. The parents also need instructions about caring for their newborn after the defect is corrected. Educate the parents about signs that need to be reported, such as weight loss, poor feeding, cyanosis, breathing difficulties, irritability, increased respiratory rate, and fever. Referrals to local support groups, national organizations, and websites also are helpful. Emphasize the importance of close supervision and follow-up care.

▶ NEURAL TUBE DEFECTS

Neural tube defect (NTD) is the common name used to describe congenital CNS structural defects. NTDs are serious malformations involving the spine (spina bifida) and brain (anencephaly). In the United States, NTDs affect 0.6 per 1,000 live births; approximately 3,000 pregnancies annually are complicated by NTDs (Jallo &

Bescke, 2007). They are the second most common major congenital anomaly worldwide, behind cardiac malformations (CDC, 2008a).

A worldwide decline in NTDs has occurred over the past few decades as a result of prevention (preconception folic acid supplementation and monitoring of maternal serum alpha-fetoprotein levels) and use of ultrasonography and amniocentesis to identify affected fetuses (Blackburn, 2007). Despite this decline, still more infants could be born free of these birth defects if all women consumed the necessary amount of folic acid (CDC, 2008a).

Pathophysiology

NTDs occur when the neural tube that develops into the brain and spinal cord fails to close properly during early embryogenesis. The neural tube normally closes between the 17th and 30th day of gestation. NTDs develop during this first month, when most women are still unaware of their pregnancy and the embryo is estimated to be about the size of a grain of rice. In pregnancies in which the fetus has a NTD, the level of alpha-fetoprotein in the amniotic fluid and maternal serum is elevated.

NTDs involve abnormalities in the region-specific neural tube closure junctions with the cranial and caudal levels of the neural tube. NTDs may be either closed (covered by skin or a membrane) or open (neural tissue exposed). These defects vary in their severity, depending on the type and level of the lesion. Common NTDs include anencephaly, spina bifida, myelomeningocele, and meningocele.

Anencephaly

Anencephaly, the most severe neural tube defect, is the congenital absence of the cranial vault, with the cerebral hemispheres completely missing or reduced to small masses. It most commonly involves the forebrain and variable amounts of the upper brain stem, where there is no brain tissue above the brain stem. The incidence is approximately 0.2 per 1,000 live births, and both genetic and environmental insults appear to be responsible (Best, 2007). Anencephaly is apparent on visual inspection after birth, with exposed neural tissue without a cranium surrounding it. Prenatally, alpha-fetoprotein levels are elevated late in the first trimester. Most newborns with anencephaly are stillborn; those born alive die within a few days.

Spina Bifida

Spina bifida is a general term used to refer to caudal defects (below the level of T12) involving spinal cord tissue. Spina bifida is the leading cause of infantile paralysis in the world today; incidence rates are about 1 per 1,000 live births (Foster, 2007).

Spina bifida may be classified by the degree of spinal cord involvement as spina bifida occulta or spinal bifida cystica (Fig. 24.8). Spina bifida occulta involves a defect

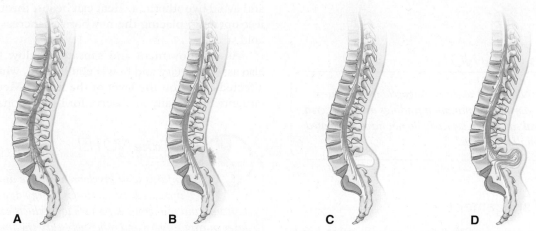

FIGURE 24.8 Neural tube defects. (**A**) Normal spine. (**B**) Spina bifida occulta. (**C**) Meningocele. (**D**) Myelomeningocele.

in the vertebrae without any protrusion or herniation of the spinal cord or meninges. It is a closed defect and is not visible externally. A hairy patch, dermal sinus tract, dimple, hemangioma, or lipoma may be noted in the thoracic, lumbar, or sacral area.

Spina bifida cystica is a more serious NTD. It includes meningocele and myelomeningocele. **Meningocele**, a less severe form of spina bifida cystica, is an opening in the spine through a bony defect (spina bifida) where a herniation of the meninges and spinal fluid has protruded. The spinal cord and nerve roots do not herniate into this dorsal dural sac. Surgical treatment to close the defect is usually warranted.

A **myelomeningocele** is a more severe form of spina bifida cystica in which the spinal cord and nerve roots herniate into the sac through an opening in the spine, compromising the meninges. It is the most common form, accounting for 94% of cases (Behrman et al., 2007). The incidence is 1 in 1,200 to 1,400 live births; it affects 6,000 to 11,000 newborns in the United States each year (Jallo & Becske, 2007). This complex condition, resulting from a neurodevelopmental disruption early in gestation, affects not just the spine but also the CNS. Hydrocephalus frequently accompanies this anomaly (Ellenbogen, 2006). This protrusion is typically covered partially or completely by skin but is very fragile and may leak CSF if traumatized.

▶ **Take** NOTE!

Myelomeningoceles can arise at any point along the vertebral column, but they most commonly occur in the lower lumbar or sacral regions, causing neurologic deficits below the level of the defect. Paralysis, bladder and bowel incontinence, and hydrocephalus are the most common complications.

Therapeutic Management

No immediate treatment is needed for spina bifida occulta. However, surgical intervention may be necessary later in life to treat complications associated with degenerative changes or spinal or nerve root involvement. For meningocele, surgery is performed to close the defect. For myelomeningocele, surgical repair is completed as soon as possible, usually within 72 hours after birth, to prevent infection and preserve neurologic function (Ellenbogen, 2006).

Nursing Assessment

Nursing assessment focuses on prevention. Assess all women of childbearing age for intake of folic acid and the use of folic acid supplementation. Review a pregnant woman's history for this supplementation throughout the pregnancy. In addition, monitor the pregnant woman's serum alpha-fetoprotein levels as indicated during pregnancy. Be alert for genetic and environmental risk factors associated with myelomeningocele, such as:

- Celtic ancestry (highest incidence)
- Female sex (accounting for 60% to 70% of affected newborns)
- Low socioeconomic status
- Maternal diabetes
- Use of anticonvulsants (valproic acid and carbamazepine)
- Previous newborn with a NTD
- Maternal obesity
- Maternal malnutrition
- Low folic acid intake (Cunningham et al., 2005)

Inspect the newborn for abnormalities of the spine and back. Look for dimpling or a tuft of hair, which would suggest spina bifida occulta. Observe for a protrusion along the back that may be partially or completely covered with skin. Note the head circumference: a newborn with myelomeningocele often exhibits hydrocephalus (Fig. 24.9).

> ▶ *Take* NOTE!
>
> *Newborns with meningocele usually have normal examination findings and a covered (closed) dural sac. They typically do not have associated neurologic malformations.*

Nursing Management

Nursing management of the newborn with spina bifida occulta is primarily supportive. Be sure that the parents understand the term used and that they do not confuse their newborn's condition with a more serious form of NTD. Teach them about the possibility of surgery in the future should complications develop.

For the child with meningocele, closely monitor the skin covering the area for evidence of CSF leakage. Prepare the newborn and parents for surgery.

Nursing management for a newborn with myelomeningocele involves the following actions to reduce the risk of infection:

- Use strict aseptic technique when caring for the defect to prevent infection.
- Avoid trauma to the sac (to prevent leakage of CSF or damage to the nerve tissue) through prone or side-lying positioning.
- Apply a sterile dressing or protective covering over the sac to prevent rupture and drying, with frequent changes to prevent the dressing from adhering to the defect.
- Frequently monitor the sac for signs of oozing fluid or drainage.
- Meticulously clean the genital area to avoid contamination of the sac.

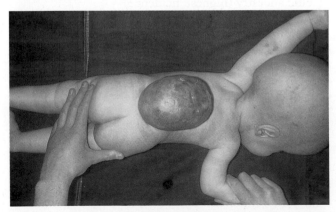

FIGURE 24.9 A newborn with myelomeningocele and hydrocephalus.

In addition, ensure a neutral thermal environment and avoid hypothermia. Heat can be lost through the defect opening, placing the newborn at increased risk for cold stress.

Assess movement and sensation below the defect; also assess urinary and bowel elimination, which may be affected based on the level of the lesion. Measure head circumference daily to observe for hydrocephalus.

> ▶ *Take* NOTE!
>
> *Infants with myelomeningocele are at increased risk for latex allergy due to their repeated and numerous exposures to products containing latex during surgery and other necessary treatments.*

Provide support and information to help the parents cope. Allow them to verbalize their feelings and ask questions. Encourage open discussions regarding the baby's prognosis and long-term care. Provide education about the care of the newborn, including measures to reduce the risk of infection and trauma to the sac. Encourage the parents to participate in their newborn's care as much as possible. As necessary, refer the parents to a support group.

▶ MICROCEPHALY

Microcephaly is a condition in which a small brain is located within a normal-sized cranium. This implies neurologic impairment. Diagnosis is confirmed by a CT scan or MRI. Care is supportive since there is no known treatment to reverse the disorder. Risk factors for this anomaly include maternal viral infections (toxoplasmosis, rubella, cytomegalovirus, herpes, and syphilis), radiation exposure, diabetes, phenylketonuria, street drug exposure, and malnutrition (DeVries, 2007). Inform parents about the potential cognitive impairment of their newborn. Ensure that appropriate community referrals are made to assist the parents and the child, who will have developmental delays.

▶ HYDROCEPHALUS

Hydrocephalus is an increase in CSF in the ventricles of the brain due to overproduction or impaired circulation and absorption. The term stems from the Greek words *hydro* (water) and *kephale* (head). It occurs in about 3 or 4 per 1,000 live births (Engelhart & Sahraker, 2007).

Pathophysiology

Congenital hydrocephalus usually arises as a result of a malformation in the brain or an intrauterine infection (toxoplasmosis or cytomegalovirus). Hydrocephalus rarely occurs as an isolated defect; it is usually associated with spina bifida or other neural tube anomalies. Normal growth of the brain is altered secondary to the increase in intracranial pressure from the CSF.

Therapeutic Management

No treatment is available that can counteract the accumulation of CSF in the brain. Therefore, surgery with the insertion of a ventricular shunt is the mainstay of treatment to relieve pressure within the cranium. Shunts are designed to maintain normal intracranial pressure by draining off excess CSF. A ventriculoperitoneal shunt is inserted from the ventricle in the brain and threaded down into the peritoneal cavity to allow drainage of excess CSF. The long-term prognosis for this condition varies and depends on the patency of the shunt, the presence of other CNS anomalies and their impact on the newborn, and the quality of care the newborn receives. However, shunting has dramatically improved the outcome of newborns with hydrocephalus (Kramer, 2007).

Nursing Assessment

Nursing assessment focuses on obtaining a health history and performing a physical examination. Be alert for risk factors in the maternal history such as intrauterine infection or preterm birth. Assess the infant's head circumference and note any increases. Also note any visible scalp veins (Fig. 24.10). Palpate the infant's head, noting any widened sutures and wide, opened fontanels. Typically the fontanels will feel tense and bulging. Also observe for other signs of hydrocephalus, including poor feeding, "setting sun" eyes, vomiting, lethargy, and irritability. A CT scan or MRI confirm the diagnosis.

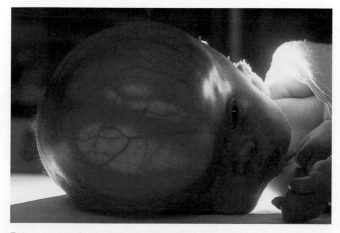

FIGURE 24.10 A newborn with hydrocephalus.

Nursing Management

Prior to shunt insertion, nursing management focuses on daily documentation of the newborn's head circumference and associated neurologic behaviors that might indicate an increase in intracranial pressure: irritability, high-pitched cry, poor feeding and sucking, vomiting, or decrease in consciousness. Gently palpate the fontanels for bulging and tenseness, and palpate the suture lines for increasing separation. Protect the enlarged head to prevent skin breakdown. Handle the head gently and use a sheepskin or a waterbed or egg-crate mattress. Change the newborn's position frequently to minimize pressure.

Postoperatively, strictly monitor the newborn's neurologic status and behavior and report any changes that might indicate increased intracranial pressure secondary to a blockage in the shunt. These findings may include pupillary dilation (increased intracranial pressure places pressure on the oculomotor nerve, producing dilation), increasing head size, bulging fontanels, and change in level of consciousness. Assess the abdomen for distention because drainage of CSF into the abdomen can cause peritonitis. Paralytic ileus is another possible postoperative complication due to distal catheter placement (Engelhart & Sahraker, 2007).

After surgery, continue to provide protective and comfort measures for the enlarged head. Position the newborn's head so that he or she does not lie on the shunt area. Educate the parents about caring for the shunt and signs of infection or blockage. A referral for follow-up home care is appropriate.

▶ CHOANAL ATRESIA

Choanal atresia is an uncommon congenital malformation of the upper airway that involves a narrowing of the nasal airway due to membranous or bony tissue. It can be unilateral or bilateral and typically presents with other anomalies involving the heart and CNS. It occurs in 1 in 8,000 live births, with a female preponderance (Tewfik, 2007).

The cause of this congenital defect is unknown, but it is thought to result from persistence of the membrane between the nasal and oral spaces during fetal development. During attempted inspiration, the tongue is pulled to the palate and obstruction of the oral airway results. If the newborn cries and takes a breath through the mouth, the airway obstruction is momentarily relieved. When the crying stops, however, the mouth closes and the cycle of obstruction is repeated (Tewfik, 2007). This structural anomaly can result in significant respiratory distress in the newborn. If the nasal airway is completely obstructed, death from asphyxia may occur at birth.

Inability to pass a suction catheter through the nose into the pharynx is highly suggestive of choanal atresia.

Other signs include respiratory distress, cyanosis unless newborn is crying, and inability to suck and breathe simultaneously. The diagnosis can be confirmed with a CT scan. Surgery to remove the obstruction and establish a patent airway is needed. Full recovery is the usual outcome.

▶ CONGENITAL DIAPHRAGMATIC HERNIA

Congenital diaphragmatic hernia (CDH) is a rare disorder (1 in 3,000 newborns) that frequently presents with significant respiratory distress in the immediate newborn period (Datin-Dorriere et al., 2008). Most hernias (85%) involve the left hemidiaphragm (Beck et al., 2008). CDH is associated with other anomalies, including congenital cardiac defects, genital or renal anomalies, NTDs, choanal atresia, or chromosomal anomalies, such as trisomy 13 and 18. The survival rate of newborns with a diaphragmatic hernia varies widely.

Pathophysiology

It is thought that the diaphragm failed to close properly during early embryonic development. The abdominal contents herniated into the thoracic cavity through a defect in the diaphragm (Fig. 24.11). The timing of the herniation and the amount of abdominal contents in the thoracic cavity greatly influence the clinical picture at birth and the survival rate. The presence of the abdominal contents in the chest compresses the lung, leads to pulmonary hypoplasia, and promotes persistent pulmonary hypertension in the newborn (Datin-Dorriere et al., 2008).

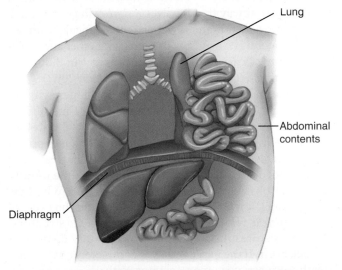

FIGURE 24.11 Congenital diaphragmatic hernia. Note how some of the abdominal contents have entered the thoracic cavity, compressing the lung.

Nursing Assessment

Assess the newborn closely for evidence of respiratory distress, including cyanosis. Affected newborns present with profound respiratory distress because at least one of the lungs cannot expand or may not have fully developed, resulting in persistent pulmonary hypertension shortly after birth. If present, institute resuscitation measures immediately.

Inspect the chest and abdomen, noting a barrel-shaped chest and scaphoid-shaped abdomen. During auscultation, note absent breath sounds on the affected side of the chest and heart sounds displaced to the right. Also listen for bowel sounds, which would be heard in the chest.

Prepare the newborn for a chest x-ray, which will reveal evidence of air-filled bowel in the chest.

> ▶ **Take** NOTE!
>
> *Prenatal diagnosis of CDH is possible through ultrasound. This diagnosis should be considered when hydramnios is present.*

Nursing Management

Nursing management focuses on maintaining optimal respiratory function until surgery is performed to correct the defect. Assist with endotracheal intubation and positive-pressure ventilation to aid in lung expansion and improvement of ventilation. Position the newborn on the affected side with the head and chest elevated to promote normal lung expansion. Monitor ventilatory pressures to prevent pneumothorax. If a pneumothorax occurs, assist with insertion of a chest tube. Monitor oxygen saturation levels to evaluate systemic perfusion status. If the infant's condition does not stabilize, anticipate use of extracorporeal membrane oxygenation (ECMO) or high-frequency oscillatory ventilation.

Administer prescribed medications as ordered. For example, give inotropics to support systemic blood pressure. Administer surfactant, steroids, and inhaled nitric oxide as ordered to correct hypoxia and acid–base imbalance.

Monitor vital signs, weight, urinary output, and serum electrolytes to identify changes early. Maintain nothing by mouth (NPO) status to prevent aspiration, and ensure a neutral thermal environment to prevent cold stress and reduce oxygen demands. Minimize environmental stimuli to reduce agitation and oxygen demand. Assist with placement of an orogastric tube for gastric decompression.

Provide the parents with continuing updates about the newborn's condition. Encourage the parents to see and touch the infant frequently to promote bonding. Assist parents with identifying newborn cues and responding to them.

◆ CLEFT LIP AND PALATE

A cleft lip involves a congenital fissure or longitudinal opening in the lip; a cleft palate involves a congenital fissure or longitudinal opening in the roof of the mouth. The defect may be limited to the outer flesh of the upper lip or it may extend back through the midline of the upper jaw through the roof of the palate. It may occur as a single defect or part of a syndrome of anomalies. It can be unilateral or bilateral. Unilateral cleft lip occurs more commonly on the left side. Bilateral cleft lip is usually accompanied by a cleft palate. Cleft palate can range from a cleft in the uvula to a complete cleft in the soft and hard palates that can be unilateral, bilateral, or in the midline (Fig. 24.12).

Cleft lip and palate is the most common craniofacial birth defect. It is more common in white and Asian males. In addition to immediate feeding difficulties, infants with cleft lip and palate may have problems with dentition, language acquisition, and hearing (March of Dimes, 2008a).

Therapeutic Management

Repairing the facial anomaly as soon as possible is important to facilitate bonding between the newborn and the parents and to improve nutritional status. Treatment of cleft lip is surgical repair between the ages of 6 to 12 weeks. Successful surgery often leaves only a thin scar on the upper lip. The outcome of surgery depends on the severity of the defect: children with more severe cases will need additional surgery in stages (March of Dimes, 2008a).

Surgical correction for cleft palate is done around 6 to 18 months of age to allow for developmental growth

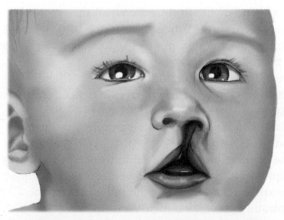

FIGURE 24.12 A newborn with a cleft lip. The defect may extend up through the roof of the palate.

to occur. A plastic palate guard to form a synthetic palate may need to be used to allow for introduction of solid foods and to prevent aspiration in the interim.

Nursing Assessment

Obtain a thorough maternal history, noting the presence of any risk factors such as maternal use of phenytoin (Dilantin), alcohol, and retinoic acid (Accutane) and cigarette smoking. Also assess for a family history of cleft lip or palate, which increases the risk.

Inspect the lip for a visible deformity. Inspect and palpate the mouth for an opening, which may be small or involve the entire palate. Also observe for any feeding difficulties, which are common in newborns with cleft lip and palate.

> ▶ *Take NOTE!*
>
> *Milk flow during feeding requires negative pressure and sucking pressure. Newborns with cleft lip and palate have feeding difficulties because they cannot generate a negative pressure in the mouth to facilitate sucking (Vieira, 2008). Use special nipples, bottles, and feeders to help meet the nutritional needs of infants with this anomaly.*

Nursing Management

Nursing management focuses on providing adequate nutrition, promoting parental bonding, and providing parental education.

Providing Adequate Nutrition

Feed the infant in an upright position to prevent aspiration, and assess for achievement of adequate suction during feeding. Use high-calorie formula to improve caloric intake. Burp the infant frequently to reduce the risk for vomiting and aspiration; burp him or her in the sitting position on your lap to prevent trauma to the mouth on your shoulder. Limit feeding sessions to avoid poor weight gain due to fatigue. After feeding, position the newborn on his or her side in an infant seat.

Promoting Parental Bonding

On first glance, parents may be upset with the appearance of their newborn. Encourage the parents to express their feelings about this highly visible anomaly. Emphasize the newborn's positive features and role-model nurturing behaviors when interacting with the infant. Encourage parents to interact with the newborn. Provide support to the parents, especially related to feeding difficulties. Allow them to vent their frustrations. Offer practical suggestions and continued encouragement for their efforts.

Providing Parental Education

Outline treatment modalities and explain the staging of surgical interventions. Show the family photos taken before and after surgical repair in other babies. These photos can alleviate some of their anxiety. Plan for discharge as soon as the parents feel comfortable with infant care. As part of the discharge plan, initiate appropriate referrals for community support and counseling as needed (Kenner & Lott, 2007).

▶ ESOPHAGEAL ATRESIA AND TRACHEOESOPHAGEAL FISTULA

Esophageal atresia and tracheoesophageal fistula are gastrointestinal anomalies in which the esophagus and trachea do not separate normally during embryonic development. Esophageal atresia is a congenitally interrupted esophagus where the proximal and distal ends do not communicate; the upper esophageal segment ends in a blind pouch and the lower segment ends a variable distance above the diaphragm (Fig. 24.13). Tracheoesophageal fistula is an abnormal communication between the trachea and esophagus. When associated with esophageal atresia, the fistula most commonly occurs between the distal esophageal segment and the trachea. The incidence of esophageal atresia is 1 per 3,000 to 4,000 live births (Blackburn, 2007).

Pathophysiology

Several types of esophageal atresia exist, but the most common anomaly is a fistula between the distal esophagus and the trachea, which occurs in 86% of newborns with an esophageal defect. Esophageal atresia and tracheoesophageal fistula are thought to be the result of incomplete separation of the lung bed from the foregut during early fetal development. A large percentage of these newborns have other congenital anomalies involving the vertebrae, kidneys, heart, and musculoskeletal and gastrointestinal systems (CDC, 2008b). Most newborns have several anomalies.

Nursing Assessment

Review the maternal history for polyhydramnios. Often this is the first sign of esophageal atresia because the fetus cannot swallow and absorb amniotic fluid in utero, leading to accumulation. Soon after birth, the newborn may exhibit copious, frothy bubbles of mucus in the mouth and nose, accompanied by drooling. Abdominal distention develops as air builds up in the stomach. In esophageal atresia, a gastric tube cannot be inserted beyond a certain point because the esophagus ends in a blind pouch. The newborn may have rattling respirations, excessive salivation and drooling,

and "the three C's" (coughing, choking, and cyanosis) if feeding is attempted. The presence of a fistula increases the risk of respiratory complications such as pneumonitis and atelectasis due to aspiration of food and secretions (Kenner & Lott, 2007).

> ▶ **Take** NOTE!
>
> The "three C's" of choking, coughing, and cyanosis in conjunction with feeding are considered the classic signs of tracheoesophageal fistula and atresia.

Prepare the newborn and parents for radiographic evaluation. Diagnosis is made by x-ray: a gastric tube appears coiled in the upper esophageal pouch, and air in the gastrointestinal tract indicates the presence of a fistula (Kenner & Lott, 2007). Once a diagnosis of esophageal atresia is established, begin preparations for surgery if the newborn is stable.

Nursing Management

Nursing management focuses on preparing the newborn and parents for surgery and providing meticulous postoperative care.

Providing Preoperative Care

Preoperative nursing interventions include the following measures:

- Initiate nothing by mouth (NPO) status.
- Elevate the head of the bed 30 to 45 degrees to prevent reflux and aspiration.
- Monitor hydration status and fluid and electrolyte balance; administer and monitor parenteral IV fluid infusions.
- Assess and maintain the patency of the orogastric tube. Monitor the functioning of the tube, which is attached to low continuous suction. Avoid irrigation of the tube to prevent aspiration.
- Have oxygen and suctioning equipment readily available should the newborn experience respiratory distress.
- Assist with diagnostic studies to rule out other anomalies.
- Use comfort measures to minimize crying and prevent respiratory distress; provide nonnutritive sucking.
- Inform the parents about the rationales for the aspiration prevention measures.
- Document frequent observations of the newborn's condition (Kenner & Lott, 2007).

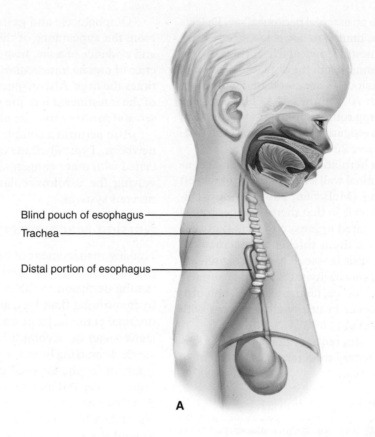

Blind pouch of esophagus —

Trachea —

Distal portion of esophagus —

A

FIGURE 24.13 Esophageal atresia and tracheoesophageal fistula. (**A**) The most common type of esophageal atresia, in which the esophagus ends in a blind pouch and a fistula connects the trachea with the distal portion of the esophagus. (**B**) The upper and distal portions of the esophagus end in a blind pouch. (**C**) The esophagus is one segment, but a portion of it is narrowed. (**D**) The upper portion of the esophagus connects to the trachea via a fistula.

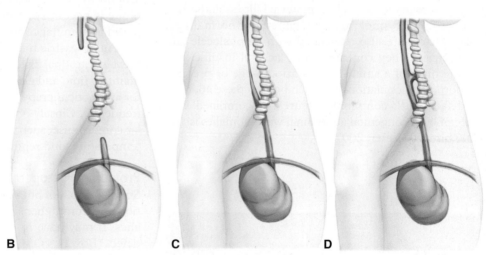

B   **C**   **D**

Providing Postoperative Care

Surgery consists of closing the fistula and joining the two esophageal segments. Postoperative care involves closely observing all of the newborn's body systems to identify any complications. Expect to administer TPN and antibiotics until the esophageal anastomosis is proven intact and patent. Then begin oral feedings, usually within a week after surgery (Blackburn, 2007). Keep the parents informed of their newborn's condition and progress. Closely assess the newborn during feeding and report any difficulty with swallowing. Provide parent teaching. Demonstrate and reinforce all teaching prior to discharge.

▶ OMPHALOCELE AND GASTROSCHISIS

Omphalocele and gastroschisis are congenital anomalies of the anterior abdominal wall. An **omphalocele** is a defect of the umbilical ring that allows evisceration of the abdominal contents into an external peritoneal sac. Defects vary in size; they may be limited to bowel loops or may include the entire gastrointestinal tract and liver (Fig. 24.14). Bowel malrotation is common, but the displaced organs are usually normal. Omphaloceles are associated with other anomalies in more than 70% of the cases. This anomaly is usually detected during routine prenatal ultrasound of the fetus or during investigation of an increased alpha-fetoprotein level (Glasser, 2007).

Gastroschisis is a herniation of the abdominal contents through an abdominal wall defect, usually to the left or right of the umbilicus (McLenan, 2007). Gastroschisis differs from omphalocele in that there is no peritoneal sac protecting the herniated organs, and thus exposure to amniotic fluid makes them thickened, edematous, and inflamed. Gastroschisis is associated with significant newborn mortality and morbidity rates. Despite surgical correction, feeding intolerance, failure to thrive, and prolonged hospital stays occur in nearly all newborns with this anomaly (Henrich et al., 2008).

Each of these diagnoses requires that a pediatric surgeon be available at delivery to determine the extent of the defect and complications.

Nursing Assessment

Review the maternal history for factors associated with high-risk pregnancies, such as maternal illness and infection, drug use, smoking, and genetic abnormalities. These factors are also associated with omphalocele and gastroschisis. They contribute to placental insufficiency and the birth of a small-for-gestational-age or preterm newborn, the populations in which both of these abdominal defects most commonly occur. The combined incidence of both congenital abdominal wall anomalies is 1 in 2,000 births (Glasser, 2007).

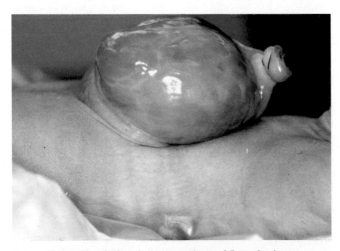

FIGURE 24.14 Omphalocele in a newborn. Note the large, protruding sac.

Omphalocele and gastroschisis are readily observed. Note the appearance of the protrusion on the abdomen and evidence of a sac. Inspect the sac closely for the presence of organs, most commonly the intestines but sometimes the liver. Also inspect the contents for any twisting of the intestines. Note the color of the organs within the sac and measure the size of the omphalocele.

Also perform a complete physical examination of the newborn. Typically these congenital conditions are associated with other congenital anomalies, such as those involving the cardiovascular, genitourinary, and central nervous systems.

Nursing Management

Nursing management of newborns with omphalocele or gastroschisis focuses on preventing hypothermia, maintaining perfusion to the eviscerated abdominal contents by minimizing fluid loss, and protecting the exposed abdominal contents from trauma and infection. These objectives can be accomplished by placing the infant in a sterile drawstring bowel bag that maintains a sterile environment for the exposed contents, allows visualization, reduces heat and moisture loss, and allows heat from radiant warmers to reach the newborn. The newborn is placed feet-first into the bag and the drawstring is secured around the torso (McLenan, 2007). Strict sterile technique is necessary to prevent contamination of the exposed abdominal contents.

An orogastric tube attached to low suction is used to prevent intestinal distention. IV therapy is administered to maintain fluid and electrolyte balance and provide a route for antibiotic therapy. Monitor the newborn's fluid status frequently. Closely observe the exposed bowel for vascular compromise, such as changes in color or a decrease in temperature, and report these immediately.

Providing Postoperative Care

Surgical repair of both defects occurs after initial stabilization and comprehensive evaluation for any other anomalies. It may have to occur in stages, depending on the defect (Box 24.4).

Postoperative care involves providing pain management, monitoring respiratory and cardiac status, monitoring intake and output, assessing for vascular compromise, maintaining the orogastric tube to suction, documenting the amount and color of drainage, and administering ordered medications and treatments (Lund, Bauer, & Berrios, 2007). Also be alert for complications, such as short bowel syndrome.

Promoting Parent–Newborn Interaction

The parents need continued support and progress reports on their newborn. They may be distraught at the sight of the anomaly, and they may be frightened to touch their newborn. Encourage the parents to touch the newborn

> **BOX 24.4** **Surgery to Repair Omphalocele and Gastroschisis**
>
> Surgical repair of gastroschisis is an emergency due to the high risk of intestinal atresia, resulting in obstruction. Primary repair of gastroschisis is usually performed without incident unless the contents are unable to fit into the abdominal cavity. This occurs more often with a large omphalocele, requiring the surgeon to do a staged closure. This involves covering the defect with a synthetic material that is sequentially squeezed like toothpaste to reduce the defect into the abdominal cavity. After enough of the defect is in the abdominal cavity, a surgical repair is then performed (Glasser, 2007). If damage to the exposed organs occurs, such as necrosis, then the necrotic sections are removed during the repair. If a significant amount of small intestine is lost, then the complication of short bowel syndrome may occur.

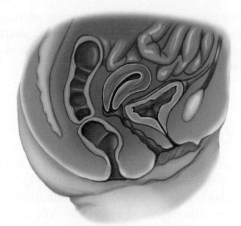

FIGURE 24.15 Imperforate anus, in which the rectum ends in a blind pouch.

and participate in care as much as possible. Because of the nature of this defect, bonding opportunities will be limited initially. However, strongly encourage frequent visiting. In addition, provide information to the parents about the defect, treatment modalities, and prognosis. After surgery, instruct the parents in care measures and give them care instructions. Anticipate the need for a referral to a home health care agency and community resources for support.

▶ IMPERFORATE ANUS

An imperforate anus is a gastrointestinal system malformation of the anorectal area that may occur in several forms. The rectum may end in a blind pouch that does not connect to the colon, or it may have fistulas (openings) between the rectum and the perineum, the vagina in girls or the urethra in boys (Fig. 24.15). The malformations occur during early fetal development and are associated with anomalies in other body systems.

Imperforate anus occurs in about 1 of every 5,000 live births (March of Dimes, 2006). The defect can be further classified as a high or low type, depending on its level. The level significantly influences fecal continence and management (Rosen & Beals, 2007).

Surgical intervention is needed for both high and low types of imperforate anus. Surgery for a high type of defect involves a colostomy in the newborn period, with corrective surgery performed in stages to allow for growth. Surgery for the low type of anomaly, which frequently includes a fistula, involves closure of the fistula, creation of an anal opening, and repositioning of the rectal pouch

into the anal opening. A major challenge for either type of surgical repair is finding, using, or creating adequate nerve and muscle structures around the rectum to provide for normal evacuation.

Nursing Assessment

In the newborn, observe for an appropriate anal opening. If the anal opening exists, observe for passage of meconium stool within the first 24 hours of life. Assess urine output to identify genitourinary problems. For the newborn with an imperforate anus, inspection of the perineal area would reveal absence of the usual opening, and meconium generally is not passed or present within 24 hours of birth.

In the infant with suspected imperforate anus, assess for common signs of intestinal obstruction, which may occur as a result of the malformation. These include abdominal distention and bilious vomiting.

Prepare the newborn and family for radiographic studies that may be ordered to assess for complications associated with imperforate anus.

Nursing Management

Nursing management focuses on preparing the newborn and parents for surgery and providing postoperative care. Preoperatively, maintain the newborn's NPO status and provide gastric decompression. Administer IV therapy and antibiotic therapy as ordered and monitor the newborn's hydration status. Provide a full explanation of the defect, surgical options, potential complications, typical postoperative course, and long-term care needed to the parents. Make sure they are aware of the available treatment modalities. Prepare them for the possibility that the newborn may require an ostomy. Provide support to the parents and family.

Postoperative care includes ensuring adequate pain relief, maintaining NPO status and gastric decompression until normal bowel function is restored, and providing colostomy care if applicable.

HYPOSPADIAS

Hypospadias is an abnormal positioning of the urinary meatus on the underside of the penis (Fig. 24.16A). Hypospadias is a relatively common birth defect that occurs in approximately 1 of every 300 male births in the United States (Gatti et al., 2007)

The malformation is the result of incomplete fusion of the urethral folds, which usually occurs between 9 and 12 weeks of gestation (Schnack et al., 2008). The cause is unknown, but it is thought to be of multifactorial inheritance because it occasionally occurs in more than one male in the same family.

The degree of hypospadias depends on the location of the opening. It is often accompanied by a downward bowing of the penis (chordee), which can lead to urination and erection problems in adulthood.

Hypospadias can be corrected surgically. Depending on the severity, the correction can be completed in one or more procedures with good results. Surgical intervention should be completed during the first year of life to prevent any body image problems in the child.

EPISPADIAS

Epispadias is a rare congenital genitourinary defect occurring in 1 of 117,000 male births and 1 of 484,000 female births (Gilbert, 2007). The condition is usually diagnosed at birth or shortly thereafter. In boys with epispadias, the urethra generally opens on the top or side rather than the tip of the penis. In females, the urinary meatus is located between the clitoris and the labia. This anomaly often occurs in conjunction with exstrophy of the bladder (Perovic & Djinovic, 2008). Surgical correction is necessary, and affected male newborns should not be circumcised (Lowdermilk & Perry, 2007; see Fig. 24.16B).

BLADDER EXSTROPHY

In bladder exstrophy, the bladder protrudes onto the abdominal wall because the abdominal wall failed to close during embryonic development (Fig. 24.17). Wide separation of the rectus muscles and the symphysis pubis accompanies this defect. Virtually all affected male infants have associated epispadias. The upper urinary tract is usually normal. The incidence is approximately 1 in 24,000 to 40,000 live births (March of Dimes, 2008b).

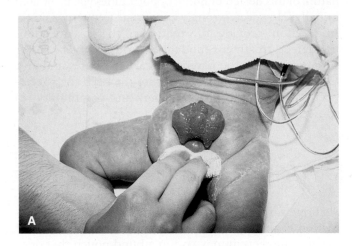

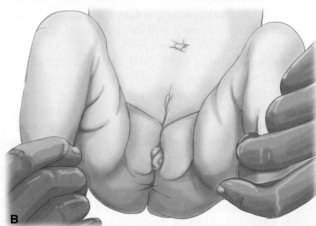

FIGURE 24.17 Bladder exstrophy. (**A**) Before surgical repair. (**B**) After surgery.

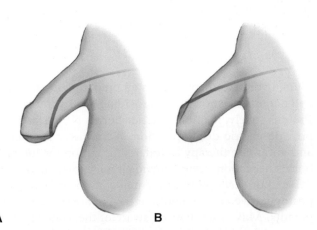

FIGURE 24.16 Genitourinary tract structural anomalies. (**A**) Hypospadias. (**B**). Epispadias.

Goals of therapy include restoring urinary continence, preserving renal function, and reconstructing functional and cosmetically acceptable genitalia. Initial bladder closure is completed within 48 hours after birth. Epispadias repair occurs at this time if possible. Further surgical reconstruction is performed in several stages at about 2 to 3 years of age (see Fig. 24.17B).

Nursing management of the newborn with bladder exstrophy includes the following activities:

- Identify the genitourinary defect at birth so that immediate treatment can be provided.
- Cover the exposed bladder with a sterile clear nonadherent dressing to prevent hypothermia and infection.
- Irrigate the bladder surface with sterile saline after each diaper change to prevent infection.
- Assist with insertion and monitoring of a suprapubic catheter to drain the bladder and prevent obstruction.
- Administer antibiotic therapy as ordered to prevent infection.
- Schedule diagnostic tests to assess for additional anomalies.
- Assess the newborn frequently for any signs of infection.
- Inspect skin surfaces frequently to ensure skin integrity.
- Maintain modified Bryant traction for immobilization after surgery.
- Administer antispasmodics, analgesics, and sedatives as ordered to prevent bladder spasm and provide comfort.
- Educate the parents about the care of the urinary catheter at home if applicable.
- Support the parents throughout.
- Promote bonding by encouraging the parents to visit and touch the newborn.
- Refer the parents to a support group to enhance their coping ability.
- Be a therapeutic listener to the family (Marvin, 2007).

▶ CONGENITAL CLUBFOOT

Clubfoot, or talipes equinovarus, is a congenital deformity that typically has four components: inversion and adduction of the forefoot, inversion of the heel and hindfoot, limitation of extension of the ankle and subtalar joint, and internal rotation of the leg (Fig. 24.18; Patel & Herzenberg, 2007). Reducing or eliminating all of the components of the deformity is the goal to ensure that the newborn has a functional, mobile, painless foot that does not require the use of special or modified shoes (Chesney, Barker, & Maffulli, 2007). The incidence of clubfoot is approximately 1 case per 1,000 live births in the United States. It is bilateral in about half of the cases and affects boys slightly more often than girls (Patel & Herzenberg, 2007).

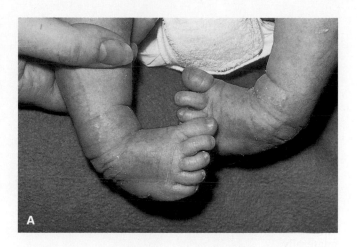

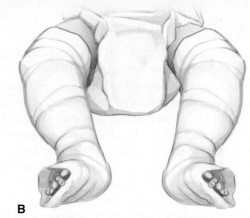

FIGURE 24.18 Clubfoot deformity. (**A**) Initial appearance. (**B**). Application of cast.

Pathophysiology

Clubfoot is a complex, multifactorial deformity with genetic and intrauterine factors. Heredity and race seem to factor into the incidence, but the means of transmission and the etiology are unknown. Most newborns with clubfoot have no identifiable genetic, syndromal, or extrinsic cause.

Clubfoot can be classified into extrinsic (supple) type, which is essentially a severe positional or soft tissue deformity, or intrinsic (rigid) type, where manual reduction is not possible.

Therapeutic Management

The type of clubfoot deformity determines the treatment course. Treatment for the extrinsic (supple) type consists of serial casting, followed by maintenance splinting. Treatment for the intrinsic (rigid) type includes initial casting followed by surgery. It is generally agreed that the initial treatment should be nonsurgical and started soon after birth.

Treatment for either type starts with serial casting, which is needed due to the rapid growth of the newborn. Casts initially are changed weekly and are applied until the deformity responds and is fully corrected. If serial casting is not successful in correcting the deformity, surgical intervention is necessary between 4 and 9 months of age (Gupta et al., 2008).

Nursing Assessment

On examination, the foot appears "down and in." It is smaller, with a flexible, softer heel because of the hypoplastic calcaneus. The heel is internally rotated, making the soles of the feet face each other when the deformity occurs bilaterally.

Nursing Management

Nursing management focuses on education, anticipatory guidance, and pain management. Educate the parents about their newborn's condition and the treatment protocol to reduce their anxiety, and provide reassurance that the clubfoot is not painful and will not hinder the child's development. Discuss challenges associated with sleep, play, and dressing. Inform them that slight modifications will be necessary to accommodate the plaster casts. Review positioning, bathing, and skin care along with pain management when new casts are applied. Stress the need to provide a calm, quiet environment to promote relaxation and sleep for their newborn.

▶ DEVELOPMENTAL DYSPLASIA OF THE HIP

Developmental dysplasia of the hip (DDH) involves abnormal growth or development of the hip that results in instability. This includes hips that are unstable, subluxated, or dislocated (luxated) or have a malformed acetabulum. The instability allows the femoral head to become easily displaced from the acetabulum. The incidence of hip instability is about 10 per 1,000 live births (Larson & Nurmi, 2008). The etiology of DDH is unclear.

Therapeutic Management

Treatment is started as soon as DDH is identified. If the newborn examination reveals DDH, the newborn is referred to an orthopaedist. The goal of treatment is to relocate the femoral head in the acetabulum to facilitate normal growth and development. The Pavlik harness is the most widely used device; it prevents adduction while allowing flexion and abduction to accomplish the treatment goal (Fig. 24.19). The harness is worn continuously

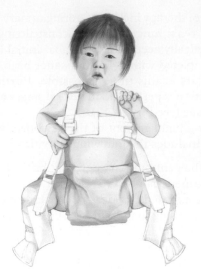

FIGURE 24.19 The Pavlik harness is used to treat developmental dysplasia of the hip.

until the hip is stable, which make take several months. If harnessing is not successful, surgery is necessary.

Nursing Assessment

Asses the history for risk factors, including racial background (Native Americans), genetic transmission (runs in families), intrauterine positioning (breech), sex (female), oligohydramnios, birth order (first-born), and postnatal infant-carrying positions (swaddling, which forces the hips to be adducted).

▶ *Take* NOTE!

DDH is frequently not identified during the newborn examination, so newborns require careful evaluation for hip dysplasia at subsequent visits throughout the first year.

Complete a physical examination. Typically, the newborn with DDH is otherwise healthy, usually without any other deformities. Pay particular attention to assessing hip instability. Perform Ortolani and Barlow manuevers (see Chapter 18 for more information on these maneuvers). Ortolani's maneuver elicits the sensation of the dislocated hip reducing; Barlow's maneuver detects the unstable hip dislocating from the acetabulum. Also observe for other physical signs of DDH, including an asymmetric number of skin folds on the thigh or buttock, an apparent or true short leg, and limited hip abduction (Fig. 24.20; Magee, 2007).

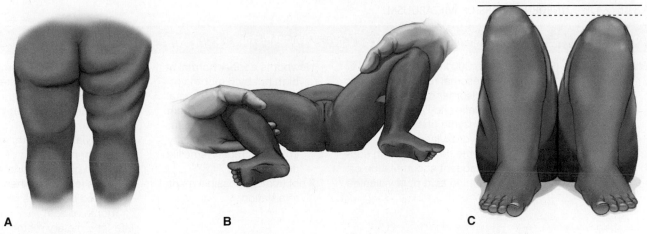

A   **B**   **C**

FIGURE 24.20 Characteristics of developmental dysplasia of the hip. (**A**) Asymmetric number of skin folds on the thigh or buttock. (**B**) Limited hip abduction. (**C**) Unequal knee height.

Nursing Management

Nursing management related to DDH starts with recognition of the disorder and early reporting to the health care provider. Early diagnosis is the crucial aspect; education also is key. Teach the parents how to care for their newborn while in the harness during treatment. Proper fit and adjustments for growth are essential for successful treatment. Frequent clinical assessment on an outpatient basis is needed to monitor progress. Through education, the nurse can be very effective in helping the parents to stay compliant with treatment.

▶ INBORN ERRORS OF METABOLISM

Inborn errors of metabolism are genetic disorders that disrupt normal metabolic function. Most are due to a defect in an enzyme or transport protein, resulting in a blocked metabolic pathway. Clinical symptoms are manifested secondary to toxic accumulations of substances before the block. When viewed individually, inborn errors of metabolism are rare, but collectively they are responsible for significant levels of infant mortality and morbidity. Table 24.6 summarizes four common inborn errors.

A successful outcome depends on early diagnosis and prompt intervention. Most inborn errors present in the newborn period with nonspecific and subtle manifestations—lethargy, hypotonia, respiratory distress, poor feeding and weight gain, vomiting, and seizures (Kwon & Tsal, 2007). Identification of an inborn error of metabolism in a newborn depends largely on the awareness of the nurse and clues from the maternal history, laboratory work, and clinical examination.

▪▪▪ Key Concepts

- Asphyxia, the most common clinical insult in the perinatal period, results in brain injury and may lead to mental retardation, cerebral palsy, or seizures.
- Transient tachypnea of the newborn occurs when the liquid in the lung is removed slowly or incompletely.
- Common risk factors for respiratory distress syndrome (RDS) include young gestational age, perinatal asphyxia regardless of gestational age, cesarean birth in the absence of labor (related to the lack of thoracic squeeze), male gender, and maternal diabetes.
- Meconium aspiration has three major pulmonary effects: airway obstruction, surfactant dysfunction, and chemical pneumonitis.
- The management of persistent pulmonary hypertension of the newborn requires meticulous attention to detail, with continuous monitoring of oxygenation, blood pressure, and perfusion.
- Retinopathy of prematurity (ROP) is a developmental abnormality that affects the immature vasculature of the retina: abnormal growth of blood vessels (neovascularization) takes place within the retina and vitreous.
- Periventricular/intraventricular hemorrhage is bleeding that usually originates in the subependymal germinal matrix region of the brain with extension into the ventricular system.
- Necrotizing enterocolitis (NEC) is a serious gastrointestinal disease of unknown etiology in newborns that can result in necrosis of a segment of the bowel.
- Infants of diabetic mothers are at risk for malformations most frequently involving the cardiovascular, skeletal, central nervous, gastrointestinal, and genitourinary systems; cardiac anomalies are the most common.
- Factors that place the newborn at risk for birth trauma include cephalopelvic disproportion, maternal pelvic anomalies, oligohydramnios, prolonged or rapid labor,

TABLE 24.6 INBORN ERRORS OF METABOLISM

Condition	Incidence and Etiology	Clinical Picture	Management
Phenylketonuria (PKU)	1:15,000 live births Autosomal recessive genetic disorder caused by a deficiency of the hepatic enzyme phenylalanine hydroxylase Enzyme deficiency with subsequent accumulation of amino acid phenylalanine	Newborns appear normal at birth but by 6 months of age signs of slow mental development are evident. Vomiting, poor feedings, failure to thrive, overactivity, irritability, musty-smelling urine If not treated, possible mental retardation	Screening of all newborns at about 48 hours after birth to ensure adequate intake of protein Dietary restriction of phenylalanine, with regular monitoring of serum phenylalanine levels (effective when started before the first month of age) Life-long dietary restriction of phenylalanine
Maple syrup urine disease (MSUR)	1:150,000 in general population; most prevalent among the Mennonite population in Lancaster, Pennsylvania Autosomal recessive inherited disorder Enzyme metabolism of certain amino acids is affected, with the buildup of acids causing ketoacidosis.	Lethargy, poor feeding, vomiting, weight loss, seizures, shrill cry, shallow respirations, loss of reflexes, coma, sweet maple syrup odor to urine	Dialysis to remove accumulated acids Life-long low-protein diet to prevent neurologic deficits of disease
Galactosemia	1:50,000 births Autosomal recessive inherited disorder in which an enzyme needed to convert galactose to glucose is missing and newborn cannot metabolize lactose	Vomiting, hypoglycemia, liver damage, hyperbilirubinemia, poor weight gain, cataracts, frequent infections	Routine newborn screening for galactosemia is performed in the majority of states. Life-long lactose-restricted diet is needed to prevent mental retardation, liver disease, and cataracts.
Congenital hypothyroidism	1:4,000 live births Multiple causes—absent or underdeveloped thyroid gland or biochemical defects in thyroid hormone	Large protruding tongue, slow reflexes, distended abdomen, large, open posterior fontanel, constipation, hypothermia, poor feeding, hoarse cry, dry skin, coarse hair, goiter, and jaundice If untreated, irreversible cognitive and motor impairment occurs. Decreased levels of thyroid hormone (T4) and elevated levels of TSH	Newborn screening program in all states Life-long thyroid replacement hormone therapy and continued monitoring of thyroid levels and clinical response to therapy

Sources: Blackburn, 2007; Fernandes, Walter, Saudubray, & Van Den Berghe, 2006; Wilcken & Wiley, 2008.

abnormal presentation, fetal prematurity, fetal macrosomia, and fetal abnormalities.
■ Women who use drugs during their pregnancy expose their unborn child to the possibility of intrauterine growth restriction, prematurity, neurobehavioral and neurophysiologic dysfunction, birth defects, infections, and long-term developmental sequelae.
■ Newborns of women who use tobacco, illicit substances, caffeine, and alcohol can exhibit withdrawal behavior.

- Physiologic jaundice is a common, normal newborn phenomenon that appears during the second or third day of life and then declines over the first week after birth. Pathologic jaundice is manifested within the first 24 hours of life when total bilirubin levels increase by more than 5 mg/dL/day and the total serum bilirubin level is higher than 17 mg/dL in a full-term infant.

- Newborn infections are usually classified according to the time of onset and grouped into three categories: congenital infection, acquired in utero by vertical transmission with onset before birth; early-onset neonatal infections, acquired by vertical transmission in the perinatal period, either shortly before or during birth; and late-onset neonatal infections, acquired by horizontal transmission in the nursery.

- Congenital conditions can arise from many etiologies, including single-gene disorders, chromosome aberrations, exposure to teratogens, and many sporadic conditions of unknown cause. Congenital structural anomalies may be inherited or sporadic, isolated or multiple, apparent or hidden, and gross or microscopic.

- Congenital heart disease is commonly classified physiologically as defects that result in increased pulmonary blood flow, defects that result in decreased pulmonary blood flow, defects that cause obstruction to blood flow out of the heart, and defects that are mixed.

- A worldwide decline in neural tube defects has occurred over the past few decades due to improved prevention secondary to preconception folic acid supplementation, maternal serum alpha-fetoprotein monitoring, and use of ultrasonography and amniocentesis.

- Congenital respiratory tract structural disorders include choanal atresia and congenital diaphragmatic hernia. Evidence of bowel sounds in the chest suggests congenital diaphragmatic hernia.

- Cleft lip and palate is the most common craniofacial birth defect. The newborn has immediate feeding difficulties and may have problems with dentition, language acquisition, and hearing.

- Esophageal atresia refers to a congenitally interrupted esophagus where the proximal and distal ends do not communicate; the upper esophageal segment ends in a blind pouch and the lower segment ends a variable distance above the diaphragm. Tracheoesophageal fistula is an abnormal communication between the trachea and esophagus.

- Omphalocele and gastroschisis are congenital anomalies of the anterior abdominal wall. An omphalocele is a defect of the umbilical ring that allows evisceration of abdominal contents into an external peritoneal sac. Gastroschisis is a herniation of abdominal contents through an abdominal wall defect, usually to the left or right of the umbilicus.

- Hypospadias and epispadias are genitourinary system structural anomalies. Epispadias often occurs in conjunction with bladder exstrophy, where the bladder protrudes onto the abdominal wall.

- Congenital clubfoot usually involves inversion and adduction of the forefoot, inversion of the heel and hindfoot, limitation of extension of the ankle and subtalar joint, and internal rotation of the leg.

- Developmental dysplasia of the hip includes dislocation, subluxation, or malformation of the acetabulum. Early recognition and prompt treatment are crucial.

- Inborn errors of metabolism are genetic disorders that disrupt normal metabolic function. Most are due to a defect in an enzyme or transport protein, resulting in a blocked metabolic pathway.

REFERENCES

American Academy of Pediatrics (AAP). (2005). AAP policy statement of breastfeeding and the use of human milk. *Pediatrics, 115*(2), 496–506.

American Academy of Pediatrics (AAP), Committee on Substance Abuse. (2005). Tobacco, alcohol, and other drugs: The role of the pediatrician in prevention, identification, and management of substance abuse. *Pediatrics, 115*(3), 816–821.

American Diabetes Association (ADA). (2007a). *Diabetic statistics for women.* Available at: http://www.diabetes.org/diabetes-statistics/women.jsp.

American Diabetes Association (ADA). (2007b). *Gestational diabetes.* Available at: http://www.diabetes.org/gestational-diabetes.jsp.

American Heart Association. (2008a). *Congenital heart defects in children fact sheet.* Available at: http://www.americanheart.org/presenter.jhtml?identifier=12012.

American Heart Association. (2008b). *Diseases, conditions, and treatments.* Available at: http://www.americanheart.org/presenter.jhtml?identifier=3028667.

American Heart Association and American Academy of Pediatrics. (2005). *Summary of major changes in the 2005 AAP/AHA Emergency Cardiovascular Care Guidelines for Neonatal Resuscitation: translating evidence-based guidelines to the NRP.* Available at: http://www.aap.org/nrp/nrpmain.html.

American Lung Association (ALA). (2007). *Respiratory distress syndrome of the newborn fact sheet.* Lung Disease Data and Minority Lung Disease Data. Available at: http://www.lungusa.org/site/pp.asp?c=dvLUK9O0E&b=35693.

Anderson-Berry, A. L., & Bellig, L. L. (2007). Neonatal sepsis. *eMedicine.* Available at: http://www.emedicine.com/ped/topic2630.htm.

Annibale, D. J., & Hill, J. (2007). Periventricular hemorrhage-intraventricular hemorrhage. *eMedicine.* Available at: http://www.emedicine.com/ped/topic2595.htm.

Arenson, J., & Drake, P. (2007). *Maternal and newborn health.* Sudbury, MA: Jones and Bartlett Publishers.

Asenjo, M. (2007). Transient tachypnea of the newborn. *eMedicine.* Available at: http://www.emedicine.com/radio/topic710.htm.

Bader, R., Huhta, J. C., & Hornberger, L. K. (2008). *The perinatal cardiology handbook: Mosby handbook series.* St. Louis: Mosby.

Barker, S. (2007). Subdural and primary subarachnoid hemorrhages: A case study. *Neonatal Network, 26*(3), 143.

Beck, C., Alkasi, Ö., Nikischin, W., Engler, S., Caliebe, A., Leuschner, I., et al. (2008). Congenital diaphragmatic hernia, etiology and management, a 10-year analysis of a single center. *Archives of Gynecology & Obstetrics, 277*(1), 55–63.

Behrman, R. E., Kliegman, R. M., & Jenson, H. B. (2007). *Nelson's textbook of pediatrics* (18th ed.). Philadelphia: Elsevier Health Sciences.

Belik, J., & Hawes, J. (2007). Neonatal abstinence syndrome. *eMedicine.* Available at: http://emedicine.com/ped/topic2760.htm.

Best, R. G. (2007). Anencephaly. *eMedicine.* Available at: http://www.emedicine.com/neuro/topic639.htm.

Blackburn, S. T. (2007). *Maternal, fetal and neonatal physiology: A clinical perspective* (3rd ed.). St. Louis: Saunders Elsevier.

Brodsky, D., & Ouellette, M. A. (2007). *Primary care of the premature infant.* Philadelphia: Elsevier Health Sciences.

Brousseau, T. J., & Sharieff, G. Q. (2007). Neonatal emergencies. *WebMD.* Available at: http://www.medscape.com/viewprogram/7232_pnt.

Burd, L. J. (2007). Interventions in FASD: We must do better. *Child: Care, Health & Development, 33*(4), 398–400.

Centers for Disease Control and Prevention (CDC). (2007a). *Surgeon General's report: Women and smoking fact sheet: tobacco use and reproductive outcomes.* Available at: http://www.cdc.gov/tobacco/sgr/sgr_forwomen/factsheet_outcomes.htm.

Centers for Disease Control and Prevention (CDC). (2007b). *Fetal alcohol syndrome: Guidelines for referral and diagnosis.* National Task Force on FAS/FAE. Atlanta: Centers for Disease Control and Prevention.

Centers for Disease Control and Prevention (CDC). (2008a). *Medical progress in the prevention of neural tube defects.* Available at: http://www.cdc.gov/ncbddd/bd/mp.htm.

Centers for Disease Control and Prevention (CDC). (2008b). *National estimates of racial and ethnic variations among selected birth defects.* Available at: http://www.cdc.gov/ncbddd/bd/keyfindings/race.htm.

Chesney, D., Barker, S., & Maffulli, N. (2007). Subjective and objective outcome in congenital clubfoot; a comparative study of 204 children. *BMC Musculoskeletal Disorders, 8,* 53.

Clark, D., & Mandal, K. (2008). Treatment of retinopathy of prematurity. *Early Human Development, 84*(2), 95–99.

Clark, D. A., & Clark, M. B. (2007). Meconium aspiration syndrome. *eMedicine.* Available at: http://www.emedicine.com/ped/topic 768.htm.

Cunningham, F. G., Leveno, K. J., Bloom, S. L., Gilstrap, L. C., Hauth, J. C., & Wenstrom, K. D. (2005). *Williams' obstetrics* (22nd ed.). New York: McGraw-Hill.

Cutz, E., & Chiasson, D. (2008). Chronic lung disease after premature birth. *New England Journal of Medicine, 358*(7), 743–746.

Datin-Dorriere, V., Rouzies, S., Taupin, P., Walter-Nicolet, E., Benachi, A., Sonigo, P., et al. (2008). Prenatal prognosis in isolated congenital diaphragmatic hernia. *American Journal of Obstetrics & Gynecology, 198*(1), 80.e1–5.

Dave, A. (2005). Absent nasal flaring in a newborn with bilateral choanal atresia. *Pediatrics, 109*(5), 989–990.

DeVries, J. (2007). Focus on the physical. The ABCs of CMV. *Advances in Neonatal Care, 7*(5), 248–257.

Driscoll, W., & Davis, J. (2007). Bronchopulmonary dysplasia. *eMedicine.* Available at: http://www.emedicine.com/ped/topic289.htm.

Ellenbogen, R. G. (2006). Neural tube defects in the neonatal period. *eMedicine.* Available at: http://www.emedicine.com/ped/TOPIC 2805.HTM#section~Epidemiology.

Engelhart, H. H., & Sahraker, K. (2007). Hydrocephalus. *eMedicine.* Available at: http://www.emedicine.com/MED/topic2884.htm.

Fanaroff, A. A., & Lissauer, T. (2008). *Neonatology at a glance.* Somerset, NJ: John Wiley & Sons.

Fernandes, J., Walter, J. H., Saudubray, J. M., & Van Den Berghe, G. (2006). *Inborn metabolic diseases: Diagnosis and treatment* (4th ed.). New York: Springer-Verlag.

Foster, M. R. (2007). Spina bifida. *eMedicine.* Available at: http://www.emedicine.com/orthoped/topic557.htm.

Gatti, J. M., Kirsch, A. J., & Snyder, H. M. (2007). Hypospadias. *eMedicine.* Available at: http://www.emedicine.com/ped/topic 1136.htm.

Gilbert, E. S. (2007). *Manual of high-risk pregnancy and delivery* (4th ed.). St. Louis: Mosby.

Glasser, J. G. (2007). Omphalocele and gastroschisis. *eMedicine.* Available at: http://www.emedicine.com/ped/topic1642.htm.

Goff, M., & O'Connor, M. (2007). Perinatal care of women maintained on methadone. *Journal of Midwifery & Women's Health, 52*(3), 23–26.

Greene, A. (2007). Retinopathy of prematurity. *Medline Plus.* Available at: http://www.nlm.nih.gov/medlineplus/ency/article/001618.htm.

Gupta, A., Patel, P., Patel, J., & Varshney, M. (2008). Evaluation of the utility of the Ponseti method of correction of clubfoot deformity in a developing nation. *International Orthopaedics, 32*(1), 75–79.

Henrich, K., Huemmer, H., Reingruber, B., & Weber, P. (2008). Gastroschisis and omphalocele: Treatments and long-term outcomes. *Pediatric Surgery International, 24*(2), 167–173.

Hermansen, C., & Lorah, K. (2007). Respiratory distress in the newborn. *American Family Physician, 76*(7), 987–994.

Huang, H. R., Tsay, P. K., Chiang, M. C., Lien, R., & Chou, Y. H. (2007). Prognostic factors and clinical features in liveborn neonates with hydrops fetalis. *American Journal of Perinatology, 24*(1), 33–38.

Jallo, G., & Bescke, T. (2007). Neural tube defects. *eMedicine.* Available at: http://www.emedicine.com/neuro/TOPIC244.HTM.

Kenner, C., & Lott, J. W. (2007). *Comprehensive neonatal care: An interdisciplinary approach* (4th ed.). St. Louis: Saunders Elsevier.

Keren, R., & Bhutani, V. K. (2007). Predischarge risk assessment for severe neonatal hyperbilirubinemia. *NeoReviews, 8*(2), 68–75.

Kramer, L. C. (2007). Management of spina bifida, hydrocephalus, and shunts. *eMedicine.* Available at: http://www.emedicine.com/ped/TOPIC2976.HTM.

Kuschel, C. (2007). Managing drug withdrawal in the newborn infant. *Seminars in Fetal & Neonatal Medicine, 12*(2), 127–133.

Kwik, M., Seeho, S. K. M., Smith, C., McElduff, A., & Morris, J. M. (2007). Outcomes of pregnancies affected by impaired glucose tolerance. *Diabetes Research & Clinical Practice, 77*(2), 263–268.

Kwon, K., & Tsai, V. (2007). Metabolic emergencies. *Emergency Medicine Clinics of North America, 25*(4), 1041–1060.

Kyle, T. (2008). *Essentials of pediatric nursing.* Philadelphia: Lippincott Williams & Wilkins.

Laroia, N. (2007). Birth trauma. *eMedicine.* Available at http://www.emedicine.com/ped/topic2836.htm.

Larson, J. P., & Nurmi, D. L. (2008). Congenital hip dysplasia. Available at: http://www.reference.com/search?q=Congenital%20Hip%20Dysplasia.

Lowdermilk, D. L., & Perry, S. E. (2007). *Maternity and women's health care* (9th ed.). St. Louis: Mosby.

Lund, C. H., Bauer, K., & Berrios, M. (2007). Gastroschisis. *Journal of Perinatal & Neonatal Nursing, 21*(1), 63–68.

Magee, D. J. (2007). *Orthopedic physical assessment* (5th ed.). St. Louis: Saunders Elsevier.

Maisels, M. J., & Newman, T. B. (2007). Kernicterus and evidence-based medicine. *Pediatrics, 119*(5), 1038–1039.

Manning, M. A., & Hoyme, E. H. (2007). Fetal alcohol spectrum disorders: A practical clinical approach to diagnosis. *Neuroscience & Behavioral Reviews, 31*(2), 230–238.

Marcellus, L. (2007). Neonatal abstinence syndrome: Reconstructing the evidence. *Neonatal Network, 26*(1), 33–40.

March of Dimes. (2006). *Birth defects.* Available at: http://search.marchofdimes.com/cgi-bin/MsmGo.exe?grab_id=0&page_id=713&query=congenital%20defects&hiword=DEFECT%20DEFECTIVE%20DEFECTOS%20congenital%20defects%20.

March of Dimes. (2007a). *Drinking alcohol during pregnancy.* March of Dimes Fact Sheets. Available at: http://www.marchofdimes.com/professionals/681_1170.asp.

March of Dimes. (2007b). *Illicit drug use during pregnancy.* MOD Quick Reference: Fact Sheets. Available at: http://www.marchofdimes.com/professionals/14332_1169.asp.

March of Dimes. (2007c). *Smoking during pregnancy.* March of Dimes Fact Sheets. Available at: http://www.marchofdimes.com/professionals/14332_1171.asp.

March of Dimes. (2008a). *Cleft lip and cleft palate.* Available at: http://www.marchofdimes.com/pnhec/4439_1210.asp.

March of Dimes. (2008b). Genital and urinary tract defects. Available at: http://www.marchofdimes.com/professionals/14332_1215.asp.

Marvin, T. (2007). Cloacal exstrophy: A case study. *Neonatal Network, 26*(1), 21–30.

Maternal & Neonatal Health (MNH). (2007). *Best practices: Detecting and treating newborn asphyxia.* MNH Program. Available at: http://www.mnh.jhpiego.org/best/detasphyxia.asp.

McLenan, D. (2007). Care of the high-risk neonate. In R. E. Rakel & E. T. Bope (Eds.), *Conn's current therapy 2007* (Section 16, pp. 1200–1210). Philadelphia: Saunders Elsevier.

Mercer, J. S., Erickson-Owens, D. A., Graves, B., & Haley, M. M. (2007). Evidence-based practices for the fetal to newborn transition. *Journal of Midwifery & Women's Health, 52*(3), 262–272.

National Center on Birth Defects and Developmental Disabilities (NCBDDD). (2007). *Fetal alcohol syndrome: Guidelines for referral and diagnosis* (p. 20). Atlanta: Centers for Disease Control and Prevention (CDC), Department of Health and Human Services (DHHS).

National Eye Institute. (2008). *Retinopathy of prematurity.* NEI Health Information. Available at: http://www.nei.nih.gov/health/rop/index.asp.

National Institute on Drug Abuse (NIDA). (2007a). *NIDA InfoFacts: Crack and cocaine.* National Institutes of Health. Available at: http://www.drugabuse.gov/infofacts/cocaine.html.

National Institute on Drug Abuse (NIDA). (2007b). *NIDA Info-Facts: Heroin.* National Institutes of Health. Available at: http://www.nida.nih.gov/Infofacts/heroin.html.

National Institute on Drug Abuse (NIDA). (2007c). *NIDA Research Report: Heroin abuse and addiction.* NIH Publication Number 05–4165. Available at: http://www.drugabuse.gov/ResearchReports/Heroin/heroin4.html.

National Institute on Drug Abuse (NIDA). (2007d). *NIDA InfoFacts: Marijuana.* National Institutes of Health. Available at: http://www.nida.nih.gov/Infofacts/marijuana.html.

National Institute on Drug Abuse (NIDA). (2007e). *NIDA InfoFacts: Methamphetamine.* National Institutes of Health. Available at: http://www.drugabuse.gov/infofacts/methamphetamine.html.

National Institute on Drug Abuse (NIDA). (2007f). *NIDA Info-Facts: Pregnancy and drug use trends.* National Institutes of Health. Available at: http://www.drugabuse.gov/Infofacts/pregnancytrends.html.

Neu, J. (2007). Gastrointestinal development and meeting the nutritional needs of premature infants. *American Journal of Clinical Nutrition, 85*(2), 629S–634S.

Ozen, N., & Mukherjee, S. (2007). Hyperbilirubinemia, unconjugated. *eMedicine.* Available at: http://www.emedicine.com/med/topic1066.htm.

Patel, M., & Herzenberg, J. (2007). Clubfoot. *eMedicine.* Available at: http://www.emedicine.com/orthoped/topic598.htm.

Pelchat, D., Lefebvre, H., Proulx, M., & Reidy, M. (2004). Parental satisfaction with an early family intervention program. *Journal of Perinatal and Neonatal Nursing, 18*(2), 128–144.

Perovic, S., & Djinovic, R. (2008). New insight into surgical anatomy of epispadiac penis and its impact on repair. *Journal of Urology, 179*(2), 689.

Rao, S. C., Ahmed, M., & Hagan, R. (2006). One dose per day compared to multiple doses per day of gentamicin for treatment of suspected or proven sepsis in neonates. *Cochrane Database of Systematic Reviews* 2006. Issue 1. Art. No.: CD005091.DOI: 10.1002/14651858.CD005091.pub2.

Rosen, N. G., & Beals, D. A. (2007). Imperforate anus. *eMedicine.* Available at: http://www.emedicine.com/ped/topic1171.htm.

Rubarth, L. B. (2008). Infant in peril: Assessing sepsis in newborns. *American Nurse Today, 3*(4), 14–16.

Rudolph, A. M. (2007). *Congenital diseases of the heart: Clinical-physiological considerations* (2nd ed.). Somerset, NJ: John Wiley & Sons.

Schnack, T., Zdravkovic, S., Myrup, C., Westergaard, T., Christensen, K., Wohlfahrt, J., et al. (2008). Familial aggregation of hypospadias: A cohort study. *American Journal of Epidemiology, 167*(3), 251–251.

Simpson, K. R. (2007). Kernicterus prevention. *MCN, 32*(2), 132.

Simpson, K. R., & Creehan, P. A. (2008). *Perinatal nursing* (3rd ed.). Philadelphia: Lippincott Williams & Wilkins.

Springer, S. C., & Annibale, D. J. (2007). Kernicterus. *eMedicine.* Available at: http://www.emedicine.com/ped/topic1247.htm.

Srinivasan, P., Brandler, M., & D'Souza, A. (2008). Necrotizing enterocolitis. *Clinics in Perinatology, 35*(1), 251–272.

Steinhorn, R. H. (2007). Pulmonary hypertension, persistent-newborn. *eMedicine.* Available at: http://www.emedicine.com/ped/topic2530.htm.

Stoll, B. J., & Kliegman, P. M. (2007). Neonatal necrotizing enterocolitis (NEC). In R. E. Behrman, R. M. Kliegman, & H. B. Jenson (Eds.), *Nelson textbook of pediatrics* (18th ed.). Philadelphia: W. B. Saunders.

Tewfik, T. L. (2007). Choanal atresia. *eMedicine.* Available at: http://www.emedicine.com/ent/TOPIC330.HTM.

Tolarova, M. M. (2006). Cleft lip and palate. *eMedicine.* Available at: http://www.emedicine.com/ped/topic2679.htm.

U.S. Department of Health and Human Services (USDHHS). (2000). *Healthy people 2010:* Volumes 1 and 2 (conference ed.). Washington, DC: U.S. Government Printing Office.

Vacchha, B., & Adams, R. (2005). Myelomeningocele, temperament patterns, and parental perceptions. *Pediatrics, 115*(1), 58–63.

Vieira, A. (2008). Unraveling human cleft lip and palate research. *Journal of Dental Research, 87*(2), 119–125.

Vision Channel (2007). *Retinopathy of prematurity.* Available at: http://www.visionchannel.net/retinopathy/index.shtml.

Wheeler, D. S., & McCaffrey, M. J. (2007). Resuscitation of the newborn. In R. E. Rakel & E. T. Bope (Eds.), *Conn's current therapy 2007* (Section 16, pp. 1193–1200). Philadelphia: Saunders Elsevier.

Wilcken, B., & Wiley, V. (2008). Newborn screening. *Pathology, 40*(2), 104–115.

Wiedmeier, S. (2008). Center differences in NEC within one healthcare system may depend on feeding protocol. *American Journal of Perinatology, 25*(1), 005–011.

Wiswell, T. E., Tin, W., & Ohler, K. (2007). Evidence-based use of adjunctive therapies to ventilation. *Clinics in Perinatology, 34*(1), 191–204.

Wood, B. P. (2007). Necrotizing enterocolitis. *eMedicine.* Available at: http://www.emedicine.com/radio/topic469.htm.

Woods, D. (2007). *Neonatal resuscitation.* International Association for Maternal and Neonatal Health (IAMANEH). Available at: http://www.gfmer.ch/Medical_education_En/PGC_RH_2004/Neonatal_asphyxia.htm.

Zaichkin, J. (2006). NPR 2006: What you should know. *Neonatal Network, 25*(2), 145–151.

WEBSITES

AHRQ's Tobacco Pathfinder: www.ahrq.gov

American Diabetes Association: www.diabetes.org

Association for the Bladder Exstrophy Community: www.bladderexstrophy.com/support.htm

Birth Defects for Children: www.birthdefects.org

Centers for Disease Control and Prevention: www.cdc.gov

Esophageal Atresia/Tracheoesophageal Fistula Family Support Connection: www.eatef.org

March of Dimes Birth Defects Foundation: www.marchofdimes.com

Narcotics Anonymous: www.na.org

National Center on Birth Defects and Developmental Disabilities: www.cdc.gov/ncbddd/fas

National Clearinghouse for Alcohol and Drug Abuse Information: www.health.org

National Institute on Alcohol Abuse and Alcoholism: www.niaaa.nih.gov

National Organization on Fetal Alcohol Syndrome: www.nofas.org

National Women's Health Information Center: www.4woman.gov

Neonatal Network: www.neonatalnetwork.com

Parental Guide for Developmentally Supportive Care: www.comeunity.com/premature/baby/supportive-care.html

Partnership for a Drug-Free America: www.drugfreeamerica.org

Physical and Developmental Environment of the High-Risk Infant: www.med.usf.edu/~tsinger

Safe Motherhood Initiative: www.safemotherhood.org

SHARE Pregnancy & Infant Loss Support, Inc.: www.nationalshareoffice.com

Substance Abuse & Mental Health Services: www.findtreatment.samhsa.gov

CHAPTER WORKSHEET

MULTIPLE CHOICE QUESTIONS

1. Which finding would lead the nurse to suspect that a newborn is experiencing respiratory distress syndrome?

   a. Abdominal distention

   b. Acrocyanosis

   c. Depressed fontanels

   d. Nasal flaring

2. When assessing the substance-exposed newborn, which finding would the nurse expect?

   a. Calm facial appearance

   b. Daily weight gain

   c. Increasing irritability

   d. Feeding and sleeping well

3. A newborn with tracheoesophageal fistula is likely to present with which assessment finding?

   a. Subnormal temperature

   b. Absent Moro reflex

   c. Inability to swallow

   d. Drooling from mouth

4. The nurse would be most alert for the development of transient tachypnea in a newborn who:

   a. Was born by cesarean birth

   b. Received no sedation

   c. Has a mother with heart disease

   d. Is small for gestational age

5. Which of the following would the nurse include in the teaching plan for an infant with cleft lip and palate?

   a. Feed the infant in a semi-lying position.

   b. Continue feeding the infant for as long as it takes.

   c. Burp the infant frequently during feedings.

   d. Avoid use of high-calorie formulas.

6. Which finding would the nurse expect to assess in an infant with developmental dysplasia of the hip?

   a. Symmetrical thigh folds

   b. Even knee height

   c. Full abduction of the hip

   d. Audible clunk on hip abduction

CRITICAL THINKING EXERCISES

1. As the nursery nurse, you receive a newborn from the labor and birth suite and place him under the radiant warmer. The nurse who gives you report states that the mother couldn't remember when her membranes broke before labor and that she ran a fever during labor for the past few hours. The Apgar scores were good, but the newborn seemed lethargic. As you begin your assessment, you note that he is pale and floppy and has a subnormal temperature; heart rate is 180 bpm and respiratory rate is 70 breaths per minute.

   a. What in the mother's history should raise a red flag to the nurse?

   b. What condition is this newborn at high risk for?

   c. What interventions are appropriate for this condition?

2. Terry, a day-old baby girl, is very fretful, and calming measures don't seem to work. As the nursery nurse you notice that she is losing weight and her formula intake is poor, even though she is manifesting hungry behavior. The mother received no prenatal care and denied drug use, but her drug screen was positive for heroin.

   a. What additional information do you need to obtain from the mother?

   b. What additional laboratory work might be needed for Terry?

   c. What specific measures need to be made for her ongoing care?

3. Baby boy Sims, a term newborn, was brought to the nursery. His mother received no prenatal care, but the newborn's Apgar scores were fine. As you carry out your newborn assessment, you note an imperforate anus and you palpate no testicles in the scrotal sac.

a. What additional assessments should you complete?

b. Are anorectal agenesis and genitourinary tract anomalies common?

c. What diagnostic tests might be ordered? What might be included in the treatment plan for this newborn?

STUDY ACTIVITIES

1. Arrange for a tour of a regional NICU to see the nurse's role in caring for sick neonates. Ask the nurse to give a quick history of each newborn's condition. Was the nurse's role like you imagined? What was your impression of the NICU, and how would you describe it to expectant parents?

2. Select a website from the list at the end of the chapter. What kind of information is given? How helpful would it be for parents with an infant diagnosed with a specific condition?

3. A herniation of a newborn's abdominal contents present at birth describes _____.

Glossary

A

Abdominal effleurage: soft massage of the abdomen

Abortion: removal of products of conception from the uterus before viable fetal life

Abruptio placentae: separation of a normally implanted placenta from the uterine wall before birth

Abstinence: voluntary self-deprivation of potential pleasures (e.g., certain foods, alcohol, or sexual activity)

Acceleration: rise in baseline fetal heart rate for a period of time

Acme: peak intensity of a uterine contraction

Acquired disorder: bodily condition not inherited genetically

Acquired immunodeficiency syndrome (AIDS): serious impairment of cell immunologic functions occurring after a long incubation time, followed by prolonged debilitating body conditions that usually result in death

Acrocyanosis: bluish color of hands or feet caused by poor peripheral circulation

Active acquired immunity: antibody responses to illness or immunization

Active phase: the second phase of labor in which the cervix dilates from 3 or 4 cm to full dilation

Afterpains: abdominal cramp-like pains caused by uterine contractions after birth; they may last for a few days and tend to be more severe during breastfeeding

Alpha-fetoprotein (AFP): glycoprotein produced by the fetal development process that crosses the placenta and can be detected in the maternal blood; can be used as a marker for Down syndrome (decreased AFP) and neural tube defects (increased AFP)

Amnion: the innermost fetal membrane that forms the sac holding the embryo/fetus and amniotic fluid

Amniotic fluid embolism: leakage of amniotic and fetal matter into the maternal circulation; blocks pulmonary circulation and causes a life-threatening situation

Amniotomy: mechanical rupturing of fetal membranes using an instrument

Ampulla: outer area of the fallopian tube where fertilization of the ovum occurs

Androgen: substance that produces testosterone and other male characteristics

Anencephaly: lack of cerebral hemispheres and skull encasing the brain due to a congenital deformation

Anovulatory cycle: menstrual cycle in which an ovum is not released

Anovulatory: absence of ovulation

Anterior fontanel: diamond-shaped area above the newborn's forehead that is formed by two frontal and two parietal bones; it typically closes between 12 and 18 months

Antiretroviral therapy: drug regimen used to destroy or suppress viruses

Apgar score: numerical assessment system for infant heart rate, respiratory effect, muscle tone, reflex irritability, and color; it is taken at 1 and 5 minutes after birth

Apnea: cessation of respirations for 15 to 20 seconds, or long enough to cause cyanosis; it is of unknown cause and occurs 24 to 48 hours after birth; it resolves spontaneously in a few days with no special treatment

Asphyxia: decrease in oxygen and accumulation of carbon dioxide due to gas exchange problems; creates a life-threatening condition

Asymmetric intrauterine growth restriction: higher percentile growth rate of fetal length to head circumference than standardized weight-based rates

Atony: absence of uterine muscle tone

Attachment: affection-forming relationship and feeling of bonding between humans that occurs over time

Augmentation of labor: pharmacologic or physical methods of labor stimulation and uterine contractions after natural labor has begun

Autosome: chromosome included in the 22 pairs that is identical in males and females

B

Babinski reflex: a normal infant response characterized by hyperextension of the toes and dorsiflexion of the great toe upon stroking of the sole of the foot

Bacterial vaginosis: a vaginal bacteria infection characterized by a grayish discharge and a foul fishy odor

Ballottement: examination technique involving finger tapping to detect a floating fetus during pregnancy; the fetus is pushed away and rebounds against the examiner's fingers

Baseline fetal heart rate: average fetal heart rate between contractions and accelerations of labor

Beat-to-beat variability: variations in fetal heart rate between one beat and the next over a short interval

Bilirubin: a yellow bile pigment associated with jaundice that is produced during the destruction of red blood cells

Biophysical profile (BPP): noninvasive fetal risk assessment based on breathing, body movement, volume of amniotic fluid, fetal heart rate, and tone

Birth rate: calculation of annual rate of births per 1,000 people

Blastocyst: inner cell mass of the morula occurring approximately 3 days after fertilization; it develops into the embryo

Bloody show: secretion of blood-tinged vaginal discharge resulting from rupture of small capillaries in the cervix as it begins to dilate about 24 to 48 hours before labor

Boggy: adjective used to describe softening of the uterus that occurs due to a lack of muscle tissue contraction; carries a risk for postpartum hemorrhage

Brachial palsy: partial or complete paralysis of arm parts resulting from prolonged labor or difficult birth

Braxton Hicks contractions: intermittent, painless uterine contractions occurring during pregnancy without cervical dilation; they are not associated with true labor but are sometimes mistaken as such and referred to as "false labor"

Breast self-examination (BSE): touching and visual inspection of the breasts to detect abnormalities such as masses, nipple discharge, or changes that could indicate malignancy or conditions needing assessment

Breech presentation: the fetal buttocks or feet appear in the maternal pelvis first instead of the head

Bronchopulmonary dysplasia (BPD): chronic pulmonary disease that occurs from the use of mechanical ventilation and high levels of oxygen in the weeks after birth

Brown adipose tissue: fetal and neonate fat deposits around the kidneys and adrenals, in the neck, between the scapulae, and behind the sternum

C

Caput succedaneum: soft tissue swelling or edema in or under the fetal scalp due to birth trauma

Carcinoma in situ: cancer contained only in the cells of an organ in which it originated without spreading to other tissue

Cardinal movements of labor: natural fetal position changes and movements that are accommodated by the maternal pelvis as the fetus moves from the abdominal region through the birth canal to delivery

Cephalhematoma: subperiosteal collection of blood in the infant's skull due to blood vessel rupture during labor and birth; lasts for a few weeks to 2 months

Cephalofetal disproportion: abnormal condition of fetal head size, shape, or position preventing descent through the maternal pelvis for delivery

Cerclage: suturing used to close a recurrent premature dilation of the cervix, which usually occurs between 14 and 20 weeks of gestation

Cervical cap: cup-shaped mechanical barrier contraceptive that is held in place over the cervix by suction

Cervical dilation: gradual widening of the cervical opening from less than 1 cm to nearly 10 cm to accommodate passage of the fetal head

Cervical funneling: recess in the cervix that is commonly associated with recurrent premature dilation of the cervix

Cervical ripening: softening and thinning of the cervix through the normal physiologic labor process or through induction of labor

Cesarean section: fetal delivery through a surgical incision in the abdominal wall and uterus

Chadwick's sign: violet or blue discoloration in the vaginal mucous membranes visible during pregnancy around the fourth week; due to vaso-congestion

Childbirth education: prenatal courses that focus on breathing, relaxation, and position techniques during labor; the goal is to minimize the need for medication and medical procedures

***Chlamydia* infection:** the most common sexually transmitted bacterial infection in the United States; caused by *Chlamydia trachomatis;* a frequent cause of sterility

Chloasma: a brown or darker pigmentation of the nose, forehead, and cheeks during pregnancy or from ingesting oral contraceptives; referred to as a "mask of pregnancy"

Chorioamnionitis: infection of the chorion, amnion, and amniotic fluid caused by organisms that can be transferred to the fetus; potentially life-threatening to the infant

Chorion: outer fetal membrane closest to the uterine wall that is lined by the trophoblast and mesoderm surrounding the amnion; forms the fetal area of the placenta

Chorionic villi: hair-like projections that carry vascular circulation to the fetus

Chorionic villus sampling: procedure to obtain fetal cells during the first trimester in order to diagnose chromosomal and congenital disorders

Chromosome: hair-like chromatin structures of the cell nucleus that contain genetic information as codes in DNA

Chronic hypertension: maternal hypertension occurring prior to week 20 of gestation, or hypertension that continues 42 days past childbirth

Circumcision: surgical removal of foreskin from the penis

Circumoral cyanosis: bluish coloration around the mouth

Clitoris: small oval-shaped area comprising erectile tissue at the anterior junction of the female vulva; homologous to the penis

Coitus interruptus: contraceptive technique in which the man withdraws his penis from the woman's vagina prior to ejaculation

Cold stress: excessive loss of body heat resulting in a compensatory mechanism such as increased respirations to maintain the core body temperature

Colostrum: yellowish breast secretion of serum and white blood cells that precedes mature breast milk; has a high level of protein and some immune and cleansing properties for the newborn's intestinal tract

Colposcopy: procedure in which a magnifying lens is inserted into the vagina for cervical and vaginal tissue examination

Conception: process in which the ovum is fertilized by union with sperm

Condom: mechanical contraceptive device that blocks sperm from entering the vagina; it is worn over the erect penis or in the female vagina; also helps prevent sexually transmitted infections

Conduction: heat transfer to a cooler area or surface through direct skin contact

Contraction stress test: method used to assess fetal reaction to natural or induced contractions

Contraction: regular or periodic tightening and shortening of the uterine muscles during natural or artificially induced labor, causing effacement and dilation of the cervix

Convection: heat transfer to cooler air from a warm body surface

Coombs test: test to check for either Rh-positive antibodies in maternal red blood cells or Rh-positive antibodies in fetal cord red blood cells

Corpus luteum: small yellow glandular mass that develops within a ruptured ovarian follicle after it has matured and discharged its ovum

Corpus: the upper two thirds of the uterus

Cotyledons: subdivisions composed of villi that are located along the uterine surface of the placenta

Crowning: appearance of the fetal head at the vulvar opening during labor

Cyanosis: blue coloration of the infant's chest, face, fingers, toes, or mucous membranes as a result of the circulatory system's inability to oxygenate the tissues fully

Cystocele: a bulge in the anterior vaginal wall as a result of downward displacement of the bladder

D

Deceleration: periodic slowing of the fetal heart rate below baseline

Decidua: nourishing cell membrane surrounding the fetus in the uterus that is shed after childbirth

Depo-Provera: progestin contraceptive that can be injected for long-term use

Descent: start of the downward movement of the fetal presenting position into the pelvis

Dilatation and curettage (D&C): dilation of the cervix and passage of a curet to scrape the endometrium; performed to eliminate the uterine contents and end pregnancy, or to obtain tissue for examination

Dilation: gradual expansion of the external os of the cervix from a few millimeters to 10 cm so that the fetus can be born

Disseminated intravascular coagulation (DIC): complex hemorrhagic disorder resulting in tissue necrosis and bleeding; possibly caused by sepsis, fetal demise, or abruptio placentae

Dizygotic: fetuses derived from two separate zygotes; referred to as fraternal twins

Doula: a companion, possibly paid, who attends to the needs of a pregnant woman through labor

Down syndrome: a genetic birth defect resulting from an extra chromosome (number 21)

Ductus arteriosus: a shunt between the pulmonary artery and the descending aorta of the fetus

Ductus venosus: a fetal shunt passing through the liver and carrying oxygenated blood between the umbilical vein and the inferior vena cava

Duration: the length of time a contraction lasts

Dysfunctional labor pattern: labor that does not exhibit normal processes

Dysfunctional uterine bleeding (DUB): any deviation from usual uterine bleeding

Dysmenorrhea: painful side effects of menstruation, including cramping in the lower abdomen, nausea, vomiting, diarrhea, and headache

Dyspareunia: pain associated with sexual intercourse

Dystocia: failed or difficult progression of labor due to physical problems between the fetus and the maternal pelvis, or from uterine or other muscular problems

E

Early-onset deceleration: fetal heart rate slowing in which the head compresses at the onset of a uterine contraction; as the contraction ends, the fetal heart rate slowly returns to baseline

Eclampsia: a major seizure complication of unknown causes that sometimes occurs after 20 weeks of gestation or within 48 hours postpartum

Ectopic pregnancy: implantation of a fertilized ovum in the fallopian tubes, ovaries, or abdomen instead of the usual location (the lining of the uterus)

EDB: estimated date of birth

EDC: estimated date of confinement or fetal due date

Effacement: process of thinning, shortening, and flattening of the cervix that occurs late in pregnancy or during labor

Ejaculation: release of seminal fluids due to stimulation of the penis

Electronic fetal monitoring: monitoring device placed on the fetus for continuous tracking and assessment of fetal heart rate characteristics

Embryo: name for the developing organism between 2 and 8 weeks of gestation

Emergency contraception: postcoital pregnancy-prevention methods

Endometrial biopsy: procedure used during a fertility workup to obtain information about the effects on the uterus of progesterone produced by the corpus luteum after ovulation and endometrial receptivity

Endometriosis: chronic condition in which endometrial tissue grows outside the uterus in the pelvic cavity; often associated with infertility

Endometritis: infection of the inner uterus lining

Endometrium: inner cellular lining of the uterus that is shed during menses

En-face positioning: parent and newborn maintain the same face-to-face vertical plane of vision

Engorgement: swelling of breast tissue from congestion due to increased blood supply and lymph supply after childbirth and before true lactation starts

Engrossment: parental (particularly paternal) sense of intense interest during early contact with the newborn

Epidural: technique used to provide local anesthesia to the lower body in which the anesthetic is instilled into the epidural space and transfers to the nerve roots exiting the dura

Episiotomy: surgical incision of the perineum to enlarge the vaginal opening to facilitate birth

Epispadias: condition in which the urethral meatus is located on the top surface of the penis

Erythema toxicum: temporary, pink, irregular, papular rash with superimposed vesicles

Erythroblastosis fetalis: hemolytic disease of the newborn caused by maternal antibodies; results in anemia, jaundice, enlarged liver and spleen, and generalized edema

Esophageal atresia: condition in which the esophagus ends in a pouch or narrows to a thin cord unconnected to the stomach

Estrogen: female sex hormone that is produced by the ovary and stored in fat cells; it influences reproduction

Evaporation: loss of heat resulting from water on the skin surface being converted to vapor

Evidence-based practice: medical decisions that are made based on conscientious problem-solving approaches from explicit, judicious use of research data, statistical analysis, and other reliable information sources

Exchange transfusion: replacement of circulating blood by withdrawal of the recipient's blood and injection of an equal amount of donor blood; done to prevent accumulation of bilirubin or other byproducts of hemolysis in the blood

External os: portion of the cervix opening into the vagina

Extremely low birthweight: neonate birth weight of 1,000 g or less

F

Face presentation: descent of fetus with hyperextension of head and neck, allowing the fetal face to descend into the maternal pelvis first

False labor: regular or irregular uterine contractions that are strong enough to be interpreted as real labor; however, they do not dilate the cervix

Female condom: thin, flexible, polyurethane contraceptive sheath placed inside the vagina to block sperm from entering the cervix

Fern test: procedure to determine the presence of amniotic fluid

Fertility awareness methods: natural family planning based on tracking the woman's ovulatory cycle; requires careful record keeping and sexual abstinence during the fertile part of the month

Fertility rate: number of annual births per 1,000 in women aged 15 to 44

Fertilization: the uniting of sperm with the outer layer of the female ovum that begins the development of a human embryo

Fetal acoustic stimulation test: process used to accelerate the fetal heart rate through use of a speaker, bell, or artificial larynx

Fetal alcohol syndrome (FAS): various fetal physical deformities and cognitive disabilities resulting from excessive alcohol consumption by the mother during pregnancy

Fetal attitude: relationship of fetal body parts to one another, characterized by normal flexion of the arms onto the chest and the legs onto the abdomen

Fetal circulation: path of fetal blood circulation

Fetal distress: problem involving the fetal heart rate or activity in response to the intrauterine environment

Fetal fibronectin testing: screening process used to predict preterm labor

Fetal heart rate (FHR): number of fetal heartbeats per minute; normal range is 110 to 160

Fetal lie: relationship of the fetal spine to the maternal spine; designated as longitudinal or transverse

Fetal movement counting: daily maternal record of fetal movements and activity within a set time period

Fetal position: presenting fetal part in relation to the left, right, front, or back of the maternal pelvis

Fetal presentation: fetal part that first enters the maternal pelvis; known as a cephalic, shoulder, or breech presentation

Fetus: unborn child from about 8 weeks of gestation until birth

Fibroadenoma: painless breast tumor or solid mass

Fibrocystic changes: age-related hormonal changes that commonly include breast tissue thickening and cyst formation

Fibroid tumor: benign tumor growing within the myometrium that can protrude into the uterine cavity and bulge through the outer uterine layer

First stage of labor: period that begins with regular uterine contractions and ends with complete dilation and effacement of the cervix; divided into latent, active, and transition phases

Flexion: position in which the fetal head is bent with chin on chest when resistance is met at the pelvic inlet and floor

Follicle-stimulating hormone: hormone produced by the anterior pituitary during the first half of the menstrual cycle; stimulates the ovary to prepare a mature ovum for release

Follicular phase: ovarian cycle phase that occurs when a follicle becomes mature and is prepared for ovulation

Fontanel: fetal membrane-filled area of strong, soft, connective tissue between the cranial bones of the skull that allows molding of the head during birth

Foramen ovale: opening between the right and left atria of the fetal heart

Forceps: obstetric instruments sometimes used on the presenting part of the fetus to aid in childbirth

Forth stage of labor: period that occurs during the first 2 to 4 hours after delivery of the placenta

Frequency: time from the beginning of one contraction to the beginning of the next

Fundus: upper section of the uterus between the fallopian tubes

G

Gavage feeding: nourishment supplied through a tube inserted into the nose or mouth and emptying into the stomach

Genetic counseling: information discussed with clients and families concerning genes and heredity

Genetic disorder: inherited gene defect passed from one generation to its offspring

Gestational diabetes: diabetes occurring with the onset of pregnancy or first diagnosed during pregnancy

Gestational trophoblastic disease: a malignant or benign (hydatidiform mole) disorder

Gonadotropin-releasing hormone (GnRH): neurohormone secreted by the hypothalamus that stimulates the pituitary to release prolactin and other hormones

Goodell's sign: softening of the cervix during the second month of pregnancy that usually indicates pregnancy

Graafian follicle: fully ripe ovum that secretes estrogen

Gravida: any pregnancy, regardless of outcome

Gravidity: state of pregnancy and number of times pregnant

Gynecoid pelvis: characteristic female pelvis with oval inlet slightly wider than it is high

H

Hegar's sign: softening and widening of the isthmus of the uterus; usually occurs in the second or third month of pregnancy and is detectable by palpitation

HELLP syndrome: changes associated with severe preeclampsia, including elevated liver enzyme levels, hemolysis, and a low platelet count

Hemolytic disease of the newborn: condition in which maternal antibodies cross the placenta and destroy fetal red blood cells due to isoimmunization; examples are ABO and Rh incompatibility, or inadequate vitamin K, leading to a lack of clotting factors and risk of hemorrhage

Hormone replacement therapy (HRT): supplemental use of hormones such as estrogen and progestin to ease menopausal symptoms

Human chorionic gonadotropin (hCG): hormone produced by the chorionic villi and secreted by the corpus luteum of the ovary after conception; detectable in the urine of pregnant women

Human immunodeficiency syndrome (HIV): a retrovirus that causes severe inability of the body to fight infection; leads to AIDS

Human placental lactogen: hormone produced by the syncytiotrophoblast cell around 3 weeks of ovulation; promotes lipolysis to increase free fatty acids during maternal metabolism; detectable in maternal serum around the first month after fertilization

Hydramnios: excess of amniotic fluid often found in pregnant diabetics; may occur even without fetal problems

Hydrocele: accumulated serous fluid in the scrotum

Hydrocephalus: excessive cerebrospinal fluid circulating in the cerebral ventricles, resulting in enlarged fetal head size

Hyperbilirubinemia: abnormally high level of bilirubin in the blood

Hyperemesis gravidarum: severe and excessive vomiting during pregnancy that may begin in the first trimester of pregnancy; can lead to dehydration and starvation

Hyperglycemia: abnormally high blood glucose level

Hypertonic contractions: uterine resting contractions of elevated strength or intensity, or occurring more than five times within 10 minutes

Hypertonic labor: condition characterized by a poor resting rate of contractions and contractions occurring too frequently during labor

Hypocalcemia: abnormally low calcium level in the blood

Hypoglycemia: abnormally low blood glucose level

Hypospadias: congenital abnormality of the penis in which the urethral meatus is on the ventral area or the shaft rather than at the end

Hypothermia: human body temperature of 97°F (37 °C) or less

Hypotonic labor: uterine contractions of insufficient intensity, frequency, or duration during labor

I

Implantation: embedding of the blastocyst into the endometrium, usually 7 to 9 days after fertilization

Infant mortality rate: annual number of infant deaths under age 1 per 1,000 live births of an identified population

Infant of a diabetic mother: at-risk infant born to a diabetic mother

Infertility: inability to conceive or produce viable offspring after regular unprotected intercourse for at least 1 year

Intensity: strength of a uterine contraction at its peak

Internal os: area of the cervix opening into the uterus that divides the cervical canal from the uterine cavity

Intrapartum: time beginning at true labor and lasting birth, until expulsion of the placenta

Intrauterine growth restriction (IUGR): fetal growth below the 10th percentile in terms of weight, length, or head circumference based on standardized gestational rates; may be due to many causes, including deficient nutrient supply, congenital malformation, or intrauterine infection

Intrauterine pressure catheter: tube placed through the cervix to monitor uterine pressure during contractions or to add warm saline to the intrauterine fluid if indicated

Intraventricular hemorrhage: bleeding into cerebral ventricles; common in preterm infants

Inversion of the uterus: condition in which the uterus turns inside out, resulting in serious hemorrhage and shock

Involution: return of the uterus to prepregnancy size and function after childbirth

J

Jaundice: yellow color of a newborn's skin, mucous membranes, and sclera caused by accumulated bilirubin

K

Kangaroo care: skin-to-skin contact between the parent and the newborn

Karyotype: set of an individual's chromosomes arranged in numeric order to assess genetic alterations

Kegel exercises: internal exercises that tighten and strengthen the perineal floor muscles

Kernicterus: a condition resulting from the deposit of excessive unconjugated bilirubin in the brain tissue; may result in impaired neurologic function or death

L

LaLeche League: an international organization that promotes breastfeeding through education and support to breastfeeding mothers

Labor induction: stimulating uterine contractions by physically rupturing the membranes or using medications

Labor: involuntary uterine contractions in which the fetus and placenta are expelled from the uterus to the external world

Laceration: a tear in the perineum or birth canal that occurs during childbirth

Lamaze childbirth: a psychoprophylactic method of childbirth

Lanugo: fine, downy hair on the fetus that develops after the fourth month of gestation

Large for gestational age (LGA): an infant whose birthweight exceeds the 90th percentile for gestational age on a growth chart; typically the weight exceeds 9 lb

Latching-on: proper position for the infant to attach to the breast during breastfeeding

Late-onset deceleration: slowing of the fetal heart rate that begins at the peak of a contraction and returns to baseline at the end of the contraction; caused by uteroplacental insufficiency and potentially inadequate oxygenation of the fetus

Latent phase: labor phase that begins with the onset of true labor and ends with cervical dilatation of 3 cm

Lecithin-sphingomyelin (L/S) ratio: amniotic fluid ratio of lecithin to sphingomyelin that changes during gestation; used to assess fetal lung maturity; an L/S ratio of 2:1 or greater indicates mature lungs and a low risk of respiratory distress syndrome if born at that time

Leopold's maneuvers: series of abdominal palpitation methods to determine presentation, position, lie, and engagement of the fetus

Let-down reflex: breast milk ejection reflex caused by emotional response to the infant or from stimulation of the breast nipple

Letting-go phase: adjustment to the maternal role

Lightening: downward movement of the fetus and uterus into the pelvic cavity

Linea nigra: a dark line of pigment sometimes appearing along the symphysis pubis during later months of pregnancy

LNMP: last normal menstrual period

Lochia alba: creamy white vaginal discharge that occurs after lochia serosa starting from 10 days postpartum to about 21 days postpartum

Lochia rubra: blood-tinged vaginal discharge that occurs for 2 to 4 days postpartum

Lochia serosa: pink, serous, vaginal discharge following lochia rubra that occurs from about 3 days postpartum to about 10 days postpartum

Lochia: normal vaginal discharge of uterine blood, mucus, and tissue after childbirth

Long-term variability: large rhythmic wave variations of the fetal heart rate occurring 2 to 6 times per minute as tracked with a monitor

Low birthweight (LBW): neonate birthweight of 2,500 g or less

Low-lying placenta: condition of an undetermined location of the placenta in relation to the cervical os, or apparent placenta previa occurring prior to the third trimester

Luteal phase: part of the ovarian cycle

Luteinizing hormone (LH): hormone secreted from the anterior pituitary to stimulate ovulation

M

Macrosomia: large newborn weighing more than 4 kg (8 lb 13 oz), or a newborn falling above the 90th percentile for gestational age and birthweight

Malposition: fetal position other than occiput anterior

Malpresentation: abnormal presenting part of the fetus into the birth canal; presentation other than the normal completely flexed head

Mastitis: breast inflammation caused by infection, usually in the milk duct

Maternal mortality rate: number of maternal deaths from any reproductive cause per 100,000 live births

Maternal role attainment: process of learning and applying maternal behaviors to gain a comfortable identity as a mother

Maternal serum alpha-fetoprotein: test of maternal blood at 16 to 22 weeks' gestation for the presence of alpha-fetoprotein to screen for neural tube disorders and genetic trisomies

Meconium aspiration syndrome: newborn respiratory distress caused when the fetus breathes meconium in the amniotic fluid into the lungs or trachea

Meconium: fecal matter present in the large intestine and passed as first the stools of newborn

Menarche: initiation of menstruation

Menopause: permanent cessation of menses for 12 consecutive months

Menorrhagia: profuse or excessive menstrual flow

Menses: vaginal bleeding that occurs approximately every 28 days in nonpregnant females in which the uterine lining is discharged

Metrorrhagia: menstrual periods that occur at irregular intervals

Milia: small, white papules appearing on the newborn's face and upper torso; caused by unopened or plugged sebaceous glands; normally disappear without treatment in a few weeks

Mittelschmerz: abdominal pain at the time of ovulation

Molding: overlapping capability of the fetal cranial bones to allow shape and size changes of the head so that it can pass through the maternal pelvis during labor

Mongolian spots: irregular dark coloration of no medical significance appearing on the lower back or buttocks of the newborn; may last until age 2

Monozygotic: originating from one zygote; identical twins

Morbidity rate: ratio of the number of cases of a given illness, disease, abnormal human quality, or condition to a given population

Mortality rate: ratio of the number of deaths from various causes to a given population

Morula: solid cell mass formed by the fertilized ovum in very early development

Mottling: temporary skin discoloration on irregular areas of the infant's body that appears as a blue or red blood vessel framework; found in combination with chills, hypoxia, or poor perfusion

Multipara: a woman having two or more pregnancies with viable fetuses of 20 weeks' gestation or more in each pregnancy

Multiple gestation: having more than one fetus in the uterus during the same pregnancy

Mutation: sudden genetic change that occurs in an individual and continues to occur in the offspring

N

Nagele's rule: a method for estimating the delivery date by determining the first day of the last menstrual period, subtracting 3 months, and adding 7 days

Necrotizing enterocolitis (NEC): acquired acute gastrointestinal disease that can be life-threatening to a newborn

Neonatal abstinence syndrome: newborn withdrawal symptoms resulting from the use of narcotics by the mother during fetal development; symptoms may include vomiting, irritability, sneezing, diarrhea, and seizures

Neonatal death: infant death at any gestational age within the first 28 days of life

Neonate: infant in the first 28 days of life

Neutral thermal environment: external conditions that sustain normal internal body temperature with minimal oxygen consumption and metabolism

Nitrazine test: indicates the presence of amniotic fluid based on alkaline content

Nonstress test: assessment of fetal heart rate in response to natural or stimulated fetal movement

O

Obstetrical conjugate: anteroposterior diameter of the pelvic inlet

Oligohydramnios: less-than-normal amount of amniotic fluid in the third trimester; may indicate a fetal urinary tract problem

Ophthalmia neonatorum: newborn eye infection usually caused by gonococci

Orgasmic phase: phase of the human sexual arousal and response process experienced as a release of intense sexual tension

Ortolani maneuver: manual procedure used to diagnose developmental dysplasia of the hip

Osteoporosis: progressively decreased bone mass that results in weak and brittle bones; common in postmenopausal women; associated with lower estrogen and androgen levels

Ovulation: normal release of a mature, unfertilized ovum by the ovary approximately 14 days before the beginning of the menstrual period

Oxytocin: hormone produced by the posterior pituitary that stimulates uterine contractions and the release of milk into the lactiferous ducts

P

Papanicolaou (Pap) smear: procedure to detect cervical cancer

Para: number of live births or stillbirths that reach viability

Parity: number of past pregnancies that have reached viability

Partial previa: category of placenta previa in which the cervical os is not completely covered by the placenta

Patent ductus arteriosus (PDA): newborn condition in which the ductus arteriosus does not close spontaneously after the first 24 hours of life

Pathologic jaundice: newborn condition characterized by an excessive breakdown of red blood cells, resulting from hematologic incompatibility

Pelvic inflammatory disease (PID): infection of the fallopian tubes, uterus, or ovaries due to vaginal bacteria; may cause pelvic abscess

Pelvic inlet: upper border of the true pelvis and entrance to the first of three pelvic planes through which the fetal head passes during delivery

Pelvic outlet: lower border of the true pelvis and opening of the third pelvic plane through which the fetal head passes during delivery

Pelvic relaxation: decline of muscle support in the pelvic region

Percutaneous umbilical blood sampling (PUB): an evaluation technique involving the direct aspiration of fetal blood from the umbilical cord in the uterus by a needle inserted through the mother's abdominal wall

Perimenopause: phase prior to menopause during which menstrual periods begin to cease

Perineum: area between the vagina and anus in women, or between the scrotum and anus in men

Phototherapy: treatment of newborn jaundice by exposure to a special ultraviolet light

Physiologic anemia of pregnancy: increased plasma volume disproportionate to red blood cells during pregnancy; results in subnormal hemoglobin and hematocrit levels

Physiologic jaundice: harmless normal breakdown and reduction of red blood cells occurring between 2 to 3 days after birth and resolving in 7 to 10 days

Pica: ingestion during pregnancy of non-food substances, such as clay, laundry starch, or ice

Placenta previa: abnormal implantation of the placenta in the lower uterus near or covering the cervical os

Plethora: red color of skin associated with hyperoxia, overheating, or polycythemia

Polycystic ovary syndrome: endocrine disorder of the ovary characterized by the failure to release an ovum for extended periods; due to excess androgens in the blood and cysts in the ovaries

Polycythemia: excessive red blood cells in the circulation

Polydactyly: development of extra digits on hands or feet

Postpartal hemorrhage: loss of more than 500 mL of blood from the birth canal within the first 24 hours of delivery ("early") or after the first 24 hours ("late")

Postpartum blues: maternal feelings of being "out of sorts" during first few days after giving birth

Postpartum depression: maternal feelings of severe depression during the first year after giving birth, with increased occurrence prior to resumed menses

Postpartum psychosis: severe maternal psychiatric condition occurring within first few months after childbirth

Postterm infant: any newborn assessed to be of more than 42 weeks' gestation

Postterm pregnancy: pregnancy that continues beyond 42 weeks of gestation

Precipitous birth: rapid labor and birth process, usually less than 3 hours in duration

Preconception care: medical information and counseling provided to a woman before she becomes pregnant; can promote optimal outcomes for the mother and infant

Pre-eclampsia: syndrome of pregnancy characterized by proteinuria, hypertension, and edema

Premature rupture of membranes (PROM): spontaneous or artificial tearing of the amniotic membranes prior to labor

Prematurity: childbirth prior to the end of 37 weeks' gestation

Premenstrual syndrome (PMS): emotional, behavioral, or physical symptoms that some women experience during the luteal phase of the menstrual cycle

Presenting part: fetal part closest to the internal os of the cervix

Preterm birth: childbirth before 37 weeks of gestation

Preterm infant: birth of an infant determined to be less than 37 weeks' gestational age

Preterm labor: any true labor occurring during 20 and 38 completed weeks of gestation

Preterm premature rupture of membranes (PPROM): spontaneous or artificial tearing of the amniotic membranes prior to labor, occurring before 37 completed weeks of gestation

Primigravida: woman in her first pregnancy

Primipara: woman in her first pregnancy who has given birth to a newborn of viability

Progesterone: hormone produced by the corpus luteum of the ovary and the adrenal cortex to prepare the uterus for implantation of the fertilized ovum

Prolactin: hormone secreted by the pituitary gland that triggers and sustains milk production in response to tactile breast stimulation

Proliferative phase: time in the menstrual cycle when the uterine lining becomes prepared for reception and implantation of the fertilized ovum

Prostaglandins: hormones synthesized by many body cells that affect uterine smooth muscle, vasodilatation, and constriction

Q

Quickening: mother's experience of first fetal movements, usually between 17 and 20 weeks' gestation

R

Radiation: transfer and loss of human body heat to cooler objects and surfaces not in direct contact

Reactive nonstress test: detection of two or more fetal heart rate changes of 15 beats or more per minute for 15 seconds or more each within a 10-minute period

Recovery stage: first 4 hours after delivery of the placenta in the fourth stage of labor

Reference daily intakes (RDIs): food content standards for vitamins and minerals

Regional anesthesia: injection of an anesthetic affecting nerve tissue by blocking neural impulses in order to obtain the loss of sensation to an area of the body

Respiratory distress syndrome (RDS): pulmonary membrane disease that causes breathing difficulty and occurs most often in preterm neonates; also known as hyaline membrane disease

Resting tone: level of uterine firmness between contractions during labor

Resuscitation: emergency procedure involving control of the airway opening, positive-pressure ventilation, chest compressions, medication, and body temperature

Retinopathy of prematurity (ROP): fibrotic disease in the blood vessels of the retina in newborns; can cause blindness

Rh incompatibility: hemolytic disease resulting from incompatibility of Rh factors of maternal and fetal blood that causes an antigen–antibody reaction; also known as isoimmunization

RhoGAM: anti-Rh (D) gamma globulin given to an Rh-negative mother after the birth of an Rh-positive child to prevent development of permanent active immunity to the Rh antigen

Rooting reflex: an infant's natural response of turning the head toward a physical stimulus of the cheek or mouth area

Rugae: transverse mucous membrane ridges lining the vagina that expand to accommodate descent of the fetal head during birth

S

Screening: a test or examination to detect a bodily condition, disorder, or disease warranting medical investigation

Second stage of labor: period from the time the cervix is completely dilated and effaced until the birth of the fetus

Secretory phase: period during the menstrual cycle following ovulation and preceding menstruation

Semen: white fluid containing sperm and their nutrient secretions ejaculated from the erect penis during orgasm

Seminiferous tubules: structures that carry sperm from the testes

Sepsis: systemic infection in the blood due to virus, parasites, or bacteria

Sexually transmitted infection (STI): disease transmitted through unprotected sexual contact with an infected individual

Short-term variability: normal changes detected between successive fetal heartbeats

Shoulder dystocia: condition during labor in which the fetal shoulder cannot freely pass beneath the maternal symphysis pubis due to either a large fetus or a small maternal pelvis

Small for gestational age (SGA): infant whose birthweight is below the 10th percentile for gestational age

Spermatogenesis: process by which mature sperm (spermatozoa) develop from spermatogonia (sperm cells)

Spermicide: chemical contraception that either destroys sperm or neutralizes vaginal secretions to immobilize sperm

Station: relationship between the presenting fetal part and an imaginary line of the pelvic ischial spines

Sterilization: surgical procedure performed on males or females to prevent reproduction

Stress incontinence: involuntary discharge of urine during exercise, sneezing, laughing, or coughing; due to loss of muscle tone at the neck of the urethra

Striae gravidarum: reddish or darkened streaks on the stretched skin of the abdomen, hips, or breasts caused by pregnancy

Subinvolution: failure of the uterus to return to normal size after pregnancy due to prolonged involution from infection, hemorrhage, or retained parts of the placenta

Sudden infant death syndrome (SIDS): the death of a healthy, properly cared for infant from unexplained causes

Surfactant: a lipoprotein that stabilizes and lowers the alveolar surface tension of fluids in the lungs, allowing gases to be exchanged in the alveoli

T

Tachycardia: rapid heart rate; in a neonate, above 160 bpm; in an adult, above 100 bpm

Tachypnea: rapid respiratory rate; in a neonate, above 70 respirations/minute

Taking-hold phase: second phase of maternal adjustment, marking maternal readiness for newborn involvement

Taking-in phase: first phase of maternal adjustment, marking maternal need for care, food, and comfort

Teratogen: nongenetic factors or environmental substances that cause physical or functional malformations of the embryo and fetus

Term infant: newborn determined by examination to be 37 to 42 weeks' gestational age

Testes: male gonads; two oval organs in the scrotum in which sperm and testosterone are produced

Testosterone: androgen (male) hormone produced in the testes, adrenal cortex, and ovary; responsible for development of secondary male characteristics

Thelarche: beginning breast development of glandular tissue behind the nipples; occurs at puberty

Thermoregulation: control of body heat production and loss through physiologic changes activated by the hypothalamus

Third stage of labor: period of labor from birth until the expulsion of the placenta

Thrush: fungal infection caused by *Candida albicans*, most common in infants; marked by white plaque patches in the mouth and on the tongue

TORCH: acronym for a pregnancy syndrome of infections (toxoplasmosis, rubella, cytomegalovirus, and herpesvirus or hepatitis); linked to potentially severe fetal or neonatal problems

Transient tachypnea of the newborn: fetal respiratory disorder characterized by mild cyanosis and increased respiratory rate, possibly caused by delayed resorption of lung fluid

Transition: third phase of the first stage of labor, in which dilation of the cervix increases from 8 to 10 cm

Transvaginal ultrasound: procedure used to monitor early pregnancy, to treat women undergoing induction cycles, and to retrieve oocytes for in vitro fertilization

Transverse lie: crosswise or horizontally positioned fetus

Trimester: one third of a normal pregnancy; pregnancy is divided into three trimesters of 3 months each

Trisomy: abnormal presence of an extra, or third, homologous chromosome rather than the normal two, resulting in 47 chromosomes per cell; Down syndrome is the most common human manifestation of this condition

True labor: regular contraction and relaxation intervals of the uterus with progressive shortening, thinning, and dilation of the cervix

Tubal ligation: method of female sterilization that involves surgical severing and tying of the fallopian tubes

U

Ultrasonography: use of high-frequency (>20,000 Hz) sound waves directed into the maternal abdomen to reflect tissue densities and outlines for visualization and diagnosis of the fetus, gestational structures, bones, and fluids

Umbilical cord compression: in utero pressure on the umbilical cord by the fetus or the uterine wall that decreases blood circulation and oxygenation of the fetus

Umbilical cord prolapse: condition in which the umbilical cord precedes the presenting fetal part through the cervix and birth canal

Urge incontinence: involuntary loss of urine associated with a sudden, strong desire to urinate

Uterine atony: inability of uterine muscle to contract after childbirth

Uterine rupture: uterine wall separation that could allow penetration of fetal parts into the abdomen

Uteroplacental insufficiency: decrease in placental function of exchange of gases, wastes, and nutrients, leading to fetal hypoxia and acidosis; evidenced by late fetal heart rate decelerations

V

Vacuum extraction: use of a vacuum suction cup applied to the fetal head to assist in birth

Vaginal birth after cesarean (VBAC): vaginal birth of an infant by a woman who has had at least one previous cesarean birth

Vaginal ring: contraceptive device used to deliver steroids through the vaginal mucosa

Variable deceleration: periodic slowing of fetal heart rate due to umbilical cord compression, and possibly unrelated to normal uterine contractions

Varicocele: varicose veins in the spermatic cord

Vasectomy: male sterilization procedure that involves removing a section of the vas deferens

Vernix caseosa: fatty, white, cheese-like substance secreted by fetal sebaceous glands and epidermal cells that covers and protects fetal skin from abrasions in utero

Vertex: crown or top of the fetal head

Vertical transmission: passing of an infection to the fetus or neonate by the mother during pregnancy, delivery, or breastfeeding

Very low birthweight: birthweight of less than 1,500 g

W

Weaning: transition from breast- or bottle-feeding to a cup

ANSWERS TO WORKSHEET QUESTIONS

CHAPTER 1

Multiple Choice Questions

1. The correct response is D. The number one cause of mortality in women is heart disease, accounting for more than one-half million deaths per year. Most women, however, believe that breast cancer is their number one concern. The mortality rate pales in comparison to that for cardiovascular deaths. Approximately 350 deaths occur secondary to childbirth complications. Statistics for injury resulting from violence would be much less than when compared with the numbers of women who die annually from heart disease.

2. The correct response is C. Lack of adequate health insurance is a major barrier to receiving adequate prenatal care. Of the millions of Americans who have no health insurance, the majority are women. Without health insurance, many have limited options to procure prenatal care. Statistics will demonstrate the better outcomes with prenatal care, and most women would want to have medical supervision for a better outcome. Most women seek care early in the pregnancy, except for teenagers who hide or are unaware of their pregnancy. The majority of women receive quality prenatal care and the outcome is positive. The mistrust of traditional medical practices may play a role in some women from different cultures since they differ in their own cultural health practices.

3. The correct response is D. Pregnancy, contraception, and mental illness treatment are provided in many states to adolescents without parental involvement. Those laws do not include the provision of care for communicable diseases such as tuberculosis, which would require parental consent and notification.

4. The correct response is B. The WIC program provided nutritional supplementation and education to low-income families; pregnant, postpartum, and lactating women; and infants and children up to age 5. Title V established a federal-state partnership and provided aid to dependent families and children, maternal-child health services, and child welfare services. The Medicaid Program under Title XIX provided state block grants to reduce financial barriers to health care for the poor and special services to pregnant women and young children. The Sheppard-Towner Act provided grants to states to establish maternal and child health division in state health care departments.

5. The correct response is B, C, and D. Factors contributing to homelessness include economic factors such as the increase in poverty, lack of affordable housing, decreases in availability of rent subsidies, unemployment, and cutbacks in public welfare programs. Personal crises such as divorce, domestic violence, and substance abuse also are factors. Deinstitutionalization of the mentally ill has played a major role, especially without the development of community centers and homes to assist these individuals during times of crisis.

Critical Thinking Exercise

a. What changes might be helpful to address this situation?

Many of the clients may have employment based on an hourly wage. If they don't work, they don't get paid, and therefore can't attend the clinic during their normal work hours. Offer evening and Saturday hours to improve their attendance at clinic appointments.

b. Outline what you might say at your next staff meeting to address the issue of clients making one clinic visit and then never returning.

Acceptance and a supportive tone are frequently set at the initial meeting, and one may need to examine how this is communicated to the client at their first encounter with the clinic staff. Offer suggestions of how the staff can set a positive, welcoming tone so clients will return for additional care.

c. What strategies might you use to improve attendance and notification?

Have a staff person call each client to remind her of her appointment the next day and offer any needed assistance to get her there. Assign a staff member to be an "outreach" person to make home visits to follow up on clients who habitually miss appointments.

d. Describe what cultural and customer service techniques might be needed.

Educate staff concerning cultural norms regarding the clientele served. Based on the culture served, devise culturally appropriate policies and procedures.

Study Activities

1. Answers will vary depending on your location and time period when researched.
2. Depending on the students' frames of reference, some will think it is a right and the government should provide it for all citizens. Others will think it

should be a privilege and should be paid for by the person and not the government. There is no right or wrong answer, but this topic can provide for a lively classroom discussion.

3. Women lack insurance to pay for services, no transportation available to get to services, language or cultural barriers, health care agency hours are in conflict with their work hours, and negative health staff attitudes.

CHAPTER 2

Multiple Choice Questions

1. The correct responses are A, B, D, and F. Secondary prevention includes early detection and treatment. Activities would include fecal occult blood testing, hearing screenings, cholesterol testing, and pregnancy testing. Smoking cessation and hygiene programs are examples of activities at the primary prevention level.

2. The correct response is C. Advantages to outpatient surgery centers include decreased risk for infection, decreased cost, decreased separation from family, and decreased disruption of family functioning. The major disadvantage associated with this site is the inability to accommodate overnight stays if necessary due to complications. The woman would need to be transferred to a hospital for continued care.

3. The correct response is B. Always assess the client's learning needs and preferred style of learning first.

4. The correct response is C. Having knowledge of the various cultural variations in health care practices helps the nurse to apply them in his or her everyday practice settings. This cultural sensitivity and application of it makes a culturally competent nurse. Knowing one's own culture does not foster tolerance and acceptance of people from different ones. Only when the nurse gains knowledge about other cultures will he or she become culturally competent. Being open to different cultural customs and beliefs is only the beginning of becoming culturally competent; application of the knowledge is critical. Playing a role in establishing policies without seeing them applied in the health care setting is not going to break down barriers to care. What is written policy may not be used in the real world. Thus, everyone can refer to the policy but attitudes and actions have not changed.

5. The correct response is A. The current emphasis is on health promotion and illness prevention. Thus, the rise in community-based care has occurred due to a movement away from an illness-oriented cure perspective to one that focuses on health promotion, with an emphasis on primary care and outpatient treatment and management. Advances in technology have allowed for improved monitoring of clients in community settings and the ability to perform complicated procedures outside of the acute care setting.

Critical Thinking Exercises

1. First, the nurse must determine who the authority figure and primary caretaker(s) of the woman are, as well as the family's support system. Determine cultural, religious, or spiritual values the family would like to have incorporated into the woman's care and the language spoken at home and by the woman. Ascertain special dietary needs or the family's desire to incorporate particular health practices or providers. Additionally, the nurse would need to assess the woman's and family's learning needs, keeping in mind the impact of culture on these needs.

2. Important areas of assessment include the woman's pregnancy and fetal status, physical condition and medical needs, home environment, other members of the family such as other children, and assessment of the teaching and learning needs of the family. The nurse needs to ensure that the woman can be cared for at home. Other assessment areas include how the family is coping with the woman's need for care and prescribed bedrest. For example, do they appear overwhelmed? Are there other children in the house that need assistance and care? How is the family functioning, and what support and resources are available? Assess whether the environment is safe and nurturing and the necessary resources are available, such as any equipment and medication that might be needed. Identify the primary care givers and include them in the assessment and development of the plan of care.

Study Activities

1. This shadowing activity will provide the student with exposure to a variety of roles and situations facing nurses in specific health care settings.

2. This visit would be very educational for nursing students to see what is happening in the real world when faced with cultural barriers in the health care setting. Hopefully, the community health center staff will be open to these students and will share their strategies. These strategies can be used by the students later in their practice.

3. Depending on the website selected, answers will vary, but most of them offer a variety of resources to learn about different cultures and could be helpful to nurses seeking information.

CHAPTER 3

Multiple Choice Questions

1. The correct response is B. FSH is secreted from the anterior pituitary gland to initiate the development of the ovarian follicles and the secretion of estrogen by them within the ovarian cycle. A is incorrect: TSH stimulates the thyroid gland and plays a limited role

in the menstrual cycle. C is incorrect: CRH is released from the hypothalamus, not the anterior pituitary gland. D is incorrect: GnRH is released from the hypothalamus to stimulate the release of FSH and LH from the anterior pituitary gland.

2. The correct response is C. Skene's glands are located close to the urethral opening and secrete mucus and lubricate during urination and sexual intercourse. A is incorrect: Cowper's glands are located on either side of the male urethra, not the female urethra. B is incorrect: Bartholin's glands are located on either side of the vaginal opening and secrete alkaline mucus that enhances the viability of the male sperm. D is incorrect: seminal glands are pouchlike structures at the base of the male urinary bladder that secrete an alkaline fluid to enhance the viability of the male sperm.

3. The correct response is B. The proliferative phase starts with the enlargement of the endometrial glands, which is stimulated by increasing amounts of estrogen. The blood vessels dilate and the endometrium increases in thickness dramatically. The proliferative phase of the menstrual cycle begins at the end of the menstrual phase and ends at ovulation. It is characterized by endometrial thickening and ovarian follicular maturation.

4. The correct response is D. Progesterone is the dominant hormone after ovulation to prepare the endometrium for implantation. A is incorrect: estrogen levels decline after ovulation, since it assists in the maturation of the ovarian follicles before ovulation. Estrogen levels are highest during the proliferative phase of the menstrual cycle. B is incorrect: prostaglandin production increases during the follicular maturation and is essential during ovulation but not after ovulation. C is incorrect: prolactin is inhibited by the high levels of estrogen and progesterone during pregnancy; when their levels decline at birth, an increase in prolactin takes place to promote lactation.

5. The correct response is C. The function of the epididymis is to store and mature sperm until ejaculation occurs. A is incorrect: the testes manufacture sperm and send them to the epididymis for storage and continued maturation. B is incorrect: the main function of the vas deferens is to rapidly squeeze the sperm from their storage site (epididymis) into the urethra. D is incorrect: the function of the seminal vesicles is to secrete an alkaline fluid rich in fructose and prostaglandins to help provide an environment favorable to sperm motility and metabolism.

Critical Thinking Exercise

a. How should the nurse respond to this question?

The nurse should respond by explaining to the student that conception is achieved only during the time of ovulation, which occurs at midcycle and not during menstruation. Further explanation might outline the phases of the menstrual cycle and how each phase contributes to the preparation of the endometrial lining if conception were to take place. If conception does not occur, sloughing of the prepared endometrial lining takes place, and this is what is shed during menstruation.

b. What factor regarding the menstrual cycle was not clarified?

The student apparently did not understand the concept of ovulation and the potential uniting of sperm and ovum. At ovulation, bodily changes occur that assist the sperm to impregnate the ovum that was released from the ovary. It is only during this midcycle period that the sperm can find the ovum and begin a pregnancy.

c. What additional topics might this question lead to that might be discussed?

Sexually transmitted infections and barrier protection; abstinence until marriage and personal responsibility; responsibilities and outcomes of becoming a young parent; self-esteem and taking pride in their bodies; future educational and career goals

Study Activities

1. This answer will vary depending on which website the student selects and which topic of interest he or she researches. With luck, a variety of topics will be presented and lend themselves to a lively class discussion.

2. The predominant hormones involved in the menstrual cycle are gonadotropin-releasing hormone (GnRH), which is responsible for reproductive hormone control and timing of the cycle; follicle-stimulating hormone (FSH), which stimulates the ovary to produce estrogen and follicles in the ovary that will mature; luteinizing hormone (LH), which induces the mature ovum to burst from the ovary and stimulate production of corpus luteum; estrogen, which induces growth and thickening of the endometrial lining; progesterone, which prepares the endometrial lining for implantation; and prostaglandins, which help to free the mature ovum inside the graafian follicle.

3. ovum or ova

4. The correct responses are F (testes) and G (seminiferous tubules). Sperm is produced in the seminiferous tubules of the testes. A is incorrect: the vas deferens is a cordlike duct that transports sperm from the epididymis and has no role in making sperm cells. B is incorrect: the penis is the organ for copulation and serves as the outlet for sperm, but it plays no role in the manufacture of sperm cells or testosterone. C is incorrect: the scrotum serves as the climate-control system for the testes to allow for normal sperm development, but it plays no direct role in their manufacture. D is incorrect: the ejaculatory ducts secrete fluids to help nourish the sperm, but do not play a part in their development. E is incorrect: the prostate gland produces fluid that nourishes

the sperm but does not participate in the production of sperm cells. H is incorrect: the bulbourethral glands (Cowper's glands) secrete a mucus-like fluid that provides lubrication during the sex act.

CHAPTER 4

Multiple Choice Questions

1. The correct response is B: the definition of infertility is the inability of a couple to conceive after 12 months of unprotected sexual intercourse. A is incorrect: 6 months is not long enough to diagnose infertility in a couple not using birth control. C is incorrect: 18 months is 6 months beyond the time needed to diagnose infertility based on the definition. D is incorrect: 24 months is double the time needed to diagnose infertility.

2. The correct response is B: if EC is taken within 72 hours after unprotected sexual intercourse, pregnancy will be prevented by inhibiting implantation. The next morning would still afford time to take EC and not become pregnant. A is incorrect: it would be too late to use a spermicidal agent to prevent pregnancy, since the sperm have already traveled up into the female reproductive tract. C is incorrect: douching with vinegar and hot water 24 hours after unprotected sexual intercourse will not change the course of events; by then it is too late to prevent a pregnancy, and this combination would not be effective anyway. D is incorrect: a laxative will stimulate the gastrointestinal tract to produce defecation but will not disturb the reproductive tract, where fertilization takes place.

3. The correct response is A: Seasonale is the only FDA-approved oral contraceptive that is packaged to provide 84 days of continuous protection. Although any oral contraceptive can be taken continuously, the FDA has not approved this, and it would be considered an "off-label" use. B is incorrect: this product has not gained FDA approval for continuous use; it is to be left in 3 weeks and then removed for 1 week to create monthly cycles. C is incorrect response: the FDA has not given approval to use this transdermal patch on a continuous basis; it is placed on the skin for 3 weeks and removed for 1 week. D is incorrect: this implantable device is protective for 5 years, but it is not a combination contraceptive; it releases synthetic progesterone only, not estrogen.

4. The correct response is D: weight-bearing exercise is an excellent preventive measure to preserve bone integrity, especially the vertebral column and hips. Walking strengthens the skeletal system and prevents breakdown that leads to osteoporosis. A is incorrect: iron does not prevent bone breakdown; while iron supplementation will build up blood and prevent anemia, it has a limited effect on bones. B is incorrect:

being in the horizontal position while sleeping is not helpful to build bone. Weight-bearing on long bones helps to maintain their density, which prevents loss of bone matrix. C is incorrect: protein gained from eating lean meats helps the body to build tissue and muscles but has a limited effect on maintaining bone integrity or preventing loss of bone density.

5. The correct response is B because smoking cigarettes causes vasoconstriction of the blood vessels, increasing peripheral vascular resistance and thus elevating blood pressure. These vascular changes increase the chances of CVD by placing additional pressure on the heart to pump blood with increasing vessel resistance. A is incorrect since fiber would be a positive diet addition and assist with elimination patterns and prevent straining, which stresses the heart. C is an incorrect response because vitamins do not cause narrowing of the vessel lumen, which places an additional burden on the heart. D is an incorrect response since alcohol produces vasodilation and reduces blood pressure. Alcohol in moderation is said to be good for the heart.

6. The correct response is C since vasomotor instability, which causes hot flashes, is directly related to declining estrogen levels. Increasing the estrogen levels by hormone replacement therapy reduces vasomotor instability and thus hot flashes. A is an incorrect response since weight gain or loss is associated with calorie intake and metabolic output in the form of energy expended through exercise. Although many women report a weight gain associated with HRT, when questioned closely they admit to a reduction in activity level. B is incorrect since estrogen has the opposite effect on bone density–it increases and/or maintains it. HRT is prescribed for post-menopausal women to prevent osteoporosis, or loss of bone density. D is incorrect since the incidence of heart disease (myocardial infarction and strokes) was found to increase in women taking HRT in the WHI research study, if hormones were taken in high doses over a long period. Based on that landmark study, women on HRT should take the lowest dose possible to relieve symptoms and should not take HRT for more than 5 years.

7. The correct response is A: exercise is heart-healthy, weight-healthy, and emotionally healthy. The motto "Keep moving" is the basis for a healthy lifestyle, since it will help maintain an ideal weight, improve circulation, and improve moods. B is incorrect: socialization does not necessarily involve physical activity and would not be proactive in preserving health. C is incorrect: quiet time alone, although needed to reduce stress, reduces movement and may result in depression and weight gain. D is incorrect: water, although needed to hydrate the body, will not maintain circulation, prevent weight gain, or improve one's emotional mindset. Exercise will accomplish all three.

8. The correct response is D. This vaginal barrier contraceptive device is a dome-shaped rubber cup with a flexible rim that needs to be inserted into the woman's vagina before sexual intercourse. The dome of the diaphragm covers the cervix and the spermicidal cream or jelly applied to the rim prevents sperm from entering the cervix. Women who use this method of contraception must be able to insert the device in their vaginas before each sex act for it to be effective. If the woman is uncomfortable "touching" herself, this is not going to be a successful method and another method should be utilized.

Critical Thinking Exercise

a. Is an IUS the most appropriate method for her? Why or why not?

In this case, based on her history of STIs, PID, and multiple partners, she is not a candidate for an IUS. This method would increase her risk of further ascending infections, which could hinder her future fertility. Unless her lifestyle choices change dramatically, she is placing herself at risk. She should be encouraged to use barrier methods for contraception.

b. What myths/misperceptions will you address in your counseling session?

This client states she isn't interested in using birth control pills because they cause cancer. That is not true, and an explanation of risk factors for cancer needs to be given, along with a discussion of the lower doses of estrogen in the birth control pills prescribed today. Positive noncontraceptive impacts such as a reduction in ovarian and colorectal cancers should also be addressed.

c. Outline the safer sex discussion you plan to have with her.

• Having a monogamous relationship reduces the incidence of STIs.
• Using barrier methods (condom, cap, diaphragm) protects against both pregnancy and STIs.
• Oral sex using a dental dam reduces the risk of STIs.
• Dry kissing with no sores or broken skin reduces the risk of STIs.
• Inform the client of the relationship between PID and infertility.
• Encourage prompt treatment of any vaginal discharge.

Study Activities

1. Teaching plan for an adolescent with PMS:
   1. Define the condition in simple terms to increase the teen's understanding of it.
   2. Cite statistics about the incidence of it to let her know it is a common entity.
   3. Assign her the task of tracking her symptoms that most profoundly bother her.
   4. Carefully study the patterns/trends of the symptoms to explain what is occurring.

5. Discuss an overall comprehensive approach to managing her symptoms:
   a. Dietary changes
      i. Resist carbohydrate cravings premenstrually
      ii. Reduce caffeine intake, which tends to increase nervous tension
      iii. Vitamins B6, A and E have shown some promise in studies
   b. Aerobic exercise throughout month helps in reducing pain
   c. Medical therapy, if lifestyle changes don't work to relive symptoms
      i. Antidepressants
      ii. Tranquilizers
      iii. Oral contraceptives
2. Typically the family planning nurse will ask the woman about any sociocultural, spiritual, and religious beliefs that will influence the decision. Lifestyle and economics also play a big role in the choice of a family planning method. Ideally this should be a decision made by both partners, but rarely is the partner involved. Important teaching involves the risks, benefits, side effects, and efficacy of each method, along with instructions on how to use it correctly. Information regarding follow-up care should be stressed.
3. Numerous websites are available, many of them sponsored by infertility health care agencies.
4. Prices will be higher in metropolitan versus rural areas of the county. Students will discover that the risk is higher for a woman undergoing a tubal ligation than a man undergoing a vasectomy. The costs will vary, but male sterilization is generally both less risky and less expensive.
5. The students will find numerous brands of male condoms and only one brand of female condom. Male condoms prices can range from 35 cents each to over $4, depending on the manufacturer. Most female condoms are priced around $2.50 to $3.50 each.
6. A, B, D, E, and G are correct responses: research studies have validated a reduced incidence of these cancers and conditions. C and F are incorrect: research has not shown a reduction, and some studies have actually found an increase in the incidence of breast cancer and deep vein thrombosis.

CHAPTER 5

Multiple Choice Questions

1. The correct response is C: it creates a mechanical barrier so that bacteria and viruses cannot gain access to the internal reproductive tract and proliferate. A is incorrect: there is no barrier or protection offered by taking an oral pill. Oral contraceptives offer protection against pregnancy by preventing ovulation, but none against STIs. B is incorrect: an infected partner can

still transmit the infection through preejaculate fluids, which may contain an active STI. D is incorrect: an IUD offers no barrier to prevent entrance of bacteria or viruses into the internal reproductive tract. Because it is an internal device, the string emerging from the external uterine os can actually enhance STI infiltration into the uterus in susceptible women.

2. The correct response is A: the HIV virus is not spread through casual contact between individuals. HIV is spread through unprotected sexual intercourse, breastfeeding, blood contact, or shared needles or sex toys. B is incorrect: HIV can be spread by sharing injection equipment because the user can come into contact with HIV-positive blood. C is incorrect: sexual intercourse (unprotected vaginal, anal, or oral) poses the highest risk of HIV transmission. D is incorrect: the newborn can receive the HIV virus through infected breast milk. HIV-positive women are advised not to breastfeed to protect their offspring from getting a HIV infection.

3. The correct response is B: the human papillomavirus (HPV) causes warts in the genital region. HPV is a slow-growing DNA virus belonging to the papilloma group. Types 6 and 11 usually cause visible genital warts. Other HPV types in the genital region (16, 18, 31, 33, and 35) are associated with vaginal, anal, and cervical dysplasia. A is incorrect: a pus-filled discharge is not typical of an HPV infection, but rather a chlamydial or gonococcal STI. C is incorrect: a single painless ulcer would be indicative of primary syphilis rather than an HPV infection. D is incorrect: multiple vesicles would indicate a herpes outbreak, not an HPV infection. The woman would also experience tingling, itching, and pain in the affected area.

4. The correct response is D: a ruptured tubal pregnancy secondary to an ectopic pregnancy can cause life-threatening hypovolemic shock. Without immediate surgical intervention, death can result. A is incorrect: involuntary infertility may be emotionally traumatic, but it is not life-threatening. B is incorrect: chronic pelvic pain secondary to adhesions is unpleasant but typically is not life-threatening. C is incorrect: depression may be caused by the chronic pain or involuntary infertility but is not life-threatening.

5. The correct response is C: the classic chancre in primary syphilis can be described as a painless, indurated ulcer-like lesion at the site of exposure. A is incorrect: a highly variable rash is characteristic of secondary syphilis, not primary. B is incorrect: this is more descriptive of a trichomoniasis vaginal infection rather than primary syphilis, which manifests with a chancre on the external genitalia. D is incorrect: a localized gumma formation on the mucous membranes, such as the lips or nose, is characteristic of late syphilis, along with neurosyphilis and cardiovascular syphilis.

Critical Thinking Exercise

a. What STI would the nurse suspect?

Based on the description of the genital lesions, the nurse would suspect genital herpes. Typically the herpetic lesions begin as erythematous papules that then develop into vesicles. The vesicles rupture and leave ulcerated lesions and then crust over. This is essentially what Sally described in her history.

b. The nurse should give immediate consideration to which of Sally's complaints?

As with any STI, treatment should aim at promoting comfort, promoting healing, preventing secondary infection, and decreasing transmission of the disease. A sample from a genital lesion should be obtained for a definitive diagnosis. A urine sample should be checked for bacteria to rule out a bladder infection. Giving information about the specific STI is important to promote understanding. Information concerning her antiviral medication therapy is paramount to reduce the viral shedding. Sitz baths and mild analgesics may be needed for pain relief.

c. What should be the goals of the nurse in teaching Sally about STIs?

Although acyclovir or another antiviral medication can reduce the symptoms of herpes, the nurse needs to point out that it is not a cure for herpes. Antiviral drugs act to suppress viral replication but do not rid the body of them. This STI is a lifetime one, and she may experience numerous episodes. The nurse should teach Sally that this condition is manageable, but she will need to be able to identify stress factors that may trigger a recurrence and reduce them. Common triggers may include hormonal changes, such as ovulation during the menstrual cycle; prolonged exposure to sunlight; emotional distress; lack of sleep; and overwork. The final goal is to make sure Sally understands how to prevent transmission of herpes and what changes in her behaviors need to take place immediately to protect her health.

Study Activities

1. Depending on which website the students select and which STI they choose to research, discussions will vary. We hope that each student will bring additional information to the discussion and will share interesting "finds" with his or her peers.

2. Statistics will vary depending on the student's location. This research will help students learn what is happening in their area and what preventive measures are being used to reduce the incidence of STIs.

3. The counseling role of the STI nurse should be one of patience and sensitivity. The nurse should be nonjudgmental and should see the client as someone who needs both treatment and education. The nurse should counsel the patient about high-risk behaviors and prevention of disease transmission.

4. chlamydia and gonorrhea

5. The correct responses are B, C, and D: all three therapies assist in reducing the viral load in the warty lesion. Treatment may reduce but does not necessarily eradicate infection. A is incorrect: penicillin is a bacteriostatic agent and is not effective against viruses. E is incorrect: antiretroviral therapy is used for HIV infections. F is incorrect: acyclovir is typically used to treat herpes infections.

CHAPTER 6
Multiple Choice Questions

1. The correct response is C: visible changes to the skin of the breast take place (dimpling, contour changes, nipple discharge) and can be seen if inspected in front of a mirror. A is incorrect: breast cancer first spreads to the axillary lymph nodes, not the cervical nodes. Palpation of the axillary lymph nodes is warranted, not the cervical ones. B is incorrect: spontaneous nipple discharge is more indicative of breast cancer than discharge produced by squeezing the nipple. D is incorrect: a mammogram is not part of a breast self-examination, which the woman does in the privacy of her home.

2. The correct response is A: the incidence of breast cancer increases with aging, especially over age 50. Only 1% of breast cancers occur in men. B is incorrect: bearing children interrupts the menstrual cycle and decreases a woman's risk of breast cancer. C is incorrect: only 7% of women have a genetic mutation resulting in breast cancer, whereas in the remaining 93% it is a sporadic occurrence. D is incorrect: colon cancer is not a risk factor for breast cancer.

3. The correct response is B: this describes the procedure for performing a sentinel node biopsy. A is incorrect: there is no dye used and a biopsy is taken of the breast mass, not the node. C is incorrect: this is an actual surgical removal of the axillary nodes and not just a biopsy, and no dye is used in this procedure. D is incorrect: an advanced breast biopsy does not use dye and involves taking a tissue sample of the breast mass, not the nodes in the axillary area.

4. The correct response is D: when the bone marrow is suppressed secondary to chemotherapy, the woman experiences bleeding tendencies (low platelets), limited immunity (low white blood cells), and anemia (low red blood cells). This myelosuppression can become life-threatening. A is incorrect: a decrease in the number of platelets in the circulating blood may cause bleeding tendencies if the body is traumatized, but it is not as life-threatening as having all bone marrow cells depressed. B is incorrect: having blood clots in deep veins is typically not a frequent response to chemotherapy, whereas myelosuppression is very common. C is incorrect: losing one's

hair, while emotionally and aesthetically traumatizing, it is not a life-threatening event, and the hair will grow back after therapy ends.

5. The correct response is B: the discomfort is usually mild and analgesics will relieve it in most cases. A is incorrect: women are advised to reduce caffeine to reduce the stimulation of breast tissue, not increase it. C is incorrect: women are advised to increase their intake of leafy vegetables, not reduce them, since this would be a part of a balanced healthy diet. D is incorrect: women are advised to wear a firm supportive bra to reduce the strain on the breast tissue, not a bra that offers no support.

6. The correct response is D: this volunteer organization offers support and practical advice to women with breast cancer; all the volunteers have had breast cancer themselves. A is incorrect: NOW does not focus on breast cancer per se, but all women's issues, especially ones of equality. B is incorrect: the FDA is concerned with the regulation, security, and safety of all foods and drugs in the United States, not breast cancer issues. C is incorrect: the March of Dimes focuses on prevention of preterm births and reduction of birth defects, not breast cancer.

Critical Thinking Exercises

1.
a. What specific questions would you ask this client to get a clearer picture?

The nurse needs to assess this client's risk factors for breast cancer by asking about:
- Her family history of breast or ovarian cancer
- Her own health history
- Her gynecologic history (menarche, parity, family planning)
- Her history of breast problems (previous benign disorders)
- Her lifestyle habits, which may be associated with cancer (e.g., smoking, high intake of fat, alcohol intake)

b. What education is needed for this client regarding breast health?

The nurse needs to reassure the client that most breast lesions are benign, but this problem will need to be explored. The fact she experiences cyclic pain suggests this problem may be fibrocystic breast changes and not cancer, but she should undergo a further workup. Stress the importance of performing monthly breast self-examinations, receiving yearly mammograms, and scheduling annual clinical breast examinations with her health care provider to assist in taking control of her health.

c. What community referrals are needed to meet this client's future needs?

During October of each year, many health care agencies honor National Breast Cancer month by offering free or reduced-cost mammograms. The nurse needs to make the client aware of this and urge her to receive a mammogram to maintain her health.

2.

a. What benign condition might the nurse practitioner suspect based on her description?

Based on her history and symptom description, the NP probably would suspect the benign breast condition duct ectasia.

b. What specific information should the nurse practitioner give Mrs. Davis about duct ectasia?

Information given should include: Duct ectasia is a disease of ducts in the subareolar zone that occurs in aging breasts. Manifestations include a palpable dilated duct; a thick, green, sticky nipple discharge; pain; itching; and inflammation. There is no association with cancer.

c. The typical treatment of this benign breast condition would include what?

Treatment for duct ectasia consists of reassurance and support. Although there is no cure for duct ectasia, antibiotics are prescribed for acute inflammatory episodes. The woman should be taught how to cleanse the breast to minimize the risk of infection. Good handwashing and personal hygiene measures are stressed. Instructing her to wear a supportive yet nonconfining bra will help reduce her discomfort.

Study Activities

1. A woman's breasts have a variety of meanings and symbolize various things to women. To some women, her breasts symbolize her female self and her ability to suckle her newborn, and separate her biologically from a man. To society, a woman's breasts can be viewed as a sex symbol and denote sexiness. Different cultures view a woman's breasts differently, dictating whether or not she is welcome to expose them for breastfeeding.
2. Feelings might include fear of cancer, anxiety, helplessness, embarrassment, denial, or depression. A nurse can help her cope with these feelings by giving her the facts and reassuring her that most breast disorders are benign. Guide the woman through the diagnostic tests needed to validate her condition.
3. Lifestyle modifications that can reduce the discomfort of fibrocystic breast changes might include taking oral contraceptives; eating a low-fat diet rich in fruits and vegetables; avoiding caffeine intake; reducing salt intake; wearing a well-fitting, supportive bra most of the time; and taking over-the-counter analgesics to reduce mild discomfort.
4. mastitis

CHAPTER 7

Multiple Choice Questions

1. The correct response is C: pressure against adjacent structures and stretching of the uterine muscle with increasing growth of the fibroid creates pain. A is

incorrect: migraines are not caused by growing fibroids, but rather a change within the vasculature in the cranium. B is incorrect: bladder pressure to cause urinary urgency would be secondary to pelvic structure relaxation, not uterine fibroids. D is incorrect: constipation would be more common in a woman experiencing pelvic organ prolapse than in one with fibroids, since fibroids usually involve the uterus, not the rectum.

2. The correct response is A: both pessaries and Kegel exercises help hold up and strengthen the pelvic floor to restore the pelvic organs to their correct anatomic position. B is incorrect: an external fixation device would not be a tolerable long-term solution; it would also be invasive and would place the woman at risk for infection. C is incorrect: weight gain is not usually a healthy intervention for women as they age. Additional weight would increase the pressure on pelvic organs and exacerbate the problem. Yoga is relaxing and could reduce the woman's stress level, but it would not be therapeutic for pelvic organ prolapse. D is incorrect: wearing firm support garments might increase intra-abdominal pressure and cause further downward descent of the pelvic organs.

3. The correct response is A: preventing constipation and straining with defecation would lessen the strain on pelvic organs. B is incorrect: sitting for long periods will not affect pelvic organ movement. Gravity will create a downward pull on all organs regardless of the position, sitting or standing. C is incorrect: exercise will help to tone muscles within the body and strengthen the pelvic floor. D is incorrect: frequent childbirth contributes to pelvic organ prolapse rather than preventing it. Spacing children only a year apart would negatively influence the pelvic-floor musculature and would be a contributing factor for prolapse.

4. The correct response is C: insulin resistance is characterized by failure of insulin to enter cells appropriately, resulting in hyperinsulinemia, a characteristic of PCOS. Factors that contribute to this include obesity, physical inactivity, and poor dietary habits. This person is at risk for developing type 2 diabetes secondary to insulin resistance. A is incorrect: osteoporosis develops in aging women because of declining estrogen and calcium levels, not due to PCOS. B is incorrect: lupus is an autoimmune condition and is not related to PCOS. D is incorrect: migraine headaches are not associated with PCOS but rather changes in cranium vessels.

5. The correct response is D: GnRH agonists block the production of estrogen, which produces menopausal symptoms. A is incorrect: osteoporosis would be a long-term result of estrogen deprivation and calcium, and typically women do not stay on GnRH agonists for long-term therapy. B is incorrect: the blocking of

estrogen would not contribute to the development of arthritis. C is incorrect: inhibiting estrogen is not a cause of depression; a change in serotonin levels in the brain is a cause of depression.

Critical Thinking Exercise

a. What condition might Faith have based on her symptoms?

The symptoms are suggestive of uterine fibroids. She presents with a typical profile.

b. What treatment options are available to address this condition?

If Faith desires to preserve her childbearing ability, she can be treated medically with oral contraceptives, gonadotropin-releasing hormones, mifepristone, or a myomectomy. If she is finished with childbearing, a vaginal hysterectomy would be advised.

c. What educational interventions should the nurse discuss with Faith?

The nurse needs to make sure that Faith understands what the disorder is and how it can be treated and should provide information to assist her in making a decision about treatment. In addition to the treatment modalities for fibroids, her iron deficiency anemia needs attention with iron preparations and dietary changes to increase her iron and vitamin C intake.

Study Activities

1. Offer an explanation of how this inconspicuous exercise can help build muscle volume. Show a picture of where this pelvic floor muscle is located. Pelvic floor relaxation comes with the aging process in women secondary to childbirth, weight gain, and the force of gravity. The easiest way to instruct a woman how to do Kegel exercises is to have her practice using the pubococcygeus muscle by starting and stopping the flow of urine. Have her tighten the pubococcygeus muscle for a count of three, then relax it. This maneuver should be done at least 10 times each day.

2. The symptoms that accompany pelvic organ prolapse might include stress incontinence, urinary frequency and urgency, a feeling of bladder fullness after voiding, constipation, rectal fullness, painful intercourse, and pelvic pressure. All of the symptoms combined would tend to keep a woman isolated from society and her partner because of the embarrassment of odor, discomfort, and accidents. A woman would not feel in control of her body functions and would thus feel vulnerable in most social or intimate circumstances. Joining a support group of women experiencing similar problems would allow her to express her feelings and find support through others. Suggestions about what works and what doesn't work and how to cope with this situation would be very helpful.

3. Symptoms common in women with uterine fibroids include low back pain, menorrhagia, anemia, dyspareunia, dysmenorrhea, bloating, and feelings of heaviness in the pelvic region. A woman might delay seeking treatment because she fears she has cancer and thus might be in denial as a protective mechanism. Many women associate irregular bleeding and pain with the diagnosis of cancer.

4. cystocele

5. rectocele

CHAPTER 8

Multiple Choice Questions

1. The correct answer is B: typically there are no glaring features of ovarian cancer. Many of the symptoms are nonspecific and can easily be explained away and rationalized as changes related to the aging process. A is incorrect: ovarian cancer is aggressive and spreads early. C is incorrect: women do not have to die to be diagnosed with ovarian cancer. D is incorrect: most women with acute pain bring it to the attention of their health care provider, but acute pain is a late symptom of cancer.

2. The correct response is D: any postmenopausal bleeding is suspicious for endometrial cancer. This event warrants immediate evaluation, which would include an endometrial biopsy. A is incorrect: postmenopausal women do not have menstrual periods unless they are taking hormone replacement therapy. B is incorrect: any postmenopausal bleeding is abnormal and needs evaluation to determine its cause. The exception would be for a woman taking hormone replacement therapy and still experiencing monthly cycles. C is incorrect: warm-water douches would not be advised for a woman experiencing postmenopausal bleeding, since it would not be therapeutic or warranted. Determining the etiology of the spotting or bleeding is imperative.

3. The correct response is A: women need clear information to make informed choices about treatment and aftercare. This information will help reduce her anxiety and chose the best course of action for her. B is incorrect: hand-holding is important if used appropriately, but having clear information about what to expect and treatment options will go a longer way to meet her psychosocial needs. C is incorrect: cheerfulness is not necessarily therapeutic in the face of a grave prognosis. D is incorrect: instilling hope is important, but giving clear information would be more of a priority.

4. The correct response is C: Pap smears are done specifically to detect abnormal cells of the cervix that might be cancerous. A is incorrect: a fecal occult blood test would be useful in detecting blood in the gastrointestinal tract and might be diagnostic of colorectal cancer, not cervical cancer. B is incorrect: this glycoprotein is

not specific for cervical cancer, but levels may rise in pancreatic, liver, colon, breast, and lung cancers. D is incorrect: a sigmoidoscopy is used to visualize the sigmoid colon to identify cancer, polyps, or blockages. It is not diagnostic of cervical cancer.

5. The correct response is B: typically ovarian cancer is not diagnosed until it is in advanced stages, when the prognosis and survival rates are poor. A is incorrect: vulvar cancer is usually recognized earlier and when treated in its early stages is curable. C is incorrect: endometrial cancer can usually be detected secondary to postmenopausal bleeding and can be treated if detected early by surgery to remove the uterus or source of cancer. D is incorrect: cervical cancer, if detected early and treated, can be eliminated. With early treatment, it does not carry a high mortality rate.

Critical Thinking Exercises

1.

a. Based on her history, which risk factors for cervical cancer are present?

This client is at high risk for several conditions, including sexually transmitted infections as well as cervical cancer, because of the following risk factors: smoking, early onset of sexual activity, multiple partners, and no previous Pap smears.

b. What recommendations would you make for her and why?

Schedule an appointment for a Pap smear and instruct her to keep it. It may save her life. The ACS strongly recommends cervical cancer screening for all women who are sexually active within 3 years of the start of sexual activity or at the age of 21. This client has not undergone any assessment and engages in high-risk behavior.

c. What are this client's educational needs concerning health maintenance?

Cigarette smoking and multiple sexual partners from an early age strongly correlate with cervical dysplasia and cancer and increase risk. This client needs to undergo a Pap smear annually, stop smoking, use barrier methods for protection, and reduce the number of sexual partners. The nurse should refer her to community social services to obtain employment and thus health insurance to continue health maintenance activities. The nurse should stress the importance of lifestyle behavioral changes that she needs to make to preserve her health.

2.

a. Is this client's profile typical for a woman with this diagnosis?

Yes, Jennifer represents the typical presentation of a woman with epithelial ovarian cancer. She was diagnosed with advanced ovarian cancer that had spread to other abdominal organs and the lymph nodes by the time she was diagnosed. She essentially experienced no symptoms of concern prior to her diagnosis. Her 5-year survival rate is poor because of her advanced cancer state.

b. What in her history might have increased her risk for ovarian cancer?

Jennifer already had been diagnosed with breast cancer, which places her at an increased risk for ovarian cancer. In addition, she had no prior pregnancies to interrupt her menstrual cycles, which would be helpful in lowering her risk of developing ovarian cancer. Finally, Jennifer has a history of perineal talc exposure, which increases her risk because of its similarity to asbestos.

c. What can the nurse do to increase awareness of this cancer for all women?

Community education can be very effective in increasing awareness of this condition. Education should focus on pertinent information about risk-reduction measures, screening options for women at high risk, and the importance of annual examinations. In addition, nurses should keep current on research concerning ovarian cancer and should be able to disseminate this information at health fairs and women's support groups.

Study Activities

1. Depending on the type of reproductive cancer the student selects, the responses will vary. Typically the symptoms described are vague, and the woman may have delayed seeking help from her health care provider. Her preoperative emotions are usually fear, denial, and anxiety regarding the unknown. Her postoperative feelings can include relief, worry, depression, and anxiety again. Her future may seem bright if the cancer was detected early, but it may be bleak if it is advanced.

2. Depending on where the student lives and what community resources are available, the responses will vary. The purpose of this field trip is to acquaint the students with their community resources and to visualize the equipment used in cancer treatment. Cancer treatment centers are very specialized, and most offer numerous modalities of care. It is important that students know what is available in their communities and be informed referral agents.

3. Most websites address the lay public and offer education about each type of cancer. Most urge clients to seek specific information concerning their symptoms or situation from their health care practitioner.

4. ovarian

5. breast and ovarian

Chapter 9

Multiple Choice Questions

1. The correct response is D: giving women the ability to gain control over their lives allows them to make the changes needed to protect themselves and their children. As long as they feel victimized, they will take little action to make change. A is incorrect: being the victim of abuse is not a mental illness, but

involves being in circumstances where her courage and self-esteem may be hindered. B is incorrect: leaving the abuser is a process, not an abrupt action, and a great deal of preparation is needed before making this move. C is incorrect: nurses don't have the resources to provide financial support to abused women, but they can make referrals to community agencies that could help with job training.

2. The correct response is B: tension builds within the abuser, and he demonstrates increased anger and violent behavior without any provocation from the woman. This tension-building phase starts the cycle of violence. A is incorrect: typically the woman doesn't provoke the abuser's violent behavior, but he blames her for his lack of anger control. C is incorrect: in the honeymoon phase, the final phase in the cycle of violence, the abuser says he is sorry, he loves her, and it will never happen again. D is incorrect: in the explosion stage of the cycle of violence, the abuser physically harms the woman. This stage follows the tension-building phase.

3. The correct response is C: women with low self-esteem and limited communication skills seem more likely to become victims of abuse than those with good communication skills and assertiveness. Women possessing these skills would be able to make changes in their life and would not fall victim to abuse. A is incorrect: cooking skills have a limited impact on abusive relationships. The woman's ability to communicate and feel strong within herself will provide her with better preventive tools than her cooking skills. B is incorrect: being a good decorator will not prevent abuse. Good self-esteem and work skills will go further to help her recover from an abusive relationship than being a good homemaker. D is incorrect: improving her appearance would not prevent her from becoming a victim again if her self-esteem remains low. Improving her appearance through weight loss and exercise would, however, improve her overall health status and ability to survive her abusive past.

4. The correct response is A: this statement promotes a sense of self-worth, which may have been destroyed by her abuser in the relationship. This statement indicates to the woman that she has a lot to offer and that she shouldn't put up with this abusive behavior. The victim may not have heard this message before; her abuser may have convinced her that she did deserve the violence. B is incorrect: many children living in violent homes are abused themselves and extremely stressed. No children should live under such stressful circumstances; a two-parent household is not healthy if one is an abuser. C is incorrect: in most cases the woman doesn't trigger the abuse; rather, the abuser has limited control over his anger and does not need to be provoked before lashing out. There is not necessarily a cause-and-effect relationship between the

woman's behavior and the violence. D is incorrect: over time the abuse typically escalates rather than lessens; thus, giving the partner more time will not bring him to his senses.

Critical Thinking Exercise

a. Outline your conversation when you broach the subject of abuse with Mrs. Boggs.

Since you suspect abuse, asking a direct question about whether she feels safe in her own home might open up the conversation and allow Mrs. Boggs to talk about the situation. If she denies that there is a problem, reassure her that you care, that you are afraid for her safety, and that she deserves better. Opening the door for discussion is the first step toward change.

b. What is your role as a nurse in caring for this family in which you suspect abuse?

Allow Mrs. Boggs to know that you are there for her when she is ready to talk about her situation and that she deserves better than this. If she is unwilling to do so at this time, continue to ask screening questions about abuse on each subsequent visit. Providing her with the National Domestic Violence Hotline number might be helpful.

c. What ethical/legal considerations are important in planning care for this family?

If you notice that Mrs. Boggs has suffered acute abuse, by law you must report it. You also need to document any injuries to strengthen this case if it were to go to trial. Accurate documentation can also be used as justification for a variety of other actions, such as restraining orders, compensation, and insurance and welfare payments. You have an ethical and legal responsibility to report the abuse and assist the woman; do not ignore it and pass it off as "a private family dispute."

Study Activities

1. This website includes postings from women in abusive relationships. It may help the students grasp the extent of violence in our society and may prompt them to lobby legislators to pass stricter laws to protect the victims of abuse.
2. This exercise may help the students put the issue of domestic violence into perspective and determine whether they live in a safe state. They may also discover what interventions might help to reduce domestic violence.
3. Campus security personnel often present safety programs for women about how to protect themselves against date rape and sexual assault. This information will serve any woman well whether she lives on the campus or not.
4. This activity should provide an eye-opening experience about the frequency of calls related to domestic violence and how much time police officers spend dealing with it.

5. Three community resources that a victim of violence might need include:
   i. Women's shelters to house women and children—United Way and local funding
   ii. Law enforcement agencies for restraining orders—county and state funding
   iii. Counseling services to empower the individual—private and local funding

Chapter 10

Multiple Choice Questions

1. The correct response to this question is C, because scientists have determined that conception/fertilization occurs in the upper portion of the fallopian tube. A is an incorrect response because this is where implantation takes place after fertilization has occurred. B is an incorrect response because this describes the inner lining of the uterus, where implantation takes place, not where fertilization of the ovum and sperm occur. D is an incorrect response because the sperm does not travel outside the fallopian tube to the ovary, but rather meets the ovum for purposes of fertilization in the fallopian tube.

2. The correct response to this question is B, because hCG is secreted by the formation of the zygote after fertilization has taken place. Its presence in the maternal urine or serum signals a pregnancy has started. Its absence denotes no pregnancy. A is an incorrect response because it is not detected until weeks later, after fertilization has taken place. It is secreted by the placenta after it is formed. C is an incorrect response because FSH stimulates ovulation, but bows out once ovulation is accomplished. D is an incorrect response because TSH, although needed to support a pregnancy, has a limited affect on fertilization and its aftermath.

3. The correct response is D. Autosomal dominant inheritance occurs when a single gene in the heterozygous state is capable of producing the phenotype. The affected person generally has an affected parent, and an affected person generally has a 50% chance of passing the abnormal gene to each of his or her children.

4. The correct response to this question is C, because uncovering an individual's family history can identify previous genetic disorders that have a high risk for recurrence in subsequent generations. A is an incorrect response because observing a patient and his or her family would be costly and unproductive in diagnosing a genetic disorder; observation would have to take place over several generations to yield results. B is an incorrect response because psychological testing might not uncover genetic predispositions to disorders. D is an incorrect response because excluding the numerous genetic conditions would be a time-consuming and tedious task.

5. The correct response is C. The family history plays a critical role in identifying genetic disorders. A history of a previous child, parents, or close relative with an inherited disease, congenital abnormalities, metabolic disorders, developmental disorders, or choromosomal abnormalities can indicate an increased risk of genetic disorders; therefore, referral to genetic counseling is appropriate.

Critical Thinking Exercise

a. What information/education should this couple consider before deciding whether to have the test?

The nurse needs to outline the facts about the genetic inheritance:
- CF is a recessive disorder that affects 1 in every 2500 babies.
- It predominantly is seen in white infants and is less common in other races.
- Because it is a recessive disorder, Mrs. Martin must also be a carrier to pass it on to their offspring.
- If Mrs. Martin is a carrier, their chance of having a child with CF is one in four.
- The risk is the same each time they have a child.
- Information about the characteristics of cystic fibrosis.

b. How can you assist this couple in their decision-making process?

Start by providing all the facts about the nature of the inheritance risk. Also, outline all options so the couple can make an informed decision. Options include the following:
- The couple does not receive genetic testing and take their chances.
- If Mrs. Martin is a CF carrier, then they could choose not to have children or adopt a baby.
- Prenatal testing could be done on the fetus to determine whether both its genes carry a CF mutation. If so, the couple could elect to abort the pregnancy.
- Use an ovum or sperm from a donor who does not carry CF.
- Make a referral to a reproductive technology health facility for the couple to become educated regarding alternatives to maximize their outcome.
- Be realistic with this couple about not having any guarantees that another genetic disorder might not occur.
- Discuss the expense involved in genetic testing and in vitro fertilization, which probably will not be covered by health insurance.

c. What is your role in this situation if you do not agree with their decision?

As a nurse, your role is to provide the facts and allow the couple to make their own decision about what they wish to do. They must live with their decision, not the nurse. Your role is to respect and support whatever this couple decides to do.

Study Activities

1. The video entitled *Miracle of Life* is a wonderful visualization of conception through fetal development and birth. A photographer was able to photograph

sperm swimming and ovum being released from the ovary. He then photographed the developing embryo and fetal development through birth. It is realistic and a true wonder of life. The title depicts the images.

2. Depending on which website the student selects, the critique will vary. Most sites are very user friendly and are geared to the lay public's understanding. Students will choose their own area of interest, depending on their frame of reference. Their information would make for an educational discussion in class.

3. Students should draw their own family pedigree to identify their past health history. This information is important to determine genetic conditions and inheritable diseases. By identifying their past health ancestry, perhaps motivation for wiser lifestyle choices might surface.

4. Results will vary depending on which fetal screening test is chosen. An example might be the fetal nuchal translucency screening test. The *purpose* of the test is to identify genetic disorders and/or physical anomalies. The *procedure* involves ultrasound measurement of fluid in the nape of the neck between 10 and 14 weeks' gestation. A nuchal translucency measurement of 3 mm or more is highly suggestive of fetal abnormalities, and diagnostic genetic testing is indicated. The student playing the role of the nurse discussing this test should be very supportive but factual with the expectant couple. They can reverse roles with a different fetal screening test to discuss.

CHAPTER 11

Multiple Choice Questions

1. The correct response is B. Progesterone is an essential hormone to maintain the pregnancy and prevent early labor. Progesterone decreases systemic vascular resistance early in pregnancy, leading to a decline in blood pressure. It causes relaxation of the uterus and gastrointestinal smooth muscle, resulting in delayed gastric emptying and calming of the uterus. This relaxation mechanism is vital to reduce uterine contractions.

2. The correct response is C. Urinary frequency occurs during early pregnancy secondary to pressure on the bladder by the expanding uterus. This is one of the presumptive signs of pregnancy. Restlessness or elevated mood is not a sign of pregnancy. As hormones increase during pregnancy, the mood might change, but it is not indicative of pregnancy. Low backache is frequently experienced by many women during the third trimester of pregnancy secondary to the change in their center of gravity, but it is not a presumptive sign of pregnancy.

3. The correct response is A. The corpus luteum secretes hCG early after conception to signal that fertilization has taken place. Without fertilization, hCG is not

detected. Thus, it is the basis for pregnancy tests. hPL is the hormone secreted by the placenta to prepare the breasts for lactation. It is also an antagonist to insulin, competing for receptor sites that force insulin secretion to increase to meet the body's demands. FSH is secreted by the anterior pituitary gland to stimulate the ovary to mature an ovum for ovulation. It is not detected during pregnancy tests. LH is secreted by the pituitary gland. An increase in LH occurs immediately before ovulation and is responsible for release of the ovum. It is not the basis for pregnancy tests.

4. The correct response is A. Consuming raw meat can increase the pregnant woman's risk of picking up toxoplasmosis, a parasitic infection that can be passed on to her fetus. Although toxoplasmosis may go unnoticed in the pregnant woman, it may cause abortion or result in the birth of an infant with the disease. Uncooked shellfish may contain high levels of mercury, which can damage the fetal central nervous system. Some raw or undercooked can also be contaminated with *Listeria,* which may result in abortion, stillbirth, or severe illness of the newborn. Raw or undercooked food items should be avoided during pregnancy.

5. The correct response is D. The feeling of ambivalence is experienced by most women when they question their ability to become a mother. Feelings fluctuate between happiness about the pregnancy and anxiety and fear about the prospect of new responsibilities and a new family member. Acceptance usually develops during the second trimester after fetal movement is felt by the mother and the infant becomes real to her. Depression is not a universal feeling experienced by most women unless there is a past history of underlying depression experienced by the woman. Jealousy is not a universal feeling of pregnant women. It can occur in partners, because attention is being diverted from them to the pregnancy and the newborn.

6. The correct response is C. Seeking acceptance of self as mother to the infant is the basis for establishing a mutually gratifying relationship between mother and infant. This "binding in" is a process that changes throughout the pregnancy, starting with the mother's acceptance of the pregnancy and then the infant as a separate entity. Ensuring safe passage through pregnancy, labor, and birth focuses on the mother initially and her concern for herself. As the pregnancy progresses, the fetus is recognized and concern for its safety becomes a priority. The mother–infant relationship is not the mother's concern yet. Seeking acceptance of this infant by others includes the world around the mother and how they will integrate this new infant into their world. The infant–maternal relationship is not the focus in this task. Learning to give of oneself on behalf of one's infant focuses on delaying maternal gratification, focusing on the infant's needs before the mother's needs.

Critical Thinking Exercises

1.

a. How should the nurse answer this question?

The feelings that the woman is describing are those of ambivalence, and they are very common in women when they first learn they are pregnant. The nurse needs to explain this to the woman, emphasizing that it is common for women to question themselves in relation to the pregnancy because it is "unreal" to them during this early period. Fetal movement helps to make the pregnancy a reality.

b. What specific information is needed to support the client during this pregnancy?

The nurse can be supportive to this woman during this time by providing emotional support and validating the various ambivalent feelings she is experiencing. Including her husband and/or family members might also provide support for her.

2.

a. What explanation can the nurse offer Sally about her discomforts?

The nurse can explain in simple terms that the new embryo needs a great deal of her glucose and nutrients to grow, and thus her energy level will be affected during early pregnancy; this is why she is feeling tired frequently. The nurse can also inform her that her energy level will increase by the second trimester and she should not feel as drained.

b. What interventions can the nurse offer to Sally?

Interventions to help Sally cope with her fatigue during her early pregnancy would be for her to plan rest periods throughout the day and make sure she gets a good night's sleep daily. Taking naps on weekends to refresh her may also help her. Also, help with meal preparation would be beneficial.

3.

What strategies can a nurse discuss with a mother when she asks how to deal with this?

Strategies to integrate a new infant into the family unit would include involving the sibling in planning the nursery for the new brother or sister, answering their questions about the new infant during the pregnancy, using age-specific books to inform the sibling of the fetus' growth and development, and providing special time set aside to be with that sibling before and after the new infant arrives into the home.

Study Activities

1. Depending on the information obtained by the interview, each symptom and/or feeling can be placed on a list and matched to the appropriate trimester. For example, fatigue, breast tenderness, urinary frequency, ambivalence = first trimester. Increased energy level, less urinary frequency, fetal movement = second trimester. Backache, frequency, introspection = third trimester.

2. The student should select about three websites and present the URLs during a post conference or in a group with a thorough description of what each site has to offer.
3. physiologic anemia of pregnancy
4. compression of the vena cava by the heavy gravid uterus

CHAPTER 12

Multiple Choice Questions

1. The correct response is C: A nonreactive fetal heart rate is one of the biophysical profile findings that indicates poor oxygenation to the fetus.
2. The correct response is C: Kegel exercises help to tighten and strengthen pelvic floor muscles to improve tone. They can help prevent stress incontinence in women after childbirth. These exercises don't strengthen the perineal area on the outside to prevent lacerations, but rather the internal pelvic floor muscles. Kegel exercises have nothing to do with the start of labor for postdate infants. A drop in progesterone levels and an increase in prostaglandins augment labor, not exercise. Kegel exercises don't burn calories.
3. The correct response is D. The uterus is constantly contracting throughout pregnancy, but the contractions are irregular and not usually felt by the woman, nor do they cause dilation of the cervix. Braxton Hicks contractions are not the start of early labor, since there aren't any measurable cervical changes. They are normal throughout the pregnancy, not an ominous sign of an impending abortion. A woman's hydration status is not related to Braxton Hicks contractions; they occur regardless of her fluid status.
4. The correct response is C: the underwater pressure incurred during scuba diving may cause oxygenation changes and a decrease in perfusion to the placenta. There is also a risk of trauma from coral reefs and boating. Swimming is an appropriate sport if the woman does not swim alone or after a heavy meal. Walking is an appropriate exercise to promote well-being. Bike riding provides good leg exercise and is appropriate if safety precautions are observed.
5. The correct response is D: using Nagele's rule, 3 months are subtracted and 7 days are added, plus 1 year from the date of the last menstrual period.

Critical Thinking Exercises

1.

a. What subjective and objective data do you have to make your assessment?

Subjective data: reports feeling extreme fatigue; sleeps 8 to 9 hours each night; eats poorly.
Objective data: pale and tired appearance; pale mucous membranes, low H & H.

b. What is your impression of this woman?

She is in her first trimester of pregnancy, when fatigue is a normal complaint due to the diversion of the maternal glucose to the developing fetus. In addition, she is anemic (low H & H) due to eating habits or perhaps pica. It is important for the nurse to report this finding to the health care professional for further investigation of the cause.

c. What nursing interventions would be appropriate for this client?

Reassure her that the fatigue is a common complaint of pregnancy in the first trimester, but her poor dietary habits are contributing to her fatigue. She is anemic and needs to improve her diet and increase the amount of iron and vitamin C she takes. She also needs to increase her fiber intake to prevent constipation. An iron supplement might be advised by the health care provider to address her anemia. Request that the client keep a food log to bring with her to the next visit to review. A referral for nutritional counseling would be appropriate.

d. How will you evaluate the effectiveness of your interventions?

To assess compliance with the iron supplement, ask her what color her stools are. If they are dark, then she is taking the iron; if not, she probably isn't. Ask what dietary changes she has made to improve her nutrition by reviewing her food log and making suggestions to increase her iron consumption. Also review the importance of good nutrition for the positive outcome of this pregnancy. Do another H & H level to monitor her anemia.

2.
a. In addition to the routine obstetric assessments, which additional ones might be warranted for this teenager?

Calculate Monica's body mass index (BMI) based on height and weight (BMI = 17.8, which places her at high risk for not gaining enough weight during pregnancy). Ask Monica if she takes drugs or alcohol, which might have a negative impact on the pregnancy. Request a 24-hour diet recall, which might reveal low calorie and calcium intake. Ascertain who does the cooking and food purchasing in her house; ask that the person accompany her to the clinic for her next visit for dietary teaching. Explore reasons why she won't drink milk, and provide her with information about other sources of calcium that she might substitute for milk, such as yogurt.

b. What dietary instruction should be provided to this teenager based on her history?

Stress the importance of gaining weight for the baby's health.
Encourage her to eat three meals each day plus three high-fiber snacks.
Go over the Food Guide Pyramid with her to show her selections from each group that she needs to consume daily.
Request that she take a peanut butter and jelly sandwich on whole-wheat bread to school to make sure she eats a good lunch each day.

Instruct her on limiting her intake of sodas and caffeinated drinks.
Encourage her to drink calcium-fortified orange juice for breakfast daily.
Reinforce the importance of taking her prenatal vitamin daily.
Send her home with printed materials for review.

c. What follow-up monitoring should be included in subsequent prenatal visits?

Increase the frequency of prenatal visits to every 2 weeks to monitor weight gain for the next few months. Refer Monica and her mother to the nutritionist in the WIC program for a more thorough dietary instruction. Request a 24-hour dietary recall at each prenatal visit to provide a basis for instruction and reinforcement.

3.
a. What additional information would the nurse need to assess her complaint?

Ask Maria for a 24-hour food intake recall to assess what other food she eats.
Ask Maria if she had this problem before becoming pregnant.
Ask Maria if she takes iron supplementation in addition to her prenatal vitamin.
Ask Maria how much and what kind of fluid intake she has in 24 hours.
Ask Maria whether she engages in any exercise consistently.

b. What interventions would be appropriate for Maria?

The nurse needs to discuss with her the reasons why she is constipated: heavy gravid uterus compressing the intestines, reduced peristalsis and smooth muscle relaxation secondary to progesterone, low fiber and fluid intake, and limited exercise. To reduce the problem, Maria will need to make changes in the areas of food, fluid, and exercise.

c. What lifestyle adaptations will Maria need to make to alleviate her constipation?

Maria will need to consume high-fiber foods (fruits and vegetables) and increase her fluid intake to 2,000 mL daily to overcome the constipation. In addition, she will need to get off the couch and get some exercise, perhaps walking. Finally, she will need to stop taking stimulant laxatives and change to bulk-forming ones if the increase in high-fiber foods and fluids doesn't work for her.

Study Activities

1–4. The answers to activities 1 to 4 are highly individualized.
5. doula

CHAPTER 13

Multiple Choice Questions

1. The correct response is A. Frequency is measured from the start of one contraction to the start of the next contraction. The duration of a contraction is

measured from the beginning of one contraction to the end of that same contraction. The intensity of two contractions is measured by comparing the peak of one contraction with the peak of the next contraction. The resting interval is measured from the end of one contraction to the beginning of the next contraction.

2. The correct response is B. A longitudinal lie places the fetus in a vertical position, which would be the most conducive for a spontaneous vaginal birth. A transverse lie does not allow for a vaginal birth because the fetus is lying perpendicular to the maternal spine. A perpendicular lie describes the transverse lie, which would not be conducive for a spontaneous birth. An oblique lie would not allow for a spontaneous vaginal birth because the fetus would not fit through the maternal pelvis in this side-lying position.

3. The correct response is C. After the placenta separates from the uterine wall, the shape of the uterus changes from discoid to globular. The uterus continues to contract throughout the placental separation process and the umbilical cord continues to pulsate for several minutes after placental separation occurs. Maternal blood pressure is not affected by placental separation because the maternal blood volume has increased dramatically during pregnancy to compensate for blood loss during birth.

4. The correct response is B. Progressive cervical changes occur in true labor. This is not the case with false labor.

5. The correct response is C. The transition phase of the first stage of labor occurs when the contractions are 1 to 2 minutes apart and the final dilation is taking place. The transition phase is the most difficult and, fortunately, the shortest phase for the woman, lasting approximately 1 hour in the first birth and perhaps 15 to 30 minutes in successive births. Many women are not able to cope well with the intensity of this short period, become restless, and request pain medications. During the latent phase, contractions are mild. The women is in early labor and able to cope with the infrequent contractions. This phase can last hours. The active phase involves moderate contractions that allow for a brief rest period in between, helping the woman to be able to cope with the next contraction. This phase can last hours. The placental expulsion phase occurs during the third stage of labor. After separation of the placenta from the uterine wall, continued uterine contractions cause the placenta to be expelled. Although this phase can last 5 to 30 minutes, the contraction intensity is less than that of the transition phase.

6. The correct response is B. Cervical dilation of 6 cm indicates that the woman is in the active phase of the first stage of labor. In this phase, the cervix dilates from 3 to 7 cm with 40% to 80% effacement occurring. During the latent phase, the cervix dilates from

0 to 3 cm. During the transition phase, the cervix dilates from 8 to 10 cm. The first stage of labor is divided into three phases: latent, active, and transition. There is no early phase.

7. The correct response is C. True labor is characterized by contractions occurring at regular intervals that increase in frequency, duration, and intensity. These contractions bring about progressive cervical dilation and effacement. Thus, a cervix dilated to 4 cm and 90% effaced indicates true labor. Rupture of membranes may occur before the onset of labor, at the onset of labor, or at any time during labor and thus is not indicative of true labor. Engagement occurs when the presenting part reaches 0 station; it typically occurs 2 weeks before term in primigravidas and several weeks before the onset of labor or at the beginning of labor for multiparas. Contractions of true labor typically last 30 to 60 seconds and occur approximately every 4 to 6 minutes.

Critical Thinking Exercises

1.

a. What additional information do you need to respond appropriately?

Ask about the frequency and duration of her contractions.

Ask about how long she has experienced "labor pains."

Ask about any other signs she may have experienced such as bloody show, lightening, backache, ruptured membranes, and so forth.

Ask if walking tends to increase or decrease the intensity of contractions.

Ask her when she last felt fetal movement.

Ask her how far away (distance) she is from the birthing center.

Ask her if she has a support person in the home with her.

b. What suggestions/recommendations would you make to her?

Stay in the comfort of her home environment as long as possible.

Advise her to walk as much as possible to see what effect it has on the contractions. Also, tell her to drink fluids to hydrate herself.

Review nonpharmacologic comfort measures she can try at home.

Tell her to keep in contact with the birthing center staff regarding her experience.

c. What instructions need to be given to guide her decision making?

Instruct her on how to time the frequency and duration of contractions.

Wait until contractions are 5 minutes apart or her membranes rupture to come to the birthing center.

Tell her to come to the birthing center when she cannot talk during a contraction.

Reinforce all instructions with her support partner.

d. What other premonitory signs of labor might the nurse ask about?

Has she experienced the feeling of the fetus dropping (lightening) lower down?

Has her energy level changed (increased) in the last day or so?

Has she noticed any reddish discharge (bloody show) from her vagina?

Has she had any episodes of diarrhea within the last 48 hours?

Has her "bag of waters" broken or does she feel any leakage?

e. What manifestations would be found if Cindy is experiencing true labor?

There would be progressive dilation and effacement of her cervix if true labor is occurring. Contraction pain also would not be relieved with walking, and the pain would start in the back and radiate around toward the front of the abdomen. Contractions also would occur regularly, becoming closer together, usually 4 to 6 minutes apart, and last 30 to 60 seconds. If she is experiencing false labor, slight effacement might be present, but not dilation.

2.

Topics to address in the community education program would include:

Information about the stages of labor, including what to expect

Explanation of risks and benefits about any interventional procedures that might be performed during the labor process

Information about the available pain relief measures

Methods of involvement and participation during the labor and birthing process by partner/doula/family member

Information about variables that may alter or influence the course of labor, including preoperative teaching for cesarean birth

Study Activities

1. This discussion should involve the passenger, powers, passageway, position, and psychological response of the student's assigned women going through labor and how each affected the length and stages of labor.

2. Answers A, B, and E are correct. The cardinal movements of labor by the fetus include engagement, descent, flexion, international rotation, extension, external rotation, and expulsion only. The other choices describe the various fetal positions.

3. This discussion will vary depending on the women's labor and birth experience. Psychological factors that could be addressed might include previous birth experiences, age, pregnancy discomforts, cultural beliefs, expectations for this birth experience, preparation for birth, and effectiveness and participation of support system.

4. See the following figure. For duration, the "X" is placed at the start of one contraction and at the end of it.

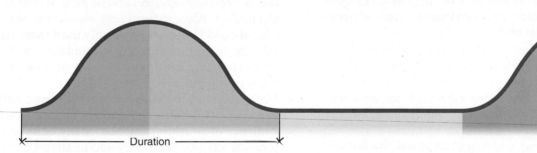

Duration

CHAPTER 14

Multiple Choice Questions

1. The correct response is D: intermittent pushing with each contraction is more effective than continuous pushing, which reduces perfusion to the placenta. Holding the breath and pushing through the entire contraction is incorrect because this action reduces blood flow and oxygenation to the uterus and to the fetus. Chest breathing is not an effective breathing pattern to increase intra-abdominal pressure, which assists the contraction to expel the fetus. Panting and blowing is used between contractions to abstain from pushing.

2. The correct response is B: a full bladder causes displacement of the uterus above it, and increased bleeding results secondary to the uncontracted status of the uterus. Massaging the uterus will help to make it firm but will not help to bring it back into the midline, since the full bladder is occupying the space it would normally assume. Notifying the primary health care provider is not necessary unless the woman continues to have difficulty voiding and the uterus remains displaced. The normal location of the uterus in the fourth stage of labor is in the midline. Displacement suggests a full bladder, which is not considered a normal finding.

3. The correct response is C: the entire focus of the labor and birth experience is for the family to make decisions, not the caretakers. The nurse's role is to respect and support those decisions. Decisions about pain management are not based on length of the various stages of labor, but rather on what provides effective pain relief for the laboring woman. Pain-relief

measures differ. Each individual responds differently and uniquely to various pain-relief measures. Not recommending nonpharmacologic measures demonstrates bias on the nurse's part; it is not the nurse's decision to make, but rather the client's.

4. The correct response is A: several professional women's health organizations have published guidelines concerning the timing of intermittent FHR assessments during the active stage of labor. The current recommendation is that intermittent FHR is assessed every 15 minutes during the active phase of labor.

5. The correct response is C: fetal accelerations denote an intact central nervous system and appropriate oxygenation levels demonstrated by an increase in heart rate associated with fetal movement. Accelerations are a reassuring pattern, so no intervention is needed. Turning the woman on her left side would be an appropriate intervention for a late deceleration pattern. Administering 100% oxygen via face mask would be appropriate for a late or variable deceleration pattern. Since fetal accelerations are a reassuring pattern, no orders are needed from the health care provider, nor does the health care provider need to be notified of this reassuring pattern.

Critical Thinking Exercises

1.

a. Based on your assessment data and the woman's request not to have medication, what nonpharmacologic interventions could you offer her?

• Progressive relaxation techniques of locating, then releasing tension from one muscle group at a time until the entire body is relaxed

• Visual imagery such as taking a journey in the woman's mind to a relaxing place that is far away from the discomfort of labor

• Music to bring about a calming effect as well as a distraction or attention focusing to divert attention away from the laboring process; focusing on sound or rhythm helps release tension and promote relaxation

• Massage/acupressure to enhance relaxation, improve circulation, and reduce pain in labor; counterpressure on the lower back to help relieve back pain

• Breathing techniques for effective attention-focusing strategies to enhance coping mechanisms during labor

b. What positions might be suggested to help facilitate fetal descent?

• Upright positions such as walking, swaying, slow-dancing with her partner, or leaning over a birthing ball will all enhance comfort and use the force of gravity to facilitate fetal descent.

• Kneeling and leaning forward will help relieve back pain.

• Pelvic rocking on hands and knees and lunging with one foot elevated on a chair may help with internal fetal rotation and speed a slow labor.

2.

a. What assessment needs to be done to determine what is happening?

The nurse should perform a vaginal examination to validate that she is in the transition phase (8 to 10 cm dilated).

b. What explanation can you offer Carrie's partner regarding her change in behavior?

Explain to her partner that she is in the transition phase of the first stage of labor and that her behavior is typical, since she is having hard contractions frequently. Reassure him not to take Carrie's comments personally, but to stay and be supportive to her.

Study Activities

1. This information will vary depending on what the woman reports to the student. Unrealistic pain-management plans need to be identified and valid evidence-based ones presented to the woman. Misconceptions can be cleared up also.

2. *Acceleration*—elevation of FHR above the baseline; a reassuring pattern

3. The findings will vary from facility to facility, but the student might find a more liberal use of nonpharmacologic techniques in the birthing center compared to the hospital setting and more frequent use of hydrotherapy and ambulation to relieve discomfort. Also, intermittent assessment using a hand-held Doppler is probably used more frequently in the birthing center compared to the hospital, where continuous electronic fetal monitoring is prevalent.

4. Many childbirth websites present very basic information about childbirth and attempt to target a wide audience of educational levels. Many of these sites promote various pregnancy and infant products.

CHAPTER 15

Multiple Choice Questions

1. The correct response is A. Engorgement refers to the swelling of the breast tissue as a result of an increase in blood and lymph supply to produce milk for the newborn. Estrogen and progesterone levels decrease considerably and are not restored until the first menses returns several weeks or months later, depending on the lactation status of the mother. Colostrum can be secreted as early as 16 weeks' gestation. The mother's body is going through profuse diuresis to restore prepregnant fluid levels to her body and therefore would not be retaining fluid in the breasts.

2. The correct response is C. According to Reba Rubin, the mother is very passive and is dependent on others

to care for her for the first 24 to 48 hours after giving birth. Gaining self-confidence would characterize a mother in the taking-hold phase, during which the mother demonstrates mastery over her own body's functioning and feels more confident in caring for her newborn. Adjustment to relationships does not occur until the third phase, letting go, when the mother begins to separate from the symbiotic relationship she and her newborn enjoyed during pregnancy and birth. Resuming control over her life would denote the second phase of taking hold, during which the mother does resume control over her life and gains self-confidence in her newborn care.

3. The correct response is D. The direct cause of afterpains is uterine contractions. Mothers experience abdominal pain secondary to contractions, especially when breast-feeding because sucking stimulates the release of oxytocin from the posterior pituitary gland, which causes uterine contractions. Manipulation of the uterus during labor would only occur during a surgical birth, and this discomfort would not be sustained weeks later. The size of the infant might cause additional stretching of the uterus, but it is not the underlying cause of the afterpains. Pregnancies spaced too close together can contribute to frequent stretching of the uterus, but this is not the cause of afterpains.

4. The correct response is B. Lochia discharge from the uterus proceeds in an orderly fashion, regardless of a surgical or vaginal birth. Its color changes from red to pink to whitish cream consistently, unless there is a complication. The correct sequence is rubra (red), then serosa (pink), and then alba (white, creamy).

5. The correct response is C. The nurse would expect light pink or brown lochia, and the uterus should be four to five fingerbreadths below the umbilicus.

6. The correct answer would be: 1, sleep and rest; 2, interaction time with the infant to facilitate bonding; 3, lessons on holding and cuddling the infant; 4, a baby bath demonstration given by the nurse.

Critical Thinking Exercises

1.

a. Is there something "wrong" with Ms Griffin's behavior? Why or why not?

No, this is typical behavior for a new mother within the first 2 days after giving birth.

b. What maternal role phase is being described by the new nurse?

This behavior is characteristic of Reba Rubin's taking-in phase, which covers the first 48 hours after childbirth. The new mother is typically focused on her own needs for rest, food, and comfort. New mothers in this phase tend to be passive and take directions/suggestions well from staff. Preoccupation with them-

selves rather than their newborns is normal during this phase. Their needs must be met before they can begin to care for others.

c. What role can the nurse play to support the mother through this phase?

The nurse can be supportive through this early phase by providing a restful, quiet environment to facilitate her recovery from childbirth. Providing her with simple guidance and suggestions of how she can care for herself and her newborn will assist the new mother in expanding her focus. Praising her for her accomplishments in care will reinforce it.

2.

a. Would you consider Mr. Lenhart's paternal behavior to be normal at this time?

Yes, inexperienced first-time fathers are anxious around their newborns because this is a new experience for them and many do not know how to handle or care for their newborns yet. Paternal attachment is a gradual process that occurs over weeks and months.

b. What might Mr. Lenhart be feeling at this time?

He is probably feeling overwhelmed with this tiny baby and, although he probably wants to help, he is anxious about how or what to do without appearing awkward.

c. How can the nurse help this new father adjust to his new role?

The nurse can help new fathers adjust to their role by taking time to listen to their concerns and demonstrating how they can become involved in the care of their newborn. Staying in the room and physically supporting the father as he tries out his new role will provide encouragement for him to become involved. The nurse can slowly introduce fathers to the care needs of their newborn and encourage their participation. This supportive role by the nurse can help reduce role strain and enhance family adjustment.

Study Activities

1. Possible Internet resources helpful to parents after childbirth are:
   a. The Center for Postpartum Health, www.postpartumhealth.com
   b. Postpartum Support International, www.chss.iup.edu/postpartum
2. The teaching plan might include the following topics:
   a. Involution of the uterus
   b. Stages and color of lochia
   c. Diaphoresis
   d. Breast changes (lactating and nonlactating)
   e. Discomforts after birth, such as perineal healing (ice packs, sitz baths), afterpains (analgesics), breast engorgement (supportive bra)
   f. Follow-up care for the mother
3. involution
4. full bladder

Chapter 16

Multiple Choice Questions

1. The correct response is C. Periodic crying and insomnia are characteristic of postpartum blues, in addition to mood changes, irritability, and increased sensitivity. Panic attacks and suicidal thoughts or anger toward self and the infant would be descriptive of postpartum psychosis, when some women turn this anger toward themselves and have committed suicide or infanticide. Women experiencing postpartum blues do not lose touch with reality. Obsessive thoughts and hallucinations would be more descriptive of postpartum psychosis.

2. The correct response is D. Nurses need first to become educated about various cultural practices to incorporate them into their care delivery. By gaining an understanding of diverse cultures different from their own, nurses can become sensitive to these different practices and not violate them. Attending a transcultural course might be beneficial, but this would take several weeks to complete and the information is needed much sooner to provide culturally sensitive care for an admitted patient and her family. Caring only for families of the nurse's cultural origin would not be possible or realistic in our global, culturally diverse population within the United States. Nurses need to care for every person regardless of their color, creed, or nationality with respect and competence. Teaching diverse cultural families Western beliefs would demonstrate ethnocentric behavior and would not be professional. Each culture needs to be respected and learned about with tolerance and understanding.

3. The correct response is B. Because weight loss is based on the principle of intake of calories and output of energy, instructing this woman to avoid high-calorie foods that yield no nutritive value and expending more energy through active exercise would result in weight loss for her. Acid-producing foods (plums, cranberries, and prunes) are typically recommended for women to prevent urinary tract infections to acidify the urine, not for weight-loss purposes. Increasing fluid intake (water) would be good for weight loss because it fills the stomach and reduces hunger sensations; however, this option does not identify which fluids should be increased. Increasing high-calorie juice and soda drinks would be counterproductive to weight-loss measures. Fluid restriction combined with a high-protein diet would increase the risk of gout and formation of kidney stones. Carbohydrates are needed by the body to make ATP and convert it to energy for cellular processes. Limiting snacks might be a good suggestion depending on which ones are selected. Raw fruits and vegetables are excellent high-fiber snacks that will help in an overall weight-loss program.

4. The correct response is C. Lactating mothers need an extra 500 calories to sustain breast-feeding. An additional 20 g of protein is also needed to help build and regenerate body cells for the lactating woman. Additional intake of carbohydrates or fiber is not suggested for lactation. An increase in fats is not recommended, nor is it needed for breast-feeding. To obtain adequate amounts of vitamins during lactation, women are encouraged to choose a varied diet that includes enriched and fortified grains and cereals, fresh fruits and vegetables, and lean meats and dairy products. An increase in vitamins via supplements is not recommended. Choosing a variety of foods from the food pyramid will provide the lactating women with adequate iron and minerals.

5. The correct response is D. A swollen, tender area on the breast would indicate mastitis, which would need medical intervention. Fatigue and irritability are not complications of childbearing, but rather the norm during the early postpartum period secondary to infant care demands and lack of sleep on the caretaker's part. Perineal discomfort and lochia serosa are normal physiologic events after childbirth and indicate normal uterine involution. Bradycardia is a normal vital sign for several days after childbirth because of the dramatic circulatory changes that take place with the loss of the placenta at birth and the return of blood back to the central circulation.

6. The correct response is A. Desiring to be in close proximity to another human being is all part of the bonding process. Bonding cannot take place with separation of individuals. Closeness is needed by the two people bonding, and not having others hold the infant. Buying or wearing expensive clothes has no emotional effect on a bonding relationship. Requesting that nurses provide care separates the parent from the infant and suggests that the parents lack the desire for closeness with their infant.

7. The correct response is C. An older sibling needs to feel they are still loved and not upstaged by the newest family member. Allowing special time for that sibling reinforces the parent's love for them also. Regression behavior is common when there is stress in that sibling's life, and punishing him brings attention to negative behavior, possibly reinforcing it. The older sibling might feel he or she is being replaced and is not wanted by the parents when he or she is sent away. Including the older sibling in the care of the newborn is a better way to incorporate the newest member into the family unit. Sharing a room with the infant could lead to feelings of displacement in the sibling. In addition, frequent interruptions during the day and night will awaken the sibling and not allow a full night's sleep or undisturbed nap.

8. The correct response is A. Home visits are usually made within the first week of discharge to assess the mother and newborn. This visit is made primarily to provide the nurse with the opportunity to recognize common biomedical and psychosocial problems or complications. Although not the primary reason, this visit also offers an opportunity to provide support and guidance to the parents in making the adjustment to the change in their lives. The home visit is not the time to complete PKU testing or complete the birth certificate.

Critical Thinking Exercises

1.

a. What is your nursing assessment of this encounter?

Nursing observations would indicate poor bonding/ attachment behaviors between mother and infant based on
- Disinterest in holding or being close to infant
- Lack of concern for infant's needs
- More concerned about phone conversation
- Negative comment about newborn ("monkey")

b. What nursing interventions would be appropriate?

Assess for risk factors in the client—age, outside family support, multiple life stressors, unrealistic expectations of newborn behaviors, level of education, family support system— and determine the client's perception of newborn behaviors and educate her about normal newborn behaviors and mothering activities needed. In addition, model parent care behaviors in caring for a newborn and ascertain the availability of any family support—extended family, neighbors, and community resources.

c. What specific discharge interventions may be needed?

Based on observations and assessment data, this client would need a referral to the discharge planner, social services department, or local health department for home visit follow-up care. Bonding/attachment behaviors are lacking, possibly placing the newborn at risk for neglect or abuse.

2.

a. Which of these assessment findings warrants further investigation?

- Tearful client pacing the floor holding her crying son
- Distended bladder upon palpation; reporting frequency
- Fundus firm and displaced to right of midline

b. What interventions are appropriate at this time and why?

It is apparent that Jennifer is overwhelmed and does not seem to be coping well with her new parenting role. She may be experiencing postpartum blues as well. She needs support during this critical period. The home care nurse needs to ascertain what family or support systems are available and make contact with them for help. Questioning Jennifer about previous crying episodes or feeling "down" recently is in order to ascertain whether she is feeling the "blues" in addition to being overwhelmed. If limited resources are available, assigning a home health aide to come daily to assist Jennifer might be needed. Counseling and active listening will be helpful during the home care visit.

The uterine fundus is displaced out of the midline as a result of a distended bladder. The bladder needs to be emptied for the uterus to assume midline positioning. Jennifer's urinary frequency may be the result of distention secondary to poor bladder tone or a developing urinary tract infection. The nurse should attempt to get Jennifer to void on her own and obtain a clean-catch urine specimen. Checking for bacteria with a chemical reagent strip ("dipstick") is appropriate. Instituting measures to promote voiding—tap water running, forcing fluids, and cranberry juice—also would be appropriate interventions. If a bacterium is found in the clean-catch urine specimen, calling Jennifer's health care provider to obtain an order for medication would be necessary. Otherwise, advising Jennifer to increase her fluid intake and voiding frequently to empty her bladder would be in order.

c. What health teaching is needed before you leave this home?

Information about postpartum blues should be discussed, emphasizing that it is benign and self-limiting. Assuring Jennifer that this is very common and allowing time for her to vent her frustrations and express her feelings can be very therapeutic. Increasing awareness about postpartum blues can bring it into focus and help her understand this event in her life. In addition, self-care and newborn care measures that allow Jennifer to rest need to be outlined. Suggesting that Jennifer nap when the baby sleeps throughout the day is a start. Attempting to cluster baby care (bathing, feeding, and dressing) might give her additional time for herself. Calling on friends and family to help out should be stressed. Other interventions would include:
- Reassurance that her mothering ability is fine and the newborn is healthy
- Referral to community home health agency to gain home health aide assistance
- Discussions concerning accepting help and support from others
- Times and dates of follow-up care appointments
- Community resources available to assist her through this time

3.

a. What response by the nurse would be appropriate at this time?

Reply in a sensitive, nonjudgmental manner that this bottle of formula has been sitting out for 3 hours since the last feeding and has not been refrigerated. It may be contaminated and would not be appropriate to feed her baby with now.

b. What action should the nurse take?

Take the old bottle of formula and tell Lisa that you will get her a fresh bottle for this feeding. Leave the room with the formula bottle and replace it with another one.

c. What health teaching is needed for Lisa prior to discharge?

A thorough explanation is needed about feeding practices, emphasizing that formula is milk and needs to be refrigerated when not being used for feeding at that time. Leaving formula sit at room temperature for long periods increases the risk of bacterial contamination and may give her infant gastroenteritis. In addition, as the infant grows, more formula will be consumed at each feeding, and making up an approximate amount that will be consumed will become easier for her to avoid waste.

Study Activities

1. How have you been feeling recently? How has your sleep been? Have you felt low in spirits and/or able to enjoy the things you usually enjoy?
2. La Leche League International: www.lalecheleague.org
3. • Wash your hands with soap and water, and dry them.
   • Fill your peribottle with warm tap water and replace the top.
   • Straddle the toilet and spray all the water from the peribottle over your perineal area.
   • Pat the area dry with a clean towel and replace your peripad from front to back.
   • Place the empty peribottle on the sink for the next time.
   • Wash your hands with soap and water before leaving the bathroom.
4. engorgement

Chapter 17

Multiple Choice Questions

1. The correct response is B. The behaviors demonstrated by the newborn, such as alertness, stabilized heart and respiratory rates, and passage of meconium are associated with the second period of reactivity. The first period of reactivity starts with a period of quiet alertness followed by an active alertness with frequent bursts of movement and crying. During the decreased responsiveness period, also called the *sleep period,* the newborn is relatively unresponsive and difficult to waken.
2. The correct response is C. Convection is loss of heat from an object to the environment. Using the portholes instead of opening the isolette door prevents rapid heat loss from the inside of the isolette. This action also protects the newborn from drafts. Evaporation is the loss of heat as water is lost from the skin to the environment. Keeping the newborn dry will prevent this type of heat loss. Conduction is the transfer of heat from one object to another when in direct contact, such as placing a newborn onto a cold scale to be weighed. Radiation is the loss of heat between objects that are not in direct contact,

such as a cold window near the newborn's isolette.
3. The correct response is D. Evaporation is the loss of heat as water is lost from the skin to the environment. Drying the newborn at birth and after bathing, keeping linens dry, and using plastic wrap blankets and heat shields will all prevent heat loss through evaporation. Placing the newborn on a warmed surface will prevent heat loss via conduction. Maintaining a warm room temperature will prevent heat loss via convection. Transporting the newborn in an isolette will prevent heat loss via radiation.
4. The correct response is A. The foramen ovale is the fetal structure within the heart that allows blood to cross immediately to the left side and bypass the pulmonary circuit. When left-side pressure gradients increase at birth, this opening closes, thereby establishing an extrauterine circulation pattern. The ductus venosus is not located in the heart; it is located between the umbilical vein and the inferior vena cava, and it shunts blood away from the liver during fetal life. The ductus arteriosus connects the pulmonary artery to the aorta to bypass the pulmonary circuit. It begins to constrict as pulmonary circulation increases and arterial oxygen tension increases. The umbilical vein, along with two umbilical arteries, is part of the umbilical cord that is cut at birth.
5. The correct answer is newborn D. Normal breathing can be described as shallow, at a rate of 36 bpm, with short periods of apnea.
6. The correct answer is C. The findings indicate a patent anus with no bowel obstruction and normal peristalsis.

Critical Thinking Exercises

1.

a. What is your impression of this behavior?

It is evident the new nurse's behaviors demonstrate a lack of awareness or knowledge about thermoregulation in newborns. Reinforcement of these principles is needed. Perhaps she needs to be reminded of newborns' inability to keep themselves warm as a result of a variety of factors, or perhaps she may feel overwhelmed with caring for more than one newborn at a time. An in-service for all nursery personnel might be a good reinforcement of this concept.

b. What principles concerning thermoregulation need to be reinforced?

All four. The nurse is subjecting the newborn to heat loss by all four methods—evaporation (bathing), radiation (leaving door open), convection (cap off), and conduction (weighing). Newborns are unable to conserve body heat and experience heat loss through four mechanisms: conduction, convection, evaporation, and radiation. Placing newborns on cold surfaces without any protection (such as a blanket or cover) will cause them to lose body heat via conduction. By exposing them while wet, such as during bathing, heat is lost through evaporation. Leaving the storage room open permits cool air flow over the newborn, allowing heat loss by convection. Placing the infant transporter near cold rooms allows for transfer of neonatal body heat via radiation.

c. How will you evaluate whether your instructions have been effective?

The effectiveness of the in-service can be evaluated by observing the behavior of the staff while caring for the newborns. Hopefully, the principles reinforced during the discussion will be applied in the handling of the newborns. For the new nurse, it would be important to observe the nurse covering the newborn when bathing, placing a warmed blanket on the scale prior to weighing, closing hallway doors to prevent drafts, and keeping a cap on the newborn's head when showing him or her to the parents. In addition, the nurse should verbalize why she is performing all these actions.

2.

A. Suction the mouth and then the nose to remove any mucus. Stimulate crying by drying the newborn immediately after birth. Assess respiratory effort to validate that it is within normal parameters. Observe for signs of respiratory distress. Auscultate chest for gas for normal gas exchange. B. Safety measures include matching identification bracelets for mother and infant; footprinting the newborn and thumbprinting the mother for identification purposes as well as prevention of abduction; handling the newborn with both hands securely to prevent dropping; positioning the newborn on his or her back to sleep; frequent handwashing when handling all newborns. C. Provide warmth by placing a hat on the newborn's head to prevent heat loss through the scalp. Take and record the newborn's axillary temperature frequently to monitor thermoregulation. Keep the newborn away from drafts and wrap in a blanket to keep warm or place under a radiant heater. After temperature stabilizes, bathe the newborn.

Study Activities

1. First period of reactivity behavior: burst of rapid, jerky movements of the extremities; sucking activity; smacking and rooting; and fine tremors of the extremities. Second period behavior: newborn's alertness gradually declines and he or she sleeps. Third period: newborns awaken and become more interactive with the environment. Movement is smoother compared with the first period of reactivity. Meconium may be passed during this period.

2. Initially the heart rate immediately on admission to the nursery would be high (120–180 bpm), but after several hours it typically will decline (120–140 bpm). The respiratory rate will be rapid (60–80 bpm), with periods of apnea lasting 5 seconds or less. After several hours, the respiratory rate will decline (30–50 bpm)

and periods of apnea will become less frequent. The temperature of the newly admitted newborn may be on the low end of normal (36.5–37° C) if there has been no hypothermia while transporting the newborn from the birthing area. After being under a radiant heat source for several hours and not exposed to drafts or moisture, the temperature should be in the mid range of temperature norms. If the temperature remains stabilized, a bath can be given.

3. American Academy of Pediatrics, www.aap.org; Neonatal Network, www.neonatalwork.com

4. evaporation

CHAPTER 18

Multiple Choice Questions

1. The correct response is D. One point would be subtracted for color (acrocyanosis) and 1 point for fair flexion of extremities. All the assessment parameters should rate 2 points, except for color and flexion. Therefore, any score except 8 points would be incorrect.

2. The correct response is D. Phototherapy reduces the bilirubin on the newborn's skin via oxidation. Phototherapy does not affect surfactant levels in the newborn's lungs, nor does it help to stabilize temperatures in the newborn. In fact, it might cause hyperthermia at times if not monitored closely. Phototherapy cannot destroy Rh antibodies attached to RBCs within the circulation.

3. The correct response is B. Vitamin K is needed for blood clotting and is a vital component of the blood-clotting cascade. The newborn's gut is sterile at birth and unable to manufacture vitamin K on its own without an outside source initially. Vitamin K has no impact on bilirubin conjugation, transport, or excretion. It is not involved in closing the foreman ovale; cutting the cord and changing gradient vascular pressures are responsible for this closure. Vitamin K has no influence over the digestive process of complex proteins.

4. The correct response is A. The eyes of newborns can be exposed to gonorrhea and/or chlamydial organisms if they are present in the mother's vagina during the birth process, possibly resulting in a severe infection and blindness. Therefore, eye prophylaxis is administered. Thrush and *Enterobacter* typically do not affect the eyes. Thrush develops in the newborn's mouth after exposure to maternal vaginal yeast infections during the birth process. Infections with *Staphylococcus* and syphilis are contracted through blood stream exposure or via the placenta and not by contact with the maternal vagina during birth. Eye treatment would not impact/treat either infectious

process. Hepatitis B and herpes are not treatable with eye ointment.

5. The correct response is C. Research has identified sleeping position and its link to SIDS. Since 1992, the AAP has recommended that all newborns be placed on their backs to sleep. This recommendation has reduced the incidence of SIDS dramatically. Respiratory distress syndrome involves a lack of surfactant in the lungs, not sleeping position. The intake of formula or juice (high lactose exposure) being allowed to sit in the infant's mouth during sleep is the cause of bottle mouth syndrome. Positioning on the back might aggravate the GI regurgitation syndrome rather than help it.

6. The correct response is D. Most newborns are started on the hepatitis B series before discharge from the hospital and receive the remaining two immunizations at 1 month and 4 to 6 months of age. The pneumococcal vaccine is given between 2 to 23 months of age, not at birth. Varicella immunization is not given until 12 to 18 months of age. Hepatitis A immunization is recommended for children and adolescents in selected states and regions and for high-risk groups. It is not a universal vaccine for all children.

7. The correct response is C. Ingestion of certain amino acids found in breast milk or formula must be accumulated in the newborn to identify a deficiency in an enzyme that cannot metabolize them. If the PKU test is done prior to 24 to 48 hours after feeding, it must be repeated after the infant has tolerated feedings for at least that length of time. Identifying hypothyroidism is not linked to ingesting protein feedings. Cystic fibrosis is a genetic inherited condition not related to protein intake. Sickle cell disease is a genetically inherited condition unrelated to protein ingestion in the newborn.

Critical Thinking Exercises

1.

a. How should the nurse respond to Ms. Scott's questions?

In a calm manner, explain to Ms. Scott that all her observations are normal variations and address each one separately:

- "Banana-shaped head"—is molding where the newborn had a slight overriding of the skull bones to navigate the bony pelvis and birth canal during the birth process
- "Mushy" feel to head—caput succedaneum, which is an edematous area of the scalp as a result of sustained pressure of the occiput against the cervix during labor and birth process
- "White spots on nose"—milia, which are plugged, distended, small, white sebaceous glands that are present in most newborns and should not be squeezed by the mother
- "Blue bruises on buttocks"—Mongolian spots, which are bluish black areas of pigmentation that are common in African-Americans and have no clinical significance, but can be mistaken for bruises

b. What additional newborn instruction might be appropriate at this time?

At this time, it might be appropriate for the nurse to unwrap the newborn and complete a thorough bedside assessment, pointing out any minor deviations to the mother and explaining their significance. This will allay any future anxiety about her newborn and will afford the opportunity to instruct Ms. Scott on various physiologic and behavioral adaptations present in her daughter.

c. What reassurance can be given to Ms. Scott regarding her daughter's appearance?

One can assume that Ms. Scott's concern is that these various normal deviations might be permanent. The nurse can identify each and provide reassurance about their approximate time of disappearance:

- Molding—transient in nature and should disappear within 72 hours
- Caput succedaneum—disappears spontaneously within 3 to 4 days
- Milia—will clear up spontaneously within the first month
- Mongolian spots—will gradually fade during the first or second year

2.

a. What impact does an infant abduction have on the family and the hospital?

The abduction of an infant is a devastating event that poses significant emotional, legal, and financial risks to both the family and the hospital. The sudden, unexpected loss of an infant followed by an infinite period of uncertainty concerning the child's well-being places the traumatized family in crisis. The hospital typically will change its security systems, policies, and procedures; heighten supervision; and increase accountability for all staff.

b. What security measure was the weak link in the chain of security?

The woman was able to pass into the hospital via the emergency room posing as a "nurse" without anyone checking her name tag. The security cameras were not working at the time of the abduction. This allowed the abductor to pass down the hall with the infant unnoticed and unrecorded. The nurses on the unit were unaware of this woman on their unit, which should not happen. There should be an alarm on the doors leading into the unit and the doors should remain locked and only be opened electronically by a staff member on the unit after the person has been identified. There was truly a breakdown of several security measures in this scenario.

c. What can hospitals do to prevent infant abduction?

Keys to infant security are awareness and education. The hospital staff should attend annual in-services on these measures and participate in a mock infant-abduction drill to heighten awareness of infant security. Specially color-coded staff badges should be worn by all obstetrics staff, and parents should be instructed not to give their newborn to anyone without that specific color badge. Parents' wristbands should match the infant's ankle and wristbands. Everyone must work together to keep all infants safe.

Study Activities

1. The discussion of newborn changes noticed will vary from student to student, depending on the interview information obtained from the new mother.
2. This discussion will vary depending on questions asked during the bath demonstration as well as each individual mother's response to it.
3. The La Leche League website is filled with helpful information with pictures to assist new mothers with breast-feeding. Each student will have his or her own opinion about how helpful the website is and what educational level it addresses.
4. The risks of neonatal circumcision include hemorrhage, infection, adhesions, dehiscence, urethral fistula, meatal stenosis, and pain. The benefits of neonatal circumcision include prevention of penile cancer, decreased incidence of UTIs and STIs, and preservation of male body consistent with father and peers where the procedure is common. Students will express their own opinions about their thoughts based on their value systems and cultural backgrounds.

CHAPTER 19

Multiple Choice Questions

1. The correct response is A. Magnesium sulfate is a central nervous system depressant that interferes with calcium uptake in the cells of the myometrium, thus reducing the muscular ability to contract. Magnesium sulfate is not used as supplementation during pregnancy because most pregnant women do not have a deficiency of this mineral. Magnesium sulfate would not be effective against constipation in pregnant women. Magnesium sulfate does not stimulate musculoskeletal tone to augment labor contractions; rather, it has the opposite effect.
2. The correct response is B. When the placenta separates from the uterine wall, it causes irritation and bleeding into the muscle fibers, which causes pain. Painless, bright-red bleeding indicates placenta previa symptomatology. Excessive nausea and vomiting would be characteristic of hyperemesis gravidarum. Hypertension and headache would be associated with gestational hypertension.
3. The correct response is A. Any time there is a pregnancy with the chance of maternal and fetal blood mixing, RhoGAM is needed to prevent sensitization or antibody production. Head injury resulting from a car crash is not a situation in which there would be mixing of fetal or maternal blood. The trauma would cause hemorrhage, but not a sensitization reaction. A blood transfusion after hemorrhage would require typing and cross-matching of the client's blood; thus, she

would receive blood with her own Rh factor, not one with Rh-positive blood. Because the artificial insemination procedure was unsuccessful, no pregnancy occurred and RhoGAM would not be necessary.
4. The correct response is C. The woman should avoid noxious stimuli such as strong flavors, odors, or perfumes because they might trigger nausea and vomiting.
5. The correct response is B. an inevitable abortion is characterized by vaginal bleeding that is greater than slight, rupture of membranes, cervical dilation, strong abdominal cramping, and possible passage of products of conception. The threatened abortion involves slight vaginal bleeding, no cervical dilation and no change in cervical consistency, mild abdominal cramping, a closed cervical os, and no passage of fetal tissue. An incomplete abortion involves intense abdominal cramping, heavy vaginal bleeding, and cervical dilation. A missed abortion involves the absence of contractions and irregular spotting with possible progression to inevitable abortion.

Critical Thinking Exercises

1.
a. What is your impression of this condition?
From her history, it appears she has hyperemesis gravidarum, because she is beyond the morning sickness time frame (6–12 weeks) and her symptoms are continual.

b. What risk factors does Suzanne have?
Her risk factors include young age and primigravida status.

c. What intervention is appropriate for this woman?
- Question Suzanne further concerning previous eating patterns and food intake.
- Ask what measures she has used at home to stop the nausea and vomiting.
- Consult the health care provider concerning hospitalization of Suzanne for IV therapy to correct hypovolemia and electrolyte imbalances.
- If home care is in order, advise her to avoid the intake of greasy or highly seasoned foods and to separate food from fluid intake; instruct her on antiemetic medication ordered and possible side effects; and instruct her to return to the clinic if symptoms do not subside within 48 hours.

2.
a. What risk factors does Gloria have that increase her risk for gestational hypertension?
Gloria is a primigravida with a family history of preeclampsia (her sister). She also is an obese woman who is older than 35 years of age. Her diet of fast foods is most likely inadequate in nutritional content. She is also African-American.

b. When assessing Gloria, what assessment findings would lead the nurse to suspect that Gloria has developed severe preeclampsia?

With severe preeclampsia, blood pressure is higher than 160/110 mm Hg on two occasions at least 6 hours apart, proteinuria is greater than 500 mg in 24 hours, and oliguria (less than 500 mL in 24 hours) is present. Other assessment findings may include pulmonary edema, cerebral or visual disturbances (altered level of consciousness, headache, blurred vision, and scotomata), hyperreflexia, and epigastric or right upper quadrant abdominal pain. Laboratory test findings would include increased hematocrit, creatinine, and uric acid levels, thrombocytopenia, and elevated liver enzymes.

Study Activities

1. Hopefully the signs and symptoms would be taught to women during their first trimester, and written material would be handed out too. During each prenatal visit, the information should be reinforced to make sure women understand what they are and what to do about them if they should occur.
2. Appropriate Internet sites might include Sidelines High Risk Pregnancy Support Office (www.sidelines.org) and Resolve through Sharing (http://www.ectopicpregnancy.com).
3. ectopic
4. choriocarcinoma
5. Various activities for the woman on prolonged bed rest at home could include watching TV, reading, visiting computer sites with chat rooms, talking on the telephone, playing cards or engaging in crafts, having visitors in frequently, and completing educational courses online. The woman could also use the time to develop lists for managing the house while on bed rest, read or play games with her other children, and expand her knowledge related to the upcoming birth of her babies.

CHAPTER 20

Multiple Choice Questions

1. The correct response is B: levels of the hormone hPL (insulin antagonist) progressively rise throughout pregnancy, and additional insulin is needed to overcome its resistance. Having a carbohydrate craving is not associated with gestational diabetes. Hyperinsulinemia in the fetus develops in response to the mother's high blood glucose levels. Glucose levels are diverted across the placenta for fetal use, and thus maternal levels are reduced in the first trimester. This lower glucose level doesn't last throughout the gestation, just the first trimester. For the remaining two trimesters, the maternal glucose levels are high because of the insulin resistance caused by hPL.
2. The correct response is D: a pregnant woman with asthma who is having an acute exacerbation will be poorly oxygenated, and thus perfusion to the placenta is compromised. Immediate treatment is needed for her well-being as well as that of the fetus. Corticosteroids are used as a first-line drug therapy for asthma treatment and management because of their anti-inflammatory properties. Having asthma has no influence on the woman's glucose levels, unless she also has diabetes. Bronchodilators usually are inhaled, not given subcutaneously, so instruction about this route of administration would not be necessary.
3. The correct response is B: extreme nausea and vomiting as part of hyperemesis gravidarum would cause fluid and electrolyte imbalances and would alter blood glucose levels tremendously. With placenta previa, the placenta is dislocated, not malfunctioning; it would not have as much of an impact on the pregnancy as would an imbalance of fluids and electrolytes. Abruptio placentae would place the mother at risk for hemorrhage, but the placenta does not govern the blood glucose levels of the mother. Rh incompatibility affects the fetus, not the mother, by causing hemolysis of the red blood cells in the fetus. This process would not influence the mother's glucose levels.
4. The correct response is C: alcohol ingested by the woman during pregnancy is teratogenic to the fetus, and the newborn can be born with fetal alcohol spectrum disorder. Drinking alcohol would decrease production of dehydrogenase, an enzyme that mobilizes the hydrogen of a substrate so that it can pass it to a hydrogen acceptor. Becoming intoxicated faster during pregnancy is not the underlying problem associated with alcohol ingestion and pregnancy. The woman's genetic makeup, how much alcohol is ingested, her amount of body fat, metabolic rate, and ingestion of food are a few of the factors that determine the metabolism of alcohol. Alcohol contains calories and if enough is ingested along with food, weight gain would occur, not weight loss.
5. The correct response is B: the highest percentage of HIV transmission results from sexual activity, followed by intravenous drug use. Transmission can occur despite a low viral load in the blood of the infected person. Pregnant women who take antiretroviral therapy during their gestation significantly reduce the chances of transmitting HIV to their newborn. The use of standard precautions will minimize the risk of transmission of HIV to health care workers. A very small percentage of nurses contract HIV through needlesticks if using appropriate precautions.

Critical Thinking Exercises

1.

a. What additional information will you need to provide care for her?

• Explore her typical daily dietary intake.
• Ask her if there is a family history of diabetes mellitus.

- Take her vital signs, weight, and fetal heart rate.
- Assess her coping abilities and capacity for managing diabetes.
- Assess her knowledge of the disease process and lifestyle changes needed.
- Ask her about symptoms of fatigue, polyuria, polyphagia, and polydipsia.
- Ask about previous pregnancy outcomes and the weight of infants.

b. What education will she need to address this new diagnosis?

- Dietary modifications to reduce the amount of simple sugars and carbohydrates
- Thorough explanation of potential complications of diabetes in pregnancy:
  - Infection: urinary tract infections and monilial vaginitis
  - Difficult labor and birth: shoulder dystocia, birth trauma, cesarean section
  - Congenital anomalies: cardiac, CNS, and skeletal anomalies
- Literature describing diet, exercise, and glucose monitoring
- Outline of hypoglycemia and hyperglycemia symptoms
- Referral to nutritionist for diet planning

d. How will you evaluate the effectiveness of your interventions?

- Schedule more frequent prenatal visits to evaluate her health status.
- Evaluate glucose values at each visit to validate that they are in the normal range.
- Monitor HbA1C to determine past glucose levels.

2.
a. What is your first approach with the client to gain her trust?

Open the conversation by asking questions about school activities and her friends. Remain nonjudgmental and bring the discussion to general questions about her monthly cycles. Finally work toward questions about when she last had her period, and assess how many months pregnant she is. Adolescents usually deny a pregnancy for several months, so she may be well into her second trimester.

b. List the client's educational needs during this pregnancy.
- Signs and symptoms of preterm labor
- Nutritional needs during pregnancy
- Need for prenatal care throughout pregnancy
- Importance of early detection of complications
- Decision about whether to involve her partner
- Reasons for the frequency of prenatal visits and importance of keeping them
- Symptoms of sexually transmitted infections
- Impact of substance abuse on fetal growth and development
- Childbearing and parenting classes
- Infant growth and development and newborn care

c. What prevention strategies are needed to prevent a second pregnancy?

- Ask about her educational goals and encourage her to complete school; perhaps refer her for vocational counseling.
- Identify her personal strengths and reinforce positive self-esteem.
- Actively involve her in her care at each visit and praise her for her efforts.
- Discuss family planning methods appropriate for her and let her decide.
- Enhance a positive perception of her ability to succeed in life.

3.
a. What aspects of this woman's history may lead the nurse to suspect that this infant is at risk for fetal alcohol spectrum disorder?

- Lack of prenatal care
- History of substance abuse (alcohol) during previous pregnancies
- Children placed in foster care from birth due to poor mothering ability
- Appearance on arrival and evidence of being malnourished
- Statement about not having any "recent" use of alcohol
- Delivery of newborn weighing 4 lb

b. What additional screening or laboratory tests might validate your suspicion?

Screening questionnaires can be used to diagnose problem drinking, along with a drug screen (urine or blood) of both her and the newborn to identify specific substances present. The social service agency can also be called to do a more thorough history on this woman.

c. What physical and neurodevelopmental deficits might present later in life if the infant has fetal alcohol spectrum disorder?

The infant might have attention-deficit/hyperactivity disorder (ADHD), poor impulse control, learning disabilities, and communication problems, as well as growth restriction/developmental problems. It is important to address this woman's alcohol dependence by offering care options such as addiction treatment, mental health therapy, and support. As a nurse, it is important to be sensitive to the client's cultural, spiritual, religious, and emotional needs during this time. Discussion of effective contraception while she is struggling with her addiction is important to prevent fetal alcohol spectrum disorder.

Study Activities

1. Responses will vary based on the woman's preexisting condition. Common themes might be changes in activity level if the woman interviewed has one of the anemias or hypertension and dietary modifications if she is diabetic; all might express concern about the pregnancy outcome.

2. This study activity is one that many college students can relate to. Confronting the friend who is in denial is the most effective way to bring the issue up. Back it up with observed behaviors that demonstrate the friend's drug or alcohol dependency. Telling the person that you care about her and her well-being can go a long way toward modifying her behavior.

3. The answers will vary depending on which side the student takes. Some of the common themes might center on civil rights and the positive aspects marijuana has had on nausea and vomiting for cancer patients and controlling glaucoma pressure. On the other side of the debate, allowing this drug to be legalized might afford many pregnant women access to it, without long-term research studies to document effects on offspring.

4. The nurse should present the facts that taking the medications will reduce the risk of transmission of HIV and should discuss how the woman and her newborn will benefit from them. Stressing the importance of lowering her viral load throughout her pregnancy and relating it to her well-being might help. Presenting her with the facts is all that the nurse can do, since the final decision will be the woman's.

5. A, B, C, E, and F. Women with all the infections listed except HIV can choose to breastfeed. An HIV-positive woman can pass the virus to her newborn through breast milk and should be discouraged from breastfeeding.

Chapter 21

Multiple Choice Questions

1. The correct response is D: fetopelvic disproportion is defined as a condition in which the fetus is too large to pass through the maternal pelvis. Cervical insufficiency would lead to an abortion, typically in the second trimester, when the heavy gravid uterus would cause pressure on the weakened cervix. A contracted pelvis might cause passageway problems, but if the fetus was small, no problem might occur. Maternal disproportion doesn't indicate where the disproportion is located.

2. The correct response is B: herpes exposure during the birth process poses a high risk for mortality to the neonate. If the woman has active herpetic lesions in the genital tract, a surgical birth is planned to avoid this exposure. Hepatitis is a chronic liver disorder, and the fetus if exposed would at most become a carrier; a surgical birth would not be expected for this woman. Toxoplasmosis is passed through the placenta to the fetus prior to birth, so a cesarean birth would not prevent exposure. HPV would be manifest clinically by genital warts on the woman, and a surgi-

cal birth would not be anticipated to prevent exposure unless the warts caused an obstruction.

3. The correct response is A: having a fetus in a posterior position would cause intense back pain secondary to the fetal head facing the maternal vertebra and causing pressure. Leg cramps are common during pregnancy and not caused by an occiput posterior position, but rather pressure from the heavy gravid uterus toward term. Fetal position would not contribute to nausea and vomiting. Going through transition in labor might cause nausea and vomiting, not the fetal position. A precipitous birth occurs rapidly and is not associated with intense back pain.

4. The correct response is D. Women with a history of preterm birth are at the highest risk for the same in subsequent pregnancies. Having had twins previously would have no bearing on this singleton pregnancy to influence preterm labor. Location of residence is not a risk for preterm labor. The woman's occupation as a computer programmer would not increase her risk of preterm labor. However, standing for long periods in a work environment might increase her risk.

5. The correct response is D: prostaglandins soften and thin out the cervix in preparation for labor induction. Although they do irritate the uterus, they aren't as effective as oxytocin in stimulating contractions. Prostaglandin gel would stimulate cervical nerve receptors rather than numb them. Prostaglandins have no power to prevent cervical lacerations.

6. The correct response is C: hypotonic labor typically occurs in the active phase; it involves ineffective contractions to evoke cervical dilation and causes secondary inertia. Hypertonic labor is characterized by painful, high-intensity contractions that usually occur in the latent phase. A precipitous labor occurs within 3 hours and cervical dilation is very fast secondary to effective, high-intensity contractions. Dysfunctional labor describes any pattern that doesn't produce dilation and effacement in a timely manner.

Critical Thinking Exercises

1.

a. Based on the nurse's findings, what might you suspect is going on?

Since Marsha is multiparous and is in the active phase of labor without progression and the contraction pattern has become less intense, a hypotonic uterine dysfunction should be suspected.

b. How can the nurse address Marsha's anxiety?

Give her, in an easily understood manner, facts about dysfunctional labor. Outline expected treatment and outcome.

Encourage questions and expression of feelings. Identify how this dysfunctional labor pattern may alter her labor plan. Reassure Marsha about the status of her fetus. Maintain a positive attitude about her ability to cope with this situation.

c. What are the appropriate interventions to change this labor pattern?

Typically some form of labor augmentation is initiated to produce more effective contractions to facilitate cervical dilatation—rupture of membranes or use of IV oxytocin to stimulate the intensity of contractions. If neither one of these interventions changes the hypotonic pattern, a surgical birth is in order.

2.
a. What might be occurring?

Based on Marsha's description, the nurse might suspect spontaneous rupture of membranes.

b. How will the nurse confirm the suspicions?

Depending on the agency protocol, the nurse may perform or assist with a sterile speculum examination to observe for evidence of fluid pooling in the posterior vagina, any discharge present, inflammation or lesions, or protrusion of the membranes through the cervix. The nurse should also document the amount, color, and consistency of any fluid found during the examination.

c. What interventions are appropriate for this finding?

- Obtain a baseline set of vital signs to assess FHR patterns for changes possibly indicating a prolapsed umbilical cord.
- Use Nitrazine paper to test for the presence of amniotic fluid: it will turn blue in the presence of amniotic fluid because it is alkaline.
- Examine a sample of fluid from the vagina under the microscope for a fern pattern once it dries.

Study Activities

1. This international website offers numerous educational and personal testimonies to assist parents who have suffered a perinatal loss. There are listings of local support groups in which they can participate.
2. Maternal/fetal risks associated with a prolonged pregnancy include maternal exhaustion, psychological depression, macrosomia, dysmaturity syndrome, fetal hypoxia, meconium aspiration syndrome, hypoglycemia, and stillbirth.
3. dystocia

CHAPTER 22

Multiple Choice Questions

1. The correct response is C: it is important to assess the situation before intervening. In addition, checking the bladder status and emptying a full bladder will correct uterine displacement so that effective contractions to stop bleeding can occur. Assessment of the situation is needed before the nurse can notify the health care provider. At this point, the nurse has no facts to report about the client's condition. Magnesium sulfate would relax the uterus and increase bleeding. Pallor and heavy bleeding are not normal findings during the postpartum period.
2. The correct response is A: psychotic persons tend to lose touch with reality and frequently attempt to harm themselves or others. This behavior may occur when a woman experiences postpartum psychosis. Anxiety typically does not induce hallucinations or cause a person to want to harm herself or others. Depression involves feelings of sadness rather than hallucinations or thoughts of harming herself or others. Feeling "down," but not to the extreme of wanting to harm herself or her newborn, is suggestive of postpartum blues.
3. The correct response is D: hemorrhage is possible if the uterus cannot contract and clamp down on the vessels to reduce bleeding. When the placenta is expelled, open vessels are then exposed and the risk of hemorrhage is great. Thrombophlebitis typically is manifested later in the postpartum period rather than within the first few hours after birth. Infection usually is manifested 24 to 48 hours after birth, not within the first few hours.
4. The correct response is C: applying compresses and giving analgesics would be helpful in providing comfort to the woman with painful breasts. Treatment for mastitis encourages frequent breastfeeding to empty the breasts. Lanolin applied to the breasts will have little impact on mastitis other than to keep them moist. Binding both breasts will not bring relief; in fact, it could cause additional discomfort. Emptying the breasts frequently through breastfeeding would be helpful. Although wearing a nursing bra will help support the heavy breasts and fresh air is helpful to prevent cracked nipples, these are ineffective once mastitis develops.
5. The correct response is C. A boggy uterus that is midline and above the umbilicus suggest that the uterus is not contracting properly. Therefore, the nurse should massage the fundus to aid in stimulating the uterine muscles to contract. In addition, the nurse should assess the client's lochia. Vital signs are taken once fundal massage has been initiated. Monitoring uterine output is important to evaluate the woman's fluid balance, but this would have no effect at all on alleviating the current situation. Since the uterus is midline, it is unlikely that a full bladder is the cause. Notifying the woman's obstetrician would be necessary if fundal massage did not alleviate the problem.

6. The correct response is D. Methergine can cause hypertension. Therefore, if the woman's blood pressure was already elevated, the nurse would need to question the order for the drug. Typically if methergine is ordered, her lochia flow would be increased, not minimal. Methergine is not used to treat mastitis, which would be evidenced by tender, inflamed breasts. A pulse rate of 68 beats per minute is not an unusual finding and would not be a reason to question the order.

Critical Thinking Exercises

1.

a. What postpartum complication is this new mother at highest risk for? Why?

Postpartum infection would be the highest risk for this client because of the risk factors present: anemia, prolonged ruptured membranes, prolonged labor before a surgical birth with an incision, the likelihood of frequent vaginal examinations during the prolonged labor, and the use of internal fetal monitoring devices.

b. What assessments need to be done to detect this complication?

Monitor the client for signs of early infection: fever, malaise, abdominal pain, foul-smelling lochia, boggy uterus, tachycardia, and anorexia. Test results would indicate an elevated white blood cell count and sedimentation rate. Assessment of her incision for drainage and approximation of edges should be done frequently.

c. What nursing measures will the nurse use to prevent this complication?

• Adhere to strict aseptic technique in providing nursing care to the incision.
• Instruct the client about self-care measures to help prevent infection such as handwashing, perineal hygiene, wiping from front to back, and hydration.
• Complete a thorough "BUBBLE=HE" assessment and record findings.
• Urge the client to change her peripads frequently and use the peri-bottle.
• Reinforce home care instructions to continue infection prevention.

2.

a. What factors place Tammy at risk for postpartum hemorrhage?

Tammy is a grand multipara with nine previous pregnancies, and thus her uterus has been stretched repeatedly with close pregnancies. She also had an epidural during labor and therefore has limited sensation to her bladder.

b. What assessments are needed before planning interventions?

If Tammy's fundus is boggy (uterine atony) and her bladder is full, intervention is needed to promote voiding. If the fundus is firm and her bladder is empty, additional evaluation is needed to rule out lacerations or retained placental fragments as a causative factor contributing to her heavy vaginal bleeding.

c. What nursing actions are needed to prevent a postpartum hemorrhage?

After the assessment is completed and the uterus is found to be boggy and the bladder is full, the next step is to get the client up to void. After Tammy empties her bladder, reassess the fundus for firmness and location. With a full bladder, the uterus is typically displaced to the right of the midline. After emptying the bladder, the fundus should return to the midline and be firm. As a result, bleeding should decrease.

3.

a. What factors/behaviors place Lucy at risk for an affective disorder?

Lucy had a previous episode of postpartum depression. Her behavior indicates limited interest in her newborn and herself by not providing care. She reports she is disappointed in the sex of this child. Lucy's inactivity and lack of appetite are also problematic since she will be going home and needs to care for herself and her newborn.

b. Which interventions might be appropriate at this time?

In a sensitive, caring manner, the nurse should approach Lucy and ask her questions to get a complete picture of her emotional status. Demonstrating concern and care might encourage Lucy to express her feelings about her situation and the newborn. Using therapeutic communication through open-ended questions might assist in gathering data. Notifying the health care provider of the findings is also crucial.

c. What education does the family need prior to discharge?

The family needs information on postpartum emotional disorders and referrals to community counseling centers to assist Lucy through this time. Providing the family with the addresses of websites that offer assistance and information about emotional disorders might also be helpful. A good social support network of family and friends will be needed to care for both Lucy and her newborn initially when she is discharged.

Study Activities

1. *Postpartum blues* are usually self-limiting and benign, occurring a few days after childbirth and ending within 2 weeks. The woman cries easily, is irritable, and is more emotionally labile than normal. This emotional disorder usually resolves without specific treatment other than reassurance and support from the family. *Postpartum depression* occurs within 6 months after childbirth and is similar to other depressive disorders. The woman feels inadequate as

a parent and has disturbances in appetite, mood, sleep, concentration, and energy. Psychotherapy and antidepressants are helpful to address this disorder, which may take months to resolve. Family patience and support are very important for her. *Postpartum psychosis* may result in suicidal or homicidal behavior and requires immediate medical and psychiatric intervention. Clinical manifestations include hallucinations, delusions, or both within 3 weeks after giving birth. Inpatient psychiatric services may be needed for this severe emotional disorder.

2. Students will offer varying opinions based on the website they select.

3. The information obtained from this interview will vary depending on the woman's experience. It is hoped that some of the comments about helpfulness will center on a nurse who was present and provided assistance to her.

4. uterine atony

5. Information the nurse needs to care for this mother and her newborn should include vital signs, fundal assessment (firm or boggy and location), lochia characteristics (color, amount, smell, consistency), appearance of perineum (episiotomy site, lacerations, swelling, bruising), breast status (wearing a soft, supportive bra; any nipple problems), and elimination status (empty or not voiding).

CHAPTER 23

Multiple Choice Questions

1. The correct response is C: a postterm infant is one born after the 42nd week of gestation. Birth between 38 and 41 weeks is considered within a normal range for a term newborn. A gestation of 44 weeks would be considered extremely long if the dates were calculated correctly.

2. The correct response is A: the fetus's body, in an attempt to compensate for the low oxygen level, produces more red blood cells to carry the limited amount of oxygen available. Thus, polycythemia will be present at birth in a fetus experiencing hypoxia in utero. Hypoglycemia is typically caused by inadequate stores of glycogen and overuse while living in a hostile environment. Low serum calcium levels are associated with perinatal asphyxia and not an increase in red blood cells. Hypothermia is associated with a decrease in body fat, particularly brown fat stores, and is not linked to increased production of red blood cells.

3. The correct response is B: subcutaneous and brown fat stores may be used by the stressed fetus to survive in utero and thus will not be available to provide extrauterine warmth. Excessive red blood cell breakdown is responsible for hyperbilirubinemia, not the breakdown of brown fat stores. Polycythemia is caused by a buildup of red blood cells in response to a hypoxic state in utero; it is not linked to loss of subcutaneous and brown fat stores. Glycogen stores are used for survival in an environment with depleted glycogen and are unrelated to brown fat stores.

4. The correct answer is D. When a newborn is born too soon, fetal circulation may persist into extrauterine life. The ductus arteriosis and foramen ovale may remain open if pulmonary vascular resistance remains high and oxygen levels remain low. This would be manifested by a heart murmur.

5. The correct response is C: the parents need to validate the experience of loss. The best way to do this is to encourage them to participate in their newborn's care so that the grieving process can take place. Avoiding the experience of loss inhibits the grieving process. Avoidance prolongs the experience of loss and does not allow the parents to vent their feelings so that they can progress through their grief. It is not the nurse's responsibility, nor is it healthy for the family, to take over decisions for a family. Family members need to support each other and need to decide what is best for their situation. Leaving the family alone can be viewed as abandonment; privacy is important, but leaving them totally alone is not therapeutic.

6. The correct response is A, B and C. Minimal handling, maintaining a neutral thermal environment, and decreasing environmental stimuli are important measures to conserve energy in newborns with variations in birth weight and gestational age. Feeding and digestion will increase energy demands. Thermal warmers may produce hypothermia and thus increase energy demands. Preventing parents from visiting their newborn is not a plan to reduce energy expenditure and could increase stress for both parents and newborn.

7. The correct response is C. Newborns feel pain and require the same level of pain assessment and pain management as adults. Pain assessment, which is comprehensive, involves observations of changes in vital signs, behavior, facial expression, and body movement. It is considered the "fifth vital sign" and should be checked as frequently as the other four signs. All newborns experience pain, not just those undergoing surgical procedures. Preterm newborns have an increased risk of pain because they are subjected to repeat procedures and exposed to noxious stimuli.

Critical Thinking Exercises

1.

a. What might these behaviors indicate?

These behaviors are clinical signs of hypoglycemia, which is common in a postterm infant after a difficult birth; glycogen stores are depleted secondary to chronic placental insufficiency.

b. For what other conditions might this newborn be at high risk?

Besides hypoglycemia, hypothermia, polycythemia, meconium aspiration, and hyperbilirubinemia are common in the post-term infant.

c. What intervention is needed to address this newborn's condition?

Feed the newborn as early as possible, or administer glucose/glucagon to counter the low blood glucose level. Decrease energy requirements to conserve glucose and glycogen stores. Maintain a neutral thermal environment to prevent cold stress, which can exacerbate the hypoglycemia.

2.

a. What might have contributed to this newborn's hypothermic condition?

The simple fact that the newborn was premature predisposes him to thermal instability because of his larger surface-to-weight ratio, immature muscle tone and decreased muscular activity to generate heat, diminished stores of subcutaneous and brown fat, and poor nutritional intake, which makes him unable to meet energy requirements for growth and development. In addition, placing the isolette close to the door might produce cold drafts, causing hypothermia.

b. What transfer mechanism may have been a factor?

This preterm newborn could experience loss of heat by convection (heat transfer via air currents).

c. What intervention would be appropriate for the nurse to initiate?

Bundle or nest the preterm newborn with warmed blankets and move the isolette away from the door to prevent heat loss by convection. Place a knitted cap on the newborn's head and monitor his temperature frequently.

3.

a. What complication might this SGA newborn be manifesting?

The signs indicate polycythemia, which is common in SGA infants.

b. What factors may have contributed to this complication?

In SGA infants, polycythemia is thought to be secondary to chronic hypoxia in utero, with resulting erythropoietin production. Complications of polycythemia are related to the increased viscosity of blood, which interferes with organ circulation.

c. What would be an appropriate intervention to manage this condition?

Obtain a venous hematocrit measurement within 4 to 6 hours after birth to validate this condition, since its manifestations are very similar to those of hypoglycemia. Hematocrit values over 65% should be brought to the health care provider's attention. Typically it is treated by a dilutional exchange transfusion.

Study Activities

1. Answers will vary depending on parents interviewed.
2. The March of Dimes web site is full of ideas on how to prevent preterm births, which include early prenatal care for all women, diagnostic tests to detect changes in the cervix, and prevention of maternal infections. The students' comments may center on the inaccessibility of health care, which precludes some pregnant women from receiving early prenatal care, and the lack of insurance to cover the cost of diagnostic tests or prescriptions for treatment of infections.
3. hypoglycemia
4. clavicle fractures, facial palsies, and brachial plexus injuries.

CHAPTER 24

Multiple Choice Questions

1. The correct response is D: nasal flaring is a cardinal sign of air hunger in respiratory distress syndrome. When an infant becomes hypoxic due to poor lung expansion, the nares expand to "search" for more oxygen to relieve the low oxygen concentration. Abdominal distention denotes air in the intestines, not hypoxia. Acrocyanosis is present only in the extremities and might indicate sluggish circulation. An infant with respiratory distress syndrome would demonstrate generalized cyanosis secondary to hypoxemia. Depressed fontanels would indicate dehydration, not respiratory distress syndrome.
2. The correct response is C: irritability is a prime symptom of drug withdrawal in newborns. As they experience physiologic withdrawal from the addictive substance, irritability with crying and the inability to be consoled are prevalent behaviors. Newborns exposed to substances are anything but calm when withdrawing from an addictive substance. They are extremely distressed, and their faces commonly exhibit that distress. Weight loss, not weight gain, is typical of the newborn exposed to substances. Although they show signs of hunger, vomiting is common and thus weight loss follows. These newborns are extremely distressed and agitated. Their feeding and sleeping patterns are disrupted and would not be described as normal.

3. The correct response is D: the newborn with this anomaly cannot handle oral secretions since the esophagus ends in a blind pouch. The secretions typically foam out of the mouth, and this becomes a clue that a fistula exists. A tracheoesophageal fistula alone doesn't affect the newborn's temperature unless an infection is present. This defect is structural, not neurologic. The newborn's ability to swallow is not related to this structural defect. There would have to be an insult to the CNS for swallowing to be affected as well as a structural defect in the pharynx.

4. The correct response is A. Transient tachypnea is commonly seen in newborns who have been born by cesarean birth. Passage through the birth canal during a vaginal birth compresses the thorax, helping remove the fluid from the fetus' lungs. This mechanism is lost with a cesarean birth. Sedation is also implicated as a contributing factor to the development of transient tachypnea. Prolonged labor, macrosmia of the fetus, and maternal asthma and smoking have also been associated with a higher incidence of this condition. Maternal heart disease and small for gestational age status are not associated with transient tachypnea.

5. The correct response is C. Instructions for the parents of a child with a cleft lip and palate should include burping the infant frequently during feedings to reduce the risk of aspiration and vomiting; feeding the infant in an upright position to prevent aspiration; limiting feeding sessions to avoid overfatigue; and using high-calorie formulas to improve caloric intake.

6. The correct response is D. An infant with developmental hip dysplasia would demonstrate an audible clunk when abducting the hip. Other findings would include asymmetric thigh folds, unequal knee height, and limited abduction of the hip.

Critical Thinking Exercises

1.

a. What in the mother's history should raise a red flag to the nurse?

Prolonged rupture of the membranes provides an avenue for bacteria to ascend into the mother's genital tract. The fact that she had a fever during labor is a key sign.

b. What condition is this newborn at high risk for?

Neonatal sepsis would be a likely diagnosis based on the mother's history and the nonspecific clinical manifestations in the newborn.

c. What interventions are appropriate for this condition?

The nurse should document the assessment findings and report them to the pediatrician so that cultures and blood work can be started to identify the offending organism. General antibiotic therapy is typically started until the offending organism is identified.

2.

a. What additional information do you need to obtain from the mother?

It is important to understand the extent and type of her drug use during pregnancy. Ask specific questions about her drug use so that you can plan care for her as well as her newborn. Place her at ease and ask direct, nonjudgmental questions.

b. What additional laboratory work might be needed for Terry?

Due to an increased risk of HIV in injection drug users, an HIV test along with a polydrug screen is needed. The mother's consent must be obtained prior to the HIV testing.

c. What specific measures need to be made for her ongoing care?

After extensive counseling regarding the perinatal risks due to her heroin use, referral to a drug detoxification center and possibly methadone maintenance may be necessary. Depending on her commitment to stop taking drugs to reduce harm to her newborn, additional social services need to be explored. Although the decision to change her lifestyle is her choice, the nurse can play a vital role in guiding the care to achieve a better outcome for the mother and her infant. Terry also will need to undergo detoxification and will require close supervision until withdrawal has been achieved. Tight wrapping, calming techniques, and reduced stimuli will help decrease the newborn's irritability.

3.

a. What additional assessments should you complete?

A spectrum of anomalies are possible, including the GI, GU, and cardiac systems. All of the systems require careful assessment for any additional disorders.

b. Are anorectal agenesis and genitourinary tract anomalies common?

Yes, genitourinary defects are the most common ones associated with anorectal agenesis since both systems share a common origin and developmental period.

c. What diagnostic tests might be ordered? What might be included in the treatment plan for this newborn?

Depending on additional anomalies found, an abdominal ultrasound, cardiac echography, and skeletal x-rays are needed to rule out associated defects. Depending on the extent of the anomalies found, surgical intervention might be in order to correct the structural defects.

Study Activities

1. This answer will vary depending on each student's perceptions, but common impressions of the role of NICU nurses would be their autonomy and the numerous types of technical equipment needed for each newborn. The students will probably note that the new parents seem overwhelmed because of the amount of equipment being used. Pointing out to expectant parents how capable and competent the nurses are will help in reducing their anxiety.

2. The students will find thorough descriptions of the specific congenital condition aimed at the level of laypeople. Many sites provide information about local support groups that parents can join.

3. gastroschisis

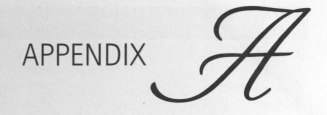

Standard Laboratory Values

Pregnant and Nonpregnant Women

Values	Nonpregnant	Pregnant
Hematologic Complete Blood Count (CBC)		
Hemoglobin, g/dL	12–16*	11.5–14*
Hematocrit, PCV, %	37–47	32–42
Red cell volume, mL	1600	1900
Plasma volume, mL	2400	3700
Red blood cell count, million/mm³	4–5.5	3.75–5.0
White blood cells, total per mm³	4500–10,000	5000–15,000
Polymorphonuclear cells, %	54–62	60–85
Lymphocytes, %	38–46	15–40
Erythrocyte sedimentation rate, mm/h	≤	30–90
MCHC, g/dL packed RBCs (mean corpuscular hemoglobin concentration)	30–36	No change
MCH (mean corpuscular hemoglobin per picogram)	29–32	No change
MCV/µm³ (mean corpuscular volume per cubic micrometer)	82–96	No change
Blood Coagulation and Fibrinolytic Activity†		
Factors VII, VIII, IX, X		Increase in pregnancy, return to normal in early puerperium; factor VIII increases during and immediately after delivery
Factors XI, XIII		Decrease in pregnancy
Prothrombin time (protime)	60–70 sec	Slight decrease in pregnancy
Partial thromboplastin time (PTT)	12–14 sec	Slight decrease in pregnancy and again during second and third stage of labor (indicates clotting at placental site)

(continued)

Values	Nonpregnant	Pregnant
Bleeding time	1–3 min (Duke) 2–4 min (Ivy)	No appreciable change
Coagulation time	6–10 min (Lee/White)	No appreciable change
Platelets	150,000 to 350,000/mm³	No significant change until 3–5 days after delivery, then marked increase (may predispose woman to thrombosis) and gradual return to normal
Fibrinolytic activity		Decreases in pregnancy, then abrupt return to normal (protection against thromboembolism)
Fibrinogen	250 mg/dL	400 mg/dL
Mineral and Vitamin Concentrations		
Serum iron, μg	75–150	65–120
Total iron-binding capacity, μg	250–450	300–500
Iron saturation, %	30–40	15–30
Vitamin B_{12}, folic acid, ascorbic acid	Normal	Moderate decrease
Serum protein		
Total, g/dL	6.7–8.3	5.5–7.5
Albumin, g/dL	3.5–5.5	3.0–5.0
Globulin, total, g/dL	2.3–3.5	3.0–4.0
Blood sugar		
Fasting, mg/dL	70–80	65
2-hour postprandial, mg/dL	60–110	Under 140 after a 100-g carbohydrate meal is considered normal
Cardiovascular		
Blood pressure, mm Hg	120/80‡	114/65
Peripheral resistance, dyne/s · cm^{-5}	120	100
Venous pressure, cm H_2O		
Femoral	9	24
Antecubital	8	8
Pulse, rate/min	70	80
Stroke volume, mL	65	75
Cardiac output, L/min	4.5	6
Circulation time (arm-tongue), sec	15–16	12–14
Blood volume, mL		
Whole blood	4000	5600
Plasma	2400	3700
Red blood cells	1600	1900
Plasma renin, units/L	3–10	10–80
Chest x-ray studies		
Transverse diameter of heart	—	1–2 cm increase
Left border of heart	—	Straightened
Cardiac volume	—	70-mL increase
Electrocardiogram	—	15° left axis deviation
V_1 and V_2	—	Inverted T-wave
kV_4	—	Low T
III	—	Q + inverted T
aVr	—	Small Q

Values	Nonpregnant	Pregnant
Hepatic		
Bilirubin total	Not more than 1 mg/dL	Unchanged
Cephalin flocculation	Up to 2+ in 48 h	Positive in 10%
Serum cholesterol	110–300 mg/dL	↑ 60% from 16–32 weeks of pregnancy; remains at this level until after delivery
Thymol turbidity	0–4 units	Positive in 15%
Serum alkaline phosphatase	2–4.5 units (Bodansky)	↑ from week 12 of pregnancy to 6 weeks after delivery
Serum lactate dehydrogenase		Unchanged
Serum glutamic-oxaloacetic transaminase		Unchanged
Serum globulin albumin	1.5–3.0 g/dL 4.5–5.3 g/dL	↑ slight ↓ 3.0 g by late pregnancy
A/G ratio		Decreased
α_2-globulin		Increased
β-globulin		Increased
Serum cholinesterase		Decreased
Leucine aminopeptidase		Increased
Sulfobromophthalein (5 mg/kg)	5% dye or less in 45 min	Somewhat decreased
Renal		
Bladder capacity	1300 mL	1500 mL
Renal plasma flow (RPF), mL/min	490–700	Increase by 25%, to 612–875
Glomerular filtration rate (GFR), mL/min	105–132	Increase by 50%, to 160–198
Nonprotein nitrogen (NPN), mg/dL	25–40	Decreases
Blood urea nitrogen (BUN), mg/dL	20–25	Decreases
Serum creatinine, mg/kg/24 hr	20–22	Decreases
Serum uric acid, mg/kg/24 hr	257–750	Decreases
Urine glucose	Negative	Present in 20% of gravidas
Intravenous pyelogram (IVP)	Normal	Slight to moderate hydroureter and hydronephrosis; right kidney larger than left kidney
Miscellaneous		
Total thyroxine concentration	5–12 µg/dL thyroxine	↑ 9–16 µg/dL thyroxine (however, unbound thyroxine not greatly increased)
Ionized calcium		Relatively unchanged
Aldosterone		↑ 1 mg/24 hr by third trimester
Dehydroisoandrosterone	Plasma clearance 6–8 L/24 hr	↑ plasma clearance tenfold to twentyfold

* At sea level. Permanent residents of higher levels (e.g., Denver) require higher levels of hemoglobin.

From Scott, J. R., et al. (2000). *Obstetrics and gynecology*. Philadelphia: Lippincott Williams & Wilkins.

† Pregnancy represents a hypercoagulable state.

‡ For the woman about 20 years of age.

10 years of age: 103/70.

30 years of age: 123/82.

40 years of age: 126/84.

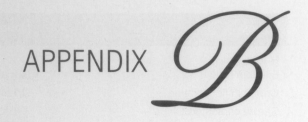

CLINICAL PATHS

LABOR AND DELIVERY CLINICAL PATH—LABOR: EXPECTED OUTCOMES

	Active Phase	Expulsion/Pushing	Recovery 1st Hour Post Partum
PATIENT EDUCATION	Patient coping with labor support Patient utilizing appropriate labor options Patient verbalizes satisfaction with plan Management interventions	Patient demonstrates effective pushing technique. Patient coping effectively with pushing. Support person coping effectively with labor.	Bonding appropriately with baby

PATIENTS STATUS	Cervix dilated 5 cm—complete
	Contraction regularly with progressive cervical change.
	Maternal/fetal well-being maintained
	Hydration maintained
	If indicated: FSE and/or IUPC placed
	   IV Pitocin started
	   Epidural placed/WE encouraged
	   Medicate with prn pain meds
		Vaginal birth	Placenta delivered
			Fundus firm
			Lochia small–moderate
			Without clots
			Perineum intact/repaired
			Hemodynamically stable
			EBL <500 cc

CONTINUUM OF CARE	Prenatal record available after 32 weeks Prenatal labs WNL Pre-registered to hospital Pediatrician identified Support after hospitalization identified Discharge plan discussed with patient/family Communicates understanding of hospital and community resources		

	Interventions		
ASSESSMENT/ TREATMENT	Assess: Continuous EFM or auscultation Q 15 of 30 minutes as indicated. Vital signs hourly/Temp Q4 hr if intact membranes/Q 2 hr if membranes ruptured Uterine by monitor or palpation Bladder for distention Hydration status Cervical dilation, effacement, station	Assess: Q 15 minutes monitoring of fetal well being (Low-Risk) and Q 5 minutes (High-Risk) Vital signs hourly Temp. Q 2–4 hr depending on membrane status Bladder for distention Hydration status Pushing effectiveness Descent of presenting part Caput	Assess: Uterus—fundus Vital signs Lochia Bladder Perineum Placenta
PATIENT EDUCATION	Reinforce comfort measures Encourage use of labor options Inform patient/support person of plan of care	Teaching of upright pushing positions Discourage prolonged maternal breath holding Encourage to assume position of choice Inform patient of progress	Baby status Breast feeding
TESTS/ PROCEDURES	Hgb or Hct (if not done recently) T & S (if ordered) VE as indicated IV therapy AROM by M.D. or CNM: assess for color, amount and odor, as appropriate FSE/IUPC placement if indicated	AROM: assess for color, amount and odor, as appropriate	Cord blood or Rhogam workup if appropriate Cord blood if O+ Mom
THERAPIES	Comfort measures/birthing ball/ambulate/telemetry/ shower IV therapy Amnio infusion for variable decelerations If appropriate, Pain Mgmt. reviewed	Perineal massage Warm soaks to perineal area Allow to rest until feels urge to push Frequent position changes Cool cloth/ice chips	Ice pack to perineum Warm blankets
MEDS	Antibiotics as indicated for + GBS Pitocin if indicated PRN pain medication (encourage WE if requesting this)	Pitocin if indicated	Pitocin IV
ACTIVITY/ SAFETY	Labor option usage Position changes	Provide wedge if supine Promote effective position for pushing: i.e., squatting, side lying, upright Breathing technique patient/ support person most comfortable with	Assist with ambulate to bathroom Infant care Assist with positioning for breast feeding Infant ID bands present

(continued)

Labor and Delivery Clinical Path—Labor: Expected Outcomes (continued)

	Interventions		
UNIQUE PATIENT NEEDS — **NUTRITION**	Clear liquids Ice chips OTHER	Clear liquids Ice chips	Return to previous diet

Integrated Plan of Care for Cesarean Delivery

	Expected Patient Outcomes			
	Phase 1 Preadmission (Cesarean Delivery)	Phase 2 Surgery/ Immediate Postop/ Day of Surgery	Phase 3 Postop Day 1	
Usual time in Phase	**N/A Date Started:**	Up to 23 hours	1 day	1–2 days
Assessment / Potential Complications	VS WNL for patient Hgb or Hct/values within normal SLH antepartum range	VS WNL for patient Systems assessment: Skin warm, dry Clear → Alert & oriented → Neg. Homans' sign → Breast soft/nipples intact → Lungs clear → Bowel sounds present → Fundus firm u/u or u 1–2 (–/+) Lochia sm—mod Dsg dry and intact No signs infiltration IV site Verbalizes comfort using pain rating scale 0–10	VS WNL for patient Afebrile Voiding without foley → Passing flatus Incision without redness or drainage Lochia small amount Fundus firm u/1–2 Verbalizes comfort using pain scale 0–10 on oral pain meds	Incision well approximated, without drainage or redness Passing flatus Lochia sm/mod amt Fundus firm u/1–2 Verbalizes comfort using pain medication as described

		Expected Patient Outcomes		
	Phase 1 Preadmission (Cesarean Delivery)	Phase 2 Surgery/ Immediate Postop/ Day of Surgery	Phase 3 Postop Day 1	
Patient / Family Knowledge	**Date All Above Met** Verbalizes understanding of condition and need for surgery Verbalizes understanding of all pre-op teaching	**Date All Above Met** Verbalizes correct use of PCA/Fentanyl pump and when to request pain medication Turn, cough & deep breath appropriately	**Date All Above Met** Can state criteria for when to call doctor for problems post discharge → ↑ bleeding ↑ Temperature → incision redness, odor or drainage →	**Date All Above Met** Verbalizes follow-up appointment date and time Verbalizes proper dosing of pain medication
ADL's / Activity	**Date All Above Met** Verbalizes understanding of NPO status	**Date All Above Met** Able to ambulate with minimal assistance Tolerating clear/full liquid diet Bonding observed with newborn— Taking-in phase →	**Date All Above Met** Ambulating without assistance Tolerating soft to regular diet	**Date All Above Met** Ambulating in hall
Unique Patient Needs	**Date All Above Met**	**Date All Above Met**	**Date All Above Met**	**Date All Above Met**
	Date All Above Met Entire Phase Outcomes Met; Progress patient to next phase	**Date All Above Met Entire Phase Outcomes Met; Progress patient to next phase**	**Date All Above Met Entire Phase Outcomes Met; Progress patient to next phase**	**Date All Above Met Entire Phase Outcomes Met; Progress patient to next phase**

		Plan of Care		
	#1 Preadmission	#2 Surgery/ Immediate Postop/ Day of Surgery	#3 Postop Day 1	#4 Postop Day 2- Discharge
Assessments	Vital Signs Fetal status immediately prior to surgery	VS per PACU then q 4 hr Systems assessment: *Skin, LOC, FROM, Homans' sign *Breasts, Lungs, Fundus, Incision *Lochia, bladder, bowel sounds, IV and site	VS q 6 hr Assess pain control 0–10 scale Incision Foley-volding Fundus/lochia Homans' sign IV site Breasts ID band on mother Activity	Assess pain control 0–10 scale Incision Volding Fundus lochia Homans' sign IV site as needed ID band on mother Activity

(continued)

INTEGRATED PLAN OF CARE FOR CESAREAN DELIVERY (continued)

	Plan of Care			
	#1 Preadmission	#2 Surgery/ Immediate Postop/ Day of Surgery	#3 Postop Day 1	#4 Postop Day 2- Discharge
		*I & O q shift *Assess pain control 0–10 scale *Assess Rhogam status *Assess Rubella titer status *ID band on mother		
Consults	Anesthesia	Social Work as needed, Anesthesia, Lactation, Dietitian as needed	Social Work, Lactation, Dietitian as needed	Social Work, Lactation, Dietitian as needed
Patient / Family Education Discharge Planning	— Need for surgery — Review Cesarean Delivery — Review procedure, postop expectations — Demonstrate/ Discuss equipment—PCA, Fentanyl pump — Tour of OR area & Nsy	Review postop expectations Review equipment us prn Instruct pt on: Hospital/Infant security systems Unity orientation Newborn orientation/care/feeding (if breastfeeding problems see decision trees)	Review dietary needs post surgery Review Bleeding/ Lochia Precautions post cesarean delivery Review follow-up care and doctor Appointments Review incision care, peri care Infant care Infant feeding	Verify follow-up appointment date and time Activity restrictions Follow-up for staple removal as needed Offer home follow-up care Discuss birth control
Tests and Procedures	PAT; Hgb or Hot (if not done recently—within one month) T & S (if ordered)			
Pharmacologic Needs		IV fluids as ordered Pain control: PCA, Fentanyl pump, IM to PO	IV lock PO pain meds Give Rhogam if indicated Give Rubella if indicated	DC IV lock as ordered

		Plan of Care		
	#1 Preadmission	#2 Surgery/ Immediate Postop/ Day of Surgery	#3 Postop Day 1	#4 Postop Day 2- Discharge
Activity / Rehabilitation	Patient's usual	Change position q 2 hr while in bed, OOB stand at bedside post-op night/dangle and transfer to chair Progress to pt. endurance Observe bonding with infant Observe family support system (if inadequate consult SW)	Progress endurance/ begin Ambulation in hall OOB in AM May shower	Ambulate in halls without assistance
Nutrition / Elimination		NPO then clear liquids to DAT Foley empty q shift	DAT to regular or pre-vious diet at home Foley DC'd	
Miscellaneous Interventions		TCDB q 2 hr while awake	Dressing removed by MD or RN with MD request	
Unique Patient Needs				

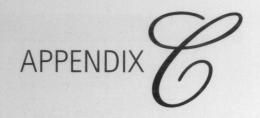

CERVICAL DILATION CHART

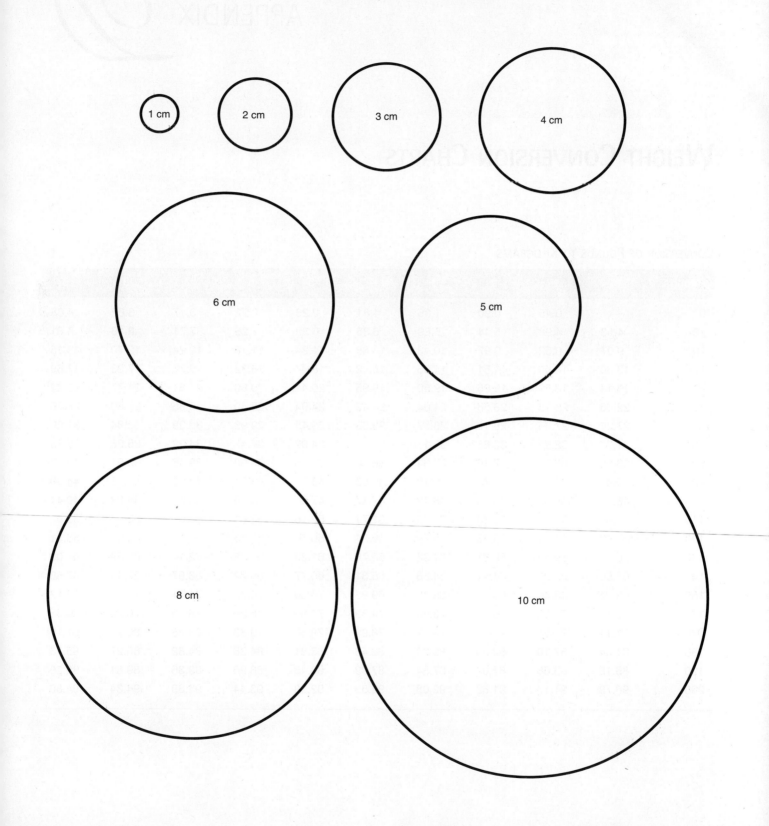

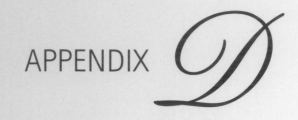

WEIGHT CONVERSION CHARTS

CONVERSION OF POUNDS TO KILOGRAMS

Pounds	0	1	2	3	4	5	6	7	8	9
0	—	0.45	0.90	1.36	1.81	2.26	2.72	3.17	3.62	4.08
10	4.53	4.98	5.44	5.89	6.35	6.80	7.25	7.71	8.16	8.61
20	9.07	9.52	9.97	10.43	10.88	11.34	11.79	12.24	12.70	13.15
30	13.60	14.06	14.51	14.96	15.42	15.87	16.32	16.78	17.23	17.69
40	18.14	18.59	19.05	19.50	19.95	20.41	20.86	21.31	21.77	22.22
50	22.68	23.13	23.58	24.04	24.49	24.94	25.40	25.85	26.30	26.76
60	27.21	27.66	28.12	28.57	29.03	29.48	29.93	30.39	30.84	31.29
70	31.75	32.20	32.65	33.11	33.56	34.02	34.47	34.92	35.38	35.83
80	36.28	36.74	37.19	37.64	38.10	38.55	39.00	39.46	39.91	40.37
90	40.82	41.27	41.73	42.18	42.63	43.09	43.54	43.99	44.45	44.90
100	45.36	45.81	46.26	46.72	47.17	47.62	48.08	48.53	48.98	49.44
110	49.89	50.34	50.80	51.25	51.71	52.16	52.61	53.07	53.52	53.97
120	54.43	54.88	55.33	55.79	56.24	56.70	57.15	57.60	58.06	58.51
130	58.96	59.42	59.87	60.32	60.78	61.23	61.68	62.14	62.59	63.05
140	63.50	63.95	64.41	64.86	65.31	65.77	66.22	66.67	67.13	67.58
150	68.04	68.49	68.94	69.40	69.85	70.30	70.76	71.21	71.66	72.12
160	72.57	73.02	73.48	73.93	74.39	74.84	75.29	75.75	76.20	76.65
170	77.11	77.56	78.01	78.47	78.92	79.38	79.83	80.28	80.74	81.19
180	81.64	82.10	82.55	83.00	83.46	83.91	84.36	84.82	85.27	85.73
190	86.18	86.68	87.09	87.54	87.99	88.45	88.90	89.35	89.81	90.26
200	90.72	91.17	91.62	92.08	92.53	92.98	93.44	93.89	94.34	94.80

CONVERSION OF POUNDS AND OUNCES TO GRAMS FOR NEWBORN WEIGHTS

Pounds	Ounces															
	0	1	2	3	4	5	6	7	8	9	10	11	12	13	14	15
0	—	28	57	85	113	142	170	198	227	255	283	312	340	369	397	425
1	454	482	510	539	567	595	624	652	680	709	737	765	794	822	850	879
2	907	936	964	992	1021	1049	1077	1106	1134	1162	1191	1219	1247	1276	1304	1332
3	1361	1389	1417	1446	1474	1503	1531	1559	1588	1616	1644	1673	1701	1729	1758	1786
4	1814	1843	1871	1899	1928	1956	1984	2013	2041	2070	2098	2126	2155	2183	2211	2240
5	2268	2296	2325	2353	2381	2410	2438	2466	2495	2523	2551	2580	2608	2637	2665	2693
6	2722	2750	2778	2807	2835	2863	2892	2920	2948	2977	3005	3033	3062	3090	3118	3147
7	3175	3203	3232	3260	3289	3317	3345	3374	3402	3430	3459	3487	3515	3544	3572	3600
8	3629	3657	3685	3714	3742	3770	3799	3827	3856	3884	3912	3941	3969	3997	4026	4054
9	4082	4111	4139	4167	4196	4224	4252	4281	4309	4337	4366	4394	4423	4451	4479	4508
10	4536	4564	4593	4621	4649	4678	4706	4734	4763	4791	4819	4848	4876	4904	4933	4961
11	4990	5018	5046	5075	5103	5131	5160	5188	5216	5245	5273	5301	5330	5358	5386	5415
12	5443	5471	5500	5528	5557	5585	5613	5642	5670	5698	5727	5755	5783	5812	5840	5858
13	5897	5925	5953	5982	6010	6038	6067	6095	6123	6152	6180	6209	6237	6265	6294	6322
14	6350	6379	6407	6435	6464	6492	6520	6549	6577	6605	6634	6662	6690	6719	6747	6776
15	6804	6832	6860	6889	6917	6945	6973	7002	7030	7059	7087	7115	7144	7172	7201	7228

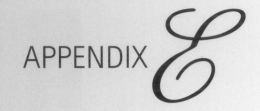

APPENDIX E

Breast-Feeding and Medication Use

General Considerations

- Most medications are safe to use while breast-feeding; however, the woman should always check with the pediatrician, physician, or lactation specialist before taking any medications, including over-the-counter and herbal products.
- Inform the woman that she has the right to seek a second opinion if the physician does not perform a thoughtful risk-versus-benefit assessment before prescribing medications or advising against breast-feeding.
- Most medications pass from the woman's bloodstream into the breast milk. However, the amount is usually very small and unlikely to harm the baby.
- A preterm or other special needs neonate is more susceptible to the adverse effects of medications in breast milk. A woman who is taking medications and whose baby is in the neonatal intensive care unit or special care nursery should consult with the pediatrician or neonatologist before feeding her breast milk to the baby.
- If the woman is taking a prescribed medication, she should take the medication just after breast-feeding. This practice helps ensure that the lowest possible dose of medication reaches the baby through the breast milk.
- Some medications can cause changes in the amount of milk the woman produces. Teach the woman to report any changes in milk production.

Lactation Risk Categories (LRC)

Location Category	Risk	Rationale
L1	Safest	Clinical research or long-term observation

Location Category	Risk	Rationale
		of use in many breast-feeding women has not demonstrated risk to the infant.
L2	Safer	Limited clinical esearch has not demonstrated an increase in adverse effects in the infant.
L3	Moderately safe	There is possible risk to the infant; however, the risks are minimal or nonthreatening in nature. These medications should be given only when the potential benefit outweighs the risk to the infant.
L4	Possibly hazardous	There is positive evidence of risk to the infant; however, in life-threatening situations or for serious diseases, the benefit might outweigh the risk.

Location Category	Risk	Rationale
L5	Contraindicated	The risk of using the medication clearly outweighs any possible benefit from breast-feeding.

Potential Effects of Selected Medication Categories on the Breast-Fed Infant

Narcotic Analgesics

• Codeine and hydrocodone appear to be safe in moderate doses. Rarely the neonate may experience sedation and/or apnea. (LRC: L3)
• Meperidine (Demerol) can lead to sedation of the neonate. (LRC: L3)
• Low to moderate doses of morphine appear to be safe. (LRC: L2)
• Trace-to-negligible amounts of fentanyl are found in human milk. (LRC: L2)

Non-narcotic Analgesics and NSAIDs

• Acetaminophen and ibuprofen are approved for use. (LRC: L1)
• Naproxen may cause neonatal hemorrhage and anemia if used for prolonged periods. (LRC: L3 for short-term use and L4 for long-term use)
• The newer COX2 inhibitors, such as celecoxib (Celebrex), appear to be safe for use. (LRC: L2)

Antibiotics

• Levels in breast milk are usually very low.
• The penicillins and cephalosporins are generally considered safe to use. (LRC: L1 and L2)
• Tetracyclines can be safely used for short periods but are not suitable for long-term therapy (e.g., for treatment of acne). (LRC: L2)
• Sulfonamides should not be used during the neonatal stage (the first month of life). (LRC: L3)

Antihypertensives

• A high degree of caution is advised when antihypertensives are used during breast-feeding.
• Some beta blockers can be used.
• Hydralazine and methyldopa are considered to be safe. (LRC: L2)

• ACE inhibitors are not recommended in the early postpartum period.

Sedatives and Hypnotics

• Neonatal withdrawal can occur when antianxiety medications, such as lorazepam, are taken. Fortunately withdrawal is generally mild.
• Phenothiazines, such as Phenergan and Thorazine, may lead to sleep apnea and increase the risk for sudden infant death syndrome.

Antidepressants

• The risk to the baby often is higher if the woman is depressed and remains untreated, rather than taking the medication.
• The older tricyclics are considered to be safe; however they cause many bothersome side effects, such as weight gain and dry mouth, which may lead to noncompliance on the part of the woman.
• The selective serotonin uptake inhibitors (SSRIs) also are considered to be safe and have a lower side effect profile, which makes them more palatable to the woman. (LRC: L2 and L3)

Mood Stabilizers (Antimanic Medication)

• Lithium is found in breast milk and is best not used in the breast-feeding woman. (LRC: L4)
• Valproic acid (Depakote) seems to be a more appropriate choice for the woman with bipolar disorder. The infant will need periodic lab studies to check platelets and liver function.

Corticosteroids

• Corticosteroids do not pass into the milk in large quantities.
• Inhaled steroids are safe to use because they don't accumulate in the bloodstream.

Thyroid Medication

• Thyroid medications, such as levothyroxine (Synthroid), can be taken while breast-feeding.
• Most are in LRC category L1.

Medications That Usually Are Contraindicated for the Breast-Feeding Woman

• Amiodarone
• Antineoplastic agents
• Chloramphenicol

- Doxepin
- Ergotamine and other ergot derivatives
- Iodides
- Methotrexate and immunosuppressants
- Lithium

- Radiopharmaceuticals
- Ribavirin
- Tetracycline (prolonged use—more than 3 weeks)
- Pseudoephedrine (found in many over-the-counter medications)

Material in this Appendix was adapted from information found on the American Academy of Pediatrics website (www.aap.org) and from Riordan, J. (2005). *Breastfeeding and human lactation* (3rd ed.). Boston: Jones and Bartlett Publishers; Hale, T. W. (2004). *Medications and mother's milk* (11th ed.). Amarillo, TX: Pharmasoft Publishing.

INDEX

Note: A *b* following a page number indicates a boxed feature; *d* indicates a display; *f* indicates a figure; and *t* indicates a table.

A

ABCDES, 224, 224*b*
ABCD's, of newborn resuscitation, 687*b*
Abdomen
  assessment of
    in newborn, 490, 492*t*
    in prenatal care, 296
  auscultation of in newborn, 490
Abdominal breathing exercises, for postpartum woman, 434*d*
Abdominal hysterectomy, 181. *See also* Hysterectomy
Abdominal ultrasonography. *See* Ultrasonography
Abdominal wall defects, omphalocele and gastroschisis, 747–749, 748*f*, 749*b*
Abdominal x-ray (KUB), in necrotizing enterocolitis, 713
ABG. *See* Arterial blood gases
ABO incompatibility, 554, 732, 733*t*
Abortion, 19, 101–103, 527
  categories of, 529*t*
  legal/ethical issues and, 19
  spontaneous, 527–528, 529*t*, 530*d*
    early amniocentesis and, 304
ABR. *See* Auditory brainstem response
Abruptio placentae, 540–543, 541*b*, 541*f*, 542*t*, 637
Abscess, Bartholin's, 183
Abstinence, 80–86, 81*t*
Abuse. *See also* Intimate partner violence
  abuser profile and, 217–218, 225
  mandated reporting and, 21
  sexual, 217, 225, 226*d*
    incest, 226
  substance. *See* Substance use/abuse
  types of, 217
  victim profile and, 217
Accelerations (fetal heart rate), 371
Acceptance, of pregnancy, 283
Accessory male reproductive glands, 58–59, 58*f*
Accidents. *See* Trauma
Acetylcholinesterase, amniotic fluid, 304*t*
Acid–base status, fetal scalp sampling in assessment of, 372

Acne, in polycystic ovary syndrome, 185, 185*d*
Acquaintance rape, 227–228, 228*d*
Acquired immune deficiency syndrome (AIDS), 595, 596*t*. *See also* HIV infection/AIDS
Acquired immunity, 466. *See also* Immunization(s)
Acrocyanosis, 485
Across-the-lap position, for breastfeeding, 509, 510*f*
Activated partial thromboplastin time (aPTT), in abruptio placentae, 542
Active immunity, 516. *See also* Immunization(s)
Active listening, 38
Active phase of stage 1 labor, 353*t*, 354
  assessments during, 389*t*
Activity/activity tolerance. *See* Exercise/activity
Acuity. *See* Auditory acuity
Acupressure, 31*t*
  for labor pain, 375
Acupuncture, for labor pain, 375
Adenocarcinoma, of endometrium, 198
Adenomyosis, 65
ADH. *See* Antidiuretic hormone
Adherence. *See* Compliance
Adipose tissue, in nonshivering thermogenesis, 463, 688
Adjunctive therapy, in breast cancer, 156–158
Adjuvant therapies. *See* Complementary and alternative medicine/therapies
Admission to hospital facility, for laboring woman, 385–388, 387*f*
Adolescence, 591. *See also* Adolescent(s)
Adolescent(s). *See also* Puberty
  HIV infection and, 134, 135*d*
  pregnant. *See* Adolescent pregnancy
  sexually transmitted infections in, 114–115, 116–119*t*. *See also* Sexually transmitted infections
Adolescent families, 12*t*. *See also* Adolescent pregnancy
Adolescent pregnancy, 591–594, 591*d*
  assessment in, 593
  developmental issues and, 592, 592*b*, 592*f*

health/social issues and, 592–593
nursing care in, 593–594, 595*f*
prevention of, 594, 594*b*
Adrenal glands, pregnancy-associated changes in hormone secretion by, 273–274
Adrenaline, in third stage of labor, 396
Adrenarche, 53
Advil. *See* Ibuprofen
Advocate (client), 41
Affective disorders
  postpartum (blues/depression/psychosis), 413, 443, 659–664, 663*d*, 664*b*
  in premenstrual dysphoric disorder, 71
AFP. *See* Alpha-fetoprotein
African-Americans
  cultural influences during postpartum period and, 431*b*
  health beliefs of, 15*t*
  sickle cell anemia and, 585
Afterbirth pains, assessment of, 422
Afterpains, 407
AGA. *See* Appropriate for gestational age
Age
  gestational, assessment of, 477–479, 478*f*
  maternal
    adolescent pregnancy and, 591–594, 591*d*
    chromosomal disorders and, 253, 254
    older pregnant woman and, 594–595
AIDS, 595, 596*t*. *See also* HIV infection/AIDS
Airway, evaluation/management of in newborn, 479
  resuscitation and, 687*b*
Alanine aminotransferase (ALT) levels, in hyperemesis gravidarum, 545
Alcohol-related birth defects, 726. *See also* Fetal alcohol spectrum disorder
Alcohol use/abuse, maternal (fetal alcohol spectrum disorder/fetal alcohol syndrome), 289, 599*t*, 600–601, 600*b*, 601*f*, 722*t*, 725–726, 726*b*
  reducing occurrence of, 702*d*
Aldomet. *See* Methyldopa